Patterson's Allergic Diseases

Sixth Edition

Patterson's Allergic Diseases

Sixth Edition

Editors

Leslie C. Grammer, M.D.
Professor of Medicine
Department of Medicine
Vice Chief, Division of Allergy-Immunology
Director, Ernest S. Bazley Asthma and Allergic Diseases Center
Northwestern University Medical School
Attending Physician
Northwestern Memorial Hospital
Chicago, Illinois

Paul A. Greenberger, M.D.
Professor of Medicine
Department of Medicine
Associate Chief, Education and Clinical Affairs
Division of Allergy-Immunology
Northwestern University Medical School
Attending Physician
Northwestern Memorial Hospital
Chicago, Illinois

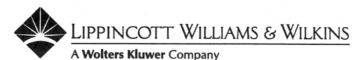

LIPPINCOTT WILLIAMS & WILKINS
A **Wolters Kluwer** Company

Philadelphia • Baltimore • New York • London
Buenos Aires • Hong Kong • Sydney • Tokyo

Acquisitions Editor: Jonathan Pine
Developmental Editor: Michael Standen
Production Editor: Tony DeGeorge
Manufacturing Manager: Colin Warnock
Cover Designer: Christine Jenny
Compositor: TechBooks
Printer: Maple Press

Printed in the USA.
Fifth Edition, 1997

Library of Congress Cataloging-in-Publication Data

Patterson's allergic diseases / editors, Leslie C. Grammer, Paul A. Greenberger.—6th ed.
   p. ; cm.
   Rev. ed. of: Allergic diseases : diagnosis and management / edited by Roy Patterson ; associate editors, Leslie Carroll Grammer, Paul A. Greenberger ; with 24 additional contributors. 5th ed. c1997.
   Includes bibliographical references and index.
   ISBN 0-7817-2386-8
   1. Allergy.   I. Patterson, Roy, 1926–   II. Grammer, Leslie Carroll.   III. Greenberger, Paul A.   IV. Allergic diseases.
   [DNLM: 1. Hypersensitivity—diagnosis. 2. Hypersensitivity—therapy. WD 300 P3185   2002]

   RC584 .A34   2002
   616.97—dc21

                                                                              2001050524

Care has been taken to confirm the accuracy of the information presented and to describe generally accepted practices. However, the authors, editors, and publisher are not responsible for errors or omissions or for any consequences from application of the information in this book and make no warranty, expressed or implied, with respect to the currency, completeness, or accuracy of the contents of the publication. Application of this information in a particular situation remains the professional responsibility of the practitioner.

The authors, editors, and publisher have exerted every effort to ensure that drug selection and dosage set forth in this text are in accordance with current recommendations and practice at the time of publication. However, in view of ongoing research, changes in government regulations, and the constant flow of information relating to drug therapy and drug reactions, the reader is urged to check the package insert for each drug for any change in indications and dosage and for added warnings and precautions. This is particularly important when the recommended agent is a new or infrequently employed drug.

Some drugs and medical devices presented in this publication have Food and Drug Administration (FDA) clearance for limited use in restricted research settings. It is the responsibility of the health care provider to ascertain the FDA status of each drug or device planned for use in their clinical practice.

10 9 8 7 6 5 4 3 2 1

In Memoriam Jacob J. Pruzansky, Ph.D.
June 20, 1921–April 5, 2001

Jack Pruzansky served as an author in five editions of Allergic Diseases. *He spent many hours mentoring fellows in the Allergy-Immunology Division during his 35-year tenure at Northwestern University. After his retirement, he still functioned as a consultant and provided scientific expertise to the division. Jack was an expert on in vitro basophil histamine release and discovered how dilute hydrochloric acid would allow for removal of IgE from basophils. This discovery allowed him to study passive transfer experimentally and led to studies of histamine releasing factors. His intellect and advice helped fellows and faculty stay out of "dark alleys" as he would say. He will be missed.*

In Memoriam Martha A. Shaughnessy, B.S.
December 3, 1943–September 9, 1997

Martha Shaughnessy was a chapter author in the last two editions of Allergic Diseases. *She had a terrific sense of humor and quick wit. Her contributions to the division included performing immunologic research, writing research papers and grants, teaching fellows, and administration of the Allergy-Immunology Division. She coauthored 71 peer-reviewed papers, 66 of which were in collaboration with other members of the Allergy-Immunology Division. She also coauthored ten book chapters, primarily in areas of allergen immunotherapy and occupational immunologic lung disease, her two major research interests. She was admired and respected by her co-investigators and all who worked with her. We, her colleagues and friends, now honor her.*

In Memory of Ernest S. Bazley

The Ernest S. Bazley Grant to Northwestern Memorial Hospital and Northwestern University has provided continuing research support that has been invaluable to the Allergy-Immunology Division of Northwestern University.

In Memoriam W. James Metzger, Jr., M.D.
October 30, 1945–November 17, 2000

Jim was a fellow at Northwestern University from 1974 to 1976 and spent his career in academic medicine at the University of Iowa and East Carolina Medical School where he was Division Chief of Allergy Asthma and Immunology and Vice-Chair of the Department of Medicine. He moved to Denver to the National Jewish Hospital in the months before he became ill. He was an author in three editions of Allergic Diseases.
Jim had many accomplishments in Allergy-Immunology including the early discovery that allergen vaccine therapy inhibited some of the late airway response to allergen.
Jim was liked by everyone and is deeply missed. It was stated, "As in so many things, Jim was the catalyst that altered and enlarged an experience, while managing to stay almost invisible himself."

Contents

Foreword

A Major Honor

I was informed by the publisher that the name Roy Patterson would be on all future editions of *Allergic Diseases: Diagnosis and Management*. I consider this a great honor and at this time I would like to acknowledge several colleagues for their contributions to my personal achievements.

As of this writing, I am 75 years old (as of 4/26/01) and am the Ernest S. Bazley Professor of Medicine of Northwestern University Medical School and the Chief of the Allergy-Immunology Division of the Department of Medicine.

I owe a debt of gratitude to the following for all their support during my academic career. I wish to thank:

The Ernest S. Bazley Trustees: Catherine Ryan of the Bank of America, Illinois, the late Ernest S. Bazley, Jr., and the late Gunnard Swanson. A major effort of the Northwestern Allergy-Immunology program has been the diagnosis and management of all forms of asthma. Research funding from the Bazley Trust has made many of our accomplishments in the area possible.

The National Institute of Allergy and Infectious Diseases: Richard Krause, M.D., Anthony Fauci, M.D., Sheldon Cohen, M.D., and Dorothy Sogn, M.D.

Full time faculty: particularly the late Jacob J. Pruzansky, Ph.D.

Voluntary faculty: particularly Richard S. DeSwarte, M.D.

Technical and support staff: Mary Roberts, R.N., Kathleen E. Harris, B.S., Margaret A. Mateja-Wieckert, and the late Martha A. Shaughnessy, B.S.

Finally, **the Graduates of the Allergy-Immunology training program.**

Roy Patterson, M.D.

Preface

The sixth edition covers allergic and immunologic problems that are encountered in the ambulatory practice or in hospitalized patients. The quantity and complexity of general and specific knowledge in the field of Allergy-Immunology continues to expand at an exciting but daunting pace. Further, the practice of Allergy-Immunology requires familiarity with many specific details. The 42 chapters contain useful, applicable, and up-to-date information on how to diagnose and manage nearly all of the conditions in Allergy-Immunology. The history of *Allergic Diseases: Diagnosis and Management* through six editions includes being a useful textbook where important, crucial information can be found and applied. Edition six has 15 new chapters, and the classic Drug Allergy chapter originated by Richard DeSwarte has been divided into three parts. The new chapters covering radiologic findings of the sinuses and lungs, role of rhinoscopy and surgery for chronic sinusitis, and work-up for immunodeficiency reflect the broadened base of knowledge required for the practice of Allergy-Immunology. In that asthma is now recognized as of one the most complicated disorders a physicians must treat, five new chapters were prepared to cover medications for asthma, inhaler devices and delivery systems, and novel approaches to treatment.

There are shortages of specialists in Allergy-Immunology in practice and even more so in academic medical centers. We hope this textbook assists physicians to provide better care for their patients, inspires medical students and residents to pursue training in Allergy-Immunology, and assists investigators in advancing our knowledge. We will always have much more to learn.

We are grateful to the authors for their superb chapters, each of which has been approved by us, should there be any oversights. We could not have completed this textbook without the love and support from our families who give us the time to continue in the Northwestern University Allergy-Immunology tradition that is now over 40 years old!

Special appreciation goes to our support staff, especially Kathleen E. Harris and Margaret Mateja Wieckert, our trainees and graduates, and our patients, from whom we can always learn.

Leslie C. Grammer, M.D.
Paul A. Greenberger, M.D.

Contributing Authors

Howard L. Alt, M.D.
Assistant Professor of Clinical Medicine
Department of Psychiatry
Northwestern University Medical School
Chicago, Illinois

Andrea J. Apter, M.D., M.Sc.
Chief
Associate Professor
Department of Allergy and Immunology
Division of Pulmonary, Allergy, and Critical
 Care
Hospital of the University of Pennsylvania
University of Pennsylvania School of Medicine
Philadelphia, Pennsylvania

Banani Banerjee, Ph.D.
Instructor of Pediatrics (Allergy/Immunology)
 and Medicine
Medical College of Wisconsin
Milwaukee, Wisconsin

Melvin Berger, M.D. Ph.D.
Professor
Departments of Pediatrics and Pathology
Case Western Reserve University
Chief
Department of Pediatrics
Rainbow, Babies and Children's Hospital
University Hospitals Health System
Cleveland, Ohio

David I. Bernstein, M.D.
Professor of Medicine
Department of Immunology
University of Cincinnati College of Medicine
Cincinnati, Ohio

Jonathan A. Bernstein, M.D.
Associate Professor
Department of Internal Medicine
University of Cincinnati
Cincinnati, Ohio

Michael S. Blaiss, M.D.
Clinical Professor
Departments of Pediatrics and Medicine
University of Tennessee, Memphis
Department of Pediatrics
Le Bonheur Children's Medical Center
Memphis, Tennessee

Bernard H. Booth III, M.D.
Clinical Professor
Department of Medicine
University of Mississippi Medical Center
Jackson, Mississippi

G. Daniel Brooks, M.D.
Department of Medicine
University of Wisconsin
Department of Medicine
University of Wisconsin Hospitals and Clinics
Madison, Wisconsin

Robert K. Bush, M.D.
Professor
Department of Medicine
University of Wisconsin-Madison
Chief
Department of Allergy
William. S. Middleton V.A. Hospital
Madison, Wisconsin

Rakesh K. Chandra, M.D.
Chief Resident
Department of Otolaryngology Head & Neck
 Surgery
Northwestern Memorial Hospital
Northwestern University
Chicago, Illinois

David B. Conley, M.D.
Assistant Professor
Department of Otolaryngology Head & Neck Surgery
Northwestern University Medical School
Chicago, Illinois

Thomas Corbridge, M.D., F.C.C.P.
Associate Professor
Department of Medicine
Northwestern University Medical School
Director
Medical Intensive Care Unit
Northwestern Memorial Hospital
Chicago, Illinois

Anne M. Ditto, M.D.
Assistant Professor
Department of Medicine
Division of Allergy-Immunology
Northwestern University Medical School
Chicago, Illinois

Jordan N. Fink, M.D.
Professor and Chief
Department of Medicine
Division of Allergy-Immunology
Milwaukee County Medical Complex
Milwaukee, Wisconsin

Leslie C. Grammer, M.D.
Professor of Medicine
Department of Medicine
Vice Chief, Division of Allergy-Immunology
Director, Ernest S. Bazley Asthma and Allergic
 Diseases Center
Northwestern University Medical School
Chicago, Illinois

Thomas H. Grant, D.O.
Associate Professor
Department of Radiology
Northwestern Memorial Hospital
Northwestern University Medical School
Chicago, Illinois

Paul A. Greenberger, M.D.
Professor of Medicine
Department of Medicine
Associate Chief, Education and
 Clinical Affairs
Division of Allergy-Immunology
Northwestern University Medical School
Chicago, Illinois

Kathleen E. Harris, B.S.
Senior Life Sciences Researcher
Department of Medicine
Division of Allergy-Immunology
Northwestern University Medical School
Chicago, Illinois

Mary Beth Hogan, M.D.
Assistant Professor
Department of Pediatrics
West Virginia University School of Medicine
Morgantown, West Virginia

Carla Irani, M.D.
Section of Allergy and Immunology
Division of Pulmonary, Allergy
Critical Care Medicine
University of Pennsylvania School of
 Medicine
Philadelphia, Pennsylvania

Kevin J. Kelly, M.D.
Professor and Chief
Department of Allergy/Immunology
Medical College of Wisconsin
Chief
Department of Medicine
Division of Allergy/Immunology
Children's Hospital of Wisconsin
Milwaukee, Wisconsin

Robert C. Kern, M.D., M.S., F.A.C.S.
Chairman
Division of Otolaryngology
Cook County Hospital
Associate Professor
Department of Otolaryngology-Head & Neck
 Surgery
Northwestern University Medical School
Chicago, Illinois

Theodore M. Lee, M.D.
Peachtree Allergy and Asthma Clinic, PC
Atlanta, Georgia

Donald Y M Leung, M.D., Ph.D.
Professor
Department of Pediatrics
University of Colorado Health Sciences Center
Head
Department of Pediatric Allergy-Immunology
National Jewish Medical and Research
 Center
Denver, Colorado

Phil Lieberman, M.D.
Clinical Professor
Department of Internal Medicine
 and Pediatrics
University of Tennessee College of Medicine
Cordova, Tennessee

Kris G. McGrath, M.D.
Associate Professor
Department of Medicine
Northwestern University Medical School
Chief
Department of Allergy-Immunology
Saint Joseph Hospital
Chicago, Illinois

Roger W. Melvold, Ph.D.
Professor and Department Chair
Department of Microbiology & Immunology
School of Medicine and Health Sciences
University of North Dakota
Grand Forks, North Dakota

W. James Metzger, M.D.
Professor and Section Head
Department of Allergy, Asthma and Immunology
East Carolina University School of Medicine
Greenville, North Carolina

Babak Mokhlesi, M.D.
Assistant Professor
Department of Medicine
Division of Pulmonary and Critical Care
Rush Medical College/Cook County Hospital
Chicago, Illinois

Michelle J. Naidich, M.D.
Department of Radiology
Northwestern Memorial Hospital
Northwestern University Medical School
Chicago, Illinois

Sai R. Nimmagadda, M.D.
Assistant Professor
Department of Pediatrics
Northwestern University Medical School
Department of Pediatrics/Allergy
Children's Memorial Hospital
Chicago, Illinois

Peck Y. Ong, M.D.
Fellow
Department of Pediatrics
Division of Allergy and Immunology
National Jewish Medical and Research Center
Denver, Colorado

Roy Patterson, M.D.
Ernest S. Bazley Professor of Medicine
Department of Medicine
Chief
Division of Allergy-Immunology
Northwestern University Medical School
Chicago, Illinois

Neill T. Peters, M.D.
Clinical Instructor
Department of Dermatology
Mercy Hospital and Medical Center
Chicago, Illinois

Jacqueline A. Pongracic, M.D.
Assistant Professor
Department of Pediatrics and Medicine
Northwestern University Medical
  School
Acting Division Head
Department of Allergy
Children's Memorial Hospital
Chicago, Illinois

Jacob J. Pruzansky, Ph.D.
Emeritus Professor of Microbiology
Department of Medicine
Division of Allergy-Immunology
Northwestern University Medical School
Chicago, Illinois

Robert E. Reisman, M.D.
Clinical Professor
Departments of Medicine and Pediatrics
State University of New York at Buffalo
Department of Medicine
  (Allergy/Immunology)
Buffalo General Hospital
Buffalo, New York

Anthony J. Ricketti, M.D.
Associate Professor of Medicine
Seton Hall University
Graduate School of Medicine
Chairman
Department of Medicine
St. Francis Medical Center
Trenton, New Jersey

Eric J. Russell, M.D., F.A.C.R.
Professor
Departments of Radiology, Neurosurgery, and
  Otolaryngology
Northwestern University
Chief of Neuroradiology
Department of Radiology
Northwestern Memorial Hospital
Chicago, Illinois

Carol A. Saltoun, M.D.
Clinical Instructor
Department of Medicine
Division of Allergy-Immunology
Northwestern University Medical School
Chicago, Illinois

Andrew Scheman, M.D.
Associate Professor of Clinical Dermatology and
*   Department of Dermatology*
Northwestern University Medical Center
Chicago, Illinois

William R. Solomon, M.D.
Professor Emeritus
Department of Internal Medicine (Allergy)
University of Michigan Medical School and
University of Michigan Medical Center
Ann Arbor, Michigan

Abba I. Terr, M.D.
Associate Professor
Department of Medicine
University of California-San Francisco
School of Medicine
San Francisco, California

Anju Tripathi, M.D.
Assistant Professor
Departments of Medicine and Allergy
Northwestern University Medical School
Chicago, Illinois

Stephen I. Wasserman, M.D.
The Helen M. Ranney Professor
Department of Medicine
University of California-San Diego
La Jolla, California
Professor and Chief of Allergic Diseases
Department of Medicine
University of California-San Diego Medical
*   Center*
San Diego, California

Carol Ann Wiggins, M.D.
Department of Allergy and Immunology
Emory University School of Medicine
Department of Allergy and Immunology
Piedmont Hospital
Atlanta, Georgia

Nevin W. Wilson, M.D.
Associate Professor
Department of Pediatrics
West Virginia University, School of Medicine
Morgantown, West Virginia

Lisa F. Wolfe, M.D.
Assistant Professor of Medicine
Clinical Instructor
Division of Pulmonary & Critical Care Medicine
*   and the Center for Sleep and Circadian Biology*
Northwestern University Medical School
Chicago, Illinois

Michael C. Zacharisen, M.D.
Assistant Professor
Departments of Pediatrics and Medicine
Medical College of Wisconsin
Children's Hospital of Wisconsin
Milwaukee, Wisconsin

C. Raymond Zeiss, M.D.
Emeritus Professor of Medicine
Department of Medicine
Division of Allergy-Immunology
Northwestern University Medical School
VA Chicago Health Care System–Lakeside
*   Division*
Chicago, Illinois

1

Review of Immunology

Roger W. Melvold

Department of Microbiology and Immunology, School of Medicine and Health Sciences,
University of North Dakota, Grand Forks, North Dakota

Although immunology is a relative newcomer among the sciences, its phenomena have long been recognized and manipulated. Ancient peoples understood that survivors of particular diseases were protected from those diseases for the remainder of their lives, and the ancient Chinese and Egyptians even practiced forms of immunization. Surgeons have also long understood that tissues and organs would not survive when exchanged between different individuals (e.g., from cadaver donors) but could succeed when transplanted from one site to another within the same individual. However, only during the past century have the mechanisms of the immune system been illuminated, at least in part. Keep in mind that the immune system, as we usually think of it, is the body's second line of defense. The first line of defense consists of a number of barriers, including the skin and mucous membranes, the fatty acids of the skin, the high pH of the stomach, resident microbial populations, and cells that act nonspecifically against infectious organisms (1).

Like the nervous and endocrine systems, the immune system is adaptive, specific, and communicative. It recognizes and responds to changes in the environment, and it displays memory by adapting or altering its response to stimuli that it has encountered previously. It can detect the presence of millions of different substances (antigens) and has an exquisite ability to discriminate among closely related molecules. Communication and interaction, involving both direct contact and soluble mediators, must occur among a variety of lymphoid and other cells for optimal function.

The complexity of the immune system is extended by genetic differences among individuals. This is because the "repertoire" of immune responses varies among unrelated individuals in an outbred, genetically heterogeneous species such as our own. Furthermore, each of us, in a sense, is "immunologically incomplete" because none of us is able to recognize and respond to all of the possible antigens that exist. Several factors contribute to this: (a) genetic or environmentally induced conditions that nonspecifically diminish immune functions, (b) variation among individuals in the genes encoding the antigen receptors of lymphocytes, (c) genetically encoded differences among individuals (often determined by the highly polymorphic genes of the human leukocyte antigen [HLA] complex) that dictate whether and how the individual will respond to specific antigens, and (d) the fact that each individual's immune system must differentiate between *self* (those substances that are a normal part of the body) and foreign, or *nonself*, in order to avoid autoimmunity. However, because self differs from one individual to the next, what is foreign also differs among individuals.

ANTIGENS

Antigens were initially defined as substances identified and bound by antibodies (immunoglobulins) produced by B lymphocytes. However, because the specific antigen receptors of

T lymphocytes are not immunoglobulins, the definition must be broadened to include substances that can be specifically recognized by the receptors of T or B lymphocytes or both. It is estimated that the immune system can specifically recognize at least 10^6 to 10^7 different antigens. These include both substances that are foreign to the body (nonself) and substances that are normal constituents of the body (self).

The immune system must distinguish between nonself and self antigens so that, under normal conditions, it can attack the former but not the latter. Thus, the immune system should be tolerant of self but intolerant of nonself. Autoimmune diseases arise when such distinctions are lost and the immune system attacks self antigens, a phenomenon originally described by Paul Erlich as *horror autotoxicus*. Well-known examples include rheumatoid arthritis, psoriasis, systemic lupus erythematosus, and some forms of diabetes.

Antigens can be divided into three general types—immunogens, haptens, and tolerogens—depending on the way in which they stimulate and interact with the immune system (2–4). An immunogen can, by itself, both stimulate an immune response and subsequently serve as a target of that response. The terms *immunogen* and *antigen* are often, but inappropriately, used interchangeably. A hapten cannot, by itself, stimulate an immune response. However, if a hapten is attached to a larger immunogenic molecule (a "carrier"), responses can be stimulated against both the carrier and the hapten, and the hapten itself can subsequently serve as the target of a response so invoked. A tolerogen is a substance that, after an initial exposure to the immune system, inhibits future responses against itself.

Because of the genetic diversity among individuals, a substance that is an immunogen for one person may be a tolerogen for another and may be ignored completely by the immune system of still others. Also, a substance that acts as an immunogen when administered by one route (e.g., intramuscularly) may act as a tolerogen when applied by a different route (e.g., intragastrically).

Antigens are usually protein or carbohydrate in nature and may be found as free single molecules or as parts of larger structures (e.g., expressed on the surface of an infectious agent).

Although some antigens are very small and simple, others are large and complex, containing many different sites that can be individually identified by lymphocyte receptors or free immunoglobulins. Each such individual part of an antigen that can be distinctly identified by the immune system is called an *epitope* or *determinant* (i.e., the smallest identifiable antigenic unit). Thus, a single large antigen may contain many different epitopes. In general, the more complex the molecule and the greater the number of epitopes it displays, the more potent it is as an immunogen.

Adjuvants are substances that, when administered together with an immunogen (or a hapten coupled to an immunogen), enhance the response against it (5). For example, immunogens may be suspended in mixtures (e.g., colloidal suspensions of mycobacterial proteins and oil) that induce localized inflammations and aid in arousal of the immune system.

MOLECULES OF THE IMMUNE SYSTEM

Immunoglobulin

B lymphocytes synthesize receptors (immunoglobulins) able to recognize and bind specific structures (antigens, determinants, epitopes). All immunoglobulins produced by a single B cell, or by a clonally derived set of B cells, have the same specificity and are able to recognize and bind only a single antigen or epitope (2–4). Immunoglobulin exists either as a surface membrane-bound molecule or in a secreted form by B cells that have been appropriately stimulated and matured.

The immunoglobulin molecule is a glycoprotein composed of two identical light chains and two identical heavy chains (Fig. 1.1) linked by disulfide bonds (6). Enzymatic cleavage of the immunoglobulin molecule creates defined fragments. Papain produces two antigen-binding fragments (Fab) and one crystallizable fragment (Fc). Pepsin produces only a divalent antigen-binding fragment termed $F(ab')_2$, and the remainder of the molecule tends to be degraded and lost.

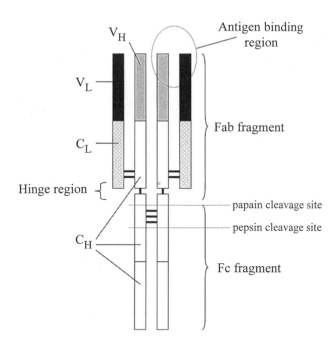

FIG. 1.1. The immunoglobulin molecule.

Each chain (heavy and light) contains one or more constant regions (C_H or C_L) and a variable region (V_H or V_L). Together, the variable regions of the light and heavy chains contribute to the antigen-binding sites (Fab) of the immunoglobulin molecule. The constant regions of the heavy chain (particularly in the Fc portion) determine what subsequent interactions may occur between the bound immunoglobulin and other cells or molecules of the immune system. When the antigen-binding sites are filled, a signal is transmitted through the immunoglobulin molecule, which results in conformational changes in the Fc portion of the heavy chain. These conformational changes permit the Fc portion to then interact with other molecules and cells. The conformationally altered Fc may be recognized by receptors (Fc receptors [FcR]) on macrophages and other cells, which allow them to distinguish bound from unbound immunoglobulin molecules (7,8), increasing their efficiency of phagocytosis. Other conformational changes in the Fc portion of bound immunoglobulin permit the binding of complement component C1q to initiate the classic pathway of complement activation. The Fab and F(ab′)$_2$

fragments are useful experimental and therapeutic tools that can bind antigens without the ensuing consequences resulting from the presence of the Fc region (9).

Immunoglobulin light chains contain one of two types of constant regions, κ or λ. The constant regions of the heavy chains exist in five major forms (Table 1.1), each associated with a particular immunoglobulin isotype or class: Cα (immunoglobulin A [IgA]), Cδ (IgD), Cϵ (IgE), Cγ (IgG), and Cμ (IgM). Some of these can be subdivided into subclasses (e.g., IgG1, IgG2, IgG3, and IgG4). Each normal individual can generate all of the isotypes. Within a single immunoglobulin molecule, both light chains are identical and of the same type (both κ or both λ), and the two heavy chains are likewise identical and of the same isotype. IgD, IgG, and IgE exist only as monomeric basic immunoglobulin units (two heavy chains and two light chains), but serum IgM exists as a pentamer of five basic units united by a J (joining) chain. IgA can be found in a variety of forms (monomers, dimers, trimers, tetramers) but is most commonly seen as a monomer (in serum) or as a dimer (in external body fluids, such as mucus, tears, and saliva).

TABLE 1.1. *Immunoglobulin isotypes*

Isotype	Molecular weight	Additional components	Serum immunoglobulin (%)	Half-life	Functions
IgA					
Monomer [a,b]	160,000	—	13–19	6 d	—
Dimer [b]	385,000	J chain, secretary piece	0.3		Provides antibodies for external body fluids including mucous, saliva, and tears. Effective at neutralizing infectious agents, agglutination, and (when bound to antigen) activation of the alternative complement pathway.
IgD					
Monomer [a,b]	180,000		<1	3 d	Almost entirely found in membrane bound form. The function is unknown, but may be related to maturational stages.
IgE					
Monomer [a,b]	190,000		<0.001	3 d	Serum level is very low because most secreted IgE is bound to mast cell surfaces. Subsequent binding of antigen stimulates mast cell degranulation, leading to immediate hypersensitivity responses (allergy).
IgG					
Monomer [a,b]	145,000–170,000		72–80	20 d	Prevalent isotype in secondary responses. In humans, subclasses are IgG1, IgG2, IgG3, IgG4
IgM					
Monomer [a]	—	—	—	—	—
Pentamer [b]	970,000	J chain	6–8	5–10 d	Prevalent isotype in primary responses. Effective at agglutination and activation of classic complement pathway.

[a] Membrane bound form.
[b] Secreted form.

The dimeric form contains two basic units, bound together by a J chain. In passing through specialized epithelial cells to external fluids, it also adds a "secretory piece," which increases its resistance to degradation by external enzymes (10).

In addition to antigen-binding specificity, variability among immunoglobulin molecules derives from three further sources: allotypes, isotypes, and idiotypes. Allotypes are dictated by minor amino acid sequence differences in the constant regions of heavy or light chains, which result from slight polymorphisms in the genes encoding these molecules. Allotypic differences typically do not affect the function of the molecule and segregate within families like typical mendelian traits. Isotypes, as already discussed, are determined by more substantial differences in the heavy chain constant regions affecting the functional properties of the immunoglobulins (11) (Table 1.1). Finally, many antigenic determinants may be bound in more than one way, and thus there may be multiple, structurally distinct, immunoglobulins with the same antigenic specificity. These differences within the antigen-binding domains of immunoglobulins that bind the same antigenic determinants are termed *idiotypes*.

Generation of Antigen Binding Diversity among Immunoglobulins

Each immunoglobulin chain, light and heavy, is encoded not by a single gene but by a series of genes occurring in clusters along the chromosome (11). In humans, the series of genes encoding κ light chains, the series encoding λ light chains, and the series encoding heavy chains are all located on separate chromosomes. Within each series, the genes are found in clusters, each containing a set of similar, but not identical, genes. All of the genes are present in embryonic and germ cells and in cells other than B lymphocytes. When a cell becomes committed to the B-lymphocyte lineage, it rearranges the DNA encoding its light and heavy chains (11,12) by clipping out and degrading some of the DNA sequences. Each differentiating B cell chooses either the κ series or the λ series (but not both). In addition, although both the maternally and paternally derived chromosomes carry these sets of genes, each B cell uses only one of them (*either* paternal *or* maternal) to produce a functional chain, a phenomenon termed *allelic exclusion*.

For the light chains, there are three distinct clusters of genes that contribute to the synthesis of the entire polypeptide: variable genes (V_L), joining genes (J_L), and constant genes (C_L) (Fig. 1.2). In addition, each V gene is preceded by a leader sequence encoding a portion of the polypeptide that is important during the synthetic process but is removed when the molecule becomes functional. The V_L and D_L

genes are used to produce the variable domain of the light chain. This is accomplished by the random selection of a single V_L gene and a single J_L gene to be united (V_L–J_L) by splicing out and discarding the intervening DNA. Henceforth, that cell and all of its clonal descendants are committed to that particular V_L–J_L combination. Messenger RNA for the light chain is transcribed to include the V_L–J_L genes, the C_L gene or genes, and the intervening DNA between them. Before translation, the messenger RNA (mRNA) is spliced to unite the V_L–J_L genes with a C_L gene so that a single continuous polypeptide can be produced from three genes that were originally separated on the chromosome.

For heavy chains, there are four distinct clusters of genes involved (Fig. 1.3): variable genes (V_H), diversity genes (D_H), joining genes (J_H), and a series of distinct constant genes (C_μ, C_δ, C_γ, C_ϵ, and C_α). As with the light chain genes, each V gene is preceded by a leader sequence (L) that plays a role during synthesis but is subsequently lost. One V_H gene, one D_H gene, and one J_H gene are randomly selected, and the intervening DNA segments are excised and discarded to bring these genes together (V_H–D_H–J_H). Messenger RNA is then transcribed to include both the V_H–D_H–J_H and constant genes, but unlike for the light chains, the processes involving constant genes are distinctly different in stimulated and unstimulated B lymphocytes.

Unstimulated B cells transcribe heavy chain mRNA from V_H–D_H–J_H through the C_μ and C_δ genes. This transcript does not contain the information from the C_γ, C_ϵ, or C_α genes. The mRNA is then spliced to bring V_H–D_H–J_H adjacent to either C_μ or C_δ, which permits the translation of a single continuous polypeptide with a variable domain (from V_H–D_H–J_H) and a constant domain (from either C_μ or C_δ). Thus, the surface immunoglobulin of naïve unstimulated B cells includes only the IgM and IgD isotypes.

After antigenic stimulation, B cells can undergo an isotype switch in which splicing of DNA, rather than RNA, brings the united V_H–D_H–J_H genes adjacent to a constant region gene (13,14). This transition is controlled by cytokines secreted by T lymphocytes. Depending on the amount of DNA excised, the V_H–D_H–J_H genes

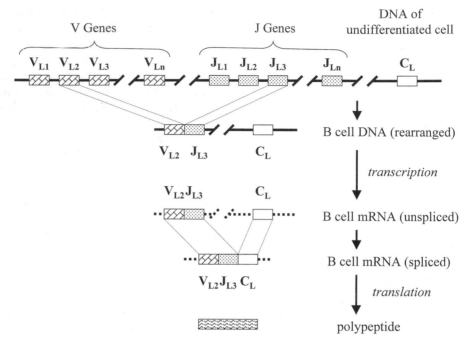

FIG. 1.2. Synthesis of immunoglobulin light chains.

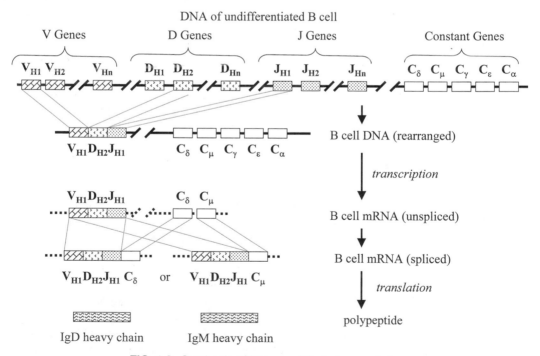

FIG. 1.3. Synthesis of immunoglobulin heavy chains.

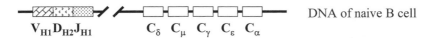

DNA of naive B cell

$V_{H1}D_{H2}J_{H1}$ C_δ C_μ C_γ C_ε C_α

After antigenic stimulation, DNA between the VDJ unit and the constant genes is excised. The length of the excision may vary, bringing VDJ adjacent to different constant genes.

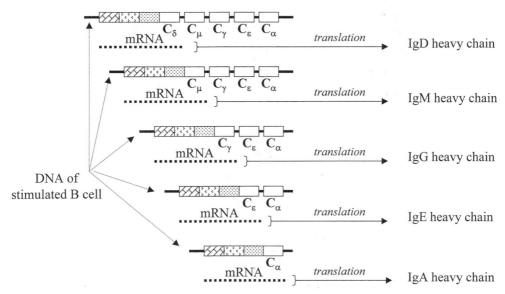

FIG. 1.4. The isotype switch.

may be joined to any of the different C_H genes (Fig. 1.4). As a result of the isotype switch, B-cell "subclones" are generated that produce an array of immunoglobulins that have identical antigen-binding specificity but different isotypes.

Two additional sources of diversity in the variable (antigen-binding) regions of light and heavy immunoglobulin chains occur. First, *junctional diversity* may result from imprecision in the precise placement of the cutting and splicing that bring V, D, and J genes together; second, *somatic mutations* may occur and accumulate in successive generations of clonally derived B lymphocytes when they undergo restimulation through later exposures to the same antigenic epitopes (15,16).

T-cell Receptor

T lymphocytes (T cells) do not use immunoglobulins as antigen receptors but rather use a distinct set of genes encoding four polypeptide chains (α, β, γ, and δ), each with variable and constant domains, used to form T-cell receptors (TCRs) (17–19). The TCR is a heterodimer, either an α β or a γ δ chain combination, which recognizes and binds antigen (Fig. 1.5). This heterodimer, which is not covalently linked together, is complexed with several other molecules (e.g., CD3, CD4, and CD8), that provide stability and auxiliary functions for the receptor (20–22). Unlike immunoglobulin, which can bind to free antigen alone, TCRs bind only to specific combinations of antigen and certain self cell surface molecules. They are therefore restricted to recognition and binding of antigen on cell surfaces and are unable to bind free antigen. In humans, the self molecules are encoded by the polymorphic genes of the HLA complex (23): class I (encoded by the HLA-A, -B, and -C loci) and class II (encoded by the -DP, -DQ, and -DR loci within the D/DR region). TCRs of T cells in which CD8 is part of the TCR complex can recognize and bind antigen

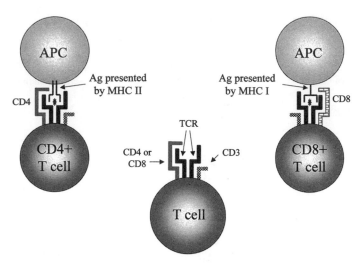

FIG. 1.5. The T-cell receptor.

only when that antigen is associated with (or presented by) class I molecules, whereas those T cells in which CD4 is part of the TCR complex can recognize and bind antigen only when the antigen is presented by class II molecules.

Like immunoglobulin, the TCR chains contain variable and constant domains. The variable domains are encoded by a series of V, J, and sometimes D (β and δ chains only) gene clusters that undergo DNA rearrangement, and the constant regions are encoded by constant genes. TCRs do not undergo any changes equivalent to the isotype switch. Junctional diversity provides an additional source of variation for the variable domains of α and β chains but not for the γ and δ chains. Somatic mutation, so important in the diversity of immunoglobulins, does not occur in TCRs and is apparently "forbidden."

Cell Determinant Molecules

Several cell surface molecules, the cell determinant (CD) molecules, indicate the functional capacities of lymphocytes and other cells (24). The most commonly used are those distinguishing T-lymphocyte subsets.

- *CD3* is a complex of several molecules associated with the T-cell antigen receptor (21,22). It provides support for the TCR and is involved in transmembrane signaling when the TCR is filled. It is found on all T cells.
- *CD4* is found on T lymphocytes of the helper T-cell (T_H) and delayed hypersensitivity (T_{dh}) subsets (25–27). CD4 molecules are found in association with the TCR and recognize class II major histocompatibility complex (MHC) molecules on antigen-presenting cells (APCs). The TCR of CD4$^+$ cells are thus restricted to recognizing combinations of antigen and class II MHC.
- *CD8* is found on T cells of the cytotoxic T-lymphocyte (CTL) and suppressor T-cell (T_s) subsets (25,27). CD8 molecules are found in association with the TCR and recognize class I MHC molecules on APCs. The TCR of CD8$^+$ cells are thus restricted to recognizing combinations of antigen and class I MHC.

All $\alpha\beta$ T cells express either CD4 or CD8 (and, during an early developmental stage, both). The $\gamma\delta$ T cells, on the other hand, often express neither CD4 nor CD8 (19).

Human Leukocyte Antigen Molecules

The HLA is the MHC of humans (23). It is a small region of chromosome 6 containing several (10 to 20) individual genes encoding proteins of three

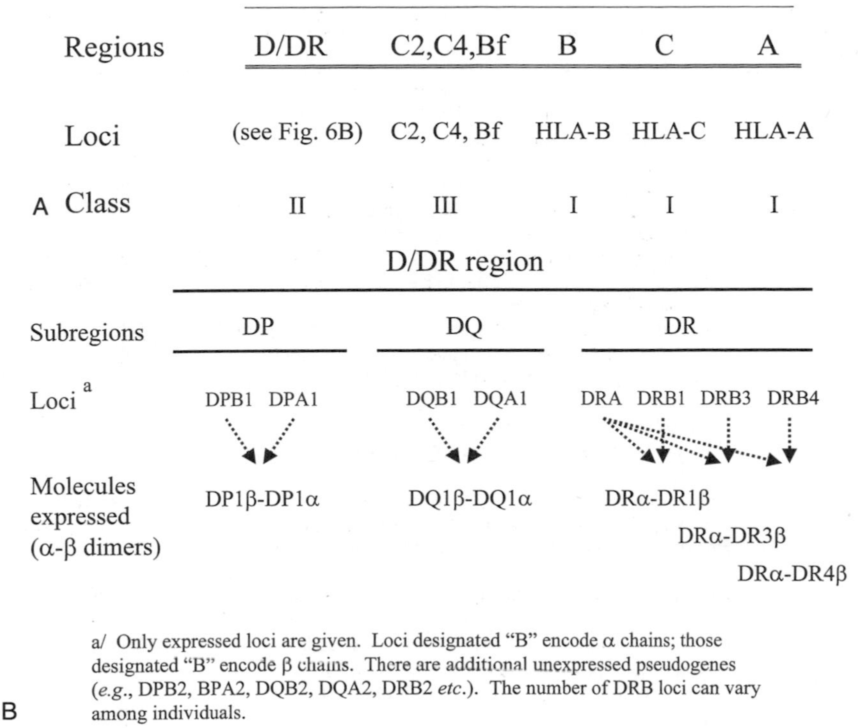

Regions	D/DR	C2,C4,Bf	B	C	A
Loci	(see Fig. 6B)	C2, C4, Bf	HLA-B	HLA-C	HLA-A
A Class	II	III	I	I	I

D/DR region

Subregions	DP	DQ	DR
Loci [a]	DPB1 DPA1	DQB1 DQA1	DRA DRB1 DRB3 DRB4
Molecules expressed (α-β dimers)	DP1β-DP1α	DQ1β-DQ1α	DRα-DR1β DRα-DR3β DRα-DR4β

a/ Only expressed loci are given. Loci designated "B" encode α chains; those designated "B" encode β chains. There are additional unexpressed pseudogenes (*e.g.*, DPB2, BPA2, DQB2, DQA2, DRB2 *etc.*). The number of DRB loci can vary among individuals.

B

FIG. 1.6. A: The HLA complex. **B**: The D/DR region.

different types, called class I, II, and III MHC molecules (Fig. 1.6A).

- *Class I molecules* are membrane-bound glyco-proteins found on all nucleated cells (28). They are a single large polypeptide (about 350 amino acids) associated with a smaller molecule (β_2-microglobulin). The HLA complex includes three distinct class I loci (HLA-A, -B, and -C), each having scores of alleles.
- *Class II molecules* are heterodimers (Fig. 1.6B) consisting of two membrane-bound, noncovalently linked chains (α and β) and show a much more limited cellular distribution than class I molecules (29). They are encoded by the DR, DP, and DQ regions of the HLA complex. They are expressed constitutively on B lymphocytes, macrophages, monocytes, and similar cells in various tissues (Kupffer cells, astrocytes, Langerhans cells of the skin). Some other cells (e.g., vascular epithelium) are able to express class II molecules transiently under particular conditions.

- *Class III molecules* are those complement molecules (e.g., C2, C4, Bf) encoded within the HLA complex (30).

Cytokines and Ligands

Cytokines are short-range acting, soluble products that are important in the cellular communication necessary for the generation of immune responses (31–37). Those produced predominantly by lymphocytes or monocytes are often referred to as *lymphokines* or *monokines*, but because so many are produced by multiple cell types, the term *cytokine* has gained favor. A large number of cytokines have been identified, although the roles of many of them are not yet well understood. Many of the cytokines are crucial in regulating lymphocyte development and the types of immune responses evoked by specific responses (37–40). Those most basically involved in common immune responses are listed in Table 1.2.

TABLE 1.2. *Cytokines*

Cytokine	Activities	Sources
Interleukin-1 (IL-1)	Stimulates the synthesis of IL-2 and of receptors for IL-2 (IL-2R) by T lymphocytes; involved in inflammatory responses. Also known as *lymphocyte-activating factor* (LAF).	Activated macrophages
Interleukin-2 (IL-2)	Stimulates proliferation and maturation of T lymphocytes; stimulates differentiation of B lymphocytes. Stimulates NK cells. Also known as *T-cell growth factor* (TCGF).	T cells, especially CD4$^+$ T_H1 cells; some CD8$^+$ T cells
Interleukin-3 (IL-3)	Stimulates proliferation and maturation of T lymphocytes and of stem cells; induces IL-1 synthesis by activated macrophages.	CD4$^+$ T cells; some CD8$^+$ T cells; eosinophils
Interleukin-4 (IL-4)	Stimulates proliferation of activated B lymphocytes and of T_H2 lymphocytes; stimulates differentiation of B lymphocytes producing IgE and IgG1. Downregulates activities of CD4$^+$ T_H1 lymphocytes. Also known as *B-cell growth factor* (BCGF).	CD4$^+$ T_H2 T cells; mast cells
Interleukin-5 (IL-5)	Stimulates differentiaton of B lymphocytes producing IgA.	CD4$^+$ T_H2 T cells
Interleukin-6 (IL-6)	Stimulates proliferation and differentiation of B lymphocytes; involved in acute-phase response.	CD4$^+$$T_H2$ T cells; macrophages
Interleukin-7 (IL-7)	Promotes growth of pre-T and pre-B lymphocytes.	Stromal cells
Interleukin-8 (IL-8)	Chemotactic factor for neutrophils and basophils.	Monocytes; eosinophils
Interleukin-10 (IL-10)	Inhibits macrophage activity, stimulates B cells and mast cells, inhibits CD4$^+$ T_H1 T cells.	CD4$^+$ T_H2 T cells
Interleukin-12 (IL-12)	Stimulates IFN-γ production by natural killer (NK) cells.	Macrophages; monocytes; B cells
Tumor necrosis factor-α (TNF-α)	Has toxic activity toward tumor cells; involved in some inflammatory responses.	T cells; activated macrophages; natural killer cells
Tumor necrosis factor-β (TNF-β)	Has toxic activity toward tumor cells. Stimulates macrophages. Also called *lymphotoxin* (LT).	CD4$^+$ T_H1 T cells; B cells
Interferon-γ (IFN-γ)	Activates macrophages, stimulates increased expression of class I and II major histocompatibility complex (MHC) molecules, inhibits viral replication, promotes the differentiation of some B lymphocytes, and stimulates activity of NK cells. Inhibits CD4$^+$ T_H2 T cells. Also known as *macrophage-activating factor* (MAF).	CD4$^+$ T_H1 T cells; CD8$^+$ T cells; natural killer cells
Interleukin-13 (IL-13)	Promotes differentiation of B cells.	CD4$^+$ T_H2 T cells
Interleukin-15 (IL-15)	Promotes proliferation of T and B cells.	T cells
Interferon-α (IFN-α)	Stimulates NK cells, promotes class I MHC expression, provides antiviral effect.	Leukocytes
Interferon-β (IFN-β)	Stimulates NK cells, promotes class I MHC expression, provides antiviral effect.	Fibroblasts

Ligands are cell surface molecules that bind molecules on the surface of other cells in order to transmit or receive signals critical to development or activation. Among those important for immune function are B7/CD28 and CD40/CD40 ligand. B7 on APCs binds CD28 or CTLA-4 (or both) on T lymphocytes to provide signals for activation and inhibition, respectively (41). CD40 ligand (CD40L) on activated T lymphocytes binds CD40 on B lymphocytes and macrophages to provide activation signals to those cells (42,43).

Complement

Complement is the composite term for a number of serum proteins (complement components) that can interact with one another, as well as with

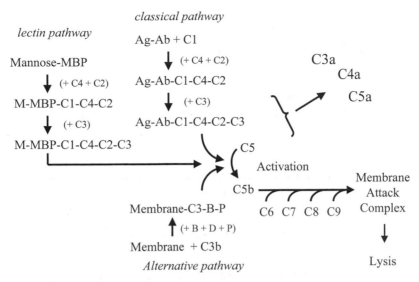

FIG. 1.7. The complement cascade.

antibodies under some circumstances, to produce several different chemical signals and destructive responses (44). The complement components (C1 through C9 plus B, D, and P) act on one another sequentially (the complement "*cascade*") (Fig. 1.7). The cascade begins with the binding of either component C1 to an antigen–antibody complex or of component C3 to a bacterial or other membrane surface (*without* the assistance of antibody). The binding of C1 initiates what is termed the *classic pathway* (involving the subsequent binding of components C4, C2, and C3), whereas the direct binding of C3 initiates the *alternative pathway* (involving the additional binding of components D, B, and P). A third pathway for complement activation, the *lectin pathway*, begins with the binding of mannose-binding protein (MBP) to mannose on bacterial cell surfaces. All three pathways eventually lead to the activation and binding of component C5, followed by components C6, C7, C8, and C9. The completion of this combination of C5 through C9 is termed the *membrane attack complex* and results in the rupture of the cell surface to which it is attached (45).

As complement components interact with one another, each is cleaved into fragments. Some become enzymatically active to continue the cascade. The smaller fragments gain hormone-like functions and are important in stimulating various inflammatory reactions (46). C5a (a fragment of C5) attracts neutrophils and macrophages to the site of interest. C3a (a fragment of C3) causes smooth muscle contraction and stimulates basophils, mast cells, and platelets to release histamine and other chemicals contributing to inflammation. C3b (another fragment of C3) stimulates the ingestion (opsonization) of the cells onto which the C3b is bound by monocytes and other phagocytic cells. C4a (fragment of C4) has activity similar to C5a, although less effective.

Antigen–Antibody Complexes

Binding of antigen with antibody is noncovalent and reversible. The strength of the interaction is termed *affinity* and determines the relative concentrations of bound versus free antigen and antibody. The formation of antigen–antibody complexes results into lattice-like aggregates of soluble antigen and antibody, and the efficiency of such binding is affected by the relative concentrations of antigen and antibody (2–4,47). This is best illustrated by the quantitative precipitin reaction (Fig. 1.8). When there is an excess of either antibody or antigen, the antigen–antibody complexes tend to remain small and in solution. The optimal binding, producing large aggregates

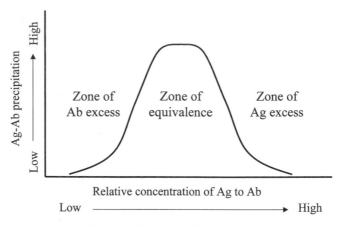

FIG. 1.8. The precipitin reactions.

that fall out of solution, occurs when the concentrations of antibody and antigen are in equivalence. The quantitative precipitin curve provides the basis of laboratory methods for determining the amount of antigen or antibody in, for example, a patient's serum.

MOLECULES FOR ADHESION, RECIRCULATION, AND HOMING

A number of surface molecules (adhesins, integrins, selectins) are used by various elements of the immune system to stabilize binding between cells to facilitate binding of antigen-specific receptors, to facilitate attachment of leukocytes to endothelial surfaces in order to leave the blood vessels and enter into the surrounding tissues, to identify and accumulate at sites of inflammation, and to identify organ- or tissue-specific sites (e.g., lymph nodes, intestinal mucosa) into which they must enter in order to undergo developmental processes or carry out other immunologic functions (48–50).

CELLS OF THE IMMUNE SYSTEM

Lymphocytes (General)

The ability of the immune system to recognize specifically a diverse range of antigens resides with the lymphocytes (2–4). The lymphocytic lineage, derived from stem cells residing within the bone marrow, includes the B lymphocytes, T lymphocytes, and null cells. B lymphocytes mature in the bone marrow, and those destined to become T lymphocytes migrate to the thymus, where they mature. The bone marrow and thymus thus constitute the primary lymphoid organs of the immune system, as opposed to the secondary organs (e.g., spleen, lymph nodes, Peyer patches), where cells later periodically congregate as they circulate throughout the body.

The ability of the immune system to identify so many different antigens is based on a division of labor—each lymphocyte (or clone of lymphocytes) is able to identify only one epitope or determinant. During its development and differentiation, each cell that is committed to becoming a B or T lymphocyte rearranges the DNA encoding its receptors (as previously described) to construct a unique antigen receptor. Thereafter, that cell and all of its clonal descendants express receptors with the same antigenic specificity. Other surface molecules and secreted products serve to define functional subsets of lymphocytes (Table 1.3). The specificity of an immune response lies in the fact that the entry of a foreign antigen into the body stimulates only those lymphocytes whose receptors recognize and bind the determinants expressed on the antigen. As a result of this specific binding and subsequent intercellular communication, a response is initiated that includes the following distinct phases:

1. Recognition of antigen by binding to the receptors of lymphoid cells—often manifested by clonal proliferation of the stimulated cells

TABLE 1.3. *Cells of the human immune system: markers and functions*

Cell	Antigen receptor	Distinctive markers[a]	Soluble products	Cell functions
B lymphocyte	Ig	Ig Class II MHC FcR C3R B7 CD40	Ig	Antibody synthesis/secretion Antigen processing/presentation
T lymphocyte				
T_H1	TCR	TCR CD2 CD3 CD4 CD28 CD40L	IL-2 IL-3 IFN-γ TNF-α, -β	Delayed-type hypersensitivity Inhibition of T_H2 T cells Help for cell-mediated immunity, including inflammatory responses
T_H2	TCR	TCR CD2 CD3 CD4 CD28	IL-3 IL-4 IL-5 IL-10 Il-13	Help for B lymphocytes producing Ig Control of "isotype switch" Stimulation of granulocytes, mast cells, and eosinophils Inhibition of T_H1 cells
Tc	TCR	TCR CD2 CD3 CD8 CD28	IL-2[a] IFN-γ[a] TNF-α, -β[a]	Lysis, by direct contact, of cells altered by infection or malignancy
NK cell	None	FcR KIR CD94/NKG2	IFN-γ	Lysis of infected or transformed cells

Macrophage,
   monocyte,
   dendritic cell
	None	Class II MHC
		FCr
		C3R
		B7
		CD40
			IL-1
			IL-6
			TNF-α, -β
				Phaocytosis, antigen processing and
				   presentation, delayed-type hypersensitivity;
				   acute-phase response

Mast cell and
   basophil
	None	FcϵRI	Histamine
			Platelet-
			   activating
			   factor
				Immediate hypersensitivity

Neutrophil	None		Enzymes	Pinocytosis, inflammation
Eosinophil	None		IL-3 IL-5 IL-8	Antiparasite activity

Ig, immunoglobulin; TCR, T-cell receptor; MHC, major histocompatibility complex; IL, interleukin; IFN, interferon; NK, natural killer; FcR, Fc receptor; FcϵRI, receptor for Fc of unbound IgE; C3R, C3 receptor.
[a] Some CD8 cells.

2. Differentiation and maturation of the stimulated cells to mature functional capacity
3. Response against the antigen, cell, or organism by any of several methods
4. Establishment of immunologic memory

Memory resides in a portion of the stimulated lymphocytes that do not carry out effector functions (51,52). Instead, they remain quiescent in the system, providing an enlarged pool of activated cells specific for the original stimulating epitope. As a result, subsequent exposures to that same epitope can produce faster and higher (secondary or anamnestic) responses than were seen in the initial (primary) response. Memory can persist for long periods of time and is primarily maintained by T lymphocytes.

B Lymphocytes

Immunoglobulins recognize and bind specific antigens and determinants. Each B cell, or clonally derived set of B cells, expresses only a single "species" of immunoglobulin and is capable of recognizing and binding to only a single epitope. Immunoglobulin can be either membrane bound or secreted, and these forms serve two different purposes:

1. When membrane-bound on a B-cell surface, immunoglobulin detects the antigen or epitope for which that particular B cell is specific. The binding of antigen to the surface immunoglobulin, together with "help" from T lymphocytes (proliferative and maturation factors), induces the B cell to proliferate and mature into a plasma cell that secretes large amounts of immunoglobulin or becomes a memory B cell (53).

2. When secreted by plasma cells, immunoglobulin binds to the antigen of interest, "tagging" it for removal or for subsequent interaction with other cells and molecules (e.g., complement or phagocytic cells). The binding specificity of the membrane-bound and secreted immunoglobulins from a single B cell or clonal set of B cells and plasma cells are essentially identical. However, as mentioned previously, mutations can occur and accumulate in the immunoglobulin-encoding genes of B lymphocytes undergoing proliferation after restimulation with antigen. Where the mutated immunoglobulins are capable of binding more tightly to the antigen, the cells producing those immunoglobulins are stimulated to proliferate more rapidly. In this way, an ongoing antibody response can generate new immunoglobulin varieties with higher affinity for the antigen in question, a process known as *affinity maturation*.

T Lymphocytes

T lymphocytes (T cells) also bear antigen-specific surface receptors. The TCR of most T cells is an α-β heterodimer, complexed with other molecules (e.g., CD3, CD4, and CD8) providing auxiliary functions. As described earlier, the TCRs bind not to antigen alone, but rather to specific combinations of antigen and class I or II MHC molecules (54,55). T cells include several different functional groups:

- *Helper T cells* initiate responses by proliferating and providing help to B cells and to other T cells (e.g., cytotoxic T lymphocytes) and participate in inflammatory responses. T-cell help consists of a variety of cytokines that are required for activation, proliferation, and differentiation of cells involved in the immune response, including the helper T cells themselves. Helper T cells, in turn, comprise two broad categories: T_H1 and T_H2 (56–59), which secrete different sets of cytokines. These two particular subsets have been best characterized in mice, and comparable subsets are being identified in humans. All helper T cells, both T_H1 and T_H2, bear the CD4 marker and receptors that recognize combinations of antigen and class II HLA molecules.

- *T_H1 cells* help other effector T cells (e.g., cytotoxic T lymphocytes) to carry out cell-mediated responses (57,58). In mice, they also help B cells producing immunoglobulins of the IgG2a isotype. T_H1 cells are characterized by the production of interleukin-2 (IL-2), tumor necrosis factor-α (TNF-α), and interferon-γ (IFN-γ) (Table 1.2). They participate in delayed-typed hypersensitivity (DTH) responses, but it is unclear whether the cells doing so are a distinct subset of T_H1. In addition to its helper functions, IFN-γ also diminishes the activity of T_H2 cells.

- *T_H2 cells* cells provide help for most B cells (with exceptions such as IgG2a in mice) and are characterized by the production of IL-4, IL-5, IL-6, and IL-10 (Table 1.2). In addition to their helper functions, IL-4 and IL-10 diminish the activity of T_H1 cells.

- *CTLs* can lyse other cells, which they identify as altered by infection or transformation, through direct contact (60–63) and using a short-range acting cytolysin, which does not damage the membrane of the CTL itself. These cells, which require help from T_H1 cells to proliferate and differentiate, bear CD8 molecules and TCRs recognizing antigen and class I HLA molecule combinations on the surface of antigen-producing cells (where they are first stimulated) and later on the surface of cells that they subsequently identify as targets for destruction. In order for a CTL to attack and lyse a potential target cell, it must see (on that target) the same combination of antigen and class I HLA molecule that provided its initial stimulation.

- *DTH T cells* (a subset of T_H1) mediate an effector mechanism whereby the T_{dh}, bearing CD4 molecules and triggered by specific combinations of antigen and class II HLA molecules, produce cytokines that attract and activate macrophages (57,58). The activated macrophages, which themselves have no specificity for antigen, then produce a localized inflammatory response arising 24 to 72 hours after antigenic challenge.

- T_s *cells* provide negative regulation to the immune system—the counterweight to T_H cells (64). These cells, classically defined as bearing CD8 markers and recognizing combinations of antigen and class I MHC molecules, are involved in keeping immune responses within acceptable levels of intensity, depressing them as the antigenic stimulation declines, and preventing aberrant immune responses against self antigens. The mechanisms by which T_s cells carry out these functions is currently a topic of intense debate, and some investigators question their existence altogether. More recently, $CD4^+$ T cells have also been implicated in some types of suppression, the mutual negative regulation of T_H1 and T_H2 cells providing one such example.

Although T lymphocytes with $\alpha\beta$ TCR also express either the CD4 or CD8 markers, those with $\gamma\delta$ TCR usually express neither. The ontogeny, distribution, and functional roles of $\gamma\delta$ T lymphocytes are still not as well understood as those of $\alpha\beta$ T lymphocytes (65). The TCRs of a lineage of T cells do not accumulate mutations and, under affinity, maturation, as do immunoglobulins.

Macrophages and Other Antigen-presenting Cells

TCRs do not usually recognize antigen alone in its natural form, but rather bind to antigen that has been processed and presented on the surface of appropriate APCs (66–68). APCs internalize antigen, enzymatically degrade it into fragments (processing), and put the fragments back onto their surface in association with class I and II MHC molecules (presentation) (7). APCs (Table 1.3) include monocytes, macrophages, and other related tissue-specific cells that express class II MHC molecules (e.g., astrocytes in the central nervous system, Langerhans cells in the skin, Kupffer cells in the liver, and so forth). In addition, B lymphocytes (which normally express class II) can efficiently process and present antigen (69,70). There are some other cells that are capable of transient expression of class II (e.g., vascular endothelium). In addition, a variety of other molecules on APCs and T cells serve to stabilize the contact between the TCR and combination of antigen and MHC molecule.

Null Cells

In addition to T and B cells, the lymphoid lineage includes a subset of cells lacking both of the classic lymphoid antigen receptors (immunoglobulin and TCR). This subset includes killer (K) and natural killer (NK) cells, and probably other cells, such as lymphokine-activated killer cells and large granular lymphocytes, which may represent differentially activated forms of K and NK cells (71,72). K cells bear receptors capable of recognizing the Fc portion of bound immunoglobulins. If the antigen is on the surface of a cell, the K cell uses the bound immunoglobulin to make contact with that cell and lyse it by direct contact, a process termed *antibody-dependent cellular cytotoxicity* (ADCC). The K cell has no specificity for the antigen that is bound to the antibody, only for the Fc portion of the bound antibody. NK cells appear to distinguish between altered (by malignant transformation or viral infection) cells and comparable normal cells and to bind preferentially and lyse the former. The means by which they make this distinction is unknown, but their activity is heightened by IFN-γ and IL-2. NK cells are able to recognize decreases in the levels of class I MHC molecules or other molecules on the surface of infected or malignant cells (71,72). Recent evidence suggests that K cells may be a subset of NK cells and that the distinction between them may simply reflect distinct stages of differentiation, or even simply the use of different assay systems.

Mast Cells and Granulocytes

A variety of other cells are involved in some immune responses, particularly those involving inflammation (Table 1.3). Mast cells and basophils bear receptors (FcεRI) for the Fc portion of unbound IgE, permitting them to use IgE on their own surface as an antigen detector (73). When antigen binds simultaneously to two or more such IgE molecules on the same mast cell (called *bridging*), a signal is transmitted into the cell, leading to degranulation and release of a variety of mediators, including histamine, resulting in immediate hypersensitivity (allergic) responses (74). Neutrophils are drawn to sites of inflammation by cytokines, where their phagocytic activity and production of enzymes and other soluble mediators contribute to the inflammation. Eosinophils (75,76) are involved in immune responses against large parasites, such as roundworms, and are apparently capable of killing them by direct contact.

PRIMARY ORGANS: BONE MARROW AND THYMUS

The primordial stem cells that ultimately produce the human immune system (and other elements of the hematopoietic system) originate in the yolk sac, about 60 days after fertilization. These cells migrate to the fetal liver and then (beginning about 80 days after fertilization) to the bone marrow, where they remain for life. These primordial hematopoietic stem cells give rise to more specialized stem cells, which lead to the erythrocytic, granulocytic, thrombocytic (platelet), myelocytic (e.g., macrophages and monocytes), and lymphocytic lineages.

Primary lymphoid organs consist of the bone marrow and thymus, where B and T lymphocytes, respectively, mature. B cells undergo their development, including generation of immunoglobulin receptors, while in the bone marrow. Cells of the T-lymphocyte lineage, however, migrate from the bone marrow to the thymus, where they undergo development and generation

of TCRs (77,78). More than 95% of the cells that migrate into the thymus perish there, failing to survive a rigorous selection process to promote the development of those relevant to the individual's MHC genotype and to eliminate potentially self-reactive cells. It is in the thymus, under the influence of thymic stroma, nurse cells, and thymic APCs, that T cells receive an initial "thymic education" with regard to what should be recognized as self (79,80).

Secondary Organs: Spleen and Lymph Nodes

The secondary organs (e.g., spleen, lymph nodes, Peyer patches) provide sites where recirculating lymphocytes and APCs enter after passage through diverse parts of the body, "mingle" in close proximity for a period of time, and then leave again to recirculate. This intimate contact between recirculating cells facilitates the close interactions needed to initiate immune responses and generate appropriately sensitized cells, whose activities may then be expressed throughout the body (2–4). Thus, most immune responses are actually initiated in the secondary organs.

INTERACTIONS IN IMMUNE RESPONSES

Antibody Responses

More than 99% of antibody responses are against T-dependent antigens, which require the involvement of T lymphocytes in generation of the responses. The relatively few T-independent (TI) antigens, which can provoke antibody production in the absence of T-cell involvement, fall into two general categories: TI-1 and TI-2. TI-1 antigens (e.g., a variety of lectins) are mitogenic, inducing proliferation and differentiation through binding of B-cell surface molecules other than immunoglobulins, whereas TI-2 antigens have regular repeating structures (e.g., dextran, with repetitive carbohydrate moieties) and are capable of cross-linking multiple immunoglobulin molecules on the surface of the same B cell.

Antibody responses to most antigens are T dependent and require interactions between APCs

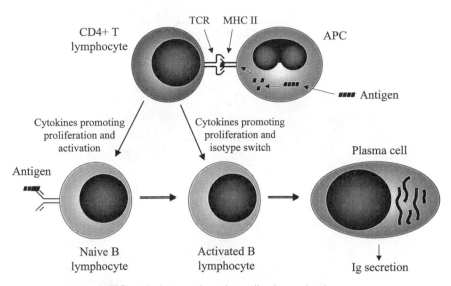

FIG. 1.9. Interactions in antibody production.

(e.g., macrophages), T lymphocytes, and B lymphocytes (53,81–84), as illustrated in Fig. 1.9. B lymphocytes responding to T-dependent antigens require two signals for proliferation and differentiation: (a) the binding of their surface immunoglobulin by appropriate specific antigen, and (b) the binding of cytokines (e.g., IL-4 and other helper factors) produced by activated helper T cells (85,86). The help provided by T cells acts only over a short range; thus, the T and B cells must be in fairly intimate contact for these interactions to occur successfully. The involvement of APCs, such as macrophages or even B cells themselves, is essential for the activation of helper T cells and provides a means of bringing T and B cells into proximity.

Cellular Responses

The mixed lymphocyte response (MLR) is an *in vitro* measure of T-cell proliferation (primarily of CD4$^+$ T cells) that is often used as a measure of the initial phase (recognition and proliferation) of the cellular response. Splenic or lymph node T cells (or both) from the individual in question (responder) are mixed with lymphocytes from another individual (sensitizer) against whom the response is to be evaluated. The sensitizing cells are usually treated (e.g., with mitomycin or

irradiation) to prevent them from proliferating. The two cell populations are incubated together for 4 to 5 days, after which time tritiated thymidine is added to the culture for a few hours. If the responder cells actively proliferate as a result of the recognition of foreign antigens on the sensitizing cells, significant increases of thymidine incorporation (over control levels) can be measured. The strongest MLR responses typically occur when the sensitizing cells bear different class II MHC molecules than the responding cells, although primary significant MLR responses can also often be observed for class I MHC differences only, and even for some non-MHC gene differences, such as the *Mls* gene in the mouse (87). If the responder was sufficiently sensitized *in vivo* before the MLR, significant responses to other non-MHC alloantigens can often be seen as well. The MLR is a special subset of T-proliferative assays, one that is directed at genetically encoded alloantigens between two populations of lymphocytes. The same principle can, however, be used to assess the proliferation of T cells against antigen in other forms, such as soluble antigen on the surface of APCs.

Cell-mediated lysis is the response function of cytotoxic T lymphocytes. After appropriate stimulation (by antigen in conjunction with class I

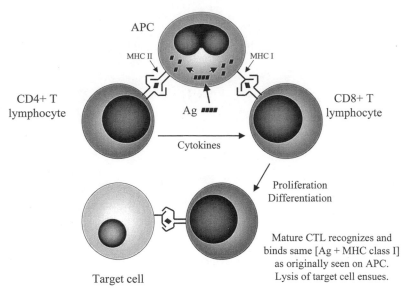

FIG. 1.10. Cytotoxic T lymphocytes.

MHC molecules on the surface of APC, together with help from T_H1 cells), CTLs proliferate and differentiate to become capable of binding and destroying target cells through direct cell–cell contact (Fig. 1.10). Clonally derived CTLs can lyse only those cells that bear the same combination of antigen and class I MHC molecules originally recognized by the originally stimulated CTL from which the clone was generated. Death of the target cell can be induced through the action of perforins secreted by the CTL or through apoptosis induced by binding of target cell receptors by ligands on the surface of CTLS or by cytokines secreted by the CTL.

DTH is an *in vivo* response by inflammatory T_H1 (or T_{dh}) cells (Fig. 1.11). Individuals presensitized against a particular antigen, then later challenged intradermally with a small amount of the same antigen, display local inflammatory responses 24 to 72 hours later at the site of challenge. Perhaps the best known example is a positive tuberculin skin test (Mantoux test). The response is mediated by $CD4^+$ T_H1 cells, previously sensitized against a particular combination of antigen and class II MHC molecules. Upon subsequent exposure to the same combination of antigen and class II MHC molecules,

the T_H1 cells respond by secreting a series of cytokines (Table 1.2) that attract macrophages to the site of interest and activate them. The activated macrophages exhibit an increased size and activity, enabling them to destroy and phagocytize the antigenic stimulus. However, because macrophages are not antigen specific, they may also destroy normal cells and tissues in the local area, referred to as *innocent bystander destruction*.

THE IMMUNE SYSTEM: A DOUBLE-EDGED SWORD

The immune system evolved to protect the body from a variety of external (infectious agents or harmful molecules) and internal (malignant cells) threats. In this regard, the immune system provides the body with a means for minimizing or preventing disease. This is most clearly illustrated by individuals who have defects in immune function (immunodeficiency disease) resulting from genetic, developmental, infective, or therapeutic causes. Because of its destructive potential, however, the immune system is also capable of causing disease when confronted with inappropriate antigenic stimulation or loss of regulatory control (88).

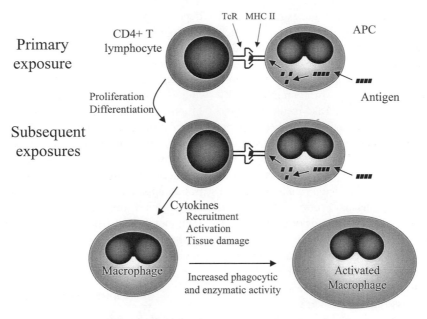

FIG. 1.11. Delayed-type hypersensitivity.

Transplantation

Transplantation involves the ability to replace damaged or diseased body parts by transplanting organs from one individual to another. Unfortunately, the immune system is exquisitely adept at recognizing nonself and rejecting transplanted organs from donors differing genetically from the recipient (89). The genetically encoded molecules that trigger the rejection response are termed *histocompatibility antigens* and are divided into two primary categories: major (encoded by class I and II MHC genes) and minor (scores, possibly hundreds, of antigens encoded by widely diverse genes scattered across the chromosomes). Because a genetically perfect match between host and donor in humans exists only between identical twins, transplantation surgeons are forced to minimize or eliminate the recipient immune response against the transplanted organ. Some of these responses can be minimized by using the closest possible genetic match between donor and recipient by tissue typing, but in humans, this is possible only for the HLA system. The alternative is the use of drugs to reduce immune responsiveness. Ideally, only the ability of the immune system to react to the antigens on the transplanted organ would be diminished (i.e., induction of antigen-specific immunologic tolerance), leaving the rest of the immune system intact. However, we currently must rely on drugs that depress the immune system in a relatively nonspecific fashion, thus leaving the patient susceptible to potentially fatal opportunistic infections. Recently, some agents (i.e., cyclosporine and FK506) have been found to diminish immune responses in a somewhat more specific fashion, but their long-term use may have secondary adverse effects on organs.

Bone marrow transplantation represents a special case in which the graft itself comprises immunocompetent tissue and the host is either immunodeficient or immunosuppressed. Thus, there is the possibility of the graft mounting an immune response against foreign host cells and tissues, leading to graft-versus-host disease (90,91)

Autoimmunity

Autoimmune diseases involve the development of antibody or cell-mediated immune responses directed against self antigens (88,92). In many autoimmune diseases, an individual's risk is affected by his or her HLA genes (2–4,93,94). There are several possible scenarios under which such undesirable responses might be initiated.

Autoimmune responses may arise when antigens that have been normally sequestered from the immune system (e.g., in immunologically privileged sites) are exposed as a result of trauma. Having never been detected previously by the immune system as it developed its sense of self versus nonself, such antigens are now seen as foreign. Second, the interaction of self molecules with small reactive chemicals (e.g., haptens) or with infectious agents may produce alterations in self molecules (altered antigens or neoantigens), resulting in their detection as nonself. Third, immune responses against determinants on infectious agents may generate clones of lymphocytes with receptors capable of cross-reacting with self antigens (cross-reactive antigens). A classic example is rheumatic fever, which results from immune responses against streptococcal antigens that are cross-reactive with molecules found on cardiac tissue. Finally, some autoimmune responses, especially those that tend to develop in later life, may result from senescence of inhibitory mechanisms, such as suppressor T lymphocytes, that keep autoimmune responses under control. For example, the onset of systemic lupus erythematosus is associated with age and an accompanying decline in suppressor T-cell function.

Immune Complex Diseases

The humoral immune response is generally efficient in eliminating antigen–antibody complexes through the phagocytic cells of the reticuloendothelial system. There are, however, situations in which antigen–antibody complexes (involving IgG and IgM antibodies) reach such high concentrations that they precipitate out of solution and accumulate in tissues, often unrelated to the source of the antigen. This may lead to systemic or localized inflammation as the complexes bind and activate serum complement components, attract phagocytic cells, and induce the release of proteolytic enzymes and other mediators of inflammation. Attempts to clear depositions of antigen–antibody complexes often damage the tissues and organs involved. Such situations most often arise as a secondary effect of situations in which there is a persistence of antigen (e.g., chronic infection, cancer, autoimmunity, or frequent repeated administration of an external reagent), leading to continual stimulation of the immune system and production of high levels of antibodies against the persisting antigen. Among the most commonly damaged sites are the kidneys, of which the filtration apparatus tends to accumulate deposited complexes (glomerulonephritis); the synovial joint membranes (rheumatoid arthritis); the skin (rashes); and the endothelial walls of blood vessels (arteritis).

Contact Dermatitis

Contact dermatitis is an example of a normally protective T-cell–mediated immune response that becomes harmful under certain circumstances. Contact dermatitis is a DTH response, usually caused by the presence of small, chemically reactive antigens (e.g., heavy metals or, as in the case of poison ivy, plant lipids such as catechol) that bind to self proteins (e.g., class II MHC molecules) on the skin and produce neoantigens.

Allergies and Anaphylaxis (Immediate Hypersensitivity)

Allergies and anaphylaxis represent antigen-specific immunologic reactions involving IgE antibodies bound (by their Fc domain) to the membranes of mast cells and basophils (95). When antigen is bound, resulting in cross-linking of the IgE molecules, the mast cells are stimulated to degranulate and release histamine, serotonin, platelet-activating factors, and other mediators of immediate hypersensitivity. The result is the rapid onset of an inflammatory response. Immediate hypersensitivity may develop against a wide array of environmental substances and may be localized (e.g., itching, tearing) or systemic (e.g., involving the circulatory system). The latter may be life-threatening if severe. Treatment involves the prompt administration of pharmaceutical agents (e.g., epinephrine, antihistamines).

TOLERANCE

In many cases, it is desirable to diminish or eliminate immune responses, thus inducing tolerance to some particular antigen. For example, autoimmune responses, asthmatic and allergic responses, and the host responses against transplanted tissues or organs all represent situations in which such tolerance would be desirable. There are two approaches: nonspecific and specific.

Immunosuppression is the elimination of all immune responses, regardless of the specificity of those responses. This may occur naturally, as in the case of individuals who are deficient in immune function for genetic reasons (e.g., severe combined immunodeficiency disease) or as the result of infection (e.g., acquired immunodeficiency syndrome). Alternatively, it may be intentionally imposed by the application of radiation, drugs, or other therapeutic reagents (e.g., antilymphocyte sera). Such procedures, however, impose a new set of risks because their nonspecificity leaves the patient (or experimental animal) open to infections by opportunistic pathogens. Attempts to diminish these consequences involve the development of reagents with narrower effects, including drugs such as cyclosporine and FK506, or the application of antibodies specific for only particular subsets of lymphocytes (96). Immunologic tolerance is the *specific* acquired inability of individuals to respond to a specific immunogenic determinant toward which they would otherwise normally respond. Tolerance is more desirable than immunosuppression because it eliminates or inactivates only those lymphocytes involved in the responses of concern, leaving the remainder of the immune system intact to deal with opportunistic infections.

The natural induction of tolerance during the development of the immune system prevents immune responses against self antigens (*self tolerance*), thus preventing autoimmunity (97,98).

Experimentally, tolerance can be induced in immunocompetent adult animals by manipulating a variety of factors, including age, the physical nature and dose of antigen, and the route of administration (99,100). Tolerance may be induced in both T and B lymphocytes, although tolerance of T cells generally requires lower doses of antigen and is effective for a longer period of time. In addition, because B lymphocytes require T-cell help, the induction of tolerance in T cells often also diminishes corresponding antibody responses.

The means by which specific tolerance is induced and maintained involve three general mechanisms, all of which probably occur in various situations. *Clonal deletion* or abortion is the actual elimination of those clones of lymphocytes that encounter the specific antigen under particular conditions. *Clonal anergy* is the functional inactivation of those clones of lymphocytes that encounter the specific antigen in a tolerogenic form. This may be reversible. *Antigen-specific suppression* relies on the presence of cells that inhibit the antigen-specific induction or expression of immune responses by other T or B lymphocytes. It is known that T_H1 cells (promoting cellular and inflammatory responses) and T_H2 cells (promoting antibody responses) directed against the same antigen may inhibit one another through the cytokines they secrete. Thus, a response against a given antigen may be dominated by cellular responses in one case and by antibody responses in another. And, for example, attempts to alleviate cellular inflammatory responses directed against a given antigen may involve the promotion of antibody responses against the same antigen. The association of autoimmune disorders with advancing age is often attributed to age-related declines in suppressor T cells.

The immune system is an amazing biologic system. Precise interactions must occur, in appropriate sequences and quantities, between a bewildering array of cells and molecules. Moreover, these highly specific cells and molecules must find one another, after patrolling throughout the entire body, in order to coordinate their activities. It is so complex that it seems incredible at times not that it all usually works so well, but that it works at all. It can malfunction, however, with potentially harmful consequences, and we still have far to go in learning how to correct and alleviate these occasions.

REFERENCES

1. Medzhitov R, Janeway C Jr. Innate immune recognition: mechanisms and pathways. *Immunol Rev* 2000; 173:89.
2. Klein J, Horejší V. *Immunology*. Malden, MA: Blackwell Scientific, 1997.
3. Roitt I. *Essential immunology*. 9th ed. Malden, MA: Blackwell Scientific, 1997.
4. Janeway CA, Travers P, Walport M, et al. *Immunobiology: the immune system in health and disease*. 4th ed. New York: Garland, 1999.
5. Audibert FM, Lise LD. Adjuvants: current status, clinical perspectives and future prospects. *Immunol Today* 1993;14:281.
6. Alzari PM, Lascombe PW, Poljak RJ. Three-dimensional structure of antibodies. *Ann Rev Immunol* 1988;6:555.
7. Van Oss CJ. Phagocytosis: an overview. *Methods Enzymol* 1986;132:3.
8. Morgan EL, Weigle WO. Biological activities residing in the Fc portion of immunoglobulin. *Adv Immunol* 1987;40:61.
9. Adair JR. Engineering antibodies for therapy. *Immunol Rev* 1992;130:5.
10. Underdown BJ, Schiff JM. Immunoglobulin A: strategic defense initiative at the mucosal surface. *Ann Rev Immunol* 1986;4:389–418.
11. Tonegawa S. Somatic generation of antibody diversity. *Nature* 1983;302:575–581.
12. Gellert M. Recent advances in understanding V(D)J recombination. *Adv Immunol* 1997;64:39.
13. Stavnezer J. Antibody class switching. *Adv Immunol* 1996;61:79.
14. Harriman W, Völk H, Defranoux N, et al. Immunoglobulin class switch recombinations. *Ann Rev Immunol* 1993;11:361.
15. Sablitzky F, Wildner G, Rajewsky K. Somatic mutation and clonal expansion of B cells in an antigen-driven immune response. *EMBO J* 1985;4:345.
16. Berek C, Milstein C. Mutation drift and repertoire shift in the maturation of the immune response. *Immunol Rev* 1987;96:23.
17. Ashwell JD, Klausner RD. Genetic and mutational analysis of the T cell antigen receptor. *Ann Rev Immunol* 1990;8:139.
18. Matis L. The molecular basis of T-cell specificity. *Ann Rev Immunol* 1990;8:65.
19. Raulet DH. The structure, function, and molecular genetics of the γ/δ T cell receptor. *Ann Rev Immunol* 1989;7:175.
20. Wilson RK, Lai E, Concannan P, et al. Structure, organization and polymorphism of murine and human T-cell receptor α and β chain gene families. *Immunol Res* 1988;101:149.
21. Clevers H, Alarcon B, Wileman T, et al. The T cell receptor/CD3 complex: a dynamic protein ensemble. *Ann Rev Immunol* 1988;6:629.
22. Chetty R, Gather K. CD3: structure, function and role of immunostaining in clinical practice. *J Pathol* 1994;73:303.
23. Morris A, Hewitt C, Young S. The major histocompatibility complex: its genes and their roles in antigen presentation. *Mol Aspects Med* 1994;15:377.
24. Lai L, Avaverdi N, Maltais L, et al. Mouse cell surface antigens: nomenclature and immunophenotyping. *J Immunol* 1998;160:3861.
25. Bierer BE, Sleckman BP, Ratnofsky SE, et al. The biological roles of CD2, CD4, and CD8 in T-cell activation. *Ann Rev Immunol* 1989;7:579.
26. Biddison WE, Shae S. CD4 expression and function in HLA class II-specific T cells. *Immunol Rev* 1989; 109:5.
27. De Vries JE, Yssel H, Spits H. Interplay between the TCR/CD3 complex and CD4 or CD8 in the activation of cytotoxic T lymphocytes. *Immunol Rev* 1989; 109:119.
28. Solheim JC. Class I MHC molecules: assembly and antigen presentation. *Immunol Rev* 1999;172:11.
29. Cresswell P. Assembly, transport and function of MHC class II MHC molecules. *Ann Rev Immunol* 1994;12:259.
30. Yu CY, Yang Z, Blanchong CA, et al. The human and mouse MHC class III region: a parade of 21 genes at the centromeric segment. *Immunol Today* 2000;21:320.
31. Dinarello CA. Interleukin-1 and its biologically related cytokines. *Adv Immunol* 1989;44:153.
32. Gardner P. IL-6: an overview. *Ann Rev Immunol* 1990;8:253.
33. Moore KW, O'Garra A, De Waal R, et al. IL-10. *Ann Rev Immunol* 1993;11:165.
34. Trinchieri G. Interleukin-12: a proinflammatory cytokine with immunoregulatory functions that bridge innate resistance and antigen-specific adaptive immunity. *Ann Rev Immunol* 1995;13:251.
35. Morel PA, Oriss TB. Crossregulation between Th1 and Th1 cells. *Crit Rev Immunol* 18:275, 1998.
36. Theze J, Alzari PM, Bertoglio J. Interleukin 2 and its receptors: recent advances and new immunological functions. *Immunol Today* 1996;17:481.
37. Billiau A. Interferon-gamma: biology and role in pathogenesis. *Adv Immunol* 1996;62:61.
38. Dallman MJ, Wood KJ, Hamano K, et al. Cytokines and peripheral tolerance to alloantigens. *Immunol Rev* 1993;133:5.
39. Sher A, Gazzinelli RT, Oswald IP, et al. Role of T-cell derived cytokines on the downregulation of immune responses in parasitic and retroviral infection. *Immunol Rev* 1992;127:183.
40. Hayday AC, Bottomly K. Cytokines in T-cell development. *Immunol Today* 1991;12:239.
41. Bousiotis VA, Freeman GJ, Gribben JG, et al. The role of B7-1/B7-2:CD28/CTLA-4 pathways in the prevention of anergy, induction of productive immunity and down-regulation of the immune response. *Immunol Rev* 1996;153:5.
42. Van Kooten C, Banchereau J. CD40–CD40 ligand: a multifunctional receptor-ligand pair. *Adv Immunol* 1996;61:1.
43. Stout RD, Suttles J. The many roles of CD40 in cell-mediated inflammatory responses. *Immunol Today* 1996;17:487.

44. Liszewski MK, Farries TC, Lublin DM, et al. Control of the complement system. *Adv Immunol* 1996;61:201.
45. Morgan BP. Regulation of the complement membrane attack complex. *Crit Rev Immunol* 1999;19:173.
46. Carroll MC. The role of complement and complement receptors in induction and regulation of immunity. *Ann Rev Immunol* 1998;16:545.
47. Colman PM. Structure of antibody-antigen complexes: implications for immune recognition. *Adv Immunol* 1988;43:99.
48. Salmi M, Jalkanen S. How do lymphocytes know where to go: current concepts and enigmas of hymphocyte homing. *Adv Immunol* 1997;64:139.
49. Kraal G, Mebius RE. High endothelial venules: lymphocyte traffic control and controlled traffic. *Adv Immunol* 1997;65:347.
50. Butcher EC, Williams M, Youngman K, et al. Lymphocyte trafficking and regional immunity. *Adv Immunol* 1999;72:209.
51. Gray D. Immunological memory. *Ann Rev Immunol* 1993;11:49.
52. Dutton RW, Bradley LM, Swain SL. T cell memory. *Ann Rev Immunol* 1996;16:201.
53. Snow EC, Pittner B, Reid S. T helper cell regulation of normal and neoplastic B cell growth. *Semin Immunol* 1994;6:311.
54. Hedrick SM. Specificity of the T cell receptor for antigen. *Adv Immunol* 1988;43:193.
55. Kourilsky P, Claverie JM. MHC-antigen interaction: what does the T cell receptor see? *Adv Immunol* 1989;45:107.
56. Murray JS. How the MHC selects Th1/Th2 immunity. *Immunol Today* 1998;19:157.
57. Romagnani S. The Th1/Th2 paradigm. *Immunol Today* 1997;18:263.
58. Street NE, Mosmann TR. Functional diversity of T lymphocytes due to secretion of different cytokine patterns. *FASEB J* 1991;5:171.
59. Fitch FW, McKisic MD, LANCKI DW, et al. Differential regulation of murine T lymphocyte subsets. *Ann Rev Immunol* 1993;11:29.
60. Henkart PA. Mechanism of lymphocyte-mediated cytotoxicity. *Ann Rev Immunol* 1985;3:31.
61. Peters PJ, Geuze HJ, Van Der Donk HA, et al. A new model for lethal hit delivery by cytotoxic T lymphocytes. *Immunol Today* 1990;11:28.
62. Miller JF, Kurts C, Allison J, et al. Induction of peripheral CD8+ T-cell tolerance by cross-presentation of self antigens. *Immunol Rev* 1998;165:267.
63. Price DA, Klenerman P, Booth BL, et al. Cytotoxic T lymphocytes, chemokines and antiviral immunity. *Immunol Today* 1999;20:212.
64. Shevach EM. Regulatory T cells in autoimmunity. *Ann Rev Immunol* 2000;18:423.
65. Hayday A. $\gamma\delta$ Cells: a right time and a right place for a conserved third way of protection. *Ann Rev Immunol* 2000;18:975.
66. Harding CV, Leyva-Cobian F, Unanue ER. Mechanisms of antigen processing. *Immunol Rev* 1988;106:77.
67. Germain RN, Margulies DH. The biochemistry and cell biology of antigen processing and presentation. *Ann Rev Immunol* 1993;11:403.
68. Geuze HJ. The role of endosomes and lysosomes in MHC class II functioning. *Immunol Today* 1998;19:282.

69. Lanzavecchia A. Receptor-mediated antigen uptake and its effect on antigen presentation to class II-restricted T lymphocytes. *Ann Rev Immunol* 1990;8:773.
70. Pierce SK, Morris JF, Grusby MJ, et al. Antigen-presenting function of B lymphocytes. *Immunol Rev* 1988;106:149.
71. Moretta L, Ciccione E, Moretta A, et al. Allorecognition by NK cells: nonself or no self? *Immunol Today* 1992;13:300.
72. Reyburn H, Mandelboim O, Vales-Gomez M, et al. Human NK cells: their ligands, receptors and functions. *Immunol Rev* 1997;155:119.
73. Metzger H. The receptor with high affinity for IgE. *Immunol Rev* 1992;125:37.
74. Stevens RL, Austin KF. Recent advances in the cellular and molecular biology of mast cells. *Immunol Today* 1989;10:381.
75. Wardlaw AJ, Moqbel R, Kay AB. Eosinophils: biology and role in disease. *Adv Immunol* 1995;60:151.
76. Haynes BF, Denning SM, Singer KH, et al. Ontogeny of T-cell precursors: a model for the initial stages of human T-cell development. *Immunol Today* 1989;10:87.
77. Nikolic-Zugic J. Phenotypic and functional stages in the intrathymic development of $\alpha\beta$ T cells. *Immunol Today* 1991;12:65.
78. Meuller DL, Jenkins MK, Schwartz RH. Clonal expansion vs functional clonal inactivation. *Ann Rev Immunol* 1989;7:445.
79. Sprent J, Lo D, Gao EK, et al. T cell selection in the thymus. *Immunol Rev* 1988;101:173.
80. Von Boehmer H, Teh HS, Kisielow P. The thymus selects the useful, neglects the useless and destroys the harmful. *Immunol Today* 1989;10:57.
81. Jelinek DF. Regulation of B lymphocyte differeniation. *Ann Allergy Asthma Immunol* 2000;84:375.
82. Liu YJ, Banchereau J. Regulation of B-cell committment to plasma cells or to memory B cells. *Semin Immunol* 1997;9:235.
83. Clark EA, Ledbetter JA. How B and T cells talk to each other. *Nature* 1994;367:425.
84. Berek C, Milstein C. The dynamic nature of the antibody repertoire. *Immunol Rev* 1988;105:5.
85. Melchers F, Anderson J. Factors controlling the B-cell cycle. *Ann Rev Immunol* 1986;4:13.
86. Hamaoka T, Ono S. Regulation of B-cell differentiation: Interactions of factors and corresponding receptors. *Ann Rev Immunol* 1986;4:167.
87. Abe R, Hodes RJ. Properties of the Mls system: a revised formulation of Mls genetics and an analysis of T-cell recognition of Mls determinants. *Immunol Rev* 1989;107:5.
88. Adams D. How the immune system works and why it causes autoimmune diseases. *Immunol Today* 1996;17:300.
89. Mason DW, Morris PJ. Effector mechanisms in allograft rejection. *Ann Rev Immunol* 1986;4:119.
90. Parkman R, Weinberg KI. Immunological reconstruction following bone marrow transplantation. *Immunol Rev* 1997;157:73.
91. Blazar BR, Korngold R, Vallera DA. Recent advances in graft-versus-host disease (GVHD) prevention. *Immunol Rev* 1997;157:79.
92. Shoenfeld Y, Isenberg DA. The mosaic of autoimmunity. *Immunol Today* 1989;10:123.

93. Horwitz MS, Sarvetnick N. Viruses, host responses, and autoimmunity. *Immunol Rev* 1999;169:241.
94. Charron D. The molecular basis of human leukocyte antigen class II disease associations. *Adv Immunol* 1989;47:187.
95. Sutton BJ, Gould HJ. The human IgE network. *Nature* 1993;366:421.
96. Kalden JR, Breedveld FC, Burkhardt H, et al. Immunological treatment of autoimmune diseases. *Adv Immunol* 1998;68:333.
97. Marrack P, Hugo P, Mccormack J, et al. Self-ignorance in the peripheral T-cell pool. *Immunol Rev* 1993;13:119.
98. Stockinger B. T lymphocyte tolerance: from thymic deletion to peripheral control mechanisms. *Adv Immunol* 1999;71:229.
99. Weiner HL. Oral tolerance: immune mechanisms and treatment of autoimmune diseases. *Immunol Today* 1997;18:335.
100. Faria AM, Weiner HL. Oral tolerance: mechanisms and therapeutic applications. *Adv Immunol* 1999;73:153.

2

Evaluation and Management of Immune Deficiency in Allergy Practice

Melvin Berger

Departments of Pediatrics and Pathology, Case Western Reserve University;
Department of Pediatrics, Rainbow Babies' and Childrens' Hospital,
University Hospitals Health System, Cleveland, Ohio

Because there is considerable overlap between the manifestations of allergy and infection (i.e., rhinorrhea, sneezing, cough, wheezing) and because allergy may be a predisposing factor in sinusitis, otitis, and other respiratory infections, the allergist is frequently called on to evaluate patients with symptoms that have been attributed to recurrent infections and in which the competence of the patient's immune system has been or should be questioned. Because half or more of all patients with primary immune defects have antibody deficiencies (1,2) and most of them have problems with recurrent sinopulmonary infections, this is not an uncommon problem in clinical practice. The intent of this chapter is to provide a practical approach to the diagnosis and management of such patients, not to provide a comprehensive review of immune deficiency disorders or their molecular bases. Readers who wish a more in-depth analysis of immune deficiency disorders should consult comprehensive texts devoted to those disorders, such as the multiauthor works edited by Ochs, Smith, and Puck (3) or Stiehm (4).

INDICATIONS FOR AN IMMUNOLOGIC WORKUP

Although many immune-deficient patients present with a clear history of distinct episodes of infection, the allergist is frequently called on to see patients with less severe, nonspecific symptoms such as nasal stuffiness, chronic and recurrent rhinorrhea, or cough, which may be due to infection, allergy, or other factors. The first step in sorting out such complaints is to try to distinguish whether the symptoms are, in fact, due to infection. Inciting factors, such as seasonality, and clearly identifiable trigger factors may suggest allergic etiologies, but changes in the weather and changes in seasons are frequently accompanied by changes in exposure to infectious diseases.

Exposure to other people with similar symptoms and characteristics, such as the presence or absence of fever, description of excessive secretions (clear and watery versus thick and purulent), and the response to antibiotics, may help to distinguish between infectious and noninfectious etiologies. After an estimate of the real incidence of infection is obtained, this can be compared with benchmarks such as the "10 warning signs of immune deficiency" (Fig. 2.1). The incidence of infection should be compared with the incidence for that age group in the community, but the exposure history also needs to be taken into consideration. For example, a 40-year-old who lives alone and sits in front of a computer screen all day would be expected to have a different degree of exposure to infectious agents than a kindergarten teacher, day care worker, or pediatric office nurse. College students moving from home to the dormitory for the first time and military recruits

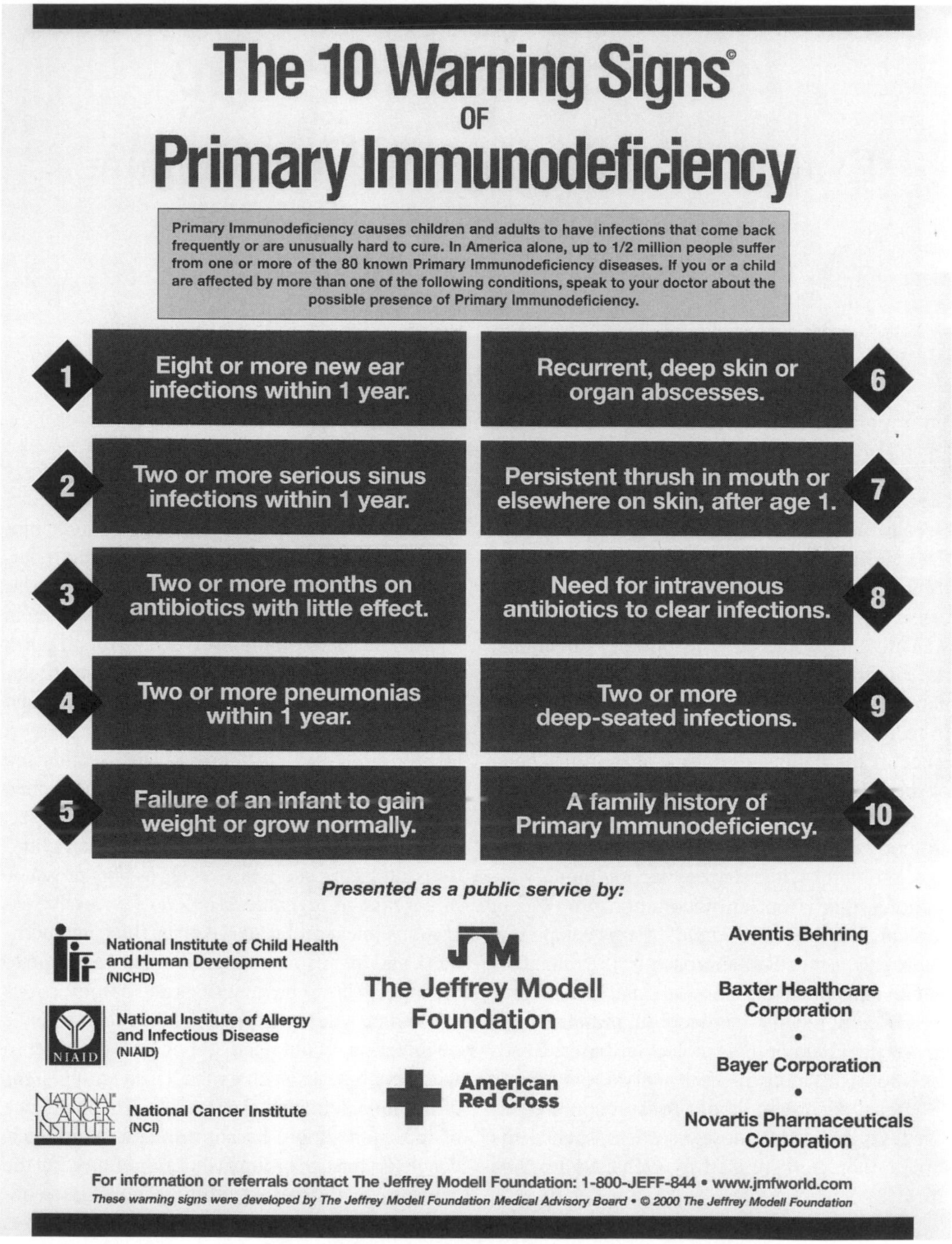

FIG. 2.1. The 10 warning signs of primary immune deficiency. (Presented as a public service by The Jeffrey Modell Foundation and American Red Cross. These warnings signs were developed by The Jeffrey Modell Foundation Medical Advisory Board.)

often have sharp increases in infectious disease exposure. Similarly, a first-born baby at home often has a very different degree of exposure than a similar-aged child in day care or with many siblings. Generally, the frequency of respiratory infection among school-aged children in the United States is about six to eight upper respiratory infections per year, but as many as one a month while school is in session is not unusual. About half of these are primary bacterial infections or secondary bacterial sequelae, such as otitis media, sinusitis, pneumonia, or bronchitis.

Patients with clear histories of more than 10 distinct episodes of infection per year, more than two documented episodes of pneumonia per year, or more than one life-threatening infection should be evaluated for possible immune deficiency or other underlying abnormality that may be contributing to this increased incidence of infection. However, the specialist must be careful in interpreting the history from the patient or parent. Frequently, antibiotics are given when the patient does not have clear evidence for bacterial infection, but the conclusion is drawn that antibiotics do not work, suggesting that there is something "wrong" with the patient's immune system. Frequent upper respiratory symptoms may represent individual viral upper respiratory infections; on the other hand, there may be prolonged symptoms from conditions, such as chronic sinusitis, that have not been adequately treated despite multiple short courses of oral antibiotics. The demonstration of densities on chest radiograph may represent atelectasis due to asthma rather than infiltrates and should not necessarily be taken as indicating recurrent pneumonia unless there is documentation of concomitant fever, elevated white blood cell count, or positive sputum Gram stain or culture.

Patients with unusually severe infections, such as those requiring parenteral antibiotics, prolonged or multiple courses of antibiotics for a single infection, or surgical intervention such as incision and drainage of abscesses or removal of seriously infected tissue (e.g., a segment of lung or infected bone), should probably also undergo at least screening (see later) to exclude immune deficiency. Patients with unusual or opportunistic infections should

also be evaluated, as should those with unusual responses, such as prostration or excessive fever, to seemingly common organisms.

Although many patients with primary immune deficiencies present with recurrent and chronic respiratory infections (2,5,6), gastrointestinal disorders are also common in these patients. The combination of recurrent respiratory infections with recurrent gastrointestinal symptoms may prompt immunologic screening even when the involvement of either organ system itself is not severe. Infection with *Giardia lamblia* (7,8) and bacterial overgrowth in the small intestine are not infrequent in patients with antibody deficiencies and may present with symptoms such as cramps or diarrhea after eating, leading to suspicion of food allergy on the part of the patient, parent (if a child), or referring physician, despite the absence of other manifestations of true allergy. In some immune deficient patients, there may be organized lymphonodular hyperplasia in the intestine or infiltration of the submucosa with scattered aggregates of lymphocytes (7); and patients with gastrointestinal workups or biopsy results not typical for recognized patterns of inflammatory bowel disease should also undergo evaluation for immune deficiencies.

The presence of nonimmunologic findings on physical examination may also provide indications for evaluation to exclude immune deficiency (Table 2.1). These may include malabsorption with failure to thrive or excessive weight loss; eczema or thrombocytopenia in Wiskott-Aldrich syndrome (9); and facial, cardiac, or skeletal features suggestive of a recognizable pattern of malformation such as that seen in DiGeorge syndrome, short-limbed dwarfism, or cartilage-hair hypoplasia (10,11). Characteristic facial and skeletal abnormalities or eczematoid dermatitis may suggest the hyper-immunoglobulin E (hyper-IgE) or Job syndrome (12), and rib or other skeletal abnormalities may be present in severe combined immune deficiency (SCID) due to adenosine deaminase (ADA) deficiency (10,13). Alopecia or endocrinopathies occur with increased frequency in chronic mucocutaneous candidiasis (14). Nystagmus, clumsiness, and other neurologic abnormalities may occur before

TABLE 2.1. *Physical findings not due to infectious disease associated with immune deficiency syndromes*

I. Facial abnormalities	
Broad nasal bridge, increased interalar distance	Hyper-IgE syndrome
Hypognathism; low, cupped ears	DiGeorge syndrome
II. Other skeletal abnormalities	
Metaphysial chrondrodysplasia	Cartilage-hair hypoplasia (Short-limbed dwarfism)
Cupped (dysplastic) costochondral junctions, abnormalities of apophyses of iliac bones and vertebrae	Adenosine deaminase deficiency
Multiple fractures	Hyper-IgE syndrome
III. Cardiac defects	
Conotruncal (great vessel) defects	DiGeorge syndrome
Single chamber, anomalous pulmonary veins	Asplenia
IV. Thymic abnormalities	
Hypoplasia or aplasia	DiGeorge syndrome
	Severe combined immunodeficiency disease
Thymoma	Chronic valvular heart disease
V. Central nervous system abnormalities	
Spasticity, retardation	Purine nucleoside phosphorylase deficiency
Ataxia (cerebellar), nystagmus	Ataxia telangiectasia
VI. Cutaneous abnormalities	
Eczematoid rashes	Hyper-IgE syndrome
	Wiskott-Aldrich syndrome
Fine, sparse hair	Cartilage-hair hypoplasia
Poor wound healing, thin scars	Leukocyte adherence deficiency
Cutaneous and ocular telangiectasias	Ataxia telangiectasia
Oculocutaneous albinism	Chédiak-Higashi syndrome
Alopecia	Chronic mucocutaneous candidiasis
VII. Endocrine defects	
Hypoparathyroidism/hypocalcemia	DiGeorge syndrome
Multiple (autoimmune) endocrinopathies	Chronic mucocutaneous candidiasis

observable telangiectasias and can suggest the diagnosis of ataxia-telangiectasia (15), and neurologic disorders are also common in purine nucleoside phosphorylase deficiency (16). Although delayed separation of the umbilical cord stump is widely recognized as an indicator of leukocyte adherence protein deficiency, in fact, there is a wide variation in the time at which the stump separates, and this should not be overemphasized in an otherwise well infant (17). Of course, patients with positive screening tests for human immunodeficiency virus (HIV) would also be candidates for immunologic evaluation.

Several immune deficiencies can clearly be hereditary. For many of these, the patterns of inheritance and the precise molecular defects have been defined (18) (Table 2.2). Family members suspected of having these disorders, perhaps because an older sibling has already been diagnosed, should undergo assessment of their

immune status. When available, tests for the specific molecular lesion should be included so that treatment aimed at correcting or compensating for the basic defect can be instituted early enough to prevent or minimize end-organ damage. Prenatal diagnosis and screening for the carrier state is now available for many of these disorders and can be used both in counseling and in ensuring that prompt and appropriate therapy is offered to affected newborns.

DOCUMENTING THE HISTORY OF INFECTION

A major goal in questioning the patient and reviewing the medical records is to develop a firm impression of the types of infections that the patient has suffered so that subsequent laboratory tests can be targeted to analyze specifically those components of the immune system whose defects

TABLE 2.2. *Inherited immune deficiencies*

Disorder	Defective gene or locus
I. X-linked	
Primarily B-cell defect or deficiency	
Bruton (X-linked) agammaglobulinemia	Bruton tyrosine kinase (BTK)
Hyper-IgM syndrome	CD40 ligand (gp39, CD154)
Wiskott-Aldrich syndrome	Wiskott-Aldrich syndrome protein (WASP)
Combined immune deficiency	
X-linked severe combined immune deficiency	Cytokine receptor common chain (γ c chain)
Phagocyte defects	
Chronic granulomatous disease (about 65%)	Gp91 phox component of cytochrome b245
Severe glucose-6-phosphatase deficiency	G-6-PD
Properdin deficiency	Properdin
II. Autosomal recessive	
Primarily B-cell defect or deficiency	
Immunoglobulin heavy chain deletion	Indicated gene on chromosome 14
κ-Light chain deletion	22p11
Autosomal agammaglobulinemia	?
Ataxia telangiectasia	*ATM*, 11q22.3
Primarily T-cell deficiency	
DiGeorge syndrome	22q11 Microdeletion
Zeta chain associated protein deficiency (ZAP-70 def)	2q12
Combined immune deficiency	
Adenosine deaminase deficiency	20q13
Janus kinase 3 (Jak 3) deficiency	19p13
Purine nucleoside phosphorylase deficiency	14q13.1
Phagocyte defects	
Chronic granulomatous disease (35%)	Gp47phox or p22phox components of neutrophil oxidase
Leukocyte adherence deficiency type I	CD18 common β chain of leukocyte integrins
Leukocyte adherence deficiency type II	Sialyl-Lewis X (ligand for E-selectin)
Other complement component defects	Various autosomes

would most likely explain the patient's symptoms. This will be best served by keeping in mind general patterns of infection that might be caused by defects in specific immunologic defense mechanisms. Thus, infections with encapsulated extracellular bacterial pathogens, particularly of the respiratory tract, are suggestive of defects in antibody production (19,20), which constitute the majority of all immune deficiencies (1). Superficial mucosal infections may particularly suggest isolated IgA deficiency (21). Infections with opportunistic pathogens, including protozoans and fungi, and recurrent episodes of chickenpox or chronic herpetic lesions, may suggest problems in cell-mediated immunity (20). Failure to clear bacteria promptly from the blood stream, resulting in bacteremia, sepsis, or hematogenously disseminated infec-

tions such as osteomyelitis, may be seen in deficiencies of C3 or early-acting components of the complement system (22), but may also indicate asplenia or poor reticuloendothelial system function, as in sickle cell disease. Problems with recurrent or disseminated neisserial infections may suggest deficiency of the later-acting complement components that form the membrane attack complex (22). Abscesses and infections with unusual bacteria or fungi may suggest neutropenia or defects in neutrophil function (19,20,23,24). Enteroviral meningoencephalitis may suggest X-linked agammaglobulinemia.

The number and types of infections and their individual and cumulative morbidity should be assessed. It is necessary to exclude carefully other causes of nonspecific symptoms; for example, is sniffling or congestion due to recurrent upper respiratory infection, allergy, or other types of rhinitis? If cough is a major complaint, it is important to determine whether this is due to sputum production, irritation, or other causes. Could it represent cough-equivalent asthma? If failure to thrive and cough are both present, could the patient have cystic fibrosis? Inflammatory bowel disease may mimic hypogammaglobulinemia in children with poor weight gain who also have recurrent rhinitis due to multiple mucosal viral infections, which by themselves would not be considered significant.

Isolation and identification of responsible organisms is clearly the gold standard for rigorous diagnosis of infection. Documentation of fever, white blood count with differential, and sensitive but nonspecific measures such as the erythrocyte sedimentation rate and C-reactive protein, can help distinguish between chronic, recurrent sinusitis and headaches due to other causes and can help with the differential diagnosis of recurrent cough or other chest symptoms. The importance of culture and examination of smears of nasal secretions for bacteria and neutrophils versus eosinophils cannot be overemphasized in distinguishing infectious from allergic and other noninfectious etiologies, particularly in small children. In some cases, the most appropriate step in the workup is to send the patient back to the primary care physician with instructions to have appropriate cultures and those simple laboratory tests performed every time an infection is suspected or the symptoms recur. Sometimes, the culture result points to the diagnosis, as in the case of *Pseudomonas aeruginosa* suggesting cystic fibrosis, invasive aspergilli suggesting neutropenia or chronic granulomatous disease (CGD) (24) or *Streptococcus pneumoniae* or *Haemophilus influenzae* suggesting an antibody deficiency (19,20).

Clues to the severity and overall morbidity resulting from infection may be obtained by asking whether hospitalization or intravenous antibiotics have been required to treat infections or whether oral antibiotics have generally been sufficient. The response to therapy should be evaluated carefully. Continued high fever or other symptoms suggesting a lack of response of culture-confirmed bacterial infec-

tion to antibiotics is more likely indicative of a significant immune deficiency than is the frequently seen pattern in which the fever and symptoms resolve promptly when antibiotic therapy is started (e.g., for otitis media) only to recur again shortly after the prescribed course of therapy is concluded. In many situations, the latter may actually represent a distinct new infection. This pattern is quite commonly seen in children in day care and in adults with frequent exposure to small children. Similarly, it is also important to distinguish inadequate or inappropriate therapy from failure to respond, and it is important to differentiate chronic infections from recurrent episodes. Absence from school or work should be quantitated if possible, and any long-term sequelae or disability should be documented.

The family history should include questions about siblings and preceding generations. Family trees with premature deaths of male infants should raise suspicion of X-linked immune deficiencies (Table 2.2). Questions should also be asked about the family history of asthma and allergy as well as other genetic diseases that may present with recurrent infection such as cystic fibrosis. In evaluating a child, it may be important to determine whether the parents have died prematurely or have known risk factors for HIV infection.

The age at onset of infections of unusual frequency or severity may yield important insights into possible underlying immune deficiencies. It must be kept in mind that term newborns have IgG levels equivalent to those of their mothers, from whom most of their IgG has been transferred across the placenta (25). Thus, babies who have problems with infections before the age of 6 months may have T-cell or phagocyte problems but are unlikely to have agammaglobulinemia or other isolated problems in antibody production. In contrast, disorders of antibody production are more likely to present after the age of 6 months. The history of exposure must be carefully considered in evaluating this issue because the frequency of common types of infections often increases after a child's exposure to infectious agents is increased after attending day care or preschool, particularly if there are no siblings in the home. Although patients with severe antibody deficiency such as that seen in Bruton agammaglobulinemia generally present between 6 months and 2 years of age (6,26), the diagnosis of the X-linked hyper-IgM syndrome is frequently delayed until later in childhood (27,28), and those with common variable immunodeficiency disease (CVID) may present at any age (5,29). It may not be clear whether this represents an early-onset deficiency that has not been previously recognized or a newly acquired problem. Just as some infants may have delayed development of the full range of immune responses (30), it seems likely that some adults may undergo premature senescence of immune responsiveness (31) and may present with recurrent bacterial infections in their 40s or 50s.

THE PHYSICAL EXAMINATION IN CASES OF SUSPECTED IMMUNE DEFICIENCY

The physical examination often provides important evidence for or against immune deficiency and may also allow the physician to assess critically the cumulative morbidity due to infection. Most importantly, the presence or absence of lymphoid tissue should be carefully documented. The absence of visible tonsils in patients who have not had them surgically removed and the absence of palpable cervical or inguinal lymph nodes should promote a strong suspicion of a significant antibody deficiency because the bulk of these tissues is composed of B-lineage lymphoid cells involved in antibody synthesis. Conversely, the presence of palpable lymph nodes and easily visible tonsils essentially excludes Bruton agammaglobulinemia and may suggest the absence of SCID but does not help one way or the other with the diagnosis of CVID or X-linked hyper-IgM syndrome. The presence of cervical or peripheral adenopathy, splenomegaly, or hepatomegaly may suggest HIV, CGD, or other abnormalities. Many anatomic findings are associated with immune defects in recognizable malformation syndromes (Table 2.1), and characteristic rashes may suggest Wiskott-Aldrich syndrome (9) or the hyper-IgE (Job) syndrome (12). Secondary effects, such as failure to thrive, weight loss, and

short stature, may suggest significant morbidity due to chronic or recurrent infection. Scars from incision and drainage of abscesses or from drainage or surgical reduction of enlarged lymph nodes may indicate significant morbidity from neutrophil defects (24).

Autoimmune phenomena (29,32) and rheumatic complaints (33,34), including infectious or chronic arthritis, are common in patients with CVID and other primary immune deficiencies and may help indicate that an evaluation for immune deficiency is warranted, even if the number or severity of acute infections has not been excessive.

Careful assessment of the tympanic membranes, paranasal sinuses, and chest is extremely important in evaluating patients suspected of having antibody deficiency syndromes, and not only should the quantity and characteristics of secretions be documented but also some attempts should be made to determine whether observed abnormalities are acute or chronic. In this regard, high-resolution (thin-slice) computed tomography (CT) scans of the chest may be very helpful because observation of bronchiectasis or areas of "ground-glass" density in the lung parenchyma may suggest the presence of subclinical chronic disease, which could be due to antibody deficiency (35,36). Clubbing of the digits may also provide an important indication of chronic lung disease.

GENERAL LABORATORY SCREENING TESTS

The Clinical and Laboratory Immunology Committee of the American Academy of Allergy, Asthma and Immunology has assembled a set of practice parameters for the diagnosis and management of immunodeficiency (37). These may help provide guidelines for the allergist-immunologist and the referring physician to those screening tests that might first be ordered and interpreted by the primary physician, as compared with situations in which referral to the specialist becomes appropriate. Often, the specialist is called by the primary care physician to determine whether a patient should be referred.

A review of laboratory tests already obtained by the primary care physician may yield important clues to the presence of an immune deficiency disorder and may save steps in the evaluation of patients by suggesting which of the more specialized tests are most likely to be informative. The complete blood count (CBC) and differential will help to exclude neutropenia or may indicate lymphopenia, which could be seen in SCID or Bruton agammaglobulinemia. Abnormal or decreased platelets may suggest Wiskott-Aldrich syndrome, and fragmented erythrocytes may suggest sickle cell disease. General blood chemistry panels will show low total protein but normal albumin in agammaglobulinemia. A low uric acid level may be indicative of ADA deficiency or purine nucleoside phosphorylase deficiency, two causes of SCID (16,38); whereas a low serum calcium level may suggest DiGeorge syndrome.

In addition to assessing the airways and lung parenchyma, the chest radiograph should be reviewed for the absence or presence of a thymus in infants and for the possibility of a thymoma, which may be associated with hypogammaglobulinemia in adults (39). Hyperinflation with patches of atelectasis, suggestive of asthma, might suggest that additional details of the past history should be carefully reviewed in patients, particularly small children, referred because of cough or recurrent pneumonia, because similar densities seen on previous films may not have actually been due to infection. The presence of old scars and active disease should be documented. Hilar adenopathy may be seen in cellular and humoral immune defects. Abnormalities of the ribs resembling those seen in rickets might suggest ADA deficiency (13), and cardiovascular abnormalities may suggest asplenia (40) or DiGeorge syndrome (41) or may steer the workup away from immune deficiency and toward Kartagener syndrome (situs inversus and ciliary dysmotility) or cystic fibrosis.

IMMUNOLOGIC SCREENING TESTS

Initial laboratory tests that may indicate that a patient has an immune deficiency can be done in most regional laboratories and community hospitals, and the results should be available in a few days. These should include measurement of the major immunoglobulins and IgG subclasses. In adults, serum protein electrophoresis should also be included because patients with monoclonal gammopathy, multiple myeloma, or chronic lymphocytic leukemia (CLL) may have antibody deficiency with a normal total level of any given class of immunoglobulin if the paraprotein is a member of that class. Interpretation of the results of measurement of the serum of concentrations of IgG and its subclasses is often less than straightforward (37,42). First of all, age-specific norms must be used, because of the marked changes in values during the first 2 years of life. Although some laboratories may report IgG concentrations as low as 200 mg/dL as normal in 3- to 6-month-old infants, concentrations of less than 400 mg/dL frequently fail to provide sufficient protective antibody levels. Second, even within a given age group, most laboratories report a normal range whose upper limit may be twofold or more higher than its lower limit. This probably reflects the fact that the total serum IgG concentration represents the sum of hundreds of separately regulated responses rather than a single variable whose physiology requires reasonably tight control, like that of an electrolyte or the blood glucose. Concentrations of IgG, and particularly its subclasses, vary not only among individuals of the same age who have different exposure histories but also in a single individual at different times. Thus, before any conclusions are reached about the diagnosis of IgG subclass deficiency, the tests should be repeated several weeks apart, and analysis of specific antibody titers should also be considered (see later).

In judging the adequacy of any given IgG concentration in a given individual, the history of exposure and the frequency of documented infections must be considered. Thus, normal individuals with frequent exposure to pathogens and those whose host defenses are compromised by conditions that do not affect lymphocyte responses, such as cystic fibrosis and chronic granulomatous disease, often have elevated total serum IgG concentrations. This may be thought of as reflecting a physiologic adaptation or as a response to increased or persistent antigen exposure by the normal immune system. IgG concentrations within the normal range, but toward its lower limit, in patients with comparably increased frequency of infection or morbidity due to infection (but without such underlying defects) may thus actually indicate relative deficiency in specific antibodies and should be evaluated further, as explained later.

In addition to those conditions in which paraproteins may conceal true antibody deficiencies within normal total IgG levels, several diseases may be associated with nonspecific polyclonal B-cell activation that may cause the total IgG or IgM level to be within the normal range or even elevated, whereas specific antibodies may actually be deficient. This occurs most often in systemic lupus erythematosus, Epstein-Barr virus infection, and HIV infection (43,44). Finding low or absent serum IgA together with low-normal or borderline levels of one or more IgG subclasses, particularly subclass 2, should also raise suspicion of more severe defects in specific antibody production than would be suggested by the total IgG concentration itself, and such patients should also be investigated further (45). Elevated serum IgE and IgA concentrations may be found coexisting with deficiency of antibodies to polysaccharides in Wiskott-Aldrich syndrome, and extremely high IgE levels may suggest, but are not by themselves diagnostic of, hyper-IgE or Job syndrome.

Analysis of lymphocyte surface antigens by flow cytometry is now widely available and should be included as a screening test in all patients in whom immune deficiency is suspected (46). A CBC with differential should always accompany lymphocyte surface marker analysis so that the absolute number of any given type of cell per cubic millimeter of blood can be calculated, in addition to ratios such as CD4/CD8 (47). As with immunoglobulin determinations, age-specific norms should be used (47). The physician should be careful about what specific test is ordered because, in the era of widespread treatment of HIV, many laboratories offer a standard lymphocyte surface marker panel, an analysis that includes only the total number of T cells (CD3$^+$) and the two major subsets of T cells (CD4$^+$ and CD8$^+$). Because antibody deficiency

due to decreased B-cell number or function is the most common type of immune deficiency overall, a complete analysis, including enumeration of natural killer (NK) and B cells, should be performed. Analysis of these lymphocyte subsets frequently provides important clues to the actual molecular defect in many cases of SCID (see later). In addition, because patients with chronic CLL may present with antibody deficiency, the ratio of lymphocytes positive for κ as opposed to λ light chains should also be determined. Flow cytometry to determine the presence of leukocyte integrins of the CD11/CD18 family can easily confirm or exclude the diagnosis of leukocyte adhesion deficiency type I (48). Similarly, flow cytometry may be used to test neutrophils for the sialyl-Lewis X antigen, whose absence establishes the diagnosis of the more rare leukocyte adhesion deficiency type II (49).

More rare deficiencies involving other arms of the immune system can also be identified and characterized at this level of testing. In patients suspected of defects in T-cell–mediated immunity, the overall functional activity of T cells is best assessed by determining the patient's ability to mount cutaneous delayed hypersensitivity reactions to recall antigens such as candida, mumps, or tetanus toxoid (37,50). Obviously, delayed hypersensitivity skin tests have little meaning in children younger than 2 years of age, who may not be adequately immunized with the antigens in question. Patients who have infections suggestive of defects in T-cell–mediated immunity should also undergo HIV screening.

The CBC will give an indication of the number of phagocytes, but assessing their function requires more specialized laboratory capabilities. Complement screening should include measurement of the serum C3 concentration and the total hemolytic activity (CH$_{50}$) because the former may be seriously reduced without affecting the latter. Although the CH$_{50}$ is the best overall screening test for complement defects and is zero in cases of late component defects, such as those that predispose to recurrent or disseminated neisserial infections (22), the serum for this test must be handled carefully or artifactually low values will be measured. In patients with a history of bacteremia, sepsis, or hematogenously spread infection, a careful review of the peripheral blood smear, looking for Howell-Jolly bodies in the erythrocytes, may suggest anatomic or functional asplenia or severely impaired reticuloendothelial system function.

DETAILED IMMUNOLOGIC LABORATORY EVALUATION

Although frank hypogammaglobulinemia, neutropenia, and complete deficiency of a component of the classic complement pathway can be detected by the screening laboratory tests described previously, more detailed testing is necessary to detect more subtle immune deficiencies. This level of testing is also frequently necessary to characterize severe defects more completely.

Because of the possibility that clinically significant antibody deficiency may be present even when the total serum concentrations of the major immunoglobulin classes and IgG subclasses are normal, specific antibody production should be assessed in all cases in which the clinical presentation suggests recurrent bacterial infections, particularly of the respiratory tract, unless the major immunoglobulin classes themselves are absent or severely depressed. Specific antibody titers should be measured against polysaccharide as well as protein antigens (51,52). Although measurement of isohemagglutinins may be used to screen for the ability to produce antibodies against polysaccharides (the A, B, or both blood group substances in patients of other blood groups), the availability of measurement of antibodies against specific bacterial antigens (see later) has decreased dependence on those assays.

In cases in which pathogens have been isolated and identified (e.g., from effusions at the time of insertion of tympanostomy tubes, endoscopic drainage of paranasal sinuses, or expectorated or induced sputum samples), antibodies against those specific organisms should also be measured. In addition, antibodies against common immunizing agents should be measured. We usually request measurement of antibodies against tetanus and diphtheria toxins and several pneumococcal polysaccharides as well as *H. influenzae* type B polysaccharide (42,51).

Testing for these and additional antibody titers are available in many commercial laboratories and are sometimes referred to as a *humoral immunity panel.*

An advantage of using these particular antigens is that they are contained in readily available, well-tested vaccines, which often have already been given to or will be clinically indicated for the patients in question, so that exposure to the antigen is definite. Obtaining titers before, as well as 4 to 8 weeks after, immunization allows comparison of the response to each antigen. The absence of a threefold rise in titer after immunization or failure to achieve protective levels indicates that the patient is unable to mount specific antibody responses. This may be seen either with protein or polysaccharide antigens and may indicate a failure to process properly or recognize an entire class of antigens, such as in what has been termed *specific polysaccharide antibody deficiency*, or certain particular antigens in what may be considered a "lacunar" defect.

In some rare cases, patients already receiving immunoglobulin infusions may require assessment of their own specific antibody production, which may be difficult because antibodies against many common antigens will have been acquired passively. In most cases, the immunoglobulin therapy can be stopped for a few months so that the patients can be immunized and their own antibody production measured while they are being reassessed clinically. If this is not possible, special test antigens, such as keyhole limpet hemocyanin and the bacteriophage ϕX174, can be obtained from specialized centers (53). Because most individuals and plasma donors have not been commonly exposed to these antigens, commercial immunoglobulin preparations do not contain antibodies against them, and they can be used to assess *de novo* specific antibody formation.

Specific T-cell function is most commonly tested by measuring the incorporation of ^{3}H-thymidine into the newly formed DNA of rapidly proliferating lymphocytes after cultures of peripheral blood mononuclear cells are stimulated *in vitro* (54). Lectins, proteins generally derived from plants that bind specific polysaccharides, commonly present in surface glycoproteins on human cells and are frequently used as the stimuli in such assays. Because these proteins stimulate most human lymphocytes, regardless of prior antigen sensitization, they are called *mitogens*, and tests using them should be referred to as *lymphocyte mitogen proliferation assays*. Plant lectins often used as stimuli for mitogen proliferation assays include concanavalin A, phytohemagglutinin, and pokeweed mitogen. Incorporation of ^{3}H-thymidine, a low-molecular-weight precursor, into high-molecular-weight cellular DNA in newly proliferating lymphocytes serves as the basis for the measurements, and the results may be expressed as the amount incorporated (in counts per minute) or as the ratio of incorporation in parallel cultures of mitogen-stimulated versus unstimulated lymphocytes, also referred to as the *stimulation index*. Mitogen stimulation tests are useful even in newborns who have not received any immunizations and may be particularly informative about lymphocyte function and immune competence in babies with partial T-cell deficiency, such as those with DiGeorge syndrome (55). Disadvantages of these tests include the requirements for several milliliters of blood, which may be prohibitive for small newborns; time constraints that may be imposed by the laboratory to facilitate isolation of the mononuclear cells during normal working hours; and the fact that the cells must be cultured for several days (usually 48 to 72 hours) before they are "pulsed" with ^{3}H-thymidine to assess its incorporation.

To surmount these difficulties, many laboratories are now using flow cytometry assays based on the appearance on the lymphocyte plasma membrane of early activation markers such as CD69 (56). Mixed lymphocyte cultures, in which a patient's (or potential donor's) T cells are stimulated by a relative's lymphocytes that have been irradiated to prevent them from proliferating, are also used to test T-cell competence and to determine histocompatability in cases in which bone marrow transplantation is contemplated. Staphylococcal enterotoxins are also often employed as stimuli in proliferation assays because they function as "superantigens," which stimulate broad families of T cells by binding to parts of their T-cell receptors other than the antigen-binding site. The response to these superantigens is thus also independent of prior antigen sensitization.

The Cowen strain of *Staphylococcus aureus* may be used as a T-cell–independent stimulus for B-cell proliferation. T-cell proliferative responses to recall antigens may also be assessed using similar techniques, although because a smaller number of T cells will respond to any given antigen than to the more broadly reacting mitogens discussed previously, these tests commonly involve 4- to 5-day incubation periods before the ^{3}H-thymidine is added and its incorporation determined.

Obviously, antigen responses can only be expected if it is documented that the patient has been exposed to the antigen in question. Thus, antigen stimulation tests are usually not useful in early infancy. However, if an older child is known to have received his or her scheduled immunizations, or if candidal infection has been obvious, the response to soluble candidal preparations and vaccine antigens such as tetanus toxoid may be useful. Thus, patients with normal responses to mitogens who fail to respond to candidal preparations may be considered to have chronic mucocutaneous candidiasis rather than a more pervasive T-cell defect, as might be seen in DiGeorge syndrome or HIV infection. In patients with opportunistic infections suggestive of AIDS or positive screening tests for HIV, confirmatory tests, such as Western blot, and quantitation of p24 antigen or viral load should be performed, and absolute CD4 number as well as T-cell function should be assessed as part of the detailed evaluation.

Detailed laboratory analysis in patients suspected of phagocyte disorders should include assessment of neutrophil chemotaxis and the oxidative respiratory burst that accompanies phagocytosis (37,57,58). Chemotaxis is assessed by measuring the migration of polymorphonuclear leukocytes through agar gels or across filters in specially designed Plexiglas (Boyden) chambers. The oxidative burst can be assessed by the nitroblue tetrazolium test, in which a soluble yellow dye is reduced to an easily visible insoluble blue intracellular precipitate (59). This is available in most hematology laboratories. Flow cytometric assays in which oxidized products are detected by fluorescence may also be employed (58). If the CH_{50} was abnormal on screening, the actual deficient component can be identified in reference laboratories that stock commercially available purified complement components and test systems. These laboratories can also screen for abnormalities of the alternative pathway, which may be indicated in patients who have recurrent bacterial infections or bacteremia and sepsis but in whom antibodies and the classic pathway have been found to be normal.

MOLECULAR DIAGNOSIS AND OTHER ADVANCED TESTING

Advanced testing designed to pinpoint the molecular lesion in cases of confirmed immune deficiency are usually performed at a university or regional research center laboratory by an immunologist specializing in such cases. However, an additional level of definition is now possible in many hospital laboratories and may aid the practitioner in providing prognostic and genetic counseling information for patients and their families. Furthermore, the practitioner should recognize the importance of defining the molecular defects in the management of immune-deficient patients because several forms of specific therapy are already available and new modalities are being developed at a rapid rate as a result in advances in understanding of the physiology of lymphocytes and cytokines as well as the genome project. Importantly, within the B-cell disorders, the pattern of X-chromosome inactivation (60) can be used to determine whether female family members are carriers of Bruton agammaglobulinemia (61). This type of analysis is also applicable to Wiskott-Aldrich syndrome, neutrophil defects, and other, but not all, X-linked disorders (60). The lack of expression on T-cells of gp-39 (CD154), the ligand for B-cell CD40, confirms the diagnosis of X-linked hyper-IgM syndrome, which might be confused with CVID in some cases (27,28).

Patients with SCID should be classified as completely as possible with flow cytometry, which may be highly suggestive of the exact molecular lesion and may have important prognostic implications (62). In particular, relative preservation of B cells in SCID patients with very low T and NK cell counts may suggest deficiency of the important signaling kinase Jak 3 or the γ c chain (62), which is an important subunit of several cytokine receptors necessary for lymphocyte development. All three cell types may be present in equal numbers in autosomal recessive SCID not due to ADA deficiency. Relatively selective deficiency of CD8 cells is characteristic of deficiency of Zap 70, a protein kinase important in signaling from the T-cell receptor. The most likely defect can then be confirmed in specialized research laboratories using assays for the specific protein (Western blot or flow cytometry) or gene that is suspect. Fluorescence *in situ* hybridization can be used to confirm the chromosome abnormality in patients suspected of having DiGeorge or velocardiofacial syndrome, overlapping sets of anomalies that may be associated with partial T-cell deficiencies and are due to microdeletions in chromosome 22q11.2 (41).

Patients with SCID, their parents, and their siblings should undergo human leukocyte antigen typing to begin to evaluate the possibility of bone marrow transplantation, which may be accompanied by minimal morbidity and may be curative in many cases (63). If there is no potential donor who matches at all loci, transplantation of T-cell–depleted marrow from a donor with a mismatch at one or more loci might be considered but is performed only at certain research centers. There may be mild or delayed presentations of SCID due to enzyme deficiencies, such as purine nucleoside phosphorylase deficiency or ADA deficiency (64). Making the correct diagnosis as early as possible is especially important in the latter because enzyme replacement with bovine ADA conjugated with polyethylene glycol (Adagen) is readily available, often results in marked amelioration of the immune defect, and can serve as a bridge until bone marrow transplantation or as long-term replacement if the patient does not have a matched donor (65,66). Anticoagulated whole blood should be sent to a research center with expertise in these assays (66) in cases of T-cell deficiency with impaired mitogen responses. Gene therapy has been used with some success in ADA deficiency and in deficiency of the γ c chain of the T-cell cytokine receptor (67); hence, early determination of the presence of the latter by flow cytometry in cases of apparent SCID in which B cells are present (62,67) is also important.

EARLY MANAGEMENT OF CELLULAR AND SEVERE COMBINED IMMUNE DEFICIENCY

Infants with significant defects in T-cell number or function and those with SCID are not only at great risk for infection with opportunistic pathogens but also may suffer from severe or overwhelming infection with attenuated live viruses normally used for immunization and may be susceptible to graft-versus-host disease (GVHD) from transfused leukocytes. For these reasons, special precautions must be initiated as soon as this type of immune defect is suspected, while the immunologic workup is proceeding and plans for referral and definitive treatment are being formulated. First, any blood products that are given must be irradiated to prevent transfusion of viable lymphocytes that could cause GVHD. Second, live virus vaccines must be avoided.

With current recommendations in the United States abandoning the use of the live attenuated oral polio vaccine and replacing it with inactivated vaccine only, polio is less of a risk. However, immunization with Bacille-Calmette-Guérin vaccine is practiced in many other countries and may lead to fatal infection. Live measles-mumps-rubella and varicella vaccines should also be avoided, and prophylaxis with varicella-zoster immune globulin should be given if infants with SCID are exposed to children with chickenpox. Trimethoprim-sulfamethoxazole or other appropriate regimens should be should be used for prophylaxis against *P. carinii* pneumonia (68), and prolonged courses of nystatin, systemic antifungal agents, or both may be necessary to control candidal infections. The use of passive immunization against respiratory syncytial virus and intravenous immune globulin (IVIG) should be considered, particularly in low-birth-weight infants and in those older than 6 months of age. This may need to be continued for more than a year, even in children who have received bone marrow transplants, because functional B-cell engraftment is often delayed.

MANAGEMENT OF ANTIBODY DEFICIENCY SYNDROMES

Because half or more of all primary immune deficiencies involve defects in antibody production, management of these patients is a common part of allergy-immunology practice. Although patients with X-linked agammaglobulinemia, X-linked hyper-IgM syndrome, and other severe immunoglobulin deficiencies generally clearly require immunoglobulin replacement (see later), others with less severe deficiencies often require complex judgment processes. In deciding which form of therapy may be most appropriate for any given patient, the practitioner must consider not only the underlying diagnosis but also the exposure history, the cumulative morbidity and future risk for end-organ damage from infection, and the risks and adverse effects of the various therapeutic options. The number of days lost from school or work and other interferences with the patient's lifestyle must also be considered. Formal pulmonary function tests and CT scans may indicate progressive yet subclinical chronic lung disease despite a relative lack of symptomatic complaints or denial on the part of the patient (69).

Often, antibody-deficient patients who present with repeated acute infections also have systemic morbidity, about which they may or may not complain. This may include fatigue, lack of stamina, poor weight gain (in infants), and musculoskeletal symptoms that have been attributed to other causes or ignored. Because these symptoms often improve with appropriate management of chronic infection and immunoglobulin replacement, they must be carefully evaluated in the review of systems and weighed in considering the options for therapy. Patients with a history of inflammatory bowel disease, recurrent problems with *Clostridium difficile,* or drug allergies may have decreased tolerance for antibiotics, which may limit the therapeutic options in their cases. Patients diagnosed with chronic obstructive pulmonary disease and those with asthma in which infection is a trigger may actually have underlying antibody deficiencies, such as the inability to respond to polysaccharides, and if so, may experience a marked amelioration of lower airway symptoms if infection is prevented with IVIG (see later) or the astute use of antibiotics.

A stepwise approach to treatment may be employed across the range of severities of antibody deficiency or sequentially in any given patient. Some patients, particularly small children, with partial antibody deficiency who have not had significant permanent end-organ damage may be managed by limiting their exposure to infectious agents (e.g., by removing them from day care or preschool) and being sure that they have received all available vaccines, including the new, conjugated heptavalent pneumococcal polysaccharide vaccine, and annual immunization against influenza. Measurement of specific antibody titers after administration of these vaccines may provide reassurance for parents and referring physicians and may suggest that additional therapy is not indicated. In some cases of partial antibody deficiency, immunization, prompt and rigorous treatment of likely bacterial infections such as sinusitis and bronchitis, and verification that these are continued until the infection has been completely resolved may provide satisfactory control of infection and freedom from chronic or progressive symptoms. In other cases, parenteral or prolonged courses of antibiotics may be initiated upon suspicion of bacterial infection, if tolerated.

The next step would be the use of prophylactic antibiotics. Many patients attain satisfactory freedom from infection by a once-daily dose of trimethoprim-sulfamethoxazole* (e.g., half of the total daily dose that would be used for otitis media). Other oral antibiotics, such as ampicillin or a cephalosporin, may also be used, especially in patients who are allergic to sulfonamides, but these agents are associated with a higher risk for resistant bacteria. Patients who develop diarrhea or other excessive gastrointestinal side effects, oral thrush, or vaginal candidiasis may be poor candidates for this approach or may not tolerate it for long. Because of the possible development

of antibiotic resistance, when patients on prophylactic antibiotics develop infections likely to be of bacterial origin, sensitivity of the organism should be confirmed, if possible, and the dose should be raised to the full treatment dose if the organism is sensitive. If isolation of the organism is not possible, or if it is not sensitive to the agent used for prophylaxis, a different agent should be used for treatment, for the full prescribed course; the prophylaxis regimen may then be resumed.

In patients with severe antibody deficiency, in those for which antibiotic therapy is problematic, and in those in whom prophylaxis has not been satisfactory, immunoglobulin replacement therapy is indicated (70–72). The introduction of preparations of pooled immunoglobulin for intravenous use has greatly facilitated administration of doses of IgG sufficient to prevent infection satisfactorily. This has become the modality of choice for most patients, particularly in the United States. Intramuscular injections of more concentrated preparations and plasma infusions have largely been abandoned, but subcutaneous infusion is also used, particularly in Scandinavian countries (73).

Most currently available preparations of immunoglobulin for intravenous use are made from the pooled plasma of thousands of donors and contain a broad spectrum of molecularly intact specific IgG antibodies of all four subclasses, with little or no IgM or IgE. The content of albumin and IgA varies. Most preparations contain sugars such as maltose, dextrose, or others, with or without glycine as a stabilizer. Because IVIG is a blood product, the possibility of transmission of blood-borne viruses must be considered. The risk for viral transmission is minimized by careful screening and selection of donors, by the processes used to purify the IgG (usually a modification of the Cohn-Oncley cold alcohol precipitation procedure), and by specific viral inactivation steps (74). These may include the use of solvent-detergent treatment, which inactivates enveloped viruses (75), pasteurization (76), or low pH (77).

Because the average half-life of IgG in the circulation is about 21 days, infusions are usually given every 3 to 4 weeks. The dose should be individualized to control infections and other

---

*Note that this would not provide satisfactory prophylaxis against *P. carinii* infection for patients with T-cell deficiencies. Recommendations for that situation may be found in reference 68.

symptoms but usually falls in a range of 300 to 600 mg/kg/dose, with the higher doses often being given at the longer dosing intervals. Serum IgG concentrations determined at the trough, just before the next infusion, can be used to provide an index and to assist decisions about the adequacy of dose and treatment interval but should not by themselves be used as an end point. This is particularly important in patients with CVID, IgG subclass deficiency, or selective antibody deficiencies, such as those who are unable to respond to polysaccharide antigens. These patients often require full replacement doses to remain free from infection despite having pretreatment serum IgG levels on the border of or within the normal range.

Antibody-deficient patients with active acute or chronic infection may experience severe systemic symptoms, including shaking chills and spiking fevers, and inflammatory reactions at the site of infection (e.g., the sinuses or airways) when they first receive IVIG. It may therefore be preferable to defer initiation of treatment until a satisfactory course of antibiotics is given in such patients. Infusions are generally initiated at the rate of 0.5 to 1 mg/kg/min (0.01 to 0.02 mL/kg/min of 5% solution) and increased in a stepwise manner at 15- to 30-minute intervals, as tolerated by the individual patient, until a maximum rate of 4 to 6 mg/kg/min is achieved. Occasional patients may tolerate rates as fast as 8 to 10 mg/kg/min. Most stable patients can thus complete their infusions within 2 to 3 hours.

A minority of patients may experience adverse reactions during infusions, which may consist of headache, backache, flushing, chills, and mild nausea (78). In severe cases, there may be dyspnea, a sense of anxiety and chest pain. These are not true anaphylactic reactions, are not mediated by IgE, and are frequently associated with increased rather than decreased blood pressure. Such reactions can usually be treated by decreasing the rate of infusion or by administration of diphenhydramine, acetaminophen, or aspirin. Patients who demonstrate consistent patterns of reactions can be kept at slower rates for subsequent infusions or pretreated with the previously mentioned drugs. In rare cases, pretreatment with corticosteroids (e.g., 0.5 to 1 mg/kg of

prednisone or intravenous methylprednisolone) may be necessary. True anaphylaxis is extremely uncommon but has been reported in a very small number of patients with IgA deficiency who have IgE antibodies against IgA (79). Because this is so rare, IgA deficiency should not be regarded as a contraindication against IVIG therapy in patients who also have significant deficiency of IgG antibodies, but slow starting rates and caution should be used with such patients.

Rarely, aseptic meningitis, thrombotic events, and acute renal failure have been caused by IVIG infusions. These have generally been cases in which high doses (>1,000 mg/kg) of IVIG have been given to achieve antiinflammatory or immunomodulatory effects in patients with underlying neurologic disease or other problems and are rare in patients receiving conventional doses as replacement therapy for immune deficiencies. Late adverse reactions include headache, which occasionally may have features of migraine; nausea, and fever, and may occur up to 48 hours after the infusion. These generally respond to acetaminophen, aspirin, or other nonsteroidal antiinflammatory drugs; however, occasionally antiemetics, serotonin receptor antagonists, or other preparations more commonly used for migraines may be required. Patients with recurrent febrile reactions should be carefully evaluated for the presence of chronic infection, which should be treated with appropriate antibiotics.

In many cases, IVIG infusions are so benign that they can be safely given in the home by a home nursing service or by a parent or spouse (80). We usually establish the safety, maximally tolerated rate, and need for premedication in our clinic before allowing the patient to go to home care. IVIG is not irritating to the veins, and conventional preparations are not viscous or difficult to administer; hence, indwelling venous access devices such as MediPort should not be required. If a patient is particularly sensitive to the pain of having the IV started, advance application of a local anesthetic, such as lidocaine or prilocaine (EMLA), which is available as a cream or presaturated disk, may be helpful. An advantage of the subcutaneous infusion method is that it makes self-administration feasible, especially if a small portable pump is used (81).

Although prevention of acute, severe bacterial infections is the major goal of antibody replacement therapy, freedom from the symptoms of chronic infections in bronchiectasis can often be achieved, and many patients report amelioration of other symptoms such as arthralgia or arthritis when appropriate replacement has been achieved. The pulmonary status, chest CT scan results, or both in all patients with significant antibody deficiencies should be carefully documented at the beginning of therapy and followed at regular intervals, even if they become asymptomatic, because recent studies show that some patients may have progressive subclinical lung disease even when they do not complain of chronic symptoms or acute exacerbations (36).

In some infants with normal lymphoid tissues and B-cell numbers in whom IVIG is started because of problems with bacterial or viral infections, the antibody deficiency may represent a maturational delay in the full range of antibody responses rather than a fixed and permanent defect. This is most likely to involve delayed development of T-independent antibody responses such as those to bacterial capsular polysaccharides. After these patients have had a satisfactory interval with a normal or decreased incidence of infections, the IVIG infusions should be stopped, and their own antibody production should be reassessed. We find it best to try such interruptions of therapy during the summer months, when the exposure to droplet-spread respiratory infection is reduced. Serum concentrations of the major immunoglobulin classes and subclasses and specific antibody titers can be redetermined after 2 to 3 months off therapy to allow sufficient catabolism of the therapeutically administered IgG so that the infant's own production can be assessed. In our experience, children whose IgG levels or specific antibody responses are not satisfactory by the time they have reached 5 years of age are not likely to improve in subsequent years, and this exercise is rarely productive above that age.

In summary, immune deficiencies include a range of disorders spanning a spectrum from SCID and X-linked agammaglobulinemia to subtle specific antibody defects. Although the former may be relatively straightforward to detect in early infancy, common variable immunodeficiency disease and specific antibody deficiencies may present with symptoms of recurrent or chronic respiratory or gastrointestinal infections at any age. Recognition of the possibility that immune deficiency may be responsible for a patient's problems is the first step in determining whether an immunologic evaluation is appropriate. The pattern of infections and the associated historical and physical features may provide important clues to the underlying diagnosis and should be kept in mind as a progression through screening and specialized and definitive laboratory tests is pursued. Therapeutic efforts aimed at minimizing the morbidity from infection or correcting the underlying problem will be suggested by the specific diagnosis and should be individualized. Because subclinical chronic infection that can lead to long-term pulmonary damage may be present (36) and because there is an increased incidence of malignancy in patients with primary immune deficiencies (5,29), close follow-up is necessary. With advances in our understanding of the basic pathogenesis of these disorders at a molecular level, additional specific therapies lie just over the horizon.

REFERENCES

1. Who Scientific Group. Primary immunodeficiency diseases: report of a WHO scientific group. *Clin Exp Immunol* 1997;109:1–28.
2. Rosen FS, Cooper MD, Wedgwood RJ. The primary immunodeficiencies. *N Engl J Med* 1995;33:431–440.
3. Ochs HD, Smith CIE, Puck JM, eds. *Primary immunodeficiency diseases: a molecular and genetic approach.* New York: Oxford University Press, 1999.
4. Stiehm ER, ed. *Immunologic disorders in infants and children.* 4th ed. Philadelphia: WB Saunders, 1996.
5. Cunningham-Rundles C. Clinical and immunologic analyses of 103 patients with common variable immunodeficiency. *J Clin Immunol* 1989;9:22–33.
6. Ochs HD, Smith CIE. X-linked agammaglobulinemia: a clinical and molecular analysis. *Medicine* 1996;75:287–299.
7. Washington K, Stenzel TT, Buckley RH, et al. Gastrointestinal pathology in patients with common variable immunodeficiency and X-linked agammaglobulinemia. *Am J Surg Pathol* 1996;20:1240–1252.
8. Ochs HD, Ament ME, Davis SD. Giardiasis with malabsorption in x-linked agammaglobulinemia. *N Engl J Med* 1972;287:341–342.

9. Sullivan KE, Mullen CA, Blaese RM, et al. A multi-institutional survey of the Wiskott-Aldrich syndrome. *J Pediatr* 1994;125:876–885.

10. Ming JE, Stiehm ER, Graham JM Jr. Syndromes associated with immunodeficiency. *Adv Pediatr* 1999;46:271–351.

11. Jones KL, ed. *Smith's recognizable patterns of human-malformation.* 5th ed. Philadelphia: WB Saunders, 1997.

12. Grimbacher B, Holland SM, Gallin JI, et al. Hyper-IgE syndrome with recurrent infections: an autosomal dominant multisystem disorder. *N Engl J Med* 1999;340:692–702.

13. Cedarbaum SD, Kautila I, Rimoin DL, et al. The chondro-osseous dysplasia of adenosine deaminase deficiency with severe combined immune deficiency. *J Pediatr* 1976;89:737–742.

14. Ahonen P, Myllamiemi S, Sipela I, et al. Clinical variation of autoimmune polyendocrinopathy-candidiasis-ectodermal dystrophy (ADECED) in a series of 68 patients. *N Engl J Med* 1990;322:1829–1836.

15. Lavin MF, Shllol Y, ed. Ataxia-telangiectasia. In: Ochs HD, ed. *Primary immunodeficiency diseases.* New York: Oxford University Press, 1999:306–323.

16. Markert ML. Purine nucleoside phosphorylase deficiency. *Immunodefic Rev* 1991;3:45–81.

17. Novak AH, Mueller B, Ochs H. Umbilical cord separation in the normal newborn. *Am J Dis Child* 1988;142:220–223.

18. Jones AM, Gaspar HB. Immunogenetics: changing the face of immunodeficiency. *J Clin Pathol* 2000;53:60–65.

19. Holland SM, Gallin JI. Evaluation of the patient with recurrent bacterial infections. *Annu Rev Med* 1998;49:185–199.

20. Stiehm ER, Chin TW, Haas A, et al. Infectious complications of the primary immunodeficiencies. *Clin Immunol Immunopathol* 1986;40:69–86.

21. Schaeffer FM, Monteiro RC, Volakis JE, et al. IgA deficiency. *Immunodefic Rev* 1991;3:15–44.

22. Figueroa JE, Densen P. Infectious diseases associated with complement deficiencies. *Clin Microbiol Rev* 1991;4:359–395.

23. Dinauer MC. Leukocyte function and nonmalignant leukocyte disorders. *Curr Opin Pediatr* 1993;5:80–87.

24. Winkelstein JA, Marino MC, Johnston RB Jr, et al. Chronic granulomatous disease: report on a national registry of 368 patients. *Medicine* 2000;79:155–169.

25. Einhorn MS, Granoff DM, Nahm MH, et al. Concentrations of antibodies in paired material and infant sera: relationship to IgG subclass. *J Pediatr* 1987;111:783–788.

26. Lederman HM, Winkelstein JA. X-linked agammaglobulinemia: an analysis of 96 patients. *Medicine* 1985;64:145–156.

27. Banatvala N, Davies J, Kanaviou M, et al. Hypogammaglobulinemia associated with normal or increased IgM (the hyper IgM syndrome): a case series review. *Arch Dis Child* 1994;71:150–152.

28. Jacov L, Boren-Espanol T, Thomas C, et al. Clinical spectrum of X-linked hyper-IgM syndrome. *J Pediatr* 1997;131:47–54.

29. Sneller MC, Strober W, Eisenstein E, et al. New insights into common variable hypogammaglobulinemia. *Ann Intern Med* 1993;118:720–730.

30. Tiller TL Jr, Buckley RH. Transient hypogammaglobulinemia of infancy: review of the literature, clinical and immunologic features of 11 new cases, and long-term follow-up. *J Pediatr* 1978;92:347–353.

31. Burns EA, Goodwin JS. Immunodeficiency of aging. *Drugs Aging* 1997;11:374–397.

32. Conley ME, Park CL, Douglas SD. Childhood common variable immunodeficiency with autoimmune disease. *J Pediatr* 1986;108:915–922.

33. Iyer M, Gorevic PD. Reactive arthropathy and autoimmunity in non-HIV-associated immunodeficiency. *Curr Opin Rheumatol* 1993;5:475–482.

34. Itescu S. Adult immunodeficiency and rheumatic disease. *Rheum Dis Clin North Am* 1996;22:53–73.

35. Curtin JJ, Webster ADB, Farrant J, et al. Bronchiectasis in hypogammaglobulinemia: a computed tomography assessment. *Clin Radiol* 1991;44:82–84.

36. Kainulainen L, Varpula M, Liippo K, et al. Pulmonary abnormalities in patients with primary hypogammaglobulinemia. *J Allergy Clin Immunol* 1999;104:1031–1036.

37. Shearer WT, Buckley RH, Engler RJM, et al. (The Clinical and Laboratory Immunology Committee of the American Academy of Allergy, Asthma, and Immunology). Practice parameters for the diagnosis and management of immunodeficiency. *Ann Allergy Asthma Immunol* 1996;76:282–294.

38. Hirschorn R. Adenosine deaminase deficiency: molecular basis and recent developments. *Clin Immunol Immunopathol* 1995;76:S219–S226.

39. Gary G, Gutowski WTI. Thymoma: a clinicopathologic study of 54 cases. *Am J Surg Pathol* 1979;3:235–249.

40. Phoon CK, Neill CA. Asplenia syndrome: insight into embryology through an analysis of cardiac and extracardiac anomalies. *Am J Cardiol* 1994;73:581–587.

41. Hong R. The DiGeorge anomaly (catch 22, DiGeorge/velocardiofacial syndrome). *Semin Hematol* 1998;35:282–290.

42. Berger M. IgG subclass determination in the diagnosis and management of antibody deficiency syndromes. *J Pediatr* 1987;110:325–328.

43. Shirai A, Consentino M, Leitman-Klinman SF, et al. Human immunodeficiency virus infection induces both polyclonal and virus-specific B-cell activation. *J Clin Invest* 1992;89:561–566.

44. Granholm NA, Cavallo T. Autoimmunity, polyclonal B cell activation and infection. *Lupus* 1992;1:63–74.

45. Oxelius V, Laurell A, Lindquist B, et al. IgG subclasses in selective IgA deficiency: importance of IgG2-IgA deficiency. *N Engl J Med* 1981;304:1476–1478.

46. Giorgi JV. Lymphocyte subset measurements: significance in clinical medicine. In: Rose NR, Friedman H, Fahey JL, eds. *Manual of clinical laboratory immunology.* 3rd ed. Washington, DC: American Society for Microbiology, 1986:236–246.

47. Comans-Bitter WM, de Groot R, van den Beemd R, et al. Immunophenotyping of blood lymphocytes in childhood. *J Pediatr* 1997;130:388–393.

48. Anderson DC, Schmalstieg FC, Finegold MJ. The severe and moderate phenotypes of inheritable Mac-1, LFA-1 deficiency: their quantitative definition and relation to leukocyte dysfunction and clinical features. *J Infect Dis* 1985;152:668–689.

49. Phillips ML, Schwartz BR, Etzionia, et al. Neutrophil adhesion in leukocyte adhesion deficiency syndrome type 2. *J Clin Invest* 1995;96:2898–2906.

50. Conley ME, Stiehm ER, eds. Skin tests. In: *Immunologic*

Disorders in Infants and Children. 4th ed. Stern ER, ed. Philadelphia: WB Saunders, 1996:221.

51. Wasserman RL, Sorensen RU. Evaluating children with respiratory tract infections: the role of immunization with bacterial polysaccharide vaccine. *Pediat Infect Dis J* 1999;18:157–163.

52. Saxon A, Kobayashi RH, Stevens RH, et al. In vitro analysis of humoral immunity in antibody deficiency with normal immunoglobulins. *Clin Immunol Immunopathol* 1980;17:235–244.

53. Wedgwood RJ, Ochs HD, Davis SD. The recognition and classification of immunodeficiency diseases with bacteriophage NX174. *Birth Defects Orig Artic Ser* 1975;11:331–338.

54. Maluish AE, Strong DM, eds. Lymphocyte proliferation. In: Rose NR, Friedman H. Fahey JL, eds. *Manual of clinical laboratory immunology.* 3rd ed. Washington, DC: American Society for Microbiology, 1986:274–281.

55. Bastian J, Law S, Vogler L, et al. Prediction of persistent immunodeficiency in the Di George anomaly. *J Pediatr* 1989;115:391–396.

56. Perfetto SP, Mickey TE, Blair PJ, et al. Measurement of CD69 induction in the assessment of immune function in asymptomatic HIV-infected individuals. *Cytometry* 1997;30:1–9.

57. Johnson CM, Rhodes KH, Katzman JA. Neutrophil function tests. *Mayo Clin Proc* 1984;59:431–434.

58. Vowells SJ, Sekhsaria S, Malech HL, et al. Flow cytometric analysis of the granulocyte respiratory burst: a comparison study of fluorescent probes. *J Immunol Methods* 1995;178:89–97.

59. Ochs HD, Igo RP. The NBT slide test: a simple method for detecting chronic granulomations disease and female carriers. *J Pediatr* 1973;83:77–82.

60. Puck JM, Willard HF. X-inactivation in females with x-linked disease. *N Engl J Med* 1998;338:325–328.

61. Allen RC, Nachtman RG, Rosenblatt HM, et al. Application of carrier testing to genetic counseling for x-linked agammaglobulinemia. *Am J Hum Genet* 1994;54:25–35.

62. Buckley RH, Schiff RI, Schiff SE, et al. Human severe combined immunodeficiency: genetic, phenotypic, and functional diversity in one hundred eight infants. *J Pediatr* 1997;130:378–387.

63. Buckley RH, Schiff SE, Schiff RI, et al. Hematopoietic stem-cell transplantation for the treatment of severe combined immunodeficiency. *N Engl J Med* 1999;340:508–516.

64. Levy Y, Hershfield MS, Fernandez-Mejia C, et al. Adenosine deaminase deficiency with late onset of recurrent infectious: response to treatment with poly ethylene glycol-modified adenosine deaminase. *J Pediatr* 1988;113:312–317.

65. Hershfield MS, Chaffee S, Sorensen RU. Enzyme replacement therapy with polyethylene glycol-adenosine deaminase in adenosine deaminase deficiency: overview and case reports of three patients, including two now receiving gene therapy. *Pediat Res* 1993;33:542–547.

66. Hershfield MS, Kurtzberg J, Aiyar VN, et al. Abnormalities in S-adenosylhomocysteine hydrolysis, ATP catabolism, and lymphoid differentiation in adenosine deaminase deficiency. *Ann N Y Acad Sci* 1985;451:78–86.

67. Cavazzana-Calvo M, Hacein-Bey S, de Saint BG, et al. Gene therapy of human severe combined immunodeficiency (SCID)-X1 disease. *Science* 2000;288:669–672.

68. Report of the committee for infectious diseases. Recommendations for *Pneumocystis carinii* pneumonia prophylaxis. In: Georges P, ed. *American Academy of Pediatrics Red Book.* 1997:423.

69. Watts WJ, Watts MB, Dai W, et al. Respiratory dysfunction in patients with common variable hypogammaglobulinemia. *Am Rev Respir Dis* 1986;134:699–703.

70. Cunningham-Rundles C, Siegal FP, Smithwick EM, et al. Efficacy of intravenous immunoglobulin in primary humoral immunodeficiency disease. *Ann Intern Med* 1984;101:435–439.

71. Roifman CM, Levison H, Gelfand EW. High-dose versus low-dose intravenous immunoglobulin in hypogammaglobulinaemia and chronic lung disease. *Lancet* 1987;1:1075–1077.

72. Buckley RH, Schiff RI. The use of intravenous immune globulin in immunodeficiency diseases. *N Engl J Med* 1991;325:110–116.

73. Gardulf A, Anderson V, Björkander J, et al. Subcutaneous immunoglobulin replacement in patients with primary antibody deficiencies: safety and costs. *Lancet* 1995;345:365–369.

74. Yap PL. The viral safety of intravenous immune globulin. *Clin Exp Immunol* 1996;104:35–42.

75. Biesert L. Virus validation studies of immunoglobulin preparations. *Clin Exp Rheumatol* 1996;104:547–552.

76. Chandra S, Cavanaugh JE, Lin CM, et al. Virus reduction in the preparation of intravenous immune globulin: in vitro experiments. *Transfusion* 1999;39:249–257.

77. Bos OJ, Sunye DG, Nieuweboer CE, et al. Virus validation of pH 4-treated human immunoglobulin products produced by the Cohn fractionation process. *Biologicals* 1998;26:267–276.

78. Misbah SA, Chapel HM. Adverse effects of intravenous immunoglobulin. *Drug Safety* 1993;9:254–262.

79. Burks AW, Sampson HA, Buckley RH. Anaphylactic reactions after gamma globulin administration in patients with hypogammaglobulinemia. *N Engl J Med* 1986;314:560–564.

80. Sorensen RU, Kallick MD, Berger M. Home treatment of antibody deficiency syndromes with intravenous immunoglobulin. *J Allergy Clin Immunol* 1987;80:810–815.

81. Berger M, Cupps TR, Fauci A. Immunoglobulin replacement therapy by slow subcutaneous infusion. *Ann Intern Med* 1980;93:55–56.

3

Immunology of IgE-mediated and Other Hypersensitivity States

C. Raymond Zeiss and Jacob J. Pruzansky

*Division of Allergy-Immunology, Department of Medicine, Northwestern University Medical School;
VA Chicago Health Care System, Lakeside Division, Chicago, Illinois*

HISTORICAL REVIEW OF IgE-MEDIATED HYPERSENSITIVITY

In 1902, Richet and Portier described the development of anaphylaxis in dogs given sea anemone toxin; subsequently, anaphylaxis was described in humans after the injection of horse serum to achieve passive immunization against tetanus and diphtheria. In 1906, Clemons von Pirquet correctly predicted that immunity and hypersensitivity reactions would depend on the interaction between a foreign substance and the immune system, and that immunity and hypersensitivity would have similar underlying immunologic mechanisms (1).

The search for the factor responsible for immediate hypersensitivity reactions became a subject of intense investigation over several years. In 1921, Prausnitz and Küstner (2) described the transfer of immediate hypersensitivity (to fish protein) by serum to the skin of a normal individual. This test for the serum factor responsible for immediate hypersensitivity reactions was termed the Prausnitz-Küstner test. Variations of this test remained the standard for measuring skin sensitizing antibody over the next 50 years.

In 1925, Coca and Grove (3) extensively studied the skin-sensitizing factor from sera of patients with ragweed hay fever. They called skin-sensitizing antibody *atopic reagin* because of its association with hereditary conditions and because of their uncertainty as to the nature of the antibody involved. Thereafter, this factor was called *atopic reagin, reaginic antibody*, or *skin-sensitizing antibody*. This antibody clearly had unusual properties and could not be measured readily by standard immunologic methods. Major research efforts from the 1920s through the 1960s defined its physical and chemical properties and measured its presence in allergic individuals (4,5).

In 1967, the Ishizakas (6) discovered that skin-sensitizing antibody belonged to a unique class of immunoglobulin, which they called immunoglobulin E (IgE). In elegant studies using immunologic techniques, they clearly demonstrated that reagin-rich serum fractions from a patient with ragweed hay fever belonged to a unique class of immunoglobulin (6). Shortly thereafter, the Swedish researchers Johansson and Bennich discovered a new myeloma protein, termed IgND, which had no antigenic relation to the other immunoglobulin classes. In 1969, cooperative studies between these workers and Ishizakas confirmed that the proteins were identical and that a new class of immunoglobulin, IgE, had been discovered (7).

PHYSIOLOGY OF IgE

IgE Structure and Receptors

The immunochemical properties of IgE are shown in Table 3.1 in contrast to those of the other immunoglobulin classes. IgE is a glycoprotein that has a molecular weight of 190,000

TABLE 3.1. *Immunoglobulin isotypes*

Isotype	No. of C$_H$ domains	Approximate size (kd)	Additional components	Percentage of serum immunoglobulin	Approximate half-life (d)	Functions
IgA						
Monomer[a]	3	160,000	J chain	13–19	6	Provides antibodies for external body fluids, including mucus, saliva, and tears; effective at neutralizing infectious agents, agglutination, and (when bound to antigen) activation of the alternative complement pathway
Dimer[b]	3	385,000	Secretory piece	0.3		
IgD						
Monomer[a,b]	3	180,000		<1	3	Found almost entirely in membrane-bound form; the function is unknown, but may be related to maturational stages
IgE						
Monomer[a,b]	4	190,000		<0.001	3	IgE is bound to mast cell surfaces; subsequent binding of antigen stimulates mast cell degranulation, leading to immediate hypersensitivity responses (allergy)
IgG						
Monomer[a,b]	3	145,000–170,000		72–80	20	Found in four subclasses: IgG1, IgG2, IgG3, and IgG4; prevalent isotype in secondary responses
IgM						
Monomer[a]	4	—	—	—	5–10	Prevalent isotype in primary responses; effective at agglutination and activation of classic complement pathway
Pentamer[b]	4	970,000	J chain	6–8	—	

C$_H$, constant heavy chain.
[a]Membrane-bound form.
[b]Secreted form.

with a sedimentation coefficient of 8S. Like all immunoglobulins, IgE has a four-chain structure with two light chains and two heavy chains. The heavy chains contain five domains (one variable and four constant regions) that carry unique, antigenic specificities termed the *epsilon (ε) determinants* (Fig. 3.1A).These unique antigenic structures determine the class specificity of this protein. Digestion with papain yields the Fc fragment, which contains the epsilon antigenic determinants, and two Fab fragments. The Fab fragments contain the antigen-combining sites. The tertiary structure of the Fc fragment is responsible for the protein's ability to fix to the FcεRI receptors on mast cells and basophils (8).

The FcεR1 receptor is the high-affinity receptor for IgE found on mast cells, basophils, eosinophils, and human skin Langerhans cells (9). Cross-linking of high-affinity receptor-bound IgE by allergen results in the release of mediators from mast cells and basophils. Molecular biologic techniques have been used to clone the gene encoding the e chain of human IgE (ND) and to determine the site on IgE that binds to its receptor (10). Recent studies have localized this site to the Cε3 heavy chain domains (11). The high-affinity receptor for IgE is composed of an α chain, a β chain, and two γ chains, and it is the α chain that binds IgE (Fig. 3.1B). The crystal structure of the α chain has been determined giving insights into the interaction of IgE with its receptor at the molecular level (12). The β and γ chains are involved in signal transduction when the receptors are aggregated by the cross-linking of IgE, resulting in mediator release (13).

Recent studies have delineated the central role that IgE molecules in the circulation play in determining the number of FcεRI receptors on mast cells and basophils (14,15) and consequently the release of mediators from these cells. With infusion of anti-IgE monoclonal antibody in allergic subjects, there was a significant reduction in serum IgE levels, with a dramatic fall in basophil FcεRI number and mediator release (14).

A low-affinity FcεRII receptor (CD23) has been localized to B lymphocytes, monocytes and macrophages, and platelets and eosinophils. The receptor has an A form found only on B lymphocytes and a B form found on all cells expressing CD23. The expression of this receptor is markedly upregulated on all cell types by interleukin-4 (IL-4) and IL-13. Binding of IgE to this receptor places IgE at the center of activation of many important effector cells (16). The role of CD23 in regulation of the IgE response is complex, having both positive and inhibitory effects (13).

Sites of IgE Production, Turnover, and Tissue Localization

With the advent of a highly specific reagent for detecting IgE, antibody against the Fc portion of IgE (anti-IgE), the sites of production of this immunoglobulin could be examined by fluorescent-labeled anti-IgE. It was found that lymphoid tissue of the tonsils, adenoids, and the bronchial and peritoneal areas contained IgE-forming plasma cells. IgE-forming plasma cells also were found in the respiratory and intestinal mucosa (17). This distribution is similar to that of IgA. However, unlike IgA, IgE is not associated with a secretory piece, although IgE is found in respiratory and intestinal secretions. The traffic of IgE molecules from areas of production to the tissues and the circulation has not been established. Areas of production in the respiratory and intestinal mucosa are associated with the presence of tissue mast cells (18).

With the development of techniques to measure total IgE in the blood and the availability of purified IgE protein, investigators were able to study the metabolic properties of this immunoglobulin in normal individuals (19). The mean total circulating IgE pool was found to be 3.3 μg/kg of body weight, in contrast to the total circulating IgG pool of about 500,000 μg/kg of body weight. IgE has an intravascular half-life of only 2.3 days. The rate of IgE production was found to be 2.3 μg/kg/day.

It had been known for several years that the half-life of reaginic antibody in human skin as determined by passive transfer studies was about 14 days. This was reconfirmed with studies that investigated the disappearance of radiolabeled IgE in human skin. The half-life in the skin was found to be between 8 and 14 days (6). The basophil and mast cell-bound IgE pool needs to be investigated thoroughly, but it has been estimated

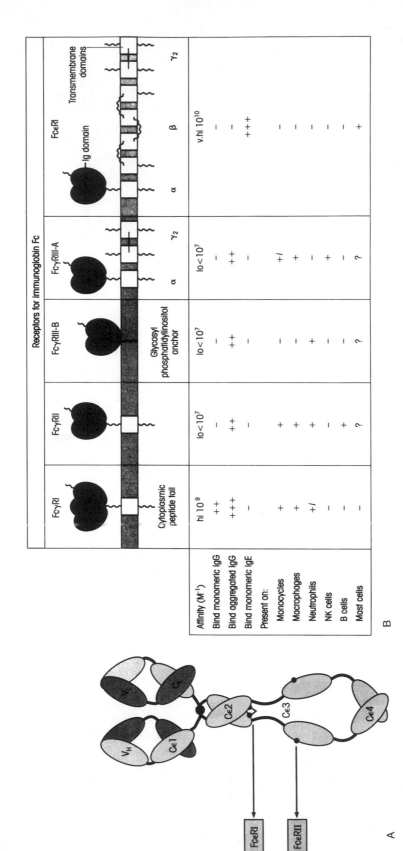

FIG. 3.1. A: The heavy chain domain structure of IgE. The binding site for the high-affinity mast cell receptor FcεRI and the low-affinity IgE receptor FcεRII is shown. **B:** The structure and characteristics of the surface receptors for immunoglobulin Fc regions. *i*, inducible; bars, disulfide bridge; NK, natural killer; v.hi, very high; Ig, immunoglobulin. (Adapted from Roitt I. *Essential immunology.* 8th ed. Oxford, UK: Blackwell Science, 1994:57, 61, with permission.)

that only 1% of the total IgE is cell bound. Direct quantification of specific IgE in the blood, in contrast to specific IgE on the basophil surface, indicates that for every IgE molecule on the basophil, there are 100 to 4,000 molecules in circulation (20).

IgE Synthesis

Major advances in the understanding of IgE synthesis have resulted from human and animal studies (21–28). Tada (21) studied the production of IgE antibody in rats and found that IgE antibody production is regulated by cooperation between T lymphocytes (T cells) and B lymphocytes (B cells). The T cells provide the helper function, and the B cells are the producers of IgE antibody.

In human systems, it became clear that IgE production from B cells required T-cell signals that were unique to the IgE system (22). In 1986, Coffman and Carty (23) defined the essential role of IL-4 in the production of IgE. The pathway to IgE production is complex, requiring not only IL-4 and IL-13 but also T- and B-cell contact, major histocompatibility complex (MHC) restriction, adhesion molecules, expression of FcϵRII (CD23) receptors, CD40 and CD40 ligand interaction, and the terminal action of IL-5 and IL-6 (24).

IL-4 acts on precursor B lymphocytes and is involved in the class switch to ϵ heavy chain production (22). IL-4 and IL-13 are not sufficient to complete the switch to functional ϵ messenger RNA, and several second signals have been described that result in productive messenger RNA transcripts (25,26). In the absence of those signals, sterile transcripts result. A key physiologic second signal is provided by CD4$^+$ helper T-cell contact. This contact signal is provided by CD40 ligand on activated T cells, which interacts with the CD40 receptor on IL-4–primed B cells and completes isotype switching to IgE (24). Recent studies indicate that IgE synthesis is critically dependent on the IL-4 receptor α chain and nuclear factors such as NF-κB and Stat 6 (27). Another cytokine, interferon-γ (IFN-γ) suppresses IgE production, acting at the same point as IL-4 (24). This complex set of interactions is shown inFig. 3.2.

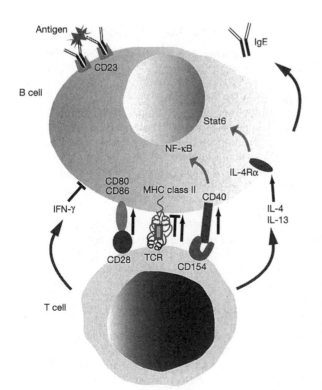

FIG. 3.2. The molecular control of the IgE response. Interleukin-4 (IL-4) and IL-13 are the most important cytokine inducers of IgE production acting at the IL-4 receptor α chain and through nuclear factor, Stat 6. Interferon-γ (IFN-γ) is the most important inhibitor of IgE synthesis. CD154, the T-cell ligand for CD40 on the B cell, promotes IgE transcription through nuclear factor, NF-κB. Antigen presented to the T-cell receptor (TCR) by class II major histocompatibility complex molecules on the B cell initiates this complex process. (Adapted from, Cory DB, Kheradmand F. Induction and regulation of the IgE response. *Nature* 1999;402s:18–23, with permission.)

During terminal differentiation of IgE B cells to plasma cells producing IgE, IgE-binding factors have been described that either enhance or suppress IgE synthesis (28). During the secondary IgE response to allergen, allergen-specific B lymphocytes capture allergen by surface IgE, internalize and degrade it, and present it to T cells as peptides complexed to class II MHC molecules. This leads to T-cell–B-cell interaction, mutual exchange of cytokine and cell contact signals, and enhanced allergen-specific IgE production.

ROLE OF IgE IN HEALTH AND DISEASE

IgE in Health

The fetus is capable of producing IgE by 11 weeks' gestation. Johansson and Foucard (29) measured total IgE in sera from children and adults. They found that cord serum contained 13 to 202 ng/mL and that the concentration of IgE in the cord serum did not correlate with the serum IgE concentration of the mother, which confirmed that IgE does not cross the placenta. In children, IgE levels increase steadily and peak between 10 and 15 years of age. Johansson and Foucard illustrate well the selection of population groups for determining the normal level of serum IgE. Studies of healthy Swedish and Ethiopian children showed a marked difference in mean IgE levels: Swedish children had a mean of 160 ng/mL, and Ethiopian children had a mean of 860 ng/mL (30). Barbee and coworkers (31) studied the IgE levels in atopic and nonatopic people 6 to 75 years of age in Tucson. IgE levels peaked in those aged 6 to 14 years and gradually declined with advancing age; male subjects had higher levels of IgE than female subjects (Fig. 3.3).

Several roles for the possible beneficial effect of IgE antibody have been postulated. The presence of IgE antibody on mast cells in the tissues that contain heparin and histamine points to a role for IgE in controlling the microcirculation, and a role for the mast cell as a "sentinel" or first line of defense against microorganisms has been advanced. The hypothesis is that IgE antibody specific for bacterial or viral antigens could

have a part in localizing high concentrations of protective antibody at the site of tissue invasion (32,33).

The role of IgE antibody has been studied extensively in an experimental infection of rats with the parasite *Nippostrongylus brasiliensis*. IgE antibody on the surface of mast cells in the gut may be responsible for triggering histamine release and helping the animal to reduce the worm burden (34). In experimental *Schistosoma mansoni* infection in the rat, IgE is produced at high levels to schistosome antigens. IgE complexed to these antigens has a role in antibody-dependent cell-mediated cytotoxicity, whereas eosinophils, macrophages, and platelets are effector cells that damage the parasite (35). IgE and IgE immune complexes are bound to these effector cells by the IgE FcϵRII receptor, which has a high affinity for IgE immune complexes. Effector cells triggered by FcϵRII receptor aggregation result in release of oxygen metabolites, lysosomal enzymes, leukotrienes, and platelet-activating factor. These observations in animals have relevance to human populations, where the IgE inflammatory cascade may protect against helminth infections (35).

IgE in Disease

The Atopic State and the T_H2 Paradigm

Extensive evidence has accumulated that may define the underlying immunologic basis for the atopic phenotype, that is, individuals with allergic asthma, allergic rhinitis, and atopic eczema (24). The atopic condition can be viewed as a T_H2 lymphocyte-driven response to allergens of complex genetic and environmental origins (36). The reciprocal action of IL-4 and IFN-γ on IgE production led to several studies on the T-cell origin of these cytokines. Mosmann and Coffman (37) described two distinct types of helper T cells in murine systems and defined them as T_H1 or T_H2 cells by the pattern of cytokine secretion. T_H1 cells produced IL-2, IFN-γ, and lymphotoxin. T_H2 cells produced IL-4, IL-5, IL-6, and IL-10.

A significant body of evidence has further defined the role of T_H2 cells in the human atopic state related to IL-4 production, IgE synthesis, and the maturation and recruitment of

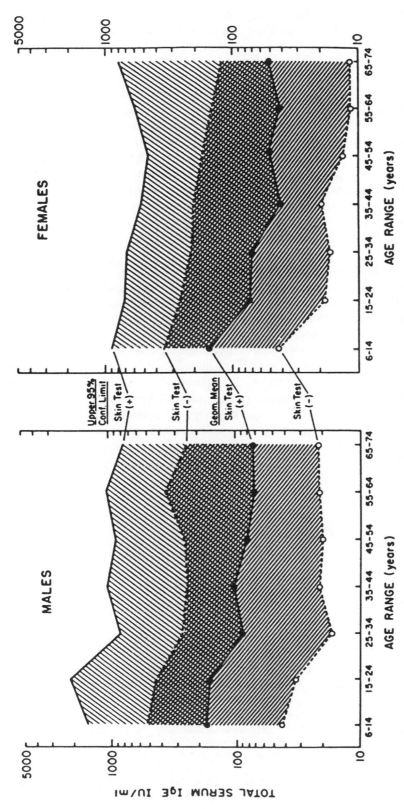

FIG. 3.3. Serum IgE as function of age and sex among whites in the United States. Geometric means and upper 95% confidence intervals are plotted against age for males and females with positive and negative results from skin tests. Double cross-hatched area represents overlap of total IgE levels between the two groups of subjects. Age-related declines in serum IgE are significant in all groups. (From Knauer KA, Adkinson NF. Clinical significance of IgE. In: Middleton E, Reed CE, Ellis EJ, eds. *Allergy principles and practice.* St. Louis: CV Mosby, 1983, with permission.)

eosinophils by IL-5 and the maturation of IgE B cells by IL-5 and IL-6 (24,36). T cells having the T_H2 cytokine profile have been cloned from individuals with a variety of atopic diseases, (24) have been identified in the airway of atopic asthmatic patients, and have been implicated as fundamental to persistent airway inflammation in asthma (38,39).

Once a T_H2 response is established, there is downregulation of T_H1 cells by the cytokines IL-4 and IL-10. T_H1 cells are capable of down-regulating T_H2 cytokine secretion through the reciprocal action of IFN-γ on T_H2 cells, a physiologic control that is abrogated by the predominant T_H2 cell response in the atopic individual (40) (Fig. 3.4).

The expression of the atopic state is dependent on genes that control the T_H2 response, total IgE production, and specific IgE responsiveness to environmental allergens. High serum IgE levels have been shown to be under the control of a recessive gene, and specific allergen responses are associated with human leukocyte antigens (41). The chromosomal location and identification of these genes are under intense investigation (42).

The recent observation that mast cells and basophils produce IL-4, leading to IgE synthesis (24), adds an amplification loop that maintains the atopic state with continued exposure to allergen, leading to mast cell and basophil activation and mediator and cytokine release with enhanced and sustained IgE production.

Studies of the interaction of histamine releasing factor (HRF) and human basophil histamine release revealed that there may be two kinds of IgE: IgE that reacts with HRF (IgE^+) and IgE that does not (IgE^-) (43). The amino acid sequence of this HRF has been determined (44). These observations may add to the role of IgE in several diseases in which no definable allergen is present.

Measurement of Total IgE

Several early studies evaluated the role of IgE in patients with a variety of allergic diseases (29–31). Adults and children with allergic rhinitis and extrinsic asthma tend to have higher total serum IgE concentrations. About half of such patients have total IgE concentrations that are two standard deviations above the mean of a normal control group. Significant overlap of total serum IgE concentrations in normal subjects and in patients with allergic asthma and hay fever has been demonstrated (Fig. 3.3). Therefore, the total

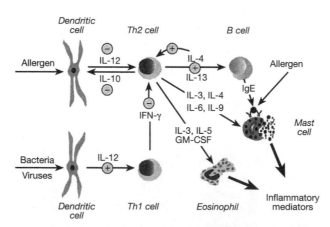

FIG. 3.4. The T_H2 cell paradigm in allergic disease. The interaction of allergen, dendritic cell, and cytokine environment causes naïve $CD4^+$ T cells to differentiate to the T_H2 phenotype with the capacity for enhanced secretion of cytokines that drive and maintain the allergic inflammatory response. The established T_H2 response downregulates the influence of T_H1 cells and the inhibitory effect of interferon-γ (IFN-γ), by the action of cytokines IL-10 and IL-4. These cytokine pathways are under complex genetic control that defines the atopic phenotype. (Adapted from Holgate ST. The epidemic of allergy and asthma. *Nature* 1999;402s:2–4, with permission.)

serum IgE concentration is neither a specific nor sensitive diagnostic test for the presence of these disorders.

Total serum IgE has been found to be markedly elevated in atopic dermatitis, with the serum IgE concentration correlating with the severity of the eczema and with the presence of allergic rhinitis, asthma, or both. Patients with atopic dermatitis without severe skin disease or accompanying asthma or hay fever may have normal IgE concentrations (45). Total IgE concentrations have been found to be markedly elevated in allergic bronchopulmonary aspergillosis.

Measurement of Specific IgE

Since the discovery of IgE in 1967, it is possible not only to measure total IgE in the serum but also to measure IgE antibody against complex as well as purified allergens. One of the first methods described by Wide and coworkers (46) was the radioallergosorbent test (RAST). Allergen is covalently linked to solid-phase particles, and these solid-phase particles are incubated with the patient's serum, which may contain IgE antibody specific for that allergen. After a period of incubation, the specific IgE present binds firmly to the solid phase. The solid phase is then washed extensively, and the last reagent added is radiolabeled anti-IgE antibody. The bound anti-IgE reflects amounts of specific IgE bound to the allergen. The results are usually given in RAST units or in units in which a standard serum containing significant amounts of IgE specific for a particular allergen is used as a reference.

Specific IgE antibody detected by RAST in the serum of patients whose skin test results are positive to an allergen has been shown to cover a wide range. Between 100-fold and 1,000-fold differences in RAST levels against a specific allergen are found in skin-reactive individuals. In studies of large groups of patients, there is a significant correlation between the RAST result, specific IgE level, and skin test reactivity. However, individuals with the same level of specific IgE antibody to ragweed allergen may vary 100-fold in their skin reactivity to that allergen (47).

The RAST concept has been extended to the use of fluorescent- and enzyme-labeled anti-IgE, which obviates the need for radiolabeled materials. Although RAST and other specific IgE measurement technologies have clarified the relationships between specific IgE in the serum and patients' clinical sensitivity, these tests do not replace skin testing with the allergens in clinical practice because skin testing is more sensitive.

It is possible to estimate the absolute quantity of specific IgE antibody per milliliter of serum against complex and purified allergens (48,49). Using one of these methods to measure IgE antibody against ragweed allergens, Gleich and coworkers (48) defined the natural rise and fall of ragweed-specific IgE over a 1-year period. In this population of ragweed-sensitive individuals, the IgE antibody specific for ragweed allergens varied from 10 to 1,000 ng/mL. A marked rise of specific IgE level occurred after the pollen season, with a peak in October followed by a gradual decrease. Specific IgE level reached a low point just before the next ragweed season in August (Fig. 3.5).It is also possible to measure basophil-bound, total, and specific IgE against ragweed antigen E. There are between 100,000 and 500,000 molecules of total IgE per basophil (50) and between 2500 and 50,000 molecules of specific IgE per basophil (20).

OTHER HYPERSENSITIVITY STATES

All immunologically mediated hypersensitivity states had been classified into four types by Gell and Coombs in 1964. This classification has been a foundation for an understanding of the immunopathogenesis of clinical hypersensitivity syndromes (51). This schema depends on the location and class of antibody that interacts with antigen resulting in effector cell activation and tissue injury.

In type I, or immediate, hypersensitivity, allergen interacts with IgE antibody on the surface of mast cells and basophils, resulting in the cross-linking of IgE, FcϵRI receptor apposition, and mediator release from these cells. Only a few allergen molecules, interacting with cell-bound IgE, lead to the release of many mediator molecules, resulting in a major biologic amplification of the allergen–IgE antibody reaction. Clinical examples include anaphylaxis, allergic rhinitis, and allergic asthma.

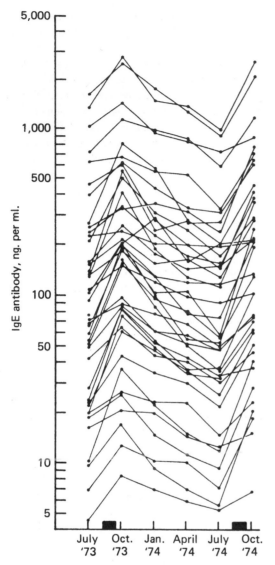

FIG. 3.5. Levels and changes of IgE antibodies to ragweed allergens in 40 untreated allergy patients. The ragweed pollination season is indicated by the *black bar* on the abscissa. (From Gleich GJ, Jacob GL, Unginger JW, et al. Measurement of the absolute levels of IgE antibodies in patients with ragweed hay fever. *J Allergy Clin Immunol* 1977;60:188, with permission.)

In type II, or cytotoxic, injury, IgG or IgM antibody is directed against antigens on the individual's own tissue. Binding of antibody to the cell surface results in complement activation, which signals white blood cell influx and tissue injury.

In addition, cytotoxic killer lymphocytes, with Fc receptors for IgG, can bind to the tissue-bound IgG, resulting in antibody-dependent cellular cytotoxicity. Clinical examples include lung and kidney damage in Goodpasture syndrome, acute graft rejection, hemolytic disease of the newborn, and certain bullous skin diseases.

In type III, or immune complex, disease, IgG and IgM antigen–antibody complexes of a critical size are not cleared from the circulation and fix in small capillaries throughout the body. These complexes activate the complement system, which leads to the influx of inflammatory white blood cells, resulting in tissue damage. Clinical examples include serum sickness (after foreign proteins or drugs), lupus erythematosus, and glomerulonephritis after common infections.

In type IV, or delayed-type, hypersensitivity, the T-cell antigen receptor on T_H1 lymphocytes binds to tissue antigens, resulting in clonal expansion of the lymphocyte population and T-cell activation with the release of inflammatory lymphokines. Clinical examples include contact dermatitis (e.g., poison ivy) and tuberculin hypersensitivity in tuberculosis and leprosy.

The classic Gell and Coombs classification has been adapted by Janeway and colleagues (52). Subsequently, Kay further expanded the adaptation (53). Type II reactions have been divided into two different subtypes. Type IIa are characterized by cytolytic reactions, such as are produced by antibodies causing immune mediated hemolytic anemia, whereas type IIb reactions are characterized by cell-stimulating reactions such as are produced by thyroid-stimulating antibody in patients with Graves disease or antibodies to the high-affinity mast cell receptor in chronic idiopathic urticaria. The latter antibodies cause mast cell activation.

Type IV reactions are divided into four subtypes. Type IVa_1 reactions are mediated by CD4$^+$ T_H1 cells causing classic delayed-type hypersensitivity reactions, such as allergic contact dermatitis or tuberculin reactions. Type IVa_2 reactions are mediated by CD4$^+$ T_H2 cells resulting in cell-mediated eosinophilic hypersensitivity as occurs in asthma. Type IVb_1 reactions are mediated by cytotoxic CD8$^+$ cells that mediate graft rejection and Stevens-Johnson syndrome. Type IVb_2 reactions are mediated by $CD8^+$ lymphocytes that can produce IL-5, resulting in cell-mediated eosinophilic hypersensitivity, usually in association with viral mucosal infection.

REFERENCES

1. Von Pirquet C. Allergie. *Münch Med Wochenschr* 1906; 53:1457.
2. Prausnitz C, Küstner H. Studien über ueberempfindlichkeit. *Centralbl Bakteriol* 1921;86:160.
3. Coca AF, Grove EF. Studies in hypersensitiveness. XIII. A study of atopic reagins. *J Immunol* 1925;10:444.
4. Stanworth DR. Reaginic antibodies. *Adv Immunol* 1963; 3:181.
5. Sehon AH, Gyenes L. Antibodies in atopic patients and antibodies developed during treatment. In: Samter M, ed. *Immunological diseases.* 2nd ed. Boston: Little, Brown, 1971:785.
6. Ishizaka K, Ishizaka T. Immunology of IgE mediated hypersensitivity. In: Middleton E, Reed CE, Ellis EJ, eds. *Allergy principles and practice.* 2nd ed. St. Louis: CV Mosby, 1983:52.
7. Bennich H, Ishizaka K, Ishizaka T, et al. Comparative antigenic study of E globulin and myeloma IgND. *J Immunol* 1969;102:826.
8. Bennich H, Johansson SGO. Structure and function of human immunoglobulin E. *Adv Immunol* 1971; 13:1.
9. Wang B, Reiger A, Kigus O, et al. Epidermal Langerhans cells from normal human skin bind monomeric IgE via FcεR1. *J Exp Med* 1992;175:1353.
10. Kenten JH, Molgaard HV, Hougton M, et al. Cloning and sequence determination of the gene for the human e chain expressed in a myeloma cell line. *Proc Natl Acad Sci USA* 1982;79:6661.
11. Henry AJ. Participation of the N-terminal region of Cepsilon3 in the binding of human IgE to its high affinity receptor FcεR1. *Biochemistry* 1997;36: 155568–15578.
12. Garman SC, Kinet JP, Jardetzky TS. Crystal structure of the human high-affinity IgE receptor. *Cell* 1998;95: 951–961.
13. Turner H, Kinet JP. Signaling through the high-affinity IgE receptor FcεR1. *Nature* 1999;402s:24–30.
14. Saini SS, MacGlashan DW, Sterbinsky SA, et al. Down-regulation of human basophil IgE and FC epsilon R1 alpha surface densities and mediator release by anti-IgE-infusions is reversible in vitro and in vivo. *J Immunol* 1999;162:5624–5630.
15. Yamaguchi M, Lantz CS, Oettgen HC, et al. IgE enhances mouse mast cell Fc(epsilon)R1 expression in vitro and in vivo: evidence for a novel amplification mechanism in IgE-dependent reactions. *J Exp Med* 1997;184: 663–672.
16. Delespesse G, Sarfati M, Wu CY, et al. The low-affinity receptor for IgE. *Immunol Rev* 1992;125:77.
17. Tada T, Ishizaka K. Distribution of gamma E-forming cells in lymphoid tissues of the human and monkey. *J Immunol* 1970;104:377.
18. Callerame ML, Londemi JJ, Ishizaka K, et al. Immunoglobulins in bronchial tissues from patients with

asthma, with special reference to immunoglobulin E. *J Allergy* 1981;47:187.
19. Waldmann TM, Iio A, Ogawa M, et al. The metabolism of IgE: studies in normal individuals and in a patient with IgE myeloma. *J Immunol* 1976;117:1139.
20. Zeiss CR, Pruzansky JJ, Levitz D, et al. The quantitation of IgE antibody specific for ragweed antigen E on the basophil surface in patients with ragweed pollenosis. *Immunology* 1978;35:237.
21. Tada T. Regulation of reaginic antibody formation in animals. *Prog Allergy* 1975;19:122.
22. Lebman DA, Coffman RL. Interleukin-4 causes isotype switching to IgE in T cell-stimulated clonal B cell cultures. *J Exp Med* 1988;168:853.
23. Coffman RL, Carty J. A T-cell activity that enhances polyclonal IgE production and its inhibition by interferon-γ. *J Immunol* 1986;136:949.
24. Leung YM. Mechanisms of the human allergic response: clinical implications. *Pediatr Clin North Am* 1994;41:727.
25. Maggi E, Romagnani S. Role of T-cells and T-cell derived cytokines in the pathogenesis of allergic diseases. *Ann N Y Acad Sci* 1994;725:2.
26. Gauchat J-F, Lebman DA, Coffman RL, et al. Structure and expression of germline e transcripts in human B cells induced by interleukin-4 to switch to IgE production. *J Exp Med* 1990;172:463.
27. Cory DB, Kheradmand F. Induction and regulation of the IgE response. *Nature* 1999;402s:18–23.
28. Ishizaka K. Regulation of the IgE antibody response. *Int Arch Allergy Appl Immunol* 1989;88:8.
29. Johansson SGO, Foucard T. IgE in immunity and disease. In: Middleton E, Reed CE, Ellis EJ, eds. *Allergy principles and practice.* 1st ed. St Louis: CV Mosby, 1978: 551.
30. Johansson SGO, Mellbin T, Vahlquist G. Immunoglobulin levels in Ethiopian preschool children with special reference to high concentrations of immunoglobulin E (IgND). *Lancet* 1968;1:1118.
31. Barbee RA, Halonen M, Lebowitz M, et al. Distribution of IgE in a community population sample: correlation with age, sex, allergen skin test reactivity. *J Allergy Clin Immunol* 1981;68:106.
32. Lewis RA, Austen KF. Mediation of local homeostasis and inflammation by leukotrienes and other mast-cell dependent compounds. *Nature* 1981;293:103.
33. Steinberg P, Ishizaka K, Norman PS. Possible role of IgE-mediated reaction in immunity. *J Allergy Clin Immunol* 1974;54:359.
34. Dineen JK, Ogilvie BM, Kelly JD. Expulsion of *Nippostrongylus brasiliensis* from the intestine of rats: collaboration between humoral and cellular components of the immune response. *Immunology* 1973; 24: 467.
35. Dessaint JP, Capron A. IgE inflammatory cells: the cellular network in allergy. *Int Arch Allergy Appl Immunol* 1989;90:28.
36. Romagnani S. The role of lymphocytes in allergic disease. *J Allergy Clin Immunol* 2000;105:399–408.
37. Mosmann TR, Coffman RL. Th1 and Th2 cells: different patterns of lymphokine secretion lead to different functional properties. *Annu Rev Immunol* 1989; 7:145.
38. Robinson DS, Hamid Q, Ying S, et al. Predominant Th2-like bronchoalveolar T-lymphocyte population in atopic asthma. *N Engl J Med* 1992;326:298.

39. Busse WW, Coffman RL, Gelfand EW, et al. Mechanisms of persistent airway inflammation in asthma: a role for T cells and T-cell products. *Am J Respir Crit Care Med* 1995;152:388.

40. Holgate ST. The epidemic of allergy and asthma. *Nature* 1999;402s:2–4.

41. Marsh DG, Huang S-K. Molecular genetics of human immune responsiveness pollen allergens. *Clin Exp Allergy* 1991;21:168.

42. Cookson W. The alliance of genes and the environment in asthma and allergy. *Nature* 1999;402s:5–11.

43. MacDonald SM, Lichtenstein LM, Proud O, et al. Studies of IgE dependent histamine releasing factors: heterogenicity of IgE. *J Immunol* 1987;139:506.

44. MacDonald SM, Rafnar T, Langdon J, et al. Molecular identification of an IgE-dependent histamine releasing factor. *Science* 1995;269:688.

45. Johnson EE, Irons JJ, Patterson R, et al. Serum IgE concentrations in atopic dermatitis:relationship to severity of disease and presence of atopic respiratory disease. *J Allergy Clin Immunol* 1974; 54:94.

46. Wide L, Bennich H, Johansson SGO. Diagnosis of allergy by an *in vitro* test for allergenic antibodies. *Lancet* 1967;2:1105.

47. Norman P. Correlations of RAST and in vivo and in vitro assays. In: Evans R III, ed. *Advances in diagnosis of allergy: RAST.* Miami: Symposia Specialists, 1975:45.

48. Gleich GJ, Jacobs GL, Yunginger JW, et al. Measurement of the absolute levels of IgE antibodies in patients with ragweed hay fever: effect of immunotherapy on seasonal changes and relationship to IgG antibodies. *J Allergy Clin Immunol* 1978;60:188.

49. Zeiss CR, Pruzansky JJ, Patterson R, et al. A solid phase radioimmunoassay for the quantitation of human reaginic antibody against ragweed antigens. *J Immunol* 1973;110:414.

50. Conroy MC, Adkinson NF, Lichtenstein LM. Measurement of IgE on human basophils: relation to serum IgE and anti-IgE induced histamine release. *J Immunol* 1977;118:1317.

51. Roitt I. Hypersensitivity. In: *Essential immunology.* 8th ed. London: Blackwell Science, 1994:313.

52. Janeway C, Travers P, eds. *Immunobiology.* 2nd ed. London: Garland Press, 1995.

53. Kay AB. Concepts of allergy and hypersensitivity in allergy and allergic diseases. In: Kay AB, ed. *Allergy and allergic diseases.* Vol. 1. Oxford, UK: Blackwell Science, 1997;23–35.

4

Biochemical Mediators of Allergic Reactions

Stephen I. Wasserman

Department of Medicine, University of California, San Diego, La Jolla, California, Department of Medicine, University of California, San Diego Medical Center, San Diego, California

Recent research has expanded the understanding of the cells and mediators relevant to diseases of immediate-type hypersensitivity. The biologically active molecules responsible have been identified, and a thorough biochemical and structural elucidation of diverse lipid mediators has been accomplished. The activity of mediator-generating cells and their diverse products has been assigned a central role in both immunoglobulin E (IgE)-mediated acute and prolonged inflammatory events. This chapter places in perspective the mediator-generating cells, the mediators themselves, and these newer concepts of their roles in pathobiologic and homeostatic events.

MEDIATOR-GENERATING CELLS

Mast cells and basophilic polymorphonuclear leukocytes (basophils) constitute the two IgE-activated mediator-generating cells (1,2). Mast cells are heterogeneous, and both connective tissue and mucosal types have been recognized (3) (Table 4.1). The latter predominate in the lamina propria of the gastrointestinal tract and in the peripheral airways and alveolar septa. Both occur in the upper airway and nose, and the connective tissue subtype dominates in the skin (4).

Mast cells are most closely related to mononuclear leukocytes (5) and are richly distributed in the deeper region of the central nervous system, the upper and lower respiratory epithelium, the bronchial lumen, the gastrointestinal mucosa and submucosa, bone marrow, and skin (6,7). They are especially prominent in bone, dense connective tissue adjacent to blood vessels (particularly small arterioles and venules), and peripheral nerves. In the skin, lungs, and gastrointestinal tract, mast cell concentrations approximate 10,000 to 20,000 cells/mm^3 (8). They develop from CD34$^+$ bone marrow precursors through the action of stem cell factor (kit-ligand SCF), which binds to a specific receptor (c-kit, CD117) (9). Precursor cells exit the marrow and terminally differentiate in tissues under a variety of local influences, such as interleukin-3 (IL-3), IL-4, IL-6, IL-9, IL-10, and factors from fibroblasts (5,10,11), but are inhibited by transforming growth factor B (12). Mast cells are large (10 to 15 mm in diameter) and possess a ruffled membrane, numerous membrane-bound granules (0.5 to 0.7 mm in diameter), mitochondria, a mononuclear nucleus, and scant rough endoplasmic reticulum. Ultrastructurally, human mast cell granules display whorl and scroll patterns (13).

Basophils, most closely related to eosinophils, are circulating leukocytes whose presence in tissue is unusual except in disease states (14). They originate in bone marrow and constitute 0.1% to 2.0% of the peripheral blood leukocytes. Basophils possess a polylobed nucleus and differ from mast cells in their tinctorial properties, their relatively smooth cell surface, and their granule morphologic makeup, which is larger and less structured than that of the mast cell. Their growth is responsive, not to SCF, but rather to IL-3

TABLE 4.1. *Human mast cell heterogeneity*

Characteristic	MC^T	MC^{TC}
Location	Lungs and gastrointestinal mucosa	Skin and gastrointestinal submucosa
Protease	Tryptase	Tryptase-chymase
Granule structure	Scrolls	Grating-lattices
Growth factor dependent	Yes	No
Formalin sensitivity	Yes	No
Proteoglycan	Heparin[a]	Heparin[a]
Secretogogue response (morphine, substance P, C5a, compound 48/80, f-met-peptide)	No	Yes
Temperature for degranulation	37°C	23°–30°C
Migratory	Yes	No

MC^T, mast cell (mucosal type); MC^{TC}, mast cell (connective tissue type).
[a] Structurally different.
Adapted from Bernstein JA, Lawrence ID. The mast cell: a comprehensive, updated review. *Allergy Proc* 1990;11:209, with permission.

and granulocyte-macrophage colony-stimulating factor (GM-CSF).

ACTIVATION OF MAST CELLS AND BASOPHILS

Mast cells and basophils possess numerous high-affinity intramembranous receptors (FcϵRI) for the Fc portion of IgE. The number of such receptors is upregulated by exposure of the mast cell or basophil to increased amounts of IgE (15). The bridging of two or more such Fc receptors by antigen cross-linking of receptor-bound surface IgE molecules leads to cell activation and rapid release of preformed granular constituents and to the generation of unstored mediators. Mast cell responsiveness may be heightened by exposure to SCF or other cytokines (16,17), whereas basophils are primed to respond by GM-CSF, IL-1, IL-3, and IL-5 (18). Other important secretagogues include a family of histamine-releasing factors (19) and complement fragments C3a and C5a.

The secretagogue-induced activation of mediator release is noncytolytic, a process termed *stimulus-secretion coupling. In vitro,* extremely complex intertwined and potentially interacting systems have been identified, some of which may play roles in cell activation (20).

An additional complexity is added as stored granule-associated mediators are regulated independently from unstored newly generated mediators. In IgE-mediated activation, receptor bridging is accompanied by protein tyrosine phosphorylation, an increase in intracellular calcium, protein kinase C translocation, G protein activation, and cyclic adenosine monophosphate generation. At the same time, membrane phospholipids are metabolized to generate monoacylglycerols, diacylglycerols, and phosphorylated inositol species, which facilitate protein kinase C function and liberate Ca^{2+} from intracellular sites. While these biochemical events are underway, adenosine triphosphate (ATP) is catabolized, and adenosine is liberated, which, in turn, activates a mast cell adenosine receptor to enhance granule release. Finally, the cell gains control over mediator release, the process stops, and the cell regranulates (21).

Although initiated at the time of IgE and antigen activation, the generation of cytokines is expressed over a time frame of hours to days. Both mast cells and basophils are important sources of a variety of inflammatory cytokines, as described later. After the initiating event of allergen binding, cytokine synthesis proceeds through activation of such signaling pathways as the STAT and NF-κB–regulated processes, with gene transcription evident within hours and protein secretion occurring subsequently (22).

Recent work has added further complexity to mast cell and basophil activation. Mast cells possess a receptor for IgG, $Fc\epsilon RII$, which can modulate mediator release (23), and these cells also respond to endotoxin through engagement of a toll-like receptor complex. The presence of these additional modulatory pathways suggests that mast cell and basophil mediators participate in inflammatory conditions in which IgE may not be present.

MEDIATORS

Whatever their final metabolic interrelationships, the early biochemical processes lead to the generation of a heterogenous group of molecules termed *mediators*. Some mediators are preformed and are stored in the granules of the cell; others are generated only after cell activation and originate in the cytosol or membrane. Mediators are classified in this chapter by their proposed actions (Tables 4.2 and 4.3), although some mediators subserve several functions.

Spasmogenic Mediators

Histamine, generated by decarboxylation of histidine, was the first mast cell mediator to be identified, and it is the sole preformed mediator

TABLE 4.2. *Mast cell vasoactive and spasmogenic mediators*

Mediator	Other actions
Histamine	Alters cell migration
	Generates prostaglandins
	Increases mucus production
	Activates suppressor T lymphocytes
Platelet-activating factor	Activates platelets
	Attracts and activates eosinophils
Prostaglandin D_2	Prevents platelet aggregation
	Alters cell migration
Sulfidopeptide leukotrienes (C_4, D_4, E_4)	Increase mucus production
	Generate prostaglandins
Adenosine	Prevents platelet aggregation
	Enhances mediator release
	Inhibits neutrophil superoxide production

TABLE 4.3. *Mast cell mediators affecting cell migration*

Mediator	Cell target
High molecular weight NCF	Neutrophils
ECF-A	Eosinophils
ECF oligopeptides	Eosinophils (secondary mononuclear)
T-lymphocyte chemotactic factors	T cells
Histamine	Nonselective
PGD_2	Eosinophils and neutrophils
Leukotriene B_4	Neutrophils
Leukotriene E_4	Eosinophils
PAF	Eosinophils and neutrophils
Lymphocyte chemokinetic factor	T and B cells

NCF, neutrophil chemotactic factor; ECF-A, eosinophil chemotactic factor of anaphylaxis; PGD_2, prostaglandin D_2; PAF, platelet-activating factor.

in this functional class. It is bound to the proteoglycans of mast cell and basophil granules (5 and $1 mg/10^6$ cells, respectively) (24,25). Histamine circulates at concentrations of about 300 pg/mL with a circadian maximum in the early morning hours (26). Histamine excretion exceeds 10 mg/24 hours; a small fraction is excreted as the native molecule, and the remainder as imidazole acetic acid or methyl histamine. Histamine interacts with specific H_1, H_2, and H_3 receptors (27,28). H_1 receptors predominate in the skin and smooth muscle; H_2 receptors are most prevalent in the skin, lungs, and stomach and on a variety of leukocytes; and H_3 receptors predominate in the brain. The biologic response to histamine reflects the ratio of these receptors in a given tissue. H_1 histamine effects include contraction of bronchial and gut musculature, vascular permeability, pulmonary vasoconstriction, and nasal mucus production (29,30). By its H_2 pathway, histamine dilates respiratory musculature, enhances airway mucus production, inhibits basophil and skin (but not lung) mast cell degranulation, and activates suppressor T lymphocytes. Both H_1 and H_2 actions are required for the full expression of pruritus, cutaneous vasodilation, and cardiac irritability (27). The H_3 actions of histamine suppress central nervous system histamine synthesis. Increased levels of histamine have been reported in the blood or urine of patients with physical urticaria, anaphylaxis, systemic mastocytosis, and antigen-induced rhinitis and asthma (31).

Platelet-activating Factor

Platelet-activating factor (PAF) is a lipid identified structurally as 1-alkyl-2-acetyl-sn-glyceryl-3-phosphorylcholine (32). This mediator is generated by mast cells, eosinophils, and monocytes. Degradation of PAF occurs by the action of acetyl hydrolase to remove acetate from the sn-2 position.

PAF causes aggregation of human platelets, wheal-and-flare permeability responses, and eosinophil chemotaxis (33); PAF also contracts pulmonary and gut musculature, induces vasoconstriction, and is a potent hypotensive agent. Effects mediated by PAF also include pulmonary artery hypertension, pulmonary edema, an increase in total pulmonary resistance, and a decrease in dynamic compliance. In addition, PAF is capable of inducing a prolonged increase in nonspecific bronchial hyperreactivity *in vivo* (34).

Oxidative Products of Arachidonic Acid

Arachidonic acid is a C20:4 fatty acid component of mast cell membrane phospholipids, from which it may be liberated by the action of phospholipase A_2 or by the concerted action of phospholipase C and diacylglycerol lipase. At least 20 potential end products may be generated from arachidonic acid by the two major enzymes, 5-lipoxygenase and cyclooxygenase, which regulate its fate.

Cyclooxygenase Products

Prostaglandin (PG) D_2 is the predominant cyclooxygenase product generated by human mast cells, whereas human basophils do not generate this molecule. The production of PGD_2 from PGH_2 is glutathione dependent and is blocked by nonsteroidal antiinflammatory drugs and dapsone. It is a potent vasoactive and smooth muscle reactive compound that causes vasodilation when injected into human skin, induces gut and pulmonary muscle contraction, and, *in vitro*, inhibits platelet aggregation (35). PGD_2 is thought to be responsible for flushing and hypotension in some patients with mastocytosis and to be an important mediator of allergic asthma (36). PGD_2 is further metabolized to PGJ_2, a natural ligand for peroxisome proliferator-activated receptor-γ (37), a nuclear receptor important in diabetes and atherosclerosis.

Immediate IgE antigen–activated PGD_2 production is dependent on the constitutive expression of cyclooxygenase 1. Later and more prolonged PGD_2 synthesis occurs after antigen challenge of sensitized cells that are stimulated with SCF and IL-10 (38).

Lipoxygenase Products

Human mast cells generate 5-lipoxygenase products of arachidonic acid, starting with an unstable intermediate, 5-HPETE (which may be reduced to the monohydroxy fatty acid), 5-HETE, or (through leukotriene synthetase) LTC_4 by addition of glutathione through the action of LTC_4 synthase. The initial product of this pathway is LTC_4, from which LTD_4 may be generated by the removal of the terminal glutamine, and LTE_4 by the further removal of glycine. A polymorphism in the LTC_4 synthase gene is thought to alter the amount of this mediator generated during biologic reactions (39). The biologic activity of the sulfidopeptide leukotrienes occurs by its binding to two specific receptors termed Cys LTR I and II (40,41). Degradation is rapid and is accomplished by various oxygen metabolites. Clinically useful inhibitors of 5-lipoxygenase or the Cys LTR I receptors are available and demonstrate efficacy in clinical asthma (42). No clinically available inhibitor of Cys LTR II has been assessed *in vivo,* and the contribution of this receptor to the physiologic manifestations of LTC_4, LTD_4, or LTE_4 remains speculative.

Leukotrienes are potent and possess a broad spectrum of biologic activity (43). They induce wheal-and-flare responses that are long lived and are accompanied histologically by endothelial activation and dermal edema. In the airway, they enhance mucus production and cause bronchoconstriction, especially by affecting peripheral units. In humans, LTD_4 is most active, LTC_4 is intermediate, and LTE_4 is the least potent. LTE_4 has been implicated as an inducer of nonspecific bronchial hyperreactivity. It has been suggested that LTD_4 augments airway remodeling (44), possibly by stimulating matrix metalloproteinase release or activity. All depress cardiac muscle performance and diminish coronary flow rates. LTC_4 and LTD_4 have been recovered from nasal washings and bronchial lavage fluids of patients with allergic rhinitis or asthma, whereas LTE_4 has been recovered from the urine.

Adenosine

The nucleoside adenosine generated from the breakdown of ATP is released from mast cells on IgE-mediated activation (45). In humans, circulating blood levels of adenosine are 0.3 μg/mL and are increased after hypoxia or antigen-induced bronchospasm. Adenosine is a potent vasodilator, inhibits platelet aggregation, and causes bronchospasm on inhalation by asthmatics. Adenosine, acting through a cell surface receptor, probably the A2b and A3 subtypes (46,47) enhances mast cell mediator release *in vitro* and potentiates antigen-induced local wheal-and-flare responses *in vivo*. Adenosine binding to its receptor is inhibited by methylxanthines.

Chemotactic Mediators

Several chemotactic molecules have been characterized by activities generated during IgE-dependent allergic responses. Most remain incompletely characterized. A new family of cytokines has been described; these cytokines, called *chemokines,* have chemoattractant activity for leukocytes and fibroblasts (Table 4.4). In the C-X-C or α chemokines, the cysteines are separated by one amino acid, whereas the cysteines are adjacent in the C-C or β chemokines. Most α chemokines attract neutrophils, whereas β chemokines attract T cells and monocytes (some also attract basophils and eosinophils). The C-X-C chemokines that attract neutrophils

TABLE 4.4. *Chemokines causing chemoattraction*

Chemokine	Cells attracted
C-X-C(α)	
GRO-α	N, T, F, M_p
GRO-β	N
IL-8	N, T, M_p, NK E, B, Mt, B_S
NAP-δ	N
PF-4	N, F
C-C(β)	
Eotaxin	M, E, T
MIP-1α	M, T, E, Mt, B, B_S
MIP-1β	M, T
MCP-1	M, T, NK, Mt, B_S
MCP-2	M, T, Mt, E, B_S
MCP-3	M, T, N, E
RANTES	M, T, NK, E, Mt, B_S

B_S, basophil; E, eosinophil; T, T cell; B, B cell; NK, NK cell; Mt, mast cell; M_P, macrophage; F, fibroblast.

include GRO-α, GRO-β, IL-8, NAP-2 and PF-4. The C-C chemokines that attract eosinophils include eotaxin, MIP-1α, MCP-2, MCP-3, and RANTES. IL-8, MIP-1α, and RANTES are also cell chemoattractants for both mast cells and basophils.

Neutrophil Chemotactic Factors

High-molecular-weight (HMW) factors are the most prominent neutrophil-directed activities noted. HMW-NCF (neutrophil chemotactic factor) is released into the circulation soon after mast cell activation (48). Its release in asthmatic patients is antigen dose dependent, inhibited by cromolyn, and accompanied by transient leukocytosis.

LTB_4 and PAF are potent chemotactic agents capable of inducing neutrophil exudation into human skin, and they induce production of oxygen radicals and lipid mediators. Histamine also alters neutrophil chemotactic responses.

Eosinophil Chemotactic Factors

The most potent and selective eosinophil-directed agent is PAF, (33) which induces skin or bronchial eosinophilia. Other, less active eosinophil-directed mast cell products include the tetrapeptides Val or ala-gly-ser-glu (eosinophil chemotactic factor of anaphylaxis

[ECF-A]) (49) and others having a molecular weight of 1,000 to 3,000. The latter ones have been found in the blood of humans after induction of physical urticaria or allergic asthma. ECF-A is capable of inducing PAF production by eosinophils (50).

Mediators with Enzymatic Properties

Two important proteases are found in human mast cells and not basophils. Tryptase (51), a tryptic protease of 140,000 daltons, is present in all human mast cells. It constitutes nearly 25% of mast cell granular protein and is released during IgE-dependent reactions. It is capable of cleaving kininogen to yield bradykinin, diminish clotting activity, and generate and degrade complement components such as C3a and a variety of other peptides. Tryptase is not inhibited by plasma antiproteases, and thus its activity may be persistent. It is present in plasma in patients experiencing anaphylaxis and in those with systemic mastocytosis. The amount and ratio of α and β subtypes have proved useful markers in these disorders (52). Its true biologic role is unclear, but it enhances smooth muscle reactivity and is a mitogen for fibroblasts, increasing their production of collagen (53,54).

A chymotryptic protease termed *chymase* is present in a subclass of human mast cells, particularly those in the skin and on serosal surfaces, and has thus been used as a marker to identify connective tissue mast cells. It cleaves angiotensinogen to yield angiotensin, activates IL-1, and is a mucus secretagogue. Other enzymes found in mast cells include carboxypeptidase and acid hydrolases.

Structural Proteoglycans

The structural proteoglycans include heparin and various chondroitin sulfates.

Heparin

Heparin is a highly sulfated proteoglycan that is contained in amounts of 5 pg/10^6 cells in human mast cell granules (55) and is released on immunologic activation. Human heparin is an anticoagulant proteoglycan and a complement inhibitor, and it modulates tryptase activity. Human heparin also may be important in angiogenesis by binding angiogenic growth factors and preventing their degradation, and it is essential for the proper packaging of proteases and histamine within the mast cell granule.

Chondroitin Sulfates

Human basophils contain about 3 to 4 pg of chondroitin 4 and 6 sulfates, which lack anticoagulant activity and bind less histamine than heparin. Human lung mast cells contain highly sulfated proteoglycans, chondroitin sulfates D and E, which accounts for the different staining characteristics of these mast cells.

Cytokines

Although cytokines traditionally have been viewed as products of monocyte-macrophages or lymphocytes, it has become clear that mast cells (56) generate many, including tumor necrosis factor-α (TNF-α), IL-1, IL-1ra, IL-3, IL-4, IL-5, IL-6, IL-9, IL-13, IL-16, and GM-CSF (57–59) in an NF-κB–dependent process (22). These molecules may be central to local regulation of mast cell growth and differentiation and may also provide new functions for mast cells in health and disease. Basophils are also a prominent source of IL-4 and IL-13 (56). The preponderance of these mast cell and basophil cytokines can be categorized as proinflammatory (IL-1, IL-6, TNF-α); possess properties important in IgE synthesis (IL-4, IL-13); stimulate eosinophil growth, longevity, localization, and activation (IL-3, IL-5, and GM-CSF); and participate in airway remodeling (IL-9).

MEDIATOR INTERACTIONS

The mediators generated and released after mast cell activation have been isolated, identified, and characterized as individual factors, whereas physiologic and pathologic events reflect their combined interactions. Given the number of mediators, the knowledge that many have yet to be purified (or even identified), and the lack of understanding of appropriate ratios of mediators generated or released *in vivo,* it is not surprising that there are no reliable data regarding these interactions in health or disease. The number and type of mast cell mediator interactions are potentially enormous, and their pathobiologic consequences are relevant to a variety of homeostatic and disease processes. The best clues to the interaction of mediators are the known physiologic and pathologic manifestations of allergic diseases. It is hoped that the valuable tool of gene knockouts in mice will elucidate critical individual and interactive roles of these molecules.

THE ROLE OF THE MAST CELL AND ITS MEDIATORS IN TISSUE

The most compelling evidence for the role of mast cells and mediators in human tissue is derived from experiments in which IgE-dependent mast cell activation in skin is caused by specific antigen (or antibody to IgE). The participation of other immunoglobulin classes and immunologically activated cells, and thus of other inflammatory pathways, is excluded in such studies by using purified IgE to sensitize nonimmune individuals passively. Activation of cutaneous mast cells by antigen results initially in a pruritic wheal-and-flare reaction that begins in minutes and persists for 1 to 2 hours, followed in 6 to 12 hours by a large, poorly demarcated, erythematous, tender, and indurated lesion (60). Histologic analysis of the initial response shows mast cell degranulation, dermal edema, and endothelial cell activation. The late reaction is characterized by edema; by infiltration of the dermis by neutrophils, eosinophils, basophils, lymphocytes, and mononuclear leukocytes; and in some instances by hemorrhage, blood vessel wall damage, and fibrin deposition of sufficient severity to warrant the diagnosis of vasculitis. Similar studies of lung tissue responses, employing passive sensitization or mast cell–deficient subjects, have only been possible in mice. In humans, a similar dual-phase reaction is experienced by allergic patients who inhale antigen, but the participation of immunoglobulins other than IgE and of activating cells other than mast cells cannot be excluded, therefore complicating assessment and prevent-

ing unambiguous assignment of any response to a particular immunologic pathway. Such challenges result in an immediate bronchospastic response followed by recovery, and, 6 to 24 hours later, by a recrudescence of asthmatic signs and symptoms (61). The mediators responsible for these pathophysiologic manifestations have not been delineated fully, but clues to their identity can be derived from knowledge of the effects of pharmacologic manipulation, by the identification of mediators in blood or tissue fluid obtained when the inflammatory response occurs, and by the known effects of isolated mediators.

Pharmacologic intervention suggests that the initial phase is mast cell dependent in both skin and lung tissues. The initial response in skin may be inhibited by antihistamines, and in the lungs by cromolyn. In both tissues, corticosteroids effectively inhibit only the late response, reflecting its inflammatory nature. Histamine, TNF-α, tryptase, LTD$_4$, PGD$_2$, IL-5, and both neutrophil and eosinophil chemotactic activity are found soon after challenge. The late response is associated with leukocyte infiltration and cytokine release, but not with a unique profile of released mediators. The exact genesis of the early and late reactions is speculative. The concerted action of the spasmogenic mediators histamine, adenosine, PGD$_2$, leukotrienes, and PAF seems sufficient to account for all of the immediate pathophysiologic (anaphylactic) responses to antigen. This concept is supported by the knowledge that the early response occurs before a significant influx of circulating leukocytes.

However, mast cell mediators or mediators from antigen-reactive T lymphocytes, epithelial cells, or macrophages may induce such changes, either directly or indirectly. In response to mediators, vascular endothelium, fibroblasts, and a variety of connective tissue and epithelial cells then could generate other inflammatory and vasoactive mediators. The late phases in lung and skin tissue are likely to represent the residue of the early response as well as the contribution of active enzymes, newly arrived plasma inflammatory cascades, various cytokines (particularly those inducing endothelial expression of adhesion molecules) (57), and the influx of activated circulating leukocytes. Of direct relevance to leukocyte recruitment are GM-CSF, IL-3, and especially IL-5, which promote eosinophil growth, differentiation, migration, adherence, and activation (62). The late inflammatory response is relevant to the progression of asthma in that patients experiencing the late responses have exacerbation of their nonspecific bronchial hyperreactivity, whereas this phenomenon does not occur after isolated early responses.

HOMEOSTATIC ROLE OF MAST CELLS

Mast cell mediators likely are important in maintaining normal tissue function and participate in the expression of innate immunity. Because mast cells are positioned near small blood vessels and at the host–environment interface, and are thus at crucial sites for regulating local nutrient delivery and for the entry of noxious materials, the potential regulatory role of mediators is obvious. They are likely to be especially important in the regulation of flow through small blood vessels, impulse generation in unmyelinated nerves, and smooth muscle and bone structural integrity and function. The ability to recruit and activate plasma proteins and cells may also provide preimmune defense against host invasion by infectious agents. Such a role is most apparent in parasitic infestation but is also likely in the case of other insults. Moreover, the recognition of mast cell heterogeneity implies that differences in mast cells relate to locally important biologic requirements.

Although the homeostatic and pathophysiologic role of mast cell mediators is understood imprecisely, the broadening understanding of their chemical nature and function provides a useful framework for addressing their role in health and disease.

REFERENCES

1. Williams CMM, Galli, SJ. The diverse potential effector and immunoregulatory roles of mast cells in allergic disease. *J Allergy Clin Immunol* 2000;105:847–859.
2. Bingham CO, Austen KF. Mast-cell responses in the development of asthma. *J Allergy Clin Immunol* 2000;105:S527–S534.
3. Bernstein JA, Lawrence ID. The mast cell: a comprehensive, updated review. *Allergy Proc* 1990;11:209.
4. Irani AA, Schechter NM, Craig SS, et al. Two types of human mast cells that have distinct neutral protease compositions. *Proc Natl Acad Sci USA* 1986;83:4464.
5. Kirshenbaum AS, Goff JP, Semerc T, et al. Demonstration that human mast cells arise from a progenitor cell population that is CD 34$^+$, cKit$^+$ and expresses aminopeptidase N (CD13). *Blood* 1999;94:2333–2342.
6. Benyon RC, Church MK, Clegg LS, et al. Dispersion and characterization of mast cells from human skin. *Int Arch Allergy Applied Immunol* 1986;79:332.
7. Fox CC, Dvorak AM, Peters SP, et al. Isolation and characterization of human intestinal mucosal mast cells. *J Immunol* 1985;135:483.
8. Mikhail GR, Miller-Milinska A. Mast cell population in human skin. *J Invest Dermatol* 1964;43:249.
9. Valent P, Bettelheim P. Cell surface structures on human basophils and mast cells. *Adv Immunol* 1992;52:333–423.
10. Thompson-Snipes L, Dhar V, Bond MW, et al. Interleukin 10: a novel stimulatory factor for mast cells and their progenitors. *J Exp Med* 1991;173:507.
11. Smith CA, Rennick DM. Characterization of a murine lymphokine distinct from interleukin-2 and interleukin-3 possessing a T-cell growth factor activity and a mast cell growth factor activity that synergizes with IL-3. *Proc Natl Acad Sci U S A* 1986;83: 1857.
12. Broide DH, Wasserman SI, Alvaro-Garcia J, et al. TGF-B selectively inhibits IL-3 dependent mast cell proliferation without affecting mast cell function or differentiation. *J Immunol* 1989;143:1591.
13. Dvorak AM. The fine structure of human basophils and mast cells. In: Holgate ST, ed. *Mast cells, mediators and disease.* London: Kluwer Academic Publishers, 1988:29.
14. Galli SJ, Austen KF. *Mast cell and basophil differentiation in health and disease.* New York: Raven Press, 1989.
15. McGlashan D, Lichtenstein LM, McKenzie-White J, et al. Upregulation of FcεRI on human basophils by IgE antibody is mediated by interaction of IgE with FcεRI. *J Allergy Clin Immunol* 1999;104:492–498.
16. Coleman JW, Holiday MR, Kimber I, et al. Regulation of mouse peritoneal mast cell secretory function by stem cell factor, IL-3, IL-4. *J Immunol* 1993;150:556.
17. Alam R, Welter JB, Forsythe PA, et al. Comparative effect of recombinant IL-1, 2, 3, 4, and 6, IFN gamma, granulocyte-macrophage colony stimulating factor, tumor necrosis factor-alpha, and histamine from basophils. *J Immunol* 1989;142:3431.
18. Lie WJ, Mue FPJ, Roos D, et al. Degranulation of human basophils by picomolar concentrations of IL-3, IL-5, or GM-CSF. *J Allergy Clin Immunol* 1998;101:683–690.
19. MacDonald SM, Lichtenstein LM, Proud D, et al. Studies of IgE dependent histamine releasing factors: heterogeneity of IgE. *J Immunol* 1987;139:506.
20. Siriganian RP. Mechanism of IgE-mediated hypersensitivity. In: Middleton E, Reed CE, Ellis EF, et al, eds. *Allergy: principles and practice.* 4th ed. St. Louis: CV Mosby, 1993.
21. Dvorak AM, Morgan ES. Ribonuclease-gold ultrastructural localization of heparin in isolated human lung mast cells stimulated to undergo anaphylactic degranulation and recovery in vitro. *Clin Exp Allergy* 1999;29:1118–1128.
22. Marquardt DL, Walker LL. Dependence of mast cell IgE-mediated cytokine production on nuclear factor-κB activity. *J Allergy Clin Immunol* 2000;105:500.

23. Kepley CL, Cambier JC, Morel PA, et al. Negative regulation of FcεRI signaling by FcγRII costimulation in human blood basophils. *J Allergy Clin Immunol* 2000;106:337–348.

24. MacGlashan DW, Lichtenstein LM. The purification of human basophils. *J Immunol* 1980;124:219.

25. Barnes P, Fitzgerald G, Brown M, et al. Nocturnal asthma and changes in circulating epinephrine, histamine, and cortisol. *N Engl J Med* 1980;303:263.

26. Black JW, Duncan WA, Durant CJ, et al. Definition and antagonism of histamine H2-receptors. *Nature* 1972;236:385.

27. Marquardt DL. Histamine. *Clin Rev Allergy* 1983;1:343.

28. West RE, Zweig A, Shih N-Y, et al. Identification of two H3-histamine receptor subtypes. *Mol Pharmacol* 1990;38:610.

29. Simons FER. Histamine and antihistamines. In: Kay AB, ed. *Allergy and allergic diseases.* Oxford, UK: Blackwell Science, 1997:421–438.

30. Naclerio R. Clinical manifestations of the release of histamine and other inflammatory mediators. *J Allergy Clin Immunol* 1999;103:S382.

31. Lin RY, Schwartz LB, Curry A, et al. Histamine and tryptase levels in patients with acute allergic reactions: an emergency department-based study. *J Allergy Clin Immunol* 2000;106:65.

32. O'Flaherty JT, Wykle RL. Biology and biochemistry of platelet-activating factor. *Clin Rev Allergy* 1983;1:353.

33. Wardlaw A, Moqbel R, Cromwell O, et al. Platelet activating factor: a potent chemotactic and chemokinetic factor for eosinophils. *J Clin Invest* 1986;78:1701.

34. Cuss FM, Dixon CM, Barnes PJ. Effects of platelet activating factor on pulmonary function and bronchial responsiveness in man. *Lancet* 1986;2:189.

35. Hardy CC, Robinson C, Tattersfield AE, et al. The bronchoconstrictor effects of inhaled prostaglandin D2 in normal and asthmatic men. *N Engl J Med* 1984;311:209.

36. Matsuoka T, Hirata M, Tanaka H, et al. Prostaglandin D2 as a mediator of allergic asthma. *Science* 2000;287:2013.

37. Kliewer SA. A prostaglandin J2 metabolite binds peroxisome proliferator-activated receptor gamma and promotes adipocyte differentiation. *Cell* 1995;88:813–819.

38. Murakami M, Bingham CO, Mastumoto R, et al. IgE-dependent activation of cytokine primed mouse cultured mast cells induces a delayed phase of prostaglandin D2 generation via prostaglandin endoperoxidase synthase 2. *J Immunol* 1995;155:4445.

39. Sanak M, Simon HU, Szezcklik A. Leukotriene C4 synthase promoter polymorphism and risk of aspirin-induced asthma. *Lancet* 1997;350:1599–1600.

40. Thivierge M, Doty J, Johnson J, et al. IL-5 upregulates cysteinyl leukotriene 1 receptor expression in HL-60 cells differentiated into eosinophils. *J Immunol* 2000;165:5221–5226.

41. Nothoeker HP, Wang Z, Zhu Y, et al. Molecular cloning and characterization of a second human cysteininyl leukotriene receptor: discovery of a subtype selective agonist. *Mol Pharmacol* 2000;58:1601–1608.

42. Sorkness CA. Leukotriene receptor antagonists in the treatment of asthma. *Pharmacotherapy* 2001;21:345–375.

43. Henderson WR Jr. The role of leukotrienes in inflammation. *Ann Intern Med* 1994;121:684.

44. Parettieri RA, Tan EM, Ciocca V, et al. Effects of LTD 4 on human airway smooth muscle cell proliferation, matrix expression, and contraction in vitro: differential sensitivity to cysteinyl leukotriene receptor antagonists. *Am J Respir Cell Mol Biol* 1998;19:453–461.

45. Marquardt DL, Gruber HE, Wasserman SI. Adenosine release from stimulated mast cells. *J Allergy Clin Immunol* 1984;73:115.

46. Gao Z, Li BS, Day YL, et al. A3 adenosine receptor activation triggers phosphorylation of protein kinase B and protects rat basophilic leukemia 2H3 mast cells from apoptosis. *Mol Pharmacol* 2001;59:76–82.

47. Feoktistov I, Polosa R, Holgate ST, et al. Adenosine A2B receptors: a novel therapeutic target in asthma? *Trends Pharmacol Sci* 1998;19:148–153.

48. Atkins PC, Norman M, Werner H, et al. Release of neutrophil chemotactic activity during immediate hypersensitivity reactions in humans. *Ann Intern Med* 1976;86:415.

49. Goetzl EJ, Austen KF. Purification and synthesis of eosinophilotactic tetrapeptides of human lung tissue: identification as eosinophil chemotactic factor of anaphylaxis (ECF-A). *Proc Natl Acad Sci USA* 1975;72:4123.

50. Lee TC, Lenihan DJ, Malone B, et al. Increased biosynthesis of platelet activating factor in activated human eosinophils. *J Biol Chem* 1994;259:5526.

51. Schwartz LB, Bradford TR, Rouse C, et al. Development of a new, more sensitive immunoassay for human tryptase: use in systemic anaphylaxis. *J Clin Immunol* 1994;14:190.

52. Kanthawatana S, Carias K, Arnaout R, et al. The potential clinical utility of serum alpha-protryptase levels. *J Allergy Clin Immunol* 1999;103:1092.

53. Ruoss SJ, Hartmann T, Caughey GH. Mast cell tryptase is a mitogen for cultured fibroblasts. *J Clin Invest* 1991;88:493.

54. Abe M, Kurosawa M, Ishikawa O, et al. Effect of mast cell-derived mediators and mast cell-related neutral proteases on human dermal fibroblast proliferation and type 1 collagen production. *J Allergy Clin Immunol* 2000;106:S78.

55. Metcalfe DD, Lewis RA, Silbert JE, et al. Isolation and characterization of heparin from human lung. *J Clin Invest* 1979;64:1537.

56. Kobayashi H, Ishizaka T, Okayama Y. Human mast cells and basophils as sources of cytokines. *Clin Exp Allergy* 2000;30:1205–1212.

57. Barata LT, Ying S, Meng O, et al. IL-4 and IL-5 positive T lymphocytes, eosinophils and mast cells in allergen induced late phase cutaneous reactions in atopic subjects. *J Allergy Clin Immunol* 1998;101:222–230.

58. Toru H, Pawanhar R, Ra C, et al. Human mast cells produce IL-13 by high affinity IgE receptor cross-linking: enhanced IL-13 production by IL-4 primed mast cells. *J Allergy Clin Immunol* 1998;102:491.

59. Wilson SJ, Shute JK, Holgate ST, et al. Localization of IL-4 but not IL-5 to human mast cell secretory granules by immunöelectron microscopy. *Clin Exp Allergy* 2000;30:493–500.

60. Dolovitch J, Hargreaves FE, Chalmers R, et al. Late cutaneous allergic responses in isolated IgE-dependent reactions. *J Allergy Clin Immunol* 1973;52:38.

61. Bentley AM, Kay AB, Durham SR. Human late asthmatic responses. In: Kay AB, ed. *Allergy and allergic diseases.* Oxford, UK: Blackwell Science, 1997:1113–1130.

62. Resnick MB, Weller PF. Mechanisms of eosinophil recruitment. *Am J Respir Cell Mol Biol* 1993;8:349.

5

Antihistamines

Jonathan A. Bernstein

Department of Internal Medicine, University of Cincinnati College of Medicine,
Cincinnati, Ohio

Histamine receptor antagonists (antihistamines) can be categorized in terms of their structure, pharmacokinetics, pharmacodynamics, and clinical utility. Second-generation, nonsedating H_1 receptor antagonists, many of which have been derived from first-generation agents, have added a new dimension to the treatment of allergic disorders. During the past several years, a new field of pharmacoepidemiology has also emerged, largely as a result of postmarketing surveillance of these newer H_1 antagonists. In fact, investigations into the adverse drug reactions associated with the second-generation agent terfenadine have served as prototypes for the design of current long-term surveillance studies monitoring the safety of drugs in a variety of clinical situations.

HISTORICAL PERSPECTIVE

Histamine, or *b*-imidazolylethylamine, was first synthesized by Windaus and Vogt in 1907 (1). The term *histamine* was adopted because of its prevalence in animal and human tissues (*hist,* relating to tissue) and its amine structure (2,3) (Fig. 5.1) Dale and Laidlaw (4), in 1910, were the first to recognize histamine's role in anaphylaxis when they observed a dramatic bronchospastic and vasodilatory effect in animals injected intravenously with this compound. Subsequently, histamine was found to be synthesized from L-histidine by L-histidine decarboxylase and metabolized by histamine *N*-methyltransferase to form *N*-methylhistadine

or by diamine oxidase to form imidazole acetic acid (5). However, only the *N*-methyltransferase pathway is active in the central nervous system (CNS). Histamine is stored in the cytoplasm of mast cells and basophils, attached to anionic carboxylate and sulfate groups on secretory granules (5). Histamine is released from mast cell and basophil secretory granules after aggregation of high-affinity immunoglobulin E (IgE) receptors. IgE receptors are coupled to G proteins, which, when activated, lead to a sequence of chemical reactions with the end result being histamine release. However, histamine can be released spontaneously by activation of mast cells and basophils by histamine-releasing factors, which include chemokines (RANTES, MCP-1, and MIP-1a) and several cytokines (interleukin-1 [IL-1], IL-3, IL-5, IL-6, IL-7) (5,6).

Originally, histamine's classic physiologic actions of bronchoconstriction and vasodilation were believed responsible for the symptoms of allergic diseases through its action on a single type of histamine receptor. Ash and Schild, in 1966, were the first to recognize that histamine-mediated reactions occurred through more than one receptor based on observations that histamine had an array of actions, including contraction of guinea pig ileal smooth muscle, inhibition of rat uterine contractions, and suppression of gastric acid secretion (7). This speculation was confirmed by Black and co-workers in 1972, who used the experimental histamine antagonists mepyramine and burimamide to block

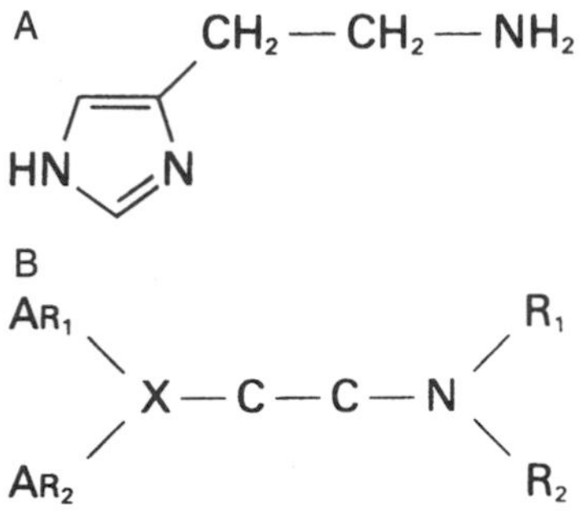

A

$CH_2 - CH_2 - NH_2$

HN — N

B

AR_1 R_1

$X - C - C - N$

AR_2 R_2

FIG. 5.1. Structure of histamine **(A)** and basic structure of H_1 receptor antagonists **(B)**.

histamine-induced reactions in animals (8). They observed that each of these antagonists inhibited different physiologic responses, suggesting that there were at least two histamine receptors, now referred to as H_1 and H_2 (8). Arrang and colleagues discovered a third histamine receptor (H_3) with unique physiologic properties, raising the possibility that additional, yet unrecognized, histamine receptors exist (9). Table 5.1 summarizes the pharmacodynamic effects after activation of the known histamine receptors and their common agonists and antagonists (3,9–12).

TABLE 5.1. *Effect of histamine on human histamine receptors*

	H_1 receptor	H_2 receptor	H_3 receptor
Location	Blood vessels, airway and gastrointestinal tract smooth muscle, heart, central nervous system	Gastric mucosa, uterus, heart, central nervous system	Neurons in central nervous system, gastrointestinal tract
Signal transduction	IP_3, DG	Activates adenylate cyclase and increases cAMP	Not known, but G proteins are involved.
Agonists	2-Methylhistamine 2-Pyridylethylamine	5-Methylhistamine (dimaprit impromidine)	(R)-a-methylhistamine SKF91606
Antagonists	Diphenhydramine Loratadine Cetirizine Fexofenadine	Cimetidine Ranitidine Famotidine Nizatidine	Thioperamide Clobenpropit Iodoproxyfan Impentamine
Function	Increases pruritus, pain, vascular permeability, hypotension, flushing, headache, and heart rate. Also causes bronchial smooth muscle constriction and activation of airway vagal afferent nerves. Increases stimulation of cough receptors, decreases atrioventricular node conduction, increases prostaglandin generation, and increases inflammatory cell recruitment and release of bioactive mediators.	Increases gastric acid secretion, hypotension, flushing, headache, heart rate and bronchial smooth muscle relaxation. Increases airway mucus production, atrial chronotropic and ventricular inotropic activity, and glycoprotein secretion. Stimulates suppressor T cells, decreases neutrophil and basophil chemotaxis and enzyme release, decreases cytotoxicity and proliferation of lymphocytes, and inhibits natural killer cell function.	Prevents excessive bronchoconstriction and inhibits gastric acid secretion.
CNS function	Sleep and wakefulness, food intake, thermal regulation	Neuroendocrine	Inhibits histamine synthesis and neurotransmitter release (histamine, dopamine, serotonin, noradrenaline, and acetylcholine)

IP_3, inositol trisphosphate; DG, diacylglycerol; cAMP, cyclic adenosine monophosphate.
From Simons FE, Antihistamines. In: Middleton E, Reed CE, Ellis EF, et al, eds. *Allergy principles and practice.* St. Louis: CV Mosby; 1998, with permission.

Characterizing histamine receptors has been essential in discovering histamine's physiologic actions on target cells, which include increased mucus secretion, increased nitrous oxide formation, endothelial cell contraction leading to increased vascular permeability, gastric acid secretion, bronchial smooth muscle contraction (H_1), and suppressor T-cell stimulation.

The first histamine antagonist was serendipitously discovered in 1937 by Bovet and Staub who found that a drug originally being studied for its adrenergic antagonistic properties in guinea pigs also had potent antihistaminic activity (3). By 1942, safe and effective antihistamines developed for human use became available. Many of these agents, such as pyrilamine maleate, tripelennamine, and diphenhydramine, are still widely prescribed today (3).

H_2 antagonists were first synthesized in 1969 for the purpose of developing a drug capable of inhibiting gastric acid secretion (13). These agents have a closer structural resemblance to histamine because most are simple modifications of the histamine molecule itself (14,15). However, histamine's affinity for H_1 receptors is 10-fold greater than for H_2 receptors (14,15).

H_1 RECEPTOR HISTAMINE ANTAGONISTS

First-generation Agents

Structure

The chemical structure of H_1 antagonists differs substantially from that of histamine (Fig. 5.1). Histamine is composed of a single imidazole heterocyclic ring linked to an ethylamine group, whereas H_1 antagonists consist of one or two heterocyclic or aromatic rings joined to a "linkage atom" (nitrogen, oxygen, or carbon) (3) (Table 5.2) The linkage atom is important in structurally differentiating these groups of agents, whereas the number of alkyl substitutions and heterocyclic or aromatic rings determines their lipophilic nature. The ethylenediamines, phenothiazines, piperazines, and piperidines all contain nitrogen as their linkage atom, whereas

TABLE 5.2. *Classification of common H_1 receptor (First-Generation) antagonists*

Structural class/linkage atom	Generic name	Trade name
Ethanolamines/"O" (oxygen)	Diphenhydramine hydrochloride	Benadryl
	Dimenhydrinate	Dramamine
	Clemastine fumarate	Tavist
Alkylamines/"C" (carbon)	Chlorpheniramine maleate	Chlortrimeton, Teldrin
	Brompheniramine maleate	Dimetane
	Dexchlorpheniramine maleate	Polaramine
	Dexbrompheniramine maleate	Drixoral[a]
	Triprolidine HCl	Actifed[a]
	Chlorpheniramine tannate; pyrilamine tannate	Rynatan[b]
	Pheniramine maleate; pyrilamine maleate	Triaminic TR+
Ethylenediamines/"N" (nitrogen)	Tripelenamine HCl	Pyribenzamine HCl (PBZ)
	Tripelenamine citrate	
	Pyrilamine maleate	Allertoc
	Antazoline phosphate	Vasocon-A
Piperazines/"N" (nitrogen)	Hydroxyzine HCl	Atarax; Vistaril
	Meclizine HCl	Antivert; Bonine
Phenothiazines/"N" (nitrogen)	Promethazine HCl	Phenergan
	Trimeprazine tartrate	Temaril
Piperidines/"N" (nitrogen)	Cyproheptadine HCl	Periactin
	Azatadine maleate	Optimine; Trinalin[a]

[a]With decongestant.
[b]Combination ethylenediamine/alkylamine compound.
From Simons FER. H_1 receptor antagonists: chemical pharmacology and therapeutics. *J Allergy Clin Immunol* 1989;84:845, with permission.

the ethanolamines contain oxygen and the alkylamines carbon as their linkage atoms (3,16).

Pharmacokinetics

Accurate pharmacokinetic data on first-generation antihistamines is now available in children and adults because of sensitive detection techniques, such as gas-liquid chromatography, mass spectrometry, and high-performance liquid chromatography (3,10,16). Generally, these compounds are rapidly absorbed orally or intravenously, resulting in peak serum concentrations within 2 to 3 hours and symptomatic relief within 30 minutes. They have large volumes of distribution, have slow clearance rates, and are metabolized primarily by hydroxylation in the hepatic cytochrome P-450 system. Most of the parent drug is excreted as inactive metabolites in the urine within 24 hours of dosing. As a rule, serum half-lives ($t_{1/2}$) are longer in adults than in children. The lipophilic nature of these antihistamines allows them to cross the placenta and the blood–brain barrier. This access into the CNS is responsible for most of the side effects experienced by patients. These agents are also excreted in breast milk (3,10,16). Table 5.3 summarizes pharmacokinetic data for the most commonly used first-generation agents (3,17–21).

Pharmacodynamics

The first-generation H_1 antagonists compete with histamine for binding to histamine receptors. This competitive inhibition is reversible and, therefore, highly dependent on free drug plasma concentrations. As these agents are metabolized and excreted into the urine as inactive metabolites, the histamine receptors become desaturated, allowing surrounding histamine to bind. This mechanism emphasizes the need to instruct patients in using these agents on a regular basis to achieve a maximal therapeutic benefit (3,22). Interestingly, smaller doses of H_1 antagonists have been found to inhibit mast cell activation *in vitro*, whereas larger doses cause mast cell activation and histamine release (23).

TABLE 5.3. *Pharmacokinetics of H_1 receptor antagonists in healthy young adults*

H_1 receptor antagonists (metabolite)	$t_{max}(hr)$[a]	$t_{1/2}(hr)$[b]
First generation		
Chlorpheniramine	2.8 ± 0.8	27.9 ± 8.7
Clemastine	4.8 ± 1.3	21.3 ± 11.6
Diphenhydramine	1.7 ± 1.0	9.2 ± 2.5
Hydroxyzine	2.1 ± 0.4	20.0 ± 4.1
Second generation		
Acrivastine	1.4 ± 0.4	1.7 ± 0.2
Astemizole (desmethylastemizole)[c]	0.5 ± 0.2 to (0.7 ± 0.3)	1.1 d (9.5 d)
Azelastine (desmethylazelastine)	5.3 ± 1.6 (20.5)	22 ± 4 (54 ± 15)
Cetirizine	1.0 ± 0.5	7.4 ± 1.6
Ebastine (carebastine)[d]	(4–6)	(13.8–15.3)
Fexofenadine	1–3	14.4
Ketotifen[e]	3.6 ± 1.6	18.3 ± 6.7
Levocabastine[e]	1–2	35–40
Loratadine (descarboethoxyloratadine)	1.0 ± 0.3 (1.5 ± 0.7)	11.0 ± 9.4 (17.3 ± 6.9)
Mizolastine[d]	0.8	8.9″2.5
Terfenadine (terfenadine carboxylic acid)[c]	0.78–1.1 (3)	16–23 (17)

Results are expressed as mean ± standard deviation.
[a]Time from oral intake to peak plasma concentration.
[b]Terminal elimination half-life.
[c]No longer sold in the United States.
[d]Currently not available in the United States.
[e]Only available in eyedrop form in the United States.
From Simons FE. Antahistamines. In: Middleton E, Reed CE, Ellis EF, et al, eds. *Allergy principles and practice.* St. Louis: CV Mosby, 1998, with permission.

TABLE 5.4. *Chemical derivations of second-generation H_1 receptor antagonists and dual-action antihistamines*

Antihistamines	Chemical family derivation
Terfenadine (Seldane)[a]	Butyrophenone related to haloperidol
Astemizole (Hismanal)[a]	Aminopiperidinyl-benzimidazole
Loratadine (Claritin)	Piperidine derivative of azatadine
Fexofenadine (Allegra)	Acid metabolite of terfenadine
Cetirizine (Zyrtec)	Cyclizine derivative of hydroxyzine
Acrivastine	Acrylic acid derivative of tripolidine
Mequitazine	Derivative of phenothiazine
Temelastine (SKF 93944)	Derivative of pyrilamine
Levocabastine (R 50547)	Stereoisomer of a cyclohexylpiperdine
Azelastine[b]	Phthalazinone derivative
Ketotifen[b]	Benzocycloheptathiophene
Oxatamide[b]	Related to cinnarizine
Norastemizole	Metabolite of astemizole
Levocetirizine	Isomer of cetirizine
Desloratadine	Metabolite of loratadine

[a]No longer available for clinical use in the United States.
[b]Dual-action antihistamines.

Pharmacy

Table 5.4 summarizes the child and adult dosing schedules of the three most commonly prescribed first-generation antihistamines (10,17,24). Before the availability of pharmacokinetic data, these agents were believed to have short half-lives, which necessitated frequent dosing intervals in order to be effective (22). Because chlorpheniramine, brompheniramine, and hydroxyzine have half-lives of longer than 20 hours in adults, it may be feasible to administer these agents only once or twice a day to achieve similar efficacy (18,19,21). The availability of sustained-release preparations of shorter half-life agents has also allowed less frequent dosing, thereby improving patient compliance and minimizing side effects. Whether treatment with sustained-released formulations of conventional agents with shorter half-lives offers any advantages over conventional agents with longer half-lives when dosed similarly remains unclear (25–27).

Second-generation Agents

Structure

Because the new nonsedating antihistamines do not fit into one of the existing structural classification categories of first-generation antagonists, they have been placed into a separate category referred to as *second-generation antagonists.* Their structural and pharmacokinetic profiles are responsible for their milder side effects and better tolerance among patients (3,28,29). Table 5.5 lists the chemical derivations of these agents in addition to other similar compounds undergoing investigation, and Fig. 5.2 illustrates their structures in comparison to first-generation agents (3,10,30,31).

The two available agents in the United States are fexofenadine, the acid metabolite of terfenadine, and loratadine. Cetirizine is considered a low-sedating antihistamine. Terfenadine and astemizole are no longer available in the United States because of safety concerns. Both of these agents were associated with serious interactions with drugs that were also metabolized by the liver cytochrome P-450 enzyme 3A4, such as erythromycin and ketoconazole. This led to accumulation of the parent compound, which caused cardiac side effects such as torsades de pointes. Although this was a rare occurrence and dose dependent, the advent of newer antihistamine drug metabolites that were not dependent on cytochrome oxidase metabolism made them expendable.

Pharmacokinetics

The pharmacokinetic data available for second-generation agents are summarized in comparison

TABLE 5.5. *Formulations and dosages of representative H_1 receptor antagonists*

H_1 receptor antagonist	Formulation	Recommended dose
First generation		
Chlorpheniramine maleate (Chlor-Trimeton)	*Tablets:* 4 mg, 8 mg, 12 mg	*Adult:* 8–12 mg b.i.d.
	Syrup: 2.5 mg/5 mL	*Child:* 0.35 mg/kg/24 hr
	Parenteral solution: 10 mg/mL	
Hydroxyzine hydrochloride (Atarax)	*Capsules:* 10 mg, 25 mg, 50 mg	*Adult:* 25–50 mg b.i.d. (or q.d. at bedtime)
	Syrup: 10 mg/5 mL	*Child:* 2 mg/kg/24 hr
Diphenhydramine hydrochloride (Benadryl)	*Capsules:* 25 mg, 50 mg	*Adult:* 25–50 mg t.i.d.
	Elixir: 12.5 mg/5 mL	
	Syrup: 6.25 mg/5 mL	*Child:* 5 mg/kg/24 hr
	Parenteral solution: 50 mg/mL	
Second generation		
Fexofenadine (Allegra)[a]	*Tablets:* 30, 60, 180 mg	*Adult:* 60 mg b.i.d. or 180 mg/d
		Child: 7–12 yr, 30 mg b.i.d.
Loratadine (Claritin)[a]	*Tablets and reditabs:* 10 mg PO or sublingual	*Adult:* 10 mg/d
	Syrup: 1 mg/mL	*Child:* (>3 yr, <30 kg = 5 mg PO q.d.; >3 yr, >30 kg = 10 mg PO q.d.)
Cetirizine hydrochloride (Zyrtec)[a]	*Tablets:* 5, 10 mg	*Adults:* 5–10 mg/d
	Syrup: 5 mg/mL	
Acrivastine (Semprex)[a]	*Tablets:* 8 mg	*Adult:* 8 mg t.i.d.
Ketotifen fumarate (Zaditor)	*Eyedrops:* 0.025%	*Allergic conjunctivitis:* 1 drop in each eye b.i.d.
Azelastine hydrochloride (Astelin)	0.1% Nasal solution 0.137-mg Spray	*Topical:* 2 sprays/nostril q.d. to b.i.d.
(Optivar)	*Eyedrops:* 0.03%	*Topical:* 1–2 drops each eye q.d. to b.i.d.
Levocabastine hydrochloride (Livostin)	*Eyedrops:* 0.05%	*Topical:* 1 drop in each eye b.i.d. to q.i.d.
Olopatadine hydrochloride (Patanol)	*Eyedrops:* 0.1%	*Topical:* 1–2 drops each eye b.i.d.

[a]Formulation available also with decongestant.
From Simons FER, Simons KJ. The pharmacology and use of H_1-receptor-antagonist drugs. *N Engl J Med* 1994;330:1663, with permission.

to first-generation agents in Table 5.3 (3,17, 29,32–37). Fexofenadine, loratadine, and cetirizine are well absorbed from the gastrointestinal tract, with peak serum concentrations occurring within 1 to 2 hours after oral administration (3,17,32,33). Data in humans on volumes of distribution for these agents is not available (3,17).

Loratadine is metabolized by the cytochrome P-450 CYP3A4 enzyme to form descarbe-

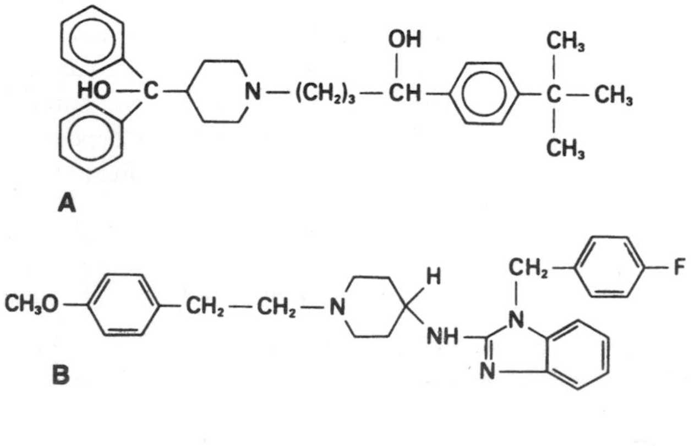

FIG. 5.2. Structures of the currently available second-generation H_1 receptor antagonists.

thoxyloratadine. However, if the CYP3A4 enzyme is inhibited, loratadine can be alternatively metabolized by the CYP2D6 enzyme, thereby preventing increased levels of the unmetabolized parent compound (38).

Astemizole undergoes oxidative dealkylation, aromatic hydroxylation, and glucuronidation through the P-450–CYP3A4 pathway to form several metabolites (39). The major active metabolite of astemizole is N-desmethylastemizole, which has a half-life of 9.5 days. Terfenadine is exclusively metabolized by oxidation and oxidative N-dealkylation through the P-450–CYP3A4 pathway to form an active acid metabolite (fexofenadine) and an inactive metabolite (MDL 4829) (3).

Astemizole is unique because it has a slower elimination half-life of 18 to 20 days, compared with terfenadine, which has a half-life of 4.5 hours, although terfenadine's antihistaminic effect lasts longer than its measured half-life (39,40). Even though the half-life of terfenadine in children is only 2 hours, it is equally effective pharmacodynamically as in adults (41). Cetirizine and fexofenadine are not extensively metabolized in the cytochrome P-450 system and are therefore less likely to compete for elimination with other medications metabolized by the same cytochrome P-450 enzyme systems. More than half of cetirizine is eliminated unchanged in the urine. Its elimination can be impaired in patients with hepatic and renal insufficiency. Most of fexofenadine is eliminated in the urine and feces unchanged. Its elimination can be also impaired in patients with renal insufficiency (3,32,40). Most (≥60%) of astemizole and terfenadine's metabolites are eliminated in the feces and bile (3,32,39).

Our understanding of drug metabolism was greatly enhanced in 1990 when the U.S. Food and Drug Administration became aware of numerous reports associating terfenadine with malignant cardiac arrhythmias such as torsades de pointes (42). By July 1992, 44 reports of adverse cardiovascular events had been reported, 9 resulting in death, 3 of which occurred after an overdose of terfenadine (42). Studies delving into this problem found that terfenadine blocked the delayed rectifier current (Ik), which prolonged normal cardiac repolarization and was manifested as an increased QTc interval on electrocardiograms (42). It was later reported that both astemizole and its active metabolite, desmethylastemizole, also inhibited the Ik, leading to QTc prolongation. Retrospective analysis of case reports citing terfenadine-induced cardiovascular events has been helpful in defining risk factors in patients prone to these cardiac side effects (42). These risk factors include drug overdose (i.e., most events and fatalities occurred at dosages 6 to 60 times the recommended dose), concomitant use of drugs that inhibit CYP3A4 (e.g., macrolide antibiotics, excluding azithromycin, and oral antifungal agents), hepatic dysfunction, alcohol abuse, electrolyte abnormalities (e.g., hypomagnesemia and hypokalemia), grapefruit juice, and several preexisting cardiovascular diseases (42). Loratadine has not been demonstrated to induce these cardiovascular side effects most likely because it is metabolized by two isoenzymes (CYP2D6 and CYP3A4) (42,43). Therefore, loratadine can be safely taken with macrolide antibiotics (e.g., erythromycin) and oral antifungal agents (e.g., ketoconazole) (42). It should be emphasized that terfenadine and astemizole were very safe and effective drugs that were able to be used in most clinical circumstances. Cetirizine and fexofenadine, the acid metabolite of terfenadine, do not affect the Ik or cause QTc prolongation.

Pharmacodynamics

In contrast to first-generation agents, second-generation agents do not operate by simple competitive inhibition. Instead, these agents bind to and dissociate from H_1 receptors slowly in a noncompetitive fashion. They are not displaced from H_1 receptors in the presence of high histamine concentrations (29,42). However, the second-generation antagonists are potent suppressors of the wheal-and-flare responses, and this feature has been established as a useful method for comparing the clinical potencies of the different agents available (38,44). Their lipophobic properties prevent them from crossing the blood–brain barrier; thus, their activity on H_1 receptors is restricted to the peripheral nervous system (30,45). They have very little affinity for non-H_1 receptors (3).

Pharmacy

Second-generation antihistamines are available only as oral formulations. They all have convenient once- or twice-daily dosing (10,17) (Table 5.4). Studies have reported that a single dose of terfenadine (120 mg) or fexofenadine (180 mg) is equally effective as 60 mg given twice a day in improving allergic rhinitis symptom scores and suppressing histamine-induced wheal-and-flare responses (46,47). Astemizole and loratadine should be injected on an empty stomach to avoid problems with absorption. All three agents have comparable antihistaminic potency to each another and to first-generation antihistamines.

DUAL-ACTION ANTIHISTAMINES

A number of agents currently not available for clinical use in the United States have been discovered to have some clinical effects in addition to their antihistaminic properties. The derivation of these compounds is summarized in Table 5.5 (3,30,31). Although many of their mechanisms of action are unknown, they have been hypothesized to act on mast cells and basophils by preventing calcium influx or intracellular calcium release, which interferes with activation and release of potent bioactive mediators (48–51). Azelastine has been demonstrated to inhibit superoxide generation by eosinophils and neutrophils, which may represent one of its important antiinflammatory mechanisms (52). These drugs can bind to H_1 receptors in a competitive and noncompetitive fashion (3,53,54). In addition to their calcium antagonistic activity, they have variable amounts of antiserotonin, anticholinergic, and antileukotriene activities (55–60).

Pharmacokinetic information on these agents is summarized in Table 5.3 (17). Cetirizine, azelastine, and ebastine, the latter of which is currently under development, may have modest antiasthma effects that are not mediated through H_1 receptors, including inhibition of eosinophil

chemotaxis, adherence to endothelial cells, and recruitment into the airways after allergen challenge (3,61,62).

OTHER AGENTS WITH ANTIHISTAMINE PROPERTIES

Tricyclic antidepressants, originally synthesized for their antihistaminic properties in the 1950s, were never fully developed as antihistamines once it was recognized that they have impressive antidepressant effects (63). Because doxepin has a very high H_1 receptor affinity, it has become an acceptable alternative agent for the treatment of chronic idiopathic urticaria (64). Interestingly, the observation that the butyrophenone antipsychotic, haloperidol, also has antihistaminic properties eventually led to the development of the derivative, terfenadine (40).

CLINICAL USE OF ANTIHISTAMINES

The ideal H_1 receptor antagonist should provide complete and rapid relief of allergic symptoms, have a moderate duration of action, and be devoid of adverse effects. Unfortunately, this type of agent does not exist (65). In general, first- and second-generation agents have fairly comparable antihistaminic effects in relieving common allergic symptoms, but they all have poor decongestant capabilities (22,66–70). H_1 antagonists have proved useful in the treatment of allergic rhinitis, allergic conjunctivitis, atopic dermatitis, urticaria, asthma, and anaphylaxis (3,10,17). The treatment of these disorders is discussed in different sections of this book.

Numerous studies have compared the antihistaminic efficacy of second-generation antagonists with that of first-generation antagonists in the treatment of allergic rhinitis. Results have uniformly shown these agents to be more effective than placebo, but just as effective as first-generation agents, such as chlorpheniramine, using comparable dosing schedules (66,71–76). Studies comparing second-generation agents to one another have found no dramatic differences in their clinical effects (77–83).

Studies have reported that a topical eye preparation of the potent H_1 antagonist, levocabastine, available in the United States as Livostin, is very effective for the treatment of allergic conjunctivitis (84). Subsequently, many novel topical antihistamine and antiinflammatory agents have become available in the United States for the treatment of this annoying and often debilitating disorder (3). Hydroxyzine and diphenhydramine are still considered by most clinicians to be the most effective agents in the treatment of allergic skin disorders because of their greater antipruritic and sedative effects (21,44,85). One exception is cold-induced urticaria, for which cyproheptadine is the treatment of choice (86). All of the second-generation agents have been found to be effective for the treatment of patients with chronic idiopathic urticaria (3,87,88).

A position paper from the American Academy of Allergy, Asthma and Immunology addressing the use of antihistamines in patients with asthma has served to clarify the controversy surrounding their use in patients with this disease (89). Previously, it had been believed that the anticholinergic properties (i.e., dryness of the airways) of these antagonists could contribute to asthma exacerbations (90). It is now known that antihistamines, including some of the dual-action compounds, may actually serve a beneficial role in the treatment of asthma because of their bronchodilator effect (90–94). Although these agents are not considered first-line therapy for asthma, they are certainly not contraindicated in asthma patients who require them for concomitant allergic problems (89). The *Physician's Desk Reference* has subsequently modified warnings stating they should be used cautiously in patients with concomitant asthma (24).

Histamine is increased during the early and late airway response after specific allergen provocation and during spontaneous asthma exacerbations. Histamine can exert many of the physiologic sequelae leading to asthma, including cough, by direct stimulation of the sensory nerves, smooth muscle constriction, mucous hypersecretion, increased permeability of the pulmonary epithelium, vasodilation, and extravasation of fluid at the postcapillary venule level (3). Many studies have shown that antihistamines are bronchoprotective depending on the stimulus. For example, antihistamines attenuate bronchospasm induced by adenosine by 80% but have little or no effect against methacholine, leukotriene agonists, or neurokinin A (3,61,62). Several current studies have demonstrated the additive effects of antihistamines and antileukotriene agents in both allergic rhinitis and asthma.

Antihistamines serve as important adjuncts in the management of anaphylaxis but should never replace the first-line therapy, which by general consensus is epinephrine (10). Antihistamines are commonly used to treat atopic dermatitis but have limited clinical utility. The sedating first-generation antihistamines, such as diphenhydramine and hydroxyzine, are often more effective than nonsedating agents for controlling pruritus because they allow the patient to sleep.

Antihistamines should be used cautiously during pregnancy to avoid the risk for teratogenicity (10). Long-term clinical experience using antihistamines during pregnancy has shown that tripelennamine, chlorpheniramine, and diphenhydramine cause no greater risk for birth defects than experienced by the normal population. Chlorpheniramine, diphenhydramine, loratadine, and cetirizine are all classified as Pregnancy Category B, indicating that no birth defects have been observed in animal models. Antihistamines are excreted in breast milk and therefore infants of nursing mothers who were taking first-generation antihistamines have been reported to experience drowsiness and irritability. The newer antihistamines, such as loratadine, cetirizine, and fexofenadine, have not been reported to cause symptoms in babies being breast-fed by mothers taking these medications.

Antihistamines are also useful in treating nonallergic disorders, such as nausea, motion sickness, vertigo, extrapyramidal symptoms, anxiety, and insomnia (3). Studies evaluating these agents in the treatment of children with otitis media and upper respiratory infections have found they offer no significant benefit when used as solo agents (95–97). However, children with recurrent otitis media and a strong family history of allergies should be evaluated by an allergist to identify potential environmental triggers. Treatment includes a combination of antihistamines, decongestants, and topical intranasal corticosteroids, cromolyn sodium, or azelastine to reduce inflammation and secretions, which could be contributing to these recurrent infections.

The use of second-generation over first-generation antagonists as first-line agents has previously been considered premature by many experts. If a first-generation agent is taken on a regular basis at bedtime, its sedative side effects are often well tolerated by many patients. Of equal importance is their substantially lower cost. However, because a large segment of patients do not tolerate these agents, they require treatment with second-generation nonsedating agents. These agents have been well documented to cause less impairment of cognitive and psychomotor skills, such as learning, reaction times, driving, memory, tracking, perception, recognition, and processing (3,42). Impairment of these functions increases indirect costs associated with the treatment of allergic rhinitis. Indirect costs include missed days from work or school and decreased concentration and performance while at work, resulting in overall decreased productivity (3,42). The Joint Task Force on Practice Parameters for the diagnosis and management of rhinitis has recently recommended that second-generation, nonsedating antihistamines should be first-line treatment of perennial and seasonal allergic rhinitis to avoid potential CNS side effects (98). However, if individuals have nonallergic rhinitis with or without an allergic component manifested as severe postnasal drainage, it may be necessary to use first-generation antihistamines with or without decongestants to take advantage of their anticholinergic drying effects. In these situations, it is best to dose the sedating antihistamine at bedtime because the sedative carryover effect the following morning of these agents does not usually significantly impair cognitive performance.

In general, it is important to educate the patient about the advantages and disadvantages of sedating and nonsedating antihistamines in the management of specific allergic diseases. Use of either or both agents should be appropriately tailored to the patient's individual needs and tolerance. Some patients become drowsy with even 2 mg of chlorpheniramine, so that second-generation antihistamines should be used instead.

ADVERSE EFFECTS OF H_1 RECEPTOR ANTAGONISTS

The numerous side effects of first-generation antihistamines have been attributed to the ability of these drugs to cross the blood–brain barrier. Side effects vary in severity among the structural subclasses. For instance, the ethylenediamines (PBZ) have more pronounced gastrointestinal side effects, whereas the ethanolamines (Benadryl) have increased antimuscarinic activity and cause a greater degree of sedation in patients. The alkylamines (Chlor-Trimeton) have milder CNS side effects and are generally the best tolerated among the first-generation agents (99).

Specific side effects of first-generation agents include impaired cognition, slowed reaction times, decreased alertness, confusion, dizziness, tinnitus, anorexia, nausea, vomiting, epigastric distress, diarrhea, and constipation. Associated anticholinergic side effects include dry mouth, blurred vision, and urinary retention (99). First-generation agents also potentiate the effects of benzodiazepines and alcohol (10,99). Cyproheptadine, a piperidine, has the unique effect of causing weight gain in some patients (16).

Intentional and accidental overdose, although uncommon, has been reported with these drugs (10,14). Adults usually manifest symptoms of CNS depression, whereas children may exhibit an excitatory response manifested as hyperactivity, irritability, insomnia, visual hallucinations, and seizures. Even with normal doses, it is not unusual for children to experience a paradoxic excitatory reaction. Malignant cardiac arrhythmias have been known to occur with overdoses, emphasizing the need to act expeditiously to counteract the toxic effect of these agents (10,14,99). Caution should be exercised using antihistamines in elderly patients or in those with liver dysfunction because of these patients' slower clearance rates and increased susceptibility to overdose (10,14,100). Because these agents are secreted in breast milk, caution should be exercised using these agents in lactating women to avoid adverse effects in the newborn (99).

The second-generation agents have substantially fewer associated side effects. Sedation and the side effects associated with first-generation agents have been noted to occur, but to no greater extent than with placebo (10,14,101). Astemizole, like cyproheptadine, was associated with increased appetite and weight gain (10). As discussed earlier, terfenadine and astemizole were associated with rare episodes of torsades de pointes leading to cardiac arrest and are no longer available in the United States (10,17,38,102). Loratadine and fexofenadine have similar side effect profiles and have not been found to cause cardiotoxicity (3). Cetirizine is considered a low sedating antihistamine but is generally well tolerated by most patients.

TOLERANCE

Tolerance to antihistamines is a common concern of patients taking these agents chronically. This phenomenon has been speculated to occur because of autoinduction of hepatic metabolism, resulting in an accelerated clearance rate of the antihistamine (103). However, studies have failed to confirm this hypothesis, and most reports of tolerance to antihistamines are now believed to be secondary to patient noncompliance because of intolerable drug side effects or breakthrough symptoms due to severity of disease (104–107). Short-term studies evaluating tolerance to second-generation agents have found no change in their therapeutic efficacy after 6 to 8 weeks of regular use (108,109). Studies up to 12 weeks found no evidence that second-generation agents cause autoinduction of hepatic metabolism leading to rapid excretion rates and drug tolerance (42). The clinical efficacy of these agents in the skin and treatment of allergic rhinitis does not decrease with chronic use.

SYMPATHOMIMETICS

Many of the first-generation antihistamines, and now the second-generation agents, have been formulated in combination with a decongestant. The decongestants used in most preparations today predominantly include phenylpropanolamine hydrochloride, phenylephrine hydrochloride, and pseudoephedrine hydrochloride. These agents have saturated benzene rings without 3- or 4-hydroxyl groups, which is the reason for their weak α-adrenergic effect, improved oral absorption, and duration of action. Compared with other decongestants, these agents have less of an effect on blood pressure and are less apt to cause CNS excitation manifested as insomnia or agitation (110).

H$_2$ RECEPTOR ANTAGONISTS

H$_2$ receptor antagonists are weak bases with water-soluble hydrochloride salts and tend to be less lipophilic than H$_1$ antagonists (3). The early agents, which were developed for their gastric acid inhibitory properties, were either not strong enough for clinical use or hazardous because of serious associated side effects (e.g., neutropenia, bone marrow suppression) (111,112). Cimetidine (Tagamet) was introduced to the United States in 1982 and has been proved safe and effective in the treatment of peptic ulcer disease (15). Cimetidine and oxmetidine resemble the earliest agents structurally because they have an imidazole ring similar to histamine's structure. The newer agents vary structurally by having different internal ring components. For example, ranitidine (Zantac) has a furan ring, whereas famotidine (Pepcid) and nizatidine (Axid) are composed of thiozole rings (15). H$_2$ antagonists act primarily by competitive inhibition of the H$_2$ receptors, with the exception of famotidine, which works noncompetitively (15). The four available H$_2$ antagonists all have potent H$_2$ antagonistic properties, varying mainly in their pharmacokinetics, and adverse effects such as drug interactions. Several of these H$_2$ antagonists are now available over the counter (3,15).

Numerous studies have been undertaken to examine the clinical utility of H$_2$ antagonists in allergic and immunologic diseases. Although several studies report that these agents have promising immunologic changes *in vitro*, these findings have not been substantiated clinically (3,22,113–117). Generally, H$_2$ antagonists have limited or no utility in treating allergen-induced and histamine-mediated diseases in humans (118–121). One notable exception to this rule may be their use in combination with H_1 antagonists in the treatment of chronic idiopathic urticaria (122). The studies evaluating the clinical efficacy of H_2 antagonists in allergic and immunologic disorders are extensively reviewed elsewhere (3,117).

H_3 RECEPTOR ANTAGONISTS

H_3 receptors were first suspected by Arrang and colleagues in 1983 when they found histamine to inhibit, by negative feedback, its own synthesis and release in the brain (3,9). These actions by histamine could not be suppressed by H_1 or H_2 antagonists, leading researchers to postulate the existence of a third class of histamine receptors. Subsequent studies have been directed toward finding a selective H_3 antagonist. Two such agents have been synthesized: (R) a-methylhistamine (a-MeHA), a chiral agonist of histamine, and thioperamide, a derivative of imidazolylpiperidine. They both have demonstrated H_3 receptor selectivity but remain strictly for experimental use (9).

CONCLUSIONS

The discovery of H_1 receptor antagonists has proved to be a significant breakthrough in the treatment of allergic diseases. Chemical modifications of these early agents have yielded the second-generation antihistamines, which are of equal antagonistic efficacy but have fewer side effects because of their lipophobic structures. Newer nonsedating antihistamines, which are metabolites or isomers of existing agents, are now under development. H_2 receptor antagonists have been found extremely useful in the treatment of peptic ulcer disease. However, they have been disappointing in the treatment of allergic and immunologic disorders in humans. Newer selective nonsedating H_1 antagonists and dual-action antihistamines, because of their lower side-effect profiles, have provided therapeutic advantages over first-generation agents for long-term management of allergic rhinitis.

Prescription of H_1 antagonists should follow a practical, stepwise approach. Because there are virtually dozens of antihistamine preparations available with or without decongestants, it is recommended that physicians become familiar with all aspects of a few agents from each structural class. Appropriate selection of one of these antihistaminic agents will satisfy the patient's clinical needs in most instances.

REFERENCES

1. Windaus A, Vogt W. Syntheses des imidazolylathylamines. *Ber Dtsch Chem Ges* 1907;3:3691.
2. Fried JP, ed. *Dorland's illustrated medical dictionary.* Philadelphia: WB Saunders, 1974.
3. Simons FE. Antihistamines. In: Middleton E, Reed CE, Ellis EF, et al, eds. *Allergy principles and practice.* St. Louis: CV Mosby, 1998.
4. Dale HH, Laidlaw PP. The physiological action of a-imidazolylethylamine. *J Physiol* 1953;120:528.
5. Pearce FL. Biological effects of histamine: an overview. *Agents Actions* 1991;33:4–7.
6. Ishizaka T. Analysis of triggering events in mast cells for immunoglobulin E-mediated histamine release. *J Allergy Clin Immunol* 1981;67:90.
7. Ash ASF, Schild HO. Receptors mediating some actions of histamine. *Br J Pharmacol Chemother* 1966;27:427.
8. Black JW, Duncan WAM, Durant CJ, et al. Definition and antagonism of histamine H_2 receptors. *Nature* 1977;236:385.
9. Arrang JM, Garbarg M, Lancelot JC, et al. Highly potent and selective ligands for histamine H_3 receptors. *Nature* 1987;327:117.
10. Simons FER. H_1 receptor antagonists: clinical pharmacology and therapeutics. *J Allergy Clin Immunol* 1989;84:845.
11. Kozlowski T, Raymond RM, Korthuis RJ, et al. Microvascular protein efflux: interaction of histamine and H_1 receptors. *Proc Soc Exp Biol Med* 1981;166:263.
12. Dobbins DE, Swindall BT, Haddy FJ, et al. Blockade of histamine-mediated increased in microvascular permeability by H_1- and H_2-receptor antagonists. *Microvasc Res* 1981;21:343.
13. Duncan WAM, Parsons ME. Reminiscences of the development of cimetidine. *Gastroenterology* 1980;78:620.
14. Ganellin CR. Medicinal chemistry and dynamic structure-activity analysis in the discovery of drugs acting as histamine H_2-receptors. *J Med Chem* 1981;24:913.
15. Lipsy RJ, Fennerty B, Fagan TC. Clinical review of histmanine_2 receptor antagonists. *Arch Intern Med* 1990;150:745.
16. Simons FER, Simons KJ. H_1 receptor antagonists: clinical pharmacology and use in allergic disease. *Pediatr Clin North Am* 1983;30:899.
17. Simons FER, Simons KJ. The pharmacology and use of H_1-receptor-antagonist drugs. *N Engl J Med* 1994;330:1663.
18. Simons FER, Luciuk GH, Simons KJ. The pharmacoki-

netics and antihistaminic effects of brompheniraine. *J Allergy Clin Immunol* 1982;70:458.

19. Simons FER, Frith EM, Simons KJ. The pharmacokinetics and antihistaminic effects of brompheniramine. *J Allergy Clin Immunol* 1982;70:458.

20. Simons KJ, Singh M, Gillespie CA, et al. An investigation of the H_1-receptor antagonist triprolidine. Pharmacokinetics and antihistaminic effects. *J Allergy Clin Immunol* 1986;77:326.

21. Simons FER, Simons KJ, Frith EM. The pharmacokinetics and antihistaminic of the H_1 receptor antagonist hydroxyzine. *J Allergy Clin Immunol* 1984;73:69.

22. Simons FER, Simons KJ. H_1 receptor antagonist treatment of chronic rhinitis. *J Allergy Clin Immunol* 1988;81:975.

23. Church MK, Gradidge CG. Inhibition of histamine release from human lung *in vitro* by antihistamines and related drugs. *Br J Pharmacol* 1980;69:663.

24. *Physicians' desk reference.* 49th ed. Montvale, NJ: Oradell Medical Economics Company Inc., 2000.

25. Fowle ASE, Hughes DTD, Knight GJ. The evaluation of histamine antagonists in man. *Eur J Clin Pharmacol* 1971;3:215.

26. Kotzan JA, Vallner JJ, Stewart JT, et al. Bioavailability of regular and controlled release chlorpheniramine products. *J Pharm Sci* 1982;71:919.

27. Yacobi A, Stoll RG, Chao GG, et al. Evaluation of sustained-action chlorpheniramine-pseudoephedrine dosage form in humans. *J Pharm Sci* 1980;69:1077.

28. Brandon ML, Weiner M. Clinical investigation of terfenadine, a non-sedating antihistamine. *Ann Allergy* 1980;44:71.

29. Laduron PM, Janssen PFM, Gommeren W, et al. *In vitro* and *in vivo* binding characteristics of a new long-acting histamine H1 antagonist, astemizole. *Mol Pharmacol* 1982;21:294.

30. Simons FER, Simons KJ. New H_1 receptor antagonists: a review. *Am J Rhinol* 1988;2:21.

31. Grant JA. Molecular pharmacology of second-generation antihistamines. *Allergy Asthma Proc* 2000;21:135–140.

32. Okerholm RA, Weiner DL, Hook RH, et al. Bioavailability of terfenadine in man. *Biopharm Drug Dispos* 1981;2:185.

33. Heykants J, Van Peer A, Woestenborghs R, et al. Dose-proportionality, bioavailability and steady-state kinetics of astemizole in man. *Drug Dev Res* 1986;8:71.

34. Rihoux JP, DeVos C, Baltes E, et al. Pharmacoclinical investigation of cetirizine, a new potent and well tolerated anti-H_1. *Ann Allergy* 1985;55:392 (abst).

35. Wood SG, John GA, Chasseaud JF, et al. The metabolism and pharmacokinetics of ^{14}C-cetirizine in humans. *Ann Allergy* 1987;59:31.

36. Watson WTA, Simons KJ, Chen XY, et al. Cetirizine: a pharmacokinetic and pharmacodynamic evaluation in children with seasonal allergic rhinitis. *J Allergy Clin Immunol* 1989;84:457.

37. Hilbert J, Radwanski E, Weglein R, et al. Pharmacokinetics and dose proportionality of loratadine. *J Clin Pharmacol* 1987;27:694.

38. Rodrigues AD, Mulford DJ, Lee RD, et al. In vitro metabolism of terfenadine by a purified recombinant fusion protein containing cytochrome p4503A4 and NADPH P450 reductase: comparison to human liver microsomes and precision cut liver tissue slices. *Drug Metab Dispos* 1995;23:765–775.

39. Richards DM, Brogden RN, Heel RC, et al. Astemizole: a review of its pharmacodynamic properties and therapeutic efficacy. *Drugs* 1984;28:38.

40. Garteiz DA, Hook RH, Walker BJ, et al. Pharmacokinetics and biotransformation studies of terfenadine in man. *Arzneimittelforschung* 1982;32:1185.

41. Simons FER, Watson WTA, Simons KJ. The pharmacokinetics and pharmacodynamics of terfenadine in children. *J Allergy Clin Immunol* 1987;80:884.

42. Meltzer EO, Baraniuk, JN, Barbey J, et al. Antihistamine update: consensus conference. *Hosp Pract* 1995;31:s1.

43. Honig PK, Wortham DC, Lazarev A, et al. Grapefruit juice alters the systemic bioavailability and cardiac repolarization of terfenadine in poor metabolizers of terfenadine. *J Clin Pharmacol* 1996;36:345–351.

44. Simons FER, et al. A double-blind, single-dose, crossover comparison of cetirizine, terfenadine, loratadine, astemizole and chlorpheniramine versus placebo: suppressive effects on histamine-induced wheals and flares during 24 hours in normal subjects. *J Allergy Clin Immunol* 1990;86:540.

45. Roth T, Roehrs T, Koshorck G, et al. Sedative effects of antihistamines. *J Allergy Clin Immunol* 1987;80:94.

46. Chu TJ, Yamate M, Biedermann AA, et al. One versus twice daily dosing of terfenadine in the treatment of seasonal allergic rhinitis: US and European studies. *Ann Allergy* 1989;63:12.

47. Russell T, Burgess G, Donahue R, et al. A comparison of peripheral H_1 blockade between single doses of fexofenadine HCl and terfenadine. *Ann Allergy Asthma Immunol* 2000;84:146.

48. Fields DA, Pillar J, Diamantis W, et al. Inhibition by azelastine of nonallergic histamine release from rat peritoneal mast cells. *J Allergy Clin Immunol* 1984;74:400.

49. Chand N, Pillar J, Diamantis W, et al. Inhibition of IgE-mediated allergic histamine release from rat peritoneal mast cells by azelastine and selected anti-allergic drugs. *Agents Actions* 1985;16:318.

50. Tasaka K, Mio M, Okamoto M. Intracellular calcium release induced by histamine releasers and its inhibition by antiallergic drugs. *Ann Allergy* 1986;56:464.

51. Lowe DA, Richardson BP, Taylor P, et al. Increasing intracellular sodium triggers calcium release from bound pools. *Nature* 1976;260:337.

52. Busse W, Randlex B, Sedgwick J. The effect of azelastine on neutrophil and eosinophil generation of superoxide. *J Allergy Clin Immunol* 1989;83:400.

53. Phillips MJ, Meyrick-Thomas RH, Moodley I, et al. A comparison of the *in vivo* effects of ketotifen, clemastine, chlorpheniramine and sodium cromoglycate on histamine and allergen induced wheals in human skin. *Br J Clin Pharmacol* 1983;15:277.

54. Armour C, Temple DM. The modification by ketotifen of respiratory responses to histamine and antigen in guinea pigs. *Agents Actions* 1982;12:285.

55. Chand N, Harrison JE, Rooney SM, et al. Inhibition of passive cutaneous anaphylaxis (PCA) by azelastine: dissociation of its antiallergic activities from antihistaminic and antiserotonin properties. *Int J Immunopharmacol* 1985;7:833.

56. Van Nueten JM, Xhouneux R, Janssen PAJ. Preliminary data on antiserotonin effects of oxatomide, a novel

antiallergic compound. *Arch Int Pharmacodyn Ther* 1978;232:217.

57. Bechel HJ, Broch N, Lenke D, et al. Pharmacologic and toxicological properties of azelastine, a novel antiallergic agent. *Arzneimittelforschung* 1981;31:1184.

58. Ney U, Bretz U, Gradwohl P, et al. Further characterization of the antianaphylactic action of ketotifen. *Allergol Immunopathol* (Madr) 1980;8:380.

59. Diamantis W, Chand N, Harrison JE, et al. Inhibition of release of SRS-A and its antagonism by azelastine, an H1 antagonist-antiallergic agent. *Pharmacologist* 1982;24:200.

60. Ohmori K, Ishii H, Kubota T, et al. Inhibitory effects of oxatomide on several activities of SRS-A and synthetic leukotrienes in guinea pigs and rats. *Arch Int Pharmacodyn Ther* 1985;275:139.

61. Van Ganse E, Kaufman L, Derde MP, et al. Effects of antihistamines in adult asthma: a meta-analysis of clinical trials. *Eur Respir J* 1997;10:2216–2224.

62. Roquet A, Dahlen B, Kumlin M, et al. Combined antagonism of leukotrienes and histamine produces predominant inhibition of allergen induced early and late phase airway obstruction in asthmatics. *Am J Respir Crit Care Med* 1997;155:1856–1863.

63. Schwartz JC, Garbarg M, Quach TT. Histamine receptors in brain as targets for tricyclic antidepressants. *TIPS* 1981.

64. Goldsobel AB, Rohr AS, Siegel SC, et al. Efficacy of doxepin in the treatment of chronic idiopathic urticaria. *J Allergy Clin Immunol* 1986;78:867.

65. Drouin MA. H$_1$ antihistamines: perspective of the use of the conventional and new agents. *Ann Allergy* 1985;55:747.

66. Connell JT, Howard JC, Dressler W, et al. Antihistamines: findings in clinical trials relevant to therapeutics. *Ann J Rhin* 1987;1:3.

67. Wong L, Hendeles L, Weinberger M. Pharmacologic prophylaxis of allergic rhinitis: relative efficacy of hydroxyzine and chlorpheniramine. *J Allergy Clin Immunol* 1981;67:223.

68. Schaaf L, Hendeles L, Weinberger M. Suppression of seasonal allergic rhinitis symptoms with daily hydroxyzine. *J Allergy Clin Immunol* 1979;3:129.

69. Empey DW, Bye C, Hodder M, et al. A double-blind crossover trial of pseudoephedrine and triprolidine: alone and in combination, for the treatment of allergic rhinitis. *Ann Allergy* 1975;34:41.

70. Diamond L, Gerson K, Cato A, et al. An evaluation of triprolidine and pseudoephedrine in the treatment of allergic rhinitis. *Ann Allergy* 1981;47:87.

71. Guill MF, Buckley RH, Rocha W, et al. Multicenter, double blind, placebo-controlled trial of terfenadine suspension in the treatment of fall-allergic rhinitis in children. *J Allergy Clin Immunol* 1986;78:4.

72. Sooknundun M, Kacker SK, Sundaran KR. Treatment of allergic rhinitis with a new long-acting H$_1$ receptor antagonist: astemizole. *Ann Allergy* 1987;58:78.

73. Kreutner W, Chapman RW, Gulbenkian A, et al. Antiallergic activity of loratadine, a nonsedating antihistamine. *Allergy* 1987;42:57.

74. Meltzer EO, Weiler JM, Widlitz MD. Comparative outdoor study of the efficacy, onset and duration of action and safety of cetirizine, loratadine and placebo for seasonal allergic rhinitis. *J Allergy Clin Immunol* 1996;97:617.

75. Juniper EF, White J, Dolovich J. Efficacy of continuous treatment with astemizole (Hismanal) and terfenadine (Seldane) in ragweed pollen-induced rhinoconjunctivitis. *J Allergy Clin Immunol* 1988;82:670.

76. Boland N. A double-blind study of astemizole and terfenadine in the treatment of perennial rhinitis. *Ann Allergy* 1988;61:18.

77. Dockhorn RJ, Bergner A, Connell JT, et al. Safety and efficacy of loratadine (Sch-29851): a new non-sedating antihistamine in seasonal allergic rhinitis. *Ann Allergy* 1987;58:407.

78. Bruttman G, Charpin D, Germouty J, et al. Evaluation of the efficacy and safety of loratadine in perennial allergic rhinitis. *J Allergy Clin Immunol* 1989;83:411.

79. Bruno G, D'Amato G, Del Giacco GS, et al. Prolonged treatment with acrivastine for seasonal allergic rhinitis. *J Int Med Res* 1989;17:41B.

80. Gervais P, Bruttman G, Pedrali P, et al. French multicentre double-blind study to evaluate the efficacy and safety of acrivastine as compared with terfenadine in seasonal allergic rhinitis. *J Int Med Res* 1989;17:47B.

81. Falliers CJ, Brandon ML, Buchman E, et al. Double blind comparisons of cetirizine and placebo in treatment of seasonal rhinitis. *Ann Allergy* 1991;66:257.

82. Skassa-Brociek W, Bousquet J, Montes F, et al. Double-blind placebo-controlled study of loratadine mequitazine, and placebo in the symptomatic treatment of seasonal allergic rhinitis. *J Allergy Clin Immunol* 1988;81:725.

83. Gutkowski A, Bedard P, Del Carpio JB, et al. Comparison of the efficacy and safety of loratadine, terfenadine and placebo in the treatment of seasonal allergic rhinitis. *J Allergy Clin Immunol* 1988;81:902.

84. Zuber P, Pecoud A. Effect of levocabastine, a new H1 antagonist, in a conjunctival provocation test with allergens. *J Allergy Clin Immunol* 1988;82:590.

85. Simons FER, Simons KJ, Becker AB, et al. Pharmacokinetics and antipruritic effects of hydroxyzine in children with atopic dermatitis. *J Pediatr* 1984;104:123.

86. Wanderer AA, St. Pierre JP, Ellis EF. Primary acquired cold urticaria: double blind study of treatment with cryproheptadine, chlorpheniramine and placebo. *Arch Dermatol* 1977;113:1375.

87. Bernstein IL, Bernstein DI. Efficacy and safety of astemizole, a long-acting and nonsedating H1 antagonist for the treatment of chronic idiopathic urticaria. *J Allergy Clin Immunol* 1986;77:37.

88. Fox RW, Lockey RF, Burkantz SC, et al. The treatment of mild to severe chronic idiopathic urticaria with astemizole: double-blind and open trials. *J Allergy Clin Immunol* 1986;78:1159.

89. Sly MR, Kemp JP, Anderson JA, et al. Position statement: the use of antihistamines in patients with asthma. *J Allergy Clin Immunol* 1988;82:481.

90. Pierson WE, Virant FS. Antihistamines in asthma. *Ann Allergy* 1989;63:601.

91. Rafferty P. The European experience with antihistamines in asthma. *Ann Allergy* 1989;63:389.

92. Rafferty P, Holgate ST. Histamine and its antagonists in asthma. *J Allergy Clin Immunol* 1989;84:144.

93. Ollier S, Gould CAL, Davies RJ. The effect of single and multiple dose therapy with azelastine on the immediate asthmatic response to allergen provocation testing. *J Allergy Clin Immunol* 1986;78:358.

94. Rafferty P, Harrison J, Aurich R, et al. The *in vivo* potency and selectivity of azelastine as an H_1 histamine-receptor antagonist in human airways and skin. *J Allergy Clin Immunol* 1988;82:1113.

95. Cantekin EL, Mandel EM, Bluestone CD, et al. Lack of efficacy of a decongestant-antihistamine combination of otitis media with effusion in children. *N Engl J Med* 1987;316:432.

96. Mandel EM, Rockette HE, Bluestone CD, et al. Efficacy of amoxicillin with and without decongestant antihistamine for otitis media with effusion in children. *N Engl J Med* 1987;316:432.

97. Gaffey MJ, Gwaltney JM, Sastre A, et al. Intranasally and orally administered antihistamine treatment of experimental rhinovirus colds. *Am Rev Respir Dis* 1987;136:556.

98. Dykewicz MS, Fineman S, Nicklas R, et al. Diagnosis and management of rhinitis. *Parameter documents of the Joint Task Force on Practice Parameters in Allergy, Asthma and Immunology* 1998;81:501.

99. Schuller DE, Turkewitz D. Adverse effects of antihistamines. *Postgrad Med* 1986;79:75.

100. Simons FER, Watson WTA, Chen XY, et al. The pharmacokinetics and pharmacodynamics of hydroxyzine in patients with primary biliary cirrhosis. *J Clin Pharmacol* 1989;29:809.

101. Nicholson AN. Antihistamines and sedation. *Lancet* 1982;2:211.

102. Simons FER, Kesselman MS, Giddens NG, et al. Astemizole-induced torsades de pointes. *Lancet* 1988;2:624.

103. Burns JJ, Conney AH, Koster R. Stimulatory effect of chronic drug administration on drug and metabolizing enzymes in liver microsomes. *Ann N Y Acad Sci* 1963;104:881.

104. Simons KJ, Simons FER. The effect of chronic administration of hydroxyzine on hydroxyzine pharmacokinetics in dogs. *J Allergy Clin Immunol* 1987;79:928.

105. Kemp JB. Tolerance to antihistamines: is it a problem? *Ann Allergy* 1989;63:621.

106. Taylor RJ, Long WF, Nelson HS. The development of subsensitivity to chlorpheniramine. *J Allergy Clin Immunol* 1985;76:103.

107. Bantz EW, Dolen WK, Chadwick EW, et al. Chronic chlorpheniramine therapy: Subsensitivity, drug metabolism and compliance. *Ann Allergy* 1987;59:341.

108. Simons FER, Watson WTA, Simons KJ. Lack of subsensitivity to terfenadine during long-term terfenadine treatment. *J Allergy Clin Immunol* 1988;82:1068.

109. Roman IJ, Kassem N, Gural RP, et al. Suppression of histamine-induced wheal response by loratadine (SCH 29851) over 28 days in man. *Ann Allergy* 1986;57:253.

110. Hendeles L. Selecting a decongestant. *Pharmacotherapy* 1993;13:129S–134S.

111. Durant GJ, Parsons ME, Black JW. Potential histamine H_2 receptor antagonists: 2N a-guanylhistamine. *J Med Chem* 1975;18:830.

112. Forest JAH, Shearman DJC, Spence R, et al. Neutropenia associated with metiamide [Letter]. *Lancet* 1975;1:392.

113. Holmberg K, Pipkorn U, Bake B, et al. Effects of topical treatment H_1 and H_2 antagonists on clinical symptoms and nasal vascular reactions in patients with allergic rhinitis. *Allergy* 1989;44:281.

114. Norm S, Permin H, Skov PS. H_2 antihistamines (cimetidine) and allergic-inflammatory reactions. *Allergy* 1980;35:357.

115. Gonzalez H, Ahmed T. Suppression of gastric H_2-receptor mediated function in patients with bronchial asthma and ragweed allergy. *Chest* 1986;4:491.

116. Ahmed T, King MM, Krainson JP. Modification of airway histamine-receptor function with methylprednisolone succinate. *J Allergy Clin Immunol* 1983;71:224.

117. Festen HPM, DePauw BE, Smeulders J, et al. Cimetidine does not influence immunological parameters in man. *Clin Immunol Immunopathol* 1981;21:33.

118. Thomas RHM, Browne PD, Kirby JDT. The effect of ranitidine, alone and in combination with clemastine, on allergen induced cutaneous wheal and flare reactions in human skin. *J Allergy Clin Immunol* 1985;76:864.

119. Nathan RA, Segall N, Schocket AL. A comparison of the actions of H_1 and H_2 antihistamines on histamine-induced bronchoconstriction and cutaneous wheal response in asthmatic patients. *J Allergy Clin Immunol* 1981;67:171.

120. Havas TE, Cole P, Parker L, et al. The effects of combined H_1 and H_2 histamine antagonists on alterations in nasal airflow resistance induced by topical histamine provocation. *J Allergy Clin Immunol* 1986;78:856.

121. Secher C, Kirkegaard J, Borum P, et al. Significance of H_1 and H_2 receptors in the human nose: rationale for topical use if combined antihistamine preparations. *J Allergy Clin Immunol* 1982;70:211.

122. Harvey RP, Schocket AL. The effect of H_1 and H_2 blockade on cutaneous histamine response in man. *J Allergy Clin Immunol* 1980;65:136.

6

Allergens and Other Factors Important in Atopic Disease

G. Daniel Brooks and *Robert K. Bush

*Department of Allergy/Immunology, University of Wisconsin, Madison, Wisconsin; *Department of Medicine, University of Wisconsin, Department of Allergy, William S. Middleton Veterans Hospital, Madison, Wisconsin*

A knowledge of the pathophysiologic mechanisms of the allergic response is essential to the understanding and proper treatment of allergic diseases. Too often, however, inadequate attention is directed to the nature of the allergen in an allergic response. The first and foremost treatment recommendation for allergies is avoidance of the trigger. Such advice is impossible to render without an intimate familiarity with the nature of common environmental allergens. This chapter presents a comprehensive yet lucid overview of allergen biology for the clinician.

An allergen is an antigen that produces a clinical allergic reaction. In atopic diseases, allergens are antigens that elicit an immunoglobulin E (IgE) antibody response. The presence of such an allergen can be demonstrated by a wheal-and-flare reaction to that antigen in a skin test, or by *in vitro* immunoassays such as the radioallergosorbent test (RAST), which measures antigen-specific IgE in serum. Other methods, usually restricted to research laboratories, also may be used to demonstrate the presence of specific IgE antibody. These include enzyme-linked immunosorbent assay (ELISA), crossed radioimmunoelectrophoresis (CRIE), immunoblotting technique, and leukocyte histamine release assay. When assessing the contribution of a particular antigen to an observed symptom, the nature of the immune response must be clarified. The clinician must differentiate the allergic (or atopic)

response from the nonallergic immune response to certain drug or microbial antigens that induce the formation of other antibody isotypes (e.g., IgG or IgA). The allergic response also demonstrates a distinct pathophysiologic mechanism compared with that seen in delayed hypersensitivity reactions, which result from contact antigens.

Allergens most commonly associated with atopic disorders are inhalants or foods, reflecting the most common entry sites into the body. Drugs, biologic products, insect venoms, and certain chemicals also may induce an immediate-type reaction. In practice, however, most atopic reactions involve pollens, fungal spores, house dust mites, animal epithelial materials, and other substances that impinge directly on the respiratory mucosa. The allergenic molecules generally are water soluble and can be easily leached from the airborne particles. They react with IgE antibodies attached to mast cells, initiating a series of pathologic steps that result in allergic symptoms. This chapter is confined to the exploration of these naturally occurring inhalant substances; other kinds of allergens are discussed elsewhere in this text.

The chemical nature of certain allergens has been studied intensively, although the precise composition of many other allergens remains undefined (1). For an increasing number of allergens, such as the major house dust mite allergen, the complementary DNA (cDNA) sequence has been derived. For others, the physiochemical characteristics or the amino acid sequence is known. Still other allergens are known only as complex mixtures of proteins and polypeptides with varying amounts of carbohydrate. Details of the chemistry of known allergens are described under their appropriate headings (2).

The methods of purifying and characterizing allergens include biochemical, immunologic, and biologic techniques. The methods of purification involve various column fractionation techniques, newer immunologic techniques such as the purification of allergens by monoclonal antibodies, and the techniques of molecular biology for synthesizing various proteins. All of these purification techniques rely on sensitive and specific assay techniques for the allergen. Specific approaches are discussed in this chapter.

AEROALLERGENS

Aeroallergens are airborne particles that can cause respiratory or conjunctival allergy (Table 6.1) The water-soluble portion of ragweed pollen, for example, affects the respiratory and conjunctival mucosa, whereas the lipid-soluble allergens of ragweed pollen may cause a typical contact dermatitis on exposed skin. This ragweed dermatitis is caused by a lymphocyte-mediated immunologic mechanism. Aeroallergens are named using nomenclature established by an International Union of Immunologic Societies subcommittee: the first three letters of the genus, followed by the first letter of the species and an Arabic numeral (3). Allergens from the same group are often given the same numeral. For example, *Lol p 1* and *Phl p 1* are both group I grass allergens.

For a particle to be clinically significant as an aeroallergen, it must be buoyant, present in significant numbers, and allergenic. Ragweed pollen is a typical example. Pine pollen, by contrast, is abundant in certain regions and is buoyant, but because it does not readily elicit IgE antibodies, it is not a significant aeroallergen. In general, the insect-pollinated plants do not produce appreciable amounts of airborne pollen,

as opposed to wind-pollinated plants, which, by necessity, produce particles that travel for miles. Fungal spores are ubiquitous, highly allergenic, and may be more numerous than pollen grains in the air, even during the height of the pollen season. The omnipresence of house dust mite needs no emphasis. The knowledge of what occurs where and when is essential to treating the allergy. The above allergens are emphasized because they are the ones most commonly encountered, and they are considered responsible for most of the morbidity among atopic patients.

Certain aeroallergens, such as animal dander, feathers, and epidermal antigens, may be localized to individual homes. Others may be associated with occupational exposures, as is the case in veterinarians who work with certain animals (e.g., cats), in farmers who encounter a variety of pollens and fungi in hay and stored grains, in exterminators who use pyrethrum, in dock workers who unload coffee beans and castor beans, and in bakers who inhale flour. Some sources of airborne allergens are narrowly confined geographically, such as the mayfly and the caddis fly, whose scales and body parts are a cause of respiratory allergy in the eastern Great Lakes area in the late summer. In addition, endemic asthma has been reported in the vicinity of factories where cottonseed and castor beans are processed.

Aeroallergen particle size is an important element of allergic disease. Airborne pollens are in the range of 20 to 60 μm in diameter; mold spores usually vary between 3 and 30 μm in diameter or longest dimension; house dust mite particles are 1 to 10 μm. Protective mechanisms in the nasal mucosa and upper tracheobronchial passages remove most of the larger particles, so only those 3 μm or smaller reach the alveoli of the lungs. Hence, the conjunctivae and upper respiratory passages receive the largest dose of airborne allergens. These are considerations in the pathogenesis of allergic rhinitis, bronchial asthma, and hypersensitivity pneumonitis as well as the irritant effects of chemical and particulate atmospheric pollutants.

The development of asthma after pollen exposure is enigmatic because pollen grains are

TABLE 6.1. *Commonly encountered allergens*

Common name	Taxonomic name	Purified/cloned allergens
Trees		
Birch	*Betula verrucosa*	*Bet v 1–5, 7*
Alder	*Alnus glutinosa*	*Aln g 1*
Hazel	*Corylus avellana*	*Cor a 1*
White oak	*Quercus alba*	*Que a 1*
Olive	*Olea curopaea*	*Ole e 1–7*
Japanese cedar	*Cryptomeria japonica*	*Cry j 1, 2*
Mountain Cedar	*Juniperus ashei*	*Jun a 1*
Weeds		
Short ragweed	*Ambrosia artemisiifolia*	*Amb a 1–7, Cystatin*
Giant ragweed	*Ambrosia trifida*	*Amb t 5*
Western ragweed	*Ambrosia psilostachya*	*Amb p 5*
Russian thistle	*Salsola pestifer*	*Sal p 1*
Mugwort	*Artemisia vulgaris*	*Art v 1, 2*
Coccharia	*Parietaria judaica, officinalis*	*Par j 1, 2, Par o 1*
Grasses		
Ryegrass	*Lolium perenne*	*Lol p 1–3, 9, 11*
Timothy grass	*Phleum pratense*	*Phl p 1, 2, 4, 5*
Orchard grass	*Dactylis glomerata*	*Dac g 1, 3, 5*
Kentucky bluegrass	*Poa pratensis*	*Poa p 1, 9*
Bermuda grass	*Cynodon dactylon*	*Cyn d 1, 7*
Fungi		
	Alternaria alternata	*Alt a 1, 2, 6, 7, 10*
	Aspergillus fumigatus	*Asp f 1–6*
	Cladosporium herbarum	*Cla h 1–3*
	Penicillium citrinum	*Pen c 1–3*
Dust mites		
	Dermatophagoides farinae	*Der f 1–3, 6*
	Pteronyssinus	*Der p 1–4, 6, 9*
Animals		
Cat	*Felis domesticus*	*Fel d 1*
Dog	*Canis familiaris*	*Can f 1, 2, albumin*
Horse	*Equus cabalus*	*Equ c 1, 2*
Mouse	*Mus musculus*	*Mus m 1*
Rat	*Rattus norvegicus*	*Rat n 1, 2*
Insects (excluding venoms)		
Nimmiti fly	*Chironomus thummi*	*Chi t 1*
German cockroach	*Blattella germanica*	*Bla g 1, 2, 4, 5*
American cockroach	*Periplaneta americana*	*Per a 1, 3*

deposited in the upper airways as a result of their large particle size. Experimental evidence suggests that rhinitis, but not asthma, is caused by inhalation of whole pollen in amounts encountered naturally (4). Asthma caused by bronchoprovocation with solutions of pollen extracts is easily achieved in the laboratory, however. Pollen asthma may be caused by the inhalation of pollen debris that is small enough to access the bronchial tree.

Evidence supports this hypothesis. Extracts of materials collected on an 8-μm filter that excludes ragweed pollen grains induced positive skin test results in ragweed-sensitive subjects. These same extracts can specifically inhibit an anti-ragweed IgG-ELISA system (5). Using an immunochemical method of identifying atmospheric allergens, *Amb a 1* was found to exist in ambient air in the absence of ragweed pollen grains (6). Positive bronchoprovocation was induced with pollen grains that had been fragmented in a ball mill, but was not induced by inhalation of whole ragweed pollen grains (7). Exposure of grass pollen grains to water creates rupture into smaller, respirable size starch granules with intact group V allergens (8), possibly explaining the phenomenon of thunderstorm asthma during grass pollen seasons (9,10).

However, despite the generally accepted limitations previously mentioned, examination of tracheobronchial aspirates and surgical lung specimens has revealed large numbers of whole pollen grains in the lower respiratory tract (11). Hence, the mechanism of pollen-induced asthma is still an open question.

Another consideration is the rapidity with which various allergens are leached out of the whole pollen grains. The mucous blanket of the respiratory tract has been estimated to transport pollens into the gastrointestinal tract in less than 10 minutes. The allergens of grass pollens and ragweed *Amb a 5* are extracted rapidly from the pollen grains in aqueous solutions and can be absorbed through the respiratory mucosa before the pollen grains are swallowed. Ragweed *Amb a 1*, however, is extracted slowly, and only a small percentage of the total extractable *Amb a 1* is released from the pollen grain in this time frame (12). This observation has not been reconciled with the presumed importance of *Amb a 1* in clinical allergy, but absorption may be more rapid in the more alkaline mucus found in allergic rhinitis (13).

The biochemical function of allergens also may contribute to their allergenicity. The enzymatic activity of *Der p 1* helps the allergen to penetrate through the respiratory mucosa and helps to promote an IgE response as described in detail later in this chapter. A similar study performed on fungal proteases also suggests the importance of enzymatic activity in the development of an allergic response (14).

Sampling Methods for Airborne Allergens

Increasing attention is being focused on the daily levels of airborne allergens detected in a particular locale. Patients commonly seek out daily reports of ragweed or *Alternaria* levels, frequently reported in newspapers and on television, to correlate and predict their allergy symptoms. The clinician must be acquainted with the various sampling techniques used to accurately assess the validity and accuracy of the readings reported. All of the methods involve averaging pollen exposure, so these pollen "predictions" are actually reports of yesterday's levels.

Aerobiologic sampling attempts to identify and quantify the allergenic particles in the ambient atmosphere, both outdoors and indoors. Commonly, an adhesive substance is applied to a microscope slide or other transparent surface, and the pollens and spores that stick to the surface are microscopically enumerated. Devices of varying complexity have been used to reduce the most common sampling errors relating to particle size, wind velocity, and rain. Fungi also may be sampled by culture techniques. Excellent resources for these methods are available (15–17). Although many laboratories use various immunoassays to identify and quantify airborne allergens, the microscopic examination of captured particles remains the method of choice. Two types of sampling devices are most commonly used: impaction and suction. Gravitational samplers were used historically, but are rarely used today because they provide qualitative data without quantitative data.

Impaction Samplers

Impaction samplers currently are the most common types of pollen samplers in use. The principle is that wind speed usually is greater than the rate of gravitational settling. Small particles carried by the wind have an inertial force that causes them to impact on an adhesive surface. If the diameter of the surface is small (e.g., 1 to several millimeters), there is little turbulence to deflect the particles. Thus, the smaller the impacting surface, the higher the rate of impaction. Small surface areas, however, are rapidly overloaded, causing a decrease in the efficiency of capture.

The rotating impaction sampler has two vertical collecting arms mounted on a crossbar, which is rotated by a vertical motor shaft. The speed of rotation is up to several thousand revolutions per minute and is nearly independent of wind velocity. The plastic collecting rods are coated with silicone adhesive. These samplers usually are run intermittently (20–60 seconds every 10 minutes) to reduce overloading. In some models, the impacting arms are retracted or otherwise protected while not in use. The Rotorod sampler (Fig. 6.1) is a commercially available impaction sampler

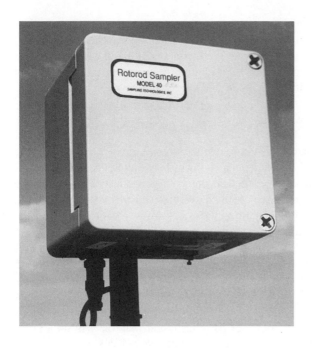

FIG. 6.1. Rotating impaction sampler: Rotorod sampler model 40 (Sampling Technologies, Minnetonka, MN). (Courtesy of Medical Media Service, Wm. Middleton Memorial Veteran's Hospital, Madison, WI.)

and has been shown to be over 90% efficient at capturing pollen particles of approximately 20 μm diameter.

Suction Samplers

Suction samplers employ a vacuum pump to draw the air sample into the device. Although suitable for pollens, they are more commonly used to measure smaller particles such as mold spores. Disorientation with wind direction and velocity skews the impaction efficiencies of particles of different sizes. For example, if the wind velocity is less than that generated by the sampler, smaller particles are collected in greater concentrations than exist in the ambient air. The reverse is true for greater wind velocities. The Hirst spore trap is an inertial suction sampler with a clock mechanism that moves a coated slide at a set rate along an intake orifice. This enables discrimination of diurnal variations. A wind vane orients the device to the direction of the wind. The Burkard spore trap collects particles on an adhesive-coated drum that takes 1 week to make a full revolution around an intake orifice. Both of these spore traps are designed to measure nonviable material. Spore traps are the most flexible

devices for sampling particles over a wide range of sizes.

The Anderson sampler is another suction device, but it is unique in its adaptability for enumerating viable fungal spores. Air passes through a series of sieve-like plates (either two or six), each containing 400 holes. Although the air moves from plate to plate, the diameter of the holes decreases. The larger particles are retained by the upper plates and the smaller ones by successive lower plates. A Petri dish containing growth medium is placed beneath each sieve plate, and the spores that pass through the holes fall onto the agar and form colonies. This method has value for identifying fungi whose spore morphologic features do not permit microscopic identification. In general, however, nonviable volumetric collection techniques more accurately reflect the actual spore prevalence than do volumetric culture methods (15). The volume of air sampled is easy to calculate for suction devices because the vacuum pumps may be calibrated. In the case of rotation impaction samplers, there are formulas that depend on the surface area of the exposed bar of slide, the rate of revolution, and the exposure time. After the adherent particles are stained and counted, their numbers can be expressed as particles per cubic meter of air. Gravitational samplers cannot be quantified volumetrically.

The location of samplers is important. Ground level is usually unsatisfactory because of liability, tampering, and similar considerations. Rooftops are used most frequently. The apparatus should be placed at least 6 m (20 feet) away from obstructions and 90 cm (3 feet) higher than the parapet on the roof.

Several adhesives are used in pollen collectors with good results (18). Silicone stopcock grease (Sampling Technologies, Minnetonka, MN) or petrolatum and Lubriseal stopcock grease (A.H. Thomas, Philadelphia) are used most often. The methods of staining, enumerating, and calculating are beyond the scope of this discussion but are detailed in the references.

Fungal Culture

Fungi also may be studied by culture techniques. This is often necessary because many spores are not morphologically distinct enough for microscopic identification. In such cases, characteristics of the fungal colonies are required. Most commonly, Petri dishes with appropriate nutrient agar are exposed to the air at a sampling station for 5 to 30 minutes. The plates are incubated at room temperature for about 5 days, then inspected grossly and microscopically for the numbers and types of colonies present. Cottonblue is a satisfactory stain for fungal morphologic identification. Potato-dextrose agar supports growth of most allergenic fungi, and rose bengal may be added to retard bacterial growth and limit the spread of fungal colonies. Specialized media such as Czapek agar may be used to look for particular organisms (e.g., *Aspergillus* or *Penicillium*).

The chief disadvantage of the culture plate method is a gross underestimation of the spore count. This may be offset by using a suction device such as the Anderson or Burkhard sampler. A microconidium containing many spores still grows only one colony. There may be mutual inhibition or massive overgrowth of a single colony such as *Rhizopus nigricans*. Other disadvantages are short sampling times, as well as the fact that some fungi (rusts and smuts) do not grow on ordinary nutrient media. Furthermore, avoiding massive spore contamination of the laboratory is difficult without precautions such as an isolation chamber and ventilation hood.

Immunologic Methods

Numerous immunologic methods of identifying and quantifying airborne allergens have been developed recently. In general, these methods are too complex to replace the physical pollen count. The immunologic assays do not depend on the morphologic features of the material sampled, but on the ability of eluates of this material collected on filters to interact in immunoassays with human IgE or IgG (19) or with mouse monoclonal antibodies (20). Studies at the Mayo Clinic have used a high-volume air sampler that retains 95% of particles larger than 0.3 μm on a fiberglass filter. The antigens, of unknown composition, are eluted from the filter sheet by descending chromatography. The eluate is dialyzed, lyophilized, and reconstituted as needed. This material is analyzed by RAST inhibition for specific allergenic activity or, in the case of antigens that may be involved in hypersensitivity pneumonitis, by interaction with IgG antibodies. The method is extremely sensitive. An eluate equivalent to 0.1 mg of pollen produced 40% to 50% inhibition in the short ragweed RAST. An equivalent amount of 24 μg of short ragweed pollen produced over 40% inhibition in the *Amb a 1* RAST (21). The allergens identified using this method have correlated with morphologic studies of pollen and fungal spores using traditional methods and with patient symptom scores. The eluates also have produced positive results on prick skin tests in sensitive human subjects (6). These techniques demonstrate that with short ragweed, different-sized particles from ragweed plant debris can act as a source of allergen in the air before and after the ragweed pollen season. Furthermore, appreciable ragweed allergenic activity has been associated with particles less than 1 μm in diameter (22).

Use of low-volume air samples that do not disturb the air and development of a sensitive two-site monoclonal antibody immunoassay for the major cat allergen (*Fel d 1*) have made accurate measurements of airborne cat allergen possible (20). These studies confirm that a high proportion of *Fel d 1* is carried on particles smaller than 2.5 μm. During house cleaning, the amount of the small allergen-containing particles in the air approached that produced by a nebulizer for bronchial provocation (40 ng/m^3). The results indicate that significant airborne *Fel d 1* is associated with small particles that remain airborne for long periods. This is in contrast to prior studies with house dust mites (23) in which the major house dust mite allergen *Der p 1* was collected on large particles with diameters greater than 10 μm. Little of this allergen remained airborne when the room was disturbed.

In other studies, nonparticulate ragweed material collected on 0.8 μm filters inhibited an antiragweed IgG-ELISA system and produced positive skin test results in ragweed-sensitive individuals (15). Liquid impingers that draw air through a liquid system also can be used to recover soluble material.

Many pollen grains may be difficult to distinguish morphologically by normal light microscopic study. Immunochemical methods may permit such distinctions. Grass pollen grains collected from a Burkard trap were blotted onto nitrocellulose; then, by using specific antisera to Bermuda grass, a second antibody with a fluorescent label, and a fluorescent microscope study, Bermuda grass pollen grains could be distinguished from grass pollens of other species (24). These newer methods show promise because they measure allergenic materials that react in the human IgE system. Currently, immunochemical assays to quantify the major house dust mite allergens *Der p 1* and *Der f 1* and the major cat allergen *Fel d 1* in settled dust samples are commercially available. Further studies with these techniques may lead to a better understanding of exposure–symptom relationships.

STANDARDIZATION OF ALLERGENIC EXTRACTS

The need to standardize allergenic extracts has been recognized for many years. Variability in antigen composition and concentration is a major problem in both allergy testing and allergen immunotherapy regimens. Without standardization of extracts, there is no accurate system of quality control. The clinician often is forced to alter immunotherapy schedules with each new vial of extract because of lot-to-lot variability. Each allergen extract supplier uses its own assays and rarely compares specific antigen concentrations with competitors. The result of this disparity is that the clinician must bring more art than science to the field of allergen immunotherapy. Fortunately, this is changing, with the requirement for standardization of ragweed pollen, house dust mite, cat dander, and grass pollen extracts. The development of purified and even cloned allergens that can be expressed in bacteria or yeast hosts have allowed the production of vast quantities of allergen extract with little or no variance between batches (25–30). With investigators, clinicians, and government agencies that license extracts demanding improved standardization, it is expected that more progress in this area of allergy will be made in the near future.

Quantitation of Allergens

The complexity of biologic material and the extreme sensitivity of the IgE system, which requires only nanogram amounts of allergen, have made standardization of aeroallergens most difficult. The traditional method of standardizing and preparing allergens for clinical use is to extract a known weight of defatted pollen in a specified volume of fluid. For example, 1 g in 100 mL of fluid would yield a 1% (1:100) solution. This weight per volume system still is one of the most commonly used in clinical practice. This solution can be concentrated or diluted as needed.

Another system of measurement, preferred by some allergists and extract manufacturers, is the protein-nitrogen unit (PNU). The basis of the PNU system is the fact that most allergenic moieties of pollens are proteins, and that the ratio of protein to dry weight of pollen varies from plant to plant. In this method, nitrogen is precipitated by phosphotungstic acid and measured by the micro-Kjeldahl technique. Total nitrogen is another method of standardization, but it offers no advantage and is used infrequently.

Both of these methods are used for other inhalant and food allergens, and clinicians generally must communicate in terms of these standards. Unfortunately, neither the weight per volume method nor the protein-nitrogen unit truly measures allergenic activity, because not all measured proteins and extractable components in the solution are allergenic. In addition, many complex allergens are destroyed during the harsh extraction procedure. Such problems have been circumvented through the use of biologic assays of "functional" allergen reactivity. Currently, ragweed pollen, grass pollen, house dust mite, and cat allergen extracts are standardized, and their activity is expressed in allergen units (AU) or biologic allergenic units (BAU). Other allergen concentrations may be added to this list in the future. It is essential for anyone devising immunotherapy regimens to have an appreciation for the biologic assays of allergenicity. These assays are described later.

Characterization of Allergens

Many methods are available to characterize an allergen. Many of these, such as the determination of protein content, molecular weight, and isoelectric point, are not unique to the study of allergenic compounds. These are simply methods of describing any protein. Several categories of tests, however, are restricted to studying molecules responsible for IgE-mediated symptoms. Both immunologic *in vitro* methods, such as RAST and Western blotting, as well as *in vivo* biologic assays, such as end-point dilution skin tests, will be considered here.

Radioallergosorbent Test

The RAST is described elsewhere in this text. Although primarily used in the quantitation of antigen-specific IgE, the test may be adapted to determine antigen concentrations. To measure potency, the unknown allergen is immobilized onto solid-phase supports (cellulose disks or beads) and reacted with a known quantity of antigen-specific IgE in a standard test system. For comparison, the extracts are compared with a reference standard, which should be carefully chosen (31). The quantity of extract required to obtain a specified degree of reactivity is determined. By definition, in this assay, the greater the binding of IgE to the antigen, the greater the allergenicity.

RAST Inhibition Assay

The most widely used assay for in vitro potency of allergenic extract is the RAST inhibition method. This test is a variation of the direct RAST. Serum from an allergic individual (containing IgE) is first mixed with the soluble unknown allergen. Next, a standard amount of the solid-phase (immobilized) allergen is added. The more "potent" the fluid phase allergen, the less IgE is free to bind to the solid-phase allergen (32). The technique and its statistical analysis have been standardized. RAST inhibition usually is the key technique to assess total allergenic activity of an extract and is used by manufacturers to calibrate new batches by comparison with the in-house reference preparation. Recently, some workers have raised concern regarding the continued use of RAST inhibition as a standard technique (33). The arguments concern the fact that the choice of antigen for the solid-phase reaction is variable and may influence results. In addition, the finite supply of allergenic reference sera limits reproducibility: without identical reference sera and immobilized allergen, comparisons are impossible. Further development of monoclonally derived IgE and recombinant allergens may help with this problem.

Assessment of Allergenicity

Biochemical methods for analyzing allergens, such as protein composition and concentration, are practical but tell nothing about the allergenicity of the extract. Immunologic reactivity with IgE antibodies as assessed *in vitro* and *in vivo* provide this information. Preparations of inhalant allergens contain more than one antigen. Of the several antigens in a mixture, usually one or more dominate in both frequency and intensity of skin reactions in sensitive persons. It is inferred from this that these antigens are the most important clinically. Not all persons allergic to a certain pollen allergen react to the same antigens from that pollen allergen extract, however. The antigens of tree, grass, and weed pollens are immunologically distinct, and this agrees with the clinical and skin test data. As more allergens are isolated and purified, it is hoped that correlations between immunogenicity and biochemical structure will emerge.

Marsh (12) proposed that a major allergen be designated when 90% of clinically allergic persons react by skin test to a concentration of 0.001 μg/mL or less of that particular extractable allergen. Others suggest that a component that binds IgE in 50% or more of sensitive patient sera tested by radioimmunoelectrophoresis (another immunologic assay) should be considered a major allergen (34). This definition currently is widely accepted. A minor allergen would be one that does not meet either of these criteria.

Naturally occurring atopic allergens have few physiochemical characteristics to distinguish them from other antigens. All are proteins or glycoproteins, although high molecular weight polysaccharides that react with IgE have been obtained from *Candida albicans*. Most protein allergens that have been identified are acidic, with molecular weights ranging from 5,000 to 60,000 daltons. It has been postulated that larger molecules cannot readily penetrate the mucous membranes. Highly reactive allergens of lower molecular weight are described in conjunction with ragweed and grass pollens. The antigenic determinants that react with IgE antibody molecules have not been clearly identified for most allergens, although it is postulated that there must be at least two such groups on each allergen molecule to trigger the allergic response. The sequence of amino acids in some determinant groups, with less regard for conformation of the protein molecule, is most important for the major codfish antigen *Gad c 1* (codfish antigen M) (35). In other allergens, such as ragweed *Amb a 3* (Ra 3) and *Amb a 5* (Ra 5), the conformation of the native protein is critical for allergenicity (36).

CLASSIFICATION OF ALLERGENIC PLANTS

The botanical considerations and taxonomic scheme given here are not exhaustive. Individual plants, their common and botanical names, geographic distributions, and relative importance in allergy are considered elsewhere in this book. Excellent sources of information on systematic botany, plant identification, and pollen morphology are listed in the references (17,37,38).

Anatomy

Seed-bearing plants produce their reproductive structures in cones or flowers. Gymnosperms ("naked seeds"; class Gymnospermae) are trees and shrubs that bear their seeds in cones. Pines, firs, junipers, spruces, yews, hemlocks, savins, cedars, larches, cypresses, retinisporas, and ginkgoes are gymnosperms. Angiosperms produce seeds enclosed in the female reproductive structures of the flower. Angiosperms may be monocotyledons, whose seeds contain one "seed leaf" (cotyledon), or dicotyledons, with two seed leaves. Leaves of monocotyledons have parallel veins, whereas leaves of dicotyledons have branching veins. Grasses are monocotyledons; most other allergenic plants are dicotyledons.

The flower has four fundamental parts:

1. *Pistils* (one or more) are the female portion of the plant and consist of an ovary at the base, a style projecting upward, and a stigma, the sticky portion to which pollen grains adhere.
2. *Stamens*, which are the male portions of the plant, are variable in number and consist of anthers borne on filaments. Pollen grains are produced in the anthers.
3. *Petals*, the colored parts of the flower, vary from three to many in number.
4. *Sepals*, the protective portion of the flower bud, are usually green and three to six in number.

The phylogenetically primitive flower had numerous separate parts, as typified by the magnolia. Fusion of flower parts and reduction of their number is a characteristic of phylogenetic advancement. As a group, dicotyledons are more primitive than monocotyledons.

A "perfect" flower contains both male and female organs; an "imperfect" flower contains only stamens or only pistils. Monoecious ("one house") plants bear both stamens and pistils;

the individual flowers may be perfect or imperfect. Dioecious ("two houses") plants have imperfect flowers, and all flowers on a particular plant are the same type (male and female). Ragweed is a monoecious plant with perfect flowers; corn is a monoecious plant with imperfect flowers; willows are dioecious plants. Like the flowering plants, gymnosperms may be either monoecious (pines) or dioecious (cypresses and ginkgoes).

Taxonomy

Plants are classified in a hierarchical system. The principal ranks, their endings, and some examples are as follows:

Class (-ae): Angiospermae, Gymnospermae
Subclass (-ae): Monocotyledonae, Dicotyledonae
Order (-ales): Coniferales, Salicales
Suborder (-ineae)
Family (-aceae): Asteraceae, Poaceae
Subfamily (-oideae)
Tribe (-eae)
Genus (no characteristic ending; italicized): *Acer*
Species (genus name plus "specific epithet"): *Acer rubrum*

Trees Gymnosperms

Trees may be gymnosperms or angiosperms. The gymnosperms include two orders, the Coniferales (conifers) and the Ginkgoales. Neither are of particular importance in allergy, but because of the prevalence of conifers and the incidence of their pollens in surveys, some comments are in order.

Conifers grow mainly in temperate climates. They have needle-shaped leaves. The following three families are germane to this discussion.

Pinaceae (Pines, Spruces, Firs, and Hemlocks)

Pines are monoecious evergreens whose leaves are arranged in bundles of two to five and are enclosed at the base by a sheath (all other members of the Pinaceae family bear leaves singly, not in bundles). The pollen grains of pines are 45 to 65 μm in diameter and have two bladders (Fig. 6.2). This pollen occasionally has been implicated in allergy (37). Spruces produce pollen grains morphologically similar to pine pollen but much larger, ranging from 70 to 90 μm exclusive of the bladders. Hemlock pollen grains may have bladders, depending on the species. The firs produce even larger pollen grains, ranging from 80 to 100 μm, not including the two bladders.

Cupressiaceae (Junipers, Cypresses, Cedars, and Savins)

Most of these trees are dioecious and produce large quantities of round pollen grains 20 to 30 μm in diameter with a thick intine (internal membrane). The mountain cedar is an important cause of allergic rhinitis in certain parts of Texas and has proliferated where the ecosystem has been disturbed by overgrazing of the grasslands.

Taxodiaceae (Bald Cypress and Redwood)

The bald cypress may be a minor cause of allergic rhinitis in Florida.

Trees: Angiosperms

Most allergenic trees are in this group. The more important orders and families are listed here with relevant notations. Other trees have been implicated in pollen allergy, but most of the pollinosis in the United States can be attributed to those mentioned here.

Order Salicales, Family Salicaceae (Willows and Poplars)

Willows are mainly insect pollinated and are not generally considered allergenic (Fig. 6.2). Poplars, however, are wind pollinated, and some (e.g., species of *Populus*) are of considerable allergenic importance. Poplar pollen grains are spherical, 27 to 34 μm in diameter, and characterized by a thick intine (Fig. 6.2). The genus *Populus* include poplars, aspens, and cottonwoods. Their seeds are borne on buoyant cotton-like tufts that may fill the air in June like a localized snowstorm. Patients often attribute their symptoms to

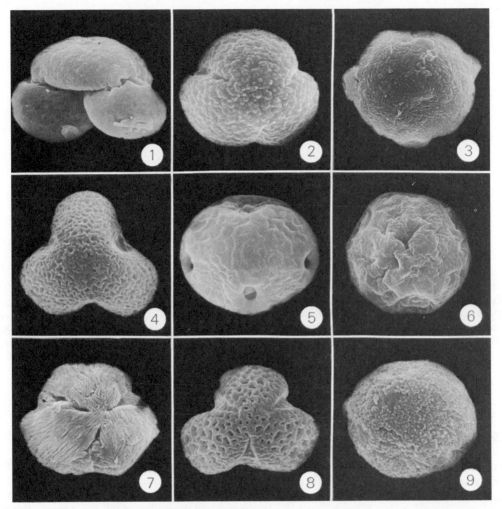

FIG. 6.2. Scanning electron photomicrographs of early spring airborne hay fever–producing pollen grains: *1*, pine (*Pinus*); *2*, oak (*Quercus*); *3*, birch (*Betula*); *4*, sycamore (*Platanus*); *5*, elm (*Ulmus*); *6*, hackberry (*Celtis*); *7*, maple (*Acer*); *8*, willow (*Salix*); *9*, poplar (*Populus*). (Courtesy of Professor James W. Walker.)

this "cottonwood," but the true cause usually is grass pollens.

Order Betulales, Family Betulaceae (Birches)

Betula species are widely distributed in North America and produce abundant pollen that is highly allergic. The pollen grains are 20 to 30 μm and flattened, generally with three pores, although some species have as many as seven (Figs. 6.2 and 6.3) The pistillate catkins may persist into winter, discharging small winged seeds.

Order Fagales, Family Fagaceae (Beeches, Oaks, Chestnuts, and Chinquapins)

Five genera of Fagaceae are found in North America, of which only the beeches (*Fagus*) and oaks (*Quercus*) are wind pollinated and of allergenic importance. The pollens of these two genera are morphologically similar but not identical. They are 40 μm in diameter, with an irregular exine (outer covering) and three tapering furrows (Figs. 6.2 and 6.4) Both produce abundant pollen; oaks in particular cause a great deal of tree pollinosis in areas where they are numerous.

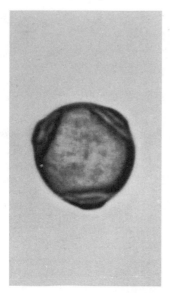

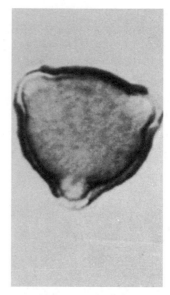

FIG. 6.3. Birch (*Betula nigra*). Average diameter is 24.5 μm. Pollen grains have three pores and a smooth exine. (Courtesy of Center Laboratories, Port Washington, NY.)

FIG. 6.4. Oak (*Quercus* species). Average diameter is 32 μm. Pollens of the various species are similar, with three long furrows and a convex, bulging, granular exine. (Courtesy of Center Laboratories, Port Washington, NY.)

Order Urticales, Family Ulmaceae (Elms and Hackberries)

About 20 species of elms are in the Northern Hemisphere, mainly distributed east of the Rocky Mountains. They produce large amounts of allergenic pollen and continue to be a major cause of tree pollinosis despite the almost total elimination of the American elm by Dutch elm disease. Elm pollen is 35 to 40 μm in diameter with five pores and a thick, rippled exine (Fig. 6.2). Hackberries are unimportant for this discussion.

Order Juglandales, Family Juglandaceae (Walnuts)

Walnut trees (*Juglans*) are not important causes of allergy, but their pollen often is found on pollen slides. The pollen grains are 35 to 40 μm in diameter, with about 12 pores predominantly localized in one area and a smooth exine (Fig. 6.5).

The Hickories (Carya)

These trees produce large amounts of highly allergenic pollen. Pecan trees in particular are important in the etiology of allergic rhinitis where they grow or are cultivated. The pollen grains are

40 to 50 μm in diameter and usually contain three germinal pores.

Order Myricales, Family Myricaceae (Bayberries)

Bayberries produce windborne pollen closely resembling the pollen of the *Betulaceae*. The wax myrtles are thought to cause pollinosis in some areas.

Order Urticales, Family Moraceae (Mulberries)

Certain members of the genus *Morus* may be highly allergic. The pollen grains are small for tree pollens, about 20 μm in diameter, and contain two or three germinal pores arranged with no geometric pattern (neither polar nor meridial).

Order Hamamelidales, Family Platanaceae (Sycamores)

These are sometimes called "plane trees." The grains of their plentiful pollen are oblate (flattened at the poles), about 20 μm in diameter, and without pores. There are three or four furrows

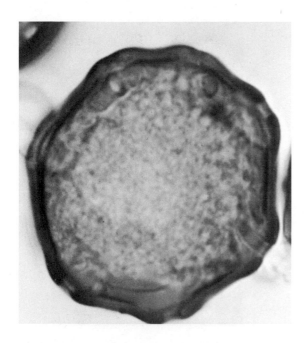

FIG. 6.5. Walnut (*Juglans nigra*). Average diameter is 36 μm. Grains have multiple pores surrounded by thick collars arranged in a nonequatorial band. (Courtesy of William P. Solomon, M.D., University of Michigan, Ann Arbor.)

on the thin, granular exine (Fig. 6.2). Regionally, sycamores may be of allergenic significance.

Order Rutales, Family Simaroubaceae (Ailanthus)

Only the tree of heaven (*Ailanthus altissima*) is of allergenic importance regionally. Its pollen grains have a diameter of about 25 μm and are characterized by three germinal furrows and three germinal pores.

Order Malvales, Family Malvaceae (Lindens)

One genus, *Tilia* (the linden or basswood tree), is of allergenic importance, although it is insect pollinated. The pollen grains are distinct, 28 to 36 μm, with germ pores sunk in furrows in a thick, reticulate exine.

Order Sapindales, Family Aceraceae (Maples)

There are more than 100 species of maple, many of which are important in allergy. Maple pollen grains have three furrows but no pores (Fig. 6.2). Box elder, a species of *Acer*, is particularly important because of its wide distribution, its prevalence, and the amount of pollen it sheds.

Order Oleales, Family Oleaceae (Ashes)

This family contains about 65 species, many of which are prominent among the allergenic trees. Pollen grains have a diameter of 20 to 25 μm, are somewhat flattened, and usually have four furrows (Fig. 6.6) The exine is coarsely reticulate.

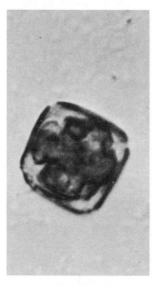

FIG. 6.6. Ash (*Fraxinus americana*). Average diameter is 27 μm. The pollen grains are square or rectangular with four furrows. (Courtesy of Center Laboratories, Port Washington, NY.)

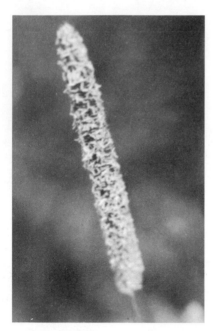

FIG. 6.7. Timothy grass (*Phleum pratense*). Morphologic features of the flowering head. (Courtesy of Arnold A. Gutman, M.D., Associated Allergists Ltd., Chicago, IL.)

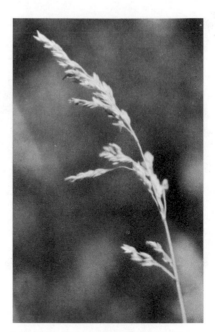

FIG. 6.8. June grass or bluegrass (*Poa pratensis*). Morphologic features of the flowering head. (Courtesy of Arnold A. Gutman, M.D., Associated Allergists Ltd., Chicago, IL.)

Grasses (Poaceae)

Grasses are monocotyledons of the family Poaceae (or Gramineae). The flowers usually are perfect (Figs. 6.7 and 6.8) Pollen grains of most allergenic grasses are 20 to 25 μm in diameter, with one germinal pore or furrow and a thick intine (Fig. 6.9) Some grasses are self-pollinated and therefore noncontributory to allergies. The others are wind pollinated, but of the more than 1,000 species in North America, only a few are significant in producing allergic symptoms. Those few, however, are important in terms of the numbers of patients affected and the high degree of morbidity produced. Most of the allergenic grasses are cultivated and therefore are prevalent where people live.

The grass family contains several subfamilies and tribes of varying importance to allergists. The most important are listed here.

Subfamily Festucoideae, Tribe Festuceae

The tribe Festuceae contains meadow fescue (*Festuca elatior*), Kentucky bluegrass (*Poa pratensis*), and orchard grass (*Dactylis glomerata*) (Fig. 6.9), which are among the most important allergenic grasses. The pollens are 30 to 40 μm in diameter.

Tribe Argostideae

The Argostideae tribe includes timothy (*Phleum pratense*) (Fig. 6.8) and redtop (*Agrostis alba*), two particularly significant grasses in terms of the amount of pollen shed, their allergenicity, and the intensity of symptoms produced. Both are cultivated as forage, and timothy is used to make hay. Other species of *Agrostis* immunologically similar to redtop are used for golf course greens. Timothy pollens are 30 to 35 μm in diameter, redtop pollens are 25 to 30 μm.

Tribe Phalarideae

Sweet vernal grass (*Anthoxanthum odoratum*) is an important cause of allergic rhinitis in areas where it is indigenous. In the total picture of grass allergy, however, it is not as important as the species previously mentioned. The pollen grains are 38 to 45 μm in diameter.

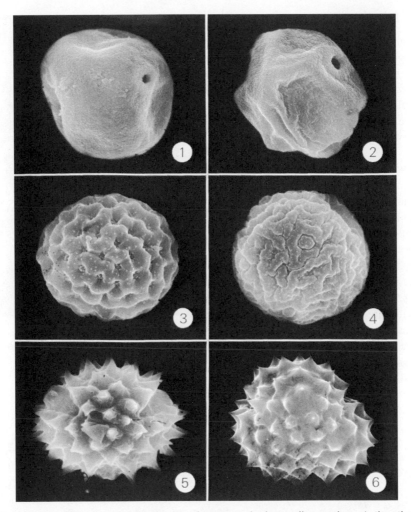

FIG. 6.9. Early and late summer airborne hay fever–producing pollen grains: *1*, timothy (*Phleum*); *2*, orchard grass (*Dactylis*); *3*, lambs quarter's (*Chenopodium*); *4*, plantain (*Plantago*); *5*, goldenrod (*Solidago*); *6*, ragweed (*Ambrosia*). (Courtesy of Professor James W. Walker.)

Tribes Triticaceae (Wheat and Wheat Grasses), Aveneae (Oats), and Zizaneae (Wild Rice)

The Triticaceae, Aveneae, and Zizaneae tribes are of only minor or local importance in allergy because they are self-pollinating or produce pollen that is not abundant or readily airborne.

Subfamily Eragrostoideae, Tribe Chlorideae

Bermuda grass (*Cynodon dactylon*) is abundant in all the southern states. It is cultivated for decorative and forage purposes. It sheds pollen almost year round and is a major cause of pollen allergy. The pollen grains are 35 μm in diameter.

Weeds

A weed is a plant that grows where people do not intend it to grow. Thus, a rose could be considered a weed if it is growing in a wheat field. What are commonly called weeds are small annual plants that grow without cultivation and have no agricultural or ornamental value. All are angiosperms and most are dicotyledons. Those of interest to allergists are wind pollinated, and thus tend to have relatively inconspicuous flowers.

Family Asteraceae (Compositae)

The composite family is perhaps the most important allergenic weed group. Sometimes called the sunflower family, it is characterized by multiple tiny flowers arranged on a common receptacle and usually surrounded by a ring of colorful bracts. There are many tribes within this family; only those of allergenic or general interest are mentioned.

Tribe Heliantheae includes sunflower, dahlia, zinnia, and black-eyed Susan. The flowers cause pollinosis mainly among those who handle them.

Tribe Ambrosieae, or the ragweed tribe, is the most important cause of allergic rhinitis and pollen asthma in North America. Other common weeds in this tribe are the cocklebur and marsh elder. *Ambrosia trifida*, giant ragweed, may grow to a height of 4.5 m (15 feet) (Fig. 6.10). The leaves are broad with three to five lobes. The staminate heads are borne on long terminal spikes, and the pistillate heads are borne in clusters at the base of the staminate spikes. The pollen grains, 16 to 19 μm in diameter, are slightly smaller than those of *Ambrosia artemisiifolia*, short ragweed.

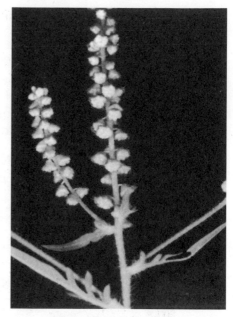

FIG. 6.11. Short ragweed (*Ambrosia artemisiifolia*). Close-up of staminate head. The anthers are full of pollen just before anthesis. (Courtesy of Arnold A. Gutman, M.D., Associated Allergists Ltd., Chicago, IL.)

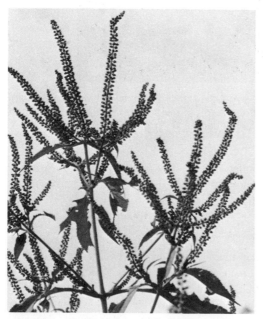

FIG. 6.10. Giant ragweed (*Ambrosia trifida*). Arrangement of staminate heads. (Courtesy of Arnold A. Gutman, M.D., Associated Allergists Ltd., Chicago, IL.)

Short ragweed grows to a height of 120 cm (4 feet) (Fig. 6.11). Its leaves are more slender and usually have two pinnae on each side of a central axis. Pollen grains range from 17.5 to 19.2 μm in diameter and are almost indistinguishable from those of giant ragweed (Figs. 6.9, 6.12, and 6.13). There is no practical reason, however, for distinguishing between the two. *Ambrosia bidentia*, southern ragweed, is an annual that grows from 30 to 90 cm (1–3 feet) tall. The pollen grains are 20 to 21 μm in diameter and resemble those of giant ragweed. *Ambrosia psilostachya*, western ragweed, grows to a height of 30 to 120(1–4 feet). It has the largest pollen grains of all the ragweeds, ranging from 22 to 25 μm in diameter. *Franseria acanthicarpa*, false ragweed, is found mainly in the South and Southwest, where it may cause allergic symptoms. *Franseria tenuifolia*, slender ragweed, is another allergenic species of this tribe.

Xanthium (cocklebur) is morphologically distinct from the ragweeds, but its pollen grains are similar. Most species of *Xanthium* produce

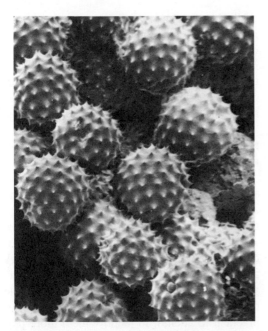

FIG. 6.12. Scanning electron photomicrograph of ragweed pollen. Notice the pore on the pollen grain (*lower right*). (Courtesy of D. Lim, M.D., and J.I. Tennenbaum, M.D.)

scanty pollen and are relatively unimportant causes of allergic rhinitis. Many patients with ragweed sensitivity also give strong skin test reactions to the cockleburs; this is probably a cross-reaction.

Cyclachaerna xanthifolia, burweed marsh elder, is antigenically distinct from ragweed, and the pollen grains are morphologically different from those of ragweed (Fig. 6.14).

Tribe Anthemideae, or the mayweed tribe, is important to allergy because it contains chrysanthemums. Pyrethrum is an insecticide made from flowers of these plants, and inhalation of this substance may cause allergic symptoms in ragweed-sensitive persons as well as in those who have been sensitized to the pyrethrum itself. The genus *Artemisia* includes the sagebrushes, mugworts, and wormwoods and is one of the most important groups of allergenic weeds. *Artemisia vulgaris* is the common mugwort, found mainly on the east coast and in the Midwest in the United States. It is indigenous to Europe and Asia. The pollen grains, like those of other *Artemisia* species, are

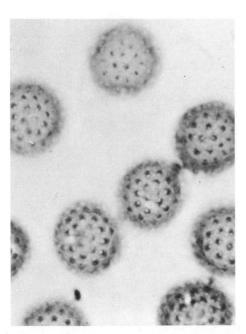

FIG. 6.13. Short ragweed (*Ambrosia artemisiifolia*). Average diameter is 20 μm. Pollen grains have spicules on the surface. (Courtesy of Schering Corporation, Kenilworth, NJ.)

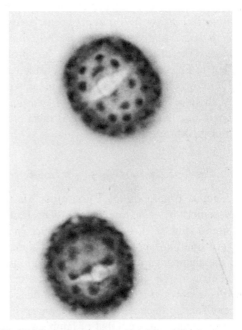

FIG. 6.14. Burweed marsh elder (*Cyclachaerna xanthifolia*). Average diameter is 19.3 μm. Three pores are centered in furrows, distinguishing it from ragweed. (Courtesy of Schering Corporation, Kenilworth, NJ.)

oblately spheroidal, 17 to 28 μm in diameter with three furrows and central pores, a thick exine, and essentially so spines. Other similar species are found on the West Coast and in the Southeast, Great Plains, and Rocky Mountains. *Artemisia tridentata* is common sagebrush, the most important allergenic plant of this tribe. It is most prevalent in the Great Plains and the Northwest, where overgrazing of grassland has increased its presence.

Polygonaceae (Buckwheat Family)

The docks, comprising the genus *Remux*, are the only allergenic members of the buckwheat family. *Rumex acetosella* (sheep sorrel), *Rumex crispus* (curly dock), and *Rumex obtusifolius* (bitter dock) are the most important species. In the whole spectrum of pollen allergy, however, the docks are of minor significance.

Amaranthaceae (Pigweed and Waterhemp Family)

The best known of the amaranths are *Amaranthus retroflexus* (red-root pigweed), *Amaranthus palmeri* (carelessweed), and *Amaranthus spinosus* (spring amaranth). They are prolific pollen producers and should be considered in the etiology of "hay fever" in the areas where they abound. Western waterhemp (*Amaranthus tamariscinus*), a potent allergen, is most prevalent in the Midwest.

Chenopodiaceae (Goosefoot Family)

The genus *Chenopodium*, "goosefoot," is best represented by *Chenopodium album* (lamb's quarters) (Fig. 6.9). Each plant produces a relatively small amount of pollen, but in some areas the abundance of plants assures a profusion of pollen in the air. *Salsola pestifer*, Russian thistle, and *Kochia scoparia*, burning bush, are other Chenopodiaceae whose allergenic presence is more significant than that of lamb's quarters. Russian thistle also is known as "tumbleweed" because in the fall the top of the plant separates from its roots and is rolled along the ground by the wind. Burning bush may be recognized

easily by the thin wing-like projections along its stems and, in the fall, by the fire engine red color of its leaves. It is often cultivated as an ornamental plant. Indigenous to Europe and Asia, these two weeds first became established in the prairie states but have migrated eastward, and are now important in the pathogenesis of pollinosis. *Atriplex* is the genus of the salt bushes, wingscale, and shadscale. These are of some allergenic significance in the Far West and Southwest.

Two crops numbered among the Chenopodiaceae are the sugar beet (*Beta vulgaris*) and spinach (*Spinacea oleracea*). The former has been implicated in allergy where it is cultivated.

Pollens of the Amaranthaceae and Chenopodiaceae are so morphologically similar that they are generally described as "chenopodamaranth" when found in pollen surveys. Although subtle differences exist, it is generally fruitless and impractical to attempt to identify them more precisely. They have the appearance of golf balls, which makes them unique and easy to identify (Fig. 6.15) Multiple pores give this peculiar

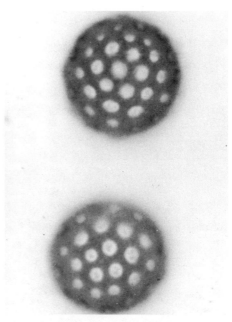

FIG. 6.15. Pigweed (*Amaranthus retroflexus*). Average diameter is 25 μm. The "golf ball" appearance of these grains is characteristic of the chenopod-amaranth group. (Courtesy of Schering Corporation, Kenilworth, NJ.)

surface appearance. The grains are 20 to 25 μm in diameter and spheroidal.

Plantaginaceae (Plantain Family)

English plantain (*Plantago lanceolata*) is the only member of this family that is important for allergy. It sheds pollen mainly in May and June, corresponding to the time when grasses pollinate. The pollen grains may be distinguished by their multiple pores (numbering 7–14) and variable size (25–40 μm) (Fig. 6.9). English plantain may be a potent cause of allergic rhinitis, which may be confused with grass pollinosis.

POLLEN ANTIGENS

Pollen grains are living male gametophytes of higher plants (gymnosperms and angiosperms). Each grain has an internal limiting cellulose membrane, the intine, and a two-layered external covering, the exine, composed of a durable substance called sporopollenin. Sporopollenin is primarily a high molecular weight polymer of fatty acids.

Morphologic studies of pollens using the scanning electron microscope disclose an intricate infrastructure. The morphologic structure varies in relation to size, number of furrows, form and location of pores, thickness of the exine, and other features of the cell wall [spines, reticulations, an operculum in grass pollens, and air sacs (bladders) in certain conifers]. Ragweed pollen is about 20 μm in diameter, tree pollens vary from 20 to 60 μm, and grass pollens, which are all morphologically similar, are usually 30 to 40 μm. The identification of pollens important in allergic disease is not difficult and is certainly within the capabilities of the physician with no special expertise in botany (37,39,40).

Some plants produce prodigious amounts of pollen. A single ragweed plant may expel 1 million pollen grains in a single day. Trees, especially conifers, may release so much pollen that it is visible as a cloud and may be scooped up by the handful after settling. The seasonal onset of pollination of certain plants (e.g., ragweed) is determined by the duration of light received daily. Pollination occurs earlier in the northern latitudes and demonstrates little year-to-year variation in terms of date. In the belt from the central Atlantic to the north-central states, August 15 is a highly predictable date for the onset of ragweed pollination. Most ragweed pollen is released between 6:00 and 8:00 A.M., and release is enhanced by high temperature and humidity. Extended dry spells in early summer inhibit flower development, reduce ragweed pollen production, and thus result in lower counts in August and September.

Most brightly colored flowering plants are of little clinical importance in inhalant allergy because their pollen generally is carried by insects (entomophilous plants) rather than the wind (anemophilous plants). Entomophilous plants have relatively scant, heavy, and sticky pollen. Roses and goldenrod are examples of plants that often are erroneously thought to cause pollinosis because of the time they bloom. Nevertheless, in isolated cases, the pollens of most entomophilous plants can sensitize and then cause symptoms if exposure is sufficient. Of the pollens of anemophilous plants, ragweed has a long range, having been detected 400 miles out at sea. The range of tree pollens is much shorter. Thus, an individual living in the center of a city is more likely to be affected by weed and grass pollens than by trees. Local weed eradication programs, more often legislated than accomplished, are futile in light of the forgoing information. Air conditioners significantly reduce indoor particle recovery because windows are shut when they operate and they largely exclude outdoor air.

Ragweed Pollen Antigens

Essentially all of the peptides and proteins in pollen extracts can elicit the formation of IgG antibodies in animals. Therefore, they are antigens. Only some of these antigens, however, are allergens [i.e., stimulate and bind IgE (in humans)]. Crossed immunoelectrophoresis shows that short ragweed pollen extract contains at least 52 antigens (as recognized by the rabbit antisera), but only 22 of these are allergens, as shown by their binding of specific IgE from the sera of ragweed-sensitive patients (41). Use of sophisticated biochemical methods has resulted in the isolation of ragweed fractions of up to 300 times the potency of crude ragweed extracts, as measured by the ability to induce positive skin test results in appropriate subjects and the ability to cause histamine release from their peripheral blood leukocytes *in vitro.*

Several investigators have studied purified ragweed antigens. The early work of King and Norman (41,42) laid the foundation for the purification and analysis of allergens. Two major allergens, *Amb a 1* (antigen E) and *Amb a 2* (antigen K), were isolated by gel filtration and ion exchange chromatography. These have certain immunologic and chemical properties in common, but differ in molecular weight and biologic activity. Recently, sophisticated molecular biology techniques have enabled workers to isolate and clone DNA sequences (cDNA) for many other ragweed allergens. This has allowed comparisons of DNA sequences. DNA sequences showing similarity (homology) are likely to correspond to proteins with similar function and structural antigenicity. In addition to the two major ragweed allergens, eight intermediate or minor allergens have been isolated. These are *Amb a 3* through *Amb a 7* and *cystatin.*

Amb a 1 is a protein contained primarily in the intine of the pollen grain (13). It accounts for about 6% of the total protein of whole ragweed extract. Quantitative studies of ragweed-sensitive patients with *Amb a 1* have shown a positive correlation with skin test reactivity and leukocyte histamine release, but no correlation with protein-nitrogen content in six commercial preparations of ragweed extract (43). Techniques are available, however, such as radial immunodiffusion, that allow direct quantitation of *Amb a 1* in allergenic extracts, and, by use of RAST inhibition, the potency of ragweed allergenic extracts can be assessed. The U.S. Food and Drug Administration (FDA) requires that ragweed allergenic extracts be labeled with their *Amb a 1* content.

Amb a 1 consists of two fragments, named A and B. These fragments are not bound covalently and are dissociated readily, which results in a significant loss of allergenic activity. Recombination of these polypeptide chains does not

restore allergenic activity, presumably because the steric conformation is not readily restored. *Amb a 1* is resistant to enzymatic degradation, suggesting that readily accessible amino or carboxyl groups are not the principal immunologic determinants. Interestingly, 10-fold more *Amb a 1* is extractable *in vitro* at the pH of nasal secretions from patients with allergic rhinitis (pH 7 to 8), than at the pH of nasal secretions from nonatopic individuals (pH 6.3) (13).

Four isoallergenic variants have been demonstrated for *Amb a 1*, both by physiochemical studies and recent cDNA analyses (44). Isoallergens have the same immunologic properties and similar chemical structures, but differ in some way such as isoelectric point, carbohydrate content, or amino acid composition (12).

It has been calculated that the maximal amount of ragweed *Amb a 1* that a person breathing outdoor air in southeastern Minnesota would inhale is approximately 0.2 μg in a season (45). The amount of *Amb a 1* produced by an individual ragweed plant appears to be determined genetically. There is considerable variation in the amount extractable by standard methods from pollen from plants grown under identical conditions (59–468 μg/mL) (46).

Amb a 2 (antigen K) constitutes about 3% of extractable ragweed pollen protein. Approximately 90% to 95% of ragweed-sensitive subjects show skin reactivity to this antigen. *Amb a 2* may cross-react slightly with *Amb a 1*, a finding reinforced by a 68% sequence homology at a DNA level (47).

Since the isolation of *Amb a 1* and 2, additional minor allergens designated *Amb a 3* (Ra 3), *Amb a 4* (Ra 4), *Amb a 5* (Ra 5) (48–50), *Amb a 6* (Ra 6) (51), *Amb a 7* (Ra 7) (52), and *cystatin* (53) have been identified. In contrast to *Amb a 1*, these low-molecular-weight fractions are rapidly extractable (<10 minutes) from pollen and have basic isoelectric points (54). *Amb a 3* has a relatively high carbohydrate content, making it similar to certain grass pollen antigens. It consists of a single peptide chain of 102 amino acids. Two variants of *Amb a 3* differing by a single amino acid residue have been described; however, this difference does not alter the allergenic specificity (55). This gene has not been cloned. *Amb a 5* consists of a single polypeptide chain whose 45 amino acids have been sequenced. The two isoallergenic forms differ at the second position by the substitution of leucine for valine in about 25% of samples. The frequency of positive skin test results to these antigens in ragweed-sensitive subjects demonstrates that approximately 90% to 95% react to *Amb a 1* and *Amb a 2*, 20% to 25% react to *Amb a 3* and *Amb a 6*, and about 10% to *Amb a 5*. The frequency of reaction to *Amb a 4* is not known. A small fraction (10%) of ragweed-sensitive patients are more sensitive to *Amb a 3* and *5* than to *Amb a 1*.

Amb a 6 and *Amb a 7* show sequence homology to other plant proteins involved in lipid metabolism and electron transport, respectively (52,56). *Cystatin*, the most recent ragweed allergen to be cloned, shows homology to a family of cysteine protease inhibitors found in other plants (53).

These various allergens have made it possible to study genetic responses in the ragweed-sensitive population. A complex antigen such as *Amb a 1* appears unrelated to total serum IgE or to any specific HLA phenotype, whereas subjects who respond to the lower molecular weight allergens such as *Amb a 3* have elevated total serum IgE levels (57). Response to *Amb a 5* requires an immune response (Ir) gene usually associated with HLA DW2 (57). Sensitivity to *Amb a 3* has been associated with increased frequency of the HLA-A2 and HLA-B12 phenotype (13). When a group of highly pollen-sensitive patients were skin-prick tested with individual purified ragweed and ryegrass allergens, each patient reacted in a distinctive pattern. This pattern was undoubtedly genetically programmed (50).

In addition to the short ragweed allergens just described, an allergen from giant ragweed (*A trifida*), *Amb t V* (Ra 5G), has been identified (58). Other allergens that cause allergic rhinitis have been purified from additional weeds. These include *Sal p 1* from *S pestifer* (Russian thistle) (59), *Par j 1* and *Par j 2* from *Parietaria judaica* pollen (Coccharia) (60,61), and *Par o 1* from *Parietaria officionalis* (62). The cDNA for *Par j 1* and *Par o 1* also have been described (63,64). *Art v 1* and *Art v 2* from *A vulgaris* (mugwort)

also have been purified (65). Mugwort has shown significant cross-reactivity with ragweed, including *Art v1* and recombinant *Bet v 1* (66).

Grass Pollen Antigens

Worldwide, grass pollen sensitivity is the most common cause of allergic disease. This is because of the wide distribution of wind-pollinated grasses. Important grass species involved in allergic reactions are *Lolium perenne* (ryegrass), *Phleum pratense* (timothy), *Poa pratensis* (June grass, Kentucky bluegrass), *Festuca pratensis* (meadow fescue), *Dactylis glomerata* (cocksfoot, orchard grass), *Agrotis tenuis* (redtop), *Anthoxanthum odoratum* (sweet vernal), *Sorghum halepense* (Johnson grass), and *Cynodon dactylon* (Bermuda grass). The last two are subtropical grasses, whereas the others are temperate grasses.

Grass pollens differ from ragweed pollen in their allergenic and antigenic properties, and offer additional immunologic perspectives because of their extensive cross-reactivity. In addition, in contrast to ragweed, grasses typically release their pollen grains in the afternoon. Among the grasses, ryegrass and timothy have been most extensively studied (12,67,68).

Examination of a number of allergenic grass pollen extracts by immunochemical methods has disclosed between 20 and 40 different antigens. Further analysis of these components has shown that some are more able than others to bind IgE from the serum of allergic patients or to produce positive skin test results. Some of these are major allergens in that they produce skin test reactivity or demonstrate IgE binding in more than 50% of grass-sensitive patients.

Several grass pollen allergens have been isolated and categorized into eight groups based on chemical and immunologic characteristics. They are as follows: I, II, III, IV, IX (V), X, XI, and the profilins. Within each group, several individual allergens have been identified that are similar immunochemically and are extensively cross-reactive.

The group I allergens are located in the outer wall and cytoplasm of the pollen grains, as well as around the starch granules (69). These small

(3 μm diameter) granules are readily released on contact with water. Two representative members of the group I grass allergens are *Lol p 1* (ryegrass) and *Phl p 1* (timothy). Despite the fact that both of these allergens have been sequenced and cloned, their biochemical identity is not known with certainty. Studies of group I allergens in maize isolated with antibody against *Lol p 1* suggest that the group I antigens may act as "cell wall–loosening agents" (70). High cross-reactivity between the group I allergens from different grass species has been observed, including similarities in IgE RAST inhibition, crossed immunoelectrophoresis (CIE), and monoclonal antibody mapping (71–73). Indeed, amino acid sequences document homologies among these group I members (74). Other studied group I members include *Poa p 1* (Kentucky bluegrass), *Cyn d 1* (Bermuda), *Dac g 1* (orchard), and *Sor h 1* (Johnson). The group I allergens are of major importance in that by skin testing and histamine release, 90% to 95% of grass pollen–allergic patients react on testing (75). Groups II and III show significant but lesser degrees of reaction, varying between 60% and 70% of patients (67).

There is a relative paucity of data regarding the group II, III, and IV grass allergens. Group II allergens include *Lol p 2*, a ryegrass allergen that has been cloned and expressed as a recombinant molecule in a bacterial vector (76). Forty-five percent of ryegrass-allergic patients react to this allergen. Profilin, a compound involved in actin polymerization, has been described as a component of several tree pollens (77). It is allergenic and also has been found to be a minor allergen in the grass allergen group II family, in addition to several weed species.

Lol p 3 and *Dac g 3* have both been sequenced and cloned. Despite 84% identity, the predicted secondary structures suggest they may not be cross-reactive (78). Group IV allergen from timothy grass has been characterized and found to have a significant cross-reactivity with *Amb a 1* (79). Only about 20% of grass pollen–sensitive patients appear to be skin test reactive to these allergens.

Groups V and IX (now grouped together as IX) are a heterogeneous group of proteins. Group IX allergens from Kentucky bluegrass, ryegrass,

and timothy grass all have been sequenced and cloned. Analysis of the cloned Kentucky bluegrass allergen, *Poa p 9*, has suggested the existence of a family of related genes. When compared with the ryegrass allergen, *Lol p 9*, a 44% homology is seen (80). No other members of group IX show this level of homology. Among the group V allergens, the most work has been done with the timothy grass allergens *Phl p 5a* and *Phl p 5b*. These allergens have been cloned and identified as novel pollen RNAses, which may play a role in host–pathogen interactions in the mature plant (81). Other group V allergens have been isolated from a number of temperate grasses, including *Dactylis glomerata* (orchard grass). The *Dac g 5b* allergen also has been cloned and coded for a fusion protein that was recognized by IgE antibodies in six of eight samples of atopic sera tested. This suggests that *Dac g 5b* may be a major allergen, but it has not been completely characterized (82).

The most recent major grass pollen to be identified, *Lol p 11*, appears to be a member of a novel allergen family (83). No sequence homology with known grass pollen allergens was found, but it does have 32% homology with soybean trypsin inhibitor (83). This allergen reacted with IgE from over 65% of grass-pollen positive sera tested. *Lol p 11* appears to share some sequences with allergens from olive pollen, as well as tomato pollen. The cDNA of *Cyn d 7* also has been cloned recently and has two calcium binding sites. Depletion of calcium causes a loss of IgE reactivity (84).

The cDNA cloning of multiple grass allergens has some potential diagnostic applications. A strategy to take advantage of the extensive cross-reactivity between species using recombinant allergens has been studied. A mixture of *Phl p 1*, *Phl p 2*, *Phl p 5*, and *Bet v 2* (birch profilin) accounted for 59% of grass-specific IgE (85). A study of purified *Lol p 1* and *Lol p 5* versus recombinant *Phl p 1* and *Phl p 5* was performed on RAST-positive patients. The *Lol p* extracts reacted with 80% of the IgE, whereas the recombinant *Phl p* reacted with 57% of the IgE (86).

One of the most innovative applications of DNA technology has been the development of rye grass plants with downregulation of the

Lol p 5 gene. This transgenic ryegrass pollen maintained its fertility, but had a significant decrease in its IgE binding capacity compared with normal pollen. This creates the possibility of genetic engineering of less allergenic grasses (87).

Tree Pollen Antigens

There seems to be a higher degree of specificity to skin testing with individual tree pollen extracts compared with grass pollens because pollens of individual tree species may contain unique allergens. Despite this observation, several amino acid homologies and antigenic cross-reactivities have been noted. Most tree pollen characterization has been done using birch (*Betula verrucosa*), alder (*Alnus glutinosa*), hazel (*Corylus avellana*), white oak (*Quercus alba*), olive (*Olea europaea*), and Japanese cedar (*Cryptomeria japonica*) allergens.

A major birch-pollen allergen, *Bet v 1*, has been isolated by a combination chromatographic technique. Monoclonal antibodies directed against this allergen have simplified the purification process (88). Both amino acid sequence as well as a cDNA clone coding for the *Bet v 1* antigen have been described (89). There is considerable ($\geq$80%) amino acid homology between *Bet v 1* and other group I tree allergens (2). *Bet v 1* is the birch tree allergen that cross-reacts with a low-molecular-weight apple allergen, a discovery that helps to explain the association between birch sensitivity and oral apple sensitivity (90). Further investigations by the same workers extend this cross-reactivity to include pear, celery, carrot, and potato allergens. Most of the 20 patients tested had birch-specific serum IgE (anti–*Bet v 1* and anti–*Bet v 2*) that cross-reacted to these fruits and vegetables. *Bet v 2* has been cloned and identified as profilin, a compound responsible for actin polymerization in eukaryotes. There is approximately 33% amino acid homology between the human and birch profilin molecules (77).

Bet v 3 and *Bet v 4* have both been cloned and further described as calcium binding molecules (91,92). Recombinant *Bet v 5* appears to have sequence homology with isoflavone reductase, but the biochemical function remains unknown (93).

Bet v 7 is the most recent to be cloned. It reacts with IgE from 20% of birch allergic patients and has been identified as a cyclophilin (94).

A major allergen has been isolated from the Japanese cedar, which contributes the most important group of pollens causing allergy in Japan. This allergen, designated *Cry j 1*, was initially separated by a combination of chromatographic techniques. Four subfractions were found to be antigenically and allergenically identical (95). There is some amino acid homology between *Cry j 1* and *Amb a 1* and 2, but the significance of this is unclear. A second Japanese cedar allergen, *Cry j 2*, also has been described (96). Allergens from mountain cedar *(Juniperus ashei)* are important in the United States. The major allergen, *Jun a 1*, has a 96% homology with *Cry j 1* and with Japanese cypress (*Chamaecyparis obtusa*) (97). Olive tree pollen is an important allergen in the Mediterranean and California. *Ole e 1* through *Ole e 7* have all been described (98).

FUNGAL ANTIGENS

The role of fungi in producing respiratory allergy is well established. In 1726, Sir John Floyer noted asthma in patients who had just visited a wine cellar; in 1873, Blackley suggested that *Chaetomium* and *Penicillium* were associated with asthma attacks; and in 1924, van Leeuwen noted the relationship of climate to asthma and found a correlation between the appearance of fungal spores in the atmosphere and attacks of asthma (99). Over the next 10 years, case reports appeared attributing the source of fungal allergies to the home or to occupational settings. In the 1930s, Prince and associates (100) and Feinberg (101) reported that outdoor air was a significant source of fungal spores and demonstrated that many of their patients had positive skin test reactivity to fungal extracts. More alarming is the association noted between elevated *Alternaria* airborne spore concentrations and risk of respiratory arrests in *Alternaria*-sensitive individuals (102).

Initially, fungal sensitivity was equated to skin test reactivity, but more direct evidence for the role of fungal sensitivity in asthma has been presented by inhalation challenge studies by

Licorish and co-workers (103). In addition to IgE-mediated reactions, sensitization to certain fungi, especially *Aspergillus*, can lead to hypersensitivity pneumonitis (104).

Although fungal spores are thought to be the causative agents in atopic disorders, other particles that become airborne (including mycelial fragments) also may harbor allergenic activity. Most fungal extracts used clinically are extracts of spore and mycelial material. They also may be derived from culture filtrates.

Alternaria is an important allergenic fungus and has been associated with significant episodes of respiratory distress. Among the *Alternaria* species, *A alternata* has been the subject of the most research. The major allergenic fraction, *Alt a 1*, has been cloned (105,106), but its biologic function remains unknown. About 90% of *Alternaria*-allergic individuals have IgE to this protein. The *Alt a 1* allergen is rich in carbohydrates, and glycosylation of proteins may be necessary for allergenic activity (107). *Alt a 1* can induce positive intradermal test results at extremely low concentrations (6 pg/mL) in *Alternaria*-sensitive subjects. Skin-prick test results are positive at concentrations as low as 0.01 mg/mL, but 1.0 mg/mL is the concentration that best identifies patients allergic to *Alternaria*. This allergen is active in RAST, leukocyte histamine release, and bronchial inhalation challenges (108,109). Interestingly, the fungus *Stemphyllium* shares at least 10 antigens with *Alternaria* and an allergen immunochemically identical to *Alt a 1* (110). Commercial *Alternaria* extracts contain widely varying amounts of *Alt a 1*, underscoring the need for improved methods of standardization (111).

Alt a 2 also has been cloned, but its function remains unknown (112). *Alt a 6*, a P_2 ribosomal protein, *Alt a 7*, a YCP4 yeast protein, and *Alt a 10*, an alcohol dehydrogenase, have all been cloned and sequenced (113). *Alt a 2* is a major allergen, recognized by 60% of *Alternaria*-sensitive patients' IgE, whereas the other three are minor allergens with less than 10% (112,113). Enolase has been obtained from both *Alternaria* and *Cladosporium*. This is a highly conserved protein among fungi. About 50% of patients reactive to *Alternaria* or *Cladosporium* have IgE to enolase. There is also evidence of further cross-reactivity with *Saccharomyces* and *Candida* (114).

Cladosporium species are among the most abundant airborne spores in the world (17). Two species, *Cladosporium cladosporoides* and *Cladosporium herbarum*, have been the focus of intense investigation. Analysis of extracts of *Cladosporium* by CIE and CRIE show complex patterns, revealing as many as 60 discrete antigens. Two major, 10 intermediate, and at least 25 minor allergens have been identified (115). Allergen content of 10 isolates of *Cladosporium* varied from 0% to 100% relative to a reference extract. Two major allergens have been isolated from *Cladosporium herbarum*: *Cla h 1* and *Cla h 2* (116). *Cla h 1* (Ag-32) was isolated by chromatographic and isoelectric focusing techniques. *Cla h 2* (Ag-54) is a glycoprotein that is reactive in a smaller percentage of patients than *Cla h 1*. Neither allergen is cross-reactive, as determined by passive transfer skin testing. Two cDNA clones of the minor allergens from *C. herbarum* have been isolated in addition to enolase. *Cla h 3* is a ribosomal P_2 protein found with RNA in the cytosol (117). Heat shock protein (hsp) 70 also has been cloned (118).

In contrast to *Cladosporium* and *Alternaria* extracts, which are traditionally prepared by extracting mycelia and spores, *Aspergillus fumigatus* extracts generally are prepared from culture filtrate material. Freshly isolated spores from *A. fumigatus* have nearly undetectable levels of the major allergen *Asp f 1*, but begin to produce it within 6 hours of germination. *A. fumigatus* and other *Aspergillus* species have been studied with particular reference to allergenic bronchopulmonary aspergillosis. This disorder is characterized by the presence of both IgE and IgG antibodies to the offending fungal antigens. Analysis by CRIE has demonstrated some components that bind IgE avidly but bind IgG poorly, whereas other components precipitate strongly (bind IgG) but react poorly with IgE (119). Another study (120) demonstrated 44 antigens by CIE and 18 allergens by CRIE. The extract used in this study was a 10-strain mixture. When the strains used in the extract were investigated individually, they varied in their quantities of the four most important allergens. Other studies demonstrated that disrupted spore antigens did not cross-react with either mycelial or culture filtrate allergens (121). Common allergens occur within the *fumigatus* and *niger* groups, which are allergenically distinct from the *versicolor*, *nidulans*, and *glaucus* groups (99).

Asp f 1 has been cloned and identified as a cytotoxin, mitogillin, which is excreted from the fungus only during growth (122,123). Approximately 50% of *Aspergillus*-sensitive patients react to *Asp f 1* (124). *Asp f 3* is a peroxisomal membrane protein, and *Asp f 5* is a metalloprotease. A combination of *Asp f 1*, *Asp f 3*, and *Asp f 5* has a sensitivity of 97% for diagnosing *Aspergillus* sensitivity (125).

Diagnostic testing for allergic bronchopulmonary aspergillosis (ABPA) may be greatly simplified in the future using recombinant *Aspergillus* allergens. *Asp f 2*, *Asp f 4*, and *Asp f 6* have all been cloned and are associated with ABPA (125,126). *Asp f 3* and *Asp f 5* are secreted proteins that are recognized by patients with *Aspergillus* sensitivity with or without ABPA, but *Asp f 4* and *Asp f 6* are nonsecreted proteins that are only recognized by patients with ABPA (125). A combination of *Asp f 4* and *Asp f 6* yielded positive skin test results in 11 of 12 ABPA patients, but in 0 of 12 patients sensitized to *Aspergillus* without ABPA. Serologic IgE determinations using ImmunoCAPs and a PharmacaciaCAP system with *Asp f 4* and *Asp f 6* also correlated well with ABPA (127).

Penicillium citrinum allergens also have been cloned. *Pen c 1* is a 33-kDa alkaline serine protease with 93% IgE reactivity among patients sensitive to *Penicillium* species (128,129). *Pen c 2* is a vacuolar serine protease (130). *Pen c 3* has 83% sequence homology with *Asp f 3* peroxisomal membrane protein allergen (131). Another allergen is hsp 70 (132).

Sensitivity to spores of the Basidiomycetes is a significant precipitant of allergic disease. Asthma epidemics have been reported in association with elevated Basidiomycetes spore counts (133). Several species have been shown to be allergenic, and extracts from these species show multiple antigens and allergens (134). Up to 20% of asthmatic individuals demonstrate positive skin test results to Basidiomycetes species (135). Only two basidiomycete allergens have been well characterized. *Cop c 1* from *Coprinus comatus* has been cloned, but only 25% of basidiomycete-allergic patients respond (136). *Psi c 2* from *Psilocybe cubensis* mycelia was also cloned and shows some homology with *Schizosaccharomyces pombe* cyclophilin (137).

Candida albicans is the most frequently isolated fungal pathogen in humans; however, its role in allergic disease is relatively minimal. [A possible role of this yeast in allergic disease is best appreciated through studies with asthmatic individuals. In studies with 149 asthmatic patients, 48% were positive for *C. albicans* on skin tests. Of these, 77% had positive inhalation provocation test results, with most demonstrating positive RAST results to *C. albicans* (138).] Two major allergens have been cloned, and one of these has been identified as a subunit of alcohol dehydrogenase (139,140). The other major allergen appears to be enolase, which cross-reacts as noted before. *Candida* also secretes an acid protease, which produces IgE antibodies in 37% of *Candida*-allergic patients (141). Candida sensitivity is also associated with eczema related to infection with the human immunodeficiency virus (142).

Estimating the extent to which a sensitive person's symptoms can be attributed to fungal allergy is a major clinical problem because exposure to fungi, like exposure to house dust mites, is continuous, usually without definite seasonal end points. Fungal spores can be roughly quantified in the air by the use of spore traps. Atmospheric fungal spore counts frequently are 1,000-fold greater than pollen counts (99), and exposure to indoor spores can occur throughout the year (143). This is in contrast to pollens, which have distinct seasons, and to animal dander, for which a definitive history of exposure usually can be obtained. Such a history is sometimes possible for fungal exposure (e.g., raking leaves, or being in a barn with moldy hay), but these exposures are not common for many patients. Some species do show distinctive seasons; nevertheless, during any season, and especially during winter, the number and types of spores a patient inhales on a given day are purely conjectural.

In the natural environment, people are exposed to more than 100 species of airborne or dust-bound microfungi. The variety of fungi is extreme, and dominant types have not been established directly in most areas. The spores produced by fungi vary enormously in size, which makes collection difficult. Moreover, both microscopic evaluation of atmospheric spores and culturing to assess viability are necessary to fully understand the allergenic potential of these organisms. Although most allergenic activity has been associated with the spores, other particles such as mycelial fragments and allergens absorbed onto dust particles may contain relevant activity. Lastly, more than half of the outdoor fungus burden (Ascomycetes and Basidiomycetes) have spores that have not been studied or are practically unobtainable.

Fungi are members of the phylum Thallophyta, plants that lack definite leaf, stem, and root structures. They are separated from the algae in that they do not contain chlorophyll and therefore are saprophytic or parasitic. Almost all allergenic fungi are saprophytes. The mode of spore formation, particularly the sexual spore, is the basis for taxonomic classification of fungi. Many fungi have two names because the sexual and asexual stages initially were described separately. Many fungi produce morphologically different sexual and asexual spores that may become airborne. Thus, describing symptom–exposure relationships becomes difficult. The Deuteromycetes ("fungi imperfecti") are an artificial grouping of asexual fungal stages that includes many fungi of allergenic importance (*Aspergillus*, *Penicillium*, and *Alternaria*). These fungi were considered "imperfect," but are now known to be asexual stages (form genera or form species of Ascomycetes). These fungi reproduce asexually by the differentiation of specialized hyphae called conidiophores, which bear the conidia or asexual spore-forming organs. The various species of these fungi are differentiated morphologically by the conidia. Other classes of fungi also can reproduce asexually by means of conidia. Hyphae are filamentous strands that constitute the fundamental anatomic units of fungi. Yeasts are unicellular and do not form hyphae. The mycelium is a mass of hyphae, and the undifferentiated body of a fungus is called a thallus. One taxonomic scheme follows, with annotations of interest to allergists. Additional resources are provided in the references (17,39,40,99,144).

CLASSES OF ALLERGENIC FUNGI

Oomycetes

This class of fungi is of little allergenic importance, but *Phytophthoria infestans* has been reported to be associated with occupational allergy (17).

Zygomycetes

The sexual forms of Zygomycetes are characterized by thick-walled spinous zygospores; the asexual forms are characterized by sporangia. Spores of this group generally are not prominent in the air, but can be found in abundance in damp basements and around composting vegetation. The order Mucorales includes the allergenic species *Rhizopus nigricans* and *Mucor racemosus*. *Rhizopus nigricans* is the black bread mold whose hyphae are colorless but whose sporangia (visible to the naked eye) are black.

Ascomycetes

The Ascomycetes are the "sac fungi." Their spores are produced in spore sacs called asci. Concentrations of ascospores reaching thousands of particles per cubic meter occur in many areas and are especially numerous during periods of high humidity. Two significant allergenic Ascomycetes are *Saccharomyces cerevisiae*, a yeast, and *Chaetomium indicum*. The former, known as baker's yeast, is seen most commonly in its asexual budding form, but under certain culture conditions it forms hyphae and asci. Skin sensitivity to conidia of a powdery mildew, *Microsphaera alni*, has been reported, but the clinical significance of this is unknown.

The conidial forms of several Ascomycetes may represent the sexual form genera of imperfect fungi. For example, *Leptosphaeria* species are prominent and represent asexual stages of *Alternaria*.

Basidiomycetes

Two major subgroups occur within the class Basidiomycetes. The subclass Homobasidiomycetidae comprises mushrooms, bracket fungi, and puffballs. The spores of these organisms constitute a significant portion of the spores found in the air during nocturnal periods and wet weather. These abundant spores are confirmed to be allergenic (134,145,146) and can provoke bronchoconstriction in sensitive asthmatic subjects (147). Numerous species, including *Pleurotus ostreatus, Cantharellus cibarius, Clavata cyanthiformis, Geaster saccatum, Pisolithus tinctorius, Scleroderma aerolatum, Ganoderma lucidum, Psilocybe cubensis, Agaricus, Armillaria,* and *Hypholoma* species, and *Merulisus lacrymans* ("dry rot") have been identified as allergens.

The Heterobasidiomycetidae include the rusts (Uredinales), smuts (Ustilaginales), and jelly fungi. The Ustilaginales and Uredinales are plant parasites of enormous agricultural importance and may cause allergy where cereal grains are grown or in the vicinity of granaries. Rust spores are encountered primarily by agricultural workers, whereas smut spores can be identified in urban areas surrounded by areas of extensive cultivation. Among the important allergenic species are *Ustilago, Urocystis,* and *Tilletia* species.

Deuteromycetes (Fungi Imperfecti)

Asexual spores (conidia) rather than sexual spores characterize the reproductive mechanism of Deuteromycetes and are the basis for subclassification into the following orders.

Sphaeropsidales

The conidiospores are grouped in spherical or flask-shaped structures called pycnidia. The genus *Phoma* is the only common allergenic fungus in this order. It frequently yields positive skin test results in patients sensitive to *Alternaria.*

Melanoconoiales

The order Melanoconoiales is not of allergenic importance.

Moniliales

The conidiophores are spread over the entire colony. Moniliales is by far the largest and most diverse order of the Deuteromycetes and contains most of the recognized and suspected fungus allergens. Three families account for most of the fungi that cause allergy in humans: Moniliaceae, Dematiaceae, and Tuberculariaceae.

The Moniliaceae are characterized by colorless or light-colored hyphae and conidia; the colonies are usually white, green, or yellow. The genera *Aspergillus* (Fig. 6.16), *Penicillium* (Fig. 6.17), *Botrytis, Monilia* and *Trichoderma* are "moniliaceous molds" associated with allergic disease.

The family Dematiaceae, one of the most important from the standpoint of allergy, is characterized by the production of dark pigment in the conidia and often in the mycelia. It contains the genera *Alternaria* (Fig. 6.18), *Cladosporium (Hormodendrum)* (Fig. 6.19), *Helminthosporium* (Fig. 6.20), *Stemphyllium*

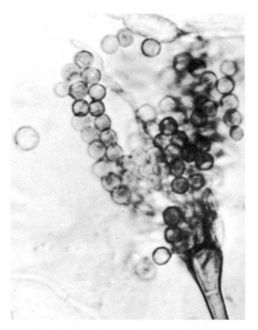

FIG. 6.16. *Aspergillus* species. Average spore diameter is 4 μm. The spores are borne in chains and have connecting collars. [Courtesy of Bayer Allergy Products (formerly Hollister-Stier Labs), Spokane, WA.]

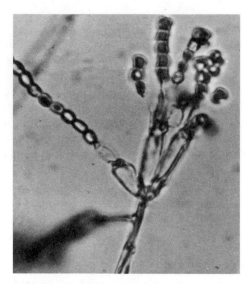

FIG. 6.17. *Penicillium chrysogenum.* Average spore diameter is 2.5 μm. The spores appear in unbranched chains on phialides, the terminal portions of the conidiophores. The phialides and chains of spores resemble a brush. [Courtesy of Bayer Allergy Products (formerly Hollister-Stier Labs), Spokane, WA.]

(Fig. 6.21), *Nigrosporia, Curvularia,* and *Aureobasidium* (*Pullularia*). The last is morphologically similar to the yeasts, and is sometimes classified with them and called the "black" yeast. This group often is described as the "dematiaceous molds."

The Tuberculariaceae produce a sporodochium, a round mass of conidiospores containing macroconidia and microconidia in a slimy substrate. The genera *Fusarium* (Fig. 6.22) and *Epicoccum* (Fig. 6.23) are important allergenic fungi in this family.

The family Cryptococcaceae contains the true yeasts, which do not produce hyphae under known cultural or natural circumstances. Allergenic genera within this family include *Rhodotorula* and *Sporobolomyces*.

This classification and list of genera are not exhaustive, but do represent most of the important allergenic fungi found in environmental surveys. The fungi listed here are a framework on which an individual allergist can build or make deletions, depending on the region or clinical judgment. Most fungal sensitivity is

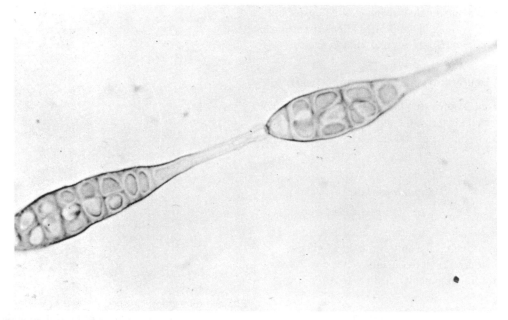

FIG. 6.18. *Alternaria alternata.* Average spore size is 12 × 33 μm. Spores are snowshoe shaped and contain transverse and longitudinal septae with pores. (Courtesy of Schering Corporation, Kenilworth, NJ.)

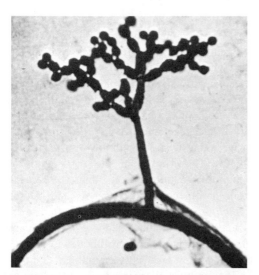

FIG. 6.19. *Cladosporium* species. Average spore size is 4 × 16 μm. Spores occur in chains and have small attaching collars at one end. The first spore buds off from the conidiophore, then the spore itself buds to form a secondary spore. [Courtesy of Bayer Allergy Products (formerly Hollister-Stier Labs), Spokane, WA.]

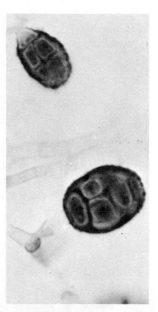

FIG. 6.21. *Stemphyllium* species. The spores superficially resemble those of *Alternaria* but lack the "tail" appendage. Also, they are borne singly rather than in chains. (Courtesy of Schering Corporation, Kenilworth, NJ.)

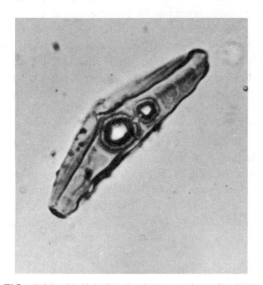

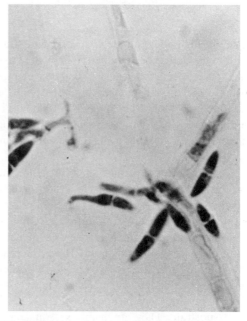

FIG. 6.20. *Helminthosporium* species. Average spore size is 15 × 75 mm. The spores, which occur in the ends of the conidiophores, are large, brownish, and have transverse septae. (Courtesy of Schering Corporation, Kenilworth, NJ.)

FIG. 6.22. *Fusarium vasinfectum.* Average spore size is 4 × 50 μm. The most prevalent spore type is the macrospore, which is sickle shaped and colorless, and contains transverse septae and a point of attachment at one end. [Courtesy of Bayer Allergy Products (formerly Hollister-Stier Labs), Spokane, WA.]

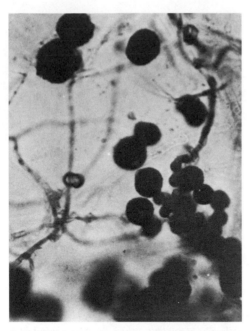

FIG. 6.23. *Epicoccum nigrum.* Average diameter is 20 μm. Large spores are borne singly on the ends of conidiophores. They are yellowish brown and rough, and develop transverse septae when old. [Courtesy of Bayer Allergy Products (formerly Hollister-Stier Labs), Spokane, WA.]

specific for genus, although species and strain differences have been reported. Where more than one species occurs for a genus, allergenic extracts usually are mixed together, as in "*Aspergillus* mixture" or "*Penicillium* mixture." It should be remembered that extracts prepared from fungi are extremely variable in allergenic content and composition.

Certain data concerning the prevalence and ecology of fungi make the list less formidable in practice. With the exception of the Pacific Northwest, *Alternaria* and *Cladosporium* (*Hormodendrum*) are the most numerous genera encountered in most surveys of outdoor air. These fungi are "field fungi" and thrive best on plants in the field and decaying plant parts in the soil. They require a relatively high moisture content (22%–25%) in their substrate. They are mainly seasonal, from spring to late fall, and diminish markedly with the first hard frost. Their spores generally disappear from air samples during the winter months when snow cover is present. *Helminthosporium*

and *Fusarium* are the other common field fungi. These and certain other fungi propagate in the soil, and their spores are released in large numbers when the soil is tilled.

Aspergillus and *Penicillium*, conversely, sometimes are called "storage fungi" because they are common causes of rot in stored grain, fruits, and vegetables. *Aspergillus* in particular thrives on a substrate with low moisture content (12%–16%). These are the two fungi most commonly cultured from houses, especially from basements, crawl spaces, and bedding. *Penicillium* is the green "mildew" often seen on articles stored in basements. *Rhizopus* causes black moldy bread and proliferates in vegetable bins in homes, especially on onions.

The foremost allergenic fungi, based not only on their incidence in atmospheric surveys, but on allergenic skin test reactivity, are *Alternaria, Aspergillus, Cladosporium*, and *Penicillium*. The prevalence of skin test reactivity to fungi in allergic patients is not known but may approach 25% of asthmatics in some surveys (148). Most patients allergic to fungi typically react on skin testing to one or more of these allergens. Many patients also react to other fungi, however, and some to fungi other than these four.

The designations "field" and "storage" fungi or "indoor" and "outdoor" fungi are not precise because exceptions are common in environmental surveys. Moreover, indoor colonization from molds varies with the season, particularly in homes that are not air conditioned (149). During the warmer months, *Alternaria* and *Cladosporium* spores are commonly found indoors, having gained entry into the home through open windows.

In contrast to field and storage fungi, yeasts require a high sugar content in their substrates, which limits their habitat. Certain leaves, pasture grasses, and flowers exude a sugary fluid that is a carbon source for the nonfermentative yeasts such as *Aureobasidium* (*Pullularia*) and *Rhodotorula*. Hundreds of millions of yeast colonies may be obtained per gram of leaf tissue. Berries and fruit also are commonly colonized. The soil is not a good habitat for yeasts unless it is in the vicinity of fruit trees. Yeasts are often cultured indoors, however.

The relationship of weather to spore dissemination is clinically important, because the symptoms of patients with respiratory allergy are often worse in damp or rainy weather. This has been attributed by some to an increase in the "fungal spore count." Absolute fungal spore counts decrease during and after a rainstorm because some spores, like pollen grains, are washed out or made less buoyant. Most of the common allergenic fungi, such as *Aspergillus* and *Cladosporium*, are of the dry spore type, the spores being released by the wind during dry periods. Alternatively, some so-called "wet weather spores," including certain yeasts such as *Aureobasidium, Trichoderma*, and *Phoma* and biologically dispersed ascospores, increase. Although these spores are loosened during wet periods and are dispersed by rain droplets, it is unlikely that they are responsible for the mass symptoms that occur during inclement weather. High spore counts are found in clouds and mist, and it is reasonable to attribute some of the symptoms encountered during long periods of high humidity to fungal allergy. Recall that other allergens, such as the house dust mite, also propagate in conditions of high humidity. Snow cover obliterates the outdoor fungal spore count, but the conditions subsequent to thawing predispose to fungal growth and propagation.

The relationship of house plants to indoor fungal exposure has been studied. Contrary to common belief, indoor plantings are associated with only a slight increase in the numbers of spores from such genera as *Cladosporium, Penicillium, Alternaria,* and *Epicoccum*. Greenhouses do show an increased number of spores, particularly when plants are agitated by watering or fanning (150). Similar studies in laboratory animal care units fail to show excessive numbers of fungal spores (151). Several reviews of fungal sensitivity and the classification of fungi are available (107,133,134,152).

HOUSE DUST AND DUST MITES

House dust has been recognized as an allergen for many centuries. In 1921, Kern (153) demonstrated that house dust extracts produced positive skin test results in many patients with asthma. In 1964, Voorhorst and co-workers reexamined and subsequently expanded the knowledge of the relationships among house dust, mites, and human allergic disorders (154). These Dutch workers are to be credited with sparking the worldwide interest in mites as allergens. Miyamoto and associates in Japan (155–159) corroborated and expanded the previous work. They discovered that the potency of house dust allergen is related to the number of mites in the dust. Skin tests, RASTs, and bronchoprovocation performed with extracts from pure cultures of mites (*Dermatophagoides pteronyssinus* and *Dermatophagoides farinae*) correlated well with the results obtained using house dust extracts. The equivalent potency of mite extracts was 10 to 100 times that of whole dust. Mites are now accepted as the major source of allergens in house dust. It has been reported that exposure to house dust mite allergen in early childhood is an important determinant in the development of asthma (160).

Mites are a subclass of arachnids that constitute several orders of Acarina. They are sightless, small (0.33 mm long), eight-legged animals. They may be identified microscopically using a low-power lens or a stereoscope. The family Pyroglyphidae contains most of the mites important in house dust allergy, but Tyroglyphidae are important in storage mite sensitivity. Mites found in houses are called domestic mites, but the term *house dust mite* is reserved for the Pyroglyphidae family of mites (161). These are free-living organisms whose natural food sources include human skin scales, fungi, and other high-protein substances in the environment. They can be cultured using human skin shavings, dry dog food, or daphnia as substrates, and can be separated from the culture medium by flotation. Mites also can be separated from dust samples by flotation in saturated salt solution, retained by a sieve with 45 μm openings, and differentiated from other retained material by crystal violet staining (162). The mites do not stain and are seen as white against a purple background.

The numerically dominant mite in European homes is *Dermatophagoides pteronyssinus*; in North American homes *Dermatophagoides farinae* predominates. There are significant overlaps, however (163,164). Other house dust mite species are *Dermatophagoides microceras*,

Euroglyphus maynei, and the tropical *Blomia tropicalis* (161,165). Other groups of mites, including *Acarus siro*, *Tyrophagus putresentiae*, *Lepidoglyphus* (*Glycyphagus*) *domesticus*, and *Lepidoglyphus destructor*, which are referred to as "storage mites," are mainly pests of stored grain, but have caused barn allergy in farm workers (166) and occasionally are associated with dust allergy in homes (167). Some of the 210 residents of London who underwent skin testing for sensitivity to a variety of mites showed strong reactions to *Acarus siro*, *Tyrophagus putresentiae*, *Lepidoglyphus destructor*, and *Lepidoglyphus domesticus*. There was some correlation between reactions to these various storage mites, but none to *Dermatophagoides pteronyssinus*. The predisposing factors for developing allergic reactions to storage mites were occupation, damp homes, and possibly the type of bedding used for household pets (168). Spider mites (*Paronychus ulmi* and *Tetranychus urticae*) have been implicated in occupational allergy among apple farmers, and citrus red mite (*Panonychus citri*) among citrus farmers (169,170).

Seasonal and geographic variation in the number of house dust mites in house dust have been observed. In North America, sharp peaks of mite growth have been observed in the summer months (165). The major factors governing mite propagation are temperature and, particularly, humidity. The key determinant for excessive mite growth seems to be an indoor absolute humidity of approximately 7 g/kg. This is equivalent to a relative humidity of 60% at 21°C (70°F) and 75% at 16°C (60°F) (165). When the relative humidity falls below 40% to 50%, mites are unable to survive more than 11 days at temperatures above 25°C (77°F), because increased transpiration of water leads to dehydration (162). The larval form (protonymph) of *Dermatophagoides farinae*, however, may survive the heating season because it is relatively resistant to desiccation. Protonymphs are the likely source of resurgence of mites in the spring. The life cycle from egg to adult is 30 days at 25°C and up to 110 days at 20°C.

Low numbers of mites are found in dust recovered from homes or other buildings at high altitude (164). At higher altitudes, the absolute humidity of the outdoor air decreases sharply, reducing indoor humidity and therefore mite growth. Environmental conditions influence not only mite growth but also the species of mites found. *Dermatophagoides farinae* tend to predominate where there are prolonged periods of dry weather (i.e., more than 3 months with a mean outdoor absolute humidity of <6 g/kg). In humid conditions, *Dermatophagoides pteronyssinus* usually predominates. *Euroglyphus maynei* has been found as a predominant species in occasional homes in damp conditions. *Blomia tropicalis* is important in the southeastern United States (e.g., Florida) as well as in Central and South America.

Mattress dust usually contains the highest concentration of mites compared with dust from rugs, clothing, closets, automobiles, and other places. Most mites are recovered from areas of the home that are occupied most commonly, including rugs, bedding, and furniture. Meticulous housekeeping or the presence of household pets does not necessarily influence the mite load. As many as 18,875 mites per gram of dust have been recovered. In Ohio, an annual average heavy density was considered 481 ± 190 mites per gram of dust; a low density was 41 ± 25 mites per gram of dust (162). The fecal particles of mites contain most of the allergenic activity in mite extracts (171). Both mite body and feces extracts, however, contain multiple antigens and allergens. A high percentage of dust mite–sensitive patients are skin test positive to both *Dermatophagoides farinae* and *Dermatophagoides pteronyssinus*. Often, in homes, one or more species may be prevalent. Studies comparing cross-reactivity by CRIE and CIE demonstrate that *D. farinae* and *D. pteronyssinus* body extracts contain numerous cross-reacting antigens and allergens. Analyses of feces extracts from the two species also demonstrate cross-reactivity. Of significance is the fact that body and fecal extracts of both species contain unique, species-specific antigens and allergens (172).

The group I allergens are small proteins recognized by most mite-sensitive individuals. These allergens are found in whole-body, fecal, and gut extracts from the various mite species. Examples of group I allergens include *Der p 1*, *Der f 1*,

Der m 1, and *Eur m 1*. Amino acid sequences of these allergens reveal 80% to 85% homology between the mite species, with moderate levels of antigenic cross-reactivity measured by IgE antibodies (2). Using sequence data, the group I allergens have tentatively been identified as members of the cysteine protease family, represented in numerous mammalian and plant species (173). Interestingly, peptides from plant cysteine proteases are potent stimulators of histamine release in allergen-stimulated human basophils (174). The enzymatic activity of this allergen may have a role in the development of asthma (175). It disrupts epithelial tight junctions in human bronchial epithelial lines, possibly explaining transepithelial delivery of antigen (176). *Der p 1* can also inactivate *in vitro* alpha 1-antitrypsin (177). The enzymatic activity of *Der p 1* has been shown to cleave the low-affinity IgE FcR CD23 from human B cells, which may augment IgE synthesis (178,179). This enzyme also cleaves CD25 from T cells favoring a Th2 type of response (180). In a mouse model, inhibition of the *Der p 1* caused decreased IgE production (181).

The group II allergens include *Der p 2* and *Der f 2*. These allergens differ from the group I members in that they are resistant to denaturing by heat and pH variations. Both allergens have been cloned and reveal over 85% sequence homology (182). The biologic function of these proteins remains uncertain.

The group III allergens, *Der p 3* and *Der f 3*, are found primarily in fecal material from the house dust mites. *Der p 3* has been cloned (183), and enzymatic studies have demonstrated serine protease activities consistent with trypsin (184) and N-terminal homology similar to *Der f 3*. In groups VI and IX, *Der p 6*, *Der f 6*, and *Der p 9* have been described as serine proteases with activity similar to chymotrypsin (185–187).

The group IV allergens Der p 4 and Eur m 4 have been cloned and identified as alpha-amylases (188). *Der p 5* and *Der p 7* have been cloned and show some cross-reactivity with each other, but their biologic function is unknown (189).

Several monoclonal antibodies have been developed against particular allergens, which have enhanced the investigator's ability to purify these antigens and determine their concentration in the atmosphere. Studies from mite feces show that 90% to 95% of the allergen content is *Der p 1*. The fecal particles have a mean diameter of 24 μm (range, 10–40 μm). They are spherical and are surrounded by a peritrophic membrane. The *Der p 1* content is about 0.1 ng per fecal particle (171). The high concentration of allergen is thought to be clinically significant in that it could cause intense local inflammatory response when inhaled into the respiratory mucosa.

In the United Kingdom, 10% of the population and 90% of allergic asthmatics have positive skin test results to house dust mite extracts. As many as 75% of the serum antibodies to mites are directed against the *Der p 1* allergen (171). In some allergic subjects, IgE antibody to *Der p 1* constitutes 9% to 21% of the total IgE, with a mean value of 12% (190). Removal of allergic children from environmental exposure to house dust mite antigen reduced both specific IgE antibodies to *Dermatophagoides pteronyssinus* and total IgE levels (164). However, whether dust mite control measures have a significant clinical effect on asthma remains a point of controversy (191–194).

In summary, the major allergens in house dust are contained in the fecal particles and bodies of mites that inhabit the dust. Because of the heterogeneous composition of crude house dust mixtures, patients should be tested and treated with house dust mite extracts rather than with crude house dust materials.

EPITHELIAL AND OTHER ANIMAL ALLERGENS

The category of animal allergens includes animal emanations: hair, dander, feathers, saliva, and urine. Because domestic animals are widespread in our society and some of their emanations are potent allergens, the topic is important for the allergist. Occupational exposure of farmers, veterinarians, and laboratory workers has economic importance. Social and family interactions may be strained severely when one person becomes allergic to a beloved family pet. The allergist often is called on to solve these problems.

Hair itself is not an important allergen because it is not buoyant or water soluble. Water-soluble proteins of epidermal or salivary origin that are attached to the hair are important allergens, however. *Dander* is a term used to describe desquamated epithelium. Desquamation is a continuous process for all animals, and the dander materials contain many water-soluble proteins that are highly antigenic and allergenic. Saliva also is rich in proteins such as secretory IgA and enzymes. People commonly develop local urticaria at the sites where they have been licked by a cat or dog or where they have been scratched by claws or teeth. Rodents excrete significant amounts of allergenic protein in their urine. All of these substances become part of the amorphous particulate matter of the air and are responsible for allergic morbidity.

Cats seemingly produce the most dramatic symptoms in sensitive individuals, particularly in those who are exposed intermittently. Whether this is caused by the concentration of cat allergens in the environs or by the potency of the allergens is unknown. Studies with cat pelts have disclosed a substance called *Fel d 1* that appears to be the major allergen, recognized by over 80% of cat-sensitive individuals (195). *Fel d 1* is produced mainly in cat saliva, but is also in the sebaceous glands of the skin, the sublingual glands, and even in the brain (196,197). The *Fel d 1* molecule has been cloned. There is still controversy over the biologic activity of *Fel d 1*.

Fel d 1 may be detected in the urine of male cats but not of female cats. Allergens other than *Fel d 1* in some sensitive individuals also have been detected in cat serum and urine, but these are minor allergens (198). Studies with individual cats show that some cats are high producers of allergen and others are not. Moreover, the rate of allergen production of individual cats varies from hour to hour. Male cats generally produce greater amounts of allergen than females. These factors may explain why some patients are more allergic to certain cats than to others (196). In addition, there does not appear to be any seasonal variation in *Fel d 1* production.

Air sampling in rooms occupied by cats has shown that the amount of *Fel d 1* allergen required to cause a 20% decrease in forced ex-

piratory volume in 1 second (FEV$_1$) on pulmonary function testing is comparable with the amounts required in conventional bronchoprovocation testings (approximately 0.09 μg/mL). Morphologic room sampling shows abundant squamous cell fragments smaller than 5 μm, enabling these fragments to reach small bronchioles and alveoli (199). This small particle size also explains why cat allergen can remain airborne in undisturbed conditions for extended periods.

Serial dust samples collected in the study of 15 homes after removal of the family cats were analyzed for *Fel d 1*. Baseline amounts of antigen ranged from 8 to 437 FDA units/gram of dust (median, 61 U/g). After removing the cats, the levels decreased to those of control homes in 20 to 24 weeks. However, significant differences occurred in the rate of decline of *Fel d 1* among homes. It may therefore be prudent to advise patients that it might take up to 6 months after removal of a cat for the bulk of the cat allergens to disappear from the home (200).

Dog allergens have been identified in dander, saliva, urine, and serum, but elegant studies like the ones described for cats have not been published. The major dog allergen, *Can f 1*, has been described and can be assayed, although most skin tests and RASTs use dander as the basis of diagnosing allergy to dogs. Using RAST inhibition, dog sera had little effect on the binding of dog dander (201). In the same experiments, using dander from 13 breeds of dogs and sera of 16 patients with documented dog allergy, the various sera showed significant breed specificity. Dander from all breeds was allergenic, including poodle. However, differences between breeds occur in the number and amount of antigens. More recently *Can f 1* and *Can f 2* have been cloned and described as lipocalins, small ligand binding proteins (202). About 30% of dog allergic patients show IgE reactivity to albumin. These patients have a high cross-reactivity with cat and other animal albumins (203). There is individual variation in the positivity of skin test results to different breeds, but in one study these variations did not correlate with the patient's perception of specific breed allergy (204). The fact that dogs tend to spend more time outdoors and are bathed more frequently may explain their decreased importance as an allergen source relative to cats.

Most patients who are demonstrably sensitive to dander are also sensitive to other perennial allergens. This complicates the determination of which allergen is responsible for their symptoms. The recommendation to eliminate a pet from a home environment places the clinician in a difficult position. Patients do not readily accept the proposition that their pet may be the cause of their allergic problem, even in light of positive skin test results. Positive bronchial provocation might be supportive, but results are not conclusive. Cat allergen is known to persist in the home for up to 24 weeks after removal of the pet, so a trial separation of the patient away from the home environment for several weeks to months is probably the best prognostic indicator at this time.

Horses resemble cats in the explosive symptoms that may occur on exposure to their dander, but this clinical situation is less common and less difficult to manage, primarily because of the absence of horse dander in the home. Horse hair has been used in the manufacture of some mattresses, furniture, and rug pads, but again, the allergic potential of hair does not approach that of dander. Some antigens are common to horse dander and serum, creating the potential for a serious problem in patients when horse serum (such as an antivenom) may be urgently needed. Tetanus antitoxin currently is available as a human antiserum. Two horse allergens have been identified so far. *Equ c 1* and *Equ c 2* have been cloned and both described as members of the lipocalin family (205,206).

Allergy to cows, goats, and sheep usually is occupational. Rabbits and small rodents such as gerbils, hamsters, guinea pigs, rats, and mice are common household pets, and their dander may induce severe reactions on skin prick testing. Significant skin test reactivity to the dander of rats and mice in persons whose homes are infested with these rodents also may be seen.

Allergic symptoms in laboratory workers exposed to immune allergens have promoted several studies on the nature of these allergens (207,208). In mouse-sensitive subjects, a major urinary protein, *Mus m 1*, appears to be the primary allergen. It is the most prominent member of a family of allergenic murine proteins collectively known as the major urinary proteins (209). The major urinary proteins are also lipocalins and have sequence homology with *Can f 2* (202). *Mus m 1* protein is synthesized in the liver, and its synthesis is stimulated by androgen, accounting for fourfold higher concentrations in male mice than in females. The urine from both sexes of mice contains 10 times more of this allergen than does the serum. *Mus m 1* is also formed in the sebaceous, parotid, and lacrimal glands, which probably explains the small quantities detected in pelt extract. The potency of this allergen in susceptible individuals was illustrated by the finding that intermittent exposure to these allergens of at least 10 days a year produced the same level of allergy in terms of IgE-related tests as daily exposure (207).

Rats and other small mammals commonly produce respiratory symptoms in laboratory workers. The airborne level of rat allergens can be high—up to 100 $\mu g/m^3$. Furthermore, urinary allergens are carried in small particles about 7 μm in diameter. Workers with intense exposure to rats develop IgG antibodies to rat urinary protein, but in the absence of IgE to these proteins, these subjects are asymptomatic. The presence of IgE antibodies to rat urinary proteins in laboratory workers usually is associated with asthma or rhinitis. Both atopic and nonatopic individuals are able to make the specific IgE (210). The two predominant rat urinary allergens are termed *Rat n 1* and *Rat n 2*. Air sampling techniques for rat allergens have reported that feeding and cleaning produce the highest airborne concentrations of the prealbumin protein *Rat n 1* (21 ng/m^3), injection and handling produce exposure to somewhat less allergen, and surgery and killing rats produce only 3.4 ng/m^3. Low concentrations of rat allergens were found outside of the handling rooms (211). Of the three layers of rat pelt, the outermost fur was most allergenic, probably because of contamination with body fluids. In one study, rat sebaceous glands were not found to be the source of allergenic secretions (212), but other studies have reported a high-molecular-weight protein (over 200 kDa), which was believed to originate from rat sebaceous glands

(213). *Rat n 2* has been definitively demonstrated in the liver, lacrimal, and salivary glands (214).

The question has been raised whether laboratory workers who deal with allergenic rodents should be screened for atopy before employment. Although it was thought initially that workers with seasonal allergic rhinitis are more likely to become allergic to laboratory animals (215), more recent studies conclude that such screening is not warranted because nonatopic individuals may become allergic when exposed to sufficient allergen loads (210,216). Of course a screening test for existing specific animal allergens may be useful, particularly if the worker has a choice of working with different animal species.

MISCELLANEOUS ALLERGENS

Included in this category of miscellaneous allergens are substances that have been shown to be allergenic in selected cases or occupations and some that may be of more general importance but are not yet accepted as such by the allergy community.

Insects

Insects were recognized as inhalant allergens long before mites (which are arachnids, not insects) came to the foreground. Cockroaches have been described as allergens based on skin test data in allergic persons (217). Kang and associates (218) extended this work to include RASTs and bronchoprovocation studies to further implicate cockroach-associated materials as asthmagenic. Asthmatics with positive skin-prick test results to cockroach extracts have been reported to have higher total serum IgE levels than their allergic counterparts with negative skin test results. Bronchoprovocation caused a transient peripheral eosinophilia in those who reacted positively.

Of the over 50 species of cockroaches described, only 8 are regarded as "indoor" pests. Allergens from the two most common species, *Blattella germanica* and *Periplanta americana*, have been the most studied. Immunoelectrophoretic studies of roach allergens have disclosed multiple antigens, with most allergens residing in the whole-body and cast-skin fractions. Feces and egg casings were less allergenic (219). Roach hemolymph also may be allergenic (220). Recombinant clones have been developed for many of the allergens, and their function has been defined. *Per a 1* and *Bla g 1* are cross-reactive and have sequence homology with a mosquito digestive protein (221). *Bla g 2* shows sequence homology to an aspartic protease (222). *Per a 3* has been defined and may have some cross-reactivity with a German cockroach allergen (223). *Bla g 4* is a lipocalin (224). *Bla g 5* is a glutathione-S-transferase (225). In addition, a tropomyosin has been identified as an allergen from *Periplanta americana*, with sequence homology to dust mite and shrimp tropomyosins (226).

Outdoor insects such as mayfly and caddis fly have been studied clinically and immunologically (227). These insects have an aquatic larval stage and therefore are found around large bodies of water such as the Great Lakes, particularly Lake Erie. These flies were reported to cause significant respiratory allergy in the summer months, but their numbers have declined, probably because of pollution of the lakes. Japanese investigators reported that 50% of asthmatics show sensitivity to the silkworm moth (*Bombyx mori*) caused by antigens found in the wings. These wing allergens cross-react almost completely on RAST inhibition with butterfly allergens, but not at all with mites (228). Finished silk products are not thought to be allergenic, but contamination of some products, such as silk-filled bed quilts, with waste products of *B. mori* and the *Antheraea pernyi* can cause asthma and rhinitis.

In the Sudan, during certain seasons, respiratory allergy has been reported from inhalation of allergens of the "green nimmiti midge." These are chironomids, nonbiting members of the order Diptera (229). Studies of these chironomid antigens by RAST show the allergenic activity of the larvae to be in the hemoglobin molecule (230). Studies on this allergen from *Chironomus thummi* have identified regions of IgE binding and T-cell epitopes (231).

Outdoor air sampling in Minnesota has disclosed allergens for the moth *Pseudaletia unipuncta* (Haworth). The levels of this moth antigen peaked in June and again in August to September, and the allergen levels were comparable with those of pollen and mold allergens. Furthermore, 45% of patients with positive skin test results to common aeroallergens had positive reactions to whole-body insect extracts. Of 120 patients with ragweed sensitivity, 5% had elevated specific IgE to moths. Hence, Lepidoptera may be considered seasonal allergens (232).

Occupational exposure to insects may cause respiratory allergy. Chironomid larvae are used as fish food, resulting in symptoms among workers in their production, laboratory personnel, and hobbyists (231). Similar symptoms, all documented with RAST and inhalation challenge, have been reported in workers handling crickets used for frog food (233) and mealworms (*Tenebrio molitor*) used as fishing bait (234). Asthma and rhinitis occur in some bee keepers and in workers involved in honey production because of inhalation of honeybee body components. In these individuals, RAST inhibition is not achieved with venom extract (235). Occupational allergy has been reported in laboratory workers dealing with locusts (236). In these workers, as in the case of murine allergen-sensitive laboratory workers, atopy was not a prerequisite for sensitization. The primary locust allergen is the peritrophic membrane that surrounds food particles when they pass through the midgut and eventually become feces. The common housefly (*Musca domestica*) also has been reported as a cause of occupational allergy in laboratory workers (237), as has the grain beetle (*Alphitobius diaperinus*). Larval, pupal, and adult stages of the life cycle of this beetle all are capable of inducing allergy, but pupal extract contains the most significant allergens (238).

Hypersensitivity to the salivary secretions of biting insects exists. Local immediate and delayed allergy to the bites of mosquitoes, fleas (papular urticaria), sand flies, deer flies, horse flies, and tsetse flies has been reported. Other case reports have described generalized reactions to multiple bites (deer fly) consisting of fever, malaise, and hypotension associated with antibodies to the offending insect. Experimental sensitization in humans with flea bites results first in the induction of delayed, and then in immediate, wheal-and-flare hypersensitivity on skin testing.

Hypersensitivity to the venom of stinging insects (Hymenoptera) is the subject of another chapter and is not discussed here.

Seeds

Seeds may be important causes of asthma and rhinitis. Cottonseed and flaxseed are exceptionally potent antigens and should be used for skin testing only by the epicutaneous method. Deaths have been reported from intradermal tests of both substances. Extreme caution should be used in skin testing.

Cottonseed is the seed of the cotton plant. After extracting the oil, which is not allergenic, the seed is ground into meal, which may be used for animal feeds or fertilizer. Cottonseed meal and flour also are used in the baking industry for certain cakes, cookies, and pan-greasing compounds. Cotton linters are the short cotton fibers that adhere to the seeds after the cotton is ginned. These are separated and used for stuffing mattresses and furniture. Enough of the water-soluble cottonseed allergen adheres to these linters to render them allergenic (239). Several cases of angioedema, urticaria, or anaphylaxis have been reported in individuals who have eaten whole-grain bread or candy containing cottonseed meal (240,241).

Flaxseed (linseed) has the same properties as cottonseed and has many of the same general uses in industry and agriculture. Additional uses are in hair preparations, poultices, electric wire insulation, and the tough backing material used in the manufacture of rugs. Linseed oil is a common household product and is found in furniture polish and printer's ink. In these forms, it produces contact rather than inhalant allergy.

Coffee bean allergy is largely confined to those who handle the green beans commercially, including longshoremen who unload the sacks of beans from ships. Chlorogenic acid has been considered an allergen in green coffee beans, castor beans, and oranges. It is a simple chemical that was thought to act as a hapten. Its importance is questionable, however, because it is destroyed by roasting and thus cannot account for allergy from drinking coffee. Castor bean (*Ricinus communis*) allergy is mainly from the pulp and hull that remain after castor oil is pressed from the bean. This castor pomace is ground into a meal that is used for fertilizer. Thus, castor bean allergy also is largely occupational. Low-molecular-weight protein fractions have been isolated, as well as a toxic substance, ricin, which is not allergenic. Castor bean allergy also may occur in neighborhoods adjacent to processing plants. Asthma and rhinitis have been reported from the protein residual in the ambient air. A study from Marseilles, France, reports the incidence of castor bean allergy to be the same in atopic and nonatopic individuals (242). Three allergenic castor bean proteins have been identified by protein electrophoresis. One of these three, *Ric c 1*, one of the "2S albumins" or storage proteins of the castor bean, has homology to both rice allergens and mustard seed allergens (243,244). The 2S albumins represent one of two common storage proteins found in a variety of seeds, including sunflower seeds, Brazil nuts, and rapeseeds. Like other sensitizing allergenic proteins, these have low molecular weights, are highly soluble in water, and generally have no toxicity for nonallergic persons (245).

Soybean allergy may be more generalized and prevalent because of the increased use of soy flour and meal in commonly encountered products. In addition to use as animal feed, soy products are used for infant formula, bakery goods, Chinese cooking, cereals, fillers in meat and candy products, and in certain topical dermatologic preparations. Occupational asthma caused by soybean flour used as a protein expander in frozen meat patties has been reported. Soybean protein consists of a globulin fraction (85%) and a whey fraction. Nine proteins bound to IgE by immunoblotting have been recognized by an allergic patient's serum (246). Asthma epidemics have occurred in Barcelona, Spain, in association with unloading soybeans from ships. Case studies of those affected show a high incidence of IgE antibodies to soybean allergens. Subsequent investigations have shown that the major allergens are glycoproteins found in the hulls

and dust, with molecular sizes less than 14 kDa (247–249).

OTHER PLANT AND ANIMAL ALLERGENS

Glues and gums are occasional causes of human allergy. Impure gelatin is the adhesive obtained from the bones and hides of terrestrial animals and fish bones. Other natural glues are made from casein, rubber, and gum arabic. Synthetic adhesives recently have minimized the glue allergy problem, although the amine hardeners used in the manufacture of epoxies have caused asthma and rhinitis in factory workers. In addition to gum arabic, other vegetable gums (acacia, chicle, karaya, and tragacanth) have been reported to cause allergy by inhalation or ingestion. These are used in candies, chewing gum, baked goods, salad dressings, laxatives, and dentifrices. They also are used as excipients in medications. Guar gum is a vegetable gum that recently has been shown to induce IgE-mediated asthma. This gum is used in the carpet industry and affects about 2% of workers in carpet-manufacturing plants. The gum is used to fix colors to carpeting. It is also used in ice cream and salad dressings and as a hardener in the manufacture of tablets in the pharmaceutical industry. Guar gum is obtained from *Cyanopsis tetragonoolobus*, a vegetable grown in India (250).

In hair-setting preparations, gums have been largely replaced by polyvinylpyrrolidine, which is not allergenic. Parenthetically, most cases of chronic pulmonary disease attributed to "hair spray allergy" or "hair spray thesaurosis" have turned out to be sarcoidosis, with no basis for attributing the cause to hair spray.

Inhalation of soap-bark dust has caused occupational asthma. This wood dust is a product of the Quillaja tree and is used in the manufacture of saponin, a surface-reducing agent. Soap-bark is chemically related to acacia and tragacanth, and these gums showed cross-reactivity in the soap-bark RAST (251).

Enzymes used in laundry detergents to enhance cleaning ability may sensitize both the workers where the product is made and the consumer who uses it (252). The enzyme subtilisin (or subtilin) is proteolytic and is derived from *Bacillus subtilis*, where it plays a role in sporulation. It may produce rhinitis, conjunctivitis, and asthma, associated with precipitating antibodies and Arthus-type reactions on skin testing. Many cases reported did not involve atopic individuals. Enzyme-containing detergents currently are not commonly used because of their sensitizing potential. Other enzymes, cellulase and macerozyme, are used to digest cell wall structures of plants. Laboratory workers have been shown to develop IgE-mediated symptoms from inhaling these enzymes (253). Papain, a cysteine protease, is obtained from the fruit of the papaya tree. It is used as a meat tenderizer, clearing agent in the production of beer, contact lens cleaner, and component of some tooth powders, laxatives, and skin lotions. Asthma has been induced by inhalation of papain, and antipapain IgE and IgG antibodies have been demonstrated in a worker in a meat tenderizer factory. In this case, the IgE-RAST result was not positive until after the other classes of immunoglobulins had been absorbed from the sera (254).

Grain mill dust and baker's flour have long been recognized as causes of occupational asthma. Positive skin test results to extracts of grain mill dust often are seen in patients who have never worked in granaries. It is generally agreed that allergens are responsible for the symptoms resulting from inhaling these substances, but it is not known if these allergens are primarily from the grains themselves or from organisms that infest them, such as molds, mites, or weevils. Enzymes have been implicated in baker's asthma. α-Amylase from *Aspergillus oryzae* (*Asp o 2*) and xylanase from *Apergillus niger* are two enzymes that are used together to increase bread volume. Bakers can have IgE reactions to both of these as well as several other *Aspergillus niger* enzymes (255,256). Flours also can produce reactions separate from the enzymes. Wheat flour (64%), rye flour (52%), and soybean flour (25%) were all more common than α-amylase in a series of bakers with workplace-related respiratory symptoms (257).

Garlic has caused asthma by inhalation (258) and ingestion (259). Both cases were documented immunologically, and one was documented by inhalation challenge. In one case (259), the capacities of onion and asparagus, other members of the Liliacee family, to inhibit the garlic RAST were two and one half to four times higher than the homologous garlic extract.

INDUSTRIAL AND OCCUPATIONAL CHEMICALS AND AIR POLLUTANTS

The isocyanates are used in the manufacture of polyurethane and are often found in the paint and printing industries. Isocyanates are the most common cause of occupational asthma in the world. Toluene diisocyanate causes asthma in some workers (5%–10%) in the plastics and electronic industries, but it does not affect members of the general public who use polyurethane. The mechanism of toluene diisocyanate asthma has been studied extensively. There is some evidence for an immune reaction, but only a proportion of people have specific immune responses (260). Other isocyanates have been associated with pulmonary syndromes of both the immediate and hypersensitivity pneumonitis types. Diphenylmethane diisocyanate is a compound in which both IgE and IgG antibodies have been shown by the polystyrene-tube radioimmunoassay (261). Hexamethylene diisocyanate in a patient with alveolitis and asthma was associated with IgG antibodies but not IgE antibodies by ammonium sulfate precipitation and an ELISA (262). All of these immunoassays were performed using human serum albumin (HSA) conjugates of the various isocyanate compounds, which are necessary for antigenic recognition. The specificity, at least for IgE antibodies, lies with both the hapten and specific portions of the carrier protein (263).

Anhydrides are commonly used in the production of resins, varnishes, and adhesives. They are simple compounds that act as haptens. Trimellitic anhydride (TMA), phthalic anhydride, and maleic anhydride can all be conjugated to HSA. IgE antibodies to TMA-HSA have been demonstrated by Prausnitz-Küstner test reactions in monkeys (264). Antibodies to the IgE, IgG, and IgA classes have been identified using the technique of solid-phase radioimmunoassay (265). TMA asthma is associated with IgE, and a late respiratory response similar to symptoms of hypersensitivity pneumonitis correlates with IgG and total antibody measured by ammonium sulfate precipitation. IgA antibody to TMA-HSA is detectable in all workers with high exposure and cannot be used to discriminate those with and without symptoms (266). A nonallergic, irritating reaction to TMA also may occur. In addition, a pulmonary disease–anemia syndrome, with an immunologic basis, has been described after TMA exposure (264). Tetrachlorophthalic anhydride is a chemical substance that produces immediate and late asthmatic reactions in a small percentage (<2%) of exposed workers. Conjugated with HSA, positive skin-prick test and RAST results were obtained in the affected workers. Cigarette smoking rather than a history of atopy appeared to be the predisposing factor (267).

Numerous other chemical and biologic materials, mainly industrial or occupational, have been implicated more recently in human asthma. It is important from practical and heuristic viewpoints to determine if the mechanisms of asthma are caused by IgE mediation, nonspecific mediator release, or irritating phenomena that are thought to act by nociceptive reflex parasympathetic stimulation. Methods used to study suspected substances include epidemiologic data, bronchoprovocation, and the ability to block bronchoprovocation by disodium cromoglycate or atropine, as well as attempts to identify antigen-specific IgE or IgG by techniques previously described. Detailed reviews have been published (268–271). Occupational asthma is reviewed in more detail elsewhere in this text.

Some examples of inhalants to which reactions are thought to be immunologically mediated are salts of platinum (269), chrome, and nickel (272). Reactions occur mainly in areas where the metals are refined or used in plating. Wood dusts, notably from western red cedar, may cause asthma in wood workers. Plicatic acid is thought to be the offending component of this wood. Asthma occurs in 5% of sawmill workers and carpenters who handle western cedar. IgE antibodies to conjugates of plicatic acid and HSA are found in 40% of symptomatic workers, but nonspecific bronchial hyperreactivity is the most constant feature of the syndrome (273). Plicatic

acid is able to activate complement and generate chemotactic activity from pooled human serum, but the role of this mechanism, if any, in red cedar asthma has not been determined (274). Only 50% of those affected eventually recover after terminating exposure to plicatic acid. Hog trypsin, used in the manufacture of plastic resins, and psyllium, a bulk laxative, may be causes of occupational asthma. The latter is related to the weed plantain.

Other examples of occupational asthma occur among snow crab processing workers and individuals who use solder. In the latter case, colophony, a component of flux, is the asthmagenic material (275).

Asthma exacerbated by direct irritation of the bronchi is common in clinical practice. Odors from perfumes and colognes, vapors from petroleum products and organic solvents, and fumes from tobacco and cooking oils cause coughing and wheezing in many patients. Metabisulfites, sulfiting agents used as preservatives agents used as preservatives and clearing agents, may act as a nonspecific irritant (276).

Meat wrapper's asthma is another occupational disorder caused by inhaling the fumes of polyvinyl chloride. The fumes are created when polyvinyl chloride is cut with a hot wire in the process of wrapping cuts of meat.

Air pollution appears to have an impact on asthma and rhinitis. Multiple epidemiologic studies have demonstrated a correlation between levels of common outdoor air pollutants and hospital admissions or emergency room visits (277,278). However, these epidemiologic studies are limited by confounding factors, including air temperature and levels of other outdoor aeroallergens. For this reason, experiments also have been performed under controlled conditions involving short exposures to individual pollutants.

The effects of ozone on lung function have been investigated extensively. Ozone is generated by the action of ultraviolet light on precursor pollutants from such sources as automobiles and power plants. Ozone causes decreased FEV_1 and forced vital capacity as well as increases in bronchial hyperresponsiveness in both asthmatics and nonasthmatics at concentrations as low as the National Ambient Air Quality Standard of

0.12 ppm (277). A few studies have suggested that ozone increases allergen responsiveness associated with both asthma and allergic rhinitis. Subjects given 3 hours of exposure to 0.25 ppm of ozone required less allergen to have a significant decrease in FEV_1 (279). A similar effect was noted after 7.6 hours of exposure to 0.16 ppm ozone (280). Nitrogen oxides from car emissions also may play a role, although the evidence in controlled exposures is less convincing than for ozone (281).

Diesel exhaust particles (DEPs) also have been implicated in allergic disease. When they are given in combination with an allergen, they promote both allergen-specific IgE production and a TH2 cytokine profile (282). One study attempted to sensitize atopic individuals to keyhole limpet hemocyanin, a protein isolated from a marine mollusk, with no known cross-reactive antibodies in humans. Exposure to this allergen with DEPs generated a specific IgE response, whereas exposure to the allergen alone did not (283).

Sulfur dioxide is a product of soft coal burned for industrial use and is the substance most closely correlated with respiratory and conjunctival symptoms. Sulfur dioxide does not come from automobile exhaust. Incompletely oxidized hydrocarbons from factories and vehicular exhaust make up the particulate matter visible in any highly populated or industrial area. Carbon monoxide impairs oxygen transport, but its concentration in ambient polluted air is probably important only for patients with marginal respiratory reserve. Traces of lead, arsenic, and formaldehyde also are found in polluted air.

Formaldehyde is primarily an indoor pollutant that emanates from particle board, insulation, furnishings, tobacco smoke, and gas stoves. Most formaldehyde symptoms occur in mobile homes, where large amounts of particle board have been used in a relatively small enclosed space. Concentrations of 1 to 3 ppm or higher may cause mucous membrane symptoms in some individuals; atopic persons may react at lower concentrations. This is thought to be largely an irritative phenomenon. Experimentally, formaldehyde can be rendered immunogenic by the formation of formaldehyde–protein complexes. However, it has not been proven that these complexes cause IgE- or IgG-mediated disease, nor has it been proven that inhalation of formaldehyde leads to the formation of formaldehyde–protein complexes (284).

The term *sick building syndrome* refers to outbreaks of acute illness among workers in a particular building or area of building. Most buildings in which this has been reported have been energy efficient, with little direct outside air exchange. The symptoms most commonly involve the conjunctivae and respiratory tract, with additional nonspecific complaints such as headache, fatigue, and inability to concentrate. Except for unusual instances of contamination with microorganisms (such as *Legionella*) or of hypersensitivity pneumonitis, the outbreaks have not resulted in serious morbidity or permanent disability. The cause in more than half of the instances studied has been inadequate ventilation, and symptoms abated when corrective measures were taken. A study in Montreal revealed that workers with *Alternaria* exposure and sensitivity were more likely to have respiratory symptoms. Exposure was correlated with less efficient filtration systems and could represent a significant avoidable exposure for some individuals (285).

Specific contamination from inside the building has been observed in 17% of "sick" buildings. Contaminants have included methyl alcohol, butyl methacrylate, ammonia, and acetic acid from various office machines; chlordane (an insecticide); diethyl ethanolamine from boilers; rug shampoos; tobacco smoke; and combustion gases from cafeterias and laboratories. Alkanes, terpenes, benzenes, and chlorinated hydrocarbons also have been identified in investigations of indoor air. In some instances, indoor contamination may occur from outside of the building: for example, the intake of automobile exhaust from an adjacent parking garage. Formaldehyde is released as a gas ("off-gassing") from a variety of sources such as foam insulation, new furniture, and carbonless carbon paper. The level in office buildings ranges from 0.01 to 0.30 ppm. In mobile homes, levels of up to 0.8 ppm have been recorded in dwellings whose occupants have no physical complaints, but levels of up to 3.6 ppm have been measured in mobile homes whose residents do have complaints.

The role of passive tobacco smoke is one of a respiratory tract irritant. Both allergic and nonallergic persons may be affected. Symptoms range from burning eyes to nasal coryza and coughing or wheezing. Additional ventilation, including outside air, may be required in smoking areas. The role of tobacco alone in the sick building syndrome is not clear when adequate ventilation is present, however. Tobacco smoke contains hundreds of toxic chemicals, including carbon monoxide, hydrogen cyanide, nitrogen dioxide, formaldehyde, acrolein, and ammonia.

Finally, the role of psychogenic suggestion in the sick building syndrome should be considered. Such instances have been reported, based on a variety of inconsistencies in the affected population and the lack of objective findings in both the patients and the building. The perception of tainted air may be induced by transitory malodors, job dissatisfaction, boredom, frustration, or other considerations (286).

REFERENCES

1. Marsh DC, Norman PS. Antigens that cause atopic disease. In: Samter M, Talmage DW, Frank MM, Austen KF, Claman HN, eds. *Immunological diseases.* Boston: Little Brown, 1988:981.
2. Stewart GA. The molecular biology of allergens. In: Busse WW, Holgate ST, eds. *Asthma and rhinitis.* Boston: Blackwell Scientific, 1995:898.
3. King TP, Hoffman D, Lowenstein H, et al. Allergen nomenclature. *Allergy* 1995;50:765–774.
4. Busse WW, Reed CE, Hoehne JH. Where is the allergic reaction in ragweed asthma? *J Allergy Clin Immunol* 1972;50:289–293.
5. Solomon WR, Burge HA, Muilenberg ML. Allergen carriage by atmospheric aerosol. I. Ragweed pollen determinants in smaller micronic fractions. *J Allergy Clin Immunol* 1983;72:443–447.
6. Agarwal MK, Swanson MC, Reed CE, et al. Immunochemical quantitation of airborne short ragweed, *Alternaria*, antigen E, and Alt-I allergens: a two-year prospective study. *J Allergy Clin Immunol* 1983;72:40–45.
7. Rosenberg GL, Rosenthal RR, Norman PS. Inhalation challenge with ragweed pollen in ragweed-sensitive asthmatics. *J Allergy Clin Immunol* 1983;71:302–310.
8. Schappi GF, Taylor PE, Pain MC, et al. Concentrations of major grass group 5 allergens in pollen grains and atmospheric particles: implications for hay fever and allergic asthma sufferers sensitized to grass pollen allergens. *Clin Exp Allergy*1999;29:633–641.
9. Suphioglu C. Thunderstorm asthma due to grass pollen. *Int Arch Allergy Immunol* 1998;116:253–260 [erratum 1999;119:37].
10. Newson R, Strachan D, Archibald E, et al. Effect of thunderstorms and airborne grass pollen on the incidence of acute asthma in England, 1990–94 [see comments]. *Thorax* 1997;52:680–685.
11. Michel FB, Marty JP, Quet L, et al. Penetration of inhaled pollen into the respiratory tract. *Am Rev Respir Dis* 1977;115:609–616.
12. Marsh D. Allergens and the genetics of allergy. In: Sela M, ed. *The antigens.* New York: Academic, 1975:271.
13. Marsh DG, Berlin L, Bruce CA, et al. Rapidly released allergens from short ragweed pollen. I. Kinetics of release of known allergens in relation to biologic activity. *J Allergy Clin Immunol* 1981;67:206–216.
14. Kauffman HF, Tomee JF, van de Riet MA, et al. Protease-dependent activation of epithelial cells by fungal allergens leads to morphologic changes and cytokine production. *J Allergy Clin Immunol* 2000;105:1185–1193.
15. Burge HA, Solomon WR. Sampling and analysis of biological aerosols. *Atmospheric Environment* 1984;21:451.
16. Solomon WR, Burge HA, Boise JR. Performance of adhesives for rotating-arm impactors. *J Allergy Clin Immunol* 1980;65:467–470.
17. Solomon WR, Mathews KP. Aerobiology and inhalant allergens. In: Middleton EJ, Reed CE, Ellis EF, Adkinson NF Jr, Yuninger JW, eds. *Allergy principles and practice.* St. Louis: CV Mosby, 1988:312.
18. Solomon WR. Aerobiology of pollinosis. *J Allergy Clin Immunol* 1984;74:449–461.
19. Reed CE. Measurement of airborne antigens. *J Allergy Clin Immunol* 1982;70:38–40.
20. Luczynska CM, Li Y, Chapman MD, et al. Airborne concentrations and particle size distribution of allergen derived from domestic cats (*Felis domesticus*). Measurements using cascade impactor, liquid impinger, and a two-site monoclonal antibody assay for Fel d I. *Am Rev Respir Dis* 1990;141:361–367.
21. Agarwal MK, Yuninger JW, Swanson MC, et al. An immunochemical method to measure atmospheric allergens. *J Allergy Clin Immunol* 1981;68:194–200.
22. Agarwal MK, Swanson MC, Reed CE, et al. Airborne ragweed allergens: association with various particle sizes and short ragweed plant parts. *J Allergy Clin Immunol* 1984;74:687–693.
23. Platts-Mills TA, Heymann PW, Longbottom JL, et al. Airborne allergens associated with asthma: particle sizes carrying dust mite and rat allergens measured with a cascade impactor. *J Allergy Clin Immunol* 1986;77:850–857.
24. Schumacher MJ, Griffith RD, O'Rourke MK. Recognition of pollen and other particulate aeroantigens by immunoblot microscopy. *J Allergy Clin Immunol* 1988;82:608–616.
25. Bousquet J, Guerin B, Michel FB. Standardization of allergens. In: Spector SL, ed. *Provocative challenge procedures: background and methodology.* Mount Kisco, NY: Futura, 1989:85.
26. Bush RK, Kagen SL. Guidelines for the preparation and characterization of high molecular weight allergens used for the diagnosis of occupational lung disease. Report of the Subcommittee on Preparation and Characterization of High Molecular Weight Allergens. *J Allergy Clin Immunol* 1989;84:814–819.

27. Dreborg S, Belin L, Eriksson NE, et al. Results of biological standardization with standardized allergen preparations. *Allergy* 1987;42:109–116.

28. Chua KY, Kehal PK, Thomas WR, et al. High-frequency binding of IgE to the *Der p* allergen expressed in yeast. *J Allergy Clin Immunol* 1992;89:95–102.

29. Reed CE, Yunginger JW, Evans R. Quality assurance and standardization of allergy extracts in allergy practice [see comments]. *J Allergy Clin Immunol* 1989;84:4–8.

30. Jeannin P, Didierlaurent A, Gras-Masse H, et al. Specific histamine release capacity of peptides selected from the modelized *Der p I* protein, a major allergen of *Dermatophagoides pteronyssinus*. *Mol Immunol* 1992;29:739–749.

31. Schroeder H. RAST-based techniques for allergen assay. In: Brede H, Going H, eds. *Regulatory control and standardization of allergenic extracts*. Stuttgart: Gustav Fisher Verlag, 1980:138.

32. Baer H, Anderson MC. Allergenic extracts. I. Allergenic extracts: sources, preparation, in vitro standardization. In: Middleton EJ, Ellis EF, Reed CE, eds. *Allergy: principles and practice*. St. Louis: CV Mosby, 1988:373.

33. Platts-Mills TA. Allergens. In: Samter M, Talmage DW, Frank MM, Austen KF, Claman HN, eds. *Immunological diseases*. Boston: Little Brown, 1993:1231.

34. Lowenstein H. Quantitative immunoelectrophoretic methods as a tool for the analysis and isolation of allergens. *Prog Allergy* 1978;25:1–62.

35. Aas K. What makes an allergen an allergen. *Allergy* 1978;33:3–14.

36. King TP. Immunochemical properties of some atopic allergens. *J Allergy Clin Immunol* 1979;64:159–163.

37. Lewis WR, Vinay P, Zenger VE. *Airborne and allergenic pollen of North America*. Baltimore: The Johns Hopkins University Press, 1983.

38. Weber RW, Nelson HS. Pollen allergens and their interrelationships. *Clin Rev Allergy* 1985;3:291–318.

39. Smith EG. *Sampling and identifying allergenic pollens and molds*. San Antonio: Blewstone, 1984.

40. Smith EG. *Sampling and identifying allergenic pollens and molds*. San Antonio: Blewstone, 1986.

41. King TP, Norman PS. Standardized extracts, weeds. *Clin Rev Allergy* 1986;4:425–433.

42. King TP, Norman PS, Lichtenstein LM. Studies on ragweed pollen allergens. V. *Ann Allergy* 1967;25:541–553.

43. Baer H, Godfrey H, Maloney CJ, et al. The potency and antigen E content of commercially prepared ragweed extracts. *J Allergy* 1970;45:347–354.

44. Rafnar T, Griffith IJ, Kuo MC, et al. Cloning of Amb a I (antigen E), the major allergen family of short ragweed pollen. *J Biol Chem* 1991;266:1229–1236.

45. Gleich GJ, Yunginger JW. Ragweed hay fever: treatment by local passive administration of IgG antibody. *Clin Allergy* 1975;5:79–87.

46. Lee YS, Dickinson DB, Schlager D, et al. Antigen E content of pollen from individual plants of short ragweed (*Ambrosia artemisiifolia*). *J Allergy Clin Immunol* 1979;63:336–339.

47. Rogers BL, Morgenstern JP, Griffith IJ, et al. Complete sequence of the allergen Amb alpha II. Recombinant expression and reactivity with T cells from ragweed allergic patients. *J Immunol* 1991;147:2547–2552.

48. Adolphson C, Goodfriend L, Gleich GJ. Reactivity of ragweed allergens with IgE antibodies. Analyses by leukocyte histamine release and the radioallergosorbent test and determination of cross-reactivity. *J Allergy Clin Immunol* 1978;62:197–210.

49. Goodfriend L. Toward structure-function studies with ragweed allergens Ra 3 and Ra 5. In: Mathov E, Sindro T, Naranjo P, eds. *Allergy and clinical immunology*. Amsterdam: Excerpta Medica, 1977:151.

50. Santilli J Jr, Potsus RL, Goodfriend L, et al. Skin reactivity to purified pollen allergens in highly ragweed-sensitive individuals. *J Allergy Clin Immunol* 1980;65:406–412.

51. Roebber M, Hussain R, Klapper DG, et al. Isolation and properties of a new short ragweed pollen allergen, Ra6. *J Immunol* 1983;131:706–711.

52. Roebber M, Marsh DG. Isolation and characterization of allergen *Amb a VII* from short ragweed pollen [Abstract]. *J Allergy Clin Immunol* 1991;87:324.

53. Rogers BL, Pollock J, Klapper DG, et al. Sequence of the proteinase-inhibitor cystatin homologue from the pollen of *Ambrosia artemisiifolia* (short ragweed). *Gene* 1993;133:219–221.

54. Hussain R, Norman PS, Marsh DG. Rapidly released allergens from short ragweed pollen. II. Identification and partial purification. *J Allergy Clin Immunol* 1981;67:217–222.

55. Goodfriend L, Roebber M, Lundkvist U, et al. Two variants of ragweed allergen Ra3. *J Allergy Clin Immunol* 1981;67:299–304.

56. Lubahnn B, Klapper DG. Cloning and characterization of ragweed allergen *Amb a VII* from short ragweed pollen [Abstract] *J Allergy Clin Immunol* 993;91:338.

57. Marsh DG, Hsu SH, Hussain R, et al. Genetics of human immune response to allergens. *J Allergy Clin Immunol* 980;65:322–332.

58. Roebber M, Klapper DG, Goodfriend L, et al. Immunochemical and genetic studies of *Amb.t. V* (Ra5G), an Ra5 homologue from giant ragweed pollen. *J Immunol* 1985;134:3062–3069.

59. Shafiee A, Yunginger JW, Gleich GJ. Isolation and characterization of Russian thistle (*Salsola pestifer*) pollen allergens. *J Allergy Clin Immunol* 1981;67:472–481.

60. Cocchiara R, Locorotondo G, Parlato A, et al. Purification of *Parj I*, a major allergen from *Parietaria, judaica* pollen. *Int Arch Allergy Appl Immunol* 1989;90:84–90.

61. Costa MA, Duro G, Izzo V, et al. The IgE-binding epitopes of *rPar j 2*, a major allergen of *Parietaria judaica* pollen, are heterogeneously recognized among allergic subjects. *Allergy* 2000;55:246–250.

62. Coscia MR, Ruffilli A, Oreste U. Basic isoforms of *Par o 1*, the major allergen of *Parietaria officinalis* pollen. *Allergy* 1995;50:899–904.

63. Duro G, Colombo P, Assunta CM, et al. Isolation and characterization of two cDNA clones coding for isoforms of the *Parietaria judaica* major allergen *Par j 1.0101*. *Int Arch Allergy Immunol* 1997;112:348–355.

64. Menna T, Cassese G, Di Modugno F, et al. Characterization of a dodecapeptide containing a dominant epitope of *Par j 1* and *Par o 1*, the major allergens of *P. judaica* and *P. officinalis* pollen. *Allergy* 1999;54:1048–1057.

65. Nilsen BM, Grimsoen A, Paulsen BS. Identification and characterization of important allergens from mugwort pollen by IEF, SDS-PAGE and immunoblotting. *Mol Immunol* 1991;28:733–742.

66. Hirschwehr R, Heppner C, Spitzauer S, et al. Identification of common allergenic structures in mugwort and ragweed pollen. *J Allergy Clin Immunol* 1998;101: 196–206.

67. Ford SA, Baldo BA. A re-examination of ryegrass (*Lolium perenne*) pollen allergens. *Int Arch Allergy Appl Immunol* 1986;81:193–203.

68. Lowenstein H, Osterballe O. Standardized grass pollen extracts. *Clin Rev Allergy* 1986;4:405–423.

69. Staff IA, Taylor PE, Smith P, et al. Cellular localization of water soluble, allergenic proteins in rye-grass (*Lolium perenne*) pollen using monoclonal and specific IgE antibodies with immunogold probes. *Histochem J* 1990;22:276–290.

70. Cosgrove DJ, Bedinger P, Durachko DM. Group I allergens of grass pollen as cell wall–loosening agents. *Proc Natl Acad Sci U S A* 1997;94:6559–6564.

71. van Ree R, Driessen MN, van Leeuwen WA, et al. Variability of crossreactivity of IgE antibodies to group I and V allergens in eight grass pollen species. *Clin Exp Allergy* 1992;22:611–617.

72. Matthiesen F, Lowenstein H. Group V allergens in grass pollens. II. Investigation of group V allergens in pollens from 10 grasses. *Clin Exp Allergy* 1991;21:309–320.

73. Mourad W, Mecheri S, Peltre G, et al. Study of the epitope structure of purified *Dac G I* and *Lol p I*, the major allergens of *Dactylis glomerata* and *Lolium perenne* pollens, using monoclonal antibodies. *J Immunol* 1988;141:3486–3491.

74. Petersen A, Schramm G, Bufe A, et al. Structural investigations of the major allergen *Phl p I* on the complementary DNA and protein level. *J Allergy Clin Immunol* 1995;95:987–994.

75. Matthiesen F, Lowenstein H. *Graminea allergens: biochemistry*. Horsholm, Denmark: ALK Research, 1990.

76. Tamborini E, Brandazza A, De Lalla C, et al. Recombinant allergen *Lol p II*: expression, purification and characterization. *Mol Immunol* 1995;32: 505–513.

77. Valenta R, Duchene M, Ebner C, et al. Profilins constitute a novel family of functional plant pan-allergens. *J Exp Med* 1992;175:377–385.

78. Guerin-Marchand C, Senechal H, Bouin AP, et al. Cloning, sequencing and immunological characterization of *Dac g 3*, a major allergen from *Dactylis glomerata* pollen. *Mol Immunol* 1996;33:797–806.

79. Fischer S, Grote M, Fahlbusch B, et al. Characterization of *Phl p 4*, a major timothy grass (*Phleum pratense*) pollen allergen. *J Allergy Clin Immunol* 1996;98: 189–198.

80. Olsen E, Zhang L, Hill RD, et al. Identification and characterization of the *Poa p IX* group of basic allergens of Kentucky bluegrass pollen. *J Immunol* 1991;147: 205–211.

81. Bufe A, Schramm G, Keown MB, et al. Major allergen *Phl p Vb* in timothy grass is a novel pollen RNase. *FEBS Lett* 1995;363:6–12.

82. Walsh DJ, Matthews JA, Denmeade R, et al. Cloning of cDNA coding for an allergen of Cocksfoot grass (*Dactylis glomerata*) pollen. *Int Arch Allergy Appl Immunol* 1989;90:78–83.

83. van Ree R, Hoffman DR, van Dijk W, et al. *Lol p XI*, a new major grass pollen allergen, is a member of a family of soybean trypsin inhibitor-related proteins. *J Allergy Clin Immunol* 1995;95:970–978.

84. Suphioglu C, Ferreira F, Knox RB. Molecular cloning and immunological characterisation of *Cyn d 7*, a novel calcium-binding allergen from Bermuda grass pollen. *FEBS Lett* 1997;402:167–172.

85. Niederberger V, Laffer S, Froschl R, et al. IgE antibodies to recombinant pollen allergens (*Phl p 1, Phl p 2, Phl p 5*, and *Bet v 2*) account for a high percentage of grass pollen-specific IgE. *J Allergy Clin Immunol* 1998;101:258–264.

86. van Ree R, van Leeuwen WA, Aalberse RC. How far can we simplify in vitro diagnostics for grass pollen allergy? A study with 17 whole pollen extracts and purified natural and recombinant major allergens. *J Allergy Clin Immunol* 1998;102:184–190.

87. Bhalla PL, Swoboda I, Singh MB. Antisense-mediated silencing of a gene encoding a major ryegrass pollen allergen. *Proc Natl Acad Sci U S A* 1999;96:11676–11680.

88. Jarolim E, Tejkl M, Rohac M, et al. Monoclonal antibodies against birch pollen allergens: characterization by immunoblotting and use for single-step affinity purification of the major allergen Bet v I. *Int Arch Allergy Appl Immunol* 1989;90:54–60.

89. Breiteneder H, Pettenburger K, Bito A, et al. The gene coding for the major birch pollen allergen *Betv1*, is highly homologous to a pea disease resistance response gene. *EMBO J* 1989;8:1935–1938.

90. Valenta R, Duchene M, Vrtala S, et al. Recombinant allergens for immunoblot diagnosis of tree-pollen allergy. *J Allergy Clin Immunol* 1991;88:889–894.

91. Ferreira F, Engel E, Briza P, et al. Characterization of recombinant *Bet v 4*, a birch pollen allergen with two EF-hand calcium-binding domains. *Int Arch Allergy Immunol* 1999;118:304–305.

92. Seiberler S, Scheiner O, Kraft D, et al. Characterization of a birch pollen allergen, *Bet v III*, representing a novel class of Ca^{2+} binding proteins: specific expression in mature pollen and dependence of patients' IgE binding on protein-bound Ca^{2+}. *EMBO J* 1994;13:3481–3486.

93. Karamloo F, Schmitz N, Scheurer S, et al. Molecular cloning and characterization of a birch pollen minor allergen, *Bet v 5*, belonging to a family of isoflavone reductase-related proteins. *J Allergy Clin Immunol* 1999;104:991–999.

94. Cadot P, Diaz JF, Proost P, et al. Purification and characterization of an 18-kd allergen of birch (*Betula verrucosa*) pollen: identification as a cyclophilin. *J Allergy Clin Immunol* 2000;105:286–291.

95. Yasueda H, Yui Y, Shimizu T, et al. Isolation and partial characterization of the major allergen from Japanese cedar (*Cryptomeria japonica*) pollen. *J Allergy Clin Immunol* 1983;71:77–86.

96. Sakaguchi M, Inouye S, Taniai M, et al. Identification of the second major allergen of Japanese cedar pollen. *Allergy* 1990;45:309–312.

97. Midoro-Horiuti T, Goldblum RM, Kurosky A, et al. Isolation and characterization of the mountain cedar (*Juniperus ashei*) pollen major allergen, *Jun a 1*. *J Allergy Clin Immunol* 1999;104:608–612.

98. Tejera ML, Villalba M, Batanero E, et al. Identification, isolation, and characterization of *Ole e 7*, a new allergen of olive tree pollen. *J Allergy Clin Immunol* 1999;104:797–802.

99. Bush RK, Yunginger JW. Standardization of fungal allergens. *Clin Rev Allergy* 1987;5:3–21.

100. Prince HE, Selle WA, Morrow MB. Molds in the etiology of hay fever. *Tex Med* 1934;30:340.
101. Feinberg SM. Mold allergy: its importance in asthma and hay fever. *Wis Med J* 1935;34:254.
102. O'Hollaren MT, Yunginger JW, Offord KP, et al. Exposure to an aeroallergen as a possible precipitating factor in respiratory arrest in young patients with asthma [see comments]. *N Engl J Med* 1991;324:359–363.
103. Licorish K, Novey HS, Kozak P, et al. Role of *Alternaria* and *Penicillium* spores in the pathogenesis of asthma. *J Allergy Clin Immunol* 1985;76:819–825.
104. Pepys J. *Hypersensitivity diseases of the lungs due to fungi and organic dusts.* Basel: S Karger, 1969.
105. Barnes CS, Pacheco F, Landuyt J, et al. Production of a recombinant protein from *Alternaria* containing the reported N-terminal of the *Alt a1* allergen. *Adv Exp Med Biol* 1996;409:197–203.
106. De Vouge MW, Thaker AJ, Curran IH, et al. Isolation and expression of a cDNA clone encoding an *Alternaria alternata Alt a 1* subunit. *Int Arch Allergy Immunol* 1996;111:385–395.
107. Horner WE, Helbling A, Salvaggio JE, et al. Fungal allergens. *Clin Microbiol Rev* 1995;8:161–179.
108. Miles RM, Parker JL, Jones RT, et al. Studies on *Alternaria* allergens. IV. Biologic activity of a purified *Alternaria* fraction (*Alt-I*). *J Allergy Clin Immunol* 1983;71:36–39.
109. Nyholm L, Lowenstein H, Yunginger JW. Immunochemical partial identity between two independently identified and isolated major allergens from *Alternaria alternata* (*Alt-I* and *Ag 1*). *J Allergy Clin Immunol* 1983;71:461–467.
110. Agarwal MK, Jones RT, Yunginger JW. Shared allergenic and antigenic determinants in *Alternaria* and *Stemphyllium* extracts. *J Allergy Clin Immunol* 1982;70:437–444.
111. Helm RM, Squillace DL, Aukrust L, et al. Production of an international reference standard alternaria extract. I. Testing of candidate extracts. *Int Arch Allergy Appl Immunol* 1987;82:178–189.
112. Bush RK, Sanchez H, Geisler D. Molecular cloning of a major *Alternaria alternata* allergen, *rAlt a 2*. *J Allergy Clin Immunol* 1999;104:665–671.
113. Achatz G, Oberkofler H, Lechenauer E, et al. Molecular cloning of major and minor allergens of *Alternaria alternata* and *Cladosporium herbarum*. *Mol Immunol* 1995;32:213–227.
114. Breitenbach M, Simon B, Probst G, et al. Enolases are highly conserved fungal allergens. *Int Arch Allergy Immunol* 1997;113:114–117.
115. Aukrust L. Allergens in *Cladosporium herbarum*. In: Oehling A, Glazer J, Mathov E, Abesman C, eds. *Advances in allergology and applied immunology.* New York: Pergamon, 1980:475.
116. Aukrust L, Borch SM. Partial purification and characterization of two *Cladosporium herbarum* allergens. *Int Arch Allergy Appl Immunol* 1979;60:68–79.
117. Zhang L, Muradia G, Curran IH, et al. A cDNA clone coding for a novel allergen, Cla h III, of *Cladosporium herbarum* identified as a ribosomal P2 protein. *J Immunol* 1995;154:710–717.
118. Zhang L, Muradia G, De Vouge MW, et al. An allergenic polypeptide representing a variable region of hsp 70 cloned from a cDNA library of *Cladosporium herbarum*. *Clin Exp Allergy* 1996;26:88–95.
119. Longbottom JL. Allergic bronchopulmonary aspergillosis: reactivity of IgE and IgG antibodies with antigenic components of *Aspergillus fumigatus* (IgE/IgG antigen complexes). *J Allergy Clin Immunol* 1983;72:668–675.
120. Wallenbeck I, Aukrust L, Einarsson R. Antigenic variability of different strains of *Aspergillus fumigatus*. *Int Arch Allergy Appl Immunol* 1984;73:166–172.
121. Kauffman HF, van der HS, Beaumont F, et al. The allergenic and antigenic properties of spore extracts of *Aspergillus fumigatus*: a comparative study of spore extracts with mycelium and culture filtrate extracts. *J Allergy Clin Immunol* 1984;73:567–573.
122. Moser M, Crameri R, Menz G, et al. Cloning and expression of recombinant *Aspergillus fumigatus* allergen I/a (*rAsp f I/a*) with IgE binding and type I skin test activity. *J Immunol* 1992;149:454–460.
123. Arruda LK, Mann BJ, Chapman MD. Selective expression of a major allergen and cytotoxin, *Asp f I*, in *Aspergillus fumigatus*. Implications for the immunopathogenesis of *Aspergillus*-related diseases. *J Immunol* 1992;149:3354–3359.
124. Moser M, Crameri R, Brust E, et al. Diagnostic value of recombinant *Aspergillus fumigatus* allergen I/a for skin testing and serology. *J Allergy Clin Immunol* 1994;93: 1–11.
125. Crameri R. Recombinant *Aspergillus fumigatus* allergens: from the nucleotide sequences to clinical applications. *Int Arch Allergy Immunol* 1998;115:99–114.
126. Banerjee B, Kurup VP, Phadnis S, et al. Molecular cloning and expression of a recombinant *Aspergillus fumigatus* protein *Asp f II* with significant immunoglobulin E reactivity in allergic bronchopulmonary aspergillosis. *J Lab Clin Med* 1996;127:253–262.
127. Hemmann S, Menz G, Ismail C, et al. Skin test reactivity to 2 recombinant *Aspergillus fumigatus* allergens in *A fumigatus*–sensitized asthmatic subjects allows diagnostic separation of allergic bronchopulmonary aspergillosis from fungal sensitization. *J Allergy Clin Immunol* 1999;104:601–607.
128. Su NY, Yu CJ, Shen HD, et al. *Pen c 1*, a novel enzymic allergen protein from *Penicillium citrinum*. Purification, characterization, cloning and expression. *Eur J Biochem* 1999;261:115–123 [erratum 1999;261:821].
129. Shen HD, Lin WL, Liaw SF, et al. Characterization of the 33-kilodalton major allergen of *Penicillium citrinum* by using MoAbs and N-terminal amino acid sequencing. *Clin Exp Allergy* 1997;27:79–86.
130. Chow LP, Su NY, Yu CJ, et al. Identification and expression of *Pen c 2*, a novel allergen from *Penicillium citrinum*. *Biochem J* 1999;341:51–59.
131. Shen HD, Wang CW, Chou H, et al. Complementary DNA cloning and immunologic characterization of a new *Penicillium citrinum* allergen (*Pen c 3*). *J Allergy Clin Immunol* 2000;105:827–833.
132. Shen HD, Au LC, Lin WL, et al. Molecular cloning and expression of a *Penicillium citrinum* allergen with sequence homology and antigenic crossreactivity to a hsp 70 human heat shock protein. *Clin Exp Allergy* 1997;27:682–690.
133. Salvaggio J, Aukrust L. Postgraduate course presentations. Mold-induced asthma. *J Allergy Clin Immunol* 1981;68:327–346.
134. Koivikko A, Savolainen J. Mushroom allergy. *Allergy* 1988;43:1–10.

135. Lehrer SB, Lopez M, Butcher BT, et al. Basidiomycete mycelia and spore-allergen extracts: skin test reactivity in adults with symptoms of respiratory allergy. *J Allergy Clin Immunol* 1986;78:478–485.

136. Brander KA, Borbely P, Crameri R, et al. IgE-binding proliferative responses and skin test reactivity to Cop c 1, the first recombinant allergen from the basidiomycete *Coprinus comatus. J Allergy Clin Immunol* 1999;104:630–636.

137. Horner WE, Reese G, Lehrer SB. Identification of the allergen *Psi c 2* from the basidiomycete *Psilocybe cubensis* as a fungal cyclophilin. *Int Arch Allergy Immunol* 1995;107:298–300.

138. Akiyama K, Yui Y, Shida T, et al. Relationship between the results of skin, conjunctival and bronchial tests and RAST with *Candida albicans* in patients with asthma. *Clin Allergy* 1981;11:343–351.

139. Bennetzen JL, Hall BD. The primary structure of the *Saccharomyces cerevisiae* gene for alcohol dehydrogenase. *J Biol Chem* 1982;257:3018–3025.

140. Shen HD, Choo KB, Lee HH, et al. The 40-kilodalton allergen of *Candida albicans* is an alcohol dehydrogenase: molecular cloning and immunological analysis using monoclonal antibodies. *Clin Exp Allergy* 1991;21:675–681.

141. Akiyama K, Shida T, Yasueda H, et al. Allergenicity of acid protease secreted by *Candida albicans. Allergy.* 1996;51:887–892.

142. Nissen D, Nolte H, Permin H, et al. Evaluation of IgE-sensitization to fungi in HIV-positive patients with eczematous skin reactions. *Ann Allergy Asthma Immunol* 1999;83:153–159.

143. Solomon WR. Assessing fungus prevalence in domestic interiors. *J Allergy Clin Immunol* 1975;56:235–242.

144. Kendrick B. *The fifth kingdom*. Waterloo, Ontario: Mycologue Publications, 1985.

145. Ibanez MD, Horner WE, Liengswangswong V, et al. Identification and analysis of basidiospore allergens from puffballs. *J Allergy Clin Immunol* 1988;82: 787–795.

146. Weissman DN, Halmepuro L, Salvaggio JE, et al. Antigenic/allergenic analysis of basidiomycete cap, mycelia, and spore extracts. *Int Arch Allergy Appl Immunol* 1987;84:56–61.

147. Lopez M, Voigtlander JR, Lehrer SB, et al. Bronchoprovocation studies in basidiospore-sensitive allergic subjects with asthma. *J Allergy Clin Immunol* 1989;84:242–246.

148. Schwartz HJ, Citron KM, Chester EH, et al. A comparison of the prevalence of sensitization to *Aspergillus* antigens among asthmatics in Cleveland and London. *J Allergy Clin Immunol* 1978;62:9–14.

149. Hirsch DJ, Hirsch SR, Kalbfleisch JH. Effect of central air conditioning and meteorologic factors on indoor spore counts. *J Allergy Clin Immunol* 1978;62:22–26.

150. Burge HA, Solomon WR, Muilenberg ML. Evaluation of indoor plantings as allergen exposure sources. *J Allergy Clin Immunol* 1982;70:101–108.

151. Burge HA, Solomon WR, Williams P. Fungus exposure risks associated with animal care units. *J Allergy Clin Immunol* 1979;64:29–31.

152. *Mold allergy*. Philadelphia: Lea & Febiger, 1984.

153. Kern RA. Dust sensitization in bronchial asthma. *Med Clin North Am* 1921;5:751.

154. Voorhorst R, Spieksma-Boezeman MI, Spieksma FT. Is a mite (*Dermatophagoides* sp.) the producer of the house-dust allergen? *Allerg Asthmaforsch* 1964; 6:329.

155. Miyamoto T, Oshima S, Domae A, et al. Allergenic potency of different house dusts in relation to contained mites. *Ann Allergy* 1970;28:405–412.

156. Miyamoto T, Oshima S, Ishizaki T. Antigenic relation between house dust and a dust mite, *Dermatophagoides farinae* Hughes, 1961, by a fractionation method. *J Allergy* 1969;44:282–291.

157. Miyamoto T, Oshima S, Ishizaki T, et al. Allergenic identity between the common floor mite (*Dermatophagoides farinae* Hughes, 1961) and house dust as a causative antigen in bronchial asthma. *J Allergy* 1968;42:14–28.

158. Miyamoto T, Oshima S, Mizuno K, et al. Cross-antigenicity among six species of dust mites and house dust antigens. *J Allergy* 1969;44:228–238.

159. Morita Y, Miyamoto T, Horiuchi Y, et al. Further studies in allergenic identity between house dust and the house dust mite, *Dermatophagoides farinae* Hughes, 1961. *Ann Allergy* 1975;35:361–366.

160. Sporik R, Holgate ST, Platts-Mills TA, et al. Exposure to house-dust mite allergen (*Der p I*) and the development of asthma in childhood. A prospective study. *N Engl J Med* 1990;323:502–507.

161. Newman LJ, Sporik R, Platts-Mills TA. The role of house-dust mite and other allergens in asthma. In: Busse WW, Holgate ST, eds. *Asthma and Rhinitis.* Boston: Blackwell Scientific Publications, 1995:933.

162. Arlian LG, Bernstein IL, Gallagher JS. The prevalence of house dust mites, *Dermatophagoides* spp, and associated environmental conditions in homes in Ohio. *J Allergy Clin Immunol* 1982;69:527–532.

163. Murray AB, Zuk P. The seasonal variation in a population of house dust mites in a North American city. *J Allergy Clin Immunol* 1979;64:266–269.

164. Vervloet D, Penaud A, Razzouk H, et al. Altitude and house dust mites. *J Allergy Clin Immunol* 1982;69: 290–296.

165. Platts-Mills TA, Chapman MD. Dust mites: immunology, allergic disease, and environmental control. *J Allergy Clin Immunol.* 1987;80:755–775 [erratum 1988;82(Part 1):841].

166. Ford AW, Platts-Mills TA. Standardized extracts, dust mite, and other arthropods (inhalants). *Clin Rev Allergy* 1987;5:49–73.

167. Warren CP, Holford-Strevens V, Sinha RN. Sensitization in a grain handler to the storage mite *Lepidoglyphus destructor* (Schrank). *Ann Allergy* 1983;50:30–33.

168. Wraith DG, Cunnington AM, Seymour WM. The role and allergenic importance of storage mites in house dust and other environments. *Clin Allergy* 1979;9:545–561.

169. Kim YK, Lee MH, Jee YK, et al. Spider mite allergy in apple-cultivating farmers: European red mite (*Panonychus ulmi*) and two-spotted spider mite (*Tetranychus urticae*) may be important allergens in the development of work-related asthma and rhinitis symptoms. *J Allergy Clin Immunol* 1999;104:1285–1292.

170. Kim YK, Son JW, Kim HY, et al. Citrus red mite (*Panonychus citri*) is the most common sensitizing allergen of asthma and rhinitis in citrus farmers. *Clin Exp Allergy* 1999;29:1102–1109.

171. Tovey ER, Chapman MD, Platts-Mills TA. Mite faeces are a major source of house dust allergens. *Nature* 1981;289:592–593.

172. Arlian LG, Bernstein IL, Vyszenski-Moher DL, et al. Investigations of culture medium- free house dust mites. IV. Cross antigenicity and allergenicity between the house dust mites, *Dermatophagoides farinae* and *D. pteronyssinus*. *J Allergy Clin Immunol* 1987;79: 467–476.

173. Chua KY, Stewart GA, Thomas WR, et al. Sequence analysis of cDNA coding for a major house dust mite allergen, Der p 1. Homology with cysteine proteases. *J Exp Med* 1988;167:175–182.

174. Cardot E, Pestel J, Callebaut I, et al. Specific activation of platelets from patients allergic to *Dermatophagoides pteronyssinus* by synthetic peptides derived from the allergen *Der p I*. *Int Arch Allergy Immunol* 1992;98: 127–134.

175. Musu T, Gregoire C, David B, et al. The relationships between the biochemical properties of allergens and their immunogenicity. *Clin Rev Allergy Immunol* 1997;15:485–498.

176. Wan H, Winton HL, Soeller C, et al. *Der p 1* facilitates transepithelial allergen delivery by disruption of tight junctions [see comments]. *J Clin Invest* 1999;104:123–133.

177. Kalsheker NA, Deam S, Chambers L, et al. The house dust mite allergen *Der p1* catalytically inactivates alpha 1-antitrypsin by specific reactive centre loop cleavage: a mechanism that promotes airway inflammation and asthma. *Biochem Biophys Res Commun* 1996;221: 59–61.

178. Hewitt CR, Brown AP, Hart BJ, et al. A major house dust mite allergen disrupts the immunoglobulin E network by selectively cleaving CD23: innate protection by antiproteases. *J Exp Med* 1995;182:1537–1544.

179. Schulz O, Laing P, Sewell HF, et al. Der p I, a major allergen of the house dust mite, proteolytically cleaves the low-affinity receptor for human IgE (CD23). *Eur J Immunol* 1995;25:3191–3194.

180. Schulz O, Sewell HF, Shakib F. Proteolytic cleavage of CD25, the alpha subunit of the human T cell interleukin 2 receptor, by *Der p 1*, a major mite allergen with cysteine protease activity. *J Exp Med* 1998;187:271–275.

181. Gough L, Schulz O, Sewell HF, et al. The cysteine protease activity of the major dust mite allergen *Der p 1* selectively enhances the immunoglobulin E antibody response. *J Exp Med* 1999;190:1897–1902.

182. Heymann PW, Chapman MD, Aalberse RC, et al. Antigenic and structural analysis of group II allergens (*Der f II* and *Der p II*) from house dust mites (*Dermatophagoides* spp). *J Allergy Clin Immunol* 1989;83:1055–1067.

183. Smith WA, Chua KY, Kuo MC, et al. Cloning and sequencing of the *Dermatophagoides pteronyssinus* group III allergen, *Der p III*. *Clin Exp Allergy* 1994;24:220–228.

184. Stewart GA, Ward LD, Simpson RJ, et al. The group III allergen from the house dust mite *Dermatophagoides pteronyssinus* is a trypsin-like enzyme. *Immunology* 1992;75:29–35.

185. Yasueda H, Mita H, Akiyama K, et al. Allergens from *Dermatophagoides* mites with chymotryptic activity. *Clin Exp Allergy* 1993;23:384–390.

186. Kawamoto S, Mizuguchi Y, Morimoto K, et al. Cloning and expression of *Der f 6*, a serine protease allergen from the house dust mite, *Dermatophagoides farinae*. *Biochim Biophys Acta* 1999;1454:201–207.

187. King C, Simpson RJ, Moritz RL, et al. The isolation and characterization of a novel collagenolytic serine protease allergen (*Der p 9*) from the dust mite *Dermatophagoides pteronyssinus*. *J Allergy Clin Immunol* 1996;98:739–747.

188. Mills KL, Hart BJ, Lynch NR, et al. Molecular characterization of the group 4 house dust mite allergen from *Dermatophagoides pteronyssinus* and its amylase homologue from *Euroglyphus maynei*. *Int Arch Allergy Immunol* 1999;120:100–107.

189. Lynch NR, Thomas WR, Garcia NM, et al. Biological activity of recombinant *Der p 2, Der p 5* and *Der p 7* allergens of the house-dust mite *Dermatophagoides pteronyssinus*. *Int Arch Allergy Immunol* 1997;114: 59–67.

190. Chapman MD, Platts-Mills TA. Purification and characterization of the major allergen from *Dermatophagoides pteronyssinus*-antigen P1. *J Immunol* 1980;125:587–592.

191. Gotzche PC, Hammarquist C, Burr M. House dust mite control measures in the management of asthma: meta-analysis. *BMJ* 1998;317:1105–1110.

192. Cloosterman SG, van Schayck OC. Control of house dust mite in managing asthma. Effectiveness of measures depends on stage of asthma. *BMJ* 1999;318:870.

193. Platts-Mills TA, Chapman MD, Wheatly LM. Control of house dust mite in managing asthma. Conclusions of meta-analysis are wrong. *BMJ* 1999;318: 870–871.

194. Platts-Mills TA, Tovey ER, Mitchell EB, et al. Reduction of bronchial hyperreactivity during prolonged allergen avoidance. *Lancet* 1982;2:675–678.

195. Ohman JL Jr, Lowell FC. IgE antibody to cat allergens in an allergic population. *J Allergy Clin Immunol* 1977;60:317–323.

196. Wentz PE, Swanson MC, Reed CE. Variability of cat-allergen shedding. *J Allergy Clin Immunol* 1990;85: 94–98.

197. Bartholome K, Kissler W, Baer H, et al. Where does cat allergen 1 come from? *J Allergy Clin Immunol* 1985;76:503–506.

198. Anderson MC, Baer H, Ohman JL Jr. A comparative study of the allergens of cat urine, serum, saliva, and pelt. *J Allergy Clin Immunol* 1985;76:563–569.

199. Van MT Jr, Marsh DG, Adkinson NF Jr, et al. Dose of cat (*Felis domesticus*) allergen 1 (*Fel d 1*) that induces asthma. *J Allergy Clin Immunol* 1986;78: 62–75.

200. Wood RA, Chapman MD, Adkinson NF Jr, et al. The effect of cat removal on allergen content in household-dust samples. *J Allergy Clin Immunol* 1989;83: 730–734.

201. Moore BS, Hyde JS. Breed-specific dog hypersensitivity in humans. *J Allergy Clin Immunol* 1980;66: 198–203.

202. Konieczny A, Morgenstern JP, Bizinkauskas CB, et al. The major dog allergens, *Can f 1* and *Can f 2*, are salivary lipocalin proteins: cloning and immunological characterization of the recombinant forms. *Immunology* 1997;92:577–586.

203. Spitzauer S, Pandjaitan B, Soregi G, et al. IgE cross-reactivities against albumins in patients allergic to animals. *J Allergy Clin Immunol* 1995;96:951–959.

204. Lindgren S, Belin L, Dreborg S, et al. Breed-specific dog-dandruff allergens. *J Allergy Clin Immunol* 1988;82:196–204.

205. Gregoire C, Rosinski-Chupin I, Rabillon J, et al. cDNA cloning and sequencing reveal the major horse allergen *Equ c1* to be a glycoprotein member of the lipocalin superfamily. *J Biol Chem* 1996;271:32951–32959.

206. Bulone V, Krogstad-Johnsen T, Smestad-Paulsen B. Separation of horse dander allergen proteins by two-dimensional electrophoresis—molecular characterisation and identification of *Equ c 2.0101* and *Equ c 2.0102* as lipocalin proteins. *Eur J Biochem* 1998;253: 202–211.

207. Schumacher MJ, Tait BD, Holmes MC. Allergy to murine antigens in a biological research institute. *J Allergy Clin Immunol* 1981;68:310–318.

208. Siraganian RP, Sandberg AL. Characterization of mouse allergens. *J Allergy Clin Immunol* 1979;63: 435–442.

209. Finlayson JS, Asofsky R, Potter M, et al. Major urinary complex of normal mice: origin. *Science* 1965;49:481.

210. Platts-Mills TA, Longbottom J, Edwards J, et al. Occupational asthma and rhinitis related to laboratory rats: serum IgG and IgE antibodies to the rat urinary allergen. *J Allergy Clin Immunol* 1987;79:505–515.

211. Eggleston PA, Newill CA, Ansari AA, et al. Task-related variation in airborne concentrations of laboratory animal allergens: studies with Rat n I. *J Allergy Clin Immunol* 1989;84:347–352.

212. Walls AF, Longbottom JL. Comparison of rat fur, urine, saliva, and other rat allergen extracts by skin testing, RAST, and RAST inhibition. *J Allergy Clin Immunol* 1985;75:242–251.

213. Longbottom JL, Austwick PK. Allergy to rats: quantitative immunoelectrophoretic studies of rat dust as a source of inhalant allergen. *J Allergy Clin Immunol* 1987;80:243–251.

214. Laperche Y, Lynch KR, Dolan KP, et al. Tissue-specific control of alpha 2u globulin gene expression: constitutive synthesis in the submaxillary gland. *Cell* 1983;32:453–460.

215. Gross NJ. Allergy to laboratory animals: epidemiologic, clinical, and physiologic aspects, and a trial of cromolyn in its management. *J Allergy Clin Immunol* 1980;66:158–165.

216. Slovak AJ, Hill RN. Does atopy have any predictive value for laboratory animal allergy? A comparison of different concepts of atopy. *Br J Ind Med* 1987;44: 129–132.

217. Bernton HS, Brown H. Insect allergy: the allergenicity of the excrement of the cockroach. *Ann Allergy* 1970;28:543–547.

218. Kang B, Vellody D, Homburger H, et al. Cockroach cause of allergic asthma. Its specificity and immunologic profile. *J Allergy Clin Immunol* 1979;63: 80–86.

219. Anderson MC, Baer H, Richman P, et al. Immunoelectrophoretic studies of roach allergens [Abstract]. *J Allergy Clin Immunol* 1983;71:1055.

220. Steinberg DR, Bernstein DI, Gallagher JS, et al. Cockroach sensitization in laboratory workers. *J Allergy Clin Immunol* 1987;80:586–590.

221. Melen E, Pomes A, Vailes LD, et al. Molecular cloning of *Per a 1* and definition of the cross-reactive group 1 cockroach allergens. *J Allergy Clin Immunol* 1999;103:859–864.

222. Arruda LK, Vailes LD, Mann BJ, et al. Molecular cloning of a major cockroach (*Blattella germanica*) allergen, *Bla g 2*. Sequence homology to the aspartic proteases. *J Biol Chem* 1995;270:19563–19568.

223. Wu CH, Wang NM, Lee MF, et al. Cloning of the American cockroach *Cr-PII* allergens: evidence for the existence of cross-reactive allergens between species. *J Allergy Clin Immunol* 1998;101:832–840.

224. Arruda LK, Vailes LD, Hayden ML, et al. Cloning of cockroach allergen, *Bla g 4*, identifies ligand binding proteins (or calycins) as a cause of IgE antibody responses. *J Biol Chem* 1995;270:31196–31201.

225. Arruda LK, Vailes LD, Platts-Mills TA, et al. Induction of IgE antibody responses by glutathione S-transferase from the German cockroach (*Blattella germanica*). *J Biol Chem* 1997;272:20907–20912.

226. Santos AB, Chapman MD, Aalberse RC, et al. Cockroach allergens and asthma in Brazil: identification of tropomyosin as a major allergen with potential cross-reactivity with mite and shrimp allergens. *J Allergy Clin Immunol* 1999;104:329–337.

227. Shulman S. Insect allergy: biochemical and immunological analysis of allergens. In: Kallos P, Waksman BH, eds. *Progress in allergy.* Basel: S Karger, 1968: 246.

228. Kino T, Oshima S. Allergy to insects in Japan. II. The reaginic sensitivity to silkworm moth in patients with bronchial asthma. *J Allergy Clin Immunol* 1979;64:131–138.

229. Gad El Rab MO, Kay AB. Widespread immunoglobulin E–mediated hypersensitivity in the Sudan to the "green nimitti" midge, *Cladotanytarsus lewisi* (diptera: Chironomidae). *J Allergy Clin Immunol* 1980;66: 190–197.

230. Baur X, Dewair M, Fruhmann G, et al. Hypersensitivity to chironomids (non-biting midges): localization of the antigenic determinants within certain polypeptide sequences of hemoglobins (erythrocruorins) of *Chironomus thummi thummi* (Diptera). *J Allergy Clin Immunol* 1982;69:66–76.

231. Mazur G, Baur X, Modrow S, et al. A common epitope on major allergens from non-biting midges (Chironomidae). *Mol Immunol* 1988;25:1005–1010.

232. Wynn SR, Swanson MC, Reed CE, et al. Immunochemical quantitation, size distribution, and cross-reactivity of lepidoptera (moth) aeroallergens in southeastern Minnesota. *J Allergy Clin Immunol* 1988;82:47–54.

233. Bagenstose AH III, Mathews KP, Homburger HA, et al. Inhalant allergy due to crickets. *J Allergy Clin Immunol* 1980;65:71–74.

234. Bernstein DI, Gallagher JS, Bernstein IL. Mealworm asthma: clinical and immunologic studies. *J Allergy Clin Immunol* 1983;72:475–480.

235. Reisman RE, Hale R, Wypych JI. Allergy to honeybee body components: distinction from bee venom sensitivity. *J Allergy Clin Immunol* 1983;71:18–20.

236. Tee RD, Gordon DJ, Hawkins ER, et al. Occupational allergy to locusts: an investigation of the sources of the allergen. *J Allergy Clin Immunol* 1988;81:517–525.

237. Tee RD, Gordon DJ, Lacey J, et al. Occupational allergy to the common house fly (*Musca domestica*): use of

immunologic response to identify atmospheric allergen. *J Allergy Clin Immunol* 1985;76:826–831.

238. Schroeckenstein DC, Meier-Davis S, Graziano FM, et al. Occupational sensitivity to *Alphitobius diaperinus* (Panzer) (lesser mealworm). *J Allergy Clin Immunol* 1988;82:1081–1088.

239. Atkins FM, Wilson M, Bock SA. Cottonseed hypersensitivity: new concerns over an old problem. *J Allergy Clin Immunol* 1988;82:242–250.

240. Malanin G, Kalimo K. Angioedema and urticaria caused by cottonseed protein in whole-grain bread. *J Allergy Clin Immunol* 1988;82:261–264.

241. O'Neil CE, Lehrer SB. Anaphylaxis apparently caused by a cottonseed-containing candy ingested on a commercial airliner [Letter]. *J Allergy Clin Immunol* 1989;84:407.

242. Thorpe SC, Kemeny DM, Panzani R, et al. Allergy to castor bean. I. Its relationship to sensitization to common inhalant allergens (atopy). *J Allergy Clin Immunol* 1988;82:62–66.

243. Izumi H, Adachi T, Fujii N, et al. Nucleotide sequence of a cDNA clone encoding a major allergenic protein in rice seeds. Homology of the deduced amino acid sequence with members of alpha-amylase/trypsin inhibitor family. *FEBS Lett* 1992;302:213–216.

244. Irwin SD, Lord JM. Nucleotide sequence of a *Ricinus communis* 2S albumin precursor gene. *Nucleic Acids Res* 1990;18:5890.

245. Thorpe SC, Kemeny DM, Panzani RC, et al. Allergy to castor bean. II. Identification of the major allergens in castor bean seeds. *J Allergy Clin Immunol* 1988;82:67–72.

246. Bush RK, Schroeckenstein D, Meier-Davis S, et al. Soybean flour asthma: detection of allergens by immunoblotting. *J Allergy Clin Immunol* 1988;82:251–255.

247. Anto JM, Sunyer J, Rodriguez-Roisin R, et al. Community outbreaks of asthma associated with inhalation of soybean dust. Toxicoepidemiological Committee [see comments]. *N Engl J Med* 1989;320:1097–1102.

248. Rodrigo MJ, Morell F, Helm RM, et al. Identification and partial characterization of the soybean-dust allergens involved in the Barcelona asthma epidemic. *J Allergy Clin Immunol* 1990;85:778–784.

249. Sunyer J, Anto JM, Rodrigo MJ, et al. Case-control study of serum immunoglobulin-E antibodies reactive with soybean in epidemic asthma. *Lancet* 1989;1:179–182.

250. Lagier F, Cartier A, Somer J, et al. Occupational asthma caused by guar gum. *J Allergy Clin Immunol* 1990;85:785–790.

251. Raghuprasad PK, Brooks SM, Litwin A, et al. Quillaja bark (soapbark)-induced asthma. *J Allergy Clin Immunol* 1980;65:285–287.

252. Belin L, Hoborn J, Falsen E, et al. Enzyme sensitisation in consumers of enzyme-containing washing powder. *Lancet* 1970;2:1153–1157.

253. Ransom JH, Schuster M. Allergic reactions to enzymes used in plant cloning experiments. *J Allergy Clin Immunol* 1981;67:412–415.

254. Novey HS, Marchioli LE, Sokol WN, et al. Papain-induced asthma—physiological and immunological features. *J Allergy Clin Immunol.* 1979;63:98–103.

255. Baur X, Chen Z, Sander I. Isolation and denomination of an important allergen in baking additives: alpha-amylase from *Aspergillus oryzae* (*Asp o II*). *Clin Exp Allergy* 1994;24:465–470.

256. Sander I, Raulf-Heimsoth M, Siethoff C, et al. Allergy to *Aspergillus*-derived enzymes in the baking industry: identification of beta-xylosidase from *Aspergillus niger* as a new allergen (*Asp n 14*). *J Allergy Clin Immunol* 1998;102:256–264.

257. Baur X, Degens PO, Sander I. Baker's asthma: still among the most frequent occupational respiratory disorders. *J Allergy Clin Immunol* 1998;102:984–997.

258. Falleroni AE, Zeiss CR, Levitz D. Occupational asthma secondary to inhalation of garlic dust. *J Allergy Clin Immunol* 1981;68:156–160.

259. Lybarger JA, Gallagher JS, Pulver DW, et al. Occupational asthma induced by inhalation and ingestion of garlic. *J Allergy Clin Immunol* 1982;69:448–454.

260. Hayes JP, Newman Taylor AJ. In vivo models of occupational asthma due to low molecular weight chemicals. *Occup Environ Med* 1995;52:539–543.

261. Zeiss CR, Kanellakes TM, Bellone JD, et al. Immunoglobulin E-mediated asthma and hypersensitivity pneumonitis with precipitating anti-hapten antibodies due to diphenylmethane diisocyanate (MDI) exposure. *J Allergy Clin Immunol* 1980;65:347–352.

262. Malo JL, Ouimet G, Cartier A, et al. Combined alveolitis and asthma due to hexamethylene diisocyanate (HDI), with demonstration of respiratory and immunologic reactivities to diphenylmethane diisocyanate (MDI). *J Allergy Clin Immunol* 1983;72:413–419.

263. Baur X. Immunologic cross-reactivity between different albumin-bound isocyanates. *J Allergy Clin Immunol* 1983;71:197–205.

264. Zeiss CR, Wolkonsky P, Pruzansky JJ, et al. Clinical and immunologic evaluation of trimellitic anhydride workers in multiple industrial settings. *J Allergy Clin Immunol* 1982;70:15–18.

265. Patterson R. Studies of hypersensitivity lung disease with emphasis on a solid-phase radioimmunoassay as a potential diagnostic aid. *J Allergy Clin Immunol* 1978;61:216–219.

266. Sale SR, Roach DE, Zeiss CR, et al. Clinical and immunologic correlations in trimellitic anhydride airway syndromes. *J Allergy Clin Immunol* 1981;68:188–193.

267. Howe W, Venables KM, Topping MD, et al. Tetrachlorophthalic anhydride asthma: evidence for specific IgE antibody. *J Allergy Clin Immunol* 1983;71:5–11.

268. Murphy RL. Industrial disease with asthma. In: Weiss EB, Segal MS, eds. *Bronchial asthma: mechanisms and therapeutics.* Boston: Little, Brown, 1976:517.

269. Pepys J. Occupational asthma: review of present clinical and immunologic status. *J Allergy Clin Immunol* 1980;66:179–185.

270. Pepys J, Davies RJ. Occupational asthma. In: Middleton EJ, Reed CE, Ellis EF, eds. *Allergy: principles and practice.* St. Louis: CV Mosby, 1978:812.

271. Salvaggio JE. Overview of occupational immunologic lung disease. *J Allergy Clin Immunol* 1982;70:5–10.

272. Novey HS, Habib M, Wells ID. Asthma and IgE antibodies induced by chromium and nickel salts. *J Allergy Clin Immunol* 1983;72:407–412.

273. Chan-Yeung M. Immunologic and nonimmunologic mechanisms in asthma due to western red cedar (*Thuja plicata*). *J Allergy Clin Immunol* 1982;70:32–37.

274. Chan-Yeung M, Giclas PC, Henson PM. Activation of complement by plicatic acid, the chemical compound responsible for asthma due to western red cedar (*Thuja plicata*). *J Allergy Clin Immunol* 1980;65: 333–337.

275. Allard C, Cartier A, Ghezzo H, et al. Occupational asthma due to various agents. Absence of clinical and functional improvement at an interval of four or more years after cessation of exposure. *Chest* 1989;96: 1046–1049.

276. Yang WH, Purchase EC, Rivington RN. Positive skin tests and Prausnitz-Kustner reactions in metabisulfite-sensitive subjects. *J Allergy Clin Immunol* 1986;78:443–449 [erratum 1987;79:15].

277. Health effects of outdoor air pollution. Committee of the Environmental and Occupational Health Assembly of the American Thoracic Society. *Am J Respir Crit Care Med* 1996;153:3–50.

278. Koenig JQ. Air pollution and asthma. *J Allergy Clin Immunol* 1999;104:717–722.

279. Jorres R, Nowak D, Magnussen H. The effect of ozone exposure on allergen responsiveness in subjects with asthma or rhinitis. *Am J Respir Crit Care Med* 1996;153:56–64.

280. Kehrl HR, Peden DB, Ball B, et al. Increased specific airway reactivity of persons with mild allergic asthma after 7.6 hours of exposure to 0.16 ppm ozone. *J Allergy Clin Immunol* 1999;104:1198–1204.

281. Health effects of outdoor air pollution. Part 2. Committee of the Environmental and Occupational Health Assembly of the American Thoracic Society. *Am J Respir Crit Care Med* 1996;153:477–498.

282. Casillas AM, Hiura T, Li N, et al. Enhancement of allergic inflammation by diesel exhaust particles: permissive role of reactive oxygen species. *Ann Allergy Asthma Immunol* 1999;83:624–629.

283. Diaz-Sanchez D, Garcia MP, Wang M, et al. Nasal challenge with diesel exhaust particles can induce sensitization to a neoallergen in the human mucosa. *J Allergy Clin Immunol* 1999;104:1183–1188.

284. Patterson R, Dykewicz MS, Grammer LC, et al. Formaldehyde reactions and the burden of proof [Editorial]. *J Allergy Clin Immunol* 1987;79:705–706.

285. Menzies D, Comtois P, Pasztor J, et al. Aeroallergens and work-related respiratory symptoms among office workers. *J Allergy Clin Immunol* 1998;101: 38–44.

286. Letz GA. Sick building syndrome: acute illness among office workers—the role of building ventilation, airborne contaminants and work stress. *Allergy Proc* 1990;11:109–116.

7

Airborne Pollen Prevalence in the United States

William R. Solomon

Department of Internal Medicine (Allergy), University of Michigan Medical School and University of Michigan Michigan Medical Center, Ann Arbor, Michigan

The dramatic appearance of windborne pollens, and resulting symptoms, are familiar events for physicians and laypersons alike. By knowing when and where symptoms occur annually, the astute allergist can deduce probable offenders with some accuracy. Therefore, appreciating the patterns of pollen prevalence confers an important advantage in providing informed patient care.

Despite this imperative, the growth of dependable information has been slow and remains incomplete. Only recently have data generated from volumetric sampling been widely based and a U.S. network of accredited North American reporting stations established. Clearly, the allergist arriving in an unfamiliar area needs to obtain or, more often, generate the information on which he or she will rely. Many difficulties attend the interpretation of traditional data and of compilations such as this chapter. First, of course, is the bias of older "gravity" data toward preferentially recovering larger bioaerosols in, at best, a semiquantitative fashion. In addition, some "conventional wisdom" reflects observations of source plants and "land use" rather than aerometric data. However, even the best available analysis can tell us only the genus or affinity group of origin for many pollens (e.g., most oaks and grasses), leaving inferences of source species to field surveys; considering this, gaps in the species listed are inevitable. Where allergen extract suppliers provide information, an

obvious conflict of interest potential, favoring overly numerous "important" candidates for testing and treatment, must be resisted. Finally, it must be appreciated that exposure levels sufficient to evoke threshold symptoms are largely unknown; exposure-induced sensitivity without disease is, thus, possible and, almost certainly, widespread.

Much of the appeal of North America's landscape arises from its climatic, and resulting floristic, diversity. This variety provides inherent challenge for the allergist, especially so because plant growth and land use rarely conform to political boundaries. Even divisions by state groupings, as attempted here, must be qualified for marked regional differences (e.g., Oregon) due especially to effects of mountain ranges and upwind bodies of water.

Although published pollen data are often treated as "revealed truth," there is little to justify such optimism. Local plantings of crops such as sugar beets, pecans, or dates may affect circumscribed populations within a perimeter. By contrast, long-distance transport (e.g., of mountain cedar pollen from west Texas) is documented and may be more common than suspected. Because bioaerosols smaller than intact grains may carry pollen allergens, their potential for more extended travel without detection is obvious. Land use practices may modify pollen exposure patterns indirectly as well as by directly providing source species. Midwestern

TABLE 7.1. *North American windborne pollen sources and their generic (Latin) names*

Familiar name	Latin genus	Familiar name	Latin genus
Alder	*Alnus*	Mugwort	*Artemisia*
Amaranth	*Amaranthus*	Mulberry	*Morus*
Ash	*Fraxinus*	Nettle	*Urtica*
Aspen, Poplar	*Populus*	Oak	*Quercus*
Beech	*Fagus*	Pecan	*Carya*
Birch	*Betula*	Pigweed	*Amaranthus*
Butternut	*Juglans*	Pine	*Pinus*
Cottonwood	*Populus*	Plantain	*Plantago*
Dock	*Rumex*	Ragweed	*Ambrosia*
Elm	*Ulmus*	Red cedar	*Juniperus*
Hackberry	*Celtis*	Sage	*Artemisia*
Hickory	*Carya*	Sorrel	*Rumex*
Juniper	*Juniperus*	Sweet gum	*Liquidambar*
Maple, Box Elder	*Acer*	Sycamore	*Platanus*
Marsh elder	*Iva*	Walnut	*Juglans*
Mesquite	*Prosopis*	Willow	*Salix*
Mountain cedar	*Juniperus*		

ragweeds, for example, selectively colonize cultivated fields and the margins of winter salted roads and are overgrown rapidly when such disturbance is removed. Changes in pollen prevalence over several decades also are referable to effects as diverse as street tree planting, reforestation (planned or as natural succession), and range extension by opportunistic species (e.g., mugwort recently in northeastern states). The last of these effects deserves special attention in a setting of climate change as well as mounting travel and commerce between continents.

Despite the aforementioned reservations, this chapter attempts to list clinically significant pollens on a state-by-state basis with their botanical names and approximate periods of peak prevalence. Where reference to two or more species of a single genus is intended, the abbreviation *spp.* is used after the generic term; *sp.* designates an uncertain species of a stated genus. Relative importance is implied by a three-level scale: + + +, generally quite important; ++, of secondary importance; +, occasionally or locally worth considering. Among the last of these, those chosen versus those excluded require, ultimately, an arbitrary decision, however refined by facts. Finally, cardinal directions, abbreviated as N, S, E, W, and L (for local occurrence) should pose no problem. Pollen sources for each state or group are listed in the following order: trees, grasses, weeds (i.e., broad-leaved, nonwoody plants or "forbs") (Tables 7.1 and 7.2).

For many prominent genera, the first letter of the Latin epithet only may be given to conserve space; Table 7.1 should allay any resulting uncertainty.

TABLE 7.2. *U.S. regions and component divisions considered in this chapter*

The Northeast
  Connecticut and New York
  Delaware and New Jersey
  Massachusetts and Rhode Island
  Pennsylvania, Maryland, District of Columbia, and West Virginia
  Maine, New Hampshire, and Vermont
The Southeast
  Kentucky and Tennessee
  North Carolina and Virginia
  Georgia, South Carolina, Alabama, and Mississippi
  Arkansas and Louisiana
  Florida
The Midwest
  Illinois and Indiana
  Ohio and Michigan
  Iowa and Missouri
  Minnesota and Wisconsin
The Great Plains
  North and South Dakota
  Kansas and Nebraska
  Oklahoma and Texas
  Colorado, Wyoming, and Montana
The Southwest
  Arizona and New Mexico
  Nevada and Utah
  California
The Pacific Northwest
  Idaho, Oregon, and Washington
The noncontiguous United States
  Alaska
  Hawaii
  Puerto Rico
  U.S. Virgin Islands

The Northeast*

Pollen type	Genus and species	Impact	Prevalence
Connecticut and New York			
Trees			
Juniper, yew	*Juniperus spp., Taxus spp.*	+	Mar–Apr
Alder	*Alnus spp.*	+(L)	Mar–Apr
Elm, white	*U. americana*	++	Apr
Birch, gray, red, etc.	*Betula spp.*	+	Apr
Cottonwood	*P. deltoides*	++	Apr
Maple, sugar, red	*A. saccharum, rubrum*	+	Apr–May
Ash, white	*F. americana*	+	Apr–May
Oak, white, red	*Q. alba, rubra*	+++	Apr–May
Hickory	*C. ovata, Carya spp.*	+	May
Beech	*F. grandifolia*	++(L)	May
Hackberry (SE)	*C. occidentalis*	+(L)	May–June
Mulberry, red, black (L)	*M. rubrum, nigra*	+	May
Grasses			
June/blue	*Poa pratensis*	+++	May–July
Orchard	*Dactylis glomerata*	+++	May–July
Timothy	*Phleum pratense*	+++	June–July
Red top	*Agrostis alba*	+	May–July
Rye	*Lolium spp.*	+	June–July
Sweet vernal	*Anthoxanthum odoratum*	++	May–July
Weeds			
Sorrel; dock	*R. acetosella, Rumex spp.*	+	May–June
Ragweed, short	*A. artemisiifolia*	+++	Aug–Sep
Ragweed, giant	*A. trifida*		
Plantain, English	*P. lanceolata*	+	June–Sep
Lambs quarters	*Chenopodium album*	+	Aug–Sep
Pigweed, amaranths	*Amaranthus spp.*	+	Aug–Sep
Mugwort	*Artemisia vulgaris*	+(L)	Aug–Sep

Sweet fern (*Myrica asplenifolia*) and bayberry (*M. caroliniana*) of sandy soils are modest local factors in pollinosis.

Pollen type	Genus and species	Impact	Prevalence
Delaware and New Jersey			
Trees			
Red cedar	*J. virginiana*	+	Mar–Apr
Alder	*Alnus spp.*	+ (L)	Mar–Apr
Elm, white	*U. americana*	++	Apr
Birch, gray, red, etc.	*B. alba, nigra, Betula spp.*	+	Apr
Cottonwood	*P. deltoides*	+	Apr
Red maple	*A. rubrum*	+	Apr
Ash, white	*F. americana*	++	Apr–May
Sycamore, eastern, hybrids	*Platanus spp.*	+	Apr–May
Oak, white, red, etc.	*Quercus spp.*	+++	Apr–May
Beech	*F. grandifolia*	+ (N)	May
Walnut, black	*J. nigra*	+ (L)	May
Hickory	*Carya spp.*	+	May
Sweet gum	*L. styraciflua*	+ (S)	May
Mulberry	*Morus spp.*	+ (L)	May

Grasses

Strongly similar to Connecticut and New York. In addition, Bermuda grass occurs in more southern areas. Others, including fescue (*Festuca elatior, Festuca spp.*)are marginal, local sources; velvet grass (*Holcus lanatus*), Johnson grass (*Sorghum halepense*), and others may evoke symptoms locally.

Weeds

Closely similar to Connecticut and New York. In addition, yellow dock (*Rumex crispus*) may contribute in June, but mugwort is less prominent.

The Northeast* (Continued)

Pollen type	Genus and species	Impact	Prevalence
Massachusetts and Rhode Island			
Trees			
Red cedar	*J. virginiana*	+	Mar–Apr
Elm, white	*U. americana*	+	Apr
Poplar, aspen(s)	*Populus spp.*	+	Apr
Willow, black	*S. nigra*	+	Apr–June
Ash, white	*F. americana*	+	Apr–May
Birch, yellow	*B. alleghaniensis, papyrifera,*	+++	Apr–May
Paper, gray	*populifolia*		
Maple, sugar	*A. saccharum*	++	Apr–May
Oak, white, red	*Q. alba, rubra*	+++	May
Beech	*F. grandifolia*	+	May
Mulberry, red, black (L)	*M. rubra, nigra*	+(L)	May
Hemlock	*Tsuga canadensis*	+(W)	May
Grasses			
Strongly similar to Connecticut and New York.			
Weeds			
Strongly similar to Connecticut and New York. Mugwort (*A. vulgaris*) is found increasingly in the east and merits clinical concern.			
Pennsylvania, Maryland, District of Columbia, and West Virginia			
Trees			
Elm, white	*U. americana*	+	Mar–Apr
Birch, yellow	*B. alleghaniensis*	++	Apr
Maple, red	*A. rubrum*	+	Apr
Cottonwood, aspen	*Populus spp.*	+	Apr
Ash, white	*F. americana*	++	Apr
Sycamore	*Platanus spp.*	+	Apr–May
Oak, white, red, etc.	*Quercus spp.*	+++	Apr–May
Hickory	*Carya spp.*	+	Apr–May
Walnut, butternut	*Juglans spp.*	+(L)	Apr–May
Sweet gum	*L. styraciflua*	+	Apr–May
Mulberry, red, black (L)	*M. rubra, nigra*	+	May
Grasses			
June (blue), orchard, timothy, and rye grasses produce abundant late May to late July pollen. Bermuda grass appears also in Maryland, D.C., and West Virginia.			
Weeds			
Strongly similar to Connecticut and New York.			
Maine, New Hampshire, and Vermont			
Trees			
Elm, white	*U. americana*	+	Apr
Ash, white	*F. americana*	+	May
Birch, yellow, paper, etc.	*B. lutea, papyrifera, Betula spp.*	++	Apr–May
Aspen, cottonwood, poplar	*P. tremuloides, grandidentata,*	++	Apr–May
	deltoides, balsamifera (N)		
Oak, red, white	*Q. rubra, alba*	++	May
Maple, sugar	*A. saccharum*	++	May
Beech	*F. grandifolia*	+	May
Hickory	*Carya spp.*	+(S)	May
Grasses			
Strongly similar to Connecticut and New York; May–July period shortens to the north.			
Weeds			
Sorrel, docks	*Rumex spp.*	+	May–June
Ragweed, short	*A. artemisiifolia*	+++	Aug–Sep
Lambs quarters	*Chenopodium album*	+	July–Sep
Pigweed, redroot	*A. retroflexus*	+	July–Sep
Plantain, English	*P. lanceolata*	+	June–Aug
Mugwort	*A. vulgaris*	+(SE)	Aug

*As the area longest intensively colonized by Europeans, the paradigm of a brief, hectic spring tree pollen season, grass pollen from late May to July, and the ragweed debacle in late summer originated here. Despite their size, metropolitan areas receive ample pollen from upwind sources and occasionally from intraurban planting of ash, oak, and sycamore. Traditional havens from ragweed exposure in northern states today offer minimal protection, at best. Rye grass–related northern grass species predominate, with Bermuda grass appearing only in the southernmost tier.

The Southeast*

Pollen type	Genus and species	Impact	Prevalence
Kentucky and Tennessee			
Trees			
Elm, white, slippery, etc.	*U. americana, rubra, Ulmus spp.*	+	Feb–Mar
Red cedar	*J. virginiana*	+(W)	Feb–Mar
Ash, white, green	*F. americana, pennsylvanica*	++	Mar–May
Red maple	*A. rubrum*	+	Feb–Mar
Oak, red, white, other	*Quercus spp.*	+++	Mar–Apr
Hornbeam, American	*Carpinus caroliniana*	+(L)	Mar–Apr
Birch, sweet, yellow	*B. lenta, alleghaniensis*	+(L)	Mar–Apr
Sweet gum	*L. styraciflua*	+	Apr
Cottonwood	*P. deltoides*	++	Mar–Apr
Hickory, pecan	*Carya spp.*	+++	Apr–May
Sycamore	*P. occidentalis*	+	Apr–May
Mulberry, red	*M. rubra*	+	Apr–May
Walnut, butternut	*Juglans spp.*	+	Apr–May
Grasses			
June (blue)	*Poa pratensis*	+++	Apr–Sep
Timothy	*Phleum pratense*	+++	May–July
Orchard	*Dactyis glomerata*	++	May–June
Bermuda	*Cynodon dactylon*	+++	May–Sep
Red top	*Agrostis alba*	+	May–July
Johnson	*Sorghum halepense*	+	June–Sep
Weeds			
Sorrel, dock	*Rumex spp.*	+	Apr–June
Plantain, English	*P. lanceolata*	+	May–Aug
Amaranths, pigweed	*Amaranthus spp.*	+	July–Sep
Burning bush	*Kochia scoparia*	+	July–Sep
Ragweed, short, giant	*A. artemisiifolia, trifida*	+++	Aug–Sep
Burweed marsh elder	*I. xanthifolia*	+(W)	Aug–Sep
North Carolina and Virginia			
Trees			
Alder, hazel	*A. serrulata*	+	Feb–Mar
Elm, white, slippery	*U. americana, rubra*	+	Feb–Apr
Maple, red	*A. rubrum*	++	Feb–Apr
Ash, white, green	*F. americana, pennsylvanica*	+	Feb–Apr
Oak, red, white, live[a]	*Quercus spp.*	+++	Mar–May
Sycamore	*P. occidentalis*	+	Apr–May
Hickory; pecan	*Carya spp.*	+++	Apr–May
Willow, black, etc.	*Salix nigra, Salix spp.*	+	Apr–May
Sweet gum	*L. styraciflua*	+	Apr–May
Hackberry	*C. laevigata*	+(S)	Apr–May
Bayberry	*Myrica spp.*	+(L)	Apr–May
Grasses			
Strongly similar to Kentucky and Tennessee, although Bermuda grass is an incrementally dominant offender.			
Weeds			
Strongly similar to Kentucky and Tennessee.			
Georgia, South Carolina, Alabama, and Mississippi			
Trees			
Red cedar	*J. virginiana*	+	Jan–Feb
Cottonwood	*P. deltoides*	+	Feb–Mar
Elm, white, slippery	*U. americana, rubra*	+	Feb–Mar
Maple, red	*A. rubrum*	+++	Mar–Apr
Birch, river	*B. nigra*	+	Mar–Apr
Mulberry	*Morus spp.*	+	Mar–Apr
Ash, white, green, etc.	*Fraxinus spp.*	+	Apr
Oak, red, white, live	*Quercus spp.*	+++	Feb–Mar
Hickory, pecan	*Carya spp.*	+++	Apr–May
Sweet gum	*L. styraciflua*	+	Mar–Apr
Bayberry	*Myrica spp.*	+(E)	Apr–May
Sugar (hack) berry	*C. laevigata*	++(L)	Apr–May

The Southeast* (Continued)

Pollen type	Genus and species	Impact	Prevalence
Grasses			
Bermuda	*Cynodon dactylon*	+++	May–Oct
June (blue)	*Poa pratensis*	++	Apr–July
Johnson	*Sorghum halepense*	++	May–Oct
Rye	*Lolium spp.*	+	May–July
Weeds			
Sorrel, dock	*Rumex spp.*	+ (N)	Apr–June
Ragweed, short, giant	*A. artemisiifolia, trifida*	+++	Aug–Oct
Pigweed, amaranths	*Amaranthus spp.*	+	May–Sep
Plantain, English	*P. lanceolata*	+	Apr–Oct
Nettle	*Urtica spp.*	+	July–Oct
Marsh elder, rough	*I. ciliata*	+(W)	July–Oct
Arkansas and Louisiana			
Trees			
Juniper; cedar	*Juniperus spp.*	+++	Jan–Mar
Elm	*Ulmus spp.*	+	Jan–Mar
Sugar (hack) berry	*C. laevigata*	++	Mar–May
Oak, white, red	*Quercus spp.*	+++	Mar–Apr
Oak, live	*Q. virginiana*	++(S)	Mar–Apr
Mulberry, red	*M. rubra*	+	Mar–Apr
Hickory, pecan	*Carya spp.*	+++	Apr–May
River birch	*B. nigra*	+	Mar–Apr
Sweet gum	*L. styraciflua*	+	Apr–May
Grasses			
Bermuda	*Cynodon dactylon*	+++	Apr–Nov
June (blue)	*Poa spp.*	++	Apr–Nov
Johnson	*Sorghum halepense*	+	Apr–Nov
Rye	*Lolium spp.*	+	May–Nov
Weeds			
Ragweed, giant, short,	*A. trifida, artemissiifolia*	+++	Aug–Oct
Marsh elder, rough	*I. ciliata*	+++	Aug–Oct
Western water hemp	*Acnida tamarascina*	++	July–Sep
Russian thistle	*Salsola pestifer*	+	June–Sep
Pigweed, amaranths	*Amaranthus spp.*	+	June–Sep

*Warmer average temperatures provide a long growing season with early appearance of common tree pollens. In certain areas, some airborne grass pollen occurs in every month; Bermuda grass is the principal source. In the south and east especially, multiple oaks contribute, including several evergreen species, e.g., live, willow and laurel oaks at lower elevations. Vast areas of yellow, long leaf, short leaf and loblolly pines produce copiously, although human effects remain uncertain. Throughout the Southeast the imported paper mulberry (*Broussonetia papyrifera*) has local importance.

[a]Live is used here as a surrogate for several evergreen oaks, including also laurel and willow.

Florida

Pollen type	Genus and species	Impact	Prevalence
Trees			
Alder	*A. serrulata*	+(N)	Dec–Feb
Juniper, cedar	*Juniperus cupressus, Juniperus spp.*	+	Jan–Mar
Bald cypress	*Taxodium distichum*	+	Jan–Apr
Australian pine	*Casuarina spp.*	++	Feb–Apr/Oct–Dec
Oak, post (N), Southern	*Q. stellata, falcata, virginiana,*	+++	Feb–Apr
red (N), live, laurel	*laurifolia*	+	Feb–Mar
Box elder	*Acer negundo*	+(N)	
Mulberry, red, white	*Morus spp.*	++(L)	Mar–Apr
Sweet gum	*L. styraciflua*	+(L)	Feb–Mar
Maple, red	*A. rubrum*	++(N)	Jan–Feb
Elm, white, etc.	*U. americana, Ulmus spp.*	+(N)	Jan–Mar
Hickory, pecan	*Carya is., Carya spp.*	++(N)	Sep–Nov
Palm, sabal, date,	Palmaceae	?+(L)	Mar–Sep
Canary, etc.			

Florida (Continued)

Pollen type	Genus and species	Impact	Prevalence
Grasses			
Bermuda	*Cynodon dactylon*	+++	Mar–Nov
Johnson	*Sorghum halepense*	+	Apr–Aug
Bahia	*Paspalum notatum*	+	Apr–Oct
June (blue)	*Poa spp.*	+	Apr–Aug
Weeds			
Sorrel; dock	*Rumex spp.*	+	May–Aug
Ragweed, short, giant (N)	*A. artemisiifolia, trifida*	++	May–Nov
Groundsel tree (shrub)	*Baccharis spp.*	+(E)	July–Sep
Nettle group	*Urtica spp.*	?+	Jan–July
Pigweed; amaranths	*Amaranthus spp.*	+	Mar–Nov

*The peninsula of Florida extends almost 600 miles into warm seas and supports a subtropical flora at its tip. Elsewhere, wind-pollinated species resemble those of Georgia and Alabama, even to major pine formations on sandy soil. A few introduced types (e.g., casuarina, eucalypts, palms) merit at least local concern and may yet be recognized as significant.

The Midwest*

Pollen type	Genus/species	Impact	Prevalence
Illinois and Indiana			
Trees			
Red cedar	*J. virginiana*	+	Feb–Mar
Cottonwood	*P. deltoides*	+	Mar–Apr
Elm, white, slippery, etc.	*U. americana, rubra, Ulmus spp.*	++	Feb–Apr
Box elder	*Acer negundo*	++	Mar–Apr
Ash, white, green, etc.	*Fraxinus spp.*	++	Apr–May
Oak, red, white, bur	*Quercus rubra, alba, macrocarpa*	+++	Apr–May
Hickory, pecan	*Carya spp.*	++(SW)	Apr–May
Mulberry, red	*M. rubra*	++(L)	Apr–May
Birch, river, etc.	*Betula spp.*	+	Apr–May
Walnut, black	*J. nigra*	+	Apr–May
Sycamore	*Platanus spp.*	+(S.L.)	Apr–May
Grasses			
June (blue)	*Poa spp.*	+++	Apr–July
Orchard	*Dactylis glomerata*	+++	May–July
Timothy	*Phleum pratense*	++	May–July
Red top	*Agrostis alba*	+	May–July
Bermuda	*Cynodon dactylon*	+++(S)	May–Aug
Johnson	*Sorghum halepense*	+(S)	May–Aug
Rye	*Lolium spp.*	+	May–Aug
Weeds			
Ragweed, short, giant	*Ambrosia spp.*	+++	Aug–Sep
Burweed marsh elder	*Iva xanthifolia*	++(S)	Aug–Sep
Burning bush[a]	*Kochia scoparia*	++	July–Oct
Russian thistle[a]	*Salsola pestifer*	+++	July–Oct
Plantain, English	*P. lanceolata*	+	May–Oct
Pigweed, amaranths	*Amaranthus spp.*	+	July–Oct
Ohio and Michigan			
Trees			
Red cedar	*J. virginiana*	+	Feb–Mar
Elm, white, etc.	*U. americana, Ulmus spp.*	++	Mar–Apr
Cottonwood, aspen (N)	*Populus spp.*	+	Mar–Apr
Box elder	*Acer negundo*	+++	Apr–May
Birch, river, gray, etc.	*Betula spp.*	+	Apr–May
Ash, white, green, etc.	*Fraxinus spp.*	+++	Apr–May
Oak, red, white, bur, etc.	*Quercus spp.*	++	Apr–May
Hickory	*Carya spp.*	+	Apr–May
Sycamore	*Platanus spp.*	+(L)	Apr–May
Walnut, butternut	*Juglans spp.*	+	Apr–May
Mulberry, red	*M. rubra*	+++(L)	Apr–May

Pollen type	Genus/species	Impact	Prevalence
Grasses			
Orchard grass	*Dactylis glomerata*	+++	May–June
June (blue)	*Poa pratensis*	+++	May–June
Timothy	*Phleum pratense*	+++	June–July
Red top	*Agrostis alba*	+	May–June
Bermuda	*Cynodon dactylon*	+++(S)	May–July
Johnson	*Sorghum halepense*	+(S)	May–July
Rye	*Lolium spp.*	+	June–July
Weeds[b]			
Ragweed, short, giant	*A. artemisiifolia, trifida*	+++	Aug–Sep
Burning Bush[a]	*Kochia scoparia*	++(L)	Aug–Sep
Pigweed; amaranths	*Amaranthus spp.*		
Plantain, English	*P. lanceolata*	+	May–Sep
Iowa and Missouri			
Trees			
Red cedar	*J. virginiana*	+	Feb–Apr
Oak, white, red, bur, etc.	*Quercus spp.*	+++	Mar–Apr
Elm, white, slippery, etc.	*Ulmus spp.*	++	Feb–Apr
Cottonwood, eastern, swamp (SE)	*P. deltoides, heterophylla*	+	Mar–Apr
Red maple	*A. rubrum*	+(SE)	Mar–Apr
Box elder	*Acer negundo*	++(N)	Mar–Apr
Willow, black, etc.	*Salix nigra, Salix spp.*	+	Mar–Apr
Ash, green, white, etc.	*Fraxinus spp.*	+(S)	Apr–May
Oak, white, red, bur, etc.	*Quercus spp.*	+++	Mar–May
Mulberry, red	*M. rubra*	++(L)	Apr–May
Hickory, pecan	*Carya spp.*	++	Apr–May
Sycamore, eastern	*P. occidentalis*	+	Apr–May
Butternut (E), black walnut	*J. cinerea, nigra*	+(L)	Apr–May
Grasses			

Both Bermuda and the rye-related, more northern species flower April–July (Aug).

Weeds

Strongly similar to Illinois and Indiana with the addition of rough marsh elder (S) and hemp (*Cannabis sativa*) in extreme NW Iowa as ++ factors as well Palmer's amaranth (++) in western Missouri.

Minnesota and Wisconsin

Trees			
Juniper, red cedar (S)	*Juniperus spp.*	++	Apr–May
Cottonwood, aspen	*Populus spp.*	+	Apr
Maple, red, sugar, black, box elder	*Acer spp.*	++	Apr–May
Birch, yellow, paper, etc.	*Betula spp.*	++	Apr–May
Ash, white, green, etc.	*Fraxinus spp.*	++	Apr–May
Oak, red, bur, pin, white, etc.	*Quercus spp.*	+++	Apr–May
Mulberry, red	*M. rubrum* (S)	++(L)	May
Hickory	*Carya spp.*	+	May
Walnut black	*J. nigra* (S)	+	May
Grasses			
June (blue)	*Poa pratensis*	+++	June–July
Orchard	*Dactylis glomerata*	+++	May–June
Timothy	*Phleum pratense*	+++	June–July
Red top	*Agrostis alba*	+	June–July
Rye	*Lolium spp.*	++	June–Aug
Weeds			
Ragweed, short, giant	*A. artemisiifolia, trifida*	+++	Aug–Sep
Burweed marsh elder	*Iva xanthifolia*	+++(W)	July–Sep
Russian thistle[a]	*Salsola kali*	++(W)	July–Sep
Ragweeds amaranths	*Amaranthus spp.*	+	July–Sep
Plantain, English	*P. lanceolata*	+	June–Aug
Hemp	*Cannabis sativa*	++(L)	July–Sep

*This broad, largely agricultural area forms the transition between the Great Plains and the (traditional) eastern forest domain. To the west, woodlands are increasingly confined to river bottoms. Bermuda becomes a principal grass pollen below central Ohio, Indiana, and Illinois, whereas the more northern types (i.e., orchard, timothy, june, red top and rye) predominate around, and west of, the Great Lakes. Sorrel and dock pollen is a variable but usually modest spring factor throughout. Nettle (-like) pollen is surprisingly abundant (July–August) in many areas, but sources such as wood nettle (*Laportea canadensis*) and a native parietaria (*P. pennsylvanica*) also may contribute.

[a]Additional chenopod sources are negligible by comparison

[b]Sorrel, dock and nettle; see introductory note.

The Great Plains*

Pollen type	Genus and species	Impact	Prevalence
North Dakota and South Dakota			
Trees			
Juniper, red cedar	*Juniperus spp.*	+	Mar–May
Cottonwood, aspen	*Populus spp.*	++	Mar–Apr
Elm, white, Siberian, etc.	*Ulmus spp.*	+++	Mar–Apr
			Aug–Oct
Ash, white, green, etc.	*Fraxinus spp.*	++(S)	Apr–May
Box elder	*Acer negundo*	++	Apr–May
Birch, paper, yellow, etc.	*Betula spp.*	+	Apr–May
Ash, white, green, etc.	*Fraxinus spp.*	+	Apr–May
Oak, bur, white (E), etc.	*Quercus spp.*	+++	Apr–May
Mulberry, red	*M. rubra*	++	May
Grasses			
June (blue)	*Poa pratensis*	+++	May–July
Timothy	*Phleum pratense*	++	June–July
Orchard (E)	*Dactylis glomerata*	+	May–July
Brome (chess)	*Bromus spp.*	+	May–July
Wheatgrass, crested, western, etc.	*Agropyron spp.*	+	June–July
Weeds			
Ragweed, short, giant, perennial, etc.	*Ambrosia spp.*	+++	Aug–Sep
Burning bush	*Kochia scoparia*	+++*	July–Sep
Russian thistle	*Salsola kali*	+++*	July–Sep
Western water hemp	*Acnida tamarascina*	++	July–Sep
Pigweed, amaranths	*Amaranthus spp.*	+	July–Sep
Nettle	*Urtica spp.*	+?	July–Aug
Hemp	*Cannabis sativa*	++(E)	July–Aug
Kansas and Nebraska			
Trees			
Red cedar, juniper	*Juniperus spp.*	++	Feb–Apr
Elm, white	*U. americana*	+	Feb–Mar
Box elder	*Acer negundo*	+	Mar–Apr
Cottonwood	*P. deltoides*	+	Mar–Apr
Oak, white, bur, post (E), etc.	*Quercus spp.*	++	Apr–May
Ash, green	*F. pennsylvanica*	+(E)	Apr–May
Mulberry, red	*M. rubra*	++(SE)	Apr–May
Grasses			
Strongly similar to North and South Dakota.			
Weeds			
Strongly similar to North and South Dakota; Palmer's amaranth is a factor in eastern Kansas.			
Oklahoma and Texas			
Trees			
Mountain cedar, Juniper	*Juniperus ashei, Juniperus spp.*	+++	Dec–Mar
Elm, white, slippery, etc.	*Ulmus spp.*	+++	Jan–Apr
Cottonwood	*P. deltoides*	+ (E)	Mar–Apr
Ash, green, white, etc.	*Fraxinus spp.*	++ (S.E.)	Feb–Mar
Sugarberry; hackberry	*Celtis spp.*	++	Feb–Apr
Box elder	*Acer negundo*	+(E)	Mar–Apr
Oak, bur, post, live (E), etc.	*Quercus spp.*	+++	Feb–May
Mulberry, red	*M. rubra*	++	Mar–Apr
Willow, black	*S. nigra*	++	Mar–June
Hickory, pecan	*Carya spp.*	+(L)	Apr–May
Osage orange	*Maclura pomifera*	++(E)	Apr–June
Mesquite	*P. glandulosa*	+(W)	Mar–May
Elm, cedar	*U. crassifolia*	+++	Aug–Oct
Grasses			
June (blue)	*Poa pratensis*	++	Apr–Aug
Orchard	*Dactylis glomerata*	+	May–July
Bermuda	*Cynodon dactylon*	+++	May–July
Rye	*Lolium spp.*	+	June–Aug
Johnson	*Sorghum halepense*	+	May–Sep

The Great Plains* (Continued)

Pollen type	Genus and species	Impact	Prevalence
Weeds			
Ragweed, short, giant, perennial, southern (E)	*Ambrosia spp.*	+++	Aug–Oct
Marsh elder, burweed (N), rough (E)	*Iva spp.*	++	June–Sep
Burning bush[a]	*Kochia scoparia*	++	June–Sep
Russian thistle[a]	*Salsola kali*	++	June–Sep
Water hemp, western[a]	*Acnida tamariscina*	++(N)	June–Sep
"Scales"[a]	*Atriplex spp.*	++(W)	June–Sep
Colorado, Wyoming, and Montana			
Trees			
Juniper, common, Utah (S), one-seeded (S), rocky mountain, etc.	*Juniperus spp.*	+++	Feb–May
Elm	*Ulmus spp.*	++	Feb–Apr
Cottonwood, eastern (E), black (NW), fremont, narrowleaf, etc; aspen, quaking (W)	*Populus spp.*	+	Mar–June
Maple, rocky mountain, etc., box elder	*Acer spp.*	+	Apr–May
Willow, pacific, peach leaf, etc.	*Salix spp.*	+	Mar–May
Alder, mountain, etc.	*Alnus spp.*	+	Mar–Apr
Oak, gambel's	*Q. gambelii*	++	Apr–June
Grasses			
June (blue)	*Poa spp.*	++	June–Aug
Brome	*Bromus spp.*	+	May–July
Fescue	*Festuca spp.*	+	June–Aug
The contribution of these and other grass genera to the modest total levels recorded, including *Koeleria, Agropyron, Buchlöe, Bouteloua,* etc., remain speculative.			
Weeds			
Russian thistle[b]	*Salsola kali*	+++	June–Oct
Burning bush[b]	*Kochia scoparia*	+++	June–Oct
Scales[b]	*Atriplex spp.*	+++ .	June–Oct
Sages	*Artemisia spp.*	++	July–Oct
Ragweeds[c]	*Ambrosia spp.*	++	July–Sep
Burweed marsh elder	*Iva xanthifolia*	+	July–Sep
Sorrel, dock (L)	*Rumex spp.*	+(N)	May–July

*This region was previously the domain of long (east) and short (west) grass prairies; however, little original cover remains, and grass pollen levels are moderate, at best. Grass pollen sources also are numerous and difficult to assign rank. Most woodland is limited to river courses and related wetlands, except in the extreme Northwest (Rocky Mountains) and South (Texas).

[a]Additional chenopods and amaranths appear to make small contributions, by comparison. Moderate levels of partly wind-pollinated composites such as *Parthenium hysterophorus* occur, but health impact remains unclear.

[b]Pollen production of types listed far exceeds that of other chenopods and amaranths.

[c]Prominently including the bur ("false") ragweeds previously designated *Franseria* (now *Ambrosia*).

The Southwest*

Pollen type	Genus and species	Impact	Prevalence
Arizona and New Mexico			
Trees			
Mountain cedar	*J. ashei*	+++(SE)	Dec–Feb
Ash, velvet, etc.	*Fraxinus spp.*	++(L)	Jan–Apr
Juniper, other cedar	*Juniperus spp.*	+++	Mar–May
Elm	*Ulmus spp.*	+++	Feb–May
Cottonwood, fremont, etc., aspen, quaking (W)	*Populus fremontii, Populus spp.*	+	Feb–May
Mulberry, white	*Morus alba*	++	Apr–June
Olive	*Olea europaea*	+++(L)	Apr–June
Box elder	*Acer negundo*	+(N,L)	Apr–May
Oak, gambel's, etc.	*Quercus gambelii, Quercus spp.*	++(L)	Apr–June
Mesquite	*Prosopis spp.*	+	Apr–June

The Southwest* (Continued)

Pollen type	Genus and species	Impact	Prevalence
Grasses			
Bermuda	*Cynodon dactylon*	++	Apr–Sep
Johnson	*Sorghum halepense*	+(L)	Apr–Aug
June (blue)	*Poa spp.*	+(L)	Apr–July
The relative contributions of other types must still be defined.			
Weeds			
Ragweed, canyon, rabbit bush, burroweed	*A. ambrosioides, deltoidea, dumosa*	+++	Mar–May
Russian thistle[a]	*Salsola kali*	++	June–Sep
Burning bush	*Kochia scoparia*	+(N)	June–Sep
Scales	*Atriplex spp.*	++	June–Sep
Sage	*Artemisia spp.*	++(L)	June–Oct
Ragweeds, short, slender, etc.	*Ambrosia spp.*	+	July–Sep
Sugar beet	*Beta vulgaris*	+(L)	Apr–June
Nevada and Utah			
Trees			
Elm	*Ulmus spp.*	+(L)	Feb–Mar
Juniper, cedar	*Juniperus spp., Cupressus spp.*	++	Feb–May
Box elder	*Acer negundo*	+(L)	Apr–May
Cottonwood, aspen	*Populus spp.*	+(L)	Apr–May
Ash, velvet, etc.	*Fraxinus spp.*	+++(L)	Apr–May
Mulberry	*Morus spp.*	+(L)	Apr–May
Mesquite	*Prosopis spp.*	+(L)	Apr–June
Grasses			
See Arizona and New Mexico listing and note.			
Weeds			
Sage	*Artemisia spp.*	+++	Aug–Sep
Ragweed, annual bur, etc.	*A. acanthacarpa, Ambrosia spp.*	+	Aug–Sep
Russian thistle[b]	*Salsola pestifer*	+++	July–Sep
Scales	*Atriplex spp.*	+++	July–Sep

*This group of states is best known for flat arid terrain and a limited variety of potent "hay fever plants." However, substantial mountains are found here, and multipurpose irrigation is increasingly extensive, creating broad "islands" of pollen exposure with a background that is neither simple nor fully described.

[a]Contribution by congeners is probably small.

[b]Additional chenopods (and amaranths), including burning bush, carelessweeds, greasewood, etc., are also variable contributors to exposure.

The Pacific Northwest*

Pollen type	Genus and species	Impact	Prevalence
Idaho, Oregon, and Washington			
Trees			
Alder, red, white	*A. rubra, rhombifolia*	+++	Feb–May
Cedar, juniper[a]	*Cupressaceae*	+++	Jan–May
Cottonwood, black, etc., aspen	*Populus spp.*	++	Feb–Apr
Birch, paper, etc.	*Betula spp.*	+++(NW)	Feb–Apr
Willow, pacific, Sitka, etc.	*Salix spp.*	+(L)	Feb–Apr
Elm	*Ulmus spp.*	+(L)	Feb–Mar
Box elder	*Acer negundo*	+++	Mar–Apr
Ash, oregon, etc.	*Fraxinus spp.*	+	Mar–Apr
Oak, Oregon white, California, black, etc.	*Q. garryana, kelloggii, Quercus spp.*	+(L)	Apr–May
Walnut, English, etc.	*Juglans regia, Juglans spp.*	++(L)	Apr–May
Grasses			
June (blue)	*Poa pratensis, Poa spp.*	+++	May–Aug
Timothy	*Phleum pratense*	+	June–Aug
Rye, perennial, etc.	*Lolium spp.*	+(L)	June–Aug
Brome	*Bromus spp.*	+(E)	May–Sep
Red top	*Agrostis alba*	+(L)	June–Sep

The Pacific Northwest * (Continued)

Pollen type	Genus and species	Impact	Prevalence
Weeds			
Nettle and related types	Urticaceae[b]	+	May–July
Sorrel, dock	Rumex spp.	+	May–July
	Salsola kali	++(E)	July–Sep
	Atriplex spp.	++(E)	July–Sep
Pigweed, amaranths	Amaranthus spp.	+	July–Sep
Sage	Artemisia spp.	+++(EL)	July–Sep
1 Additional chenopods appear to contribute little, by comparison			

*The north–south course of the Cascades Mountain Range is the arbiter of moisture here, with well-watered western slopes, a dryer region downwind, and, ultimately, high desert to the east. Regional features include red alder as a preeminent tree pollen source, a grass flora recalling the Northeast and heightened grass pollen levels in the Willamette valley of Oregon where seed is produced commercially. Idaho presents a mountainous spine with a patchwork of dry and moist, agricultural lowlands.

[a]May include other sources, among them incense cedar (Calocedrus decurrens), Douglas fir (Pseudotsuga menziesii), etc.; hence, the family is listed.

[b]Contributions of types other than nettle (Urtica spp.) are uncertain; hence the family name is used here.

California *

Pollen type	Genus and species	Impact	Prevalence
Trees			
Alder, red, white, etc.	A. rubra, rhombifolia, Alnus spp.	+(W)	Jan–Feb
Cedar; juniper	Cupressus spp., Juniperus spp.	++	Jan–Apr
Cottonwood, Fremont	Populus fremontii	++	Feb–Apr
Oak, black, interior live, coast live (W), etc.	Q. Kelloggii, wislizenii, agrifolia, Quercus spp.	+++	Jan–May
Ash, velvet (S) Oregon, etc.	F. velutina, latifolia, Fraxinus spp.	++	Jan–Apr
Acacia (S)	Acacia spp.	+(L)	Feb–Oct
Sycamore, california	P. racemosa	+	Feb–Apr
Mulberry, white, etc.	Morus alba, morus spp.	+++	Mar–May
Australian pine (Casuarina)	Casuarina spp.	+	Mar–May
Walnut, English, etc.	J. regia, Juglans spp.	+	
Olive (S)	Olea europaea	+++(L)	Apr–June
Castor bean[a]	Ricinus communis	+(L)	Apr–July
Elm, Siberian, etc.	Ulmus pumila spp.	+++(L)	Aug–Oct
Grasses			
Bermuda	Cynodon dactylon	+++	Apr–Oct
Rye	Lolium spp.	+(N)	May–Aug
Brome	Bromus spp.	+	Apr–Sep
Fescue	Festuca spp.	+	May–Sep
Johnson	Sorghum halepense	+(S)	May–Sep
June (blue)	Poa spp.	+	Apr–Sep
Diverse additional species are noted and may contribute.			
Weeds			
Sage	Artemisia spp.	+++(S)	June–Oct
Russian thistle[b]	Salsola kali	+++(L)	June–Sep
Scale[b]	Atriplex spp.	++(E)	June–Sep
Ragweed (L)	Ambrosia spp.	++(E, L)	July–Sep
Pigweed, amaranth	Amaranthus spp.	+	July–Sep
Nettle	Urticaceae	?+(L)	Apr–Sep
Burning bush[b]	Kochia scoparia	++(S)	Mar–July

*The diversity of life zones that California presents argues for separate treatment as well as care in discriminating the many circumscribed pollen sources. A complex oak flora is prominent and (northern) conifer pollens of uncertain significance abound. Bermuda is the dominant grass offender, with many more minor sources recognized. To the south, seasonal rains determine pollen output, both varying between extremes. Clinical reactivity to eucalypts, bottle brush, maples, and mesquite probably is uncommon, although skin test reactivity is documented.

[a]Additional shrubby species, including pepper-tree (Schinus spp.) chamise (Adenostoma) and blue blossom or California lilac (Ceanothus spp.) produce appreciable windborne pollen of uncertain significance clinically.

[b]Pollen output by other chenopods is comparatively minor.

The Noncontiguous United States

Alaska
A somewhat limited wind-pollinated flora, sources with pollen output limited, at best, and a short growing season serve to allow relief for many "stateside" sufferers. Throughout the state, birch (*B. papyrifera*) pollen is paramount, and grasses and sedges are secondary sources, with Sitka and mountain alders (*A. sinuata and A. tenuifolia*) locally significant. Quaking aspen, balsam poplar, and black cottonwood are factors in moist areas, where brief pollination by several scrubby willows also is recognized. Primarily in the south, limited shedding by docks, chenopods, amaranth, and sages is recognized, but probably none have clinical impact, and ragweeds are absent.

Hawaii
With its unfailing pleasant temperatures and high humidity, Hawaii provides perennially favorable conditions for much plant growth. However, like many other tropical sites, abundant, wind-pollinated species are distinctly limited. Bermuda grass pollen is present potentially at all times, but other sources including sugar cane (*Sorghum vulgare var.*) Johnson grass (*Sorghum halepense*) panic grasses (*Panicum spp.*) and pennisetum appear minimal. Sufficient weed pollen to elicit symptoms also must be rare, indeed. When grouped, mesquite (*Prosopis spp.*) casuarina (*Casuarina spp.*) and several palms (Palmaceae) have been implicated as occasional offenders.

BIBLIOGRAPHY

Anderson EF, Dorsett CS, Fleming EO. Airborne pollens of Walla Walla, Washington. *Ann Allergy* 1978;41;232–235.

Anderson JH. Allergenic airborne pollens and spores in Anchorage, Alaska. *Ann Allergy* 1985;54:390–399.

Bucholtz GA, Hensel AE III, Lockey RF, Serbousek D. Australian pine (*Casuarina equistifolia*) pollen as an aeroallergen. *Ann Allergy* 1987;59:52–56.

Bucholtz GA, Lockey RF, Serbousek D. Bald cypress tree (*Taxodium distichum*) pollen, an allergen. *Ann Allergy* 1985;55:805–810.

Bucholtz GA, Lockey RF, Wunderlin RP, et al. A three year aerobiologic pollen survey of the Tampa Bay area, Florida. *Ann Allergy* 1991;67:534–543.

Buck P, Levetin E. Airborne pollens and mold spores in a subalpine environment. *Ann Allergy* 1985;55:794–801.

Durham OC, LaFalla H. A study of the air-borne allergens of the Virgin Islands National Park and adjacent parts of St. John Islands. *J Allergy* 1961;32:27–29.

Ellis MH, Gallup J. Aeroallergens of Southern California. *Immunol Allergy Clin North Am* 1989;9:365–380.

Freeman GL. Pine pollen allergy in northern Arizona. *Ann Allergy* 1993;70:491–494.

Gergen PJ, Turkeltaub PC, Kovar MG. The prevalence of allergic skin test reactivity to eight common aeroallergens in the US population: results from the second National Health and Nutritional Examination Survey. *J Allergy Clin Immunol* 1987;80:669–679.

Girsh L. Ragweed pollen in the United States: utilization of graphic maps. *Ann Allergy* 1982;49:23–28.

Jelks ML. Aeroallergens of Florida. *Immunol Allergy Clin North Am* 1989;9:381–397.

Leavengood DC, Renard RL, Martin BG, Nelson HS. Cross allergenicity among grasses determined by tissue threshold changes. *J Allergy Clin Immunol* 1986;76:789–794.

Levetin E, Buck P. Evidence of mountain cedar pollen in Tulsa, Oklahoma. *Ann Allergy* 1986;56:295–299.

Lewis WH, Dixit AB, Wedner HJ. Asteraceae aeropollen of the western United States Gulf Coast. *Ann Allergy* 1991;67:37–46.

Lewis WH, Imber WE. Allergy epidemiology in the St. Louis Missouri area. II. Grasses. *Ann Allergy* 1975;35:42–50.

Lewis WH, Imber WE. Allergy epidemiology in the St. Louis Missouri area. III. Trees. *Ann Allergy* 1975;35:113–119.

Lewis WH, Imber WE. Allergy epidemiology in the St. Louis Missouri area. IV. Weeds. *Ann Allergy* 1975;35:180–187.

Mansfield LE, Harris NS, Rael E, Goldstein P, et al. Regional individual allergen based miniscreen to predict IgE-mediated airborne allergy. *Ann Allergy* 1988;61:259–261.

McLean AC, Parker L, von Reis J, et al. Airborne pollen and fungal spore sampling on the central California coast: the San Luis Obispo pollen project. *Ann Allergy* 1991; 67:441–449.

Newark FM. The hayfever plants of Colorado. *Ann Allergy* 1978;40:18–24.

Phillips JW, Bucholtz GA, Fernandez-Caldas E, et al. Bahia grass pollen, a significant aeroallergen: evidence for the lack of clinical cross-reactivity with timothy grass pollen. *Ann Allergy* 1989;63:503–507.

Prince HE, Meyers GH. Hayfever from the southern wax myrtle (*Myrica cerifera*): a case report. *Ann Allergy* 1977; 38:252–254.

Reid MJ, Moss RB, Hsu Y-P, et al. Seasonal asthma in northern California: allergic causes and efficacy of immunotherapy. *J Allergy Clin Immunol* 1986;78:590–600.

Reiss NM, Kostic SR. Pollen season severity and meteorologic parameters in central New Jersey. *J Allergy Clin Immunol* 1976;57:609–614.

Roth A, Shira J. Allergy in Hawaii. *Ann Allergy* 1966;24:73–78.

Samter M, Durham OC. *Regional allergy of the United States, Canada, Mexico, and Cuba.* Springfield, IL: Charles C. Thomas, 1955.

Seggev JS, Cruz-Perez P, Naylor MH, et al. Outdoor aeroallergens in the Las Vegas Valley [Abstract]. *Ann Allergy* 1997;78:145.

Silvers WS, Ledoux RA, Dolen WK, et al. Aerobiology of the Colorado Rockies: pollen count comparisons between Vail and Denver, Colorado. *Ann Allergy* 1992;69:421–426.

Sneller MR, Hayes HD, Pinnas JL. Pollen changes during five decades of urbanization in Tucson, Arizona. *Ann Allergy* 1993;71:519–524.

Solomon WR. Volumetric studies of aeroallergen prevalence. I. Pollens of weedy forbs at a midwestern station. *J Allergy* 1976;57:318–327.

Statistical report of the pollen and mold committee. Milwaukee, WI: American Academy of Allergy, Asthma & Immunology 1978–1999.

Street DH, Hamburger RN. Atmospheric pollen and spore sampling in San Diego, California. I. Meteorological correlations and potential clinical relevance. *Ann Allergy* 1976;37:32–40.

Vaughan WT, Black JH. *Practice of allergy,* 3rd ed. St. Louis: CV Mosby, 1954.

Weber R. Cross reactivity among pollens. *Ann Allergy* 1981;46:208–215.

Wodehouse RP. *Hayfever plants.* Waltham MA: Chronica Botanica, 1945.

Yoo T-J, Spitz E, McGerrity JL. Conifer pollen allergy: studies of immunogenicity and cross antigenicity of conifer pollens in rabbits and man. *Ann Allergy* 1975;34:87–93.

8

Diagnosis of Immediate Hypersensitivity

Anju Tripathi and *Bernard H. Booth

*Division of Allergy-Immunology, Department of Medicine, Northwestern University Medical School, Chicago, Illinois; *Department of Medicine, University of Mississippi Medical Center, Jackson, Mississippi*

Immediate hypersensitivity is one of the explanations for conjunctivitis, rhinitis, and asthma. In addition, it may be responsible for some cases of atopic dermatitis and urticaria. Many other causative explanations are possible for each of these conditions. Consequently when a patient has been troubled enough with one of these conditions to consult a physician, it is necessary to perform a complete medical evaluation.

First, it must be determined if the symptoms are allergic in origin or if they have another cause. If the symptoms are considered to be allergic in origin, a more specific diagnostic evaluation must be completed by identifying the antigen or antigens responsible for producing the symptoms. In addition, various other factors must be evaluated. The degree of sensitivity to an antigen may vary, as may the degree of exposure to a clinically significant antigen. Many patients are sensitive to multiple antigens, and cumulative effects of exposure to several antigens may be important. The influence of nonimmunologic phenomena on symptoms also must be evaluated. Infections, inhaled irritants, fatigue, and emotional problems may be significant factors independently or cumulatively, and may fluctuate widely in degree of significance. Considering the large number of variables, it is not surprising that the most important portion of any clinical evaluation is the expertly taken history.

PATIENT HISTORY

Many techniques have been used in obtaining a history, and these include completion of forms by the patient or the interviewer (Fig. 8.1). These may be useful, but they can only facilitate and not replace the careful inquiries of a skilled historian. The significant information can be obtained in some cases with relative ease, but adequate information usually can be obtained only after considerable time and energy has been invested.

The history not only provides most of the information necessary for diagnosis, but it is necessary before further diagnostic tests can be selected that will help confirm the diagnosis and not be dangerous to a patient with an extreme degree of sensitivity.

HISTORY TO ESTABLISH PRESENCE OF IMMEDIATE HYPERSENSITIVITY

The history of the patient is taken in the same way as an ordinary medical history. The patient is asked to state his or her major complaint and to describe the symptoms. During the history, the presence or absence of symptoms of nonallergic conditions must be determined and evaluated. Certain details of the allergic history are so characteristic that they should be always be specifically asked and noted:

Allergy Survey Sheet

Name_____Age_____Sex_____Date_____

I.   **Chief compliant:**
II.   **Present illness:**
III. **Collateral allergic symptoms**

Eyes:	Pruritus_____	Burning _____	Lacrimation _____
	Swelling _____	Infection_____	Discharge_____
Ears:	Pruritus _____	Fullness _____	Popping _____
	Frequent infections _____		
Nose:	Sneezing _____	Rhinorrhea _____	Obstruction _____
	Pruritus _____	Mouth breathing _____	
	Purulent discharge _____		
Throat:	Soreness _____	Postnasal discharge _____	
	Palatal pruritus _____	Mucus in the morning _____	
Chest:	Cough _____	Pain _____	Wheezing _____
	Sputum _____	Dyspnea_____	
	Color _____	Rest _____	
	Amount _____	Exertion_____	
Skin:	Dermatitis_____	Eczema_____	Urticaria _____

IV. **Family allergies**
V.   **Previous allergic treatment or testing:**
Prior skin test:
Drugs:

Antihistamines	Improved _____	Unimproved _____
Bronchodilators	Improved _____	Unimproved _____
Nose drops	Improved _____	Unimproved _____
Immunotherapy	Improved _____	Unimproved _____
Duration _____		
Antigens _____		
Reactions_____		
Antibiotics	Improved _____	Unimproved _____
Steroids	Improved _____	Unimproved _____

VI. **Physical agents and habits:**   **Bothered by:**

Tobacco for _____years	Alcohol _____	Air cond. _____
Cigarettes _____ packs/day	Heat _____	Muggy
Cigars _____per day	Cold _____	weather _____
Pipe _____per day	Perfumes_____	Weather _____
Never smoked _____	Paints_____	changes _____
Bothered by smoke _____	Insecticides _____	Hair spray _____
Illicit drugs_____	Cosmetics _____	Newspapers_____

Time and circumstances of 1st episode:
Prior health:
Course of illness over decades: progressing _____ regressing_____

Time of year   Exact dates
        Perennial _____
        Seasonal _____
        Seasonally exacerbated _____
Monthly variations (menses, occupation): _____
Time of week (weekends vs weekdays):_____
Time of day or night: _____
After insect stings: _____

FIG. 8.1. Diagnosis of immediate hypersensitivity.

VII.   **Where symptoms occur:**

Living where at onset: _____

Living where since onset:_____

Effect of vacation or major geographic change:_____

Symptoms better indoors or outdoors: _____

Effect of school or work: _____

Effect of staying elsewhere nearby: _____

Effect of hospitalization:_____

Effect of specific environments:_____

Do symptoms occur around:_____

old leaves_____ hay _____ lakeside _____ barns _____

summer homes_____ damp basement _____ dry attic _____

lawn mowing _____ animals _____ other _____

Do symptoms occur after eating:

melons _____

bananas _____ fish _____ nuts _____ citrus fruits _____

other foods (list) _____

Home: city _____ rural _____ house _____ age _____

       apartment _____ basement_____ damp _____ dry _____

       heating system _____

       pets (how long) _____ dog _____ cat _____ other _____

Bedroom:	Type	Age	**Living Room:**	Type	Age
Pillow	____	____	Rug	_____	_____
Mattress	____	____	Matting	_____	_____
Blankets	____	____	Furniture	_____	_____
Quilts	____	____			
Furniture	____	____			

Anywhere in home symptoms are worse:_____

VIII.   **What does patient think makes symptoms worse:** _____

IX.   **Under what circumstances is he or she free of symptoms:**

_____

X.   **Summary and additional comments:**

FIG. 8.1. (*Continued*)

1. *Are there other symptoms in addition to the presenting complaint that may be allergic in origin?* The presence of urticaria, atopic dermatitis, sneezing, rhinorrhea, nasal congestion and itching, ocular irritation, intermittent hearing loss, wheezing, dyspnea, or cough should always be determined. Several allergic symptoms frequently exist simultaneously even though the patient has not associated them with a common cause. If several of these symptoms are present, it is more likely that they all have an allergic origin. Conversely, a single symptom in a single system such as isolated nasal obstruction probably is not allergic.

2. *Are the symptoms bilateral?* Unilateral symptoms, whether ocular, nasal, or pulmonary, suggest the presence of nonallergic conditions, often anatomic in nature.

3. *Is there a family history of atopic disease?* Most allergic patients have a positive history in this respect. Specifically ask about allergic diseases in parents, grandparents, siblings, aunts, uncles, cousins, and children.

4. *How has the patient responded to previous treatment?* Information about previous therapy is useful. A good response to antihistamines would increase the likelihood that the symptoms have an allergic origin. Response to bronchodilator, antimediator, or steroid therapy, either systemically or by inhalation, may give valuable information regarding the presence or absence of reversible airway obstruction. A prior good response to immunotherapy would strongly implicate an allergic problem.

5. *Are symptoms continuous or intermittent?* Allergic symptoms are often intermittent, and

even in those cases in which they are continuous, there may be intermittent exacerbations.

6. *Are there specific triggers?* A careful history can often narrow the list of suspected allergens responsible for the symptoms of allergic diseases. This facilitates selection of further diagnostic tests and minimizes the amount of testing performed. A detailed survey of the patient's home, work, or school environment may identify potential triggers. All medications taken for any reason should be elicited and their role evaluated. For example, sympathomimetic nasal sprays, oral contraceptives, other medications, and (for historical purposes) reserpine can cause nasal obstruction. β-Adrenergic blockers rarely can be responsible for wheezing and dyspnea. Angiotensin-converting enzyme (ACE) inhibitors can produce a severe persistent cough or angioedema. Awareness of these reactions can prevent unnecessary and expensive allergic evaluations.

CHARACTERISTICS OF ANTIGENS

See Table 8.1 for a review of the important antigens. Some general characteristics of the antigens responsible for allergic illnesses must be appreciated before an adequate clinical history can be obtained or interpreted. Although foods may be important in cases of infantile eczema, urticaria, angioedema, or anaphylaxis, they are almost never important in cases of allergic conjunctivitis, allergic rhinitis, or allergic asthma. The antigens most important in those conditions are usually airborne. Several different groups of these aeroallergens are of major clinical significance, including pollens, fungi, house dust mite, cockroach, and animal danders.

Pollens

The grains of pollen from plants are among the most important antigens that cause clinical sensitization.

Most plants produce pollen that is rich in protein, and therefore potentially antigenic. Whether a specific pollen regularly causes symptom or not depends on several factors. The pollens that routinely cause illness usually fulfill four criteria: they are produced in large quantities by a plant that is common; they depend primarily on the wind for their dispersal; they are 2 to 60 μm in diameter; and the pollen itself is antigenic.

Many plants produce pollens that are large, thick, and waxy. Under natural conditions,

TABLE 8.1. *Symptoms characteristically produced by common antigens*

Antigens	Symptoms
Pollens	Seasonal symptoms or seasonal exacerbation or symptoms
Mold spores	Perennial symptoms in warm climates Seasonal exacerbations in some moderate climates Reduced symptoms when living or vacationing in dry climates Symptoms that decrease with snow Sudden increase in symptoms if exposed to basements, moldy hay or leaves, barns or silos, dairies, breweries, food storage areas, buildings with contaminated air conditioning systems, rotting wood or any location that might have high humidity Rarely may have exacerbation after ingesting mold products
House dust mite	Characteristically perennial symptoms Exacerbations when making beds, cleaning or dusting the home Occasional exacerbations when entering older homes with older furnishings
Animal danders	Perennial symptoms Marked improvement in symptoms when leaving home for several days or weeks, if animal lives in the home Sudden exacerbations of symptoms after a new pet has been introduced to the home Sudden increase in symptoms when visiting a home where animals live Less frequently, sudden increase in symptoms when playing with an animal Worsening of symptoms at work and clearing of symptoms on weekends or vacations if exposure is occupational

transfer of the pollen between flowering plants is accomplished chiefly by insects. These pollens are not widely dispersed in the air; therefore, they are rarely clinically significant. Goldenrod, which is popularly considered to cause hay fever, has little significance because its pollen rapidly falls from the air before it can be dispersed widely and reach the hay fever patient. In contrast, the ragweed plant pollinates at the same time, and its pollen is small, light, widely dispersed by the wind, and highly antigenic. Ragweed plants also grow abundantly in many geographic areas of the United States and Canada.

In the United States, many trees, grasses, and weeds produce large quantities of highly antigenic, windborne pollen. The seasonal occurrence of tree, grass, and weed pollens varies with the geographic location. Even though many factors may alter the total amount of pollen produced in any year, the season of pollination of a plant remains remarkably constant in any one area from year to year. This is because pollen release is determined by length of day, which is so remarkably consistent, year to year. The physician treating allergies must know which windborne pollens are abundant in the area and their seasons of pollination. The major clinically significant pollens vary with geographic location and are discussed in Chapter 7

Fungi and Molds

Many thousands of different fungi exist. The role of many of them in producing allergic symptoms is speculative, but some species have been definitely implicated. Because fungi can colonize almost every possible habitat and reproduce spores prolifically, the air is seldom free of spores. Consequently, they are important in some patients with perennial symptoms. However, seasonal or local influences can greatly alter the number of airborne spores.

Periods of warm weather with relatively high humidity allow optimal growth of molds. If this period is followed by hot, dry, windy weather, the spores often become airborne in large concentration. A frost may produce a large amount of dying vegetation, but the decreased temperature may reduce the growth rate of fungi. In contrast, spring and fall provide the relative warmth, humidity, and adequate substrate necessary for the growth of fungi.

High local concentrations of mold spores also are encountered frequently. Deep shade may produce high humidity because of water condensing on cool surfaces. High humidity may occur in areas of water seepage such as basements, refrigerator drip trays, or garbage pails. Food storage areas, dairies, breweries, air conditioning systems, piles of fallen leaves or rotting wood, and barns or silos containing hay or other grains may provide nutrients as well as a high humidity, and therefore may have high concentrations of mold spores.

Insects

The contents of house dust are usually very heterogeneous and contain many potential antigens, including fungi, insect debris, debris from small mammals as well as humans, food remnants, fibrous materials from plants, and inorganic substances. The role of insects, fungi, and mammals as indoor antigens has been definitely established.

House dust mites (*Dermatophagoides* species) are now recognized as the major source of antigen in house dust (1,2). Carpeting, bedding, upholstered furniture, and draperies are the main sanctuaries of dust mites in a home. They are discussed in another chapter. In tropical climates, storage mites such as *Lepidus destructor* and *Blomia tropicalis* are important indoor allergens.

Dust mite–sensitive patients may have perennial symptoms, although these may be somewhat improved outdoors with less humidity or during summer months. They may have a history of sneezing, lacrimation, rhinorrhea, or mild asthma whenever the house is cleaned or the beds are made. In many dust mite–sensitive patients, the history is not so obvious, and the presence of perennial symptoms is the only suggestive feature.

In the inner city, cockroaches are an important allergen. A child with a positive skin test to cockroaches is more likely to develop asthma. Both mite and cockroach allergen are airborne in rooms with activity. In the absence of activity, airborne levels decline rapidly.

Animal Danders

Particles of skin and the urinary proteins of animals can act as potent antigens. When warm-blooded pets live inside a home, these products can reach high concentrations and completely permeate the furniture, bedding, rugs, and air. Household pets often are entirely responsible for severe disabling asthma. A short-haired pet does not eliminate this hazard. Although cats and dogs are involved most frequently, many other animals are occasionally responsible. A remarkable number of homes have hamsters, gerbils, rabbits, parakeets, parrots, rabbits, or mice. Certain occupational groups such as laboratory workers, veterinarians, ranchers, farmers, or pet shop owners may be exposed to an unusual variety of animal dander.

A patient with clinical sensitivity to a household pet may have a history similar to that of dust mite–sensitive patients. In addition, they may have rapid, marked symptomatic improvement when leaving home or being hospitalized. Symptoms may persist outside the home, however, and patients may use this as inappropriate evidence that animals that they do not wish to eliminate from the environment are not a cause of their problem. Many patients may relate a history of wheal and erythema at a skin site that was scratched or bitten by the animal. Sensitivity to animals always should be suspected when a patient develops fairly severe asthma as an adult. In contrast to mite or cockroach antigens, cat and dog antigens remain airborne many hours after activity in a room has ceased.

A patient with an inhalant allergy may respond well to treatment for many months, only to have a sudden increase in symptoms. Frequently, this increase may be associated with the introduction of a pet into the home. If a physician does not inquire about the presence of a new pet, the patient's symptoms may be completely misinterpreted and improper therapy may be prescribed.

NONIMMUNOLOGIC FACTORS

Certain nonimmunologic factors so frequently aggravate allergic conditions that they should always be evaluated. Primary irritants such as tobacco smoke, paint, hair spray, perfumes, colognes, or other strong odors or more generalized air pollution may precipitate flares of allergic conditions. The effects of infection, weather, temperature, psychic stress, and exercise should be ascertained.

While the history is being taken, it is also appropriate to evaluate in detail the severity of the illness. The severity of the symptoms determines the extent of the diagnostic evaluation and the intensity of the therapy. Later, this will also allow an objective evaluation of the results of therapy. Whether the symptoms are nasal, ocular, dermatologic, or pulmonary, it is necessary to judge the degree of discomfort they cause. This judgment of necessity is subjective, and depends on the personality of the patient and the physician. More objective evaluation can determine the frequency of the symptoms. The number of days that symptoms occur, number of hours that they persist, and number of days lost from work or school should be determined. In severe cases, the number of days hospitalized also should be noted, as should whether the illness has ever been life threatening.

PHYSICAL EXAMINATION

Every patient should have a complete physical examination. Particular attention obviously must be directed to sites affected by the common allergic diseases: the eyes, nose, oropharynx, ears, chest, and skin.

Conjunctivitis

Physical findings of allergic conjunctivitis are hyperemia and edema of the conjunctiva. Occasionally, a pronounced chemosis occurs associated with clear, watery discharge. Periorbital edema may be present, and, rarely, a bluish discoloration about the eyes may occur. If chemosis is severe, acute allergic conjunctivitis may be confused with atopic keratoconjunctivitis.

Rhinitis

The examination of the nose requires good exposure and adequate light. In a patient with allergic rhinitis, the inferior turbinates usually appear to be swollen and actually may meet the nasal septum. They may have a uniform bluish or pearly gray discoloration, but more frequently there may be adjacent areas where the membrane is red, giving a mottled appearance. Polyps may or may not be seen within the nose. The skin of the nose, and particularly of the upper lip, may show irritation and excoriation produced by the nasal discharge and continuous nose wiping. Tenderness over the paranasal sinuses may be present if concomitant infection is present. In patients with nasal allergic disease, the ears should be examined for evidence of acute or chronic otitis media, either serous or infectious in nature. Nasal secretions also may be observed draining into the posterior pharynx.

Asthma

Physical findings in asthmatic patients are highly variable, not only between patients but also in the same patient at different times. The rapidity with which symptoms and physical findings can appear or disappear is one of the characteristic features of the illness.

During an acute attack of asthma, the patient is often tachycardic and tachypneic. The patient appears to be in respiratory distress and usually uses the accessory muscles of respiration. Mechanically, these muscles are more effective if the patient stands or sits and leans slightly forward. During an acute attack, the patient rarely will lie down unless severely exhausted. Intercostal, subcostal, and supraclavicular retraction, as well as flaring of the alae nasi, may be present with inspiratory effort. On auscultation, musical wheezes may be heard during both inspiration and expiration, and the expiratory phase of respiration may be prolonged. These auscultory findings tend to be present uniformly throughout the lungs in uncomplicated asthma exacerbation. Asymmetry of auscultory findings might be caused by concomitant disease such as pneumonia, or by a complication of the asthma itself, such as occlusion of a large bronchus with a mucous plug. In severely ill patients, extreme bronchial plugging and loss of effective mechanical ventilation may be associated with disappearance of the wheezing and a marked decrease in all audible breath sounds.

In these critically ill patients, alveolar ventilation has almost disappeared, and they may be cyanotic.

When the asthmatic patient is not having an acute exacerbation, there may be no demonstrable abnormalities on auscultation even when evidence of reversible airway obstruction can be demonstrated with pulmonary function studies. In many instances, asthma is chronic, and wheezes may be heard even while the patient is feeling subjectively well. In some cases, wheezes will not be heard during normal respiration but can be heard if the patient exhales forcefully.

Atopic Dermatitis

The findings on physical examination of a patient with atopic dermatitis also vary widely. The findings depend on the age of the patient and stage of the disease. In an infant 4 to 6 months of age, the initial manifestation usually is erythema and edema. Initial lesions are most likely to occur on the cheeks, in the antecubital fossa, the popliteal spaces, or about the neck and ears. The distribution in other age groups is discussed in Chapter 15. Generalized skin involvement may occur, and any area of the body can be involved. After the initial erythema, a fine papular rash may appear. The papules then may form small vesicles, and when these vesicles rupture there may be oozing and crusting. Different areas of the skin may have erythema, papules, vesicles, or oozing and crusting, indicating that there are multiple lesions in varying stages of development. Secondary bacterial infection is frequently present.

In the chronic form, lichenification of the skin is the predominant cutaneous finding. The skin appears thickened, coarse, and dry. There may be moderate scaling and alteration in pigmentation. Pruritus may not be as severe as during the acute phases, but is still present. The cosmetic effects of the chronic form are often very disturbing to the patient.

OTHER EXAMINATIONS

Abnormalities of red cells or of the sedimentation rate are not associated with atopic disease. If such abnormalities are present, other illnesses or complications should be suspected. The differential white blood cell count is usually normal, with the frequent exception of eosinophilia that may range from 3% to 10%. Eosinophilia of 12% to 20% is seldom present in allergies to extrinsic antigens unless there is also an infection. Higher eosinophil counts are not ordinarily seen in atopic diseases. The evaluation of eosinophilia is reviewed in Chapter 33.

Chest radiographs may be necessary to rule out concomitant disease or complications of asthma. Chest radiographs in patients with asthma may reveal hyperinflation or bronchial cuffing; however, most often they are normal (3). A screening sinus computed tomography (CT) scan without contrast material may be required in the evaluation of upper airways of patients with chronic or recurrent sinus infections (4). Conventional radiographs of the sinuses provide limited information and may have high false-positive and false-negative rates.

Sputum Gram stains, cultures, and cytology; rhinoscopy, bronchoscopy, bronchial lavage, and electrocardiograms; as well as CT and magnetic resonance imaging (MRI) of the chest aid in the diagnosis of some patients. All or some of these procedures may be necessary to establish the correct diagnosis. Gross and microscopic findings in nasal secretions and in sputum have been described in allergic patients. These changes include eosinophils, Curschmann spirals, Charcot-Leyden crystals, and Creola bodies. Although interesting findings, their presence or absence may or may not be of diagnostic value.

EVALUATION OF RESPIRATORY FUNCTION

Quantitative tests of ventilation can be of great value. They may yield some insight into the type and severity of the functional defect and, more importantly, may provide an objective means for assessing changes that may occur with time or may be induced by treatment. These tests are described in detail elsewhere. It must be remembered that single sets of values describe conditions at designated points in time, and conditions such as asthma have rapid pathophys-

iologic changes. Asymptomatic patients with asthma usually have normal lung volumes. A flow–volume loop may demonstrate extrathoracic obstruction such as vocal cord dysfunction.

Provocation Tests

Although nasal or bronchial challenges with specific antigens to confirm immediate sensitivity are rarely performed in routine practice, they are nevertheless important tools in research studies. Nonspecific bronchial reactivity may be assessed with methacholine or histamine and is occasionally used in the diagnosis of asthma. Methacholine challenge needs to be interpreted cautiously because it can be falsely positive in patients with a variety of disorders, including allergic rhinitis, upper respiratory infections, chronic obstructive airway diseases, and sarcoidosis, as well as in smokers (5).

Food challenges may be necessary in the diagnosis of food allergies and are performed on a regular basis in clinical practice. Double-blind placebo-controlled food challenges are the gold standard in the diagnosis of food allergies and may occasionally be required. Provocation testing should be performed in a supervised setting with emergency treatment available.

Skin Tests

Skin tests are the diagnostic test of choice for allergic diseases. Used in the evaluation of conjunctivitis, rhinitis, asthma, and anaphylaxis, skin tests confirm or exclude allergic factors, such as airborne allergens, reactions to foods, certain drugs, and venom.

Pathogenesis of Skin Testing

Immediate response elicited by skin testing peaks in 15 to 20 minutes and involves production of the wheal and flare reaction characteristic of atopic sensitization. Mast cell degranulation and subsequent release of histamine is responsible for the immediate reaction (6). The wheal and erythema reaction can be reproduced by injection of histamine into the skin.

Skin Testing Techniques

Currently, two methods of skin testing are widely used: prick/puncture tests and intracutaneous tests. Both are easy to perform, fairly reproducible, reliable, and relatively safe. The tests should be read in 20 to 30 minutes, but if a large wheal reaction occurs before that time, the test site should be wiped free of antigen to reduce the possibility of a systemic reaction.

Prick/Puncture Test

Prick/puncture tests are more specific than intracutaneous tests in corroborating allergic disease (7,8). These tests can be performed with a minimum of equipment and are the most convenient and precise method of eliciting the presence of immunoglobulin E (IgE) antibodies. A drop of the allergen extract to be tested is placed on the skin surface and a needle is gently penetrated into the epidermis through the drop. The epidermis is then gently raised without causing any bleeding. If appropriate antigen concentrations are used, there is relatively little risk of anaphylaxis, although rare large local skin reactions may occur.

Intracutaneous Test

If the skin-prick test result is negative, an intracutaneous test is performed by injecting the allergen into the dermis. The skin is held tense and the needle is inserted almost parallel to its surface, just far enough to cover the beveled portion. Allergen (0.01–0.02 mL) is injected using a 26-gauge needle to form a small bleb. Because there is a risk of a systemic reaction, preliminary prick tests with the same antigen are advisable, and dilute concentrations of the antigen are used. If the skin-prick test is positive, the intracutaneous test is not needed and should be avoided. Intracutaneous tests are more sensitive but less specific compared to prick/puncture tests. Intracutaneous testing for food allergies is avoided because it has rarely been shown to provide useful information, so the risk to patients is not justified (9).

Variables Affecting Skin Testing

Site of Testing

The skin tests may be performed on the back or on the volar surface of the forearm. The back is more reactive than the forearm (10), but the clinical significance of the greater reactivity of the back is considered to be minimal.

Age

Although all ages can be skin tested, skin reactivity has been demonstrated to be reduced in infants and the elderly (11,12).

Gender

There is no significant difference in skin test reactivity between males and females (12).

Medications

Antihistamines reduce skin reactivity to histamine and allergens, and thus should be withheld for a period of time corresponding to three half-lives of the drug. Histamine (H_2) antagonists also may blunt dermal reactivity, although this is usually not clinically significant (13,14). Other medications, such as tricyclic antidepressants and chlorpromazine, can block skin test reactivity for extended periods of time and may need to be avoided for up to 2 weeks before testing (15).

Short courses of oral corticosteroids do not affect skin reactivity (16). Long-term systemic corticosteroid therapy may affect mast cell response; however, it does not appear to affect skin testing with airborne allergens (17). Topical corticosteroid preparations may inhibit skin reactivity and should not be applied at the site of testing for at least 1 week before testing (18). β Agonists, theophylline, decongestants, cromolyn, and inhaled or nasal corticosteroids have no effect on skin reactivity.

Immunotherapy

Individuals who have previously received allergen immunotherapy can have diminished skin reactivity to aeroallergens when repeat testing is performed (19,20). The domination is less than 10-fold on end-point titration and therefore rarely clinically relevant.

Circadian Rhythm and Seasonal Variation

There is conflicting data whether cutaneous reactivity changes during the day (21,22). Testing during certain times of the year also may influence skin reactivity (23,24). These variations, however, are of no clinical significance.

Extracts

Skin testing should be performed with clinically relevant and potent allergens. Currently a number of standardized allergenic extracts are available and should be used when possible. Standardized extracts decrease lot-to-lot variability and facilitate cross-comparison among extracts from different physicians. Factors that decrease stability of extracts include storage duration, increasing temperature, and presence of proteases. Refrigeration of extracts and addition of glycerine diminishes loss of potency (25).

Grading of Skin Tests

Currently no standardized system exists for recording and interpreting skin test results. Many systems for grading positive reactions have been devised. A simple semiquantitative system that measures wheal and erythema is shown in Table 8.2 (26).

Both positive and negative controls are essential for the proper interpretation and the assessment of individual variability in skin reactivity. Histamine is the preferred agent for positive control. Saline or extract diluent may be used for the negative control. Because large reactions at adjacent test sites might coalesce, the test sites should be at least 2 to 5 cm apart (10). In cases of dermographism, there may be reactivity at the control site. This should be noted when the results of the tests are recorded. Interpretation of the tests is then more difficult. Tests that do not clearly have a greater reaction than the negative control must be considered indeterminate.

TABLE 8.2. *Grading system for skin testing*

Grade	Skin appearance
0	No reaction or a reaction no different than negative control
1+	Erythema less than 21 mm and larger than negative control
2+	Erythema larger than 21 mm and larger than negative control
3+	Erythema and wheal formation without pseudopod
4+	Erythema and wheal formation with pseudopod formation

Adapted from Doan T, Zeiss CR. Skin testing in allergy. *Allergy Proc* 1993;14:110–111; with permission.

Late Phase Response

Occasionally delayed reactions characterized by erythema and induration will occur at the site of skin tests. They become apparent 1 to 2 hours after application, peak at 6 to 12 hours, and usually disappear after 24 to 48 hours (27). In contrast to the immediate reactions, they are inhibited by conventional doses of corticosteroids but not by antihistamines (28,29). It is uncertain if the presence of a cutaneous late phase response (LPR) to an antigen will predict occurrence of LPR in the nose or lung of the same patient. Some investigators believe there is a correlation and others do not (30–34).

Adverse Reactions from Skin Testing

Large local reactions at the site of testing are the most common adverse reaction from skin testing. These usually resolve with cold compresses and antihistamines. Systemic reactions are rare and usually occur within 20 minutes of testing (35,36). Emergency treatment should be available during testing, and patients should be kept under observation for at least for 20 minutes after testing. Patients with unstable asthma are at a greater risk of an adverse reaction from skin testing and should not be tested until their asthma is stabilized.

Interpretation of Skin Tests

Table 8.3 provides a guide for the interpretation of skin tests. Both false-negative and

TABLE 8.3. *Interpretation of skin tests*

If:	And:	Then:
History suggests sensitivity,	skin tests are positive,	strong possibility that antigen is responsible.
History does not suggest sensitivity,	skin test results are positive,	may want to observe patient during time of high natural exposure.
History suggests sensitivity,	skin tests are negative,	1. Review medications the patient has taken: antihistamines, antidepressants 2. Review other reasons for false negative tests such as poor quality of testing materials or poor technique 3. Observe patient during a period of high natural exposure 4. Perform provocative challenge (rarely)

false-positive skin test results may occur because of improper technique or material. Improperly prepared or outdated extracts may contain nonspecific irritants or may not be physiologic with respect to pH or osmolarity, and therefore produce false-positive results. The injection of an excessive volume can result in mechanical irritation of the skin and false-positive results.

Population studies have demonstrated that asymptomatic individuals may have positive skin test results (37,38). A positive skin test result only demonstrates the presence of IgE antibody that is specifically directed against the test antigen. A positive result does not mean that a person has an allergic disease, or that an allergic person has ever had a clinically significant reaction to the specific antigen. The number and variety of prick tests performed depend on clinical aspects of the particular case. The antigens used may vary because of the prevalence of particular antigens in any geographic location. Satisfactory information usually can be obtained with a small number of tests if they are carefully chosen. With inhalant antigens, correlating positive skin tests with a history that suggests clinical sensitivity may strongly incriminate an antigen. Conversely, a negative skin test and a negative history exclude the antigen as being clinically significant.

Interpretation of skin tests that do not correlate with the clinical history or physical findings is much more difficult. If there is no history suggesting sensitivity to an antigen, and the skin test result is positive, the patient can be evaluated again during a period of maximal exposure to the antigen. At that time, if there are no symptoms or physical findings of sensitivity, the skin test result may be ignored. Positive results may predict future symptomatology (38). A three-year study of college students demonstrated that asymptomatic students who were skin test positive were more likely to develop allergic rhinitis 3 years later than skin test–negative asymptomatic students.

Patients with a history that strongly suggests an allergic disease or clinical sensitivity to specific antigens may have negative skin test results for the suspected antigens. It is difficult to make an allergic diagnosis in these cases because, when properly done, negative results indicate that no specific IgE antibody is present. These patients may be requestioned and reexamined, and the possibility of false-negative skin test results must be excluded.

IN VITRO MEASUREMENT OF IgE ANTIBODIES

Total Serum IgE

Total serum IgE is generally elevated in atopic individuals, especially patients with asthma who also have atopic dermatitis. However concentrations fluctuate widely around a mean of 300 ng/mL (125 IU/mL) among atopic and nonatopic individuals (39–42). Because there is no normal limit for IgE concentrations, measuring total IgE is not of diagnostic significance and rarely provides useful information (43,44).

Total serum IgE determinations are indicated in patients suspected of having allergic bronchopulmonary allergic aspergillosis, both in the diagnosis and monitoring of the course of the disease (45). High IgE concentrations in infants may predict future allergic diseases and occasionally are checked in infants with frequent respiratory infections. IgE concentrations are also necessary in the evaluation of certain immunodeficiencies such as hyper-IgE syndrome.

Specific IgE

In vitro procedures such as radioallergosorbent tests and enzyme-linked immunosorbent assays detect allergen-specific IgE antibodies in the patient's serum. Skin testing is the diagnostic test of choice for IgE-mediated diseases and is generally reported to be more sensitive and specific than *in vitro* tests (46). In addition, skin testing is less expensive and provides immediate results. High quality *in vitro* tests are comparable with skin tests in diagnostic value, especially for demonstration of aeroallergen and food sensitivity (46–50).

The same clinical problems observed in skin testing are present when the results of *in vitro* tests are interpreted. In addition, there are a number of technical problems over which the clinician has no control that can influence the test results. Both *in vitro* testing and skin testing can yield false-negative, false-positive, or equivocal results, depending on a number of variables. If performed optimally, both methods detect specific IgE antibody accurately and reproducibly.

In vitro testing may be indicated in some circumstances:

1. Some patients may not be able to omit medications that interfere with skin testing. Because no medications interfere with *in vitro* testing, it may be useful in these patients.
2. Some patients may have a history of extreme sensitivity to allergens. *In vitro* tests would avoid the possibility of anaphylaxis or even uncomfortable local reactions.
3. In contrast to skin testing, dermographism and widespread skin diseases, do not interfere with *in vitro* testing, and therefore may be useful in patients with these problems.

Irresponsible promotion of any testing method is inappropriate. Commercial firms and individual physicians may misrepresent the value of any testing method. The results of any tests must correlate with the production of allergic symptoms and signs by a specific antigen to have any meaning. Consequently, the history and physical examination personally performed by the physician remain the fundamental investigative procedure for the diagnosis of allergic disease.

REFERENCES

1. Platts-Mills TAE, Chapman MD. Dust mites: immunology, allergic diseases, and environmental control. *J Allergy Clin Immunol* 1987;80:755–775.
2. Platts-Mills TAE, de Weck AL. Dust mite allergens and asthma: a worldwide problem. *J Allergy Clin Immunol* 1989;83:416–427.
3. Findley LJ, Sahn SA. The value of chest roentgenograms in acute asthma in adults. *Chest* 1981;80:535–536.
4. Wippold II FJ, Levitt RG, Evens RG, et al. Limited coronal CT: an alternative screening examination for sinonasal inflammatory disease. *Allergy Proc* 1995; 16:165–169.
5. Smith L, McFadden ER Jr. Bronchial hyperreactivity revisited. *Ann Allergy Asthma Immunol* 1995;74:545–470.
6. Friedman MM, Kaliner M. Ultrastructural changes in human skin mast cells during antigen-induced degranulation in vivo. *J Allergy Clin Immunol* 1988;82: 988–1005.
7. Nelson HS, Oppenheimer J, Buchmeier A, et al. An assessment of the role of intradermal skin testing in the diagnosis of clinically relevant allergy to timothy grass. *J Allergy Clin Immunol* 1996;97:1193–1201.
8. Idrajana T, Spieksma FTM, Vorrhorst R. Comparative study of the intracutaneous, scratch, and prick tests in allergy. *Ann Allergy* 1971;29:639–660.
9. Bock SA, Lee WY, Remigio L, et al. Appraisal of skin tests with food extracts for diagnosis of food hypersensitivity. *Clin Allergy* 1978;8:559–564.
10. Nelson HS, Knoetzer J, Bucher B. Effect of distance between sites and region of the body on results of skin prick tests. *J Allergy Clin Immunol* 1996;97: 596–601.
11. Menardo JL, Bousquet J, Rodiere M, et al. Ski test reactivity in infancy. *J Allergy Clin Immunol* 1985;75:646–651.
12. Skassa-Brociek W, Manderscheid JC, Michel FB, et al. Ski test reactivity to histamine from infancy to old age. *J Allergy Clin Immunol* 1987;80:711–716.
13. Harvey RP, Schocket AL. The effect of H_1 and H_2 blockage on cutaneous histamine response in man. *J Allergy Clin Immunol* 1980;65:136–139.
14. Miller J, Nelson HS. Suppression of immediate skin tests by ranitidine. *J Allergy Clin Immunol* 1989;84:895–899.

15. Rao KS, Menon PK, Hilman BC, et al. Duration of the suppressive effect of tricyclic antidepressants on histamine-induced wheal-and-flare reactions in human skin. *J Allergy Clin Immunol* 1988;82:752–757.

16. Slott RJ, Zweiman B. A controlled study of the effects of corticosteroids on immediate skin test reactivity. *J Allergy Clin Immunol* 1974;54:229–235.

17. Olson R, Karpink MH, Shelanki S, et al. Skin reactivity to codeine and histamine during prolonged corticosteroid therapy. *J Allergy Clin Immunol* 1990;86:153–159.

18. Pipkorn U, Hammerlund, Enerbaeck L. Prolonged treatment with topical corticosteroids results in an inhibition of the allergen-induced wheal-and-flare response and a reduction in skin mast cell numbers and histamine content. *Clin Exp Allergy* 1989;19:19–27.

19. Garcia-Ortega P, Merelo A, Marrugat J, et al. Decrease of skin and bronchial sensitization following short-intensive schedule immunotherapy in mite-allergic asthma. *Chest* 1993;103:183–187.

20. Graft DF, Schuberth KC, Kagey-Sobotka A, et al. The development of negative skin tests in children treated with venom immunotherapy. *J Allergy Clin Immunol* 1984;73:61–68.

21. Paquet F, Boulet LP, Bedard G, et al. Influence of time of administration on allergic skin prick tests response. *Ann Allergy* 1991;67:163–166.

22. Seery JP, James SM, Ind PW, et al. Circadian rhythm of cutaneous hypersensitivity reactions in nocturnal asthma. *Ann Allergy Asthma Immunol* 1998;30:329–330.

23. Haahtela T, Jokela H. Influence of the pollen season on immediate skin test reactivity to common allergens. *Allergy* 1980;35:15–21.

24. Nahm DH, Park HS, Kang SS, et al. Seasonal variation of skin reactivity and specific IgE antibody to house dust mite. *Ann Allergy Asthma Immunol* 1997;78:589–593.

25. Bernstein L, Storms WW. Practice parameters for allergy diagnostic testing. *Ann Allergy Asthma Immunol* 1995;75:553–625.

26. Doan T, Zeiss CR. Skin testing in allergy. *Allergy Proc* 1993;14:110–111.

27. Reshef A, Kagey-Sobotka A, Adkinson N Jr, et al. The pattern and kinetics in human skin of erythema and mediators during the acute and late-phase response (LPR). *J Allergy Clin Immunol* 1989;84:678–687.

28. Umemoto L, Poothullil J, Dolovich J, et al. Factors which influence late cutaneous allergic responses. *J Allergy Clin Immunol* 1976;58:60–68.

29. Poothullil J, Umemoto L, Dolovich J, et al. Inhibition by prednisone of late cutaneous allergic response induced by antiserum to human IgE. *J Allergy Clin Immunol* 1976;57:164–167.

30. Atkins PC, Martin GL, Yost R, Zweiman B. Late onset reactions in humans: correlation between skin and bronchial reactivity. *Ann Allergy* 1988;60:27–30.

31. Price KF, Hey EN, Soothill JF. Antigen provocation to the skin, nose, and lung in children with asthma: immediate and dual hypersensitivity reactions. *Clin Exp Immunol* 1982;47:587–594.

32. Warner JO. Significance of late reactions after bronchial challenge with house dust mite. *Arch Dis Child* 1976; 51:905–911.

33. Boulet LP, Robert RS, Dolovich JE, et al. Prediction of late asthmatic responses to inhaled allergen. *Clin Allergy* 1984;14:379–385.

34. Taylor G, Shivalkor PR. Arthus-type reactivity in the nasal airways and skin in pollen sensitive subjects. *Clin Allergy* 1971;1:407–414.

35. Lin MS, Tanner E, Lynn J, et al. Nonfatal systemic allergic reactions induced by skin testing and immunotherapy. *Ann Allergy* 1993;71:557–562.

36. Lockey RF, Benedict LM, Turkeltaub PC, et al. Fatalities from immunotherapy (IT) and skin testing (ST). *J Allergy Clin Immunol* 1987;79:660–677.

37. Droste JHJ, Kerkhof M, de Monchy JGR, et al. Association of skin reactivity, specific IgE, total IgE, and eosinophils with nasal symptoms in a community based population study. *J Allergy Clin Immunol* 1996;97:922–932.

38. Hagy GW, Settipane GA. Prognosis of positive allergy skin tests in asymptomatic population. A three year followup of college students. *J Allergy Clin Immunol* 1971;48:200–212.

39. Klink M, Cline MG, Halonen M, et al. Problems in defining normal limits for serum IgE. *J Allergy Clin Immunol* 1990;85:440–444.

40. Sunyer J, Anto JM, Castellsague J, et al. Total serum IgE is associated with asthma independently of specific IgE levels. *Eur Respir J* 1996;9:1880–1884.

41. Luoma R, Koivikko A, Viander M. Development of asthma, allergic rhinitis and atopic dermatitis by the age of five years. *Allergy* 1983;38:339–346.

42. Peat JK, Toelle BG, Dermand J, et al. Serum IgE levels, atopy, and asthma in young adults: results from a longitudinal cohort study. *Allergy* 1996;51:804–810.

43. Ezeamuzie CI, Ali-Ali AF, Al-Dowaisan A, et al. Reference values of total serum IgE and their significance in the diagnosis of allergy among the young adult Kuwaiti population. *Clin Exp Allergy* 1999;29:375–381.

44. Wittig HJ, Belloit J, De Fillippi L, et al. Age-related serum immunoglobulin E levels in healthy subjects and in patients with allergic disease. *J Allergy Clin Immunol* 1980;66:305–313.

45. Roberts ML, Greenberger PA. Serologic analysis of allergic bronchopulmonary aspergillosis. In: Patterson R, Greenberger PA, eds. *Allergic bronchopulmonary aspergillosis.* Providence, RI: Oceanside Publications, 1995:11–15.

46. Position statement. The use of in vitro tests for IgE antibody in the specific diagnosis of IgE-mediated disorders and in the formulation of allergen immunotherapy. *J Allergy Clin Immunol* 1992;90:263–267.

47. Plebani M, Borghesan F, Faggian D. Clinical efficiency of in vitro and in vivo tests for allergic diseases. *Ann Allergy Asthma Immunol* 1995;74:23–28.

48. Williams PB, Dolen WK, Koepke JW, et al. Comparison of skin testing and three in vitro assays for specific IgE in the clinical evaluation of immediate hypersensitivity. *Ann Allergy* 1992;68:35–42.

49. Kam KL, Hsieh KH. Comparison of three in vitro assays for serum IgE with skin testing in asthmatic children. *Ann Allergy* 1994;73:329–336.

50. Kelso JM, Sodhi N, Gosselin VA, et al. Diagnostic performance characteristic of the standard Phadebas RAST, modified RAST, and Pharmacia CAP system versus skin testing. *Ann Allergy* 1991;67:511–514.

9

Allergic Rhinitis

Anthony J. Ricketti

Department of Medicine, Seton Hall University, Graduate School of Medicine

The term *rhinitis* is used to describe disease that involves inflammation of the nasal membrane and is characterized by periods of nasal discharge, sneezing, and congestion that persist for a period of at least 1 hour per day. It is also considered pathologic when a subject occasionally has symptoms of such intensity to require therapy or when an individual's nasal reaction to certain stimuli differs fundamentally from that of other people. Rhinitis may be classified into two types, infectious and noninfectious (Table 9.1). Infectious rhinitis is characterized predominantly by cloudy (white, yellow, or green) nasal secretions, with many neutrophils, and less commonly, bacteria (1). Noninfectious rhinitis is characterized by clear (watery or mucoid) discharge that often contains eosinophils. The noninfectious group can be subdivided into seasonal allergic rhinitis, perennial allergic rhinitis, and perennial nonallergic rhinitis.

Perennial nonallergic rhinitis comprises a heterogeneous group consisting of at least two subgroups (2). One subgroup is characterized by nasal eosinophilia, frequent occurrence of polyps, abnormal sinus radiographs, concurrent asthma, and good response to therapy, whereas these characteristics usually are lacking in the other subgroup. This subdivision of patients with nonallergic rhinitis may not always be possible in a particular case and therefore may not be an entirely suitable system for clinical routine.

SEASONAL ALLERGIC RHINITIS

Definition

Seasonal allergic rhinitis is a specific allergic reaction of the nasal mucosa to allergens and is characterized mainly by watery rhinorrhea, nasal congestion, sneezing, and pruritus of the eyes, nose, ears, and throat. These symptoms are periodic in nature and occur during the pollinating season of the plants to which the patient is sensitive.

Incidence

Although allergic rhinitis may have its onset at any age, the incidence of onset is greatest in children at adolescence, with a decrease in incidence seen in advancing age. Occasionally, however, symptoms may appear first in middle or advanced age. Although it has been reported in infants as young as 6 months of age (3), in most cases, an individual requires two or more seasons of exposure to a new antigen before exhibiting the clinical manifestations of allergic rhinitis (4).

One community study of allergic rhinitis reported that 75% of patients resided inside the city (5), but other studies have not reported variation in the prevalence of allergic rhinitis based on geographic location (6). In addition, there does not appear to be any correlation between socioeconomic status or race and the prevalence of allergic rhinitis (6). Boys tend to have an increased

TABLE 9.1. *Classification of rhinitis*

Type	Skin test	Predominant cells in secretions
Infectious (purulent)	−	
Common cold		Neutrophils
Rhinosinusitis (various organisms)	−	Neutrophils
Noninfectious (nonpurulent)		
Seasonal allergic rhinitis	+	Eosinophils
Perennial allergic rhinitis	+	Eosinophils
Perennial nonallergic rhinitis		
Eosinophilic subgroup	−	Eosinophils
Noneosinophilic subgroup	−	Few cells
Nasal polyps	+/−	Eosinophils
Atrophic rhinitis	−	Few cells

incidence of allergic rhinitis in childhood, but the sex ratio becomes even in adulthood.

Although the prevalence of allergic rhinitis has been estimated to range from as low as 4% to more than 40% (5,7,8), an accurate estimate of the incidence of allergic rhinitis is difficult to obtain. Some obstacles in obtaining accurate estimates of allergic disease include variability in geographic pollen counts, misinterpretation of symptoms by patients, and inability of the physician to recognize the disorder. Epidemiology studies suggest that the prevalence of allergic rhinitis in the United States and around the world is increasing (9). The cause of this increased prevalence of allergic rhinitis is unknown. However, contributing factors may include higher concentrations of airborne pollution, such as diesel exhaust particles (10); rising dust mite populations (11); less ventilation in homes and offices; dietary factors (12); and a trend toward more sedentary lifestyles (13).

With the increased prevalence of allergic rhinitis, the disorder has increased in importance, and the suffering and annoyance that many experience should not be underestimated. In allergy-specific questionnaires (14,15), subjects with allergic rhinitis consistently reported lower quality of life than nonallergic controls. In a large health outcomes study of patients with moderate to severe allergic rhinitis symptoms, 70% of untreated patients reported being embarrassed or frustrated by their allergy symptoms, and 98% reported being troubled by practical problems (15).

Considerable expenditures are involved in medications, physician fees, and economic loss secondary to absenteeism and inefficient performance at work. Seasonal and perennial allergic rhinitis account for the loss of 1.5 million school days per year and may be responsible for 3.4 million missed work days per year. Ross estimated that the cost of decreased productivity in the United States labor force due to allergic rhinitis totaled $2.4 billion in men and $1.4 billion in women (16). Conservative estimates report that prescription medication costs are greater than $1 billion per year, and over-the-counter medications are at least twice that amount (17).

The disease tends to persist indefinitely after clinical symptoms appear. The severity of symptoms, however, may vary from year to year depending on the quality of pollen released and patient exposure during the specific pollinating seasons. Occasionally, the disease undergoes a spontaneous remission without specific therapy.

Etiology

Pollen and mold spores are the allergens responsible for seasonal allergic rhinitis (Table 9.2). The pollens important in causing allergic rhinitis are from plants that depend on the wind for cross-pollination. Many grasses, trees, and weeds produce lightweight pollen in sufficient quantities to sensitize individuals with genetic susceptibility. Plants that depend on insect pollination, such as goldenrod, dandelions, and most other plants with obvious flowers, do not cause allergic rhinitis symptoms.

The pollination season of the various plants depends on the individual plant and on the

TABLE 9.2. *Major aeroallergens in allergic rhinitis*

Outdoor (generally seasonal)
  Pollens
    Weeds (ragweed)
    Grasses (rye, timothy, orchard)
    Trees (oak, elm, birch, alder, hazel)
  Molds (*Alternaria, Cladosporium* species)—March, April, May
Indoor (generally perennial)
  House dust mites
    Dermatophagoides farinae
    Dermatophagoides pteronyssinus
  Warm-blooded pets
  Pests
    Mice
    Cockroaches
    Rats
  Molds
    Aspergillus species
    Penicillium species
  Occupational allergens
    Laboratory animals

various geographic locations. For a particular plant in a given locale, however, the pollinating season is determined by the relative amount of night and day and is constant from year to year. Weather conditions, such as temperature and rainfall, influence the amount of pollen produced but not the actual onset or termination of a specific season.

Ragweed pollen, a significant cause of allergic rhinitis, produces the most severe and longest seasonal rhinitis in the eastern and midwestern portions of the United States and Ontario, Canada. In those areas, ragweed pollen appears in significant amounts from the second or third week of August through September. Occasionally, sensitive patients may exhibit symptoms as early as the first few days of August, when smaller quantities of pollen first appear. Although ragweed is the dominant airborne allergen in North America during the late summer and early fall, there are also other important weed pollens, such as sheep sorrel in the spring and plantain during the summer months. Western ragweed and marsh elder in the western states, sagebrush and franseria in the Pacific areas, and careless weed, pigweed, and franseria in the southwestern United States are important allergens in the late summer and early fall. In the northern and eastern United States, the earliest pollens to appear are tree pollens, usually in March, April, or May. Late spring and early summer allergic rhinitis in this locale is caused by grass pollens, which appear from May to late June or early July. During this season, patients may complain of "rose fever," which, like "hay fever," is a misnomer. Roses coincidentally are in full bloom during the grass-pollinating season, and this accounts for the misconception. About 25% of pollinosis patients have both grass and ragweed allergic rhinitis, and about 5% have all three allergies. In other geographic locations, these generalizations are not correct, because of the particular climate and because some less common plants may predominate. For example, grass pollinates from early spring through late fall in the southwestern regions and accounts for allergic rhinitis that is almost perennial.

Airborne mold spores, the most important of which throughout the United States are *Alternaria* and *Cladosporium* species, also cause seasonal allergic rhinitis. Warm, damp weather favors the growth of molds and thereby influences the severity of the season. Generally, molds first appear in the air in the spring, become most significant during the warmer months, and usually disappear with the first frost. Thus, patients with marked hypersensitivity to molds may exhibit symptoms from early spring through the first frost, whereas those with a lesser degree of hypersensitivity may have symptoms from early summer through late fall only.

Clinical Features

The major symptoms of allergic rhinitis are sneezing, rhinorrhea, nasal pruritus, and nasal congestion, although patients may not have the entire symptom complex. When taking the patient's history, record the specific characteristics of symptoms, as follows:

1. Define onset and duration of symptoms and emphasize any relationship to seasons or life events, such as changing residence or occupation or acquiring a new pet.
2. Define current symptoms, including secretions, degree of congestion, sneezing and nasal itching, or sinus pressure and pain.

Obtain history regarding ocular symptoms, such as itching, lacrimation, puffiness, and chemosis; pharyngeal symptoms of mild sore throat, throat clearing, and itching of the palate and throat; and associated systemic symptoms of malaise, fatigue, or sleep disturbances.

3. Identify exacerbating factors, such as seasonal or perennial allergens and nonspecific irritants (e.g., cigarette smoke, chemical fumes, cold air).

4. Identify other associated allergic diseases, such as asthma or atopic dermatitis, or a family history of allergic diathesis.

5. Obtain a complete medication history, including both prescription and over-the-counter medications.

Sneezing is the most characteristic symptom, and occasionally one may have paroxysms of 10 to 20 sneezes in rapid succession. Sneezing episodes may arise without warning, or they may be preceded by an uncomfortable itching or irritated feeling in the nose. Sneezing attacks result in tearing of the eyes because of activation of the nasal lacrimal reflex. During the pollinating season, nonspecific factors, such as dust exposure, sudden drafts, air pollutants, or noxious irritants, may also trigger violent sneezing episodes.

The rhinorrhea is typically a thin discharge, which may be quite profuse and continuous. Because of the copious nature of the rhinorrhea, the skin covering the external nose and the upper lip may become irritated and tender. Purulent discharge is never seen in uncomplicated allergic rhinitis, and its presence usually indicates secondary infection. Nasal congestion resulting from swollen turbinates is a frequent complaint. Early in the season, the nasal obstruction may be intermittent or more troublesome in the evening and at night, only to become almost continuous as the season progresses. If the nasal obstruction is severe, interference with aeration and drainage of the paranasal sinus or the eustachian tube may occur, resulting in complaints of headache or earache. The headache is of the so-called vacuum type, presumably caused by the development of negative pressure when air is absorbed from the obstructive sinus or middle ear. Patients also complain that their hearing is decreased and that sounds seem muffled. Patients also may notice a crackling sensation in the ears, especially when swallowing. Nasal congestion alone, particularly in children, occasionally may be the major or sole complaint. With continuous severe nasal congestion, the senses of smell and taste may be lost. Itching of the nose also may be a prominent feature, inducing frequent rubbing of the nose, particularly in children. Eye symptoms (pruritus erythema and lacrimation) often accompany the nasal symptoms. Patients with severe eye symptoms often complain of photophobia and sore, "tired" eyes. Sclera and conjunctival injection and chemosis often occur. Occasionally, there may be marked itching of the ears, palate, throat, or face, which may be extremely annoying. Because of irritating sensations in the throat and the posterior drainage of the nasal secretions, a hacking, nonproductive cough may be present. A constricted feeling in the chest, sometimes severe enough to cause the patient to complain of shortness of breath, may accompany the cough. This sensation of tightness in the chest is particularly bothersome to the patients with severe nighttime cough. The diagnosis of coexisting asthma should be considered in such patients. Some patients have systemic symptoms of seasonal allergic rhinitis. Complaints may include weakness, malaise, irritability, fatigue, and anorexia. Certain patients relate that nausea, abdominal discomfort, and poor appetite appear to occur with swallowing excess mucous.

A characteristic feature of the symptom complex is the periodicity of its appearance. Symptoms usually recur each year for many years in relation to the duration of the pollinating season of the causative plant. The most sensitive patients exhibit symptoms early in the season, almost as soon as the pollen appears in the air. The intensity of the symptoms tends to follow the course of pollination, becoming more severe when the pollen concentration is highest and waning as the season comes to an end, when the amount of pollen in the air decreases. In some patients, symptoms disappear suddenly when the pollination season is over, whereas in others, symptoms may disappear gradually over a period of 2 or 3 weeks after the pollination season is completed. There may be an increased reactivity of the nasal mucosa after repeated exposure to the pollen (18). This local and nonspecific increased reactivity has been termed the *priming effect.* The nonspecificity of this effect was suggested by demonstration under experimental conditions that a patient may respond to an allergen not otherwise considered clinically significant if he or she had been exposed or primed to a clinically significant allergen. This effect may account for the presence of symptoms in some patients beyond the termination of the pollinating season because an allergen not important clinically by itself may induce symptoms in the "primed" nose. For example, a patient with positive skin tests to mold antigens and ragweed, and no symptoms until August, may have symptoms until late October, after the ragweed-pollinating season is over. The symptoms persist because of the presence of molds in the air, which affect the primed mucous membrane. In most patients, however, this does not appear to occur (19). The presence of a secondary infection, or the effects of nonspecific irritants on inflamed nasal membranes, may also prolong rhinitis symptoms beyond a specific pollinating season.

To a lesser degree, the symptoms of allergic rhinitis may exhibit periodicity within the season. Many patients tend to have more intense symptoms in the morning because most windborne pollen is released in greatest numbers between sunrise and 9:00 AM. Other specific factors modify the intensity of rhinitis symptoms. These symptoms may diminish while it is raining because of the clearing of the pollen from the air. Dry, windy days aggravate the symptoms because a higher concentration of pollen may be distributed over larger areas.

In addition to specific factors, nonspecific factors may also influence the degree of rhinitis symptoms. Some of these include tobacco smoke, paints, newspaper ink, and soap powders. Rapid atmospheric changes may aggravate symptoms in predisposed patients. Nonspecific air pollutants may also potentiate the symptoms of allergic rhinitis, such as sulfur dioxide, ozone, carbon monoxide, and nitrogen dioxide.

Overall, allergic rhinitis tends to increase in severity for 2 or 3 years until a stabilized condition is reached. Symptoms then recur year after year. Occasionally, patients spontaneously lose their hypersensitivity, for reasons that are not well understood.

Physical Examination

The most abnormal physical findings are present during the acute stages of the patient's seasonal complaints. The following common physical findings appear in allergic rhinitis patients during a seasonal exacerbation:

- Nasal obstruction, associated mouth breathing
- Pale to bluish nasal mucosa and enlarged (boggy) inferior turbinates
- Clear nasal secretions (whitish secretions may be seen in patients experiencing severe allergic rhinitis.)
- Clear or white secretions along the posterior wall of the nasopharynx
- Conjunctival erythema, lacrimation, puffiness of the eyes

The physical findings, which are usually confined to the nose, ears, and eyes, aid in the diagnosis. Rubbing of the nose and mouth breathing are common findings in children. Some children will rub the nose in an upward and outward fashion, which has been termed the allergic salute. The eyes may exhibit excessive lacrimation, the sclera and conjunctiva may be reddened, and chemosis is often present. The conjunctivae may be swollen and may appear granular in nature. In addition, the eyelids are often swollen. The skin above the nose may be reddened and irritated because of the continuous rubbing and blowing of the nose. Examination of the nasal cavity discloses a pale, wet, edematous mucosa, frequently bluish in color. A clear, thin nasal secretion may be seen within the nasal cavity. Swollen turbinates may completely occlude the nasal passageway and severely affect the patient. Nasal polyps may be present in individuals with allergic rhinitis. Occasionally, there is fluid in the middle ear, resulting in decreased hearing. The pharynx is usually normal. The nose and eye examination are normal during asymptomatic intervals.

Pathophysiology

The nose has five major functions:

1. An olfactory organ
2. A resonator for phonation
3. A passageway for airflow in and out of the lungs
4. A means of humidifying and warming inspired air
5. A filter of noxious particles from inspired air

Allergic reactions occurring in the nasal mucous membranes markedly affect the nose's major functions. The nose can initiate immune mechanisms, and the significance of mediator release from nasal mast cells and basophils in immediate-type allergic reaction is well established. Patients with allergic rhinitis have immunoglobulin E (IgE) antibodies that bind to high-affinity receptors on mast cells and basophils and to low-affinity receptors on other cells, such as monocytes, eosinophils, and platelets (20–23). On nasal reexposure to antigen, the mast cells degranulate, releasing a number of mediators of inflammation. Mediators released include histamine, leukotrienes, prostaglandins, platelet-activating factor, and bradykinin. These mediators are responsible for vasodilation, increased vascular permeability, increased glandular secretion, and stimulation of afferent nerves (24–26), which culminate in the immediate-type rhinitis symptoms.

Mast cells and their mediators are central to the pathogenesis of the early response, as indicated by the demonstration of mast cell degranulation in the nasal mucosa and the detection of mast cell–derived mediators, including histamine, leukotriene C-4 (LTC-4), and prostaglandin D_2 (PGD_2) in nasal washings (27). In addition to mast cell mediators, the early response is associated with an increase in neuropeptides, such as calcitonin gene–related peptide, substance P, and vasoactive intestinal peptide, and increasing numbers of cytokines, such as interleukin-1 (IL-1), IL-3, IL-4, IL-5, IL-6, granulocyte-macrophage colony-stimulating factor (GM-CSF), and tumor necrosis factor-α (TNF-α) (27). With continuation of allergic inflammation, one sees an accumulation of CD4[+] T lymphocytes, eosinophils, neutrophils, and

basophils (28,29). Eosinophils release major basic protein, which may further disrupt the respiratory epithelium and promote further mast cell mediator release. There are strong correlations between the number of basophils and the level of histamine in the late reaction and between the number of eosinophils and the amount of eosinophil major basic protein (30), which suggest that these cells may participate in allergic inflammation by not only entering the nose but also degranulating. Other evidence for the participation of eosinophils in allergic inflammation is that eosinophils increase during the seasonal exposure (31,32), and the number of eosinophil progenitors in nasal scrapings increases after exposure to allergens and correlates with the severity of seasonal disease (33). Basophils may also participate in the late-phase allergic response because cell counts have confirmed increases of basophils from nasal lavage fluids. Recent studies involving nasal mucosal biopsy confirm an increase in CD4[+] CD25 T cells, in addition to neutrophils and eosinophils, during late responses (34). These CD4 T lymphocytes help promote the late-phase allergic reaction because they express messenger RNA for IL-3, IL-4, IL-5, and GM-CSF. IL-5 participates in eosinophil chemotaxis and growth, whereas IL-4 helps mediate IgE production and upregulates adhesion molecules, such as vascular cell adhesion molecule, on vascular endothelium. Although neutrophils enter the nose in larger numbers than eosinophils, their role in allergic inflammation is unknown. Overall, the late-phase reaction of allergic rhinitis is characterized by the infiltration of the nasal cavity with basophils, lymphocytes, eosinophils, and neutrophils, as well as the release of the same mediators involved in the early response, except PGD_2 and tryptase. The absence of the mast cell–derived mediators PGD_2 and tryptase during the late-phase reaction is consistent with basophil-derived histamine release rather than mast cell involvement.

The heating and humidification of inspired air is an important function of the nasal mucosa. The highly vascularized mucosa of the turbinates in the septum provides an effective structure to heat and humidify air as it passes over them. The blood vessels are under the direction of the autonomic nervous system, which controls reflex adjustments for efficient performance of this function. The sympathetic nervous system provides for vascular constriction with a reduction of secretions. The parasympathetic nervous system enables vascular dilation and an increase in secretions. These two systems are in a constant state of balance to meet any specific demand.

The protecting and cleansing role of the nasal mucosa is also an important function. Relatively large particles are filtered out of the inspired air by the hairs within the nostrils. The nasal secretions contain an enzyme, lysozyme, which is bacteriostatic. The pH of the nasal secretions remains relatively constant at 7. Lysozyme activity and ciliary action are optimal at this pH. The major portions of the nose, septum, and paranasal sinuses are lined by ciliated cells.

The cilia beat at a frequency of 10 to 15 beats per minute, producing a streaming mucus blanket at an approximate rate of 2.5 to 7.5 mm per minute. The mucus is produced by mucous and serous glands and epithelial goblet cells in the mucosa. The mucus blanket containing the filtered materials is moved toward the pharynx to be expectorated or swallowed.

Laboratory Findings

The only characteristic laboratory finding in allergic rhinitis is the presence of large numbers of eosinophils in a Hansel-stained smear of the nasal secretions obtained during a period of symptoms. In classic seasonal allergic rhinitis, this test is usually not necessary to make a diagnosis. Its use is limited to questionable cases and more often in defining chronic allergic rhinitis. Peripheral blood eosinophilia of 4% to 12% may or may not be present in active seasonal allergic rhinitis. The presence or absence of eosinophilia should not be relied on in making the diagnosis of seasonal allergic rhinitis. A significantly elevated level of serum IgE may occur in the serum of some patients with allergic rhinitis (35) but is not a prerequisite for this diagnosis.

Diagnosis

The diagnosis of seasonal allergic rhinitis usually presents no difficulty by the time the patient has had symptoms severe enough to seek medical attention. The seasonal nature of the condition, the characteristic symptom complex, and the physical findings should establish a diagnosis in almost all cases. If the patient is first seen during the initial or second season, or if the major symptom is conjunctivitis, there may be a delay in making the diagnosis from the history alone.

Additional supporting evidence is a positive history of allergic disorders in the immediate family and a collateral history of other allergic disorders in the patient. After the history is taken and the physical examination is performed, skin tests should be performed to determine the reactivity of the patient against the suspected allergens. For the proper interpretation of the meaning of a positive skin test, it is important to remember that patients with allergic rhinitis may exhibit positive skin tests to allergens other than those that are clinically important. In seasonal allergic rhinitis, it has been demonstrated that prick puncture testing is adequate for diagnostic purposes and that intradermal testing when positive may not clinically correlate with allergic disease (36). Skin testing should be performed and interpreted by trained personnel because results may be altered by the distance placed between allergens (37), the application site (back versus arm), the type of device used for testing (38), the season of the year tested (39), and the quality of extracts used for testing (40). The radioallergosorbent test (RAST), an *in vitro* procedure for assessing the presence of specific IgE antibodies to various allergens, has been employed as a diagnostic aid in some allergic diseases. RAST determination of circulating IgE antibody can be used instead of skin testing when high-quality extracts are not available, when a control skin test with the diluents is consistently positive, when antihistamine therapy cannot be discontinued, or in the presence of a widespread skin disease such as atopic dermatitis. The serum RAST appears to correlate well with other measures of sensitivity, such as skin tests, end-point titration, histamine release, and provocation tests (41–44). Although occasional patients may have an elevated nasal secretion RAST, relative to serum RAST levels, one usually finds a good correlation between specific IgE measurements of skin tests, nasal secretion RAST, and serum RAST levels. These findings usually reflect the fact that specific IgE, regardless of where it is synthesized, is in equilibrium with the skin, nose, and serum of allergic rhinitis patients (45). Clinical symptoms usually correlate well with skin tests, nasal RAST, and serum RAST. The frequency of positive reactions obtained from skin testing is usually greater than that found on serum or nasal RAST.

In view of these findings, the serum or nasal RAST may be used as a supplement to skin testing, but skin testing is the diagnostic method of choice to demonstrate IgE antibodies. When the skin test is positive, there is little need for other tests. When the skin test is dubiously positive, the RAST will, as a rule, be negative. Therefore, the information obtained by examining serum IgE antibody by RAST usually adds little to the information obtained by critical evaluation of skin testing with high-quality extracts.

Another procedure, nasal provocation, is a useful research tool but not a generally recognized diagnostic procedure. Skin testing should be performed because, in contrast to the nasal test, the skin test is quick, inexpensive, safe, and without discomfort to the patient, and it has the additional advantage of possessing better reproducibility.

The major clinical entity that enters into the differential diagnosis of allergic rhinitis is that of infectious rhinitis. Fever, sore throat, thick purulent rhinorrhea, erythematous nasal mucosa, the absence of pruritus, and the presence of cervical lymphadenopathy are helpful differential findings in infectious rhinitis. Stained smears of the nasal secretions usually show a predominance of polymorphonuclear neutrophils. The total duration of symptoms, 4 to 10 days, is another helpful sign, because pollination seasons are usually much longer.

PERENNIAL ALLERGIC RHINITIS

Definition

Perennial allergic rhinitis is characterized by intermittent or continuous nasal symptoms resulting from an allergic reaction without seasonal variation. Some clinicians have used the term *perennial allergic rhinitis* to include both allergic and nonallergic forms of nonseasonal rhinitis, but it should be applied to those cases in which an allergic etiology is known to exist. The term *allergic* in this book is used only for those responses mediated by, or presumed to be mediated by, an immunologic reaction. Although many aspects related to the etiology, pathophysiology, symptomatology, and diagnosis have been discussed in the preceding section, separate consideration of perennial allergic rhinitis is warranted because of certain complexities of the disease with particular reference to the diagnosis, management, and complications.

Etiology

Perennial allergic rhinitis has the same mechanisms as seasonal allergic rhinitis. The difference is only that chronic antigen challenge results in recurring, almost continuous, symptoms throughout the year. Inhalant allergens are the most important cause of perennial allergic rhinitis. The major perennial allergens are house dust mites, mold antigens, feather pillows, animal dander, and cockroaches (Table 9.2). Pollen allergy may contribute to seasonal exacerbations of rhinitis in patients with perennial symptoms. Occasionally, perennial allergic rhinitis may be the result of exposure to an occupational allergen. Symptoms are perennial but not constant in such cases because there is a clear, temporal association with workplace exposure. Occupational allergic rhinitis has been described in flour industry workers (46), detergent workers (47), and wood workers (48).

Although some clinicians believe that food allergens may be significant factors in the cause of perennial allergic rhinitis, a direct immunologic relationship between ingested foods and persistent rhinitis symptoms has been difficult to establish. Rarely, hypersensitivity to dietary proteins may induce the symptoms of nonseasonal allergic rhinitis. Such reactions are usually confirmed by double-blind food challenges (49). Cow's milk, both on an allergic and nonimmunologic basis, has been the food most associated with precipitating or aggravating upper respiratory symptoms (50). Usually, however, the overwhelming majority of patients with proven food allergies exhibit other symptoms, including gastrointestinal disturbances, urticaria, angioedema, asthma, and anaphylaxis, in addition to rhinitis, after ingestion of the specific food.

Nonspecific irritants and infections may influence the course of perennial allergic rhinitis. Children with this condition appear to have a higher incidence of respiratory infections that tend to aggravate the condition and often lead to the development of complications (51). Irritants such as tobacco smoke, air pollutants, and chemical fumes can aggravate the symptoms. Drafts, chilling, and sudden changes in temperature also tend to do so and, in this event, may also indicate that the patient has nonallergic vasomotor rhinitis.

Pathophysiology

The alterations of normal physiology that have been described for seasonal allergic rhinitis are present to a lesser degree in the perennial form of the disease but are more persistent. These changes are more chronic and permanent in nature and are significant factors in the development of many of the complications associated with nonseasonal allergic rhinitis. The histopathologic changes that occur are initially identical to those found in seasonal allergic rhinitis. With persistent disease, more chronic and irreversible changes may be noted, such as thickening and hyperplasia of the mucosal epithelium, more intense mononuclear cellular infiltration, connective tissue proliferation, and hyperplasia of adjacent periosteum.

Clinical Features

The symptoms of perennial allergic rhinitis are similar to those of seasonal allergic rhinitis, although they frequently are less severe. This is due to the constant exposure to low concentrations of an allergen, such as house dust mite. The decreased severity of symptoms seen in these patients may lead them to interpret their symptoms as resulting from "sinus trouble" or "frequent colds." Nasal obstruction may be the major or sole complaint, particularly in children, in whom the passageways are relatively small. Sneezing; clear rhinorrhea; itching of the nose, eyes, ears, and throat; and lacrimation may also

occur. The presence of itching in the nasopharyngeal and ocular areas is consistent with an allergic cause of the chronic rhinitis. The chronic nasal obstruction may cause mouth breathing, snoring, almost constant sniffling, and a nasal twang to the speech. The obstruction has been reported to be severe enough to cause a form of sleep apnea in children. Because of the constant mouth breathing, patients may complain of a dry, irritated, or sore throat. Loss of the sense of smell may occur in patients with marked chronic nasal obstruction. In some patients, the nasal obstruction is worse at night and may interfere with sleep. Sneezing episodes on awakening or in the early morning hours are a complaint. Because the chronic edema involves the opening of the eustachian tube and the paranasal sinuses, dull frontal headaches and ear complaints, such as decreased hearing, fullness in the ears, or popping in the ears, are common. In children, there may be recurrent episodes of serous otitis media. In addition, chronic nasal obstruction may lead to eustachian tube dysfunction. Persistent, low-grade nasal pruritus leads to almost constant rubbing of the nose and nasal twitching. In children, recurrent epistaxis may occur because of the friability of the mucous membranes, sneezing episodes, forceful nose blowing, or nose picking. After exposure to significant levels of an allergen, such as close contact with a pet or when dusting the house, the symptoms may be as severe as in the acute stages of seasonal allergic rhinitis. Constant, excessive postnasal drainage of secretions may be associated with a chronic cough or a continual clearing of the throat.

Physical Examination

Physical examination of the patient with perennial allergic rhinitis will aid in diagnosis, particularly in a child, who may constantly rub his nose or eyes. A child may have certain facial characteristics that have been associated with chronic allergic disease (52). These include a gaping appearance due to the constant mouth breathing and a broadening of the midsection of the nose. In addition, there may be a transverse nasal crease across the lower third of the nose where the soft cartilaginous portion meets the rigid bony bridge. This is a result of the continual rubbing and pushing of the nose to relieve itching. The mucous membranes are pale, moist, and boggy and may have a bluish tinge. Polyps may be present in cases of chronic perennial allergic rhinitis of long duration. Their characteristic appearance is smooth, glistening, and white. They may take the form of grapelike masses. Polyps may also occur in patients without allergic rhinitis, and thus causality cannot be inferred. The nasal secretions are usually clear and watery but may be more mucoid in nature and may show large numbers of eosinophils when examined microscopically.

Dark circles under the eyes, known as allergic shiners, appear in some children. These are presumed to be due to venous stasis secondary to constant nasal congestion. The conjunctiva may be injected or may appear granular. In children affected with perennial allergic rhinitis early in life, narrowing of the arch of the palate may occur, leading to the Gothic arch. In addition, these children may develop facial deformities, such as dental malocclusion or gingival hypertrophy. The throat is usually normal on examination, although the posterior pharyngeal wall may exhibit prominent lymphoid follicles.

Laboratory Findings

A nasal smear examined for eosinophils may be of value when diagnosing perennial allergic rhinitis. It is particularly useful in cases in which there is no clear clinical relationship of symptoms to positive skin tests. The presence of large numbers of eosinophils suggests an allergic cause for the chronic rhinitis, although nonallergic rhinitis with eosinophilia syndrome (NARES) certainly occurs. Their absence does not exclude an allergic cause, especially if the test is done during a relatively quiescent period of the disease, or in the presence of bacterial infection when large numbers of polymorphonuclear neutrophils obscure the eosinophils. There is no particular diagnostic relationship between the presence or absence of low-grade peripheral blood eosinophilia and the presence of the disease, although eosinophilia is suggestive evidence. An elevated level of serum IgE also tends to support the diagnosis.

Diagnosis

Positive skin tests to aeroallergens are important confirmatory findings in patients whose history and physical examination suggest chronic allergic rhinitis. The RAST may be a useful diagnostic aid in conjunction with an appropriate history when skin testing cannot be performed. In rare patients in whom food allergy might play a significant role, a food elimination diet is indicated, although food allergy as a hidden cause of allergic rhinitis is almost never seen. Only by avoidance of suspected food substances and a consequent reduction or complete abatement of the symptoms, which then reoccur with reintroduction of the food, can one be assured of a specific food allergy. It should be emphasized that food allergy is rarely an important factor in perennial allergic rhinitis, particularly in adults. Therefore, good medical judgment must be used to avoid the overdiagnosis of food allergy.

Differential Diagnosis

Incorrect diagnosis may result in expensive treatments and alterations of the patient's environment; therefore, the diagnosis must be established carefully. Major disease entities that may be confused with perennial allergic rhinitis are chronic sinusitis, recurrent infectious rhinitis, abnormalities of nasal structures, and nonseasonal, nonallergic, noninfectious rhinitis (Table 9.3). In addition, skin tests in these conditions are usually negative or do not correlate clinically with the symptoms. In infectious rhinitis and chronic rhinitis, eosinophilia is not common in nasal secretions. The predominant cell found in the nasal secretions in these conditions is the neutrophil, unless there is a coexistent allergic rhinitis. These entities are discussed in greater detail in the last section of this chapter.

Causes of chronic nasal congestion and discharge include rhinitis medicamentosa, drugs, pregnancy, nasal foreign bodies, other bony abnormalities of the lateral nasal wall, concha bullosa (air cell within the middle turbinate), enlarged adenoids, nasal polyps, cerebrospinal fluid (CSF) rhinorrhea, tumors, hypothyroidism, ciliary dyskinesia from cystic fibrosis, primary

TABLE 9.3. *Known causes of nonallergic rhinitis*

Associated drugs
  Topical α-adrenergic agonists
  α-adrenergic blockers
  Oral estrogens
  Ophthalmic and oral β-blockers
Infections
  Chronic sinusitis
  Tuberculosis
  Syphilis
  Fungal infection
Systemic conditions
  Cystic fibrosis
  Immunodeficiencies
  Immotile cilia syndrome
  Hypothyroidism
  Rhinitis of pregnancy
Structural abnomalities
  Marked septal deviation
  Concha bullosa
  Nasal polyps
  Adenoidal hypertrophy
  Foreign body
Neoplasms
  Squamous cell carcinoma
  Nasopharyngeal carcinoma
Granulomatous diseases
  Wegener's granulomatosis
  Sarcoidosis
  Midline granuloma
Other
  Atrophic rhinitis

---

ciliary dyskinesia or Kartagener syndrome, granulomatous diseases such as sarcoidosis, Wegener granulomatosis, midline granuloma, nasal mastocytosis, congenital syphilis, or atrophic rhinitis.

Rhinitis Medicamentosa

A condition that may enter into the differential diagnosis is rhinitis medicamentosa, which results from the overuse of vasoconstricting nose drops. Every patient who presents with the complaint of chronic nasal congestion should be questioned carefully as to the amount and frequency of the use of nose drops.

Drugs

Patients taking antihypertensive agents such as propranolol, clonidine, α blockers such as terazosin and prazosin, α-methyldopa, reserpine, guanabenz, hydralazine, and certain psychoac-

tive drugs may complain of marked nasal congestion, which is a common side effect of these drugs. A medical history of current drug therapy will suggest a diagnosis. Discontinuing these drugs for a few days results in marked symptomatic improvement. Contraceptives have been incriminated as a cause of perennial rhinitis (53,54) but the evidence for this is meager, except in cases in which other history factors strongly implicate causality. It is not presently recommended that women with rhinitis stop using oral contraceptives. Cocaine sniffing can also produce rhinorrhea.

Pregnancy

Congestion of the nasal mucosa is a normal physiologic change in pregnancy. This is presumably a major factor in the development in some women of "rhinitis of pregnancy," a syndrome of nasal congestion and vasomotor instability limited to the gestational period (55). The rhinitis characteristically begins at the end of the first trimester and then disappears immediately after delivery. Patients with or without a history of chronic nasal symptoms may develop rhinitis medicamentosa or acute pharyngitis or sinusitis during pregnancy. In one series, 32% of 79 pregnant women surveyed reported frequent or constant nasal problems during pregnancy (56).

Foreign Body

On rare occasions, a patient with a foreign body in the nose may be thought to have chronic allergic rhinitis. Foreign bodies usually present as unilateral nasal obstruction accompanied by a foul, purulent nasal discharge. Children may put foreign bodies into the nose, most commonly peas, beans, buttons, and erasers. Sinusitis is often diagnosed if the nose is not examined properly. Examination is best done after secretions are removed so that the foreign body may be visualized.

Physical Obstruction

Careful physical examination of the nasal cavity should be performed to exclude septal deviation, enlarged adenoids, choanal atresia, and nasal polyps as the cause of nasal congestion.

Cerebral Spinal Fluid Rhinorrhea

CSF rhinorrhea may follow a head injury. CSF is clear and watery in appearance, simulating that seen in allergic rhinitis. In most cases, the CSF rhinorrhea is unilateral. Because spinal fluid contains sugar, and mucus does not, testing for the presence of glucose should be done to make the diagnosis. CSF rhinorrhea results from a defect in the cribriform plate that requires surgical repair.

Tumor

Several tumors and neoplasms may occur in the nasopharyngeal area. The most important are encephalocele, inverting papilloma, squamous cell carcinoma, sarcoma, and angiofibroma. Encephaloceles are generally unilateral. They usually occur high in the nose and occasionally within the nasopharynx. They increase in size with straining, lifting, or crying. They may have a pulsating quality. If a biopsy is done, CSF rhinorrhea and meningitis may ensue.

Inverting papillomas have a somewhat papillary appearance. They are friable and more vascular than nasal polyps, and they bleed more readily. They occur either unilaterally or bilaterally and frequently involve the nasal septum as well as the lateral wall of the nose. A biopsy is necessary to confirm the diagnosis.

Angiofibromas are the most common in preadolescent boys. They arise in the posterior choana of the nasopharynx. They have a polypoid appearance but are usually reddish blue in color. They do not pit on palpation. Angiofibromas are highly vascular tumors that bleed excessively when injured or when a biopsy is done. Larger tumors may invade bone and extend into adjacent structures (57).

Carcinomas and sarcomas may stimulate nasal polyps. They are generally unilateral in location, may occur at any site within the nasal chamber, are firm, and usually bleed with manipulation. As the disease progresses, adjacent structures are involved.

Hypothyroidism

A careful review of systems is important to exclude hypothyroidism as a cause of nasal congestion.

Syphilis

Congenital syphilis can cause rhinitis in infancy.

Ciliary Disorders

With the dyskinetic cilia syndrome, patients may experience rhinitis symptoms secondary to abnormalities of mucociliary transport. The criteria for diagnosis include (a) absence or near absence of tracheobronchial or nasal mucociliary transport, (b) total or nearly total absence of dynein arms of the cilia in nasal or bronchial mucosa, or rarely one may see defective radial spokes or transposition of a peripheral microtubular doublet to the center of the axoneme, and (c) clinical manifestations of chronic upper and lower respiratory tract infections, such as sinusitis, bronchitis, and bronchiectasis (58). Rare patients may have the triad of bronchiectasis, sinusitis, and situs inversus known as Kartagener syndrome (59). In some patients, cilia, although abnormal in structure, may in fact be motile. The cilia in patients with this syndrome can be distinguished from those in patients with asthma, sinusitis, chronic bronchitis, and emphysema, who may have nonspecific abnormalities in cilia structure (60).

COURSE AND COMPLICATIONS

Allergic rhinitis accounts for the largest number of patients with respiratory allergy. Most patients develop symptoms before the age of 20 years, with the highest rate of increase of onset of symptoms occurring between the ages of 12 and 15 years (8). Because of a variety of factors, including geographic location, allergen load, weather conditions, and emotions, the course and prognosis for any single patient cannot be predicted. One study suggests that more than one third of patients with allergic rhinitis were better over a 10-year period, but most were worse (61).

In another study, 8% of those with allergic rhinitis had remissions for at least 2 years' duration. A chance for remission was better in those with seasonal allergic rhinitis and if the disease was present for less than 5 years (62).

The possibility of developing asthma as a sequela to allergic rhinitis may worry the patient or the parents. It has been generally stated that about 30% of patients with allergic rhinitis not treated with specific immunotherapy eventually develop allergic asthma. A survey of an entire city, however, showed that only 7% of those with allergic rhinitis developed asthma as a late sequela (63). In most patients with both allergic rhinitis and asthma, the asthmatic condition develops before the onset of allergic rhinitis, or the two conditions appear almost simultaneously. If asthma develops, the patient's concern for the symptoms of asthma usually overshadows the symptoms of allergic rhinitis. It is frequently stated that the individual with more severe allergic rhinitis has a greater risk for developing asthma, but clear evidence for this is lacking.

Patients with allergic rhinitis may develop complications because of chronic nasal inflammation, including recurrent otitis media with hearing loss, impaired speech development, acute and chronic sinusitis, recurrence of nasal polyps, abnormal craniofacial development, sleep apnea with its related complications, aggravation of asthma, and increased propensity to develop asthma. In patients with allergic rhinitis, a continuous allergen exposure results in persistent inflammation that upregulates the expression of intercellular adhesion molecule-1 (ICAM-1)/CD54 and vascular cell adhesion molecule-1 (VCAM-1) in the inflamed epithelium. Because ICAM-1 is the ligand for almost 90% of rhinoviruses, its upregulation may be responsible for the increased viral respiration infections in these patients. Poorly controlled symptoms of allergic rhinitis may contribute to sleep loss, secondary daytime fatigue, learning impairment, decreased overall cognitive functioning, decreased long-term productivity, and decreased quality of life.

The symptoms of allergic rhinitis and skin test reactivity tend to wane with increasing age. In most patients, however, skin tests remain positive despite symptomatic improvement; therefore, symptomatic improvement is not necessarily directly correlated with skin test conversion to negative.

TREATMENT

There are three types of management of seasonal allergic or perennial allergic rhinitis. These methods are avoidance therapy, symptomatic therapy, and immunotherapy.

Avoidance Therapy

Complete avoidance of an allergen results in a cure when there is only a single allergen. For this reason, attempts should be made to minimize contact with any important allergen, regardless of what other mode of treatment is instituted.

Allergic rhinitis associated with a household pet can be controlled completely by removing the pet from the home. If the patient is allergic to feathers, he or she should be advised to change the feather pillow to a Dacron pillow, or to cover the pillow with encasings. Mold-sensitive patients occasionally note their precipitation or aggravation of symptoms after ingestion of certain foods having a high mold content. Avoidance of beer, wine, cantaloupe, melons, mushrooms, and various cheeses may be helpful. Tips for controlling allergic rhinitis are listed in Table 9.4.

In most cases of allergic rhinitis, complete avoidance therapy is difficult, if not impossible, because aeroallergens are so widely distributed. Attempts to eradicate sources of pollen or molds have not proved to be significantly effective. Mold-sensitive patients should avoid damp, musty basements, raked or burning leaves, barns, moldy hay, and straw, and they should disinfect or destroy mold articles.

In the case of house dust mite allergy, complete avoidance is not possible in most climates, but certain measures decrease the exposure to antigen. Instructions for a dust-control program also should be given to the patient with house dust mite sensitivity. There should be a least one room in the house that is relatively dust free. The most practical program is to make the bedroom as dust free as possible, so that the patient may have the

TABLE 9.4. *Tips for patients with allergic rhinitis*

1. Keep pets out of the bedroom and preferably outside of the house.
2. Avoid smoking and secondhand smoke.
3. Routinely clean areas of the home that promote mold growth, such as shower stalls, basements, and window sills (mold sensitivity).
4. Have cooking systems in the home checked periodically for mold growth.
5. Avoid locations that promote the growth of molds, such as damp, poorly ventilated areas. Avoid sleeping in a bedroom located in a basement or attic.
6. Use air conditioning to reduce humidity and decrease temperature. Keep windows closed to avoid contact with outdoor allergens (house dust mite and pollen sensitivity).
7. Encase pillows, mattresses, and even box springs in zippered protective encasings (house dust mite sensitivity).
8. Replace heavily mite-infected mattresses and pillows. Use foam pillows instead of down or feather pillows (house dust mite sensitivity), but use encasing on the pillows.
9. Launder bedding regularly, including mattress pads and blankets, in hot water (140°F) (house dust mite sensitivity).
10. Vacuum carpets and clean floors regularly. If possible, remove carpeting from bedroom, or treat carpet with acaricide (house dust mite sensitivity).
11. Minimize dust-collecting surfaces, such as shelves, stuffed animals, books, stored blankets, and woolens.

sleeping area as a controlled environment. Certain measures to decrease house dust exposure are relatively easy to perform. The patient should wear a mask when house cleaning if such activity precipitates significant symptoms. Bed linens should be washed in very hot water (140°F). Both the mattress and box spring should be encased in mite-proof casings. Upholstered furniture, wall-to-wall carpeting, chenille spreads, bed pads, and stuffed toys can be eliminated from the bedroom for more complete control. These simple measures are often enough to enable the patient to have fewer and milder symptoms.

Pharmacologic Therapy

Antihistamines

Antihistamines are the foundation of symptomatic therapy for allergic rhinitis and are most useful in controlling the symptoms of sneezing, rhinorrhea, and pruritus that occur in allergic rhinitis. They are less effective, however, against the nasal obstruction and eye symptoms in these patients. Antihistamines are compounds of varied chemical structures that have the property of antagonizing some of the actions of histamine (63). Histamine acts through three receptors, referred to as H_1, H_2, and H_3. Activation of H_1 receptors causes smooth muscle contraction, increases vascular permeability, increases the production of mucus, and activates sensory nerves to induce pruritus and reflexes such as sneezing (64). Activation of H_2 receptors primarily causes gastric acid secretion and some vascular dilation and cutaneous flushing. The H_3 receptors located on histaminergic nerve endings in brain tissue control the synthesis and release of histamine (65). They may also decrease histamine release from mast cells and release of proinflammatory tachykinins from unmyelinated C fibers in the airways. The antihistamines used in treating allergic rhinitis are directed against the H_1 receptors and thus are most effective in preventing histamine-induced capillary permeability. They may also inhibit mediator release (azatadine, terfenadine, ketotifen) (66), inhibit tissue eosinophil influx (cetirizine) (67), and act as a mild bronchodilator (terfenadine, astemizole, cetirizine) (68). In clinical use, these drugs are most effective when given early, at the first appearance of symptoms, because they do not abolish existing effects of histamine, but rather prevent the development of new symptoms caused by further histamine release. The antihistamines may also exhibit sedative, antiemetic, or local anesthetic effects, depending on the particular antihistamine, route of administration, and dosage used. Many of the first-generation antihistamines also result in anticholinergic effects, which account for side effects such as blurred vision or dry mouth.

All the antihistamines are readily absorbed after oral administration. They vary in speed, intensity, and duration of effect. Because so many are available, it is best to become familiar with selected antihistamines for use. In practice, clinical choice should be based on effectiveness of antihistaminic activity and the limitation of side effects. However, contrary to previous belief, pharmacologic tolerance to antihistamines does not occur, and poor compliance is considered to be a major factor in treatment failures (69). Thus, there is no rationale for the practice of rotating patients through the various pharmacologic classes of antihistamines. In general, elimination half-life values of antihistamines are shorter in children than older adults. Dryness of the mouth, vertigo, gastrointestinal upset, irritability in children, and drowsiness account for more than 90% of the side effects reported with these drugs. The depressed effect on the central nervous system (CNS) is the major limiting side effect. Drowsiness in some patients with antihistamines is mild and temporary and may disappear after a few doses of the drug. Because patients exhibit marked variability in response to various antihistamines, individualization of dosage and frequency of administration are important. Recent studies have reported that these drugs may be administered less frequently than previously recommended because of the prolonged biologic actions of these medications in tissues (70,71).

Because the newer second-generation antihistamines do not appreciably penetrate the CNS, most studies show that the incidence of sedation and other abnormal measures of CNS function are similar to placebo with loratadine (72), fexofenadine (73), astemizole (74), and terfenadine (75). Another major advantage of the nonsedating antihistamines is that these medications are free of anticholinergic side effects, such as dry mouth, constipation, difficulty voiding, and blurry vision (76). These drugs are usually tolerated by older patients, who may have benign prostatic hypertrophy or xerostomia as complicating medical problems. Because fatal cardiac arrhythmias occurred when terfenadine and astemizole were given concomitantly with erythromycin (macrolide antibiotics), imidazole antifungal agents (ketoconazole and itraconazole), or medications that inhibit the cytochrome P-450 system (71), these drugs have been removed from the United States market. A major factor in the emergence of these arrhythmias is the prolongation of the QTc interval. Patients with hepatic dysfunction, cardiac disorders associated with a prolonged QTc interval, or metabolic disorders such as hypomagnesemia or hypokalemia were also predisposed to the adverse cardiac effects. This side effect has not been seen with fexofenadine (the active carboxylic acid metabolite of terfenadine). Bernstein (77) noted no electrocardiogram abnormalities, including QTc prolongation, even at dosages of 480 mg/day of fexofenadine. This side effect has not been reported with loratadine or cetirizine (78).

Loratadine is a selective peripheral H_1 receptor antagonist. Loratadine has been reported to be 10 times less potent against central than peripheral H_1 receptors (79). In adults, a 10-mg dose is approved for treatment of seasonal allergic rhinitis, but higher doses may have greater bronchoprotective effects for histamine-induced bronchospasm. The half-life of loratadine is 7 to 11 hours, which makes it appropriate for once-daily dosing, especially because the clinical half-life of blockage of the histamine-induced wheal response for loratadine is 24 hours. The serum half-life is prolonged in elderly patients, and drug levels may be increased when administered with macrolide antibiotics or imidazole antifungal agents.

In contrast to its parent compound hydroxyzine, the carboxylic acid metabolite of hydroxyzine cetirizine has poor penetration into the CNS and therefore is relatively nonsedating. Cetirizine is highly selective for H_1 receptors in the brain and does not bind to serotonin, dopamine, or α-adrenergic and calcium antagonist receptors in the brain (80). The drug is not metabolized by the hepatic cytochrome system and is excreted unchanged in the urine (81). Therefore, the half-life of cetirizine may be prolonged in patients with renal failure. Cetirizine has been studied in seasonal and perennial rhinitis and has been reported to have bronchodilating activity in addition to antiinflammatory properties (82,83).

Azelastine nasal spray is an effective topical management for the symptoms of seasonal allergic rhinitis. The active ingredient, azelastine hydrochloride, is a selective, high-affinity, H_1 receptor antagonist with structural and chemical differences that distinguish it from currently available antihistamines. Azelastine is about 10 times more potent than chlorpheniramine at the H_1 receptor site (84). In addition to this H_1-blocking action, azelastine has demonstrated an inhibitory response on cells and chemical mediators of the inflammatory response. Azelastine prevents leukotriene generation from mast cells and basophils (85,86) and modulates the activity of eosinophils and neutrophils (87), macrophages (88), monocytes, and cytokines (89). Azelastine has a low incidence of somnolence and does not seem to result in psychomotor impairment. Azelastine is free of drug interactions and may also be used as an alternative to oral antihistamines. In certain patients, this drug may be used as a replacement for the antihistamine–intranasal corticosteroid combination (90).

Sympathomimetic Agents

Sympathomimetic drugs are used as vasoconstrictors for the nasal mucous membranes. The current concept regarding the mechanism of action of these includes two types of adrenergic receptors, called α and β receptors. Activation of the α receptors results in constriction of smooth muscle in the vessels of the skin, viscera, and mucous membranes, whereas activation of β receptors induces dilation of vascular smooth muscle, relaxation of bronchial smooth muscle, and cardiac stimulation. By taking advantage of drugs that stimulate α receptors, the edema of the nasal mucous membranes in allergic rhinitis can be reduced by topical or systemic administration. In large doses, these drugs induce elevated blood pressure, nervousness, and insomnia. Although there may be differences in blood pressure response to the various preparations (91,92), these agents should be used with caution in patients who have hypertension, organic heart disease, angina pectoris, and hyperthyroidism. In addition to their use as decongestants, the sympathomimetic drugs are also combined with antihistamines in many oral preparations to decrease the drowsiness that often accompanies antihistamine therapy.

Nose drops or nasal sprays containing sympathomimetic agents may be overused. The topical application of these drugs is often followed by a "rebound" phenomenon in which the nasal mucous membranes become even more congested and edematous as a result of the use of the drugs. This leads the patient to use the drops or spray more frequently and in higher doses to obtain relief from nasal obstruction. The condition resulting from the overuse of topical sympathomimetics is called *rhinitis medicamentosa*. The patient must abruptly discontinue their use to alleviate the condition. Other measures, including a course of topical corticosteroids for a few weeks, are often helpful to decrease the nasal congestion until this distressing side effect disappears. Because of the duration of seasonal or perennial allergic rhinitis, it is best not to use topical vasoconstrictors in the allergic patient, except temporarily during periods of infectious rhinitis. The systemic use of sympathomimetic drugs has not been associated with rhinitis medicamentosa. Phenylephrine, pseudoephedrine, isoephedrine, phenylpropanolamine, and cyclopentamine are some of the more common vasoconstricting agents used in association with various antihistamines and oral preparations. Phenylpropanolamine, but not the other decongestants, has been associated with stroke within 3 days of use in women using doses of this agent in appetite suppression.

Topical Corticosteroids

Cortisone and its derivatives have marked beneficial effects in managing various allergic processes. Corticosteroids are generally considered the most effective medications for the management of the inflammatory component of allergic rhinitis. The effectiveness of corticosteroids for the management of allergic rhinitis is most likely related to multiple pharmacologic actions. Corticosteroids have been demonstrated to have specific effects on the inflammatory cells and chemical mediators involved in the allergic process.

Corticosteroids have been considered to increase the synthesis of lipocortin-1, which has an inhibitory effect on phospholipase A_2 and therefore may inhibit the production of lipid mediators (91–93). However, other actions may be more relevant. Corticosteroids reduce the number of circulating T lymphocytes and inhibit T-lymphocyte activation (94), IL-2 production, IL-2 receptor generation (95), and IL-4 production (96). They reduce circulating numbers of eosinophils and eosinophil influx in the late-phase reaction (97), inhibit IL-5–mediated eosinophil survival (98), and inhibit GM-CSF production (99). Corticosteroids reduce seasonally induced increases in nasal mast cells (100) and histamine levels (101), reduce the number of circulating basophils, and inhibit neutrophil influx after allergen challenge (102). Corticosteroids cause reductions in the numbers of circulating macrophages and monocytes and inhibit the release of cytokines, including IL-1, interferon-1 (IFN-1), TNF-α, and GM-CSF (103).

Studies in patients with allergic rhinitis have demonstrated that these effects of intranasal steroids on rhinitis symptoms are dependent on local activity of the steroids (104,105). When administered topically, the steroid molecule diffuses across the target cell membrane and enters the cytoplasm, where it binds to the glucocorticoid receptor (106). After the association of corticosteroid and receptor, the activated glucocorticoid receptor enters the cell nucleus, where it attaches as a dimer to specific binding sites on DNA in the promotor region of steroid-responsive genes. The effect of this interaction is to either induce or suppress gene transcription. The messenger RNA transcripts induced during this process then undergo posttranscriptional processing and are transported to the cytoplasm for translation by ribosomes, with subsequent production of new proteins. After post-translational processing occurs, the new proteins are either released for extracellular activity or retained by the cell for intracellular activity (107–109). In addition, the activated glucocorticoid receptors may interact directly with other transcription factors in the cytoplasm and alter the steroid responsiveness of the target cell (110).

At the present time, several nasal corticosteroids are available for treating patients with allergic rhinitis, including beclomethasone dipropionate, flunisolide, triamcinolone acetonide, budesonide, fluticasone propionate, and mometasone furoate. With the exception of beclomethasone dipropionate, these drugs are quickly metabolized to less active metabolites, have minimal systemic absorption, and have been associated with few systemic side effects. The total bioavailability of an intranasal dose of mometasone is reported at 0.1% (111) and that of fluticasone at 0.5% to 2% (112). The total bioavailability of intranasal budesonide is reported to be 20% (113), and that of flunisolide is reported to be 40% to 50%. The intranasal bioavailability of intranasal triamcinolone acetonide is unknown. There are no reliable data regarding the bioavailability of beclomethasone dipropionate by any route. Unlike other intranasal steroids, beclomethasone dipropionate is metabolized to an active metabolite, beclomethasone-17-monoprionate, and relatively inactive metabolites, beclomethasone-21-monopropionate and beclomethasone (114).

Intranasal steroids have been helpful in relieving the common allergic symptoms of the upper airway, such as sneezing, congestion, and rhinorrhea. In addition, they may be of value in relieving throat pruritus and cough associated with allergic rhinitis and may also improve concomitant seasonal allergic asthma (115).

The major side effects of intranasal steroids include local dryness or irritation in the form of stinging, burning, or sneezing (116) (Table 9.5). With prolonged administration of intranasal steroids, periodic examination of the nasal cavity is warranted, especially in patients who experience nasal crusting or bleeding (117,118). Hemorrhagic crusting and perforation of the nasal septum are more common in patients who improperly point the spray toward the septal wall, and this complication can be reduced by (a) careful education, (b) using a mirror when spraying into the nose, and (c) the new actuators used for steroid sprays, or having the right hand spray the device into the left nostril and left hand spray the device into the right nostril. The incidence of local irritation with intranasal steroids has been reduced by the development of aqueous formulations of these drugs (119,120), and the subsequent reduction in local irritation with these preparations has increased their use in children.

TABLE 9.5. *Complications of topical steroids sprays*

Systemic reactions
Common (>5% incidence)
  Headaches
Uncommon (<5% incidence)
  Nausea and vomiting
  Loss of sense of taste and smell
  Dizziness and light-headedness
Rare
  Increased intraocular pressure (high doses)
  Anaphylaxis, urticaria, angioedema,
    bronchospasm
Local reactions
  Nasal burning and stinging
  Sneezing, sinus congestion, watery eyes, throat
    irritation, bad taste in mouth
  Drying of the mucous membranes with epistaxis or
    bloody discharge
  Perforation of nasal septum (more likely from
    sinusitis or after septal repair)

Long-term use of intranasal steroids does not appear to cause any significant risk for adverse morphologic effects in the nasal mucosa. In a study of patients with perennial rhinitis treated with mometasone for 12 months, nasal biopsy specimens showed a decrease in focal metaplasia, no change in epithelial thickness, and no sign of atrophy (121). In a study of intranasal steroid treatment in 90 patients with perennial rhinitis, nasal biopsy specimens revealed normalization of the nasal mucosa at the end of the 12-month study period (122).

Systemic side effects are generally not considered a serious risk associated with intranasal steroids, although early studies of intranasal dexamethasone administration at dosages used in allergic rhinitis produced mild to moderate adrenal suppression (123,124). However, clinical experiences with intranasal fluticasone (125), triamcinolone (126), and mometasone have indicated no reports of systemic side effects.

Bilateral posterior subcapsular cataracts have been reported in association with nasal or oral inhalation of beclomethasone dipropionate, although many of these patients had used higher-than-recommended doses or had received concomitant oral steroid therapy (127). In a case-control study, nasal steroids were not associated with an increased risk for ocular hypertension or open-angle glaucoma, whereas prolonged administration of high doses of inhaled steroids

increased the risk for these adverse effects (128).

Initially, some patients may require topical decongestants before administering intranasal steroids. In some patients, the congestion is so severe that a 3- to 5-day course of oral corticosteroids is required to allow delivery of the intranasal steroids. In contrast to decongestant nasal sprays, patients should be informed that intranasal steroids should be used prophylactically and that maximum benefit is not immediate and may take weeks. Although a delayed onset of action with the intranasal steroids may occur in some patients, well-controlled studies (129–132) have shown that many patients have a clinically evident onset of effect during the first day of administration. Some studies suggest that intranasal steroids can be used on an as-needed basis by many patients, but for some patients, optimal effectiveness can be achieved only with regular use (133,134).

Intranasal Corticosteroid Injection

Intranasal corticosteroid injections have been used for clinical practice in the management of patients with common allergic and nonallergic nasal conditions such as nasal polyposis. With the advent of newer and safer intranasal steroids, the use of this technique has decreased in recent years. Turbinate injections have two major adverse effects that are not seen with intranasal corticosteroid sprays: (a) adrenal suppression secondary to absorption of the steroid, and (b) absorption of steroid emboli, which may lead to transient or permanent loss of vision (135).

Systemic Corticosteroids

Systemic corticosteroids are regarded by many allergists as inappropriate therapy for patients with mild to moderate allergic rhinitis. Although rhinitis is not a threat to life, it can seriously impair the quality of it, and some patients respond only to corticosteroids. Also, when the topical steroid cannot be adequately distributed in the nose because of marked obstruction, it will not be effective. In such cases, the blocked nose can be opened by giving a systemic corticosteroid for 3 to 7 days, and the improvement can then be maintained by the topical corticosteroid spray. It is essential always to relate the risk for side effects to the dosage given, and especially to the length of the treatment period. When short-term systemic steroid treatment is given for 1 to 2 weeks, it can be a valuable and safe supplement to topical treatments in the management of severe allergic rhinitis or nasal polyposis. As in the use of topical corticosteroids, however, systemic steroids should be reserved for severe cases that cannot be controlled by routine measures and should be used for a limited period and never on a chronic basis.

Anticholinergics

Ipratropium is an anticholinergic drug that was released in recent years for treatment of chronic bronchitis and chronic obstructive lung disease. It has a quaternary ammonia structure, which gives this medication high topical activity, but because of its structure, there is no appreciable absorption of this medication across mucosal barriers. Therefore, the unpleasant anticholinergic side effects commonly associated with atropine are not experienced with this medication.

Because cholinergic mechanisms in the nose may lead to hypersecretion and blood vessel dilation, interest in this medication has increased. Ipratropium decreases the watery rhinorrhea in patients with perennial rhinitis (136) and reduces nasal drainage in patients with the common cold or vasomotor rhinitis (137). Unfortunately, it has no appreciable effect on obstruction or sneezing in patients with rhinitis.

Intranasal Cromolyn

Cromolyn sodium is a derivative of the natural product khellin. The proposed mechanism of action of cromolyn in allergic rhinitis is to stabilize mast cell membranes, apparently by inhibiting calcium transmembrane flux and thereby preventing antigen-induced degranulation. It has been reported to be effective in the management of seasonal and perennial allergic rhinitis (138,139). Cromolyn can be effective in reducing sneezing, rhinorrhea, and nasal pruritus (140,141) but is minimally useful in nonallergic types of rhinitis and nasal polyps (142) and has little effect on mucociliary transport. Cromolyn often prevents the symptoms of both seasonal and perennial allergic rhinitis, and diligent prophylaxis can significantly reduce both immediate and late symptoms after allergen exposures (143).

Adverse effects occur in fewer than 10% of patients and most commonly include sneezing, nasal stinging, nasal burning, transient headache, and an unpleasant aftertaste. Patients also may experience mucosal irritation due to the preservatives benzalkonium chloride and ethylenediaminetetraacetic acid. For management of seasonal rhinitis, treatment should begin 2 to 4 weeks before contact with the offending allergens and should be continued throughout the period of exposure. Because cromolyn has a delayed onset of effect, concurrent antihistamine therapy is usually necessary to control symptoms. It is essential for the patient to understand the rate and extent of response to be expected from intranasal cromolyn and that, because the product is prophylactic, it must be used on a regular basis for maximum benefit. In the United States, cromolyn nasal spray is available without prescription.

Several studies have compared the therapeutic efficacy of cromolyn nasal solution with that of the intranasal corticosteroids in allergic rhinitis. In both perennial (144,145) and seasonal allergic rhinitis (146,147), intranasal steroids have been reported to be more effective than cromolyn. Nedocromil sodium is a pyranoquinolone dicarboxylic acid derivative that is reported to be effective against both mucosal and connective tissue–type mast cells. In contrast, cromolyn sodium appears to be effective only against connective tissue–type mast cells. Nedocromil has been reported to be effective in seasonal and perennial allergic rhinitis (148). Like cromolyn, nedocromil is recommended primarily for prophylactic use, and therapy should be instituted 2 to 4 weeks before the allergy season. It is not available in the United States as a nasal spray.

Immunotherapy

Immunotherapy is a treatment that attempts to increase the threshold level for symptom appearance after exposure to the aeroallergen. This altered degree of sensitivity may be the result of either the induction of a new antibody (the so-called blocking antibody), a decrease in allergic antibody, a change in the cellular histamine release phenomenon, or an interplay of all three possibilities. Other immunologic changes reported with immunotherapy include change from T_H2 to T_H1 $CD4^+$ cells, induction of the generation of antigen-specific suppressor cells, and reduction in the production of a mononuclear cell-derived histamine-releasing factor.

The severity of allergic rhinitis and its complications is a spectrum varying from minimal to marked symptoms and from short to prolonged durations. Indications for immunotherapy, a fairly long-term treatment modality, are relative rather than absolute. For example, a patient who has mild grass pollinosis for only a few weeks in June may be managed well by symptomatic therapy alone. On the other hand, those with perennial allergic rhinitis or allergic rhinitis in multiple pollen seasons who require almost daily symptomatic treatment for long periods may be considered candidates for specific therapy. The advantages of long-term relief of such therapy, which is relatively expensive, should be considered in relationship to the cost of daily medication. In addition, specific therapy may help to deter the development of some of the complications of chronic rhinitis. Antigens used for immunotherapy should be those that cannot be avoided (e.g., pollens, molds, and house dust mite). Animal dander injection therapy should be restricted to veterinarians and laboratory personnel whose occupation makes avoidance practically and financially impossible. Patients are generally not cured of their disease but rather have fewer symptoms that are more easily controlled by symptomatic medication.

A frequent cause of treatment failure is that a patient expects too much, too soon, and thus prematurely discontinues the injection program because of dissatisfaction. Another important cause of failure is seen in patients with nonallergic rhinitis who have positive but clinically insignificant skin tests or RAST, and have received immunotherapy based on those tests. Immunotherapy based on positive skin tests or RAST alone should not be expected to be beneficial.

There is no adequate laboratory method of indicating to a patient how long immunotherapy must be continued. Therefore, the clinical response to therapy dictates that decision concerning the duration of specific treatment. A minimum of 3 years of immunotherapy should be given to avoid the rapid recurrence of symptoms in uncomplicated allergic rhinitis. A recent study (149) reported that traditional allergen immunotherapy with a grass pollen extract, administered for 3 to 4 years, induced a clinical remission that persisted for at least 3 years after treatment was discontinued. However, it is unknown whether remission of symptoms is maintained after longer periods of observation.

REFERENCES

1. Pederson N, Mygind N. Rhinitis, sinusitis and otitis media in Kartagener's syndrome. *Clin Otolaryngol* 1982;52:189.
2. Mygind N. *Nasal allergy.* 2nd ed. Oxford: Blackwell, 1979.
3. Hill LW. Certain aspects of allergy in children. *N Engl J Med* 1961;265:1194.
4. Phillips EW. Time required for production of hayfever by a newly encountered pollen. *J Allergy* 1939;11:28.
5. Broder I, Higgins MW, Matthews KP, et al. Epidemiology of asthma and allergic rhinitis in a total community, Tecumseh, Michigan. 3. Second Survey of the community. *J Allergy Clin Immunol* 1974;53:127.
6. Nathan RA, Meltzer EO, Selner JC, et al. Prevalence of allergic rhinitis in the United States. *J Allergy Clin Immunol* 1997;99:S808–814.
7. Haahtela R, Heiskala M, Suonemi I. Allergic disorders and immediate skin test reactivity in Finnish adolescents. *Allergy* 1980;35:433.
8. Hagy GW, Settipane GA. Bronchial asthma, allergic rhinitis and allergy skin tests among college students. *J Allergy Clin Immunol* 1969;44:323.
9. Sly RM. Changing prevalence of allergic rhinitis and asthma. *Ann Allergy Asthma Immunol* 1999; 82:233–248.
10. Platts-Mills TA. How environment affects patients with allergic diseases: indoor allergens and asthma. *Ann Allergy* 1994;72:381–384.
11. Platts-Mills. Airborne allergen exposure, allergen avoidance and bronchial hyperactivity. In: Kay AB, Austen KF, Lichtenstein LM, eds. *Asthma: physiology, immunopharmacology, and treatment.* Third International Symposium. London: Academic Press, 1984:297–314.
12. Hodge L, Salome CME, Peat JK, et al. Consumption of oily fish and childhood asthma risk. *Med J Aust* 1996;164:137–140.
13. Mallol J, Clayton T, Asher I, et al. ISSAC finding in children aged 13–14 years: an overview. *Allergy Clin Immunol Int* 1999;11:176–182.

14. Juniper EF, Guyatt GH. Development and testing of a new measure of health status for clinical trials in rhinoconjunctivitis. *Clin Exp Allergy* 1991;21:77–83.

15. Meltzer ED, Nathan RA, Seiner JC, et al. Quality of life and rhinitis symptoms: results of a nationwide survey with the SF-36 and RQLQ questionnaires. *J Allergy Clin Immunol* 1997;99:S15–19.

16. Ross RN. Hayfever: an expensive disease for American business. *Am J Man Care* 1996;2:285–290.

17. Malone DC, Lawson KA, Smith DH, et al. A cost of illness study of allergic rhinitis in the United States. *J Allergy Clin Immunol* 1997;99:22–27.

18. Connell JT. Quantitative intranasal pollen challenges. III. The priming effect in allergic rhinitis. *J Allergy* 1969;43:33.

19. Grammer L, Wiggins C, Shaughnessy MA, et al. Absence of nasal priming as measured by rhinitis symptoms scores of ragweed allergic patient during seasonal exposure to ragweed pollen. *Allergy Proc* 1990;11:243.

20. Tada T, Ishizaka K. Distribution of gamma E-forming cells in lymphoid tissues of human and monkey. *J Immunol* 1970;194:377.

21. Grangette C, Grunt V, Ouaissi MA, et al. IgE receptor on human eosinophils: comparison with B cell CD23 and association with the adhesion molecule. *J Immunol* 1989;143:3580.

22. Melewicz FM, Spiegelberg HL. Fc receptors for IgE on a subpopulation of human peripheral blood monocytes. *J Immunol* 1980;125:1026.

23. Clines DB, Vander Keyl H, Levinson AI. In vitro binding of an IgE protein to human platelets. *J Immunol* 1986;136:3433.

24. Proud D, Reynolds CH, Lacapra S, et al. Nasal provocation with bradykinin induces symptoms of rhinitis and sore throat. *Am Rev Respir Dis* 1988;187:613.

25. Karim SMM, Adaikian PG, Kumaratnam N. Effects of topical prostaglandins on nasal potency in man. *Prostaglandins* 1978;15:457.

26. Okuda M, Watase T, Mezawa A, et al. The role of leukotriene D4 in allergic rhinitis. *Ann Allergy* 1988;39:537.

27. White MV, Kalimer MA. Mediators of allergic rhinitis. *J Allergy Clin Immunol* 1992;90:699–704.

28. Bascom R, Wachs M, Naderio RM, et al. Basophil influx occurs after nasal antigen challenge: effects of topical corticosteroid pretreatment. *J Allergy Clin Immunol* 1988;81:580.

29. Bascom R, Pipkorn U, Lichtenstein LM, et al. The influx of inflammatory cells into nasal washings during the late response to antigen challenge: effect of systemic steroid pretreatment. *Ann Rev Respir Dis* 1988;138:406.

30. Linder A, Venge P, Deusch LH. Eosinophil cationic protein and myeloperoxidase in nasal secretion as markers of inflammation in allergic rhinitis. *Allergy* 1987;42:583.

31. Svensson C, Andersson M, Persson CGA, et al. Albumin, bradykinins, and eosinophil cationic protein on the nasal mucosa surface in patients with hay fever during natural allergen exposure. *J Allergy Clin Immunol* 1990;85:828.

32. Furin MJ, Norman PS, Creticos PS, et al. Immunotherapy decreases antigen-induced eosinophil migration into the nasal cavity. *J Allergy Clin Immunol* 1991;88:27.

33. Denburg JA, Dolovich J, Harnish D. Basophil mast cell and eosinophil growth and differentiation factors in human allergic disease. *Clin Exp Allergy* 1989;19:249.

34. Varney VA, Jacobson MR, Robinson DS, et al. Immunohistology of the nasal mucosa following allergen-induced rhinitis. *Am Rev Respir Dis* 1992;146:170.

35. Ishizaka T, Ishizaka K. Biology and immunoglobulin E: molecular basis of reaginic hypersensitivity. *Prog Allergy* 1976;19:60.

36. Nelson HS, Oppenheimer J, Buchmeier A. An assessment of the role of intradermal skin testing in the diagnosis of clinically relevant allergy to timothy grass. *J Allergy Clin Immunol* 1996;97:1193–1201.

37. Nelson HS, Kroetzer AB, Bucher B. Effect of distance between sites and region of the body on results of skin prick tests. *J Allergy Clin Immunol* 1996;97:596–601.

38. Nelson HS, Lahr J, Buchmeier A. Evaluation of devices for skin prick testing. *J Allergy Clin Immunol* 1998;101:153–156.

39. Oppenheimer J, Nelson HS. Seasonal variation in immediate skin test reactions. *Ann Allergy* 1993;71(3):227–229.

40. Lavins BJ, Dolen WK, Nelson HS. Use of standardized and conventional allergen extracts in prick skin testing. *J Allergy Clin Immunol* 1992;89(3):658–666.

41. Berg T, Bennich II, Johansson SGO. In vitro diagnosis of atopic allergy. I. A comparison between provocation tests and the RAST test. *Int Arch Allergy* 1971;40:770.

42. Fouchard T, Aas K, Johansson SGO. Concentration IgE antibodies, P-K titers and chopped lung titers in sera from children with hypersensitivity to cod. *J Allergy Clin Immunol* 1973;51:39.

43. Norman P. RAST. In: Evans R, ed. *Advances in the diagnosis of allergy.* Miami: Symposia Specialists, 1970:45.

44. Reddy PM, Nagaga H, Pascual HE, et al. Reappraisal of intracutaneous tests in diagnosis of reaginic allergy. *J Allergy Clin Immunol* 1978;61:36.

45. Schatz M, Incaudo F, Yamamoto F, et al. Nasal serum, and skin-fixed IgE in perennial rhinitis patients treated with flunisolide. *J Allergy Clin Immunol* 1978;61:150.

46. Baur X. Baker's asthma: causes and prevention. *Int Arch Occup Environ Health* 1999;72(5):292–296.

47. Newhouse M, Tagg B, Polock S, et al. An epidemiological study of workers producing enzyme washing powders. *Lancet* 1970;1:689.

48. Fernandez-Rivas M, Perez-Carral C, Senent CJ. Occupational asthma and rhinitis caused by ash *(Fraxinus excelsior)* wood dust. *Allergy* 1997;52(2):196–199.

49. Bock SA. Prospective appraisal of complaints of adverse reaction to foods in children during the first three years of life. *Pediatrics* 1987;79:683.

50. Perlman DS. Chronic rhinitis in children. *Clin Rev Allergy* 1984;2:197.

51. Settipane RA. Complications of allergic rhinitis. *Allergy Asthma Proc* 1999;20(4):209–213.

52. Marks MB. Physical signs of allergy on the respiratory tract in children. *Ann Allergy* 1969;25:310.

53. Ammat-Kohja A. Influence des contraceptifs oranux sur las muqenuse nasal. *Rev Laryngol Otol Rhinol* (Board) 1971;92:40.

54. Chilla R, Haubrich J. Vasomotorische rhinitis: Eine nebenwirkung homonaler kontrazeption. *HNO* 1975;23:202.

55. Sorri M, Hortikamen-Sorri AL, Karja J. Rhinitis during pregnancy. *Rhinology* 1980;18:83.

56. Mabry RL. Intranasal steroid injection during pregnancy. *South Med J* 1980;73:1176.

57. English GM, Henenway WG, Cundy RI. Surgical treatment of invasive angiofibroma. *Arch Otolaryngol* 1972;96:312.

58. Rossman CM, Lee RM, Forrest JB, et al. Nasal ciliary ultrastructure and function in patient with primary ciliary dyskinesia compared with that in normal subjects and in subjects with various respiratory diseases. *Ann Rev Respir Dis* 1984;129:161.

59. Eliasson R, Mossberg B, Cammer P, et al. The immotile-cilia syndrome: a congenital ciliary abnormality as an etiologic factor in chronic airway infections and male sterility. *N Engl J Med* 1977;197:1.

60. Afzelius BA. Immotile-cilia syndrome and ciliary abnormalities induced by infection and injury. *Am Rev Respir Dis* 1981;124:107.

61. McKnee WD. The incidence and familial occurrence of allergy. *J Allergy* 1966;38:226.

62. Broder I, Higgings MN, Matthews KP, et al. Epidemiology of asthma and allergic rhinitis in a total community. Tecumseh, Michigan. IV. Natural history. *J Allergy Clin Immunol* 1974;54:10.

63. Broder I, Barlow PP, Horton RJM. The epidemiology of asthma and hayfever in a total community, Tecumseh, Michigan. 2. The relationship between asthma and hayfever. *J Allergy* 1962;33:524.

64. Douglus WW. Histamine and serotonin and their antagonists. In: Gilman AG, Goodman LS, Rall TW, et al, eds. *Goodman and Gilman's the pharmacological basis of therapeutics*. 7th ed. New York: Macmillan, 1985:605.

65. Arrang J, Garbarg M, Lancelot J, et al. Highly potent and selective ligands for histamine H_3 receptors. *Nature* 1987;327:117.

66. Togias AG, Naclerio RM, Warner J, et al. Demonstration of inhibition of mediator release from human mast cells by azatadine base. *JAMA* 1986;255:225.

67. Massey WA, Lichtenstein LM. The effects of antihistamines beyond H_1 antagonism in allergic inflammation. *J Allergy Clin Immunol* 1990;86:1019.

68. Gong H Jr, Lashkin DP, Dauphinee B, et al. Effects of oral cetirizine, a selective H_1 antagonist on allergen and exercise induced bronchoconstriction in subjects with asthma. *J Allergy Clin Immunol* 1990;85:632.

69. Kemp JP, Buckley CE, Gershwin ME, et al. Multicenter, double-blind placebo controlled trial of terfenadine in seasonal allergic rhinitis and conjunctivitis. *Ann Allergy* 1985;54:502.

70. Simmons FER. H_1 receptor antagonists: clinical pharmacology and therapeutics. *J Allergy Clin Immunol* 1989;84:845.

71. Simons FER, Simons KJ. The pharmacology and use of H_1 receptor antagonist drugs. *N Engl J Med* 1994;330:1663–1670.

72. Loratadine: a new antihistamine. *Med Lett* 1993;35:71.

73. DuBuske LM. Clinical comparison of histamine H1-receptor antagonist drugs. *J Allergy Clin Immunol* 1996;98:S307–318.

74. Richards DM, Brogden RN, Heel RC, et al. Astemizole: a review of its pharmacodynamic properties and therapeutic efficacy. *Drugs* 1984;28:38.

75. Surkin EM, Heel RC. Terfenadine: a review of its pharmacodynamic properties and therapeutic efficacy. *Drugs* 1985;29:34.

76. Barnes CL, McKenzi CA, Webster KD, et al. Cetirizine: a new nonsedating antihistamine. *Ann Pharmacother* 1993;27:464.

77. Bernstein DI, Shoenwetter W, Nathan R, et al. Fexopenadine: a new nonsedating antihistamine is effective in the treatment of seasonal allergic rhinitis. *J Allergy Clin Immunol* 1996;97:435.

78. Woosley RL, Barby JT, Yeh J, et al. Lack of electrocardiographic effects of cetirizine in healthy humans. *J Allergy Clin Immunol* 1993;91:258(abst).

79. Mauser PJ, Kreutner W, Egan RW, et al. Selective inhibition of peripheral histamine responses by loratadine and terfenadine. *Eur J Pharmacol* 1990;182:125–129.

80. Synder, Solomon H, Snowman AM. Receptor effects of cetirizine. *Ann Allergy* 1987;59:4.

81. Wood SG, John BA, Chasseared LF, et al. The metabolism and pharmacokinetics of cetirizine in humans. *Ann Allergy* 1987;59:31.

82. Wasserfallen JB, Levenberger P, Pecoud A. Effect of cetirizine, a new H1 antihistamine, on the early and late allergic reactions in a bronchial provocation test with allergen. *J Allergy Clin Immunol* 1993;91:1189–1197.

83. Grant JA, Nicodemus CF, Findlay SR, et al. Cetrizine in patients with seasonal rhinitis and concomitant asthma: prospective, randomized, placebo controlled trial. *J Allergy Clin Immunol* 1995;95:923–932.

84. Casale TB. The interaction of azelastine with human lung histamine H1, beta, and musarinic receptor-binding sites. *J Allergy Clin Immunol* 1989;83:771–776.

85. Chand N, Pillar J, Nolan K, et al. Inhibition of allergic and nonallergic leukotriene C4 formation and histamine secretion by azelastine: implication for its mechanism of action. *Int Arch Allergy Appl Immunol* 1989;90:67–70.

86. Hamaski Y, Shafigeh M, Yamamoto S, et al. Inhibition of leukotrienesynthesis by azelastine. *Ann Allergy Asthma Immunol* 1996;76:469–475.

87. Busse W, Randley B, Sedgwick, J et al. The effect of azelastine on neutrophil and eosinophil generation of superoxide. *J Allergy Clin Immunol* 1989;83:400–405.

88. Nakamura T, Nishizawa Y, Sato T, et al. Effect of azelastine on intracellular Ca^{2+} mobilization in guinea pig peritoneal macrophages. *Eur J Pharmacol* 1988;148:35–41.

89. Werner U, Schmidt J, Szelenyi I. Influence of azelastine on IL-lb generation in vitro and IL-16 induced effect in vivo. *Agents Actions* 1991;32[Suppl]:243–247.

90. Berger WE, Fineman SM, Lieberman P, et al. Double-blind trials of azelastine nasal spray monotherapy versus combination therapy with loxatadine tablets and beclomethasone nasal spray in patients with seasonal allergic rhinitis. *Ann Allergy Asthma Immunol* 1999;82:535–541.

91. Blackwell GJ, Carnuccio R, DiRosa M, et al. Macrocortin: a polypeptide causing the anti-phospholipase effect of glucorticoids. *Nature* 1980;287:147–149.

92. Siegel SC. Topical corticosteroids in the management of rhinitis. In: Settipane GA, ed. *Rhinitis*. 2nd ed. Providence, Rhode Island: Oceanside Publications, 1991:232.

93. Barnes PJ, Petersen S, Busse WW. Efficacy and safety of inhaled corticosteroids: new developments. *Am J Respir Crit Care Med* 1998;157[Suppl 1]:53–55

94. Rak S, Jacobson MR, Sudderick RM, et al. Influence of prolonged treatment with topical corticosteroids (fluticasone propionate) on early and late phase nasal responses and cellular infiltration in the nasal mucosa after allergen challenge. *Clin Exp Allergy* 1994;24:930–939.

95. Reed JC, Abidi AH, Alpers JD, et al. Effect of cyclosporin A and dexamethasone on interleukin 2 receptor gene expresssion. *J Immunol* 1986;137:150–154.

96. Masuyama K, Jacobson MR, Rak S, et al. Topical glucorticosteroid (fluticasone propionate) inhibits cells expressing cytokine on RNA for interleukin-4 in the nasal mucosa in allergen-induced rhinitis. *Immunology* 1994;82:192–199.

97. Van As A, Bronsky EA, Dockhorn RJ, et al. Once daily fluticasone propionate is as effective for perennial allergic rhinitis as twice daily beclomethasone dipropionate. *J Allergy Clin Immunol* 1993;91:1146–1154.

98. Wallen N, Kita H, Weiler D, et al. Glucorticoids inhibit cytokine mediated eosinophil survival. *J Immunol* 1991;147:3490–3495.

99. Kato M, Schleimer RP. Antiinflammatory steroids inhibit GM-CSF production by human lung tissue. *Lung* 1994;172:113–124.

100. Gomez E, Claque JE, Galland D, et al. Effect of topical corticosteroids on seasonally induced increases in nasal mast cells. *Br Med J* 1988;296:1572–1573.

101. Meltzer EO, Jalowayski AA, Field EA, et al. Intranasal fluticasone propionate reduces histamine and tryptase in the mucosa of allergic rhinitis. *J Allergy Clin Immunol* 1993;91:298.

102. Bascom R, Wachs M, Naclerio RM, et al. Basophil influx occurs after nasal antigen challenge: effects of topical corticosteroid pretreatment. *J Allergy Clin Immunol* 1988;81:580–589.

103. Guyre PM, Munck A. Glucocorticoid action on monocytes and macrophages. In: Schleimer RP, Claman HN, Oronsky AR, eds. *Antiinflammatory steroid action: basic and clinical aspects.* New York: Academic Press, 1991:199–225.

104. Lindquist N, Andersson M, Bende M, et al. The clinical efficacy of budesonide in hay fever treatment is dependent on topical nasal application. *Clin Exp Allergy* 1989;19:71–76.

105. Howland WC. Fluticasone propionate: topical or systemic effects? *Clin Exp Allergy* 1996;26[Suppl 3]:18–22.

106. Barnes PJ. Molecular mechanisms of steroid action in asthma. *J Allergy Clin Immunol* 1996;97:159–168.

107. Townley RG, Suliaman F. The mechanism of action of corticosteroids in treating asthma. *Ann Allergy* 1987;58:1–8.

108. Schleimer RP. The mechanisms of antiinflammatory steroid action in allergic diseases. *Ann Rev Pharmacol Toxicol* 1985;25:381–412.

109. Pauwels R. Mode of action of corticosteroids in asthma and rhinitis. *Clin Allergy* 1986;16:281–288.

110. Barnes PJ, Adcock I. Anti-inflammatory actions of steroids: molecular mechanisms. *Trends Pharmacol Sci* 1993;14:436–441.

111. *Nasonex Product Monograph.* Schering Corporation, Kenilworth, NJ, 1998.

112. McDowall JE, Mackie AE, Ventresca GP, et al. Pharmacokinetics and bioavailability of intranasal fluticasone in humans. *Clin Drug Invest* 1997;14:44–52.

113. *Physician's Desk Reference.* Montvale, NJ: 52nd ed. Medical Economics Company, 1998:572–574.

114. Falcoz C, Kirby SM, Smith J, et al. Pharmacokinetics and systemic exposure of inhaled beclomethasone dipropionate. *Eur Respir J* 1996;9[Suppl 23]:162S.

115. Welsh PW, Strickwe WE, Chu CP, et al. Efficacy of beclomethasone nasal solution, flunisolide, and cromolyn in relieving symptoms of ragweed allergy. *Mayo Clin Proc* 1987;62:125.

116. Mygind N. Topical steroid treatment for allergic rhinitis and allied conditions. *Clin Otolaryngol* 1982;7:343.

117. Soderberg-Warner ML. Nasal septal perforation associated with topical corticosteroid spray. *J Pediatr* 1984;105:840.

118. Schoelzl EP, Menzel ML. Nasal sprays and perforation of the nasal septum. *JAMA* 1985;253:2046.

119. Ratner P, van Bauel J, Gross G, et al. New formulation of aqueous flunisolide nasal spray in the treatment of allergic rhinitis: comparative assessment of safety, tolerability, and efficacy. *Allergy Asthma Proc* 1996;17:149–156.

120. Munk ZM, LaForce C, Furst JA, et al. Efficacy and safety of triamcinolone acetonide aqueous nasal spray in patients with seasonal allergic rhinitis. *Ann Allergy Asthma Immunol* 1996;77:277–281.

121. Minshall E, Ghaffar O, Cameron L, et al. Assessment by nasal biopsy of long-term use of mometasone furoate aqueous nasal spray in the treatment of perennial rhinitis. *Otolaryngol Head Neck Surg* 1998;118:648–654.

122. Orgel HA, Meltzer EO, Bierman CW, et al. Intranasal fluocortin butyl in patients with perennial rhinitis: a 12-month efficacy and safety study including nasal biopsy. *J Allergy Clin Immunol* 1991;88:257–264.

123. Norman PS, Winkerwerder WL, Agbayani BF, et al. Adrenal function during the use of dexamethasone aerosols in the treatment of ragweed hay fever. *J Allergy* 1967;40:57–61.

124. Michels MI, Smith RE, Heimlich EM. Adrenal suppression and intranasally applied steroids. *Ann Allergy* 1967;24:569–574.

125. Wiseman LR, Benfield P. Intranasal fluticasone propionate: a reappraisal of its pharmacology and clinical efficacy in the treatment of rhinitis. *Drugs* 1997;53:885–907.

126. Jeal W, Faulds D. Triamcinolone acetonide: a review of its pharmacologic properties and therapeutic efficacy in the management of allergic rhinitis. *Drugs* 1997;53:257–280.

127. Fraunfelder FT, Myer SM. Posterior subcapsular cataracts associated with nasal or inhalation corticosteroids. *Am J Ophtalmol* 1990;109:489–490.

128. Garbe E, Lelorier J, Boivin JF, et al. Inhaled and nasal glucocorticoids and the risks of ocular hypertension or open-angle glaucoma. *JAMA* 1997;277:722–727.

129. LaForce DF, Dockhorn RJ, Findlay SR, et al. Fluticasone propionate: an effective alternative treatment for seasonal allergic rhinitis in adults and adolescents. *J Fam Pract* 1994;38:145–152.

130. Selner JC, Weber RW, Richmond GW, et al. Onset of action of aqueous beclomethasone dipropionate

nasal spray in seasonal allergic rhinitis. *Clin Ther* 1995;17:1099–1109.

131. Day JH, Buckeridge DL, Clark RH, et al. A randomized, double-blind placebo controlled antigen delivery study in subjects with ragweed-induced allergic rhinitis. *J Allergy Clin Immunol* 1996;97:1050–1057.

132. Davies RJ, Nelson HS. Once-daily mometasone furoate nasal spray: efficacy and safety of a new intranasal glucocortoid for allergic rhinitis. *Clin Ther* 1997;19: 27–38.

133. Juniper EF, Guyatt GH, O'Byrne PM, et al. Aqueous beclomethasone dipropionate nasal spray: regular versus as required use in the treatment of seasonal allergic rhinitis. *J Allergy Clini Immunol* 1990;86:380–386.

134. Juniper EF, Guyatt GJ, Archer B, et al. Aqueous beclomethasone dipropionate in the treatment of ragweed pollen-induced rhinitis: further exploration of as needed use. *J Allergy Clin Immunol* 1993;92:66–72.

135. Mabry RL. Practical applications of intranasal corticosteroid injection. *Ear Nose Throat J* 1981;60:23.

136. Sjogren I, Johasz J. Ipratropium in the treatment of patients with perennial rhinitis. *Allergy* 1984;39:457.

137. Borum P, Olsen L, Winther B, et al. Ipratropium nasal spray: a new treatment for rhinorrhea in the common cold. *Am Rev Respir Dis* 1981;123:418.

138. Pelikan Z, Pelikan-Filipek M. The effect of disodium-cromoglycate and beclomethasone diproprionate on the immediate response of the nasal mucosa to allergic challenge. *Ann Allergy* 1982;49:283.

139. Coffman DA. A controlled trial of disodium cromoglycate in seasonal allergic rhinitis. *Br J Clin Pract* 1971;25:403.

140. Jenssen AO. Measurement of resistance to airflow in the nose in a trial with sodium cromoglycate (BP) solution in allergen induced nasal stenosis. *Clin Allergy* 1983;3:277.

141. Hasegawa M, Watanabe K. The effect of sodium cromoglycate on the antigen-induced nasal reaction in allergic rhinitis as measured by rhinomanometry and symptomatology. *Clin Allergy* 1976:6:359.

142. Nelson BL, Jacobs RL. Responses of the nonallergic rhinitis with eosinophilia syndrome to 4% cromolyn sodium nasal solution. *J Allergy Clin Immunol* 1982;70:125.

143. Okunda M, Ohnishi M, Ohstuka H. The effects of cromolyn sodium on the nasal mast cells. *Ann Allergy* 1985;55:721.

144. Hillas J, Booth RJ, Somerfield S, et al. A comparative trial of intranasal beclomethasone diproprionate and sodium cromoglycate in patients with chronic perennial rhinitis. *Clin Allergy* 1980;10:53.

145. Tanilon MK, Strahan EG. Double-blind cross-over trial comparing beclomethasone diproprionate and sodium cromoglycate in perennial allergic rhinitis. *Clin Allergy* 1980;10:450.

146. Brown HM, Engler C, English JR. A comparative trial of flunisolide and sodium cromoglycate nasal sprays in the treatment of seasonal allergic rhinitis. *Clin Allergy* 1981;11:169.

147. Pelikan Z, Pelikan EM. The effect of disodium cromoglycate and beclomethasone diproprionate on the immediate response of the nasal mucosa to allergen challenge. *Ann Allergy* 1982;49:283.

148. Ruhno J, Derburg J, Dolovich J. Intranasal nedocromil sodium in the treatment of ragweed-allergic rhinitis. *J Allergy Clin Immunol* 1988;81:571.

149. Durham SR, Walker SM, Vanga EM. Long term clinical efficacy of grass pollen immunotherapy. *N Engl J Med* 1999;341(7)468–475.

10

Principles of Immunologic Management of Allergic Diseases Due to Extrinsic Antigens

Leslie C. Grammer

Department of Medicine, Division of Allergy-Immunology, Ernest S. Bazley Asthma and Allergic Diseases Center, Northwestern University Medical School; Northwestern Memorial Hospital, Chicago, Illinois

Three principal modalities are available to treat allergic diseases: avoidance of allergens, pharmacologic intervention, and immunotherapy. Pharmacologic intervention is discussed in the chapters relating to specific allergic diseases and in the chapters devoted to specific pharmacologic drug classes. The immunologic interventions—avoidance of allergens and immunotherapy—are the subjects of this chapter.

ALLERGEN EXPOSURE RISK

Sensitization to a variety of allergens has been associated with asthma among children and young adults in numerous studies, with odds ratios ranging from 3 to 19 (1). The particular associated allergen varies with geographic location. Sensitization to house dust mite as a risk factor for asthma has been reported in the United Kingdom (2), Australia (3), New Zealand (4), Virginia (5), and Atlanta (6). In drier climates such as Sweden (7) and New Mexico (8), sensitization to cat and dog dander has been associated with increased risk for asthma. Children in the inner city who become sensitized to cockroach allergens are at increased risk for asthma (9). All of these studies suggest that avoidance of sensitization might reduce the predisposition to asthma. Unfortunately, avoidance is not always simple. For instance, even if cockroaches and pets can be avoided at home, school dust may have very

high levels of these allergens (10,11), resulting in sensitization.

AVOIDANCE OF ANTIGENS

Allergic diseases result from antigen–antibody interaction that subsequently results in release of mediators and cytokines that affect target organs. If exposure to the antigen or allergen can be avoided, no antigen–antibody interaction takes place, and thus there are no allergic disease manifestations. Consequently, the first tenet of allergic management is to remove the allergen if possible.

In the case of certain allergens, removal can be accomplished fairly well. For instance, an individual who is sensitive to cat or dog dander or other animal protein should not have the animal in the home if complete control of symptoms is the goal of management. Another example would be an individual who is sensitive to certain foods or drugs. That individual should avoid the ingestion of those agents.

House Dust Mite

In the case of house dust mite allergy, complete avoidance is not possible in most climates, but the degree of exposure to this allergen can be diminished. House dust mite control measures that are evidence based are listed in Table 10.1.

TABLE 10.1. *Control measures to reduce house dust mite exposure*

Encase mattress, box springs, and pillow in allergen nonpermeable cover.
Wash bed linens weekly in water ≥130°F or tumble dry linens at ≥130°F for 10 minutes.
Reduce indoor humidity to ≤50%.
Inform patients that carpets are reservoirs for mites; polished floors (e.g., linoleum, hardwood, terrazzo) are not and are therefore the flooring of choice, if feasible. This is especially important in the bedroom.
Do not sleep on upholstered furniture.

The effectiveness of controlling mite allergens in beds by using encasings is well established (12,13). Covers should be chosen that are sturdy and easily cleaned. Washing linens in hot water (>130°F) or tumble-drying at a temperature of more than 130°F for 10 minutes will essentially kill all mites (14,15). It is well recognized that carpet is a reservoir for mites; polished floors are preferable, especially in the bedroom (14). Several studies have reported the association between indoor humidity and dust mite allergen levels (16,17). For this reason, the relative humidity in the home should be kept below 50%.

Relative to ionizers or filtration devices, including HEPA filters, the data are conflicting. Although steam cleaning of carpets or use of acaricides can kill mites, the reduction tends to be incomplete and short lived. Freezing stuffed animals, blankets, or clothes will kill mites. However, washing is required to remove the allergen from these items. Vacuum cleaning does help to reduce the overall allergen burden but is not likely to result in control of allergen from reservoirs like carpet and stuffed furniture (14).

Mold Spores

Exposure to mold spores may also be reduced by environmental precautions (18). The patient should avoid entering barns, mowing grass, and raking leaves because high concentrations of mold spores may be found there. Indoor molds are particularly prominent in humid environments. Bathrooms, kitchens, and basements require adequate ventilation and frequent cleaning. If the patient's home has a humidifier, it should be cleaned regularly so that mold does not have an opportunity to grow. Humidity should ideally be 25% to 50%. Water-damaged furnishings or structural elements should be completely replaced to avoid mold growth. Certain foods and beverages, such as aged cheese, canned tomatoes, and beer, may produce symptoms in some mold-sensitive patients. These foods and beverages should be avoided in highly sensitive subjects.

Cockroach Allergens

Control of cockroach allergen exposure may be very difficult, especially in the inner city. The National Co-operative Inner-City Asthma Study Group reported that intervention using abamectin applied by professional exterminators resulted in decreased *Bla g 1* levels in the kitchen, only for a short time. Moreover, even the reduced levels were above those considered clinically significant (19). In another study of the effect of professional extermination using 0.05% abamectin and house-cleaning measures, there was also a decrease in the cockroach population in inner-city homes of Baltimore. However, at the end of the 8-month study, levels of *Bla g 1* were still above the clinically significant level of 20 units per gram of house dust (20). In a study of cockroach extermination with hydramethylnon, there was persistence of elevated *Bla g 1* and *Bla g 2* 6 months after treatment (21). Taken together, the results of these studies indicate that pesticides applied by professional pest control technicians are effective. Sustained cockroach elimination in the inner city will therefore likely require regular extermination in all rooms, coupled with cleaning measures such as addressing reservoirs of allergen in carpets and furniture and keeping food sources such as leftovers, snacks, pet food, and garbage in tightly sealed containers.

Animal Dander

Compared with house dust mite and cockroach allergen, animal aeroallergens are associated with smaller particles that remain airborne for hours; thus, there is a rationale for using air filtration. However, the extent to which exposure to cat allergen can be effectively controlled by methods such as removing reservoirs like carpet and HEPA filtration is not clear. There are conflicting studies (22–26). Two studies reported clinical efficacy using the combination of removal of reservoirs, keeping the cat out of one room (preferably the bedroom), air filtration, and washing the cat (24,26).

Other Inhalant Allergens

Other airborne allergens, such as tree, grass, and ragweed pollens, cannot be avoided except by staying out of geographic areas where they pollinate. For most individuals, this is impractical socially and economically. Air-conditioning and air-filtration systems reduce but do not eliminate exposure to these pollens.

IMMUNOTHERAPY

Immunotherapy is known by various other names: "allergy shots" to the lay public; hyposensitization or desensitization in older medical literature. These terms are not strictly correct in that they imply a mechanism that has not been proved. Desensitization applies to clinical situations in which antigens are administered in a few hours in sufficient quantity to neutralize available immunoglobulin E (IgE) antibody rapidly (27). This type of true desensitization may be necessary in treating patients with allergy to an antibiotic. It is not the operative mechanism in immunotherapy.

Immunotherapy, a term introduced by Norman and co-workers (28), does not imply a mechanism. It consists of injections of increasing amounts of allergen to which the patient has type I immediate hypersensitivity. As a result of these injections, the patient is able to tolerate exposure to the allergen with fewer symptoms. The mechanism by which this improvement occurs has not been definitely established. However, over the years, several mechanisms have been postulated to account for the improvement. Immunotherapy was first used by Noon and Freeman, who observed that pollen was the etiologic agent of seasonal rhinitis and that immunization was effective in the treatment of

TABLE 10.2. *Immunologic changes with immunotherapy*

Increase in allergen-specific IgG
Decreased allergen-specific IgE after prolonged therapy
Decrease in seasonal rise of specific IgE
Increase in antiidiotypic antibodies
Decreased allergen-induced basophil histamine release
Increased suppressor T cells
Decrease in histamine-releasing factors
Change of $CD4^+$ cells from the T_H2 to the T_H1 phenotype

various infectious diseases, including tetanus and diphtheria.

Immunotherapy was used empirically by physicians over the ensuing 40 years. Cooke (29) observed that cutaneous reactivity was not obliterated by allergy injections. Cooke also discovered a serum factor, which he called "blocking antibody," in the serum of patients receiving immunotherapy (30). This serum factor could inhibit the passive transfer of allergic antibody described by Prausnitz and Küstner. However, there was not a constant relationship between blocking antibody titers and symptom relief.

The first controlled study of the efficacy of immunotherapy was published in 1949 (31). Within a short time *in vitro* techniques were developed to assess objectively the immunologic results of immunotherapy. Many immunologic changes occur as a result of immunotherapy (32,33) (Table 10.2). Which changes are responsible for the efficacy of immunotherapy is unknown.

In general, immunotherapy is indicated for clinically significant disease when the usual methods of avoidance and medication are inadequate to control symptoms (34) (Table 10.3). It is considered to be effective in ameliorating

TABLE 10.3. *Indications for allergen immunotherapy*

IgE-mediated disease (allergic rhinitis or allergic asthma)
Significant symptomatology, in terms of duration and severity
Avoidance not possible
Pharmacologic therapy unsatisfactory
Availability of high-potency extract, appropriate dosage schedule, and compliant patient

TABLE 10.4. *Examples of double-blind placebo-controlled allergen immunotherapy studies reporting efficacy*

Investigator, year (ref.)	Allergen	Patients	Controls
Allergic rhinitis			
Van Metre et al, 1982 (35)	Ragweed	33	11
Ortolani et al, 1984 (36)	Grass	8	7
Pence et al, 1976 (37)	Mountain cedar	17	15
Des Roches et al, 1997 (38)	House dust mite	22	22
Horst et al, 1990 (39)	Alternaria	13	11
Dreborg et al, 1986 (40)	Cladosporium	14	16
Asthma			
Reid et al, 1986 (41)	Grass	9	9
Rak et al, 1990 (42)	Birch	20	20
Bousquet et al, 1988 (43)	House dust mite	171	44
Haugaard et al, 1993 (44)	House dust mite	55	19
Malling et al, 1986 (45)	Cladosporium	11	11
Dreburg et al, 1986 (40)	Cladosporium	14	16

symptoms of allergic rhinitis, allergic asthma, and Hymenoptera sensitivity. These topics are discussed in Chapters 9, 22, and 12, respectively. There are many examples of studies reporting the efficacy of immunotherapy in treating allergic rhinitis or allergic asthma caused by various inhalants, including ragweed, grass, and tree pollens, mold spores, and house dust mites (35–45) (Table 10.4). Assessment of efficacy in these studies is difficult because the diseases being treated are chronic and have variations based on geography, climate, and individuals. Assessments are generally made from subjective daily symptom and medication reports by the patient. In some studies, objective clinical evaluation by physicians or by nasal or bronchial challenge was also a part of the assessment. In one study, children who were monosensitized to house dust mite and who received allergen immunotherapy developed fewer new sensitivities than those who did not receive immunotherapy (38). This encouraging finding requires confirmation. A metaanalysis of immunotherapy studies in asthma concluded that immunotherapy was efficacious (46).

There is no indication for immunotherapy in food allergy or chronic urticaria, nor is there sufficient evidence to support the use of bacterial vaccine (18,47).

Choice of Allergens

The aeroallergens that are commonly used in immunotherapy of allergic rhinitis or allergic asthma include extracts of house dust mites, mold spores, and pollen from trees, grasses, and weeds. The pollen species vary to some extent with geographic location, and this information can be obtained from Chapter 7. Because the population is quite mobile, it is usual practice to perform a skin test and treat with common, important allergens outside a physician's geographic location (48). For instance, there is no Bermuda grass in Chicago. However, it is a potent allergen in the southern United States, where people often vacation. Thus, it is used in skin testing and treatment of patients in Chicago. In the allergic evaluation, a patient undergoes skin testing with various allergens. Radioallergosorbent tests (RAST) and other *in vitro* assays are less sensitive and more expensive than skin testing; therefore, skin tests are preferred for the diagnosis of IgE-mediated sensitivity (49). If the patient's history of exacerbations temporally corresponds to the skin test reactivity, the patient probably will benefit from immunotherapy. For example, a patient having a positive grass skin test, rhinorrhea, and palatal itching in May and June in the Midwest will benefit from grass pollen immunotherapy. In contrast, a patient with an isolated positive grass skin test and with perennial symptoms of rhinorrhea and nasal congestion probably has vasomotor rhinitis and will not benefit from immunotherapy.

Many patients have allergic rhinitis or allergic asthma from various types of animal dander. Avoidance is the most appropriate therapeutic maneuver for such patients. In rare instances,

TABLE 10.5. *Allergy extract unitage*

Unitage	Derivation of unit
Weight-to-volume ratio (W/V)	Weight (in grams) extracted per volume (in milliliters)
Protein nitrogen unit (PNU)	0.01 μg of protein nitrogen
Biologic allergy unit (BAU)	Based on average skin test end point of allergic individuals
Major allergen unit	Based on the amount of a major allergen in the extract
Biologic unit (BU)	Based on skin tests end point relative to histamine
International unit (IU)	Based on *in vitro* assays relative to World Health Organization standard allergenic preparations

avoidance is unacceptable; for example, a blind person with a seeing-eye dog or a veterinarian whose livelihood depends on animal exposure cannot be expected to avoid these animals. In these rare instances, immunotherapy with animal dander may be given. Patients who are very sensitive to dander extracts may have difficulties with local or systemic reactions, such that it is difficult to attain clinically efficacious doses (50).

Technical Aspects

Allergen Extract Potency and Dosage Schedules

The preparation and distribution of allergen extracts, also called *vaccines,* is regulated by the U.S. Food and Drug Administration (FDA) Center for Biologics Evaluation and Research (CBER). This agency has developed reference standards for a number of allergen vaccines and reference serum pools to be used by manufacturers to standardize their vaccines. The potency is initially established by an end-point titration technique called the ID_{50} EAL method. Based on these results, the extract is assigned a biologic allergy unit (BAU) potency. Subsequently, allergen extract manufacturers use *in vitro* assays to compare their extracts to the CBER references, and a BAU potency is assigned on the basis of these tests, most commonly RAST inhibition or enzyme-linked immunosorbent assay (ELISA) inhibition (51,52). Two dust mite extracts and eight grass extracts are standardized in this way. Short ragweed and cat extracts (both hair and pelt) are standardized by major allergen content, unit per milliliter of *Amb a 1* or unit per milliliter of *Fel d 1*, respectively. Other aeroallergen preparations made in the United States are not required to be standardized. Several unitage systems are currently in use (Table 10.5).

Neither of the common unitages, protein nitrogen unit (PNU) or weight per volume (W/V), is necessarily an indicator of potency. Potency can be measured practically in various ways: cutaneous end-point titration, radioimmunoassay inhibition, or content of a known major allergen like antigen E (*Amb a 1*) in ragweed, or *Fel d 1* in cat extracts (51). Standard extracts, including short ragweed and *Dermatophagoides pteronyssinus,* have been developed by the Allergen Standardization Subcommittee of the International Union of Immunologic Societies (53,54). These extracts have been extensively tested for allergen content and immunologic properties and have been assigned an arbitrary unitage, international units (IU). Until reference standards and exact quantitation of potency can be established for all extracts, less exact methods such as W/V will continue to be used.

Allergen extracts may be given individually or may be mixed in one vial. That is, a patient receiving immunotherapy to grass pollen and tree pollen could receive two injections, one of grass and one of tree, or could receive one injection containing both grass and tree pollens. The latter is almost always preferable for patient comfort. Because mold extracts contain proteases that may influence other extracts like pollens and dust mite, some recommend giving mold as a separate injection (51). Most clinicians in the United States administer allergen immunotherapy subcutaneously, beginning with weekly or twice-weekly injections (55). Current evidence suggests that treatment with higher doses of pollen extracts results in better long-term reduction of clinical symptoms and greater immunologic

TABLE 10.6. *Example of an allergy treatment tentative dosage schedule*

Date	Extract concentration (W/V) (approx.)	Extract concentration (BAU/mL)	Volume	Remarks
	1:100,000	1	0.1	
			0.2	
			0.4	
			0.8	
	1:10,000	10	0.05	
			0.10	
			0.15	
			0.20	
			0.30	
			0.40	
			0.50	
	1:1,000	100	0.05	
			0.10	
			0.20	
			0.30	
			0.40	
			0.50	
	1:100	1000	0.05	
			0.10	
			0.15	
			0.20	
			0.25	
			0.30	
			0.35	
			0.40	
			0.45	
			0.50	

BAU, biologic allergy unit; W/V, weight-to-volume ratio.

changes than low-dose therapy. There is evidence that dosage based on the Rinkel technique, a low-dose protocol, is not effective (56).

There are no clear data on the optimal length of time immunotherapy should be continued. Most patients who are maintained on immunotherapy and show improvement through three annual pollen seasons continue to maintain improvement even when their injections are discontinued (57). Patients who do not respond after receiving maintenance doses of immunotherapy for 1 year are unlikely to improve with further treatment. Therefore, immunotherapy should be discontinued in patients who have not had appreciable improvement after an entire year of maintenance doses.

The most common method of administering perennial immunotherapy is subcutaneously using a dose schedule similar to that in Table 10.6.

Very sensitive patients must begin at 1:100,000 W/V. The injections are given weekly until the patient reaches the maintenance dose of 0.50 mL of 1:100 W/V. At that point, the interval between injections may be gradually increased to 2 weeks, 3 weeks, and ultimately monthly. When a new vial of extract is given to a patient receiving a maintenance dose of 0.50 mL of 1:100 W/V, the volume should be reduced to about 0.35 mL and increased by 0.05 mL each injection to 0.50 mL. The reason for this is that the new vial may be more potent. There are patients whose achievable maintenance dose is lower than the standard shown in Table 10.6.

Other types of dosage schedules have also been published. In *rush immunotherapy* schedules, the starting doses are similar to those in Table 10.6, but patients receive injections more frequently, at least twice a week. In *cluster immunotherapy* schedules, the initial dosages are similar to those in Table 10.6, and the visit frequency is usually weekly; however, at each visit, more than one injection is administered, with the interval between injections varying from 30 minutes to 2 hours. The advantage of both rush and cluster regimens is that the maintenance dose can be achieved more quickly; the cluster regimen can be especially useful in treating a patient who resides at a significant distance from the physician's office. The disadvantage of both cluster and rush regimens is that the reaction rate is probably somewhat higher than with more conventional schedules (58). For patients on those regimens, initial doses from new vials should also be reduced. Allergen extracts should be kept refrigerated at 4°C for retention of maximum potency. If a vial freezes or heats above 4°C, it should be discarded because the allergens may be altered.

A RAST-based method for determining patient sensitivity and first injection doses has been proposed (59). However, there is not sufficient evidence to support the use of this expensive technique instead of history and properly interpreted skin tests (60). In position statements by the American Academy of Allergy and Immunology (61) and the American College of Asthma, Allergy, and Immunology (49), it was noted that *in vitro* tests may be abused. Abuses of particular concern included the screening of unselected populations, remote formulation of allergen extracts, and the use of *in vitro* test results for translation into immunotherapy prescriptions without an appropriate clinical evaluation.

Procedures for Injections

Immunotherapy injections should be given only after the patient, the patient's dose schedule, and the patient's vial have been carefully identified because improper dose is a common cause of allergic reactions to immunotherapy. Injections should be given with a 1-mL syringe so that the appropriate dose can be given accurately. The injection should be subcutaneous with a 26-gauge needle. Before injecting material, the plunger of the syringe should be withdrawn; if blood appears, the needle and syringe should be withdrawn and discarded. Another needle and syringe should be used for the injection. Patients should be observed at least 20 minutes after their injections for evidence of reactions.

Reactions

Small local reactions with erythema and induration less than 20 mm are common and are of no consequence. Large local reactions and generalized reactions (e.g., rhinitis, conjunctivitis, urticaria, angioedema, bronchospasm, and hypotension) are cause for concern. Large local reactions generally can be treated with antihistamines and local application of ice. Rarely, significant swelling occurs such that 2 days of oral steroids are indicated. Generalized reactions consisting of bronchospasm, angioedema, or urticaria usually respond to 0.3 mL of 1:1,000 epinephrine subcutaneously. The dose for children weighing up to 30 kg is 0.01 mL/kg. This may be repeated every 10 or 15 minutes for up to 3 doses.

Practice parameters for the diagnosis and management of anaphylaxis have been published (62). If the patient has laryngeal edema and is unresponsive to epinephrine, intubation or tracheostomy is necessary. If the patient has hypotension unresponsive to epinephrine, the administration of intravenous fluids and pressors is necessary. Any physician who administers allergen injections must be prepared to treat serious anaphylactic reactions should they occur. If a patient has a large local reaction, the dose should be reduced or repeated, based on clinical judgment. If a systemic reaction occurs, the dose should be reduced to one half to one tenth the dose atwhich the reaction occurred before subsequent slow increase. The management of local and systemic reactions is outlined in Table 10.7. Because of local or systemic reactions, there are patients who are unable to tolerate usual maintenance doses and must be maintained on a smaller dose, for instance, 0.20 mL of 1:100 W/V.

The safety of immunotherapy has been questioned. In one report, five of nine patients who developed polyarteritis nodosa had received immunotherapy (63). Asthma, however, may be

TABLE 10.7. *Management of reactions to immunotherapy*

Local reactions
1. Oral antihistamine
2. Local application of cold
3. Review of dosage schedule

Systemic reactions (including generalized erythema, urticaria, angioedema, bronchospasm, laryngeal edema, shock, and cardiac arrest)
1. 0.01 mL/kg up to 0.2 mL aqueous adrenalin, 1:1,000 subcutaneously, at site of immunotherapy injection to slow absorption of antigen
2. 0.01 mL/kg up to 0.3 mL aqueous adrenalin, 1:1,000 subcutaneously, at another site
3. Diphenhydramine intravenously or intramuscularly, 1.25 mg/kg to 50 mg
4. Tourniquet above the site of injection of allergen.
5. Specific reaction
   a. Bronchospasm: inhaled β-adrenergic bronchodilator. Intravenous aminophylline 4 mg/kg up to 500 mg given over 20 min, aqueous hydrocortisone 5 mg/kg up to 200 mg oxygen
   b. Laryngeal edema: oxygen, intubation, tracheostomy
   c. Hypotension: vasopressors, fluids, corticosteroids
   d. Cardiac arrest: resuscitation, sodium bicarbonate, defibrillation, antiarrhythmia medications.
6. Review of dosage schedule

---

the first symptom of polyarteritis nodosa, and the latter disease may have been present subclinically before the start of the injection therapy. If the polyarteritis nodosa were directly related to immunotherapy, an immunologic mechanism must be postulated, the likely one being antigen–antibody complex damage. However, the amount of antigen used in standard immunotherapy is far less than that producing antigen–antibody complex damage in experimental animals.

Another study compared a group of atopic patients receiving immunotherapy for at least 5 years with a group of atopic patients not on injection therapy (64). The treated group did not show an increased incidence of autoimmune, collagen vascular, or lymphoproliferative disease. There were no adverse effects on immunologic reactivity as measured by several laboratory immunologic tests. Appropriate immunotherapy is accepted as a safe therapy.

Special Considerations

Pregnancy

Patients doing well on maintenance doses of immunotherapy who become pregnant can be continued on immunotherapy (65). However, if a pregnant patient is not on immunotherapy, the risks and benefits need to be evaluated and the decision when to initiate immunotherapy individualized.

Medications

Because patients who receive immunotherapy may require treatment with epinephrine, the risks and benefits of concomitant drug therapy must be considered. For example, the *Physician's Desk Reference* cautions that monoamine oxidase inhibitors should not be administered in conjunction with sympathomimetics (66). Also, β-blocking agents and possibly angiotensin-converting enzyme inhibitors make the treatment of anaphylaxis more difficult in some cases (62).

Failure

If a patient has been on maintenance doses of immunotherapy for 12 months and has no improvement, the clinical allergy problem should be reassessed. Perhaps a new allergen such as an animal has been introduced into the environment. Perhaps the patient has developed new sensitivities for which he or she is not receiving immunotherapy. Perhaps the patient's disease is not allergic in origin but is nonallergic rhinitis or nonallergic asthma, neither of which is altered by immunotherapy. Or, the patient may have misunderstood the benefits of immunotherapy. That is, symptom reduction, not symptom eradication, is all that can be expected from immunotherapy. It is important that the patient understand this at the initiation of therapy.

Alternate Administration Routes

In addition to the administration of allergen through the subcutaneous route, several other routes have been suggested. Local nasal immunotherapy (LNIT) consists of extracts that are sprayed into the nasal cavity by the patient at specified dosages at specified time intervals. There are reported clinical successes, but local side effects may be very bothersome and make LNIT relatively unpalatable (67). Pretreatment with nasal cromolyn does reduce the severity of the local reaction (68).

The efficacy of oral immunotherapy with birch pollen in capsules has been reported (69). Sublingual immunotherapy in a trial of low-dose house dust mite extract has been reported to be efficacious (70). In a trial of sublingual immunotherapy with a standardized cat extract, efficacy was not demonstrated (71). International consensus is that there is not a sufficient number of convincing controlled studies that show effectiveness of sublingual or oral immunotherapy (18).

Modified Allergens

Except for in the United States, most immunotherapy in industrialized nations is given as some type of modified allergen. Although immunotherapy with aqueous antigens has demonstrated efficacy, it is still a long, expensive process with a risk for severe systemic reactions. Therefore, polymerized allergens, formaldehyde-treated allergens, allergens conjugated to alginate, and other forms of modified immunotherapy are used, except in the United States, where such allergens could not be characterized to the satisfaction of CBER.

Administration of purified antigens, for instance, antigen E of short ragweed, was tried as a possible improvement of immunotherapy. Improvements similar to those obtained with whole extracts but with fewer reactions and injections were found with antigen E. The expense of the antigen E purification process has made this sort of administration impractical. Recombinant allergens have also been produced (72). Mixtures of recombinant allergens could be used for allergen immunotherapy but would be unlikely to improve safety or efficacy of current immunotherapy. Recombinant allergens can be engineered to produce proteins that no longer bind IgE but do retain T-cell epitopes that could result in efficacy with improved safety (73).

At present, there are two basic avenues of research to improve immunotherapy. The first is to attempt to inhibit IgE antibody production to a given allergen. Several compounds devised individually by Katz, Sehon, and Ishizaka and colleagues have been successful in animal models, but not in humans. Immunotherapy with T-cell epitope containing peptides has been reported to induce T-cell anergy and clinical efficacy, but trials have been discontinued for commercial reasons (74).

Administration of a neuropeptide, substance P with allergens, has reduced immediate cutaneous and airway responses in a subhuman primate model (75). Mechanistic studies are underway to assess this promising therapy. Others have reported that substance P and allergen cause a switch from the helper T-cell subtypes T_H2 to T_H1 cytokines (76,77).

The other avenue is to reduce allergenicity of allergens while maintaining immunogenicity. The absorption of the antigen from the injection site can be slowed by using an aluminum-precipitated, buffered, aqueous extract of pollen antigen. Patients receiving this extract have shown significant clinical response and immunologic changes with fewer injections and reactions. This is the only modified immunotherapy available in the United States.

Aqueous antigens were used in a mineral oil emulsion to delay the absorption of antigen from the injection site. Problems with this method of treatment include persistent nodules, sterile abscesses, and granulomas. Mineral oil induces tumors in animals, and mineral oil emulsions are not licensed in the United States for human use. Use of liposomes as a form of repository therapy has been considered.

Norman and co-workers treated allergens with formalin to alter antigenic determinants (78). This reduced the allergenicity of the original extract and the skin test reactivity. There are data that demonstrate an efficacy of formaldehyde-treated grass allergens equivalent to that of standard allergy therapy in grass rhinitis. This therapy is available in countries other than the United States.

Glutaraldehyde-modified tyrosine–adsorbed short ragweed extracts have been reported to result in only a modest reduction in symptoms.

Patterson and colleagues polymerized ragweed and other pollen proteins with glutaraldehyde. Because there are fewer molecules of polymer on a weight basis compared with monomer allergens, there are fewer molecules to react with histamine-containing cells. There are data that demonstrate an efficacy of polymer equivalent to that of monomer with fewer injections and fewer systemic reactions. There are also data demonstrating efficacy of polymerized ragweed in double-blind histamine placebo-controlled trials (79). This therapy is also available in countries other than the United States.

Other Novel Therapies

Other novel therapies, such as anti-IgE, anti–interleukin-5 (anti–IL-5), sIL-4, immunostimulatory sequences of DNA, T-cell epitopes, human recombinant engineered proteins, and interferons are discussed in Chapter 38.

REFERENCES

1. Platts-Mills TAE, Rakes G, Heymann PW. The relevance of allergen exposure to the development of asthma in childhood. *J Allergy Clin Immunol* 2000;105:S503–508.
2. Sporik RB, Holgate ST, Platts-Mills TAE, et al. Exposure to house dust mite allergen (*Der p* I) and the development of asthma in childhood: a prospective study. *N Engl J Med* 1990;323:502–507.
3. Peat JK, Tovey E, Toelle BE, et al. House dust mite allergens: a major risk factor for childhood asthma in Australia. *Am J Respir Crit Care Med* 1996;153:141–146.
4. Sears MR, Hervision GP, Holdaway MD, et al. The relative risks of sensitivity to grass pollen, house dust mite, and cat dander in the development of childhood asthma. *Clin Exp Allergy* 1989;19:419–424.
5. Squillace SP, Sporik RB, Rakes G, et al. Sensitization to dust mites as a dominant risk factor for asthma among adolescents living in central Virginia: multiple regression analysis of a population-based study. *Am J Respir Crit Care Med* 1997;156:1760–1764.
6. Call RS, Smith TF, Morris E, et al. Risk factors for asthma in inner city children. *J Pediatr* 1992;121:862–866.
7. Ronmark E, Lundback B, Jonsson E, et al. Asthma, type-1 allergy and related conditions in 7- and 8-years-old children in Northern Sweden: prevalence rates and risk factor patterns. *Respir Med* 1998;92:316–324.
8. Sporik R, Ingram JM, Price W, et al. Association of asthma with serum IgE and skin-test reactivity to allergens among children living at high altitude: tickling the dragon's breath. *Am J Respir Crit Care Med* 1995;151:1388–1392.
9. Rosenstreich DL. The role of cockroach allergy and exposure to cockroach allergen causing morbidity among inner-city children with asthma. *N Engl J Med* 1997;336:1356–1363.
10. Sarpong SB, Wood RA, Karrison T, et al. Cockroach allergen (Bla g 1) in school dust. *J Allergy Clin Immunol* 1997;99:486–492.
11. Warner JA. Environmental allergen exposure in homes and schools. *Clin Exp Allergy* 1992;22:210–216.
12. Custovic A, Taggart SCO, Francis HC, et al. Exposure to house dust mite allergens and the clinical activity of asthma. *J Allergy Clin Immunol* 1996;98:64–72.
13. Frederick JM, Warner JO, Jessop WJ, et al. Effect of a bed covering system in children with asthma and dust mite sensitivity. *Eur Respir J* 1997;10:361–363.
14. Platts-Mills TAE, Vervloet D, Thomas WR, et al. Indoor allergens and asthma: report of the Third International Workshop. *J Allergy Clin Immunol* 1997;100:S1–S24.
15. Manjra A, Berman D, Toerien A, et al. The effects of a single treatment of an acaricide, Acarosan, and a detergent, Metsan, on *Der p* 1 allergen levels in the carpets and mattresses of asthmatic children. *S Afr Med J* 1994;84:278–280.
16. Kuehr J, Frischer T, Karmaus W, et al. Natural variation in mite antigen density in house dust and relationship to residential factors. *Clin Exp Allergy* 1994;24:229–237.
17. Sundell J, Wickman M, Pershagen G, et al. Ventilation in homes infested by house-dust mites. *Allergy* 1995;50:106–112.
18. *NHLBI 1992 International Consensus report on diagnosis and management of asthma.* NIH Pub No. 92-3091. Bethesda, MD, NHLBI.
19. Gergen PJ, Mortimer KM, Eggleston PA, et al. Results of the National Cooperative Inner-city Asthma Study (NCICAS) environmental intervention to reduce cockroach allergen exposure in inner-city homes. *J Allergy Clin Immunol* 1999;103:501–506.
20. Eggleston PA, Wood RA, Rand C, et al. Removal of cockroach allergen from inner city homes. *J Allergy Clin Immunol* 1999;104:842–846.
21. Williams LW, Reinfried P, Brenner RJ. Cockroach extermination does not rapidly reduce allergen in settled dust. *J Allergy Clin Immunol* 1999;104:702–703.
22. Koren LGH, Janssen E, Willemse A. Cat allergen avoidance: a weekly cat treatment to keep the cat at home. *J Allergy Clin Immunol* 1995;95:322.
23. Avner D, Perzanowski MS, Platts-Mills TAE, et al. Evaluation of different techniques for washing cats: quantitation of allergen removed from the cat and the effect on airborne Fel d 1. *J Allergy Clin Immunol* 1997;100:307–312.
24. Soldatov D, de Blay P, Griess P, et al. Effects of environmental control measures on patient status and airborne Fel d 1 levels with a cat in situ. *J Allergy Clin Immunol* 1995;95:263.
25. Klucka CV, Ownby D, Green J, et al. Cat shedding of Fel d I is not reduced by washings, Allerget-C spray, or acepromazine. *J Allergy Clin Immunol* 1995;95:1164–1171.
26. de Blay F, Chapman MD, Platts-Mills TAE. Airborne cat allergen (Fel d I). *Am Rev Respir Dis* 1991;143:1334–1339.
27. Patterson R, Mellies CJ, Roberts M. Immunologic reactions against insulin. II. IgE anti-insulin, insulin allergy and combined IgE and IgG immunologic insulin resistance. *J Immunol* 1973;110:1135–1145.
28. Norman P. The clinical significance of IgE. *Hosp Pract* 1975;10:41–49.

29. Cooke RA. Studies in specific hypersensitiveness. IX. On the phenomenon of hyposensitization (the clinically lessened sensitiveness of allergy). *J Immunol* 1922;7:219–242.

30. Cooke RA, Barnard JH, Hebald S, et al. Serologic evidence of immunity with coexisting sensitization in a type of human allergy (hayfever). *J Exp Med* 1935;62:733–750.

31. Bruun E. Control examination of the specificity of specific desensitization in asthma. *Acta Allergologica* 1949;2:122–128.

32. Durham SR, Varney VA. Mechanisms. In: Kay AB, ed. *Allergy and allergic diseases.* London: Blackwell Science, 1997:1227–1233.

33. Bousquet J, Lockey RF, Malling HJ. WHO Position Paper. Allergen immunotherapy: therapeutic vaccines for allergic diseases. *Eur J Allergy Clin Immunol* 1998;53:1–42.

34. Immunotherapy Subcommittee of the European Academy of Allergology and Clinical Immunology. Immunotherapy position paper. *Allergy* 1988;43 [Suppl 6]:9–33.

35. Van Metre Jr TE, Adkinson NF, Amodio FJ, et al. A comparison of immunotherapy schedules for injection treatment of ragweed pollen hay fever. *J Allergy Clin Immunol* 1982;69:181–193.

36. Ortolani C, Pestorello E, Moss RB. Grass pollen immunotherapy: a single year double blind placebo controlled study in patients with grass pollen induced asthma and rhinitis. *J Allergy Clin Immunol* 1984;73:283–290.

37. Pence HL, Mitchell DQ, Greely RL, et al. Immunotherapy for mountain cedar pollinosis: a double-blind controlled study. *J Allergy Clin Immunol* 1976;58:39–50.

38. Des Roches A, Paradis L, Menardo J-L, et al. Immunotherapy with a standardized *Dermatophagoides pteronyssinus* extract. VI. Specific immunotherapy prevents the onset of new sensitizations in children. *J Allergy Clin Immunol* 1997;99:450–453.

39. Horst M, Hejjaoui A, Horst V, et al. Double-blind placebo controlled rush immunotherapy with a standardized *Alternaria* extract. *J Allergy Clin Immunol* 1990;85:460–472.

40. Dreborg S, Agrell B, Foucard T, et al. A double-blind, multicenter immunotherapy trial in children, using a purified and standardized *Cladosporium Herbarum* preparation. *Allergy* 1986;41:131–140.

41. Reid MJ, Moss RB, Hsu YP, et al. Seasonal asthma in northern California: allergic causes and efficacy of immunotherapy. *J Allergy Clin Immunol* 1986;78:590–600.

42. Rak S, Hakanson L, Venge P. Immunotherapy abrogates the generation of eosinophil and neutrophil chemotactic activity during pollen season. *J Allergy Clin Immunol* 1990;86:706–713.

43. Bousquet J, Hejjaoui A, Clauzel A-M, et al. Specific immunotherapy with a standardized *Dermatophagoides pteronyssinus* extract. II. Prediction of efficacy of immunotherapy. *J Allergy Clin Immunol* 1988;82:971–977.

44. Haugaard L, Dahl R, Jacobsen L. A controlled dose-response study of immunotherapy with standardized, partially purified extract of house dust mite: Clinical efficacy and side effects. *J Allergy Clin Immunol* 1993;91:709–722.

45. Malling HJ, Dreborg S, Weeke B. Diagnosis and immunotherapy of mould allergy. V. Clinical efficacy and side effects of immunotherapy with *Cladosporium herbarum. Allergy* 1986;41:507–519.

46. Abramson MJ, Puy RM, Weiner JM. Is allergen immunotherapy effective in asthma? A meta-analysis of randomized controlled trials. *Am J Respir Crit Care Med* 1995;151:969–974.

47. Ledford DK. Efficacy of immunotherapy. In: Lockey RF, Bukantz SC, eds. *Allergens and allergen immunotherapy.* 2nd ed. New York: Marcel Dekker, 1999:359–380.

48. Schatz M. An approach to diagnosis and treatment in the migrant allergic population. *J Allergy Clin Immunol* 1977;59:254–262.

49. Bernstein IL, Storms WW. Practice parameters for allergy diagnostic testing. *Ann Allergy Asthma Immunol* 1995;75:543–615.

50. Varney VA, Edward J, Tabbah K. Clinical efficacy of specific immunotherapy to cat dander, a double-blind placebo controlled trial. *Clin Exp Allergy* 1997;27:860–867.

51. Nelson HS. Preparing and mixing allergen vaccines. In: Lockey RF, Bukantz SC, eds. *Allergens and allergen immunotherapy.* 2nd ed. New York: Marcel Dekker, 1999:401–422.

52. Yunginger JW, Swanson MC. Quantitation and standardization of allergens. In: Rose NR, de Macario EC, Folds JD, et al, eds. *Manual of clinical laboratory immunology.* 5th ed. Washington, DC: American Society for Microbiology, 1997:868–874.

53. Helm RM, Gauerke MB, Baer H, et al. Production and testing of an international reference standard of short ragweed pollen extract. *J Allergy Clin Immunol* 1984;73:790–800.

54. Ford A, Seagroatt V, Platts-Mills TAE, et al. A collaborative study on the first international standard of *Dermatophagoides pteronyssinus* (house-dust mite) extract. *J Allergy Clin Immunol* 1985;75:676–686.

55. Bernstein IL, Nicklas RA, Greenberger PA, et al. Practice parameters for allergen immunotherapy. *J Allergy Clin Immunol* 1996;98:1001–1011.

56. Hirsch SR, Kalbfleisch JH, Golbert TM, et al. Rinkel injection therapy: a multicenter controlled study. *J Allergy Clin Immunol* 1981;68:133–155.

57. Druham SR, Walker SM, Varga EM, et al. Long-term clinical efficacy of grass-pollen immunotherapy. *N Engl J Med* 1999;341:468–475.

58. Van Metre TE Jr, Adkinson NF Jr, Amodio FJ, et al. A comparison of immunotherapy schedules for injection treatment of ragweed hay fever. *J Allergy Clin Immunol* 1982;69:181–193.

59. Fadal RG, Nalebuff DJ. A study of optimum dose immunotherapy in pharmacological treatment failures. *Arch Otolaryngol* 1980;106:38–43.

60. Adkinson NR Jr. The radioallergosorbent test: uses and abuses. *J Allergy Clin Immunol* 1980;65:1–4.

61. American Academy of Allergy and Immunology. The use of in vitro tests for IgE antibody in the specific diagnosis of IgE mediated disorders and in the formulation of allergen immunotherapy. *J Allergy Clin Immunol* 1992;90:263–267.

62. Practice parameters for the diagnosis and management of anaphylaxis. *J Allergy Clin Immunol* 1998;101:S465–S528.

63. Phanupak P, Kohler PF. Recent advances in allergic vasculitis. *Adv Allergy Pulmonary Dis* 1978;5:19–28.

64. Levinson AI, Summers RJ, Lawley TJ, et al. Evaluation of the adverse effects of long term hyposensitization. *J Allergy Clin Immunol* 1978;62:109–114.

65. Metzger WJ, Turner E, Patterson R. The safety of immunotherapy during pregnancy. *J Allergy Clin Immunol* 1978;61:268–272.

66. *Physician's desk reference.* 54th ed. Montvale, NJ: Medical Economics, 2000.

67. Passalacqua G, Albano M, Ruffoni S, et al. Nasal immunotherapy to prietaria: evidence of reduction of local allergic inflammation. *Am J Respir Crit Care Med* 1995;152:461–466.

68. Hasegawa M, Saito Y, Watanabe K. The effects of sodium cromoglycate on the antigen induced nasal reaction in allergic rhinitis as measured by rhinomanometry and symptomology. *Clin Allergy* 1976;6:359–363.

69. Taudorf E, Laursen LC, Lanner A, et al. Oral immunotherapy in birch pollen hay fever. *J Allergy Clin Immunol* 1987;80:153–161.

70. Scadding GK, Brostoff J. Low dose sublingual therapy in patients with allergic rhinitis due to house dust mite. *Clin Allergy* 1986;16:483–491.

71. Nelson HS, Opperheimer J, Vatsio GA, et al. A double-blind, placebo-controlled evaluation of sublingual immunotherapy with standardized cat extract. *J Allergy Clin Immunol* 1993;92:229–236.

72. Smith AM, Chapman MD. Allergen-specific immunotherapy: new strategies using recombinant allergens. In: Bousquet J, Yssel H, eds. *Immunotherapy in asthma.* New York: Marcel Dekker 1999:99–118.

73. Schramm G, Kahlert H, Suck R, et al. "Allergen engineering": variants of the timothy grass pollen allergen Ph1 p 5b with reduced IgE-binding capacity but conserved T cell reactivity. *J Immunol* 1999;162:2406–2414.

74. Norman PS, Ohman Jr, JL, Long AA, et al. Treatment of cat allergy with T cell reactive peptides. *Am J Respir Crit Care Med* 1996;154:1623–1628.

75. Patterson R, Harris KE, Grammer LC, et al. Potential effect of the administration of substance P and allergen therapy on immunoglobulin E-mediated allergic reactions in human subjects. *J Lab Clin Med* 1999: 189–199.

76. Carucci JA, Herrick CA, Durkin HG. Neuropeptide-mediated regulation of hapten-specific IgE responses in mice. II. Mechanisms of substance P-mediated isotype-specific suppression of BPO-specific IgE antibody-forming cell responses induced in vitro. *J Neuroimmunol* 1994;49:89–95.

77. Kincy-Cain T, Bost KL. Substance P-induced IL-12 production by murine macrophages. *J Immunol* 1997;158:2334–2339.

78. Norman PS, Lichtenstein LM. Comparisons of alum-precipitated and unprecipitated aqueous ragweed pollen extracts in the treatment of hayfever. *J Allergy Clin Immunol* 1978;61:384–389.

79. Grammer LC, Zeiss CR, Suszko IM, et al. A double-blind placebo-controlled trial of polymerized whole ragweed for immunotherapy of ragweed allergy. *J Allergy Clin Immunol* 1982;69:494–499.

11

Allergic Diseases of the Eye and Ear

Phil Lieberman and Michael S. Blaiss

Division of Allergy and Immunology, Departments of Medicine and Pediatrics
University of Tennessee, Memphis

THE EYE

The allergic eye diseases are contact dermatoconjunctivitis, acute allergic conjunctivitis, vernal conjunctivitis, and atopic keratoconjunctivitis (allergic eye diseases associated with atopic dermatitis). Several other conditions mimic allergic disease and should be considered in any patient presenting with conjunctivitis. These include the blepharoconjunctivitis associated with staphylococcal infection, seborrhea and rosacea, acute viral conjunctivitis, chlamydial conjunctivitis, keratoconjunctivitis sicca, herpes simplex keratitis, giant papillary conjunctivitis, and the "floppy eye syndrome." Each of these entities are discussed in relationship to the differential diagnosis of allergic conjunctivitis. The allergic conditions themselves are emphasized.

In addition to the systematic discussion of these diseases, because the chapter is written for the nonophthalmologist, an anatomic sketch of the eye (Fig. 11.1) is included.

Diseases Involving the External Eye Surfaces

Contact Dermatitis and Dermatoconjunctivitis

Because the skin of the eyelid is thin (0.55 mm), it is particularly prone to develop both immune and irritant contact dermatitis. When the causative agent has contact with the conjunctiva and the lid, a dermatoconjunctivitis occurs.

Clinical Presentation

Contact dermatitis and dermatoconjunctivitis affect women more commonly than men because women use cosmetics more frequently. Vesiculation may occur early, but by the time the patient seeks care, the lids usually appear thickened, red, and chronically inflamed. If the conjunctiva is involved, there is erythema and tearing. A papillary response with vasodilation and chemosis occurs. Pruritus is the cardinal symptom; a burning sensation may also be present. Rubbing the eyes intensifies the itching. Tearing can occur. An erythematous blepharitis is common, and in severe cases, keratitis can result.

Causative Agents

Contact dermatitis and dermatoconjunctivitis can be caused by agents directly applied to the lid or conjunctiva, aerosolized or airborne agents contacted by chance, and cosmetics applied to other areas of the body. In fact, eyelid dermatitis occurs frequently because of cosmetics (e.g., nail polish, hair spray) applied to other areas of the body (1). Agents applied directly to the eye are probably the most common causes. Contact dermatitis can be caused by eye makeup, including eyebrow pencil and eyebrow brush-on products, eye shadow, eye liner, mascara, artificial lashes, and lash extender. These products contain coloring agents, lanolin, paraben, sorbitol, paraffin, petrolatum, and other substances such as vehicles and perfumes (1). Brushes and pads used to

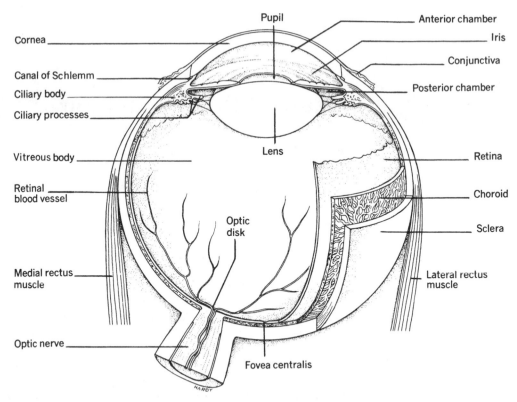

FIG. 11.1. Transverse section of the eye. (From Brunner L, Suddarth D. *Textbook of medical-surgical nursing.* 4th ed. Philadelphia: JB Lippincott, 1980, with permission.)

apply these cosmetics also can produce dermatitis. In addition to agents applied directly only to the eye, soaps and face creams can also produce a selective dermatitis of the lid because of the thin skin in this area. Cosmetic formulations are frequently altered (1). Therefore, a cosmetic previously used without ill effect can become a sensitizing agent.

Any medication applied to the eye can produce a contact dermatitis or dermatoconjunctivitis. Ophthalmic preparations contain several sensitizing agents, including benzalkonium chloride, chlorobutanol, chlorhexidine, ethylenediaminetetraacetate (EDTA), and phenylmercuric salts. EDTA cross-reacts with ethylenediamine, so that patients sensitive to this agent are subject to develop dermatitis as a result of several other medications. Today, neomycin and idoxuridine are probably the major cause of iatrogenic contact dermatoconjunctivitis. Several other topically applied medications,

however, have been shown to cause dermatoconjunctivitis. These include antihistamines, such as antazoline, as well as atropine, chloramphenicol (Chloromycetin), pilocarpine, gentamicin, phenylephrine, epinephrine, and topical anesthetics.

Of increasing importance is the conjunctivitis associated with the wearing of contact lenses, especially soft lenses. Reactions can occur to the lenses themselves or to the chemicals used to treat them. Both toxic and immune reactions can occur to contact lens solutions. Thimerosal, a preservative used in contact lens solutions, has been shown to produce classic, cell-medicated contact dermatitis (2). Other substances found in lens solutions that might cause either toxic or immune reactions are the bacteriostatic agents (methylparaben, chlorobutanol, and chlorhexidine) and EDTA, which is used to chelate lens deposits. With the increasing use of disposable contact lenses, the incidence of contact allergy to lenses and their cleansing agents appears to be declining.

Dermatitis of the lid and conjunctiva can also result from exposure to airborne agents. Hair spray, volatile substances contacted at work, and the oleoresin moieties of airborne pollens have all been reported to produce contact dermatitis and dermatoconjunctivitis. Hair preparations and nail enamel frequently cause problems around the eye while sparing the scalp and the hands. Finally, *Rhus* dermatitis can affect the eye, producing unilateral periorbital edema, which can be confused with angioedema.

Diagnosis and Identification of Causative Agents

The differential diagnosis includes seborrheic dermatitis and blepharitis, infectious eczematous dermatitis (especially chronic staphylococcal blepharitis), and rosacea. Seborrheic dermatitis usually can be differentiated from contact dermatitis on the basis of seborrheic lesions elsewhere and the lack or pruritus. Also, pruritus does not occur in staphylococcal blepharitis or rosacea. If the diagnosis is in doubt, an ophthalmology consultation should be obtained.

In some instances, the etiologic agents may be readily apparent. This is usually the case in dermatitis caused by the application of topical medications. However, many cases present as chronic dermatitis, and the cause is not readily apparent. In such instances, an elimination-provocation procedure and patch tests can identify the offending substance. The elimination-provocation procedure requires that the patient remove all substances under suspicion from the environment. This is often difficult because it requires the complete removal of all cosmetics, hair sprays, spray deodorants, and any other topically applied substances. It should also include the cessation of visits to hair stylists and day spas during the course of the elimination procedure. The soaps and shampoo should be changed. A bland soap (e.g., Basis) and shampoo free of formalin (e.g., Neutrogena, Ionil) should be employed. In recalcitrant cases, the detergent used to wash the pillowcases should also be changed. The

elimination phase of the procedure should continue until the dermatitis subsides, or for a maximum of 1 month. When the illness has cleared, cosmetics and other substances can be returned at a rate of one every week. On occasion, the offending substances can be identified by the recurrence of symptoms upon the reintroduction of the substance in question.

Patch tests can be helpful in establishing a diagnosis. However, the skin of the lid is markedly different from that of the back and forearm, and drugs repeatedly applied to the conjunctival sac concentrate there, producing high local concentrations of the drug. Thus, false-negative results from patch tests are common (1). Testing should be performed, not only to substances in standard patch test kits, but also to the patient's own cosmetics. In addition to the cosmetics themselves, tests can be performed to applying agents, such as sponges and brushes. Both open- and closed-patch tests are indicated when testing with cosmetics (1). Fisher describes a simple test consisting of rubbing the substances into the forearm three times daily for 4 to 5 days, and then examining the sites. Because of the difficulty involved in establishing the etiologic agent with standard patch test kits, an ophthalmic patch test tray (Table 11.1) has been suggested (3).

Therapy

The treatment of choice is removal of the offending agent. On occasion, this can be easily accomplished. An example of this is the switch from chemically preserved to heat-sterilized systems in patients with contact lens–associated contact conjunctivitis. The offending agent, however, frequently cannot be identified, regardless of the diagnostic procedures applied. In these instances, chronic symptomatic therapy, possibly in conjunction with an ophthalmologist, is all that can be offered to the patient.

Symptomatic relief can be obtained with topical corticosteroid creams, ointments, and drops. Corticosteroid drops should be employed only under the direction of the ophthalmologist. Cool tap-water soaks and boric acid eye baths may help.

TABLE 11.1. *Suggested ophthalmic tray for patch testing*

Compound	Patch test concentration (%)	Vehicle
Preservatives		
Benzalkonium chloride	0.1	aq
Benzethonium chloride	1	aq
Chlorhexidine gluconate	1	aq
Cetalkonium chloride	0.1	aq
Sodium EDTA	1	aq
Sorbic acid	2.5	pet
Thimerosal	0.1;1	pet
β-Adrenergic blocking agents		
Befunolol	1	aq
Levobunolol HCl	1	aq
Metipranolol	2	aq
Metoprolol	3	aq
Timolol	0.5	aq
Mydriatics		
Atropine sulfate	1	aq
Epinephrine HCl	1	aq
Phenylephrine HCl	10	aq
Scopolamine hydrobromide	0.25	aq
Antibiotics		
Bacitracin	5	pet
Chloramphenicol	5	pet
Gentamicin sulfate	20	pet
Kanamycin	10	pet
Neomycin sulfate	20	pet
Polymyxin B sulfate	20	pet
Antiviral drugs		
Idoxuridine	1	pet
Trifluridine	5	pet
Antihistamines or antiallergic drug		
Chlorpheniramine maleate	5	pet
Sodium cromoglycate	2	aq
Anesthetics		
Benzocaine	5	pet
Procaine	5	aq
Oxybuprocaine	0.5	aq
Proxymetacaine	0.5	aq
Enzymatic cleaners		
Papain	1	pet
Tegobetaine	1	aq
Miotics		
Pilocarpine	1	aq
Tolazoline	10	aq
Echothiophate iodide	1	aq
Other		
Epsilon aminocaproic acid	1	aq

aq, aqueous; pet, petrolatum.
From Mondino B, Salamon S, Zaidman G. Allergic and toxic reactions in soft contact lens weavers. *Surv Ophthalmol* 1982;26:337–344, with permission.

Acute Allergic Conjunctivitis

Pathophysiology

Acute allergic conjunctivitis is the most common form of allergic eye disease (4). It is produced by IgE-induced mast cell and basophil degranulation. As a result of this reaction, histamine, kinins, leukotrienes, prostaglandins, interleukins, chemokines, and other mediators are liberated (5–7). Patients with allergic conjunctivitis have elevated amounts of total IgE in their tears (8–10), and tear fluid also contains IgE specific for seasonal allergens (11). Eosinophils are found in ocular scrapings (12–14). These eosinophils are activated, releasing contents such as eosinophil cationic protein from their granules. These contents appear in tear fluid (14). Ocular challenge with pollen produces both an early- and a late-phase ocular response (15). In humans, the early phase begins about 20 minutes after challenge. The late phase is dose dependent, and large doses of allergen cause the initial inflammation to persist and progress (15). The late phase differs from that which occurs in the nose and lungs in that it is usually continuous and progressive rather than biphasic (15). It is characterized by the infiltration of inflammatory cells, including neutrophils, eosinophils, and lymphocytes. The eosinophil is the predominant cell (15). In addition, during the late-phase reaction, mediators are continually released, including histamine, leukotrienes, and eosinophil contents (16).

Subjects with allergic conjunctivitis demonstrate a typical T_H2 (allergic) profile of cytokines in their tear fluid showing excess production of interleukin-4 (IL-4) and IL-5 (17–19). If the illness becomes chronic, however, there may be a shift in cytokine profile to a T_H1 pattern with excess production of interferon-γ, as seen in atopic keratoconjunctivitis (19).

Subjects with allergic conjunctivitis have an increased number of mast cells in their conjunctivae (20), and they are hyperresponsive to intraocular histamine challenge (21). Of interest is the fact that there is evidence of complement activation. Elevated levels of C3a des-Arg appear in tear fluid (4). The consequences of this immune reaction are conjunctival vasodilation and edema. The clinical reproducibility of the reaction is dependable. Instillation of allergen into the conjunctival sac was once used as a diagnostic test (22).

Clinical Presentation

Acute allergic conjunctivitis is usually recognized easily. Itching is always a prominent feature. Rubbing the eyes intensifies the symptoms. The illness is almost always bilateral. However, unilateral acute allergic conjunctivitis can occur secondary to manual contamination of the conjunctiva with allergens such as foods and animal dander. Ocular signs usually are minimal despite significant symptoms. The conjunctiva may be injected and edematous. In severe cases, the eye may be swollen shut. These symptoms of allergic conjunctivitis may be so severe as to interfere with the patient's sleep and work.

Allergic conjunctivitis rarely occurs without accompanying allergic rhinitis. Occasionally, the eye symptoms may be more prominent than nasal symptoms and can be the patient's major complaint. However, if symptoms or signs of allergic rhinitis are totally absent, the diagnosis of allergic conjunctivitis is doubtful. Allergic conjunctivitis also exists in a chronic form. Symptoms are usually less intense. As in acute allergic conjunctivitis, ocular findings may not be impressive (8).

Diagnosis and Treatment

The diagnosis of allergic conjunctivitis can usually be made on the basis of history. There is an atopic personal or family history; the disease is usually seasonal. At times, the patient may be able to define the offending allergen accurately. Skin tests are confirmatory. Stain of the conjunctival secretions may show numerous eosinophils, but the absence of eosinophils does not exclude the condition (23). Normal individuals do not have eosinophils in conjunctival scrapings; therefore, the presence of one eosinophil is consistent with the diagnosis (23). The differential diagnosis should include other forms of acute conjunctivitis, including viral and bacterial conjunctivitis, contact dermatoconjunctivitis, conjunctivitis sicca, and vernal conjunctivitis.

Treating allergic conjunctivitis is the same as for other atopic illness: avoidance, symptomatic relief, and immunotherapy, in that order. When allergic conjunctivitis is associated with respiratory allergic disease, the course of treatment is usually dictated by the more debilitating respiratory disorder. Avoiding ubiquitous aeroallergens is impractical, but avoidance measures outlined elsewhere in this text can be employed in the treatment of allergic conjunctivitis.

Effective symptomatic therapy for allergic conjunctivitis can usually be achieved with

TABLE 11.2. *Representative topical agents used to treat allergic eye disorders*

Drug class	Representative trade name examples	Dosage	Comments
Vasoconstrictors			
Tetrahydrozoline, phenylephrine, oxymetazoline, naphazoline	Naphcon, Vasocon, Visine	1–2 drops q4h p.r.n. (not more than q.i.d.)	Only helpful for eye redness. Does not relieve itch. Available without prescription. Some concern about "rebound." Contraindicated in narrow-angle glaucoma.
Antihistamines			
Levocabastine	Livostin	1 drop q.i.d.	Effective for itching. Available by prescription only. May be more potent than antihistamines available without prescription.
Emedastine	Emadine	1 drop q.i.d.	
Combinations			
Vasoconstrictor antihistamines			
Antazoline, naphazoline	Vasocon-A	1 drop q.i.d.	Effective for eye redness and itch. Available without prescription.
Mast cell stabilizers			
Lodoxadine	Alomide	1 drop q.i.d.	Best when initiated before onset of symptoms
Cromolyn	Crolom, Opticrom	1 drop q.i.d.	
Nedocromil	Allocril	1 drop q.i.d.	
Pemirolast	Alamast	1 drop q.i.d.	
Nonsteroidal antiinflammatory			
Ketorolac	Acular	1 drop q.i.d.	Indicated for itching
Drugs with multiple antiallergic activities			
Olopatadine	Patanol	1–2 drops b.i.d. every 6–8 hr	Antihistamine, mast cell stabilizing, and antieosinophil activities
Ketotifen	Zaditor	1 drop every 8–12 hr	

topical medications. The most significant change in the management of allergic eye disorders since the last edition of this text is the release of new topical agents to treat these disorders. Six classes of topical agents are now available. These are vasoconstrictors, "classic" antihistamines, "classic" mast cell stabilizers, new agents with multiple "antiallergic" activities, nonsteroidal antiinflammatory agents, and corticosteroids. Selected examples of these agents are noted in Table 11.2. Corticosteroids are not discussed here because, as a result of their well-known side effects, patients should use them only when prescribed by the ophthalmologist.

Several preparations contain a mixture of a vasoconstrictor combined with an antihistamine (Table 11.2). These drugs can be purchased over the counter. The antihistamine is most useful for itching but also reduces vasodilation. Vasoconstrictors only diminish vasodilation and have little effect on pruritus. The two most frequently employed decongestants are naphazoline and phenylephrine. The two most common antihistamines available in combination products are antazoline and pheniramine maleate.

Levocabastine (Livostin) is an antihistamine available only by prescription. Levocabastine was specifically designed for topical application. In animal studies, it is 1,500 times more potent than chlorpheniramine on a molar basis (24). It has a rapid onset of action (25), is effective in blocking intraocular allergen challenge (26), and appears to be as effective as other agents, including sodium cromoglycate (27) and terfenadine (28).

Emedastine (Emadine) is also a high-potency selective H_1 antagonist with a receptor-binding affinity even higher than levocabastine (29). It appears to have a rapid onset of action (within 10 minutes) and a duration of activity of 4 hours (29).

As a rule, vasoconstrictors and antihistamines are well tolerated. However, antihistamines may be sensitizing. In addition, each preparation contains several different vehicles that may produce transient irritation or sensitization (13). Just as vasoconstrictors in the nose can cause rhinitis medicamentosa, frequent use of vasoconstrictors in the eye results in conjunctivitis medicamentosa. As a rule, however, these drugs are effective and well tolerated (30).

Four mast cell stabilizers are available for therapy. They are cromolyn sodium, nedocromil sodium, lodoxamide, and pemirolast. All are efficacious and usually well tolerated (29,31–33). They are more effective when started before the onset of symptoms and used regularly four times a day (34), but they can relieve symptoms within 2 minutes after ocular allergen challenge (35). They are also useful in preventing symptoms caused by isolated allergen challenge such as occurs when visiting a home with a pet or mowing the lawn. In these instances, they should be administered immediately before exposure.

Ketorolac tromethamine (Acular) is the first nonsteroidal antiinflammatory drug to be used in this country for the therapy of allergic conjunctivitis. It is most effective in controlling itching but also ameliorates other symptoms (36). Its effect results from its ability to inhibit the formation of prostaglandins, which cause itching when applied to the conjunctiva (37).

Two agents for the treatment of allergic eye disorders have broad-based antiallergic or antiinflammatory effects in addition to their antihistamine activity. These are olopatadine (Patanol) and ketotifen (Zaditor). They prevent mast cell degranulation, reduce eosinophil activity, and downregulate the expression of adhesion molecules as well as inhibit the binding of histamine to the H_1 receptor (38–41).

Allergen immunotherapy can be helpful in treating allergic conjunctivitis. A study designed to assess the effect of immunotherapy in allergic rhinitis demonstrated improvement in ocular allergy symptoms as well (42). Immunotherapy can also exert an added beneficial effect to pharmacotherapy (43). Finally, immunotherapy has been demonstrated to reduce the sensitivity to ocular challenge with grass pollen (44).

Vernal Conjunctivitis

Clinical Presentation

Vernal conjunctivitis is a chronic, bilateral, catarrhal inflammation of the conjunctiva most commonly arising in children during the spring and summer. It can be perennial in severely affected patients. It is characterized by an intense itching. Burning and photophobia can occur.

The illness is usually seen during the preadolescent years and often resolves at puberty. Male patients are affected about three times more often than female patients when the onset precedes adolescence, but when there is a later onset, female patients predominate. In the later-onset variety, the symptoms are usually less severe. The incidence is increased in warmer climates. It is most commonly seen in the Middle East and along the Mediterranean Sea.

Vernal conjunctivitis presents in palpebral and limbal forms. In the palpebral variety, which is more common, the tarsal conjunctiva of the upper lid is deformed by thickened, gelatinous vegetations produced by marked papillary hypertrophy. This hypertrophy imparts a cobblestone appearance to the conjunctiva, which results from intense proliferation of collagen and ground substance along with a cellular infiltrate (45). The papillae are easily seen when the upper lid is everted. In severe cases, the lower palpebral conjunctiva may be similarly involved. In the limbal form, a similar gelatinous cobblestone appearance occurs at the corneal–scleral junction. Trantas' dots—small, white dots composed of eosinophils—are often present. Usually, there is a thick, stringy exudate full of eosinophils. This thick, ropey, white or yellow mucous discharge has highly elastic properties and produces a foreign-body sensation. It is pathognomonic for vernal conjunctivitis (45). It is usually easily distinguished from the globular mucus seen in seasonal allergic conjunctivitis or the crusting of infectious conjunctivitis. The patient may be particularly troubled by this discharge, which can string out for more than 2.5 cm (1 inch) when it is removed from the eye. Widespread punctate keratitis may be present. Severe cases can result in epithelial ulceration with scar formation.

Pathophysiology and Cause

The cause and pathophysiologic mechanisms of vernal conjunctivitis remain obscure. Several features of the disease, however, suggest that the atopic state is related to its pathogenesis. The seasonal occurrence, the presence of eosinophils, and the fact that most of the patients have other atopic disease (46) are circumstantial evidence supporting this hypothesis. In addition, several different immunologic and histologic findings are consistent with an allergic etiology. Patients with vernal conjunctivitis have elevated levels of total immunoglobulin E (IgE) (47), allergen-specific IgE (48), histamine (47), and tryptase (49) in the tear film. In addition, histologic study supports an immune origin. Patients with vernal conjunctivitis have markedly increased numbers of eosinophils, basophils, mast cells, and plasma cells in biopsy specimens taken from the conjunctiva (50). The mast cells are often totally degranulated (47). Elevated levels of major basic protein are found in biopsy specimens of the conjunctiva (51). Also, in keeping with the postulated role of IgE-mediated hypersensitivity is the pattern of cytokine secretion and T cells found in tears and on biopsy specimens. A T_H2 cytokine profile with increased levels of IL-4 and IL-5 has been found (16,52). Finally, ocular shields, designed to prevent pollen exposure, have been reported to be therapeutically effective (53,54).

A role for cell-mediated immunity has also been proposed and is supported by the findings of increased $CD4^+/CD29^+$ helper T cells in tears during acute phases of the illness (52). Also in keeping with this hypothesis is the improvement demonstrated during therapy with topical cyclosporine.

Fibroblasts appear to be operative in the pathogenesis as well. They may be activated by T-cell or mast cell products. When stimulated with histamine, fibroblasts from patients with vernal conjunctivitis produce excessive amounts of procollagen I and II (55). In addition, they appear to manufacture constitutively increased amounts of transforming growth factor-β (TGF-β, IL-1, IL-6, and tumor necrosis factor-α (TNF-α) *in vitro*. The increased levels of cytokines noted *in vitro* are accompanied by increased serum levels of IL-1 and TNF-α as well (56). This overexpression of mediators both locally and systemically probably accounts for the upregulation of adhesion molecules (57) on corneal epithelium noted in this disorder.

Also of interest is the hypothesis that complement, perhaps activated by IgG–allergen immune complexes, plays a role in producing vernal conjunctivitis. Pollen-specific IgG antibodies (58) and complement activation products (C3 des-Arg) occur in tears of patients with vernal conjunctivitis (59). The specific IgG antipollen found in the tear film may not be acting through the complement system, however, because much of it appears to be IgG4 (58), a non–complement-fixing subclass with putative reaginic activity. Also, patients with vernal conjunctivitis have decreased tear lactoferrin, an inhibitor of the complement system (60).

Diagnosis and Treatment

Vernal conjunctivitis must be distinguished from other conjunctival diseases that present with pruritus or follicular hypertrophy. These include acute allergic conjunctivitis, conjunctivitis and keratoconjunctivitis associated with atopic dermatitis, the giant papillary conjunctivitis associated with soft contact lenses and other foreign bodies, the follicular conjunctivitis of viral infections, and trachoma (rarely found in the United States).

In most instances, the distinction between acute allergic conjunctivitis and vernal conjunctivitis is not difficult. However, in the early phases of vernal conjunctivitis or in mild vernal conjunctivitis, giant papillae may be absent. In such instances, the distinction may be more difficult because both conditions occur in atopic individuals, and pruritus is a hallmark of each. However, in vernal conjunctivitis, the pruritus is more intense, the tear film contains a significantly greater concentration of histamine and greater amounts of eosinophils, and the conjunctival epithelium has more abundant mast cells (47). Also, the cornea is not involved in acute allergic conjunctivitis.

The conjunctivitis and keratoconjunctivitis associated with atopic dermatitis can be similar to vernal conjunctivitis. In atopic dermatitis, the conjunctivitis can produce hypertrophy and opacity of the tarsal conjunctiva (61,62). A form of keratoconjunctivitis with papillary hypertrophy and punctate keratitis can occur (63). Many of these patients have signs and symptoms typical of vernal conjunctivitis, including giant follicles and pruritus. In addition, vernal conjunctivitis and atopic dermatitis can occur together in the same patient. However, because the treatment of both conditions is similar, the distinction, except for its prognostic value, may not be essential.

The giant papillary conjunctivitis caused by wearing of soft contact lenses is similar to that of vernal conjunctivitis. Patients complain of itching, mucous discharge, and a decreasing tolerance to the lens. Symptoms usually begin 3 to 36 months after lenses are prescribed (64). The syndrome can occur with hard and soft lenses and can be seen with exposed sutures (64) and plastic prostheses (65). Thus, chronic trauma to the lid appears to be the common inciting agent. Several features distinguish this entity from vernal conjunctivitis. Lens-associated papillary conjunctivitis causes less intense itching and shows no seasonal variation. It resolves with discontinuation of lens use.

Viral infections can be distinguished from vernal conjunctivitis by their frequent association with systemic symptoms and the absence of pruritus. A slit-lamp examination can produce a definitive distinction between these two entities.

Patients with mild vernal conjunctivitis can be treated with cold compresses and topical vasoconstrictor-antihistamine preparations. Levocabastine has been shown to be effective in a double-blind, placebo-controlled trial of 46 patients over a period of 4 weeks (66). Oral antihistamines may be of modest help. Cromolyn sodium has been used effectively not only for milder but also for more recalcitrant, chronic forms of the condition (67–70). Cromolyn has been shown to decrease conjunctival injection, punctate keratitis, itching, limbal edema, and tearing when administered regularly. It may be more effective in patients who are atopic (69). In a multicenter, double-blind 28-day study, another mast cell stabilizer, lodoxamide, was found to be more effective than cromolyn sodium (71).

Aspirin (72,73) has been found to be helpful in a dose of 0.5 to 1.5 g daily. Ketorolac tromethamine has not been approved for use in vernal conjunctivitis, but based on the studies of aspirin, it might be an effective agent in this regard. Acetylcysteine 10% (Mucomyst) has been suggested as a means of counteracting viscous secretions. In severe cases, cyclosporine has been used (74).

None of the above medications is universally effective, however, and topical corticosteroids often are necessary. If topical corticosteroids are needed, the patient should be under the care of an ophthalmologist. A sustained-release, hydrocortisone epiocular depository has also been successfully employed (75). Fortunately, spontaneous remission usually occurs at puberty.

Eye Manifestation Associated with Atopic Dermatitis

Atopic dermatitis is associated with several manifestations of eye disease. These include lid dermatitis, blepharitis, conjunctivitis, keratoconjunctivitis, keratoconus, cataracts, and a predisposition to develop ocular infections, especially with herpes simplex and vaccinia viruses (76).

Atopic dermatitis patients with ocular complications can be distinguished from those without ocular disease in that they have higher levels of serum IgE and more frequently demonstrate IgE specific to rice and wheat. Those with associated cataract formation have the highest levels of IgE. Patients with ocular complications also have increased tear histamine and LTB-4 levels compared with atopic dermatitis subjects without ocular complications (77).

As with other allergic eye conditions, subjects with atopic keratoconjunctivitis have cells in ocular tissue that express a T_H2 cytokine profile with increased expression of messenger RNA for IL-4 and IL-5. Subjects with allergic keratoconjunctivitis, however, are different from those with vernal conjunctivitis in that they also expressed increased levels of interferon-γ and IL-2, indicating that in later stages of this disease, an element of delayed hypersensitivity is involved in the pathogenesis (16). Lid involvement can resemble contact dermatitis. The lids become thickened, edematous, and coarse; the pruritus may be intense.

Conjunctivitis may vary in intensity with the degree of skin involvement of the face (61). It resembles acute allergic conjunctivitis and to some extent resembles vernal conjunctivitis. It actually may be allergic conjunctivitis occurring with atopic dermatitis.

Atopic keratoconjunctivitis usually does not appear until the late teenage years. The peak incidence is between 30 and 50 years of age. Male patients are affected in greater numbers than female patients.

Atopic keratoconjunctivitis is bilateral. The major symptoms are itching, tearing, and burning. The eyelids may be red, thickened, and macerated. There is usually erythema of the lid margin and crusting around the eyelashes. The palpebral conjunctiva may show papillary hypertrophy. The lower lid is usually more severely afflicted and more often involved. Punctate keratitis can occur and the bulbar conjunctiva is chemotic.

Atopic keratoconjunctivitis must be differentiated from blepharitis and vernal conjunctivitis. This may be difficult in the case of blepharitis. Indeed, staphylococcal blepharitis often complicates this disorder. Vernal conjunctivitis is usually distinguished from atopic keratoconjunctivitis by the fact that it most often involves the upper rather than lower lids and is more seasonal. It also occurs in a younger age group. The papillae in vernal conjunctivitis are also larger. Cromolyn sodium is helpful in treating atopic keratoconjunctivitis (78). Topical corticosteroids often are needed, however. Their use should be under the direction of the ophthalmologist.

Keratoconus occurs less frequently than conjunctival involvement. The cause of the association between atopic dermatitis and keratoconus is unknown, but there appears to be no human leukocyte antigen (HLA) haplotype that distinguishes atopic dermatitis patients with keratoconjunctivitis from patients without it or from controls (62).

The incidence rate of cataract formation in atopic dermatitis has been reported to range from 0.4% to 25% (62). These cataracts may be anterior or posterior in location, as opposed to those caused by administering corticosteroids, which are usually posterior. They have been observed in both children and adults. They may be unilateral or bilateral. Their presence cannot be correlated with the age of onset of the disease, its severity, or its duration (79). The pathophysiology involved in the formation of cataracts is unknown, but patients with atopic cataracts have higher serum IgE levels (80) and have elevated levels of major basic protein in aqueous fluid and the anterior capsule, which is not found in senile cataracts (80).

Eyelid disorders may be the most common ocular complaint in patients with atopic dermatitis (81). Dermatitis of the lid produces itching with lid inversion. The skin becomes scaly, and the skin of the eyes around the lid may become more wrinkled. The skin is extremely dry. The lesion is pruritic, and the disorder can be confused with contact dermatitis of the lid.

Herpes keratitis is more common in patients with atopic dermatitis. This condition may be recurrent, and recalcitrant epithelial defects can occur (82).

Blepharoconjunctivitis (Marginal Blepharitis)

Blepharoconjunctivitis (marginal blepharitis) refers to any condition in which inflammation of the lid margin is a prominent feature of the disease. Conjunctivitis usually occurs in conjunction with the blepharitis. Three illnesses are commonly considered under the generic heading of blepharoconjunctivitis: staphylococcal blepharoconjunctivitis, seborrheic blepharoconjunctivitis, and rosacea. They often occur together.

Staphylococcal Blepharoconjunctivitis

The staphylococcal organism is probably the most common cause of conjunctivitis and blepharoconjunctivitis. The acute bacterial conjunctivitis is characterized by irritation, redness, and mucopurulent discharge with matting of the eyelids. Frequently, the conjunctivitis is present in a person with low-grade inflammation of the eyelid margins.

In the chronic form, symptoms of staphylococcal blepharoconjunctivitis include erythema of the lid margins, matting of the eyelids on awakening, and discomfort, which is usually worse in the morning. Examination frequently shows yellow crusting of the margin of the eyelids, with collarette formation at the base of the cilia, and disorganized or missing cilia. If the exudates are removed, ulceration of the lid margin may be visible. Fluorescein staining of the cornea may show small areas of dye uptake in the inferior portion. It is believed that exotoxin elaborated by *Staphylococcus* organisms is responsible for the symptoms and signs. Because of the chronicity of the disease and the subtle findings, the entity of chronic blepharoconjunctivitis of staphylococcal origin can be confused with contact dermatitis of the eyelids and contact dermatoconjunctivitis. The absence of pruritus is the most important feature distinguishing staphylococcal from contact dermatoconjunctivitis.

Seborrheic Dermatitis of the Lids

Staphylococcal blepharitis can also be confused with seborrheic blepharitis. Seborrheic blepharitis occurs as part of seborrheic dermatitis. It is associated with oily skin, seborrhea of the brows, and usually scalp involvement. The scales, which occur at the base of the cilia, tend to be greasy, and if these are removed, no ulceration is seen. There is no pruritus.

Rosacea

The blepharoconjunctivitis of rosacea often occurs in combination with seborrhea. Patients with blepharoconjunctivitis exhibit the classic hyperemia with telangiectasia over the malar area. Symptoms are often worsened by the ingestion of spicy foods.

Diagnosis and Treatment of Blepharoconjunctivitis

In all three forms of blepharoconjunctivitis, the cardinal symptoms are burning, redness, and irritation. True pruritus is usually absent or minimal. The inflammation of the lid margin is prominent. The discharge is usually mucopurulent, and matting in the early morning may be an annoying feature. In the seborrheic and rosacea forms, cutaneous involvement elsewhere is present.

All three forms are usually chronic and are often difficult to manage. In staphylococcal blepharoconjunctivitis, lid scrubs using a cotton-tipped applicator soaked with baby shampoo and followed by the application of a steroid ointment may be helpful. Control of other areas of seborrhea is necessary. Tetracycline can be beneficial in the therapy of rosacea. Ophthalmologic and dermatologic consultation may be needed.

Viral Conjunctivitis

Viral conjunctivitis is usually of abrupt onset, frequently beginning unilaterally and involving the second eye within a few days. Conjunctival injection, slight chemosis, watery discharge, and enlargement of a preauricular lymph node help to distinguish viral infection from other entities. Clinically, lymphoid follicles appear on the conjunctiva as elevated avascular areas, which are usually grayish. These correspond to the histologic picture of lymphoid germinal centers. Viral conjunctivitis is usually of adenoviral origin and is frequently associated with a pharyngitis and low-grade fever in pharyngoconjunctival fever.

Epidemic keratoconjunctivitis presents as an acute follicular conjunctivitis, with a watery discharge and preauricular adenopathy. This conjunctivitis usually runs a 7- to 14-day course and is frequently accompanied by small corneal opacities. Epidemic keratoconjunctivitis can be differentiated from allergic conjunctivitis by the absence of pruritus, the presence of a mononuclear cellular response, and a follicular conjunctival response.

The treatment of viral conjunctivitis is usually supportive, although prophylactic antibiotics are frequently used. If significant corneal opacities are present, the application of topical steroid preparations has been suggested.

Chlamydial (Inclusion) Conjunctivitis

In adults, inclusion conjunctivitis presents as an acute conjunctivitis with prominent conjunctival follicles and a mucopurulent discharge. There is usually no preceding upper respiratory infection or fever. This process occurs in adults who may harbor the chlamydial agent in the genital tract, but with no symptoms referable to this system.

A nonspecific urethritis in men and a chronic vaginal discharge in women are common. The presence of a mucopurulent discharge and follicular conjunctivitis, which lasts more than 2 weeks, certainly suggests inclusion conjunctivitis. A Giemsa stain of a conjunctival scraping specimen may reveal intracytoplasmic inclusion bodies and helps to confirm the diagnosis. The treatment of choice is systemic tetracycline for 10 days.

Keratoconjunctivitis Sicca

Keratoconjunctivitis sicca is a condition characterized by a diminished tear production. This is predominately a disorder of menopausal or postmenopausal women and may present in patients with connective tissue disease, particularly rheumatoid arthritis. Although keratoconjunctivitis sicca may present as an isolated condition affecting the eyes only, it may also be associated with xerostomia or Sjögren syndrome.

Symptoms may begin insidiously and are frequently confused with a mild infectious or allergic process. Mild conjunctival injection, irritation, photophobia, and mucoid discharge are present. Corneal epithelial damage can be demonstrated by fluorescein or rose Bengal staining, and hypolacrimation can be confirmed by inadequate wetting of the Schirmer test strip. Frequent application of artificial tears usually provides relief.

Herpes Simplex Keratitis

A primary herpetic infection occurs subclinically in many patients. However, acute primary keratoconjunctivitis may occur with or without skin involvement. The recurrent form of the disease is seen most commonly. Patients usually complain of tearing, ocular irritation, blurred vision, and occasionally photophobia. Fluorescein staining of the typical linear branching ulcer (dendrite) of the cornea confirms the diagnosis. Herpetic keratitis is treated with antiviral compounds or by débridement. After the infectious keratitis has healed, the patient may return with a geographic erosion of the cornea, which is known as *metaherpetic (trophic) keratitis*. In this stage, the virus is not replicating, and antiviral therapy is usually not indicated. If the inflammation involves the deep corneal stroma, a disciform keratitis may result and may run a rather protracted course, leaving a corneal scar. The exact cause of disciform keratitis is unknown, but it is thought that immune mechanisms play an important role in its production (83,84). It is important to distinguish herpetic keratitis from allergic conjunctivitis. The absence of pruritus and the presence of photophobia, blurred vision, and a corneal staining area should alert the clinician to the presence of herpetic infection. Using corticosteroids in herpetic disease only spreads the ulceration and prolongs the infectious phase of the disease process.

Giant Papillary Conjunctivitis

Giant papillary conjunctivitis, which is characterized by the formation of large papillae (larger than 0.33 mm in diameter) on the upper tarsal conjunctiva, has been associated with the wearing of contact lenses, prostheses, and sutures (85,86). Although it is most commonly caused by soft contact lenses (87), it can also occur with gas-permeable and rigid lenses. Patients experience pruritus, excess mucus production, and discomfort when wearing their lenses. There is decreased lens tolerance, blurred vision, and excessive lens movement (frequently with lens displacement). Burning and tearing are also noted.

The patient develops papillae on the upper tarsal conjunctiva. These range from 0.3 mm to greater than 1 mm in diameter. The area involved correlates with the type of contact lens worn by the patient (45).

The mechanism of production of giant papillary conjunctivitis is unknown. One hypothesis is that the reaction is caused by an immunologic response to deposits on the lens surface. Deposits consist not only of exogenous airborne antigens but also of products in the tear film such as lysozyme, IgA, lactoferrin, and IgG (88,89). However, the amount of deposits does not clearly correlate with the presence of giant papillary conjunctivitis, and all lenses develop deposits within 8 hours of wear (90). More than two thirds of soft lens wearers develop deposits within 1 year of wear. Evidence suggesting an immune mechanism in the production of giant papillary conjunctivitis is based on several observations. The condition is more common in atopic subjects. Patients with giant papillary conjunctivitis have elevated, locally produced tear IgE (91). Eosinophils, basophils, and mast cells are found in giant papillary conjunctivitis in greater amounts than in acute allergic conjunctivitis (45). There are elevated levels of major basic protein in conjunctival tissues of patients with giant papillary conjunctivitis (51) and elevated levels of LTC-4 (92), histamine (93), and tryptase in their tears (45). Further evidence for an IgE-mediated mechanism is the observation that ocular tissues from patients with giant papillary conjunctivitis exhibit increased messenger RNA for IL-4 and IL-5 (17) and have increased levels of major basic protein and eosinophilic cationic protein in tears (90).

Non–IgE-mediated immune mechanisms have also been incriminated in the production of this disorder. IgG levels are elevated, but the IgG is bloodborne rather than locally produced (91). There is also evidence for complement activation, and there is decreased lactoferrin in the tears of patients with giant papillary conjunctivitis (59,60). Neutrophil chemotactic factor is present in tear fluids in amounts exceeding levels found in nonaffected soft contact lens wearers (94).

Treatment of giant papillary conjunctivitis is usually carried out by the ophthalmologist. Early recognition is important because discontinuation of lens wear early in the stage of the disease and prescription of appropriate lens type and edge design can prevent recurrence. It is also important to adhere to a strict regimen for lens cleaning and to use preservative-free saline. Enzymatic cleaning with papain preparations is useful to reduce the coating of the lenses by antigens. Disposable lenses may also be beneficial. Both cromolyn sodium and nedocromil sodium have been found to be helpful (95).

Floppy Eye Syndrome

Floppy eye syndrome is a condition characterized by lax upper lids and a papillary conjunctivitis resembling giant papillary conjunctivitis. Men older than 30 years of age constitute the majority of patients. The condition is thought to result from chronic traction on the lax lid produced by the pillow at sleep. It may be unilateral or bilateral (96).

Approach to the Patient with an Inflamed Eye

The physician seeing a patient with acute or chronic conjunctivitis should first exclude diseases (not discussed in this chapter) that may be acutely threatening to the patient's vision. These include conditions such as acute keratitis, uveitis, acute angle-closure glaucoma, and endophthalmitis. The two most important symptoms pointing to a threatening condition are a loss in visual acuity and pain. These are signs that the patient could have an elevated intraocular pressure, keratitis, endophthalmitis, or uveitis. On physical examination, the presence of circumcorneal hyperemia (dilation of the vessels adjacent to the corneal edge limbus) is present in four threatening conditions, including keratitis, uveitis, acute angle-closure glaucoma, and endophthalmitis. This contrasts with the pattern of vasodilation seen in acute allergic conjunctivitis, which produces erythema that is more pronounced in the periphery and decreases as it approaches the cornea.

If the physician believes that the patient does not have a threatening eye disease, the next step is to differentiate between allergic and nonallergic diseases of the eye (Table 11.3). The differential diagnosis between allergic and nonallergic diseases of the eye can usually be made by focusing on a few key features. Five cardinal questions should be asked in this regard:

1. Does the eye itch? This is the most important distinguishing feature between allergic and nonallergic eye disorders. All allergic conditions are pruritic. Nonallergic conditions usually do not itch. The physician must be certain that the patient understands what is meant by itching because burning, scratching, sandy eyes are often described as "itchy" by the patient.

TABLE 11.3. *Differential features to be considered in diagnosing allergic eye disease*

Clinical feature	Seasonal	Itching	Scratchy (sandy) irritation	Skin of lids and/or margin involved	Bilateral	Tearing	Discharge	Remarks
Acute allergic conjunctivitis	Yes	Prominent	Not usual	No	Yes	Increased	Mucoid	Itching is cardinal feature; rhinitis is present
Vernal conjunctivitis	Yes	Prominent	Not usual	No	Yes	Slightly increased	Stringy and tenacious	Seasonal—spring and summer, more common in children
Conjunctivitis sicca	No	No	Prominent	No	Yes	Markedly decreased	Slight mucoid	Dry mouth, associated with autoimmune disease, especially Sjögren's syndrome
Acute viral conjunctivitis	Variable, usually is not	No	Variable	No	Variable	Normal to slightly increased	Watery	Follicular conjunctivitis, prominent injection, may have preauricular node enlargement
Acute bacterial conjunctivitis	No	No	Variable	Matting	Variable	Normal to increased	Mucopurulent	Exudate most prominent feature
Dermatoconjunctivitis	No	Yes	No	Variable	Usually	Normal to increased	Variable	Itching usually is a helpful diagnostic feature
Chronic staphylococcal blepharoconjunctivitis	No	No	No	Yes	Usually	Normal	Early morning matting	Crusting of lids, loss of cilia
Seborrheic dermatitis	No	No	No	Yes	Yes	Normal	None	Signs of seborrheic dermatitis elsewhere

2. What type of discharge, if any, is present? A purulent discharge with early morning matting is not a feature of allergic disease and points toward infection.
3. Is the lid involved? Lid involvement indicates the presence of atopic dermatitis, contact dermatitis, or occasionally seborrhea or rosacea. Often, the patient complains of "eye irritation," which may mean the lid, conjunctiva, or both. The physician should be careful to ascertain which area of the eye is involved.
4. Are other allergic manifestations present? Examples include atopic dermatitis, asthma, and rhinitis.
5. Are there other associated nonallergic conditions? Nonallergic conditions include dandruff and rosacea.

THE EAR: OTIC MANIFESTATIONS OF ALLERGY

The most common otologic problem related to allergy is otitis media with effusion (OME). The potential role of allergic disease in the pathogenesis of OME is explored in the following discussion.

Otitis media is a general term defined as any inflammation of the middle ear with or without symptoms and usually associated with an effusion. It is one of the most common medical conditions seen in children by primary care physicians (97). It is estimated that total costs for otitis media in the United States range from $3 to $4 billion dollars and $600 million in Canada (98). The classification of otitis media can be confusing. The First International Symposium on Recent Advances in Middle Ear Effusions (99) includes the following types of otitis media: (a) acute purulent otitis media, (b) serous otitis media, and (c) mucoid or secretory otitis media. Chronic otitis media is a condition displaying a pronounced, retracted tympanic membrane with pathologic changes in the middle ear, such as cholesteatoma or granulation tissue. The acute phase of otitis media occurs during the first 3 weeks of the illness, the subacute phase between 4 and 8 weeks, and the chronic phase begins after 8 weeks. For this review, *acute otitis media* (AOM) applies to the classic ear infection, which is rapid in onset and associated with a red, bulging, and painful tympanic membrane. Fever and irritability usually accompany AOM. The presence of middle ear fluid without signs or symptoms of infection is OME. In many of these patients, hearing loss accompanies the condition. Other commonly used names for OME are serous otitis media and secretory otitis media.

In the United States, about 10 million children are treated with OME annually (100), and this condition results in the one of the most commonly performed surgeries in the United States: tympanostomy tube placement (101). OME is of major importance in children because the effusion can lead to a mild to moderate conductive hearing loss of 20 dB or more (102). It has been theorized that chronic conductive hearing loss in the child may lead to poor language development and learning disorders. There are many epidemiologic factors in the development of recurrent and chronic OME in children, with age at first episode being a major risk factor (103) (Table 11.4). In a study of 2,565 children by Teele and co-workers (104), half of all infants have had one or more episodes of OME in the first year of life, with 75% having at least one episode of OME by the age of 6 years. One third had three or more episodes of OME by the age of 3 years. The study further showed that after the first episode, 40% of the children had middle ear effusion that persisted for 4 weeks, and 10% had effusions that were still present after 3 months. Zeisel and

TABLE 11.4. *Risk factors for chronic and recurrent otitis media with effusion (OME)*

1. Age—children with OME in the first year of life have increased incidence of recurrence
2. Males > females
3. Bottle-fed infants
4. Passive smoking exposure
5. Allergy
6. Lower socioeconomic status
7. Race—Native Americans and Eskimos > whites > African Americans
8. Day care centers
9. Season—winter > Summer
10. Genetic predisposition—if siblings have OME, higher risk
11. Down syndrome
12. Primary immunodeficiency disorders
13. Primary and secondary ciliary dysfunction
14. Craniofacial abnormalities

colleagues reported that persistent bilateral OME occurred commonly between 6 and 18 months of age in African American infants who enter group child care during the first year of life (105). The proportion of child examinations revealing bilateral OME ranged from 76% between 6 and 12 months of age to 30% between 21 and 24 months of age. In this study, spontaneous resolution of bilateral effusion by 2 years of age was typical. In a British study of schoolchildren aged 5 to 8 years, Williamson reported that OME was more common in 5-year-old patients with an annual prevalence of 17%, compared with 6% in 8-year-olds; it is also more common in the winter months (106). A study from Malaysia involving 1,097 preschool-aged children aged between 5 and 6 years reported that the overall prevalence rate of OME was 13.8% (107).

Other major factors in development of OME include male gender, exposure to parental cigarette smoke (108,109), race, and allergy. Numerous studies have documented that day care center attendance increases the incidence of OME (110–113). Children who are breast-fed tend to have a lower rate of OME than bottle-fed infants (114,115). Race appears to increase the risk for OME, with the highest incidence in Native Americans and Eskimos. Diseases of the antibody-mediated immune system, primary ciliary dyskinesia, Down syndrome, and craniofacial abnormalities, especially cleft palate, can all contribute to chronic OME. In evaluation of the patient with recurrent or chronic OME, each of these conditions needs to be investigated.

Pathogenesis of Otitis Media with Effusion

It appears that multiple factors influence the pathogenesis of OME. Most studies link OME with eustachian tube dysfunction, viral and bacterial infections, abnormalities of mucociliary clearance, and allergy.

Eustachian Tube Anatomy and Physiology

The nasopharynx and middle ear are connected by the eustachian tube. The production of middle ear effusions appears to be related to functional or anatomic abnormalities of this tube. Under normal conditions, the eustachian tube has three physiologic functions: (a) ventilation of the middle ear to equilibrate pressure and replenish oxygen; (b) protection of the middle ear from nasopharyngeal sound pressure and secretions; and (c) clearance of secretions produced in the middle ear into the nasopharynx.

The eustachian tube of the infant and the young child differs markedly from that of the adult. These anatomic differences predispose infants and young children to middle ear disease. In infancy, the tube is wide, short, and more horizontal in orientation. As growth occurs, the tube narrows, elongates, and develops a more oblique course (Fig. 11.2). Usually after the age of 7 years, these physical changes lessen the frequency of middle ear effusion (116). In the normal state, the middle ear is free of any significant amount of fluid and is filled with air. Air is maintained in the middle ear by the action of the Eustachian tube. This tube is closed at the pharyngeal end except during swallowing, when the tensor veli palatini muscle contracts and opens the tube by lifting its posterior lip (Fig. 11.3A). When the eustachian tube is opened, air passes from the nasopharynx into the middle ear, and this ventilation system equalizes air pressure on both sides of the tympanic membrane (Fig. 11.3B).

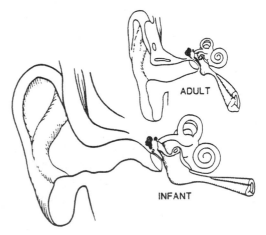

FIG. 11.2. Illustration showing difference in angles of eustachian tubes in infants and adults.

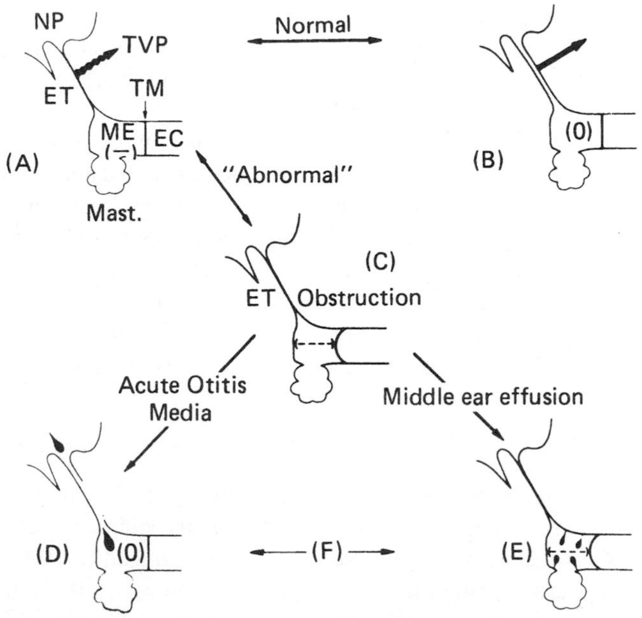

FIG. 11.3. Proposed pathogenic mechanisms of middle ear effusion. NP, nasopharynx; ET, eustachian tube; TVP, tensor veli palatini muscle; ME, middle ear; Mast., mastoid; TM, tympanic membrane; EC, external canal. (From Bluestone CD. Eustachian tube function and allergy in otitis media. *Pediatrics* 1978;61:753, with permission.)

When the eustachian tube is blocked by either functional or anatomic defects, air cannot enter the middle ear, and the remaining air is absorbed. This results in the formation of negative pressure within the middle ear and subsequent retraction of the tympanic membrane (Fig. 11.3C). High negative pressure associated with ventilation may result in aspiration of nasopharyngeal secretions into the middle ear, producing acute otitis media with effusion (Fig. 11.3D). Prolonged negative pressure causes fluid transudation from the middle ear mucosal blood vessels (Fig. 11.3E). With chronic OME, there is infiltration of lymphocytes and macrophages, along with production of different inflammatory mediators. Also, there is an increased density of goblet cells in the epithelium of the eustachian tube. It is thought that many children with middle ear effusions, without a demonstrable cause of eustachian tube obstruction, have a growth-related inadequate action of the tensor veli palatini muscle. Another possibility is functional obstruction

from persistent collapse of the tube owing to increased tubal compliance.

Nasal obstruction, either from adenoid hypertrophy or from infectious or allergic inflammation, may be involved in the pathogenesis of middle ear effusion by the Toynbee phenomenon (117). Studies have reported that, when the nose is obstructed, there is an increased positive nasopharyngeal pressure followed by a negative nasopharyngeal pressure upon swallowing. The increased positive nasopharyngeal pressure may predispose to insufflation of secretions into the middle ear, and the secondary negative pressure in the nasopharynx may further be a factor in the inadequate opening of the eustachian tube, thereby causing obstruction.

Infection

Respiratory bacterial and viral infections are significant contributors to the pathogenesis of otitis media. Bacteria have been cultured in about 70%

of middle ear effusions during tympanocentesis for otitis media in children (118). The three most common bacterial isolates in AOM and OME in are *Streptococcus pneumoniae*, nontypable *Haemophilus influenzae* (NTHI), and *Moraxella catarrhalis* (119). *Streptococcus pyogenes* and anaerobic cocci are isolated in less than 5% of the patients with AOM. Recently, *Alloiococcus otitis* has been found to be a significant bacterial pathogen in relationship with otitis media with effusion (120). The predominant anaerobes are gram-positive cocci, pigmented *Prevotella* and *Porphyromonas* species, *Bacterioides* species, and *Fusobacterium* species. The predominant organisms isolated from chronic otitis media are *Staphylococcus aureus*, *Pseudomonas aeruginosa*, and anaerobic bacteria. In neonates, group B streptococci and gram-negative organisms are common bacterial pathogens causing otitis media (121). Most patients with chronic OME have sterile middle ear effusions.

Post and associates used a polymerase chain reaction (PCR) to detect bacterial DNA in middle ear effusions in children undergoing myringotomy and tube placement who had failed multiple courses of antibiotics (122). Of the 97 specimens, 75 (77.3%) were PCR positive for one or more of the following bacteria: *Streptococcus pneumoniae*, NTHI, and *Moraxella catarrhalis*. This suggests that active bacterial infection may be occurring in many children with chronic OME.

Viral agents are not commonly found in middle ear effusions but are probably important in the pathogenesis of otitis media (123). Most studies demonstrate viral isolates in less than 5% of the aspirates from the middle ear, with the most common being respiratory syncytial virus (RSV) (124). Even though viruses are rarely cultured from middle ear aspirates, immunoassays have found viral antigens in about 10% to 20% of the samples. Ciliary dysfunction secondary to viral infections in the upper respiratory tract can predispose to OME. Viral infections have been shown to increase bacterial adhesion in the upper respiratory tract (125). This may allow for colonization of the upper respiratory tract with bacteria and increase the risk for otitis media. Influenza A infection has been demonstrated to contribute

to the pathogenesis of experimental pneumococcal AOM (126). Another possible mechanism for viral infections in the pathogenesis of otitis media is the production of viral-specific IgE. Welliver reported that most of the 42 RSV-infected infants demonstrated anti-RSV IgE bound to exfoliated nasopharyngeal epithelial cells in the acute phase of the infection (127). With RSV being the most common viral agent in middle ear effusion, IgE-mediated reactions triggered by this virus may be a contributory factor of the development of OME in many patients.

Mucociliary Dysfunction

Mucociliary dysfunction from either a genetic defect or an acquired infectious or environmental condition can lead to OME. Investigations suggest that the mucociliary transfer system is an important defense mechanism in clearing foreign particles from the middle ear and the eustachian tube (128). Goblet and secretory cells provide a mucous blanket to aid ciliated cells in transporting foreign particles toward the nasopharynx for phagocytosis by macrophages, or to the lymphatics and capillaries for clearance. Respiratory viral infections are associated with transient abnormalities in the structure and function of cilia (129). Primary ciliary dyskinesia, an autosomal recessive syndrome, has been linked to more than 20 different structural defects in cilia, which lead to ciliary dysfunction (130). Both of these conditions can lead to inefficient ciliary transport, which results in mucostatics and can contribute to eustachian tube obstruction and the development of middle ear effusion.

Allergy and Immunology

There is considerable debate about whether allergic disorders are a factor in the pathogenesis of OME. Many investigators believe that allergic disorders do play a prominent role, either as a cause or contributory factor; whereas others state that there is no convincing evidence that allergy leads to otitis media (131). Allergy has been implicated as a causative factor in otitis media with effusion by (a) double-blind placebo-control nasal challenge studies with histamine and allergens; (b) studies on allergic children; and (c) studies on randomly selected children with OME referred to specialty clinics (132,133). Kraemer compared risk factors of OME among children with tympanostomy tubes compared with controls matched for age and reported atopy as a risk factor (134). In a series of 488 new patients referred to a pediatric allergy clinic, 49% had documented middle ear dysfunction (135). In a prospective study, Bierman and Furukawa have demonstrated that allergic children have a high incidence of OME with conductive hearing loss (136). Half of their patients developed chronic effusion or acute otitis media in a 6-month follow-up. Japanese investigators evaluated 605 children with allergic rhinitis and found 21% with OME. They also determined that 50% of 259 children with diagnosed OME had allergic rhinitis (137). Bernstein and Reisman reviewed the clinical course of 200 randomly selected children with OME who had at least one tympanostomy with tube insertion (138). Twenty-three percent were considered allergic by history, physical examination, and allergy skin testing. Other studies have failed to demonstrate atopy as a risk factor for otitis media (139,140).

The evidence that middle ear effusions are produced as a direct consequence of the mucosa of the middle ear or eustachian tube being an allergic shock organ is conflicting. Animal experiments suggest that the middle ear can serve as a shock organ. Miglets and co-workers sensitized squirrel monkeys with human serum containing ragweed antibodies (141). Forty-eight hours later, sensitized animals and control animals were injected with Evans blue dye. Their eustachian tube orifices then were infiltrated with liquid ragweed antigen. Only the sensitized animals developed dark blue stains at the injected area. This was postulated to occur secondary to an increase in capillary permeability owing to an antigen–antibody interaction. Twelve of the 15 sensitized animals developed a middle ear effusion. Histologically, there was an early polymorphonuclear response followed by a plasma cell infiltration. The authors concluded that the middle ear mucosa of the squirrel monkey has the capacity to act as a shock organ. Labadie and associates demonstrated that allergen presentation to the middle ear of sensitized Brown-Norway rats causes functional disruption of the eustachian tube predisposing to the development of OME (142). In contrast, Yamashita and colleagues challenged ovalbumin-sensitized guinea pigs through the nose (143). In this study, there was an absence of histopathologic changes in the middle ear space when only the nose was challenged. This study fails to support the theory that immediate hypersensitivity is commonly associated with middle ear effusion.

In human studies, Friedman and co-workers evaluated eight patients, aged 18 to 29 years, with seasonal rhinitis but no middle ear disease (144). Patients were blindly challenged with the pollen to which the patient was sensitive or to a control. Nasal function was determined by nasal rhinomanometry and eustachian tube function by the nine-step-deflation tympanometric test. The results from this and other studies (4,145) showed that eustachian tube dysfunction can be induced by antigen and histamine challenge (146), although no middle ear effusions occurred. Osur evaluated 15 children with ragweed allergy and measured eustachian tube dysfunction before, during, and after a ragweed season (145). There was a significant increase in eustachian tube dysfunction during the pollen season, but it did not lead to OME. It appears that other variables need to be present for effusion to develop.

Many studies of OME have involved immunoglobulin analysis of effusions (147–149). The most prominent immunoglobulin found in effusions is secretory IgA, although IgG and IgE are found to be elevated in some patients. In most of these investigations, patients failed to demonstrate an elevated effusion IgE level compared with the serum IgE level (150). Although allergen-specific IgE can be found in effusions, the specificity is usually the same as that of serum. A definitive interpretation of these data is impossible, but it appears as if they, on the whole, fail to support the concept of the middle ear as a shock organ in most patients. There may be exceptions to this because IgE antibodies against ragweed (151), *Alternaria* species (55), and mite (152) have been reported in effusions but not in sera, in isolated instances. Khan and co-workers compared the IgE, IgM, and

IgA levels of the serum and tympanic fluid in 16 pediatric patients with OME and in 32 normal children (153). Seven of 10 patients with OME had elevated levels of specific IgE to common inhalants, as compared with only 4 of 32 control patients. The elevated specific IgE found in this study may be an "innocent bystander," but it does provide some support for the importance of the allergic diathesis in OME.

Recent work by Hurst and co-workers has provided the most conclusive evidence of the role of allergy in OME. These researchers evaluated 89 patients for allergy who required the placement of tympanostomy tubes because of persistent effusion. Radioallergosorbent test (RAST), serum IgE levels, and skin tests were performed. Atopy was present in 97% of the patients with OME by skin testing. Significant levels of eosinophil cationic protein and eosinophils were found in the effusions, suggesting allergic inflammation in the middle ear (154). These researchers also determined that IgE in middle ear effusion is not a transudate but more likely reflects an active localized process in atopic patients (155) and that tryptase, a reflection of mast cell activity, is found in most ears of patients with chronic effusion who were atopic (156). These findings support the hypothesis that middle ear mucosa is capable of an allergic response and that the inflammation within the middle ear of most OME patients is allergic in nature.

Much speculation on the role of allergy in the development of OME centers on the possibility of nasal obstruction due to allergic rhinitis causing the Toynbee phenomenon, as previously described. This may predispose to insufflation of secretions into the middle ear (4,50). Georgitis and associates failed to show that allergen and histamine-induced challenge leads to total nasal obstruction by the use of an anterior rhinomanometry (157). Bernstein and colleagues (158) failed to demonstrate eustachian tube dysfunction by the nine-step eustachian tube test in 24 adults who had the test performed with nasal packing because of septoplasty for deviated septum. These studies leave in doubt that nasal obstruction from allergic rhinitis increases the likelihood of OME. Allergy appears to be more often a contributory factor in the development of middle ear effusions. One possible mechanism is the release of chemical mediators from mast cells and basophils in allergic rhinitis that could lead to eustachian tube inflammation and obstruction. It is clear that, as the tube changes and improved muscle action of the tensor veli palatini develops in older children, the incidence of middle ear effusion dramatically decreases. The facts that the incidence of middle ear effusion declines dramatically with age and that the incidence of allergic rhinitis rises with age suggest that age-related factors may be more important than allergic factors in the development of middle ear effusion.

Another controversy in the pathogenesis of OME is the possible role of food allergy (159). Nsouli studied 104 children to assess the role food allergy might play in recurrent OME (160). These children had no history of food sensitivity and were assessed by prick skin tests, RAST, and open food challenges. Physical examination, tympanometry, and audiometry were used to assess middle ear effusions. Seventy-eight percent of the children had positive food skin tests and went through a 16-week period of elimination of the offending food followed by open challenge. Middle ear effusion resolved in 86% of the children when the offending food was eliminated from the diet. On open food challenge, 94% of children redeveloped OME. This study has been criticized because it was not controlled or blinded by the researchers (161). The study failed to include a group of children with food allergy and OME who did not participate in an elimination diet to determine the number of children who would have had spontaneous resolution of their effusion.

Bernstein measured IgG and IgE antibodies to food substances by enzyme-linked immunosorbent assay (ELISA) in the serum and middle ear of otitis-prone children younger than 2 years of age and compared them with a age-related control group. There were significantly higher levels of IgG antibodies to milk, wheat, and egg white in the serum and middle ear of the otitis prone children, but no difference in IgE levels (162). Immune complexes have been demonstrated in middle ear fluid by using anti-C3 solid-phase ELISA (163). Mravec and co-workers produced an acute local inflammatory response by injecting immune complexes from rabbit and goat antirabbit sera into the bullae of chinchillas (164). Bernstein and co-workers demonstrated positive immune complexes in only 2 of 41 samples of middle ear effusion using three assays: the Raji cell radioimmunoassay, direct immunofluorescence, and inhibition of anti-antibody (165). In studies with chinchillas, Ueyama found that formation of immune complexes in the tympanic cavity plays an important role in the occurrence of persistent middle ear effusion after pneumococcal otitis media (166). The literature is conflicting on whether immune complexes are fundamental in the development in middle ear effusion. There is no convincing body of evidence to invoke clearly the role of IgE hypersensitivity and IgG immune complexes to foods in the etiology of OME.

Acute and chronic suppurative otitis media are commonly part of a primary or secondary immunodeficiency syndrome. The middle ear is usually one of many locations for infection in immunodeficient patients. Of the primary immunodeficiency conditions, otitis media is more common in the humoral or B-cell disorders, such as X-linked hypogammaglobulinemia, common variable immunodeficiency, and selective IgA deficiency. A patient's incapacity to produce antibodies against pneumococcal polysaccharide antigens and a related IgG2 subclass deficiency has been associated with the development of recurrent otitis media in children (167).

Diagnosis

Acute otitis media usually presents with fever, otalgia, vomiting, diarrhea, and irritability. In young children, pulling at the ear may be the only manifestation of otalgia. Otorrhea, discharge from the middle ear, may occur if spontaneous perforation of the tympanic membrane occurs. It is not uncommon for AOM to be preceded by an upper respiratory infection. The pneumatic otoscope is an important tool for making accurate diagnosis of AOM. Classically, the tympanic

membrane is erythemic and bulging without a light reflex or the ossicular landmarks visualized. Pneumatic testing fails to elicit any movement of the tympanic membrane on applying positive and negative pressure.

Most children with OME do not have symptoms. Others may complain of stopped-up or popping ears or a feeling of fullness in the ear. Older children may even note a hearing loss. Their teachers and parents detect the condition in many younger children because they are noted to be inattentive, loud talkers, and slow learners. Other children may be discovered with OME in screening tests done for hearing at school. When middle ear effusions become chronic, there may be significant diminution of language development and auditory learning, with resultant poor academic achievement. On pneumatic otoscopic examination of patients with OME, the tympanic membrane may appear entirely normal. At other times, air-fluid levels and bubbles may be apparent. There is often retraction of the tympanic membrane, and the malleus may have a chalky appearance. As the disease progresses, the tympanic membrane takes on an opaque amber or bluish gray color. Alteration of the light reflex is commonly present. Mild retraction of the tympanic membrane may indicate only negative ear pressure without effusion. In more severe retraction, there is a prominent lateral process of the malleus with acute angulation of the malleus head. Tympanic membrane motility is generally poor when positive and negative pressures are applied by the pneumatic otoscopy.

Tympanometry is commonly used as a confirmatory test for OME. It is a tool for indirect measuring of the compliance or mobility of the tympanic membrane by applying varying ear canal pressure from 200 to −400 mm H_2O. Patients with OME have a flat (type B) curve because of failure of the tympanic membrane to move with the changing pressure. Audiometric examination in OME often discloses a mild to moderate degree of conduction hearing impairment of 20 to 40 dB. The guidelines for the treatment of OME in young children from the Agency for Health Care Policy and Research recommends that an otherwise healthy child with bilateral OME for

3 months should have a hearing evaluation (168). Acoustic reflectometry, a test that involves a tone sweep in the patient's ear and measuring reflected sound pressure to assess effusion, and tuning fork tests can also be used in the diagnosis and evaluation of OME.

The physical examination of the patient with OME should not stop at the tympanic membrane. Craniofacial anomalies, such as Down syndrome, submucous cleft palate, and bifid uvula, may be present that predispose to OME. Stigmata of an allergic diathesis should be sought in each patient. Eye examination may illustrate injected conjunctiva seen in patients with allergic conjunctivitis. Pale, boggy turbinates with profuse serous rhinorrhea are commonly found with allergic rhinitis. When chronic middle ear effusions are associated with the signs and symptoms of allergic disease, a standard allergic evaluation is indicated. A nasal smear for eosinophils, peripheral eosinophil count, and cutaneous tests for specific allergens may be of diagnostic importance.

In patients with recurrent or chronic otitis media in whom middle ear disease is just one of many sites of infection, screening of the immune system should be considered. Laboratory studies, such as IgG, IgA, and IgM, naturally occurring antibodies such as isohemagglutinins, and specific antibody titers to antigens previously given in vaccines, such as tetanus, are useful in evaluation of humoral immune status. Measuring specific antibody levels before and after administration of a pneumococcal polyvalent vaccine is an effective means of evaluating humoral immune function. Another possible condition to consider in children with multiple sites of recurrent infection is primary ciliary dyskinesia. Examination of the cilia by electron microscopy can illustrate abnormalities of the cilia ultrastructure, which can lead to ciliary dysfunction and its related chronic otitis.

Management

Management of the patient with OME requires appropriate pharmacologic and surgical intervention. It is important to understand the natural history of AOM and OME. Usually, the symptoms of AOM resolve in 48 to 72 hours if the organism is sensitive to the prescribed antibiotic. Two weeks into treatment, 70% of patients have a middle ear effusion. One month after treatment, 40% continue to have effusion, but after 3 months, only 10% of patients continue to have a persistent effusion (8). In patients with OME in which allergy may be a contributing factor, appropriate allergy treatment of avoidance of particular allergens, medication, and immunotherapy may be indicated.

Pharmacotherapy

Antimicrobial agents are the first-line therapy in AOM and may be beneficial in OME because bacteria are found in many cases. Amoxicillin is recommended as the first-line agent to treat uncomplicated AOM. For clinical treatment failures after 3 days of amoxicillin, recommended antimicrobial agents include oral amoxicillin or clavulanate, cefuroxime axetil, cefprozil, cefpodoxime proxetil, and intramuscular ceftriaxone. Intramuscular ceftriaxone should be reserved for severe cases or patients in whom noncompliance is expected. Tympanocentesis for identification of pathogens, and susceptibility to antimicrobial agents is recommended for selection of third-line agents (169). Resistant bacteria are an increasing problem in the management of children with otitis media. Sutton found penicillin resistance in the middle ear fluid of 38.2% of *S. pneumoniae* cultures at the time of tympanostomy tube surgery (170). β-Lactamase production was found in 65.1% and 100% of *H. influenzae* and *M. catarrhalis* specimens, respectively, in that study. The Agency of Health Care Policy and Research, in their guidelines on OME in young children, revealed by metaanalysis of the literature that there was a 14% increase in the probability that OME would resolve when antibiotic therapy was given as compared with no treatment (72). Another management option advocated for OME is observation of the patient for up to 4 months because of the natural history of resolution of OME in most patients. In patients with recurrent episodes of otitis media, several studies have confirmed that prophylactic regimens may be effective (171–173). The suggested duration for prophylactic antibiotics is 3 to 6 months with amoxicillin 20 mg/kg given once a day or sulfisoxazole 75 mg/kg given once a day.

Another therapeutic modality frequently prescribed in patients with OME is oral corticosteroids. The proper role for this agent in OME therapy is not clear. Many studies have evaluated corticosteroids alone and in combination with antibiotics in clearing of middle ear effusions. Berman and associates performed a metaanalysis comparing studies with the use of corticosteroids alone and with antibiotics and placebo (174). These authors reported that clearance of middle ear effusion occurred in 64% of patients treated with combination therapy, in contrast to 39% of patients treated with antibiotics only and 15% of those treated with placebo. Berman has recommended a 7-day trial of prednisone, 1 mg/kg/day divided into two doses, along with antibiotic therapy (175). The panel from the Agency of Health Care Policy and Research Guidelines on OME in young children reviewed 10 studies on the use of oral corticosteroids with and without antibiotics in OME and came to the conclusion that corticosteroid therapy is not effective in treating these children (72). It appears that additional data need to be obtained before a clear recommendation about the use of oral corticosteroids can be given.

At present, the data do not support the use of intranasal corticosteroids in the management of OME. Schwartz and colleagues gave intranasal beclomethasone to 10 children with OME, and only 3 improved (176). Shapiro and associates reported that dexamethasone nasal spray in children with OME did not affect the ultimate outcome but did facilitate rapid improvement in eustachian tube dysfunction (177).

Studies on the effectiveness of antihistamines and decongestants in randomly selected pediatric populations have shown no significant effect of these agents on resolution of OME (178,179). Mandel and associates compared antibiotic, antibiotic with antihistamine-decongestant, and placebo in the treatment of OME (180). The addition of an antihistamine-decongestant did not significantly affect the resolution of OME compared with antibiotic alone. In an animal study, Suzuki and co-workers demonstrated in guinea pigs that treatment with azelastine, an H_1 antihistamine, promoted the evacuation of middle ear fluid associated with nasal allergy (181). Antihistamine-decongestant combinations are not indicated for the treatment of otitis media with effusion in nonallergic patients, but studies need to be performed to determine their benefit in patients with allergic rhinitis and concomitant OME.

Environmental Control

When allergic rhinitis is associated with OME, environmental control of allergens and irritants should be advised. The most significant irritant is cigarette smoke. The parents must be urged to avoid exposure of their children to cigarette smoke in the home, car, restaurant, and day care facilities. Environmental inhalant allergens are more important to younger children because of the greater time spent in the home. Specific instructions for the avoidance of house dust mites, cockroaches, animal dander, and house mold spores should be given when indicated.

Vaccination

The heptavalent pneumococcal conjugate vaccine has been effective in significantly decreasing the number of episodes of otitis media in children. Black and colleagues demonstrated that children who received the pneumococcal conjugate vaccine were 20.1% less likely to require insertion of tympanostomy tubes than were controls (182). It is estimated to prevent up to 1,000,000 episodes of AOM a year, leading to cost savings of $160 per otitis media episode prevented (183).

Surgical Treatment

Refractory cases that continue to have middle ear fluid after a 4-month trial of observation or medical management often need surgical intervention.

Chronic middle ear effusion has been associated with the development of cholesteatomas, atrophy of the tympanic membrane, facial paralysis, and retention pockets. The Agency of Health Care Policy and Research Guidelines recommend myringotomy with the insertion of tympanostomy tubes for children with OME between the ages of 1 and 3 years who have bilateral hearing loss of at least 20 dB for 4 to 6 months. This procedure is effective in removing the effusion and restoring normal hearing in the child. A number of studies (184–186) have demonstrated the beneficial effect of tympanostomy tubes in OME. Tympanostomy tubes have been documented to improve the quality of life of the child with otitis media (187). It is usually recommended that tympanostomy tubes remain in place for 6 to 18 months. The longer the tube remains in the tympanic membrane, the greater the chance of complications. These include tympanosclerosis, persistent perforation, otorrhea, and occasionally cholesteatoma. Adenoidectomy has been suggested in the treatment of OME to remove blockage of the eustachian tube and improve ventilation. The Agency of Health Care Policy and Research Guidelines do not recommend adenoidectomy for children between 1 and 3 years of age with OME, although older children may benefit from the surgery. Gates and co-workers demonstrated that adenoidectomy improved and reduced recurrence of OME in children older than 4 years of age (188). They reported that the size of the adenoids did not relate to improvement of OME with adenoidectomy. Recently, the use of CO_2 laser myringotomy has been shown to be more efficacious than incisional myringotomy with adenoidectomy in OME (189). Tonsillectomy is not recommended in the management of children with OME (190). In a study of 150 children between 2 and 9 years of age with OME, adenotonsillectomy was no more effective than adenoidectomy alone (191).

Immunotherapy

Immunotherapy has been proved to be effective in the therapy for allergic rhinitis, when avoidance of the allergen is not possible or the symptoms are uncontrolled by medication. Many have the clinical impression that immunotherapy may be of help in OME in children with allergic rhinitis. However, there have been no controlled studies to verify this clinical impression.

In conclusion, the prognosis in OME is usually good. As the child gets older, the incidence of OME tends to decrease. The medical and surgical intervention outlined for OME helps to control the condition until the child "outgrows" this disease.

REFERENCES

1. Bashir SJ, Maibach HI. Compound allergy: an over view. *Contact Dermatitis* 1997;36:179–183.
2. Marsh R, Towns S, Evans K. Patch testing in ocular drug allergies. *Trans Ophthalmol Soc UK* 1978;98:278–280.
3. Mondino B, Salamon S, Zaidman G. Allergic and toxic reactions in soft contact lens wearers. *Surv Ophthalmol* 1982;26:337–344.
3a. Fisher AA, ed. *Contact dermatitis* 3rd ed. Philadelphia: Lea & Febiger, 1986.
4. Herbst R, Maibach H. Contact dermatitis caused by allergy to ophthalmic drugs and contact lens solutions. *Contact Dermatitis* 1991;25:305–312.
5. Friedlaender M. Conjunctivitis of allergic origin: clinical presentation and differential diagnosis. *Surv Ophthalmol* 1993;38[Suppl]:105–114.
6. Bonini S, Bonini S, Berruto A, et al. Conjunctival provocation test as a model for the study of allergy and inflammation in humans. *Int Arch Allergy Appl Immunol* 1988;998:1–5.
7. Proud D, Sweet J, Stein P, et al. Inflammatory mediator release on conjunctival provocation of allergic subjects with allergen. *J Allergy Clin Immunol* 1990;85(5):896–905.
8. Fukagawa K, et al. Chemokine production in conjunctival epithelial cells. In: Sullivan EA, ed. *Lacrimal gland, tear film, and dry eye syndromes*. 2nd ed. New York: Plenum, 1998.
9. Brauninger G, Centifanto Y. Immunoglobulin E in human tears. *Am J Ophthalmol* 1971;72:588–561.
10. Liotet S, Warnet V, Arrata M. Lacrimal immunoglobulin E and allergic conjunctivitis. *Ophthalmologica* 1983;186:31–34.
11. Nomura K, Takamura E. Tear IgE concentrations in allergic conjunctivitis. In: *Eye*. Tokyo: Tokyo College of Ophthalmologists, 1998:296–298.
12. Donshik P. Allergic conjunctivitis. *Int Ophthalmol Clin* 1988;28:294–302.
13. Miller S. Hypersensitivity diseases of the cornea and conjunctiva with a detailed discussion of phlyctenular disease. *Ophthalmic Semin* 1977;2:119–165.
14. Bonini S, Bonini S, Vecchione A, et al. Inflammatory changes in conjunctival scrapings after allergen provocation in humans. *J Allergy Clin Immunol* 1988;82:462–469.
15. Bonini S, et al. The eosinophil has a pivotal role in allergic inflammation of the eye. *Int Arch Allergy Immunol* 1992;99:354–358.

16. Bonini S, Bonini S. IgE and non-IgE mechanisms in ocular allergy. *Ann Allergy* 1993;71:296–299.

17. Bonini S, et al. Conjunctival provocation test as a model for the study of allergy and inflammation in humans. *Int Arch Allergy Appl Immunol* 1989;88:144–148.

18. Bonini S, Bonini S. Pathogenesis of allergic conjunctivitis. In: Denburg JA, ed. *Allergy and allergic diseases: the new mechanisms and therapeutics.* Totowa, NJ: Humana, 1996:509–519.

19. Leonardi A. Pathophysiology of allergic conjunctivitis. *Acta Ophthalmol Scand* 1999:21–23.

20. Metz D, et al. T-cell cytokines in chronic allergic eye disease. *J Allergy Clin Immunol* 1997;100:817–824.

21. Morgan S, et al. Mast cell numbers and staining characteristics in the normal and allergic human conjunctiva. *J Allergy Clin Immunol* 1991;87[1 Pt 1]:111–116.

22. Ciprandi G, et al. Ocular challenge and hyperresponsiveness to histamine in patients with allergic conjunctivitis. *J Allergy Clin Immunol* 1993;91:1227–1230.

23. Woods A. Ocular allergy. *Am J Ophthalmol* 1949;32:1457–1461.

24. Friedlaender M, Ohashi Y, Kelley J. Diagnosis of allergic conjunctivitis. *Arch Ophthalmol* 1984;102:1198–1199.

25. Dechant K, Goa K. Levocabastine: a review of its pharmacological properties and therapeutic potential as a topical antihistamine in allergic rhinitis and conjunctivitis. *Drugs* 1991;41:202–224.

26. Stokes T, Feinberg G. Rapid onset of action of levocabastine eyedrops in histamine-induced conjunctivitis. *Clin Exp Allergy* 1993;23:791–794.

27. Abelson M, et al. Evaluation of the new ophthalmic antihistamine, 0.05% levocabastine, in the clinical allergen challenge model of allergic conjunctivitis. *J Allergy Clin Immunol* 1994;94[3 Pt 1]:458–464.

28. Frostad A, Olsen A. A comparison of topical levocabastine and sodium cromoglycate in the treatment of pollen-provoked allergic conjunctivitis. *Clin Exp Allergy* 1993;23:406–409.

29. Shoel P, et al. Topical levocabastine compared with orally administered terfenadine for the prophylaxis and treatment of seasonal rhinoconjunctivitis. *J Allergy Clin Immunol* 1993;92:73–81.

30. El-Defrawy S, Jackson W. New directions in therapy for ocular allergy. In: *International ophthalmology clinic.* Philadelphia: Lippincott-Raven, 1996:25–44.

31. Lanier B, Tremblay N, Smith JP, et al. A double-masked comparison of ocular decongestants as therapy for allergic conjunctivitis. *Ann Allergy* 1983;50:174–177.

32. Friday G, Biglan AW, Hiles PA, et al. Treatment of ragweed conjunctivitis with cromolyn sodium 4% ophthalmic solution. *Am J Ophthalmol* 1983;95:169–174.

33. Greenbaum J, Cockcroft D, Hargreave FE, et al. Sodium cromoglycate in ragweed-allergic conjunctivitis. *J Allergy Clin Immunol* 1977;59:437–439.

34. Melamed J, et al. Evaluation of nedocromil sodium 2% ophthalmic solution for the treatment of seasonal allergic conjunctivitis. *Ann Allergy* 1994;73:57–66.

35. Juniper E, et al. Sodium cromoglycate eye drops: regular versus as needed use in the treatment of seasonal allergic conjunctivitis. *J Allergy Clin Immunol* 1994;94(1):36–43.

36. Montan P, et al. Topical sodium cromoglycate (Opticrom) relieves ongoing symptoms of allergic conjunctivitis within 2 minutes. *Allergy* 1994;49:637–640.

37. Ballas Z, et al. Clinical evaluation of ketorolac tromethamine 0.5% ophthalmic solution for the treatment of seasonal allergic conjunctivitis. *Surv Ophthalmol* 1993;38[Suppl]:141–148.

38. Woodward D, et al. Acular: studies on its mechanism of action in reducing allergic conjunctival itching. *J Allergy Clin Immunol* 1995;95:360.

39. Yanni J, et al. Comparative effects of topical ocular antiallergy drugs on human conjunctival mast cells. *Ann Allergy Asthma Immunol* 1997;79:541–545.

40. Sharif N, Xu S, Yanni J. Olopatadine (AL-4943A): ligand binding and functional studies on a novel, long acting H1-selective histamine antagonist and anti-allergic agent for use in allergic conjunctivitis. *J Ocular Pharmacol* 1996;12(4):401–407.

41. Grant S, et al. Ketotifen, a review of its pharmocodynamic and pharmacokinetic properties, and therapeutic use in asthma and allergic disorders. *Drugs* 1990;40(3):412–440.

42. Nabe M, et al. The effect of ketotifen on eosinophils as measured at LTC4 release and by chemotaxis. *Allergy Proc* 1991;12(4):267–271.

43. Taudorf E, et al. Oral immunotherapy in birch pollen hayfever. *J Allergy Clin Immunol* 1987;80:153–161.

44. Moages R, Hassan H, Wenzel M. Optimal use of topical agents for allergic conjunctivitis. In: *BioDrugs.* 1997:250–262.

45. Arsovski Z, et al. The effect of immunotherapy on grass pollen allergic conjunctivitis. *J Allergy Clin Immunol* 1995;95:318.

46. Abelson M, George M, Garofalo C. Differential diagnosis of ocular allergic disorders. *Ann Allergy* 1993;70:95–113.

47. Allansmith M, Frick O. Antibodies to grass in vernal conjunctivitis. *J Allergy* 1963;34:535–538.

48. Allansmith M, Baird RS, Higginbotham EJ, et al. Technical aspects of histamine determination in human tears. *Am J Ophthalmol* 1980;90:719–724.

49. Ballow M, Mendelson L. Specific immunoglobulin E antibodies in tear secretions of patients with vernal conjunctivitis. *J Allergy Clin Immunol* 1980;66:112–118.

50. Fukagawa K, et al. Histamine and tryptase levels in allergic conjunctivitis and vernal keratoconjunctivitis. *Cornea* 1994;13(4):345–348.

51. Allansmith M, Baird R. Mast cells, eosinophils and basophils in vernal conjunctivitis. *J Allergy Clin Immunol* 1978;61:154.

52. Trocme C, et al. Conjunctival deposition of eosinophil granule major basic protein in vernal keratoconjunctivitis and contact lens-associated giant papillary conjunctivitis. *Am J Ophthalmol* 1989;108:57–63.

53. Avunduk A, et al. A flow cytometric study about the immunopathology of vernal keratoconjunctivitis. *J Allergy Clin Immunol* 1998;101:821–824.

54. Huntley C, Fletcher W. Current concept in therapy: vernal conjunctivitis—simple treatment. *South Med J* 1973;66:607–608.

55. Little EC. Keeping pollen at bay. *Lancet* 1968;2:512–513.

56. Leonardi A, et al. Histamine effects on conjunctival fibroblasts from patients with vernal conjunctivitis. *Exp Eye Res* 1999;68:739–746.

57. Leonardi A, et al. Procollagens and inflammatory cytokine concentrations in tarsal and limbal vernal keratoconjunctivitis. *Exp Eye Res* 1998;67:105–112.
58. Gill K, et al. ICAM-1 expression in corneal epithelium of a patient with vernal keratoconjunctivitis: case report. *Cornea* 1997;16(1):107–111.
59. Ballow M, et al. IgG specific antibodies to rye grass and ragweed pollen antigens in the tear secretions of patients with vernal conjunctivitis. *Am J Ophthalmol* 1983;95:161–168.
60. Ballow M, Donshik P, Mendelson L. Complement proteins and C3 anaphylatoxin in tears of patients with conjunctivitis. *J Allergy Clin Immunol* 1985;76: 463–476.
61. Ballow M, et al. Tear lactoferrin levels in patients with external inflammatory ocular disease. *Invest Ophthalmol Vis Sci* 1987;28:543–545.
62. Karel I, Myska V, Kvicaolva E. Ophthalmological changes in atopic dermatitis. *Acta Derm Venerol* 1965;45:381–383.
63. Oshinskie L, Haine C. Atopic dermatitis and its ophthalmic complications. *J Am Ophthalmic Assoc* 1982; 53:889–894.
64. Jay JL. Clinical features and diagnosis of adult atopic keratoconjunctivitis and the effect of treatment with sodium cromoglycate. *Br J Ophthalmol* 1981;65:335–340.
65. Reynolds RM. Giant papillary conjunctivitis. *Trans Ophthalmol Soc N Z* 1980;32:92–95.
66. MacIvor J. Contact allergy to plastic artificial eyes. *Can Med Assoc J* 1950;62:164–166.
67. Goes F, Blockhuys S, Janssens M. Levocabastine eye drops in the treatment of vernal conjunctivitis. *Doc Ophthalmol* 1994;87:271–281.
68. Hyams S, Bialik M, Neumann E. Clinical trial of topic disodium cromoglycate in vernal and allergic keratoconjunctivitis. *J Ophthalmol* 1975;12:116.
69. Collum L, Cassidy H, Benedict-Smith A. Disodium cromoglycate in vernal and allergic keratoconjunctivitis. *Ir Med J* 1981;74:14–18.
70. Foster C, Duncan J. Randomized clinic trial of topically administered cromolyn sodium for vernal keratoconjunctivitis. *Am J Ophthalmol* 1980;90:175–181.
71. Foster C, and the T.C.S.C.S. Group. Evaluation of topical cromolyn sodium in the treatment of vernal keratoconjunctivitis. *Ophthalmology* 1988;95:194–201.
72. Caldwell D, et al. Efficacy and safety of iodoxamide 0.1% vs. cromolyn sodium 4% in patients with vernal keratoconjunctivitis. *Am J Ophthalmol* 1992;113:632–637.
73. Abelson M, Butrus S, Weston J. Aspirin therapy in vernal conjunctivitis. *Am J Ophthalmol* 1983;95:502–505.
74. Meyer E, Kraus E, Zonis S. Efficacy of antiprostaglandin therapy in vernal conjunctivitis. *Br J Ophthalmol* 1987;71:497–499.
75. Trocme S, Raizman M, Bartley G. Medical therapy for ocular allergy. *Mayo Clin Proc* 1992;67:557–565.
76. Friedlander MH, Allansmith M. Ocular allergy. *Ann Ophthalmol* 1975;7:1171–1174.
77. Foster C, Calonge M. Atopic keratoconjunctivitis. *Ophthalmology* 1990;97(8):992–1000.
78. Uchio E, et al. Systemic and local immunological features of atopic dermatitis patients with ocular complications. *Br J Ophthalmol* 1998;82:82–87.
79. Oster H, Martin R, Dawson C. The use of disodium cormoglycate in the treatment of atopic disease. In: Leopold J, Burns R, eds. *Symposium on ocular therapy.* New York: John Wiley & Sons, 1977:99–108.
80. Amemiya T, Matsuda H, Vehara M. Ocular findings in atopic dermatitis with special reference to the clinical feature of atopic cataract. *Ophthalmologica* 1980;180:129–132.
81. Yokoi N, et al. Association of eosinophil granule major basic protein with atopic cataract. *Am J Ophthalmol* 1996;122:825–829.
82. Garrity J, Liesegang T. Ocular complications of atopic dermatitis. *Can J Ophthalmol* 1984;19:21–24.
83. Easty D, et al. Herpes simplex keratitis and keratoconums in the atopic patient: a clinical and immunological study. *Trans Ophthalmol Soc UK* 1975;95:267–276.
84. Meyers R. Immunology of herpes virus infection. *Int Ophthalmol Clin* 1975;15:37.
85. Pavan-Langston D. Diagnosis and management of herpes simplex ocular infection. *Int Ophthalmol Clin* 1975;15:19–35.
86. Allansmith M, Korb DR, Greiner JV, et al. Giant papillary conjunctivitis in contact lens wearers. *Am J Ophthalmol* 1977;83:697–708.
87. Culbertson W, Ostler B. The floppy eyelid syndrome. *Am J Ophthalmol* 1981;92:568–574.
88. Stenson S. Contact lenses: guide to selection, fitting, and management of complications. East Norwalk, CT: Appleton-Lange, 1987:215–217.
89. Gudmonsson O, et al. Identification of proteins in contact lens surface deposits by immunofluorescence microscopy. *Arch Ophthalmol* 1985;103:196–197.
90. Tripathy R, Tripathy B. Soft lens spoilage. *Ophthalmic Forum* 1984;2:80–92.
91. Katelaris C. Giant papillary conjunctivitis: a review. *Acta Ophthalmol Scand* 1999;77:17–20.
92. Barishak Y, et al. An immunologic study of papillary conjunctivitis due to contact lenses. *Curr Eye Res* 1984;3(10):1161–1168.
93. Irkec M, Orhan M, Erdener U. Role of tear inflammatory mediators in contact lens-associated giant papillary conjunctivitis in soft contact lens wearers. *Ocular Immunol Inflam* 1999;7(1):35–38.
94. Tan M, et al. Presence of inflammatory mediators in the tears of contact lens wearers and non-contact lens wearers. *Aust N Z J Ophthalmol* 1997;25[Suppl 1]:S27–S29.
95. Donshik P, et al. The detection of neutrophil chemotactic factors in tear fluids of contact lens wearers with active papillary conjunctivitis. *Invest Ophthalmol Vis Sci* 1988;29:230.
96. Bailey C, Buckley R. Nedocromil sodium in contact-lens-associated papillary conjunctivitis. *Eye* 1993;7[Suppl]:29–33.
97. Schappert S. Office visits for otitis media: United States, 1975–90, advance data from vital and health statistics. Hyattsville, MD: National Center for Health Statistics: 1992.
98. Elden L, Coyte P. Socioeconomic impact of otitis media in North America. *J Otolaryngol* 1998;27[Suppl 2]: 9–16.
99. Paparella M. Middle ear effusions: definitions and terminology. *Ann Otol Rhinol Laryngol* 1976;85 [Suppl 25]:8–11.
100. Cotton R. Serous otitis in children: medical and surgical

aspects, diagnosis and management. *Clin Rev Allergy* 1984;2:319–328.

101. Gates G, et al. Chronic secretory otitis media: effects of surgical management. *Ann Otol Rhinol Laryngol* 1989;138:2–32.

102. Dempster J, MacKenzie K. Tympanometry in the detection of hearing impairments associated with otitis media with effusion. *Clin Otolaryngol* 1991;16:157–159.

103. Engel J, et al. Risk factors of otitis media with effusion during infancy. *Int J Pediatr Otorhinolaryngol* 1999;48(3):239–249.

104. Teele O, Klein J, Rosner B. Epidemiology of otitis media in children. *Ann Otol Rhinol Laryngol* 1980;89:5–6.

105. Zeisel S, et al. Prospective surveillance for otitis media with effusion among black infants in group child care. *J Pediatr* 1995;127(6):875–880.

106. Williamson I, et al. The natural history of otitis media with effusion: a three-year study of the incidence and prevalence of abnormal tympanograms in four South West Hampshire infant and first schools. *J Laryngol Otol* 1994;108(11):930–934.

107. Saim A, et al. Prevalence of otitis media with effusion amongst pre-school children in Malaysia. *Int J Pediatr Otorhinolaryngol* 1997;41(1):21–28.

108. Strachan D, Cook D. Health effects of passive smoking. 4. Parental smoking, middle ear disease and adenotonsillectomy in children. *Thorax* 1998;53:50–56.

109. Ely J, et al. Passive smoke exposure and otitis media in the first year of life. *Pediatrics* 1995;95(5):670–677.

110. Rovers M, et al. Prognostic factors for persistent otitis media with effusion in infants. *Arch Otolaryngol Head Neck Surg* 1999;125(11):1203–1207.

111. Daly K, et al. Determining risk for chronic otitis media with effusion. *Pediatr Infect Dis J* 1988;7(7):471–475.

112. Zielhuis G, et al. Environmental risk factors for otitis media with effusion in preschool children. *Scand J Prim Health Care* 1989;7(1):33–38.

113. Sorensen C, Holm-Jensen S. Middle ear effusion and risk factors. *J Otolaryngol* 1982;11(10):46–51.

114. Duncan B, Ey J, Holberg C. Exclusive breast-feeding for at least 4 months protects against otitis media. *Pediatrics* 1993;91:867–872.

115. Aniansson G, et al. A prospective cohort study on breast-feeding and otitis media in Swedish infants. *Pediatr Infect Dis J* 1994;13(3):183–188.

116. Strong M. The eustachian tube: basic considerations. *Otol Clin North Am* 1972;5:19–27.

117. Bellioni P, Cantani A, Salvinelli F. Allergy: a leading role in otitis media with effusion. *Allergol Immunopathol* (Madr) 1987;15(4):205–208.

118. Riding K, et al. Microbiology of recurrent and chronic otitis media with effusion. *J Pediatr* 1978;93(5):739–743.

119. Brook I. Otitis media: microbiology and management. *J Otolaryngol* 1994;23(4):269–275.

120. Hendolin P, et al. High incidence of alloiococcus otitis in otitis media with effusion. *Pediatr Infect Dis J* 1999;18(10):860–865.

121. Bluestone C, Klein J. *Otitis media in infants and children.* Philadelphia: WB Saunders, 1988.

122. Post J, Preston R, Aul J. Molecular analysis of bacterial pathogens in otitis media with effusion. *JAMA* 1995;273:1598–1604.

123. Heikkinen T, Chonmaitree T. Increasing importance of viruses in acute otitis media [In process citation]. *Ann Med* 2000;32(3):157–163.

124. Brook I, Van de Heyning P. Microbiology and management of otitis media. *Scand J Infect Dis* 1994; [Suppl 93](1):20–32.

125. Fainstein V, Musher D, Cate T. Bacterial adherence to pharyngeal cells during viral infection. *J Infect Dis* 1980;141:172–176.

126. Giebink G, Wright P. Different virulence of influenza A virus strains and susceptibility to pneumococcal otitis media in chinchillas. *Infect Immunol* 1983;41:913–920.

127. Welliver R, Kaul T, Orga P. The appearance of cell-bound IgE in respiratory tract epithelium after respiratory tract viral infection. *N Engl J Med* 1980;303:1198–1202.

128. Ohashi Y, Nakai Y. Current concepts of mucociliary dysfunction in otitis media with effusion. *Acta Otolaryngol* 1991;[Suppl 486]:149–161.

129. Carson J, Collier A, Hu S. Acquired ciliary defects in nasal epithelium of children with acute viral upper respiratory infections. *N Engl J Med* 1985;312:463–468.

130. Schidlow D. Primary ciliary dyskinesia (the immotile cilia syndrome). *Ann Allergy* 1994;73(6):457–468; quiz, 468–470.

131. Hall L, Lukat R. Results of allergy treatment on the eustachian tube in chronic serous otitis media. *Am J Otol* 1981;3:116–121.

132. Bernstein J. The role of IgE-mediated hypersensitivity in the development of otitis media with effusion: a review. *Otolaryngol Head Neck Surg* 1993; 109(3 Pt 2):611–620.

133. Caffareli C, et al. Atopy in children with otitis media with effusion. *Clin Exp Allergy* 1998;28(5):591–596.

134. Kraemer M, et al. Risk factors for persistent middle-ear effusions: otitis media, catarrh, cigarette smoke exposure, and atopy. *JAMA* 1983;249(8):1022–1025.

135. Marshall S, Bierman C, Shapiro G. Otitis media with effusion in childhood. *Ann Allergy* 1984;53(5):370–378.

136. Bierman C, Furukawa C. Medical management of serous otitis in children. *Pediatrics* 1978;61:768–774.

137. Tomonaga K, Kurono Y, Mogi G. The role of nasal allergy in otitis media with effusion: a clinical study. *Acta Otolaryngol* 1988;[Suppl 458]:41–47.

138. Bernstein J, Reisman R. The role of acute hypersensitivity in secretory otitis media. *Trans Am Acad Ophthalmol Otolaryngol* 1974;78:120–127.

139. Senturia B. Allergic manifestations and otologic disease. *Laryngoscope* 1960;70:285–287.

140. Black N. The aetiology of glue ear: a case control study. *Int J Pediatr Otorhinolaryngol* 1985;9:121–133.

141. Miglets A, Spiegel J, Bronstein H. Middle ear effusion in experimental hypersensitivity. *Ann Otol Rhinol Laryngol* 1976;85(2)[Suppl 25](Pt 2):81–86.

142. Labadie R, et al. Allergy increases susceptibility to otitis media with effusion in a rat model. Second place, Resident Clinical Science Award 1998. *Otolaryngol Head Neck Surg* 1999;121(6):687–692.

143. Yamashita T, Okazaki N, Kumazawa T. Relation between nasal and middle ear allergy: experimental study. *Ann Otol Rhinol Laryngol* 1980;[Suppl 89](3 Pt 2):147–152.

144. Friedman R, Doyle WJ, Casselbrant ML, et al. Immunologic-mediated eustachian tube obstruction: a

double-blind crossover study. *J Allergy Clin Immunol* 1983;71:442–447.

145. Osur S, Volovitz B, Bernstein J. Eustachian tube dysfunction in children with ragweed hayfever during natural pollen exposure. *Allergy Proc* 1989;10:133–139.

146. Kraemer M, Ochs H, Lindgren C. Etiology factors in the development of chronic middle ear effusions. *Clin Rev Allergy* 1984;2:319–328.

147. Lim D, et al. Immunoglobulin E in chronic middle ear effusions. *Ann Otol Rhinol Laryngol* 1976; 85(2)[Suppl 25](Pt 2):117–123.

148. Sipila P, et al. Secretory IgA, secretory component and pathogen specific antibodies in the middle ear effusion during an attack of acute and secretory otitis media. *Auris Nasus Larynx* 1985;12[Suppl 1]:S180–S182.

149. Bernstein J, Ogra P. Mucosal immune system: implications in otitis media with effusion. *Ann Otol Rhinol Laryngol* 1980;[Suppl 89](3 Pt 2):326–332.

150. Bernstein J, et al. The role of IgE mediated hypersensitivity in recurrent otitis media with effusion. *Am J Otol* 1983;5(1):66–69.

151. Reisman R, Bernstein J. Allergy and secretory otitis media: clinical and immunologic studies. *Pediatr Clin North Am* 1975;22:2517.

152. Mogi G. Secretory IgA and antibody activities in middle ear effusions. *Ann Otol Rhinol Laryngol* 1976; 85[2 Suppl][25 Pt 2]:97–102.

153. Khan J, Marcus P, Cummings S. S-carboxymethylcysteine in otitis media with effusion (a double-blind study). *J Laryngol Otol* 1981;95(10):995–1001.

154. Hurst D. Association of otitis media with effusion and allergy as demonstrated by intradermal skin testing and eosinophil cationic protein levels in both middle ear effusions and mucosal biopsies. *Laryngoscope* 1996;106(9 Pt 1):1128–1137.

155. Hurst D, Weekley M, Ramanarayanan M. Evidence of possible localized specific immunoglobulin E production in middle ear fluid as demonstrated by ELISA testing. *Otolaryngol Head Neck Surg* 1999;121(3):224–230.

156. Hurst D, et al. Evidence of mast cell activity in the middle ears of children with otitis media with effusion. *Laryngoscope* 1999;109(3):471–477.

157. Georgitis J, Gold W, Bernstein J. Eustachian tube function associated with histamine-induced and ragweed-induced rhinitis. *Ann Allergy* 1988;61: 234–238.

158. Bernstein J, et al. The role of IgE mediated hypersensitivity in recurrent otitis media with effusion. *Am J Otol* 1983;5:66–69.

159. Host A. Mechanisms in adverse reactions to food: the ear. *Allergy* 1995;50(20):64–67.

160. Nsouli T, et al. Role of food allergy in serous otitis media. *Ann Allergy* 1994;73(3):215–219.

161. James J. Role of food allergy in serous otitis media [Letter to the editor]. *Ann Allergy Asthma Immunol* 1995;74:277.

162. Bernstein J, Brentjens J, Vladutiu A. Are immune complexes a factor in the pathogenesis of otitis media with effusion ? *Am J Otolaryngol* 1982;3:20–26.

163. Yamanaka N, et al. Immune complexes in otitis media with effusion. *Auris Nasus Larynx* 1985;12 [Suppl 1]:S70–S72.

164. Mravec J, Lewis D, Lim D. Experimental otitis media with effusion: an immune-complex-mediated response. *Otolaryngology* 1978;86(2):ORL258–268.

165. Bernstein J, Brentjens J, Vladutiu A. Are immune complexes a factor in the pathogenesis of otitis media with effusion ? *Am J Otolaryngol* 1982;3(1):20–25.

166. Ueyama S, et al. The role of immune complex in otitis media with effusion. *Auris Nasus Larynx* 1997;24(3):247–254.

167. Umetsu D, Ambrosino D, Quinti I, et al. Recurrent sinopulmonary infection and impaired antibody response to bacterial capsular polysaccharide antigen in children with selective IgG-subclass deficiency. *N Engl J Med* 1985;313:1247–1251.

168. Stool S, Berg A, Berman S. Otitis media with effusion in young children. In: *Clinical Practice Guidelines*. 1994(12), DHHS publication no (AHCRP) 94-0622.

169. Aronovitz G. Antimicrobial therapy of acute otitis media: review of treatment recommendations. *Clin Ther* 2000;22(1):29–39.

170. Sutton D, et al. Resistant bacteria in middle ear fluid at the time of tympanotomy tube surgery. *Ann Otol Rhinol Laryngol* 2000;109(1):24–29.

171. Principi N, et al. Prophylaxis of recurrent acute otitis media and middle-ear effusion: comparison of amoxicillin with sulfamethoxazole and trimethoprim [published erratum appears in *Am J Dis Child* 1990;144 (11):1180]. *Am J Dis Child* 1989; 143(12): 1414–1418.

172. Biedel C. Modification of recurrent otitis media by short-term sulfonamide therapy. *Am J Dis Child* 1978; 132:681–683.

173. Williams R, Chambers T, Stange K. Use of antibiotics in preventing recurrent acute otitis media and in treating otitis media with effusion: a meta-analytic attempt to resolve the brouhaha. *JAMA* 1993;270:1344–1351.

174. Berman S, Roark R, Luckey D. Theoretical cost effectiveness of management options for children with persisting middle ear effusions. *Pediatrics* 1994;93: 353–363.

175. Berman S. Otitis media in children. *N Engl J Med* 1995;332:1560–1565.

176. Schwartz R, Schwartz D, Grundfast K. Intranasal beclomethasone in the treatment of middle ear effusion: a pilot study. *Ann Allergy* 1980;45(5):284–287.

177. Shapiro G, Bierman CW, Furukawa CT, et al. Treatment of persistent eustachian tube dysfunction in children with aerosolized nasal dexamethasone phosphate versus placebo. *Ann Allergy* 1982;49:81–85.

178. Cantekin E, Mandel E, Bluestone C. Lack of efficacy of a decongestant-antihistamine combination for otitis media with effusion ("secretory" otitis media) in children: results of a double-blind randomized trial. *N Engl J Med* 1983;308:297–301.

179. Dusdieker L, Smith G, Booth B. The long-term outcome of nonsuppurative otitis media with effusion. *Clin Pediatr* 1985;24:181–186.

180. Mandel E, Rockette H, Bluestone C. Efficacy of amoxicillin with and without decongestant-antihistamine for otitis media with effusion in children: results of a double-blind, randomized trial. *N Engl J Med* 1987(316):432–437.

181. Suzuki M, et al. Efficacy of an antiallergic drug on otitis media with effusion in association with allergic rhinitis: an experimental study. *Ann Otol Rhinol Laryngol* 1999;108(6):554–558.

182. Black S, et al. Efficacy, safety and immunogenicity of heptavalent pneumococcal conjugate vaccine in children. *Pediatr Infect Dis J* 2000;19:187–195.

183. Lieu T, et al. Projected cost-effectiveness of pneumococcal conjugate vaccination of healthy infants and young children. *JAMA* 2000;283(11):1460–1468.

184. Maw A, Bawden R. The long term outcome of secretory otitis media in children and the effects of surgical treatment: a ten year study. *Acta Otorhinolaryngol Belg* 1994;48(4):317–324.

185. Maw R, et al. Surgical treatment of chronic otitis media with effusion [In process citation]. *Int J Pediatr Otorhinolaryngol* 1999;49[Suppl 1]:S239–S241.

186. Biedlingmaier J. Otitis media in children: medical versus surgical treatment. *Postgrad Med* 1993;93(5): 153–155.

187. Rosenfeld R, et al. Impact of tympanostomy tubes on child quality of life. *Arch Otolaryngol Head Neck Surg* 2000;126(5):585–592.

188. Gates G, et al. Effectiveness of adenoidectomy and tympanostomy tubes in the treatment of chronic otitis media with effusion. *N Engl J Med* 1987;317(23):1444–1451.

189. Szeremeta W, Parameswaran M, Isaacson G. Adenoidectomy with laser or incisional myringotomy for otitis media with effusion [In process citation]. *Laryngoscope* 2000;110(3 Pt 1):342–345.

190. Stewart I. Evaluation of factors affecting outcome of surgery for otitis media with effusion in clinical practice. *Int J Pediatr Otorhinolaryngol* 1999;49(Suppl 1):S243–S245.

191. Maw A. Chronic otitis media with effusion and adenotonsillectomy: a prospective randomized controlled study. *Int J Pediatr Otorhinolaryngol* 1983;6(3): 239–246.

12

Allergy to Stinging Insects

Robert E. Reisman

*Departments of Medicine and Pediatrics, State University of New York at Buffalo,
Department of Medicine (Allergy/Immunology),
Buffalo General Hospital, Buffalo, New York*

Allergic reactions to insect stings constitute a major medical problem, resulting in about 50 recognized fatalities annually in the United States, and are likely responsible for other unexplained sudden deaths. People at risk are often very anxious about future stings and modify their daily living patterns and lifestyles. Major advances in recent years have led to appreciation of the natural history of insect sting allergy and appropriate diagnosis and treatment for people at risk for insect sting anaphylaxis. For most affected people this is a self-limited disease; for others, treatment results in a "permanent cure."

THE INSECTS

The stinging insects are members of the order Hymenoptera of the class Insecta. They may be broadly divided into two families: the vespids, which include the yellow jacket, hornet, and wasp; and the apids, which include the honeybee and the bumblebee. People may be allergic to one or all of the stinging insects. The identification of the culprit insect responsible for the reactions is thus important in terms of specific advice and specific venom immunotherapy discussed later.

The honeybee and bumblebee are quite docile and tend to sting only when provoked. The bumblebee is a rare offender. Because of the common use of the honeybee for the production of honey and in plant fertilization, exposure to this insect is quite common. Multiple stings from honeybees may occur, particularly if their hive, which

may contain thousands of insects, is in danger. The honeybee usually loses its stinging mechanism in the sting process, thereby inflicting self-evisceration and death.

The problem of multiple insect stings has recently been intensified by the introduction of the Africanized honeybee, the so-called killer bee, into the southwestern United States (1). These bees are much more aggressive than the domesticated European honeybees that are found throughout the United States. Massive stinging incidents have occurred, resulting in death from venom toxicity. The Africanized honeybees entered South Texas in 1990 and are now present in Arizona and California. It is anticipated that these bees will continue to spread throughout the southern United States. They are unable to survive in colder climates but may make periodic forays into the northern United States during the summer months.

The yellow jacket is the most common cause of allergic insect sting reactions. These insects nest in the ground and are easily disturbed in the course of activities, such as lawn mowing and gardening. They are also attracted to food and commonly found around garbage and picnic areas. They are present in increasing numbers in late summer and fall months of the year. Hornets, which are closely related to the yellow jacket, nest in shrubs and are also easily provoked by activities such as hedge clipping. Wasps usually build honeycomb nests under eaves and rafters and are relatively few in number in such nests.

However, in some parts of the country, such as Texas, they are the most common cause for insect stings.

In contrast to stinging insects, biting insects such as mosquitoes rarely cause serious allergic reactions. These insects deposit salivary gland secretions, which have no relationship to the venom deposited by stinging insects. Anaphylaxis has occurred from bites of the deer fly, kissing bug, and bed bug. Isolated reports also suggest that, on a rare occasion, mosquito bites have caused anaphylaxis. It is much more common, however, for insect bites to cause large local reactions, which may have an immune pathogenesis (2).

REACTIONS TO INSECT STINGS

Normal Reaction

The usual reaction after an insect sting is mild redness and swelling at the sting site. This reaction is transient and disappears within several hours. Little treatment is needed other than analgesics and cold compresses. Insect stings, in contrast to insect bites, always cause pain at the sting site.

Large Local Reactions

Extensive swelling and erythema, extending from the sting site over a large area is a fairly common reaction. The swelling usually reaches a maximum in 24 to 48 hours and may last as long as 10 days. On occasion, fatigue, nausea, and malaise may accompany the large local reaction. Aspirin and antihistamines are usually adequate treatment. When severe or disabling, administration of steroids, such as prednisone, 40 mg daily for 2 to 3 days, may be very helpful. These large local reactions have been confused with infection and cellulitis. Insect sting sites are rarely infected and antibiotic therapy rarely indicated.

Most people who have had large local reactions from insect stings will have similar large local reactions from subsequent re-stings (3). The risk for generalized anaphylaxis is very low, less than 5%. Thus, people who have had large local reactions are not considered candidates for venom immunotherapy (discussed later) and do not require venom skin tests.

Anaphylaxis

The most serious reaction that follows an insect sting is anaphylaxis. Retrospective population studies suggest that the incidence of this acute allergic reaction from an insect sting ranges between 0.4% and 3% (4–6). Allergic reactions can occur at any age; most have occurred in individuals younger than 20 years of age, with a male-to-female ratio of 2:1. These factors may reflect exposure rather than any specific age or sex predilection. Several clinical studies suggest that about one third of individuals suffering systemic reactions have a personal history of atopic disease. Stings around the head and neck most commonly cause allergic reactions, but reactions may occur from stings occurring on any area of the body (7–11).

In most patients, anaphylactic symptoms occur within 15 minutes after the sting, although there have been rare reports of reactions developing later. Clinical observations suggest that the sooner the symptoms occur, the more severe the reactions may be. The clinical symptoms vary from patient to patient and are typical of anaphylaxis from any cause. The most common symptoms involve the skin and include generalized urticaria, flushing, and angioedema. More serious symptoms are respiratory and cardiovascular. Upper airway edema involving the pharynx, epiglottis, and trachea has been responsible for numerous fatalities. Circulatory collapse with shock and hypotension also has been responsible for mortality. Other symptoms include bowel spasm and diarrhea and uterine contractions (9,12).

Severe anaphylaxis, including loss of consciousness, occurs in all age groups. Most deaths from sting anaphylaxis occur in adults. The reason for this increased mortality rate in adults might be the presence of cardiovascular disease or other pathologic changes associated with age. Adults may have less tolerance for the profound biochemical and physiologic changes that accompany anaphylaxis (13–15).

There are no absolute criteria that will identify people at risk for acquiring venom allergy. Most people who have venom anaphylaxis have tolerated stings without any reaction before the first episode of anaphylaxis. Even individuals who have died from insect sting anaphylaxis usually had no history of prior allergic reactions. The occurrence of venom anaphylaxis after first known insect sting exposure is another confusing observation, raising the issue of the etiology of prior sensitization or the pathogenesis of this initial reaction. People who have had large local reactions usually have positive venom skin tests and often very high titers of serum venom-specific immunoglobulin E (IgE); thus, these tests do not discriminate the few potential anaphylactic reactors. Anecdotal observations suggest that the use of β-blocking medication, which certainly potentiates the seriousness of any anaphylactic reaction, may also be a risk factor for subsequent occurrence of anaphylaxis in people who have had large local reactions.

Many simultaneous stings (greater than 100) may sensitize a person, who then might be at risk for anaphylaxis from a subsequent single sting. Exposure to this large amount of venom protein can induce IgE production. This potential problem is now recognized more often because of the many stings inflicted by the so-called killer bees. After experiencing a large number of stings with or without a toxic clinical reaction, people should be tested to determine the possibility of potential venom allergy.

After an uneventful insect sting, some people may develop a positive skin test, which is usually transient in occurrence. A report from Johns Hopkins suggested that if the skin test remains positive for a long period of time, 5 to 10 years, 17% of people have a systemic reaction after a subsequent sting (16). The authors made no specific therapeutic recommendations to address this issue. If these data were verified, it would raise the question of venom skin tests for individuals who have tolerated insect stings. If the test remains positive, people might be advised to have medication available for treatment of an allergic reaction. Obviously, the efficiency and economics of this approach are debatable. Currently, skin testing of people who have

no allergic reaction from a single sting is not recommended.

The natural history of insect sting anaphylaxis has now been well studied and is most intriguing. People who have had insect sting anaphylaxis have an approximate 60% recurrence rate of anaphylaxis after subsequent stings (17). Viewed from a different perspective, not all people presumed to be at risk react to re-stings. The incidence of these re-sting reactions is influenced by age and severity of the symptoms of the initial reaction. In general, children are less likely to have re-sting reactions than are adults. The more severe the anaphylactic symptoms, the more likely it is to reoccur. For example, children who have had dermal symptoms (hives, angioedema) as the only manifestation of anaphylaxis have a remarkably low re-sting reaction rate (17,18). On the other hand, individuals of any age who have had severe anaphylaxis have an approximate 70% likelihood of repeat reactions (17,19). When anaphylaxis does reoccur, the severity of the reaction tends to be similar to the initial reaction. No relationship has been found between the occurrence and degree of anaphylaxis and the intensity of venom skin test reactions. Thus, factors other than IgE antibodies modulate clinical anaphylaxis.

Unusual Reactions

Serum sickness–type reactions, characterized by urticaria, joint pain, malaise, and fever have occurred about 7 days after an insect sting. On occasion, these reactions have also been associated with an immediate anaphylactic reaction. People who have this serum sickness–type reaction are subsequently at risk for acute anaphylaxis after repeat stings and thus are considered candidates for venom immunotherapy (20).

There have been isolated reports of other reactions, such as vasculitis, nephritis, neuritis, and encephalitis, occurring in a temporal relationship to an insect sting. The basic etiology for these reactions has not been established (21).

Toxic Reactions

Toxic reactions may occur as a result of many simultaneous stings. Insect venom contains a number of potent pharmacologic agents, and as a result of the properties of these substances, vascular collapse, shock, hypotension, and death may occur (22). The differentiation between allergic and toxic reactions sometimes can be difficult. As noted, after a toxic reaction, individuals may develop IgE antibody and then be at risk for subsequent allergic sting reactions following a single sting.

IMMUNITY

Studies of immunity to insect venoms were initially carried out with beekeepers, who are stung frequently and generally have minor or no local reactions (23). Beekeepers have high levels of serum venom-specific IgG, correlating to some extent with the amount of venom exposure (stings). These IgG antibodies are capable of blocking *in vitro* venom-induced histamine release from basophils of allergic individuals. In addition, administration of hyperimmune gammaglobulin obtained from beekeepers provided temporary immunity from venom anaphylaxis in sensitive individuals (24). Successful venom immunotherapy is accompanied by the production of high titers of venom-specific IgG. These observations suggest that IgG antibodies reacting with venom have a protective function.

DIAGNOSTIC TESTS

Individual honeybee (*Apis mellifera*), yellow jacket (*Vespula* species), yellow hornet (*Vespula arenaria*), bald-face hornet (*Vespula maculata*), and wasp (*Polistes* species) extracts are available for the diagnosis and therapy of stinging insect allergy. Honeybee venom is obtained by electric stimulation. The vespid venoms (yellow jacket, hornet, and wasp) are obtained by dissecting and crushing the individual venom sacs. People with relevant stinging insect histories should undergo skin tests with the appropriate dilutions of each of the available five single Hymenoptera venom preparations. Venom dilutions must be made with a special diluent that contains human serum albumin. Testing is initiated with venom concentrations of 0.01 to 0.0001 μg/mL. The initial studies of venom skin tests concluded that an immunologically specific reaction suggesting that the

patient is sensitive is a reaction of 1+ or greater at a concentration of 1 μg/mL or less, provided the 1+ reaction is greater than that of a diluent control (25). Reactions to only 1 μg/mL must be evaluated carefully because another study of skin test reactions in an insect nonallergic population showed that 46% of individuals reacted to this concentration of at least one venom (26). This study suggested that 0.1 μg/mL might be a better cutoff point between immunologically specific and irritative skin tests reactions. Venom concentrations higher then 1 μg/mL cause nonspecific or irritative reactions and do not distinguish the insect-nonallergic from the insect-allergic population.

In vitro tests have been used for the diagnosis of stinging insect allergy. IgE antibodies have been measured by the radioallergosorbent test (RAST) (27,28) and by histamine release from leukocytes (29). In general, about 15% to 20% of people who had positive venom skin tests do not react to the RAST. This may be a reflection of the sensitivity of the test. Conversely, the RAST results are affected by other factors, including the type and concentration of venom used for coupling and the presence of serum venom-specific IgG that could interfere by competing for the radiolabeled antisera. The RAST remains an excellent procedure for quantifying antibody titers over time. Rare patients have been reported who have negative skin tests and positive RASTs, usually in low titer, and are clinically allergic (30). Currently, there is no explanation to resolve this apparent discrepancy in the sensitivity of the *in vivo* and *in vitro* tests. This issue has practical significance because many allergists, including myself, believe that a negative skin test reaction indicates lack of or loss of clinical venom allergy. Further insight into this problem will require more analyses of this specific RAST, which is done at one laboratory.

Histamine release from leukocytes is basically a laboratory procedure too cumbersome for routine diagnostic evaluation.

THERAPY

People who have a history of systemic reactions after an insect sting and have detectable venom-specific IgE (positive skin tests or

RAST) are considered at risk for subsequent reactions. Recommendations for therapy include measures to minimize exposure to insects, availability of emergency medication for medical treatment of anaphylaxis, and specific venom immunotherapy.

Avoidance

The risk for insect stings may be minimized by the use of simple precautions. Individuals at risk should protect themselves with shoes and long pants or slacks when in grass or fields and should wear gloves when gardening. Cosmetics, perfumes, and hair sprays, which attract insects, should be avoided. Black and dark colors also attract insects; individuals should choose white or light-colored clothes. Food and odors attract insects; thus, garbage should be well wrapped and covered, and care should be taken with outdoor cooking and eating.

Medical Therapy

Acute allergic reactions from the insect stings are treated in the same manner as anaphylaxis from any cause. See Chapter 20 for specific recommendations. Patients at risk are taught to self-administer epinephrine and are advised to keep epinephrine and antihistamine preparations available. Epinephrine is available in preloaded syringes (Ana-Kit, Bayer Corporation, West Haven, CT; EpiPen, Dey Pharmaceuticals, Napa, CA) and can be administered easily. Consideration should be given to having an identification bracelet describing their insect allergy.

Venom Immunotherapy

Venom immunotherapy has been shown to be highly effective in preventing subsequent sting reactions (31,32). Successful therapy is associated with the production of venom-specific IgG, which appears to be the immunologic corollary to clinical immunity. Current recommendations are to administer venom immunotherapy to individuals who have had sting anaphylaxis and have positive venom skin tests. As discussed previously, recent studies of the natural history of the disease process in untreated patients have led to observations that modify this recommendation.

TABLE 12.1. *Indications for venom immunotherapy in patients with positive venom skin tests[a]*

Insect sting reaction	Venom immunotherapy
"Normal"—transient pain, swelling	No
Extensive local swelling	No
Anaphylaxis—severe	Yes
Anaphylaxis—moderate	Yes[b]
Anaphylaxis—mild; dermal only	
Children	No
Adults	Yes[b]
Serum sickness	Yes
Toxic	Yes

[a] Venom immunotherapy is not indicated for individuals with negative venom skin tests.
[b] Patients in these groups might be managed without immunotherapy. See text.

The presence of IgE antibody in an individual who has had a previous systemic reaction does not necessarily imply that a subsequent reaction will occur on reexposure. Observations relevant to the decision to use venom immunotherapy include age, interval since the sting reaction, and the nature of the anaphylactic symptoms. Immunotherapy guidelines are summarized in Tables 12.1 through 12.3.

Patient Selection

Children who have dermal manifestations alone as the sole sign of anaphylaxis do not require

TABLE 12.2. *General venom immunotherapy dosing guidelines*

Initial dose	Dose of 0.01 to 0.1 μg, depending on degree of skin test reaction
Incremental doses	Schedules vary from "rush" therapy, administering multiple venom injections over several days, to traditional once-weekly injections.
Maintenance dose	Dose of 50 to 100 μg of single venoms, 300 μg of mixed vespid venom
Maintenance interval	4 wk, 1st yr 6 wk, 2nd yr 8 wk, 3rd yr
Duration of therapy	Stop if 1) skin test becomes negative, 2) finite time; 3 to 5 yr (see text).

TABLE 12.3. *Representative examples of venom immunotherapy dosing schedules[a]*

	Traditional	Modified rush	Rush	
Day				
1	0.1	0.1	0.1[b]	3.0
		0.3	0.3	5.0
		0.6	0.6	10.0
			1.0	
			20.0	
2			35.0	
			50.0[c]	
			75.0	
3			100.0	
Week				
1	0.3	1.0		
		3.0		
2	1.0	5.0	100	
		10.0	Repeat every 4 wk	
3	3.0	20.0		
4	5.0	35.0		
5	10.0	50.0[c]		
6	20.0	65.0		
7	35.0	80.0		
8	50.0[c]	100.0		
9	65.0			
10	80.0	100.0		
11	100.0	Repeat every 4 wk		
12				
13	100.0			
	Repeat every 4 wk			

[a] Starting dose may vary depending on patients' skin test sensitivity. Subsequent doses modified by local or systemic reactions. Doses expressed in micrograms.
[b] Sequential venom doses administered on same day at 20- to 30-min intervals.
[c] 50 μg may be used as top dose.

venom immunotherapy and can be treated with keeping symptomatic medication available (Table 12.1). Adults who have had mild symptoms of anaphylaxis, such as dermal reactions only, probably could be managed similarly. However, because the documentation for the benign prognosis in adults has not been as well substantiated, this decision requires full patient discussion and concurrence. The recommendation to have epinephrine available is not a benign one. There is often great concern, justifiably so, that epinephrine is always available, such as in school, the work environment, and recreational areas, and that personnel have been trained to administer the medication. An equally important aspect is the duration of this recommendation, especially in children—how long is it necessary to prescribe epinephrine? The results of venom skin tests may resolve this question. If venom skin tests are negative, there should be no risk for anaphylaxis, and epinephrine availability should be unnecessary. It is reasonable to repeat skin tests every 2 to 3 years in this situation.

All people who have had more severe symptoms of anaphylaxis, such as respiratory distress, hypotension, or upper airway edema, should receive venom immunotherapy, regardless of the time interval since the sting reaction. There is a small minority of people who have had venom anaphylaxis but do not have positive venom skin tests (33). They are not considered candidates for venom immunotherapy. The mechanism for their reaction remains unclear. As mentioned previously, after uneventful stings, a small percentage of individuals have positive skin tests, which are usually transient. In this situation, venom immunotherapy is not recommended.

Because of this discrepancy in the actual incidence of re-sting reactions as compared with the number of individuals who are considered at potential risk, a diagnostic sting challenge has been suggested as a criterion for initiating venom immunotherapy. In a large study by van derLinden and associates (34), sting challenges elicited reactions in 25% to 52% of people potentially at risk. This reaction rate is even lower than that described in earlier studies. In this study, the selection of patients for these sting challenges was dependent on a history of an insect sting reaction and a positive skin test. The volume of venom used for intradermal testing was 0.1 mL, which is about five times the volume usually recommended. For this reason, it is not clear that all of the patients enrolled in the study would have been considered clinically potentially allergic by our usual criteria.

Safety, reliability, and practicality are pertinent to the general application of the sting challenge. Observations after both field stings and intentional sting challenges have shown that 20% of potentially allergic individuals who initially tolerate an insect re-sting will react to a subsequent re-sting (17,35). Thus, the credibility of a single sting challenge can be questioned. The issue is further confused by recent observations by Kagey-Sobotka and colleagues (36), who found differences in the incidence of sting challenge reactions induced by stings of two different yellow jacket species. Also, safety is a serious concern because life-threatening reactions have occurred after these intentional diagnostic sting challenges. Testing must be carefully monitored, and medication must be available for treatment of possible acute anaphylaxis. It is very impractical, if not impossible, to suggest that all candidates for venom immunotherapy have a sting challenge. Unfortunately, there are no clinical or immunologic data from these challenge studies that can reliably identify potential reactors or nonreactors.

Venom Selection

The commercial venom product brochure recommends immunotherapy with each venom to which the patient is sensitive, as determined by the skin test reaction. Applying this criterion, one or multiple venoms may be administered. A mixed vespid venom preparation composed of equal parts of yellow jacket, yellow hornet, and bald-face hornet venoms, is available.

The area of venom selection is also controversial. The issue is whether multiple positive skin tests indicate specific individual venom allergy or reflect cross-reactivity between venoms. Extensive studies have been carried out on cross-reactivity among venoms. The honeybees (apids) and yellow jackets, hornets, and wasps (vespids) are in different families. Within the vespid family, there is extensive cross-reactivity between the two hornet venoms (37), extensive cross-reactivity between the yellow jacket and hornet venoms (38), and limited cross-reactivity between wasp venom and other vespid venoms (39). In our experience, most patients who have had yellow jacket sting reactions have positive skin test reactions to hornet venom and occasionally to *Polistes* species venom. Thus, it is very common to find multiple vespid skin test reactions in individuals who have reacted to one of the vespids. The product brochure recommends treatment with each of these vespid venoms. In our experience, when the causative insect can be positively identified (particularly, the yellow jacket), single vespid venoms may be given with satisfactory protection (32).

The relationship between honeybee venom and yellow jacket venom is more complex (40). RAST inhibition studies using serum from patients with coexisting titers of honeybee venom and yellow jacket venom-specific IgE have shown different patterns of reactivity, ranging from no cross-reaction to fairly extensive cross-reaction. For an individual patient, this procedure is too tedious and not available to define the pattern. Knowledge of these results, however, may help suggest that single venom therapy would be adequate.

Dosing Schedule

The basic approach to venom immunotherapy is similar to other forms of allergy immunotherapy (Tables 12.2 and 12.3). Therapy is initiated in small doses, usually from 0.01 to 0.1 μg, and incremental doses are given until a recommended dose of 100 μg is reached. Several dosing schedules have been used. The usual schedule suggests two or three injections during early visits, with doses being doubled or tripled at 30-minute intervals. When higher doses are reached, a single dose is given each week. Other schedules call for more traditional dosing, with one injection per week throughout the buildup period. At the other end of the spectrum, rush desensitization has been given, with multiple doses administered to patients in a hospital setting over a period of 2 to 3 days to 1 week. The most important goal of venom therapy is to reach the recommended 100-μg dose of a single venom or 300-μg of mixed vespid venom. Maintenance doses are given every 4 weeks during the first year. Thereafter, the maintenance interval usually can be extended to 6 or even 8 weeks with no loss of clinical effectiveness or increase in immunotherapy reactions (41,42).

In our experience, 50 μg may be used as the top venom dose. Using this maximum dose and primarily single-venom therapy, results with immunotherapy have been excellent, with an approximate 98% success rate (32).

The more rapid schedules appear to be accompanied by a more rapid increase in venom-specific IgG production, and thus this schedule might provide protection earlier (43). Reaction rates to venom administered by both rapid and slower schedules vary in different studies but are not significantly different.

Reactions to Therapy

As with other allergenic extracts, reactions can occur from venom immunotherapy. The usual reactions are fairly typical large local reactions lasting several days, and immediate systemic reactions. These reactions may present more of a problem, however, because to ensure clinical protection, it is necessary to reach full maintenance doses of venom. With other allergenic extracts, such as pollen, doses are usually decreased and maintained at lower levels. Treatment of local reactions includes splitting of doses, thus limiting the amount of venom delivered at one site, cold compresses, and antihistamines.

In the large study of insect sting allergy conducted by the American Academy of Allergy and Immunology, the incidence of venom systemic reactions was about 10% (44). There were no identifiable factors predicting these reactions. After a systemic reaction, the next dose is reduced by about 25% to 50%, depending on the severity of the reaction, and subsequent doses are slowly increased. If patients are receiving multiple venom therapy, it might be useful to give individual venom on separate days. This may help identify the specific venom responsible for the reaction.

Another adverse reaction occasionally noted after injections of other allergenic extracts but more frequently with venom is the occurrence of generalized fatigue and aching often associated with large local swelling. Prevention of these reactions can usually be accomplished with aspirin, 650 mg, given about 30 minutes before the venom injection and repeated every 4 hours as needed. If this therapy is ineffective, steroids may be administered at the same time as venom injection.

Most people who have had reactions to venom immunotherapy are ultimately able to reach maintenance doses. On rare occasions, systemic reactions have necessitated cessation of treatment.

There have been no identified adverse reactions from long-term venom immunotherapy. Venom injections appear to be safe during pregnancy, with no adverse effect to either pregnancy or the fetus (45).

Monitoring Therapy

Venom immunotherapy is associated with immunologic responses, which include rising titers of serum venom-specific IgG and, over a period of time, decreasing titers of serum venom-specific IgE. One criterion for stopping venom immunotherapy (discussed later) is the conversion to a negative venom skin test. For this reason, venom-treated patients should have repeat venom skin tests about every 2 years.

As discussed earlier, serum venom-specific IgG is associated with the development of immunity to insect stings. Initial evidence for the role of venom-specific IgG came from studies of beekeepers, who are a highly immune population, the antithesis of the allergic individual. More specific documentation of this protective role was provided by the results of passive administration of hyperimmune gammaglobulin, obtained from beekeepers, to honeybee-allergic people and the subsequent inhibition of allergic reactions following a venom challenge. Studies of people receiving venom immunotherapy have suggested that, at least in early months, this antibody might be responsible for the loss of clinical sensitivity.

Golden and colleagues (46) compared people who failed venom immunotherapy treatment continued to have sting-induced systemic reactions with successfully treated people and suggested that the difference was related to lower titers of serum venom-specific IgG. A group of patients with a serum IgG antibody level greater than 3 μg/mL had a 1.6% re-sting reaction rate, compared with a group of patients with serum levels less than 3 μg/mL who had a 16% reaction rate. These data applied only to yellow jacket venom-allergic people treated for less than 4 years. There was no correlation between honeybee-specific IgG and re-sting reaction rates. The authors recommended periodic monitoring of serum venom-specific IgG in order to detect potential treatment failures, which then would dictate an increase in the venom immunotherapy dose. Careful review of individual data suggested, however, that there was not a close relationship between treatment failure and IgG response (47). There was lack of reproducible reactions to sting challenges in people with low antibody titers. There was no documentation that increased antibody responses induced by higher venom doses were clinically effective. The data could not be applied to yellow jacket–allergic people treated for more than 4 years or to honeybee-allergic people. Thus, in my opinion, review of this study and other relevant data, particularly the remarkable success rate of venom immunotherapy, does not support the routine measurement of venom-specific IgG. From a practical viewpoint, there is little clinical reason to measure venom-specific IgG as part of the overall management and treatment of venom-allergic people.

Cessation of Venom Immunotherapy

The adequate duration of venom immunotherapy (i.e., the timing of its cessation) is probably the most common concern and question raised by allergists. Germane to this question are two major observations. First, for many individuals, insect sting allergy is a self-limiting process. This is the only explanation for the 50-year-old belief that whole insect body extracts, now recognized as impotent, seemed to be effective treatment. Second is the clinical observation that not all individuals with positive venom skin tests and a history of venom-induced anaphylaxis will continue to have clinical reactions when re-stung. Thus, in analyzing the appropriate criteria for discontinuing therapy, this spontaneous loss of clinical allergy must be appreciated.

Two major criteria have been suggested as guidelines for discontinuing treatment:

1. Conversion to a negative venom skin test
2. A finite period of treatment, usually 3 to 5 years, despite the persistence of a positive venom skin test

The second criterion is influenced by a number of issues, such as the nature of the initial anaphylactic symptoms, reactions during venom immunotherapy, perhaps the specific insect causing the reaction, and the general physical health of the individual, particularly the presence of significant cardiovascular disease. These issues are reviewed in detail in a position paper from the Insect Committee of the American Academy of Allergy, Asthma and Immunology (48).

Conversion to a negative venom skin test should be an absolute criterion for stopping venom immunotherapy. This conclusion is supported by several studies and is obviously a rational decision. If the immunologic mediator of venom anaphylaxis, an IgE antibody, is no longer present, there should no longer be any risk for anaphylaxis. In individuals who have had severe anaphylactic reactions, the lack of specific IgE can be confirmed with a serum antibody assay. As noted, there have been rare anecdotal reports of individuals who apparently had allergic reactions from insect stings despite a negative venom skin test. These observations need much further

TABLE 12.4. *Re-sting reactions after stopping venom immunotherapy—selected reports*

Investigators (ref.)	No. of patients	Results (venom immunotherapy duration)	Reaction
Lerch & Müller (49)	200	>3 yr	25 (12.5%)
Haugaard et al (50)	25	3–7 yr	0
Golden et al (51)	74	5 yr	7 (10%)
Reisman (52)	113	2–5 yr	10 (9%)

analysis before concern is raised that conversion to a negative skin test should not be an acceptable absolute criterion to stop treatment.

Because a positive skin test does not necessarily imply continued clinical sensitivity, a number of studies have explored the efficacy of a finite period of treatment, usually 3 to 5 years, in the presence of a persistently positive skin test. The skin test is a very sensitive test, as exemplified by people with burned-out ragweed hayfever who continue to have a positive test indefinitely. In venom studies, the re-sting reaction rate after cessation of venom immunotherapy in this setting is usually low, generally in the range of 5% to 10%. Four of the studies that reported re-sting reactions after cessation of venom immunotherapy are summarized in Table 12.4. Lerch and Müller (49), Haugaard and associates (50), and Golden and colleagues (51) reported the results of intentional sting challenges in patients off immunotherapy, usually for 1 to 2 years. The re-sting reaction rates ranged from 0% to 12.5%. Our studies used field re-stings and found a 9% re-sting reaction rate; these data were further analyzed in relationship to the severity of the initial anaphylactic reaction (52). There were 25 patients who had initial mild anaphylaxis; no reactions occurred after re-stings. Forty-one patients had had initial moderate reactions; three had re-sting reactions. In the group of 47 patients who had severe anaphylaxis, as defined by loss of consciousness, respiratory distress, hypotension, or upper airway edema, there was a 15% re-sting reaction rate. Unfortunately, the severity of the allergic reaction, when it did occur, was often the same as the initial reaction preceding venom immunotherapy. In our study (52) and that of Lerch and Müller (49), no re-sting reactions occurred in the presence of a negative venom skin test. For

most individuals, the loss of clinical sensitivity is permanent, with no reactions to subsequent re-stings once therapy is stopped for the appropriate reasons.

In one study (53) in which we examined a decrease in serum antibody levels to insignificant levels as a criterion for stopping treatment, the control group included patients who stopped by self-choice. It was interesting to see that the average time of therapy was about 2 years both in the patients who stopped because of a decreased RAST and in those patients who stopped by self-choice. The re-sting reaction rate was very close in both groups, about 10%. Thus, 2 years of treatment may significantly reduce the risk for reactions from about 60% in untreated individuals to only 10%.

Other factors have been suggested as related to increased risk for a re-sting reaction after stopping therapy and are outlined in Table 12.5. There is no association with gender or presence of atopy. As already noted, more severe initial reactions are associated with increase risk. Re-sting reaction risk may be higher in adults, in honeybee-allergic people, in people who have had systemic reactions to venom immunotherapy, and in people whose degree of skin test reactivity is unchanged during immunotherapy.

My current recommendations for stopping treatment are as follows:

1. Conversion to a negative venom skin test is an absolute criterion for stopping treatment. This may occur at any time whether treatment has been given for 1 or 5 years.
2. For people who have had mild to moderate anaphylactic symptoms and retain positive venom skin tests, 3 years of treatment is sufficient. This decision is influenced by

TABLE 12.5. *Potential risk factors related to risk of re-sting reaction after stopping therapy*

Parameter	Re-sting risk
Age	Increased in adults
Atopy	No association
Sex	No association
Insect species	Increased with honeybee
Initial anaphylaxis	Increased with more severe reaction
Venom immunotherapy tolerance	Increased with reactions to therapy
Skin test reactivity	Increased if unchanged during therapy

consideration of other medical problems, concomitant medication, patient lifestyle, and patient preference.

3. For individuals who have had severe anaphylaxis as exemplified by hypotension, loss of consciousness, or upper airway edema, therapy is administered indefinitely as long as the skin test remains positive. It is important to point out that maintenance venom therapy is given every 8 weeks and even at longer intervals after 3 years.

FIRE ANT AND HARVESTER ANT STINGS

Systemic reactions to the stings of the fire ant have been reported with increasing frequency (54,55). This insect is present in growing numbers in the southeastern United States, particularly in states bordering the Gulf Coast, and has now spread into Virginia and California. The fire ant attaches itself to its victim by biting with its jaws and then pivots around its head, stinging in multiple sites in a circular pattern with a stinger located on the abdomen. Within 24 hours of the sting, a sterile pustule develops that is diagnostic of the fire ant sting. Allergic symptoms occurring after stings are typical of acute anaphylaxis. Fatalities have occurred in children and adults. Recently, indoor massive sting attacks by fire ants have been reported.

Skin tests with extracts prepared from whole bodies of fire ants appear to be reliable in identifying allergic individuals, with few false-positive reactions in nonallergic controls. Fire ant venom, not commercially available at present, has been collected and compared with fire ant whole-body extract. The results of skin tests and *in vitro* tests show that the venom is a better diagnostic antigen. Whole-body extracts can be prepared, however, that apparently contain sufficient allergen and are reliable for skin test diagnosis. These results suggest that the antigens responsible for allergic reactions can be preserved in the preparation of whole-body extracts. Unfortunately, the potency of different commercial fire ant whole-body extracts has been variable. Future availability of fire ant venom will provide a potent, reliable extract.

Fire ant venom has been well studied and differs considerably from other Hymenoptera venoms. Studies have shown four allergenic fractions in the fire ant venom (56).

Immunotherapy with whole-body fire ant extract appears to be quite effective. Because the whole-body fire ant extract can be a good diagnostic agent, this therapeutic response might be anticipated. It is important, however, that control observations studying the response of subsequent stings in allergic individuals not receiving venom immunotherapy have been limited. There has been one study comparing the results of fire ant re-stings in whole-body extract–treated patients and untreated patients (57). In the treated group, there were 47 re-stings, with one systemic reaction. In contrast, of the 11 untreated patients, 6 patients had 11 re-stings, all of which resulted in systemic reactions. Serologic studies defining the nature of the immunity to fire ant stings have not been conducted.

In vitro studies suggest there is some cross-reaction between the major allergens in fire ant venom and the winged Hymenoptera venoms. The clinical significance of this observation is still unclear; there appears to be limited clinical application. Individuals allergic to bees and vespids do not appear to be at major risk for fire ant reactions, and similarly, fire ant–allergic individuals are not at major risk for reactions from the winged Hymenoptera.

Anaphylaxis from the sting of the harvester ant, another nonwinged Hymenoptera present in the southwestern United States, has been described (58). Specific IgE antibodies have been detected with direct skin tests and leukocyte histamine release using harvester ant venom.

In summary, hypersensitivity reactions to ants, especially fire ants, have become clinically important. Fire ant venom has been analyzed, and many of the antigens are cross-reactive among the species. Fire ant whole-body extract has also been characterized and is known to contain venom antigens. Fire ant allergy will likely become a more important clinical problem as the ants spread, as the human population grows in the southern United States, and as the land is cultivated to favor their habitation.

REFERENCES

1. McKenna WR. Killer bees: what the allergist should know. *Pediatr Asthma Allergy Immunol* 1992;4:275–285.
2. Brummer-Korvenkontio H, Lappalainen P, Reunala T, et al. Detection of mosquito saliva-specific IgE and IgG$_4$ antibodies by immunobloting. *J Allergy Clin Immunol* 1994;93:551–555.
3. Mauriello PM, Barde SH, Georgitis JW, et al. Natural history of large local reactions (LLR) to stinging insects. *J Allergy Clin Immunol* 1984;74:494–498.
4. Golden DBK. Epidemiology of allergy to insect venoms and stings. *Allergy Proc* 1989;10:103–107.
5. Chaffee FH. The prevalence of bee sting allergy in an allergic population. *Acta Allergol* 1970;25:292–293.
6. Settipane GA, Boyd GK. Prevalence of bee sting allergy in 4,992 boy scouts. *Acta Allergol* 1970;25:286–297.
7. Brown H, Bernton HS. Allergy to the Hymenoptera. *Arch Intern Med* 1970;125:665–669.
8. Frazier CA. Allergic reactions to insect stings: a review of 180 cases. *South Med J* 1964;57:1028–1034.
9. Mueller HL. Further experiences with severe allergic reactions to insect stings. *N Engl J Med* 1959;261:374–377.
10. Mueller HL, Schmid WH, Rubinsztain R. Stinging insect hypersensitivity: a 20 year study of immunologic treatment. *Pediatrics* 1975;55:530–535.
11. Schwartz HJ, Kahn B. Hymenoptera sensitivity. II. The role of atopy in the development of clinical hypersensitivity. *J Allergy* 1970;45:87–91.
12. Barnard JH. Nonfatal results in third degree anaphylaxis from Hymenoptera stings. *J Allergy* 1970;45:92–96.
13. Jensen OM. Sudden death due to stings from bees and wasps. *Acta Pathol Microbiol Scand* (A) 1962;54:9–29.
14. O'Connor R, Stier RA, Rosenbrook W Jr, et al. Death from "wasp" sting. *Ann Allergy* 1964;22:385–393.
15. Schenken JR, Tamisiea J, Winter FD. Hypersensitivity to bee sting. *Am J Clin Pathol* 1953:23:1216–1221.
16. Golden DBK, Marsh DG, Freidhoff LR, et al. Natural history of Hymenoptera venom sensitivity in adults. *J Allergy Clin Immunol* 1997;100:760–766.
17. Reisman RE. Natural history of insect sting allergy: relationship of severity of symptoms of initial sting anaphylaxis to re-sting reactions. *J Allergy Clin Immunol* 1992;90:335–339.
18. Valentine MD, Schuberth KC, Kagey-Sobotka A, et al. The value of immunotherapy with venom in children with allergy to insect stings. *N Engl J Med* 1991;23:1601–1603.
19. Lantner R, Reisman RE. Clinical and immunologic features and subsequent course of patients with severe insect sting anaphylaxis. *J Allergy Clin Immunol* 1989;84:900–906.
20. Reisman RE, Livingston A. Late onset reactions including serum sickness, following insect stings. *J Allergy Clin Immunol* 1989;84:331–337.
21. Light WC, Reisman RE, Shimizu M, et al. Unusual reactions following insect stings. *J Allergy Clin Immunol* 1977;59:391–397.
22. Hoffman DR. Hymenoptera venoms: composition, standardization, stability. In: Levine MI, Lockey RF, ed. *Monograph on insect allergy.* American Academy of Allergy and Immunology, 1995:27–38.
23. Light WC, Reisman RE, Wypych JI, et al. Clinical and immunological studies of beekeepers. *Clin Allergy* 1975;5:389–395.
24. Lessof MH, Sobotka AK, Lichtenstein LM. Effects of passive antibody in bee venom anaphylaxis. *Johns Hopkins Med J* 1978;142:1–7.
25. Hunt KJ, Valentine MD, Sobotka AK, et al. Diagnosis of allergy to stinging insects by skin testing with Hymenoptera venoms. *Ann Intern Med* 1976;85:56–59.
26. Georgitis JW, Reisman RE. Venom skin tests in insect-allergic and insect non-allergic populations. *J Allergy Clin Immunol* 1985;76:803–807.
27. Reisman RE, Wypych JI, Arbesman CE. Stinging insect allergy: detection and clinical significance of venom IgE antibodies. *J Allergy Clin Immunol* 1975;56:443–449.
28. Sobotka AK, Adkinson JF Jr, Valentine MD, et al. Allergy to insect stings. V. Diagnosis by radioallergosorbent tests (RAST). *J Immunol* 1978;121:2477–2484.
29. Sobotka AK, Valentine MD, Benton AW, et al. Allergy to insect stings. I. Diagnosis of IgE-mediated Hymenoptera sensitivity by venom induced histamine release. *J Allergy Clin Immunol* 1974;53:170–184.
30. Golden DBK, Kagen-Sobotka A, Bailey D, et al. Sting challenge (sc) trial IV: the history positive skin test negative patient. *J Allergy Clin Immunol* 2000;104:S376–377.
31. Valentine MD. Insect venom allergy: diagnosis and treatment. *J Allergy Clin Immunol* 1984;73:299–304.
32. Reisman RE, Livingston A. Venom immunotherapy (VIT): ten years experience with administration of single venoms and fifty micrograms maintenance doses. *J Allergy Clin Immunol* 1992;89:1185–1189.
33. Clayton WF, Georgitis JW, Reisman RE. Insect sting anaphylaxis in patients without detectable serum venom specific IgE. *J Allergy Clin Immunol* 1983;71(II):141.

34. van derLinden PWH, Hack CE, Struyvenberg A, et al. Insect-sting challenge in 324 subjects with a previous anaphylactic reaction: current criteria for insect-venom hypersensitivity do not predict the occurrence and severity of anaphylaxis. *J Allergy Clin Immunol* 1994;94: 151–159.

35. Franklin HH, DuBois EAJ, Minkema HJ, et al. Lack of reproducibility of a single negative sting challenge response in the assessment of anaphylactic risk in patient with suspected yellow jacket hypersensitivity. *J Allergy Clin Immunol* 1994;93:431–435.

36. Sobotka AK, Golden DBK, Guralnick M, et al. Sting challenge (sc) trial III: variables affecting the outcome of insect sting. *J Allergy Clin Immunol* 2000;104:5377.

37. Mueller U, Elliott W, Reisman RE, et al. Comparison of biochemical and immunologic properties of venoms from the four hornet species. *J Allergy Clin Immunol* 1981;67:290–298.

38. Reisman RE, Mueller U, Wypych J, et al. Comparison of the allergenicity and antigenicity of yellow jacket and hornet venoms. *J Allergy Clin Immunol* 1982;69: 268–274.

39. Reisman RE, Wypych JI, Mueller UR, et al. Comparison of the allergenicity and antigenicity of Polistes venom and other vespid venoms. *J Allergy Clin Immunol* 1982;70:281–287.

40. Reisman RE, Mueller UR, Wypych JI, et al. Studies of coexisting honeybee and vespid venom sensitivity. *J Allergy Clin Immunol* 1983;73:246–252.

41. Goldberg A, Reisman RE. Prolonged interval maintenance venom immunotherapy. *Ann Allergy* 1988;61: 177–119.

42. Golden DBK, Kagey-Sobotka A, Valentine MD, et al. Prolonged maintenance interval in Hymenoptera venom immunotherapy. *J Allergy Clin Immunol* 1987;67: 482–484.

43. Golden DBK, Valentine MD, Sobotka AK, et al. Regimens of Hymenoptera venom immunotherapy. *Ann Intern Med* 1980;92:620–624.

44. Lockey R, Peppe B, Barid I, et al. Hymenoptera venom study, safety. *J Allergy Clin Immunol* 1983;71:141(abst).

45. Schwartz HJ, Golden DBK, Lockey RF. Venom immunotherapy in the Hymenoptera allergic pregnant patient. *J Allergy Clin Immunol* 1990;85: 709–712.

46. Golden DBK, Lawrence ID, Hamilton RH, et al. Clinical correlations of the venom specific IgG antibody level during maintenance venom immunotherapy. *J Allergy Clin Immunol* 1992;90:386–393.

47. Reisman RE. Should routine measures of serum venom specified IgG be a standard of practice in patients receiving venom immunotherapy? *J Allergy Clin Immunol* 1992;90:282–284.

48. Position Statement. Report from the Committee on Insects. American Academy of Allergy, Asthma and Immunology. *J Allergy Clin Immunol* 1998;101:573–575.

49. Lerch E, Müller UR. Long-term protection after stopping venom immunotherapy: results of restings in 200 patients. *J Allergy Clin Immunol* 1998;101:606–612.

50. Haugaard L, Norregaard OFH, Dahl R. In-hospital sting challenge in insect venom-allergic patients after stopping venom immunotherapy. *J Allergy Clin Immunol* 1991;87:699–702.

51. Golden DBK, Kwiterovich KA, Kagey-Sobotka A, et al. Discontinuing venom immunotherapy: extended observations. *J Allergy Clin Immunol* 1998;101:298–305.

52. Reisman RE. Duration of venom immunotherapy: relationship to the severity of symptoms of initial insect sting anaphylaxis. *J Allergy Clin Immunol* 1993;92: 831–836.

53. Reisman RE, Lantner R. Further observations on discontinuation of venom immunotherapy: comparisons of patients stopped because of a fall in serum venom specific IgE to insignificant levels with patients stopped "prematurely" by self-choice. *J Allergy Clin Immunol* 1989;83:1049–1054.

54. Stafford CT, Hypersensitivity to fire ant venom. *Ann Allergy Asthma Immunol* 1996;77:87–95.

55. Kemp SF, deShazo RD, Moffitt JE, et al. Expanding habitat of the imported fire ant (Solenopsis invicta): a public health concern. *J Allergy Clin Immunol* 2000;105: 683–691.

56. Hoffman DR. Fire ant venom allergy. *Allergy* 1995;50: 535–544.

57. Freeman TM, Hylander R, Ortiz A, et al. Imported fire ant immunotherapy: effectiveness of whole body extracts. *J Allergy Clin Immunol* 1992;90:210–215.

58. Pinnas JL. Strunk RC, Wang TM, et al. Harvester ant sensitivity: in vitro and in vivo studies using whole body extracts and venom. *J Allergy Clin Immunol* 1977;59:10.

13

Urticaria, Angioedema, and Hereditary Angioedema

Carol A. Saltoun and *W. James Metzger

*Division of Allergy-Immunology, Department of Medicine, Northwestern University Medical School, Chicago, Illinois; *Allergy, Asthma and Immunology, The Brody School of Medicine at Eastern Carolina University, Greenville, North Carolina*

The earliest texts called urticaria and angioedema "a vexing problem" (1). Little has changed since that assessment. Today's clinician is still faced with a common syndrome that affects 20% of the population at some time in their lives (2), but there is no cohesive understanding of the many clinical mechanisms, presentations, or clinical management of the urticarias. For the clinician, this requires a broad knowledge of the many clinical forms of urticaria and an even more extensive familiarity with the creative ways that medications and treatment can be applied. Modern concepts of allergen-induced cellular inflammation, late-phase cutaneous responses, adhesion molecules, cytokines, and inflammatory autocoids, are leading to a better understanding of pathogenesis and treatment. Meanwhile, clinicians should formulate a rational approach to the care of patients with these conditions.

Urticarial lesions can have diverse appearances. Generally they consist of raised, erythematous skin lesions that are markedly pruritic, tend to be evanescent in any one location, are usually worsened by scratching, and always blanch with pressure. Individual lesions typically resolve within 24 hours and leave no residual skin changes. This description does not cover all forms of urticaria, but it includes the features necessary for diagnosis in most clinical situations. Angioedema is frequently associated with urticaria, but the two may occur independently. Angioedema is similar to urticaria, except that it occurs in deeper tissues and is often asymmetric. Because there are fewer mast cells and sensory nerve endings in these deeper tissues, pruritus is less common with angioedema, which more typically involves a tingling or burning sensation. Although urticaria may occur on any area of the body, angioedema most often affects the perioral region, periorbital regions, tongue, genitalia, and extremities. In this review, angioedema and urticaria are discussed jointly except where specified.

The incidence of acute urticaria is not known. Although it is said to afflict 10% to 20% of the population at some time during life, it is most common in young adults (1). Chronic urticaria occurs more frequently in middle-aged persons, especially women. In a family practice office, its prevalence has been reported to be 30% (3). If patients have chronic urticaria for more than 6 months, 40% will continue to have recurrent wheals 10 years later (4). It is possible that the true prevalence of urticaria is higher than reported owing to many acute, self-limited episodes that do not come to medical attention.

Acute urticaria is arbitrarily defined as persisting for less than 6 weeks, whereas chronic urticaria refers to episodes lasting more than 6 to 8 weeks. When considering chronic urticaria, an

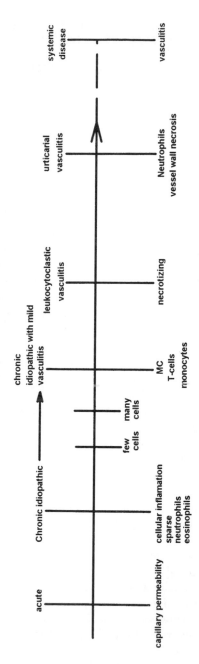

FIG. 13.1. A hypothetical model for describing the range of histology of chronic idiopathic urticaria.

etiologic agent or precipitating cause such as a physical urticaria is established in up to 30% of patients who are thoroughly evaluated (5). However, most chronic urticaria is idiopathic. Success rates of determining an inciting agent are higher in acute forms. Because of the sometimes extreme discomfort and cosmetic problems associated with chronic urticaria, a thorough evaluation to search for etiologic factors is recommended. This evaluation should rely primarily on the history and physical examination and response to therapy; limited laboratory evaluation may be indicated (see Fig. 13.2).

PATHOGENESIS

There is no unifying concept to account for all forms of urticaria. Histamine plays a major role in many forms, based first on the observations by Lewis (6) of a cutaneous "triple response" characterized by erythema, edema, and flare due to an axon reflex, possibly mediated by substance P. Erythema and edema are mimicked by intracutaneous injection of histamine, causing localized pruritus, a major characteristic of urticaria. The hypothesis that histamine is the central mediator of urticaria is bolstered by (a) the cutaneous response to injected histamine; (b) the frequent clinical response of various forms of urticaria to therapeutic antihistamines; (c) the documented elevation of plasma histamine or local histamine release from "urticating" tissue in some forms of the condition; and (d) the apparent degranulation of skin mast cells. An association with histamine release, however, has not been made in many forms of urticaria.

Various forms of chronic urticaria have now been associated with eosinophil granule proteins presumed to be capable of causing prolonged inflammation of the skin (7). Cytokines, such as interleukin-5 (IL-5), may be responsible for the attraction to and maintenance of activated eosinophils at the skin site (7,8). Platelet activating factor (PAF) (9,10) also may be integral to certain urticarias because of its potent eosinophil-chemotactic properties (11), and because very effective medications such as doxepin have PAF antagonist activity among other inhibitory effects (12).

If any central hypothesis for pathogenesis can be formulated, histamine and the skin mast cell certainly play a crucial role in several forms of urticaria (8,13,14). Whether certain subtypes of skin mast cells are characterized by their content of tryptase and/or chymase (8,15) requires further investigation. Although helper T cells are increased (16), activation of T cells is not demonstrable. Dysregulation of E-selectin, intracellular adhesion molecule type 1, and VCAM-1 may account for the former and be precipitated by mast cell–released cytokines (3,16). Autoactivation by discharged substance P may perpetuate the urticaria (9).

Several potential mechanisms for mast cell activation in the skin are summarized in Table 13.1 and include (a) IgE immediate hypersensitivity such as occurs with penicillin or foods, (b) activation of the classical or alternative complement cascades such as occurs in immune complex disease like serum sickness or collagen vascular disease, and (c) direct mast cell membrane activation such as occurs with injection of morphine or radio contrast media. The presence of major basic protein in biopsy samples of chronic urticaria (7) makes the eosinophil suspect as an effector cell. Prolonged response to histamine, but not leukotrienes, in the skin of patients with chronic urticaria may suggest abnormal clearance of mediators locally (17).

Studies attempting to find the etiology of histamine release in chronic urticaria reported that 14% of patients with chronic idiopathic urticaria (CIU) had antithyroid antibodies (18). Treatment of these patients with thyroid hormone has not changed the natural course of the disease, but it may have variable benefit to severity and duration of urticarial lesions. Because of the association between autoimmune thyroid disease and urticaria, researchers began to look for other autoantibodies in patients with chronic urticaria. Greaves (19) reported a 5% to 10% incidence of anti–immunoglobulin E (IgE) antibodies in these patients. Next, the high affinity IgE receptor (FcεRI) was identified and isolated. Shortly thereafter, it was reported that 45 to 50% patients with CIU have anti–IgE receptor antibodies that bind to the α subunit of the IgE receptor, causing activation of mast cells or basophils (20).

TABLE 13.1. *Potential mechanisms of mast cell activation in urticaria or angioedema*

Type	Cause	Mediators
IgE immediate hypersensitivity	Allergens (21) Modified IgE IgG (64) Autoimmune anti-IgE or FcϵRIα FcϵRII (CD23) on platelets, lymphocytes or eosinophils	Histamine leukotrienes PGD2, PAF (9), ECF-A (22), HRF (23)
Activation of classical pathway of complement	Antigen-antibody complexes (IgM IgG1, IgG2, or IgG3)	C3a, C4a, C5a (anaphylatoxins) cause release of MC mediators
Activation of alternative pathway of complement	IgA-antigen complexes, complex polysaccharides, lipopolysaccharides	C3a, C4a, C5a (anaphylatoxins) cause release of MC mediators
Direct activation of mast cell membrane	Morphine, codeine, d-turbocuarine, polymyxin antibiotics, thiamine, certain foods causing histamine release (strawberries)	Opiates act through specific receptors to release histamine Others nonspecifically activate cell membrane to release or generate MC mediators
Plasma-kinin generating system	Activation of plasma and/or tissue Kallikrein or coagulation pathway Negatively charges surfaces, collagen vascular basement membrane or endotoxin	Bradykinin; thrombin activation; especially for HAE (8,27)

Presence and clinical relevance of these autoantibodies can be identified by cutaneous injections of autologous serum resulting in a wheal and flare.

Products from the kinin-generating system have been thought to be important in hereditary angioedema (HAE) (24) and angioedema resulting from angiotensin-converting enzyme (ACE) inhibitors (8). In addition, bradykinin has been reported to be capable of causing a wheal and flare reaction when injected into human skin. Aspirin and nonsteroidal antiinflammatory drugs (NSAIDs) are capable of altering arachidonic acid metabolism and can result in urticaria without specific interaction between IgE and the pharmacologic agent.

Nonspecific factors that may aggravate urticaria include fever, heat, alcohol ingestion, exercise, emotional stress, premenstrual or postmenopausal status, and hyperthyroidism. Anaphylaxis and urticaria due to progesterone have been described (25) but seem to be exceedingly rare, and progesterone has been used to treat chronic cyclic urticaria and eosinophilia (26). Certain food preservatives have been reported to aggravate chronic urticaria (8,27). Many experts experienced in urticaria believe that progesterone is not a cause or a treatment and that food preservatives do not aggravate chronic urticaria.

BIOPSY

Biopsy of urticarial lesions has accomplished less than expected to improve our understanding of the pathogenesis of urticaria. Three major patterns are currently recognized (Table 13.2). Acute and physical urticarias show only dermal edema without cellular infiltrate, whereas chronic urticaria typically shows a perivascular mononuclear or lymphocytic infiltrate with an increased number of mast cells. Urticarial vasculitis—in which lesions last more than 24 hours, may be purpuric, and may heal with residual hyperpigmentation—show neutrophil infiltration and vessel wall necrosis with or without immunoprotein deposition. Further longitudinal and pathogenetic studies may determine if these several pathologic forms of urticaria represent a continuum of disease (Fig. 13.1) or separate pathophysiologic entities.

TABLE 13.2. *Biopsy patterns of urticarial and angioedema lesions*

Type	Description
Acute urticaria/ angioedema	Dilation of small venules and capillaries in superficial dermis (urticaria) or subcutaneous tissue (angioedema); flattening of rete pegs; swollen collagen fibrils (8)
Chronic idiopathic urticaria	Mild cellular inflammation including activated T-lymphocytes, monocytes, and mast cells; delayed-onset urticaria may be mediated by cytokines; eg., IL-1, 3, 5 or HRF (23)
Urticarial vasculitis	Neutrophil infiltration with vessel wall necrosis; occasional deposition of immunoglobulin and complement (8,28)

CLASSIFICATION

Classification in terms of known causes is helpful in evaluating patients with urticaria. Table 13.3 presents one classification that may be clinically useful. Additional knowledge of pre-

cipitating events or mechanisms may simplify this classification (29).

Nonimmunologic

Dermographism

Dermographism literally means "write on skin." This phenomenon may be detected unexpectedly on routine examination, or patients may complain of pruritus and rash, frequently characterized by linear wheals. When questioned carefully, they may state that itching precedes the rash, causing them to scratch and worsen the condition. The cause of this lesion is unknown. Because it appears in approximately 5% of people, it may be a normal variant. Its onset has been described following severe drug reactions and may be confused with vaginitis in evaluating genital pruritus (30). A delayed form has been recognized with onset of lesions three to eight hours after stimulus to the skin, which may be related to delayed pressure urticaria (DPU). It may accompany other forms of urticaria. The lesion is readily demonstrated by lightly stroking the skin of an affected patient with a pointed instrument.

TABLE 13.3. *Classification of urticaria*

Dermographism	Hereditary urticaria	Miscellaneous
Nonimmunologic		
Idiopathic	Hereditary angioedema	Infections
Cutaneous mastocytosis	Hereditary vibratory angioedema	Vasculitis
Adrenergic	Urticaria, deafness, amyloidosis syndrome	Neoplasm
Physical urticaria	Familial localized heat urticaria	Anaphylaxis
Pressure	C3b inactivator deficiency	Recurrent idiopathic
Vibratory	Porphyria	Exercise induced
Solar	Papular urticaria	
Cholinergic	Urticaria pigmentosa	
Local Heat		
Cold		
Immunologic		
Food	Transfusion reactions	
Drugs	Schnitzler's syndrome (89)	
Autoimmune Anti-IgE and/or anti-FcεRI	Atopy	
Insect stings	Acquired C1 INH deficiency	
Identifiable agents (uncertain mechanisms)		
Aspirin	Metabisulfites	
Opiates	Tartrazine	

A dermatographometer (Hook & Tucker Ltd, Croydon, England) can be used to quantify this response. This produces erythema, pruritus, and linear streaks of edema or wheal formation. No antigen, however, has been shown to initiate the response, but dermographism has been passively transferred with plasma. Antihistamines usually ameliorate symptoms if they are present. Cutaneous mastocytosis may be considered under the heading of dermographism, because stroking the skin results in significant wheal formation (Darier sign). This disease is characterized by a diffuse increase in cutaneous mast cells. The skin may appear normal, but is usually marked by thickening and accentuated skin folds.

Physical Urticaria

The physical urticarias are a unique group that constitute up to 17% of chronic urticarias and several reviews have been published (13,31,32). They are frequently missed as a cause of chronic urticaria, and more than one type may occur together in the same patient. Most forms, with the exception of DPU, occur as simple hives without inflammation, and individual lesions resolve within 24 hours. As a group, they can be reproduced by various physical stimuli that have been standardized in some cases (Table 13.4). A new form of "autonomic" urticaria called adrenergic urticaria has been described and can be reproduced by intracutaneous injection of noradrenaline (0.5×10^{-6} M) (33). This unique form of urticaria is characterized by a "halo" of white skin surrounding a small papule. It may have been previously misdiagnosed as cholinergic urticaria because of its small lesions and its association with stress. In this case, however, relief can be provided with β blockers.

Delayed pressure urticaria, with or without angioedema, is clinically characterized by the gradual onset of wheals or edema in areas where pressure has been applied to the skin. Onset is usually 4 to 6 hours after exposure, but wide variations may be noted. An immediate form of pressure urticaria has been observed. The lesion of DPU can be reproduced by applying pressure with motion for 20 minutes (34). DPU may be associated with malaise, fevers, chills, arthralgias,

TABLE 13.4. *Test procedures for physical and chronic idiopathic urticaria*

Test	Procedure
Dermographism	Firmly stoke interscapular skin with tongue blade or dermatographometer
Delayed pressure urticaria	Hang 15-pound weight across shoulder while walking for 20 min
Solar urticaria	Expose skin to defined wavelengths of light
Cholinergic urticaria	1. Methacholine skin test 2. Immersion in hot bath (42°C) to raise body temperature 0.7°C
Local heat urticaria	Apply warm compress to forearm.
Cold urticaria	1. Apply ice cube to forearm for 4 min; observe rewarming for 10 min 2. Exercise in cold and observe for cholinergic-like urticaria (cold-induced cholinergic urticaria)
Aquagenic	Apply water compress (35°C) for 30 min
Vibratory	Laboratory vortex applied gently to mid-forearm for 4 min
Autoimmune	Intradermal injection of autologous serum

and leukocytosis. When chronic urticaria is also present, foods have been rarely reported to precipitate episodes. The mechanism of these reactions is unknown, but biopsy samples of lesions closely resemble aspects of the late cutaneous response (35). Treatment is based on avoidance of situations that precipitate the lesions. Antihistamines are generally ineffective, and a low-dose, alternate-day corticosteroid is usually necessary for the more severe cases. NSAIDs (36) and the addition of a histamine (H_2) blocker have occasionally been helpful.

Solar urticaria is clinically characterized by development of pruritus, erythema, and edema within minutes of exposure to light. The lesions are typically present only in exposed areas, and have been classified into six types according to the wavelength of light that elicits the lesions: I, 2,800 to 3,200 nm; II, 3,200 to 4,000 nm; III, 4,000 to 5,000 nm; IV, 4,000 to 5,000 nm; V, 2,800 to 5,000 nm; and VI, 4,000 nm. The mechanism of these lesions is not known. Types I and IV can be passively transferred with plasma. Type VI is a metabolic abnormality recognized as erythropoietic protoporphyria. Diagnosis can be established by using broad-spectrum light with various filters or a spectrodermograph to document the eliciting wavelength. Treatment includes avoidance of sunlight and use of protective clothing and various sunscreens or blockers, depending on the wavelength eliciting the lesion. An antihistamine taken 1 hour before exposure may be helpful in some forms, and induction of tolerance is possible.

Cholinergic urticaria (generalized heat), a common form of urticaria (5%–7%), especially in teenagers and young adults (11.2%), is clinically characterized by small, punctate hives surrounded by an erythematous flare, the so-called "fried egg" appearance. These lesions may be clustered initially, but can coalesce and usually become generalized in distribution, primarily over the upper trunk and arms. Pruritus is generally severe. The onset of the rash is frequently associated with hot showers, sudden temperature change, exercise, sweating, or anxiety. A separate entity with similar characteristic lesions induced by cold has been described (37). Rarely, systemic symptoms may occur. The mechanism of this reaction is not certain, but cholinergically mediated thermodysregulation resulting in a neurogenic reflex has been postulated, because it can be reproduced by increasing core body temperature by 0.7° to 1°C (38). Histamine and other mast cell mediators have been documented in some patients (39) and increased muscarinic receptors have been reported in lesional sites of a patient with cholinergic urticaria (40). The appearance and description of the rash are highly characteristic and are reproduced by an intradermal methacholine skin test, but only in one third of the patients. Exercise in an occlusive suit or submersion in a warm bath is a more sensitive method of reproducing the urticaria. Passive heat can be used to differentiate this syndrome from exercise anaphylaxis. Hydroxyzine is considered the treatment of choice, but if it is ineffective or not tolerated, other antihistamines or combinations may be more efficacious.

Local heat urticaria, a rare form of heat urticaria (41), may be demonstrated by applying localized heat to the skin. A familial localized heat urticaria also has been reported (42) and is manifested by a delay in onset of urticarial lesions of 4 to 6 hours following local heat exposure.

Cold urticaria is clinically characterized by the rapid onset of urticaria or angioedema after cold exposure. Lesions are generally localized to exposed areas, but sudden total body exposure, as in swimming, may cause hypotension and result in death (43). Although usually idiopathic, cold urticaria has been associated with cryoglobulinemia, cryofibrinogenemia, cold agglutinin disease, and paroxysmal cold hemoglobinuria. The mechanism of cold urticaria is not known. Release of histamine and several other mediators has been demonstrated in selected patients following cold exposure (18). In patients with abnormal proteins, passive transfer of the cold sensitivity has been accomplished using plasma (44,45). Some cryoprecipitates can fix complement, and thus may induce anaphylatoxin production. Diagnosis of cold urticaria frequently can be confirmed by placing an ice cube on the forearm for 4 minutes (Table 13.4). Several coexisting cold-induced urticarias do not respond to an ice cube test (46). Treatment should consist of limited cold exposure (e.g., the patient should enter swimming pools cautiously), proper clothing, and oral cyproheptadine (47), although other antihistamines such as doxepin may be useful (48). In cases in which an abnormal protein is present, treatment of the underlying disease may be indicated and curative. Delayed-onset hypersensitivity to cold also has been reported (49).

Inherited Angioedema

Hereditary angioedema (HAE) is clinically characterized by recurrent episodes of angioedema involving any part of the body. Urticaria is not a feature of this disease. Laryngeal edema is common and is the major cause of death. Angioedema of the gastrointestinal tract may cause abdominal discomfort and can mimic an acute abdomen. HAE type I (Table 13.5) is inherited as an autosomal codominant trait, manifested by the absence of C1 inhibitor. HAE type II is characterized by

TABLE 13.5. *Forms of hereditary and acquired angioedema*

	Mechanism	Diagnosis
HAE type I	Autosomal codominant Deficiency of C1 inhibitor (C1 INH) Bradykinin (27) and possible C2b-derived kinin (38)	Low C4 (50); undetectable during an attack Low or absent C2 (54) when symptomatic Normal C1 level
HAE type II	Anaphylatoxin-generated histamine	Normal C1 level Low C4
	Functionally inactive C1 INH (20%) of HAE	Present, but inactive C1 INH (functional assay necessary)
Acquired angioedema (55,56)	Reduced C1q levels by excessive activation of C1 (e.g., lymphoma) through autoimmune immunoglobulin	Low C1q levels Low C1 INH
Autoimmune acquired angioedema (57)	Autoantibody (IgG) against C1 INH	Normal C1 level Low C4, C1 INH Absent family history

the functional absence of this inhibitor, which allows activation of the complement cascade and results in the clinical features noted in Table 13.5. The diagnosis usually is established by a history of angioedema, a family history of similar disease or early death because of laryngeal obstruction, and appropriate complement studies. The usual forms of treatment for angioedema, including epinephrine, are generally ineffective for HAE. Tracheostomy may be necessary in urgent situations where laryngeal edema has occurred. Supportive therapy, such as intravenous fluids or analgesics, may be required for other manifestations of the disease.

Danazol (51) and stanozolol (52), which is less expensive, have been used successfully on a chronic basis to treat HAE. Each of these attenuated androgens appears to upregulate the synthetic capability of hepatic cells that make C1 inhibitor, thus raising the C4 level and reducing the number and severity of acute exacerbations. Often, sufficient clinical improvement may be obtained with minimal doses such that the C4 level is normalized, but the C1 inhibitor level is not significantly increased. Long-term low (minimal) dose stanozolol at 2 mg/day or 4 to 6 mg every other day or danazol at 200 mg/day is remarkably safe. Side effects include abnormal liver function, lipid abnormalities, weight gain, amenorrhea, and hirsutism. One woman given attenuated androgens during the last 8 weeks of pregnancy experienced no ill effects, and virilization of the infant was transient (53). Esterase-

inhibiting drugs such as epsilon amino caproic acid (5 g every 6 hours) and tranexamic acid have been used to slow complement activation during severe attacks. Currently, C1 inhibitor pooled from plasma is being used in trials (55,56) for intermittent attacks, prophylaxis in surgery, and in children and pregnant women. Its use is limited by infectious disease issues that are of concern with all blood products, such that a C1 inhibitor bioengineered protein is being developed (57).

Acquired forms of C1 inhibitor deficiency result from increased destruction or metabolism of C1 inhibitor. Destruction occurs when autoantibodies directed against the C1 inhibitor are produced, bind to its active site, and cause inactivation (58). Alternatively, antiidiotypic antibodies are produced against specific B-cell surface immunoglobulins, leading to immune complex formation and continuous C1 activation (59). Large quantities of C1 inhibitor are subsequently consumed, causing a deficit and thus the symptoms of C1 inhibitor deficiency. This acquired type of deficiency is usually associated with rheumatologic disorders or B-cell lymphoproliferative disorders such as multiple myeloma, leukemia, and essential cryoglobulinemia. These patients may require larger doses of androgens to control symptoms, but therapy should be directed at the underlying lymphoproliferative or autoimmune disorder. As in the hereditary form of the disease, C1 inhibitor, C2, and C4 are low, but only in the acquired form is C1q also depressed.

Hereditary vibratory angioedema is clinically characterized by localized pruritus and swelling in areas exposed to vibratory stimuli (60). It appears to be inherited as an autosomal-dominant trait, and generally is first noted in childhood. The mechanism is not certain, but histamine release has been documented during experimental induction of a lesion (61). Treatment consists of avoidance of vibratory stimuli and use of antihistamines in an attempt to reduce symptoms.

Other Forms of Urticaria Angioedema

Papular urticaria is clinically characterized by slightly erythematous, highly pruritic linear papular lesions of various sizes. Each lesion tends to be persistent, in contrast to most urticarial conditions. The lower extremities are involved most often, although the trunk also may be affected, especially in young children. The mechanism is unknown, but the rash is thought to be caused by hypersensitivity to the saliva, mouth parts, or excreta of biting insects such as mosquitoes, bedbugs, fleas, lice, and mites. Treatment is supportive: antihistamines are given, often prophylactically, in an attempt to reduce pruritus. Good skin care is essential to prevent infection caused by scratching. Examination of a person's sleeping quarters and children's play areas for insects may provide a clue to the etiology. Pruritic urticaria papules and plaques of pregnancy (PUPP) are an extremely pruritic condition of primigravida women that occurs in the third trimester. Lesions begin in the striae distensae and spread up and around the umbilicus, thighs, and buttocks. In some atypical cases, biopsy should be performed to distinguish the diagnosis from herpes gestationis (8).

Urticaria Pigmentosa

Urticaria pigmentosa is characterized by persistent, red-brown, maculopapular lesions that urticate when stroked (Darier sign). These lesions generally have their onset in childhood. Rare familial forms have been described. Biopsy shows mast cell infiltration. The diagnosis may be established by their typical appearance, Darier sign, and skin biopsy. Occasionally, it has been noted to complicate other forms of anaphylaxis such as *Hymenoptera* venom sensitivity, causing very severe reactions with sudden vascular collapse. These cutaneous lesions may occur in patients with systemic mastocytosis, a generalized form of mast cell infiltration into bone, liver, lymph nodes, and spleen.

The remaining forms of urticaria are associated with many diverse etiologies (Table 13.3). Diagnosis is established by history and physical examination based on knowledge of the possible causes. Laboratory evaluation is occasionally helpful in establishing a diagnosis and identifying the underlying disease. Treatment is based on the underlying problem, and may include avoidance, antihistamines, and corticosteroid therapy or other forms of antiinflammatory drugs.

Clinical Approach

History

The clinical history is the single most important aspect of evaluating patients with urticaria. The history generally provides important clues to the etiology; therefore, an organized approach is essential.

If the patient has no rash at the time of evaluation, urticaria or angioedema usually can be established historically with a history of hives, welts, or wheps resembling mosquito bite–like lesions; raised, erythematous, pruritic lesions; evanescent symptoms; potentiation of lesions by scratching; and lesions that may coalesce. By contrast, angioedema is asymmetric, often involves nondependent areas, recurs in different sites, is transient, and is associated with little pruritus. Urticaria and angioedema may occur together. Cholinergic or adrenergic urticaria, papular urticaria, dermographism, urticaria pigmentosa, jaundice with urticaria, and familial cold urticaria, however, do not fit the typical pattern.

Both papular urticaria and urticaria pigmentosa most often arise in childhood. HAE and hereditary vibratory angioedema also may occur during childhood, but are readily recognized by the absence of urticaria in both diseases. Other etiologic factors in childhood urticaria have been reviewed (62,63).

Once the diagnosis of urticaria is established on the basis of history, etiologic mechanisms should be considered. The patient with dermographism usually reports a history of rash after scratching. Frequently, the patient notices itching first, scratches the offending site, and then develops linear wheals. Stroking the skin with a pointed instrument without disrupting the integument confirms the diagnosis. With most patients, the physical urticarias may be eliminated quickly as a possible diagnosis merely by asking about the temporal association with light, heat, cold, pressure, or vibration, or by using established clinical tests (Table 13.4). Cholinergic urticaria is usually recognized by its characteristic lesions and relationship to rising body temperature or stress. Hereditary forms of urticaria are rare. Familial localized heat urticaria is recognized by its relationship to the local application of heat, and familial cold urticaria by the unusual papular skin lesions and the predominance of a burning sensation instead of pruritus. Porphyria is a light-sensitive reaction. C3b inactivator deficiency is rare, and can be diagnosed by special complement studies. Thus, after a few moments of discussion with a patient, a physical urticaria or hereditary form usually can be suspected or established.

The success of determining an etiology for urticaria is most likely a function of whether it is acute or chronic, because a cause is discovered much more frequently when it is acute. Each of the items in Table 13.3 may be involved. Food may be identified in acute urticaria. Great patience and effort are necessary, along with repeated queries to detect drug use. Over-the-counter preparations are not regarded as drugs by many patients, and must be specified when questioning the patient. Penicillins are common, but aspirin or other NSAIDs are frequently recognized both as a cause and an aggravator of urticaria. Drug-induced episodes of urticaria are usually of the acute variety. Another recognized offender causing angioedema is the group of ACE inhibitor drugs used primarily for hypertension or heart failure. Reactions to ACE inhibitors usually occur within 1 week of initiating therapy, but can occur at any time. The newer class of antihypertensive therapy, the angiotensin II receptor blockers, are believed to have no effect on bradykinin production. Although theoretically they should not cause angioedema, several case reports have been published (64). Infections documented as causes of urticaria include infectious mononucleosis, viral hepatitis (both B and C), and fungal and parasitic invasions. Chronic infection as a cause of chronic urticaria is a rare event, although chronic hepatitis has been postulated to cause chronic urticaria (65). If the history does not reveal significant clues, the patient's urticaria generally is labeled chronic idiopathic urticaria (CIU). Most patients with chronic urticaria fall into this category.

Physical Examination

A complete physical examination should be performed on all patients with urticaria. The purpose of the examination is to identify typical urticarial lesions, if present; to establish the presence or absence of dermographism; to identify the characteristic lesions of cholinergic and papular urticaria; to characterize atypical lesions; to determine the presence of jaundice, urticaria pigmentosa (Darier sign), or familial cold urticaria; exclude other cutaneous diseases; exclude evidence of systemic disease; and establish the presence of coexisting diseases.

Diagnostic Studies

It is difficult to outline an acceptable diagnostic program for all patients with urticaria. Each diagnostic workup must be individualized, depending on the results of the history and physical examination. An algorithm may become a useful adjunct in this often unrewarding diagnostic endeavor (Fig. 13.2).

Foods

Five diagnostic procedures may be considered when food is thought to be a cause of urticaria (Table 13.6). These include (a) avoidance, (b) restricted diet, (c) diet diary, (d) skin testing with food extracts or fresh foods, and (e) food challenge.

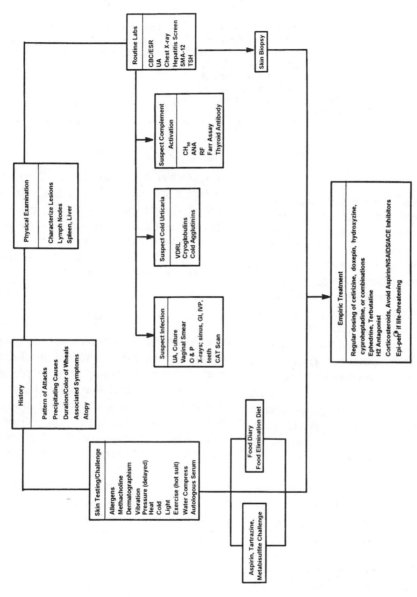

EVALUATION OF CHRONIC URTICARIA

History
Pattern of Attacks
Precipitating Causes
Duration/Color of Wheals
Associated Symptoms
Atopy

Physical Examination
Characterize Lesions
Lymph Nodes
Spleen, Liver

Skin Testing/Challenge
Allergens
Methacholine
Dermatographism
Vibration
Pressure (delayed)
Heat
Cold
Light
Exercise (hot suit)
Water Compress
Autologous Serum

Aspirin, Tartrazine, Metabisulfite Challenge

Food Diary
Food Elimination Diet

Suspect Infection
UA, Culture
Vaginal Smear
O & P
X-rays; sinus, GI, IVP, teeth
CAT Scan

Suspect Cold Urticaria
VDRL
Cryoglobulins
Cold Agglutinins

Suspect Complement Activation
CH_{50}
ANA
RF
Farr Assay
Thyroid Antibody

Routine Labs
CBC/ESR
UA
Chest X-ray
Hepatitis Screen
SMA-12
TSH

Skin Biopsy

Empiric Treatment
Regular dosing of cetirizine, doxepin, hydroxyzine, cyproheptadine, or combinations
Ephedrine, Terbutaline
H2 Antagonist
Corticosteroids, Avoid Aspirin/NSAIDS/ACE Inhibitors
Epi-pen if life-threatening

FIG. 13.2. This algorithm suggests a potential method for evaluating and treating chronic urticaria. The method includes challenge procedures and laboratory data. Empiric treatment should generally follow the cumulative, sequential use of the medications shown. Avoidance of aspirin, nonsteroidal antiinflammatory drugs, and angiotensin-converting enzyme inhibitors is essential. Corticosteroids may be useful for a brief time during the initial treatment until the severity of the urticaria is controlled.

TABLE 13.6. *Diagnostic studies of food-induced urticaria*

Avoidance (acute)	Use patient history	Eliminate 1 or 2 foods; urticaria should clear
Restricted diet (chronic relapsing)	Use standardized rice/ lamb or other restrictive diets; elemental diet may be useful	Reinstitute one food every 3–5 days; duplicate, if successful
Diet diary intermittent episodes for extended period	List all foods and events for 24 h prior to episode on several occasions	Eliminate suspected food; duplicate, if successful
Skin tests (chronic unknown etiology)	Use a brief battery of food skin tests based on patient's history; certain inhalant or latex allergens may suggest cross-reacting foods	Eliminate suspected test positive foods; a battery of negative skin tests suggests no food hypersensitivity
Double-blind, placebo-controlled food challenge	Gold standard; especially useful when the patients' perceptions may bias accurate symptom assessment	

Skin Tests

Routine food skin tests used in evaluating urticaria are of unproven value at best. Because the etiology of chronic urticaria is established in only an additional 5% of patients (38), and only some of these cases will be related to food, the diagnostic yield from skin testing is very low. In unselected patients, the positive predictive value of skin tests is low. Important studies of food-induced atopic dermatitis (66) have revealed a few selected foods that are most commonly associated with symptoms. These include eggs, peanuts, fish, soy, pork, milk, wheat, beef, and chicken. If no food skin test results are positive, then foods are probably not a cause. If all food skin test results are positive, dermatographism is probably present. Second, for patients in whom a mixed food (combination of ingredients) is thought to be the problem, food tests may isolate the particular item (e.g., soybeans). At present, an extensive battery of food tests cannot be recommended on a routine basis, and must be used with clinical discretion. Commercially prepared extracts frequently lack labile proteins responsible for IgE-mediated sensitivity to many fruits and vegetables. If the clinical history is convincing for a food allergy, but skin testing with a commercially prepared extract is negative, testing should be repeated with the fresh food before concluding that food allergen-specific IgE is absent (67). Additionally, certain foods have been shown to cross-react with pollen allergens (68) or latex allergens (69) to which a patient may be exquisitely sensitive. Radioallergosorbent testing (RAST) may be used in place of skin testing. Although it is considered less sensitive, it may be necessary when a patient has an exquisite sensitivity to a certain food or significant dermographism.

Drugs

With the exception of penicillins, foreign sera, and recombinant proteins such as insulin, there are no reliable diagnostic tests for predicting or establishing clinical sensitivity to a drug. In patients with urticaria, drugs must always be considered as etiologic agents. The only evaluation of value is avoidance of the drug. This can be accomplished safely and effectively in most patients, even when multiple drugs are involved and coexisting diseases are present. Substitute drugs with different chemical structures are frequently available and may be used. Not all drugs need to be stopped simultaneously unless the allergic reaction is severe.

Infections

As noted previously, viral infections, fungal infections, and parasites may cause urticaria. Patients with infectious mononucleosis or hepatitis generally have other symptoms, and appropriate laboratory studies confirm the diagnosis.

Routine physical examination should include a search for tinea pedis, capitas, or thrush to rule out fungal infection as the possible cause. Many of the parasitic infections will be associated with peripheral blood eosinophilia, high serum IgE concentrations, or positive stool specimens. An extensive search for occult infection is of no value. If history or examination suggests undiagnosed infection, appropriate laboratory studies should be undertaken (Fig. 13.2).

Penetrants

The medical literature is filled with numerous case reports of urticaria following contact. The only tests to be performed involve actual contact with the agent and demonstration of a localized skin eruption in the area of contact. Usually, these cases of urticaria result from penetration of the skin by antigen or a mediator-releasing substance from animal hairs or stingers. Examples of agents causing such urticaria include latex, drugs, and occupationally used chemicals (70).

Insect Stings

Urticaria may present as a result of insect stings, and this history generally is obtained easily. Appropriate skin tests with *Hymenoptera* venoms may be indicated in cases of generalized urticaria and anaphylaxis to demonstrate immediate hypersensitivity. One should consider fire ant stings due to their continued migration into more northern latitudes. Whole body extract skin testing or a RAST for venom may be helpful diagnostically.

Neoplasm

If neoplasm is suspected by history or examination, standard evaluation should be undertaken and perhaps repeated on several occasions.

Vasculitis

In a patient who has urticarial lesions that last for more than 24 hours, leave residual scarring, or appear petechial in nature, vasculitis should be suspected. A complete blood count (CBC),

sedimentation rate, urinalysis, and tissue biopsy are indicated. Tests for antinuclear antibody and rheumatoid factor, complement studies, and screening for hepatitis and mononucleosis are generally indicated. A highly sensitive test for thyroid-stimulating hormone (TSH) also should be performed because of the association with autoimmune thyroiditis (71,72). Urticarial vasculitis must be differentiated from CIU (8).

Serum Sickness

Acute urticaria in association with arthralgias, fever, and lymphadenopathy developing 1 to 3 weeks following drug exposure, insect sting, or heterologous serum administration is suspicious for serum sickness. CBC, urinalysis, and a sedimentation rate are indicated. Serum concentrations of C3, C4, and total hemolytic complement are depressed, indicating that immune complexes are involved in the pathogenesis of this disease.

Idiopathic Chronic Urticaria

The more difficult and more common problem regarding diagnostic tests relates to those patients who appear to have idiopathic disease. Laboratory studies are probably unnecessary in the absence of abnormal features in the history or physical examination. Most of these episodes are self-limited and resolve spontaneously.

In patients with CIU, the discomfort, inconvenience, and disfigurement of the disease generally warrant further evaluation. The following tests should be considered but not necessarily performed in all patients: CBC with differential; urinalysis; chest radiography; sedimentation rate; complement studies; examination of stool for ova and parasites; antinuclear antibody; Venereal Disease Research Laboratory (VDRL) testing; hepatitis screen; and skin biopsy. Because thyroid disease (particularly Hashimoto thyroiditis) is more common in chronic urticaria, thyroid function testing (T3, T4, ultrasensitive TSH; antibodies for thyroglobulin and microsomes) may be considered in anyone with a palpable goiter, family history of thyroid disease, or evidence of thyroid dysfunction (22).

Urinalysis (cells or protein), CBC (anemia, leukocytosis, or eosinophilia), and chest radiography are most likely to demonstrate significant abnormalities. The sedimentation rate may be elevated in active vasculitis. Circulating hepatitis-related antibodies may indicate acute or chronic disease. Although complement abnormalities are common in reports of CIU, the underlying mechanisms are unclear and their relevance is uncertain. Thus, the need for complement assays should be reserved for difficult to treat cases.

Skin biopsy is currently suggested for CIU that is difficult to manage, and it is probably indicated in patients with connective tissue disease or a complement abnormality. Acute urticaria probably does not warrant biopsy when laboratory studies are normal.

Therapy

Pharmacologic therapy is the main form of treatment for urticaria and angioedema (Table 13.7). However, as in other forms of allergic disease, if an allergen has been identified, avoidance is the most effective treatment. Avoidance techniques for specific forms of urticaria have been reviewed previously (8). For most urticaria patients, three types of drugs are adequate to obtain symptomatic control: sympathomimetic agents, antihistamines, and corticosteroids.

The sympathomimetic agents, notably epinephrine and ephedrine, have α agonist properties that cause vasoconstriction in superficial cutaneous and mucosal surfaces, which directly opposes the effect of histamine on these end organs. Normally, they are used for severe acute urticaria or in conjunction with antihistamines.

Antihistamines (H_1 blockers) are useful in most cases of urticaria. They are competitive

TABLE 13.7. *Treatment of chronic idiopathic urticaria*

Avoidance of triggers
Keep diary of flares
Regular use of antihistamines, 3–6 mo
Add ketotifen
Add ephedrine or β agonists
Add leukotriene modifiers
β blockers (adrenergic urticaria only)
Cautious use of corticosteroids

inhibitors of histamine, reducing the end-organ effect of histamine even if histamine release continues. Although documentation of histamine release is not available for all forms of urticaria, antihistamines are the mainstay of symptomatic improvement or control of urticaria. Notably, low-dose antidepressants, especially doxepin, are unique in having very potent H_1 and H_2 antagonist effects and inhibit other mediators such as platelet-activating factor. Their main side effect is sedation, but when administered in small doses (10–25 mg) at bedtime, this may be avoided. A trial of therapy with representative agents from the different classes of antihistamines may be required to select the proper drug.

The newer antihistamines offer some valuable options because they are long acting and cause little sedation (73,74). Fexofenadine (75) and cetirizine (76–78) are well tolerated and effective in most cases of chronic urticaria. Ketotifen (79) is another effective alternative for the treatment of chronic urticaria and physical urticarias (14) because in addition to being a histamine antagonist, it can inhibit mast cell degranulation. Unfortunately, ketotifen is not available in the United States but is available in 2-mg tablets in many countries.

Hydroxyzine has clinical antihistaminic effects as well as experimental anticholinergic and antiserotoninergic effects. This agent is considered the drug of choice for cholinergic urticaria, and is also very effective in many other forms of chronic urticaria. Often, the initially effective dose can be reduced or used only at night for chronic therapy. A combination of a nonsedating second-generation antihistamine given in the morning with a first-generation agent given at night might be necessary in patients with more persistent urticaria.

Cyproheptadine is thought to be a serotonin and histamine antagonist, and to have anticholinergic effects. Its mechanism of action in urticaria is uncertain, but it appears to be effective in some cases. It is most commonly used to treat cold urticaria (47), but it can stimulate the appetite and result in significant weight gain. Leukotriene modifiers such as montelukast and zafirlukast have been reported to help control chronic urticaria as well as reduce corticosteroid requirements in an undefined subset of patients (80,81). These agents work best when given in combination with antihistamines. Limited benefit has been reported from using a combination of H_1 and H_2 antihistamines for both acute and chronic urticaria (82).

Corticosteroids, such as oral prednisone, may be necessary in the management of urticaria. Because of their potential for significant long-term side effects, these drugs should be used to control urticaria only after a demonstrated failure of both high-dose and combination antihistamine therapy. Based on clinical experience, moderate-dose steroid therapy (30–40 mg prednisone) may be required initially to control the urticaria. Thereafter, alternate-day therapy generally provides control on a long-term basis, often with decreasing doses. As in all forms of therapy, the risk:benefit ratio must be assessed when using steroid therapy for long-term treatment. Short-term prednisone has limited side effects, and is often useful for control of acute urticaria not responding to antihistamines. DPU frequently may require the use of low-dose or every other day corticosteroids to maintain the patient's activity, and a cautious trial of a nonsteroidal anti-inflammatory drug may be helpful.

The choice of agents and the route of administration of drugs is dependent on the clinical situation. The adult patient who presents in an emergency room or physician's office within hours of the onset of significant urticaria can be treated with epinephrine 0.3 mL (1:1,000) subcutaneously, as well as hydroxyzine 25 to 50 mg or cetirizine 10 mg orally. Such an approach gives prompt relief from symptoms in many patients. After evaluation for a precipitating agent (e.g., drug or food), the patient may be released with instructions to take hydroxyzine or cetirizine for 24 to 48 hours. A brief "burst" of corticosteroids and prolonged observation may be judicious, and is essential if there have been associated signs of anaphylaxis. Ambulatory medical follow-up should be required.

The patient who presents with urticaria of several days' duration may be treated with regular doses of antihistamines. The combination of cetirizine 10 mg every morning and hydroxyzine 25 mg at bedtime is quite useful. Ephedrine, oral albuterol, or H_2 antagonist may be prescribed with the initial antihistamine. Failure to respond in a few days to this therapy may indicate the need for a short course of prednisone. Many patients respond to this therapy, but the antihistamines should be continued for a period after the prednisone is stopped.

The patient with a history of chronic urticaria presents a more complicated therapeutic-problem. Following evaluation for an etiology, therapy is usually initiated with regular dosing of a potent antihistamine (often hydroxyzine cetirizine or doxepin) and possibly a leukotriene modifier. Failure to respond suggests that moderate-dose prednisone should be initiated if the symptoms are sufficiently severe. Every effort to use alternate day therapy should be made, but this is often initially inadequate. When control is achieved, the steroids are slowly withdrawn to determine whether chronic steroid therapy is required.

Other antiinflammatory medications have been reported to be useful in refractory patients (Table 13.8). Stanozolol (83), nifedipine (84), and other antiinflammatory drugs, including cyclosporine (85), methotrexate (86), and azathioprine have been used experimentally for inflammatory urticaria. Sulfasalazine (87,88) has been effective in case studies for DPU and angioedema.

Patients with urticaria can be very uncomfortable, have difficulty sleeping, and complain of facial swelling. Aggressive and consistent therapy for at least several months provides relief in many cases.

In summary, CIU may be unpleasant, frustrating, and frightening to a patient. Often these

TABLE 13.8. *Treatment of chronic idiopathic urticaria: use of secondary options*

Cautiously use corticosteroids (low dose or every other morning)
Add stanozolol to corticosteroid
Add sulfasalazine
Add nifedipine
Antiinflammatory drugs
Consider immunosuppressive therapy

patients seek help from various physicians for an allergen that does not exist. At times, they undergo expensive, inappropriate tests and treatments that are of no value and perhaps dangerous. These patients need reassurance. Treatment with prednisone in doses that will induce a remission followed by 3 to 6 months of a nightly dose of a potent antihistamine often yields a good outcome.

REFERENCES

1. Sheldon JM, Mathews KP, Lovell RG. The vexing urticaria problem: present concepts of etiology and management. *J Allergy* 1954;25:525.
2. Mathews KP. Urticaria and angioedema. *J Allergy Clin Immunol* 1983;72:1–14.
3. Cooper KD. Urticaria and angioedema: diagnosis and evaluation. *J Am Acad Dermatol* 1991;25:166–176.
4. Champion RH, Roberts SOB, Carpenter RG, et al. Urticaria and angioedema: a review of 554 patients. *Br J Dermatol* 1969;81:588–597.
5. Green GR, Koelsche GA, Kierland RR. Etiology and pathogenesis of chronic urticaria. *Ann Allergy* 1965;23:30–36.
6. Lewis T. *The blood vessels of the human skin and their responses.* London: Shaw & Sons, 1927.
7. Peters MS, Schroeter AL, Kaphart GM, et al. Localization of eosinophilic granule major basic protein in chronic urticaria. *J Invest Dermatol* 1983;81:39–43.
8. Charlesworth EN. The spectrum of urticaria. *Immunol Allergy Clin North Am* 1995;15:641.
9. Bressler RB. Pathophysiology of chronic urticaria. *Immunol Allergy Clin North Am* 1995;15:659.
10. Grandel KE, Farr RS, Wanderer AA, et al. Association of platelet activation factor with primary, acquired cold urticaria. *N Engl J Med* 1985;313:405–409.
11. Juhlin L. Late-phase cutaneous reactions to platelet activating factor and kallikrein in urticaria. *Clin Exp Allergy* 1990;90:9–10.
12. Goldsobel AB, Rohr AS, Siegel SC, et al. Effect of doxepin in the treatment of chronic idiopathic urticaria. *J Allergy Clin Immunol* 1986;78:867–873.
13. Greaves MW. The physical urticarias. *Clin Exp Allergy* 1991;21(suppl 1):284–289.
14. Fox RW. Update on urticaria and angioedema (hives). *Allergy Proc* 1995;16:289–292.
15. Smith CH, Kepley C, Schwartz LB, et al. Mast cell membrane and phenotype in chronic urticaria. *J Allergy Clin Immunol* 1995;96:360–364.
16. Barlow RJ, Ross EL, MacDonald DM, et al. Mast cells and T lymphocytes in chronic urticaria. *Clin Exp Allergy* 1994;25:317–322.
17. Maxwell DL, Atkinson BA, Spur BW, et al. Skin responses to intradermal histamine and leukotrienes C4, D4 and E4 in patients with chronic idiopathic urticaria and in normal subjects. *J Allergy Clin Immunol* 1990;86:759–765.
18. Lexnoff A, Sussman GL. Syndrome of idiopathic chronic urticaria and angioedema with thyroid autoimmunity: a study of 90 patients. *J Allergy Clin Immunol* 1989; 84:66–71.
19. Greaves MW. Chronic urticaria. Current concepts. *N Engl J Med* 1995;332:1767–1772.
20. Tong Li Juan, Balakrishman G, Kochan JP, et al. Assessment of autoimmunity in patients with urticaria. *J Allergy Clin Immunol* 1997;99:461–465.
21. Zavadak D, Tharp MD. Chronic urticaria as a manifestation of the late phase reaction. *Immunol Allergy Clin North Am* 1995;15:745.
22. Wasserman SI, Austen KF, Soter NA. The functional and physicochemical characterization of three eosinophilotactic activities released into the circulation by cold challenge of patient with cold urticaria. *Clin Exp Immunol* 1982;47:570–578.
23. Lichtenstein LM. Histamine releasing factors and IgE heterogeneity. *J Allergy Clin Immunol* 1988;81:814–820.
24. Fields T, Ghebrehiwet B, Kaplan AP. Kinin formation in hereditary angioedema plasma: evidence against kinin derivation from C2 and in support of "spontaneous" formation of bradykinin. *J Allergy Clin Immunol* 1983;72:54–60.
25. Meggs WJ, Pescovitz OR, Metcalfe DD, et al. Progesterone sensitivity as a cause of recurrent anaphylaxis. *N Engl J Med* 1984;311:1236–1238.
26. Mittman RJ, Berstein DI, Steinberg DR, et al. Progesterone-responsive urticaria and eosinophilia. *J Allergy Clin Immunol* 1989;84:304–310.
27. Goodman DL, McDonnell JT, Nelson HS, et al. Chronic urticaria exacerbated by the antioxidant food preservatives, butylated hydroxyanisole (BHA) and butylated hydroxytoluene (BHT). *J Allergy Clin Immunol* 1990;86:570–575.
28. Dohl MV. Clinical pearl: diascopy helps diagnose urticarial vasculitis. *J Am Acad Dermatol* 1994;30:481.
29. Vaughn MP, DeWalt AC, Diaz JD. Urticaria associated with systemic disease and psychological factors. *Immunol Allergy Clin North Am* 1995;15:725–743.
30. Sherertz EF. Clinical pearl: symptomatic dermatographism as a cause of genital pruritus. *J Am Acad Dermatol* 1994;31:1040–1041.
31. Casale TB, Sampson HA, Honifan J, et al. Guide to physical urticarias. *J Allergy Clin Immunol* 1988;82:758–763.
32. Schafer CM. Physical urticaria. *Immunol Allergy Clin North Am* 1995;15:679–699.
33. Shelley WB, Shelley EO. Adrenergic urticaria: a new form of stress induced hives. *Lancet* 1985;2:1031–1033.
34. Ryan TJ, Shim-Young N, Turk JL. Delayed pressure urticaria. *Br J Dermatol* 1968;80:485–490.
35. Mekori YA, Dobozin BS, Schocket AL, et al. Delayed pressure urticaria histologically resembles cutaneous late phase reactions. *Arch Dermatol* 1988;124:230–235.
36. Sussman GL, Harvey RP, Schocket AL. Delayed pressure urticaria. *J Allergy Clin Immunol* 1982;70:337–342.
37. Kaplan AP, Garofalo J. Identification of a new physically induced urticaria. Cold- induced cholinergic urticaria. *J Allergy Clin Immunol* 1981;68:438–441.
38. Kaplan AP. Urticaria and angioedema. In: Middleton E Jr et al., eds. *Allergy: principles and practice,* 4th ed. St. Louis: CV Mosby, 1993:1553.
39. Kaplan AP, Gray L, Shaff RE. *In vivo* studies of mediator release in cold urticaria and cholinergic urticaria. *J Allergy Clin Immunol* 1975;55:394–402.

40. Shelley WB, Shelley ED, Ho AK. Cholinergic urticaria: acetylcholine-receptor–dependent immediate-type hypersensitivity reaction to copper. *Lancet* 1983;843–846.
41. Greaves MW, Kaplan AP. Urticaria and angioedema. In: Samter M et al., eds. *Immunological diseases,* 4th ed. Boston: Little, Brown, 1988:1187.
42. Michaelson G, Ros A. Familial localized heat urticaria of delayed type. *Acta Derm Venereal (Stockh)* 1971;51: 279.
43. Horton BT, Brown GE, Roth GM. Hypersensitivities to cold with local and systemic manifestations of a histamine-like character: its amenability to treatment. *JAMA* 1936;107:1263.
44. Costanzi JJ, Coltman JR Jr, Donaldson VH. Activation of complement by a monoclonal cryoglobulin associated with cold urticaria. *J Lab Clin Med* 1969;74:902–910.
45. Costanzi JJ, Coltman JR Jr. Kappa chain precipitable immunoglobulin G (IgG) associated with cold urticaria. I. Clinical observations. *Clin Exp Immunol* 1967;2:167.
46. Kaplan AP. Urticaria and angioedema. In: Kaplan AP, ed. *Allergy.* New York: Churchill Livingstone, 1985:439.
47. Sigler RW, Evans R, Hoarkova Z, et al. The role of cyproheptadine in the treatment of cold urticaria. *J Allergy Clin Immunol* 1980;65:309–312.
48. Bentley B II. Cold-induced urticaria and angioedema: diagnosis and management. *Am J Emerg Med* 1993;11:43–46.
49. Sarkany I, Turk JL. Delayed type hypersensitivity to cold. *Proc R Soc Med* 1965;58:622.
50. Sim TC, Grant JA. Hereditary angioedema: its diagnosis and management perspective. *Am J Med* 1990;88:656–664.
51. Gelfand JA, Sherins RJ, Alling DW, et al. Treatment of hereditary angioedema with danazol: reversal of clinical and biochemical abnormalities. *N Engl J Med* 1976;295:1444–1448.
52. Sheffer AL, Fearon DT, Austen KF. Clinical and biochemical effects of stanozolol therapy for hereditary angioedema. *J Allergy Clin Immunol* 1981;68:181–187.
53. Cicardi M, Bergamaschini L, Cugno M, et al. Long-term treatment of hereditary angioedema with attenuated androgens: a survey of a 13-year experience. *J Allergy Clin Immunol* 1991;87:768–773.
54. Austen KF, Sheffer AL. Detection of hereditary angioneurotic edema by demonstration of a reduction in the second component of human complement. *N Engl J Med* 1965;272:649.
55. Bork K, Witzke G. Long-term prophylaxis with C1-inhibitor (C1 INH) concentrate in patients with recurrent angioedema caused by hereditary and acquired C1-inhibitor deficiency. *J Allergy Clin Immunol* 1989;83:677–682.
56. Gadek JE, Hosea SW, Gelfand JA, et al. Replacement therapy in hereditary angioedema: successful treatment of acute episodes of angioedema with partially purified C1 inhibitor. *N Engl J Med* 1980;302:542–546.
57. Finn AF. Urticaria and angioedema. In: Kaliner MA, ed. *Current review of allergic diseases.* Philadelphia: Current Medicine, 2000:168–178.
58. Gelfand JA, Boss GR, Conley CL, et al. Acquired C1 esterase inhibitor deficiency and angioedema: a review. *Medicine* 1979;58:321–328.
59. Frigas E. Angioedema with acquired deficiency of the C1 inhibitor: a constellation of syndromes. *Mayo Clin Proc* 1989;64:1269–1275.
60. Patterson R, Mellies CJ, Blankenship ML, et al. Vibratory angioedema: a hereditary type of physical hypersensitivity. *J Allergy Clin Immunol* 1972;50:174–182.
61. Metzger WJ, Kaplan AP, Beaven MA, et al. Hereditary vibratory angioedema: confirmation of histamine release in a type of physical hypersensitivity. *J Allergy Clin Immunol* 1976;57:605–608.
62. Ghosh S, Kanwar AJ, Kaur S. Urticaria in children. *Pediatr Dermatol* 1993;10:107–110.
63. Volonakis M, Katsarou-Katsari A, Stratigos J. Etiologic factors in childhood chronic urticaria. *Ann Allergy* 1992;69:61–65.
64. Pylypchuk GB. ACE inhibitor–versus angiotensin II blocker–induced cough and angioedema. *Ann Pharmacother* 1998;32:1060–1066.
65. Vaida, GA, Goldman MA, Blockk KJ. Testing for hepatitis B in patients with chronic urticaria and angioedema. *J Allergy Clin Immunol* 1983;72:193–198.
66. Sampson HA. The role of food allergy and mediation release in atopic dermatitis. *J Allergy Clin Immunol* 1988;81:635–645.
67. Sampson H. Food allergy. Part 2: diagnosis and management. *J Allergy Clin Immunol* 1999;103:987–989.
68. Bush RK, Helfe SL. Lessons and myths regarding cross-reacting foods. *Allergy Proc* 1995;16:245–246.
69. Dompmartin A, Szczurko C, Michel M, et al. 2 cases of urticaria following fruit ingestion, with cross-sensitivity to latex. *Contact Dermatitis* 1994;30:250–252.
70. Vonkrog HG, Maiback HI. Contact urticaria. In: Adams RM, ed. *Occupational skin disease.* New York: Grune & Stratton, 1983:58–69.
71. Altus P, Blandon R, Wallach PM, et al. Case report: the spectrum of autoimmune thyroid disease with urticaria. *Am J Med Sci* 1993;306:379–380.
72. Rumbyrt JS, Katz JL, Schocket AL. Resolution of chronic urticaria in patients with thyroid autoimmunity. *J Allergy Clin Immunol* 1995;96:901–905.
73. Ormerod AD. Urticaria: recognition, causes and treatment. *Drugs* 1994;48:717–730.
74. Soter NA. Treatment of urticaria and angioedema: low-sedating H_1-type antihistamines. *J Am Acad Dermatol* 1991;24:1084–1087.
75. Nelson HS, Reynolds R, Mason J. Fexofenadine HC1 is safe and effective for the treatment of chronic idiopathic urticaria. *Ann Allergy Asthma Immunol* 2000;84:517–522.
76. Campoli-Richards DM, Buckley MM, Fitton A. Cetirizine: a review of its pharmacological properties and clinical potential in allergic rhinitis, pollen-induced asthma, and chronic urticaria. *Drugs* 1990;40:762–781.
77. Breneman D, Bronsky EA, Bruce S, et al. Cetirizine and astemizole therapy for chronic idiopathic urticaria: a double-blind, placebo-controlled, comparative trial. *J Am Acad Dermatol* 1995;33:192–198.
78. Townley RG. Cetirizine: a new H_1 antagonist with antieosinophilic activity in chronic urticaria. *J Am Acad Dermatol* 1991;25:668–674.
79. Hutson DP, Bressler RB, Kaliner M, et al. Prevention of mast-cell degranulation by ketotifen in patients with physical urticarias. *Ann Intern Med* 1986;104:507–510.
80. Ellis MH. Successful treatment of chronic urticaria with leukotriene antagonist. *J Allergy Clin Immunol* 1998;102:876–877.
81. Bensch G, Borish L. Leukotriene modifiers in chronic urticaria. *Ann Allergy Asthma Immunol* 1999;83:348.

82. Lin RV, Curry A, Pesola GR, et al. Improved outcomes in patients with acute allergic syndromes who are treated with combined H_1 and H_2 antagonists. *Ann Emerg Med* 2000;36:5:462–468.
83. Brestel EP, Thrush LB. The treatment of glucocorticosteroid-dependent chronic urticaria with stanozolol. *J Allergy Clin Immunol* 1988;82:265–269.
84. Bressler RB, Sowell K, Huston DP. Therapy of chronic idiopathic urticaria with nifedipine: demonstration of beneficial effect in a double-blinded, placebo-controlled, crossover trial. *J Allergy Clin Immunol* 1989;83:756–763.
85. Fradin MS, Ellis CN, Goldfarb MT, et al. Oral cyclosporine for severe chronic idiopathic urticaria and angioedema. *J Am Acad Dermatol* 1991;25:1065–1067.
86. Weiner MJ. Methotrexate in corticosteroid-resistant urticaria. *Ann Intern Med* 1989;110:848.
87. Engler RJ, Squire E, Benson P. Chronic sulfasalazine therapy in the treatment of delayed pressure urticaria and angioedema. *Ann Allergy Asthma Immunol* 1995; 74:155–159.
88. Jaffer AM. Sulfasalazine in the treatment of corticosteroid-dependent chronic idiopathic urticaria. *J Allergy Clin Immunol* 1991; 88:964–965.
89. Berdy SS, Bloch KJ. Schnitzler's syndrome: a broader clinical spectrum. *J Allergy Clin Immunol* 1991;87:849–854.

14

Food Allergy

Anne M. Ditto and Leslie C. Grammer

Division of Allergy-Immunology, Department of Medicine, Ernest S. Bazley Asthma and Allergic Diseases Center, Northwestern University Medical School, Chicago, Illinois

The term *adverse food reaction* includes a variety of untoward reactions to food, only some of which are the result of a true food *allergy*. The American Academy of Allergy and Immunology and the National Institutes of Health have defined food reactions in an attempt to standardize the nomenclature used in scientific literature (1). An *adverse food reaction* is defined as any untoward reaction to food or food additive ingestion. This can be further subdivided into food allergy and food intolerance. Food allergy is any adverse food reaction due to an immunologic mechanism. Food intolerance is any adverse reaction due to a nonimmunologic mechanism. This may be the result of pharmacologic properties of the food (e.g., caffeine in irritable bowel, tyramine-induced nausea, emesis, and headache), toxins in the food, usually from improper food handling (e.g., histamine generation in scombroid fish poisoning, *Staphylococcus* food poisoning), or metabolic disorders (lactose deficiency, phenylketonuria).

PREVALENCE

The true prevalence of food allergy is not known but the public perception exceeds the prevalence noted in several clinical studies. According to one prospective survey, at least one in four atopic adults report an adverse reaction to food they have ingested or handled (2). Similarly, 28% of mothers in one study perceived their children to have had at least one adverse reaction to food (3). Only 8% of these children had reactions confirmed by double-blind placebo-controlled food challenge (DBPCFC) (3)—one third of the patients whose history was suggestive of food allergy. A study of an unselected population of over 1,700 Danish children reported that 6.7% had symptoms suggestive of cow's milk allergy in the first year of life, with 2.2% confirmed by open challenge (4). Recently, the prevalence of peanut and tree nut allergy in the United States, as determined by a nationwide telephone survey, was estimated to be approximately 1.1% (1.6% in adults, 0.6% in children <18 years old) (5). Food allergy prevalence in the general population, as reported by Buckley, is estimated to be 0.3% to 7.5%, and less common in adults (6). Prevalence, however, appears to be much higher in children with moderate-severe, refractory atopic dermatitis. One study reported that one third of the 63 such patients recruited had immunoglobulin E (IgE)-mediated food allergy (7). Studies like those mentioned above have not been systematically conducted in adults, but some surveys suggest the prevalence of food allergy in adults to be 1% to 2%.

FATAL FOOD ANAPHYLAXIS

The most easily recognized food hypersensitivity reactions and the best characterized are the IgE-mediated type I reactions in the Gell and Coombs rubric (8). These account for the majority of food allergies. They are notable for their immediate onset—most within 1 hour but frequently within minutes. As with other IgE-mediated reactions they can have a late-phase response 4 to 6 hours later. Protracted anaphylaxis, relatively resistant to epinephrine, has been noted and also has been described with venom anaphylaxis (9). Reactions can be severe, even fatal. Recent studies have reported foods to be the number one cause of anaphylaxis (10,11).

Historically, the incidence of fatal and near-fatal food-induced anaphylaxis has been difficult to ascertain, primarily due to a lack of coding in the International Classification of Disease. Sampson et al. reported a series of 13 children and adolescents who had fatal and near-fatal reactions to foods (12). Peanuts, tree nuts, fish, and shellfish were the foods responsible for the most severe, life-threatening anaphylactic reactions. The four factors that appeared to contribute to a fatal outcome were a concomitant diagnosis of asthma, a delay in the administration of epinephrine, previous allergic reactions to the responsible food, and not recognizing food allergen in the meal. Of note, only one child of the six who died had cutaneous manifestations. The latter was also described in a study by Yunginger et al. (13) of seven adult patients whose deaths were also correlated with denial of symptoms and treatment with antihistamines alone.

PATHOPHYSIOLOGY

The gastrointestinal (GI) tract is exposed to many foreign proteins, including bacteria, parasites, and viruses, as well as food. Its function is to digest food into forms more easily absorbed and available for energy and cell growth. In this process it must provide a defensive barrier against any pathogens entering by this route and simultaneously tolerate the many foreign proteins in foods to which it is exposed. The fact that the GI tract is exposed to a multitude of potentially allergenic proteins daily, yet food hypersensitivity is rare, attests to the efficiency with which this process is executed.

There are multiple nonimmunologic as well as immunologic barriers within the GI tract that operate to reduce systemic exposure to foreign antigens. Nonimmunologic or mechanical barriers include gastric acid secretions and proteolytic enzymes. These digest proteins into molecules that are less antigenic, either by reducing the size (14) or by altering the structure (4,14), as described below in the section on tolerance. Other physical barriers include peristalsis, mucus production, and mucus secretion. These barriers decrease contact of potential allergens with the GI mucosa (14). The gut epithelium itself provides a barrier against significant macromolecular absorption (15). Physical factors that increase the rate of absorption are alcohol ingestion and decreased gastric acid secretion. Increased acid production and food ingestion both decrease the rate of absorption (16).

In addition to the physical barriers, there are immunologic barriers. The GI tract is supplied with a local immune system referred to as the gut-associated lymphoid tissue (GALT) (17). GALT is composed of the following four components: discrete aggregates of lymphoid follicles distributed throughout the intestinal mucosa (i.e., Peyer's patches and the appendix); intraepithelial lymphocytes; lymphocytes, plasma cells, and mast cells throughout the lamina propria; and mesenteric lymph nodes (17). There can be an increased production and release of antibodies within the gut following food ingestion; however, the predominant response is increase in IgA production (18), with suppression of IgG, IgM, and IgE (14,19,20). Dimeric secretory IgA accounts for most of the increase in IgA production and serves to bind proteins, forming complexes and thereby decreasing the rate of absorption (21). It is found in high quantities in the mucus, aiding in barrier protection. The functional significance of other antibodies is not known. For the macromolecules that do get absorbed as intact antigens—approximately 2% (19)—there is the development of oral tolerance. Tolerance is an immunologic unresponsiveness to a specific antigen, in this case food proteins (23).

Both the local and systemic immune system appear to play a significant role in the development of oral tolerance (22), although the exact mechanisms are not well understood. The processing of antigens by the gut into a non-allergenic or "tolerogenic" form is important (24). This form has a slightly different structure and appears to cause a decreased immune response in cell-mediated immunity through stimulation of CD8$^+$ T cells (25). This has been reported in studies of mice fed ovalbumin, which is immunogenic when administered parenterally. Within 1 hour after ingestion, a form similar in molecular weight to native ovalbumin was recovered from the serum. This "tolerogenic" form of ovalbumin induced suppression of cell-mediated responses but not antibody responses to native ovalbumin in recipient mice (24). This intestinally processed ovalbumin is distinct from systemic antigen processing (24). Lymphoid cells seem to be necessary for this process. Mice that were first irradiated were unable to process the ovalbumin into a "tolerogenic" form. However, with infusion of spleen cells, they regained this ability (25). Antigen-presenting cells also appear to play an important role. With an increase in antigen presentation, there is reported to be a decrease in CD8$^+$ T cells and a decrease in tolerance (26). Depletion of CD8$^+$ T cells with cyclophosphamide prevents the development of oral tolerance (27), with resultant cell-mediated immune responses, further supporting a role for CD8$^+$T cells in the development of tolerance.

Ia$^+$cells, initially reported in inflamed bowel, have been demonstrated in the normal bowel in humans (28). These cells were reported to function as antigen-presenting cells and, in particular, to stimulate CD8$^+$ suppressor T cells (29). In this way, they may contribute to the development of oral tolerance.

Food hypersensitivity is the result of a loss of or lack of tolerance, the cause of which is likely multifactorial. An increased incidence is noted in infants and children, and this may be due to immaturity of both the immune system and the physiologic functions of the GI tract. Until recently some of this immaturity was thought to lead to increased absorption of macromolecules from the gut of infants, but studies now indicate that this is not likely (30,31). There is, however, a lower level of IgA in the immature gut (32), and perhaps this, combined with a relatively low number of CD8$^+$ T cells or suppressor macrophage activity (33–35), may contribute to the increased incidence of food allergy in genetically prone children (36). The importance of local IgA is further supported by the finding of an increase in incidence of food allergy associated with IgA deficiency (36). Also, as compared with adults, infants have decreased acid secretion (37), less effective mucus secretion with differences in both chemical and physical properties of the glycoproteins (38), and decreased enzymatic activity (9), factors that when combined with immunologic immaturity may increase the risk of development of allergies. Mast cells that play a significant role in the food allergy reaction also appear to play a role in the maturation of the gut associated with weaning (40), a process affected by the mucosal immune system. This is evidenced by inhibition of small intestinal maturation and decreased numbers of intraepithelial lymphocytes with the addition of cyclosporine A (41).

Interruption of the physical barrier of the GI tract could lead to increased absorption. It has been noted that there is an increase in systemic antibody production, generally food-specific IgM, and IgG in patients with inflammatory bowel disease and celiac disease (36). However, the significance of these antibodies is not known because the patients often tolerate these foods well (42,43). Food-specific antibodies are also found in normal individuals, although usually of lower level (42). They may reflect dietary intake and not specific allergenicity.

The handling of food by the GI tract is complex, and the development of food hypersensitivity is likely multifactorial. In order for sensitization to occur, an antigen must come in contact with lymphocytes in the lamina propria, Peyer's patches, lymph nodes, spleen, or circulation (44). Any disruption of the immunologic or nonimmunologic barriers could alter the handling of antigen and lead to an increased production of systemic antibodies. In individuals with genetic predisposition to atopy, this could lead to IgE production and resultant food hypersensitivity reactions on reexposure (45). Many more human studies need to be performed in order to elucidate the mechanisms.

ALLERGENS

Proteins, carbohydrates, and fats comprise food content. The glycoprotein in food is the component that is most implicated in food allergies. Glycoproteins that are allergenic have molecular weights of 10,000 to 67,000 daltons. They are water soluble, predominantly heat stable, and resistant to acid and proteolytic digestion (46). Although many foods are potentially antigenic, the vast majority of food allergies involve only a few foods (47).

The combined results of double-blind placebo-controlled food challenges performed in the United States (primarily in children) showed that eight foods were responsible for 93% of reactions (39). These foods listed in order of frequency are eggs, peanuts, milk, soy, tree nuts, fish, crustacea, and wheat (47). Of note, allergy to chocolate, previously thought to be responsible for food reactions, was not found in any of the 710 patients tested (47) and likely is explained by hazelnut, walnut, or peanuts that flavor the chocolate. In adults and older children, peanuts, crustacea, tree nuts, and fish (in order of frequency) were reported to be responsible for the majority of fatal anaphylactic reactions (13). There have not been any well-studied DBPCFCs in this age group.

The prevalence of specific allergens may vary for different countries, depending on exposure patterns. For example, fish allergy is more common in Scandinavian countries, where fish is introduced early in life, whereas peanut allery is much more prevalent in the United States, where peanut butter and jelly sandwiches are a staple of young children. Allergens found commonly in children but not in adults (eggs, soy, milk and wheat) are usually outgrown with strict elimination for 1 or more years (48), although evidence of IgE antibodies may persist (49). Those with histories of severe reactions may take longer to develop clinical tolerance, up to several years (48,50). The others [peanuts (51), tree nuts, crustacea (52), and fish (53)] tend to be lifelong and thus are common to both populations.

Food processing can alter antigenicity in certain foods. Some whey proteins found in milk are denatured by heating and routine processing, whereas others are rendered more allergenic (54). Fish allergens may be changed with the canning process, and a patient who cannot tolerate fresh fish may tolerate canned tuna and other processed fish (55). Lyophilization also can change fish allergens. Because this is the process often used in food preparation for DBPCFC, great caution should be taken in interpreting a negative result of a DBPCFC to fish (55). A different preparation may be needed. Beef has been reported to have heat-labile allergens; therefore, cooking may abrogate sensitivity (56). Peanut allergen is remarkably resistant to any kind of processing, retaining its allergenicity (57). Peanut oil has been tolerated by 10 peanut-allergic individuals (58), but there have not been adequate studies ensuring its safety. In fact, cold-pressed peanut oils may contain peanut allergen (59).

Allergen cross-reactivity is readily demonstrated by skin test, radioallergosorbent testing (RAST), RAST inhibition, and immunoblotting techniques and varies with the different food groups (1,60–63). It does not, however, always reflect clinical cross-reactivity. For example, immunologic cross-reactivity between peanuts and other legumes is common (62), but clinical allergic reactions (as demonstrated by DBPCFC) to more than one legume is rare (61).

In a study of 11 patients with multiple positive skin-prick test reactions to fish, 7 patients reacted to only one fish when challenged with DBPCFC (63). Extensive cross-reactivity among cereal grains (wheat, rye, oat, barley, rice, and corn) was noted *in vitro*, with less than 25% confirmed by DBPCFC in one study (64). Crustacea also show considerable cross-reactivity (65) but the clinical significance remains unknown due to a lack of controlled food challenges. Many children with allergy to cow's milk protein also react to milk from goats (66), and *in vitro* studies have reported cross-reactivity between eggs from different poultry (67).

IgE-MEDIATED REACTIONS

Food hypersensitivity IgE-mediated reactions are the result of mast cell and basophil mediator release. Food-specific IgE bound to mast cells or basophils via the high-affinity FcεRI is cross-linked by the food allergen, resulting in the release of preformed mediators such as histamine and newly formed mediators such as leukotrienes and prostaglandins. These result in smooth muscle contraction, vasodilation, microvascular leakage, and mucus secretion. Cytokines are also generated over several hours and thought to play a significant role in the late-phase response. Eosinophils, monocytes, and lymphocytes are recruited to the area affected in the late-phase response and release a variety of cytokines and inflammatory mediators. Clinical manifestations of IgE-mediated food allergy depend on the organ systems involved. Reactions can be isolated, in combination, or as part of a generalized anaphylactic reaction.

Cutaneous Manifestations

Cutaneous manifestations are the most common reaction, but the absence of skin symptoms does not exclude food-induced anaphylaxis (12). These cutaneous reactions range from acute urticaria or angioedema to a morbilliform pruritic dermatitis. Chronic urticaria is almost never caused by food allergy (68). Contact dermatitis also has been reported to various foods (69). In children with atopic dermatitis, food allergies have been confirmed by DBPCFC in about one third of the children (70). In one study of 210 children evaluated and followed to determine a relationship between food allergy and exacerbations of their atopic dermatitis, 62% of children had a reaction to at least one food. Of all reactions that occurred within 2 hours of a DBPCFC, 75% were cutaneous (71). Urticaria was rare, and cutaneous manifestations were predominantly erythema and pruritus leading to scratching and exacerbation of the atopic dermatitis.

Sampson and Broadbent reported an increase in histamine releasabililty in patients with atopic dermatitis who repeatedly ingest a food allergen (72). This is probably due to the stimulation of mononuclear cells to secrete histamine-releasing factors (HRFs), some of which interact with IgE molecules bound to the surface of basophils. Increased HRF production has been associated

with an increase in symptoms as well as increased lung and skin hyperreactivity.

Gastrointestinal Manifestations

Gastrointestinal symptoms are the second most frequently noted manifestation of food allergy. Clinical presentations include nausea, vomiting, diarrhea, and abdominal pain and cramping. These symptoms may occur alone or in combination with symptoms from other organ systems. Studies in humans have elucidated some possible mechanisms but there is still much that is not known. There is considerable evidence that many of these symptoms result from the activation of mast cells (73). Radiologic data have shown alteration in GI motility in allergic individuals in response to specific foods (74), as well as hypotonia and retention of the allergen test meal and prominent pylorospasm (75). Direct visualization of the gastric mucosa during food allergen challenge revealed hyperemia, edema, petechiae, increased mucus, and decreased peristalsis (76). Studies of passive sensitization of rectal mucosa, ileostomies, and colostomies in nonatopic patients revealed local erythema, edema, and increased mucus secretion within minutes of the patient ingesting the allergen (77,78).

The oral allergy syndrome is considered to be a form of contact urticaria with symptoms resulting from contact of the food allergen with the oral mucosa. Symptoms include pruritus with or without angioedema of the lips, tongue, palate, and posterior oropharynx. It is associated with the ingestion of fresh fruits and vegetables and is the result of cross-allergenicity between the fruit or vegetable and some pollen. Shared allergen sensitivities have been reported between ragweed and the gourd family (watermelon, cantaloupe, honeydew melon, zucchini, and cucumbers) and banana (79). Oral allergy syndrome has been described with ingestion of apples (80), carrots, parsnips, celery, hazelnuts, potatoes (81,82), celery (83), and kiwi (84) in patients sensitive to birch pollen, and with ingestion of apples, tree nuts, peaches, oranges, pears, cherries, fennel, tomatoes, and carrots in patients allergic to tree and grass pollens (85). Oral allergy symptoms resolve rapidly and rarely involve any other target organs. However, ingestion of celery tuber (celery root), which cross-reacts with birch pollen, may cause more severe systemic symptoms in pollen-allergic patients (83). This may be explained by the presence of both heat-labile and heat-stable proteins (86). Pruritus of the mouth and lips, however, can be the initial symptoms of more severe food allergy, especially in those foods most commonly implicated in food anaphylaxis (i.e., tree nuts, peanuts, nuts, and shellfish). Therefore, in the setting of known food anaphylaxis, these symptoms should not be trivialized.

Allergic eosinophilic gastroenteropathy is manifested by eosinophilic infiltration of the GI tract. Symptoms depend on the layers of GI tract involved and are intermittent. Often this is associated with peripheral eosinophilia and rarely may involve other organs. Yet these patients do not meet criteria for hypereosinophilic syndrome (87). Eosinophilic infiltration of the mucosal layer is most common and can be seen in any part of the GI tract. Clinical symptoms include abdominal pain, postprandial nausea, vomiting, diarrhea, weight loss, failure to thrive, occult or gross blood loss in the stools, anemia, hypoalbuminemia, and peripheral edema (87,88). Involvement of the submucosal and muscular regions is more common in the prepyloric region of the gastric antrum and the distal small intestine (89). These patients also may have symptoms of gastric outlet obstruction, a mass lesion with epigastric tenderness, and even perforation of the intestinal wall (87,90). Rarely, eosinophilic infiltration involves the serosal surface, presenting with prominent ascites (87–89). Patients in whom eosinophilic gastroenteropathy is thought to be IgE mediated (approximately 50% of adult cases) tend to have a history of atopy, including asthma and allergic rhinitis, and tend to have elevated IgE levels. These patients tend to have multiple food intolerances and positive skin test results to multiple foods (91). Repeated degranulation of mast cells resulting from multiple food allergies is thought to be the cause of this disease in these atopic patients. Food-induced symptoms are thought to more

common in children, although the prevalence is not known (92).

Infantile colic is a syndrome that occurs in infants less than 3 months of age, and is characterized by recurrent attacks of fussiness, inconsolable crying, drawing up of the legs, abdominal distension, and excess gas. Symptoms often appear to be relieved with the passage of feces and flatus (93). Symptoms commonly occur in the late afternoon or evening (after feeding) and last for several hours. Several double-blind crossover trials have supported IgE-mediated food hypersensitivity as a mechanism in a minority of cases (94–96), in both breast-fed and formula-fed babies. However, the syndrome is poorly defined and is likely multifactorial with no treatment that consistently relieves symptoms. Social factors, emotional factors, environment, feeding techniques, and over- and underfeeding have all been frequently implicated. True food allergy is thought to be responsible for only 10% to 15% of cases (97). Although not thought to be due to food hypersensitivity, there is evidence mast cells may be involved in irritable bowel syndrome (IBS) (98). A majority of patients with IBS have increased number of mast cells demonstrated in the terminal ileal mucosa and in the colonic muscular layer (99). This observation supports a possible role for the mast cell in IBS.

Respiratory Manifestations

Respiratory manifestations of food allergy usually present as part of a generalized anaphylactic reaction. Symptoms include sneezing; rhinorrhea; ocular, otic, and palatal pruritus; bronchospasm; and laryngeal edema. Isolated airway symptoms as a manifestation of food allergy are exceedingly rare (100).

NON–IgE-MEDIATED REACTIONS

Food-Induced Enterocolitis

Food-induced enterocolitis syndrome presents as protracted vomiting and diarrhea in children 2 days to 3 months of age. Symptoms occur 1 to 8 hours after ingestion of the allergen, leading to a clinical picture of chronic diarrhea, eosinophilia, and malabsorption. Severe symptoms can lead to dehydration (101). Allergy to cow's milk protein is the most common cause, although soy allergy also has been implicated. Occasionally, this condition is seen in breast-fed infants due to the antigens passed on through the mother's milk. Children who develop cow's milk–induced enterocolitis can subsequently develop soy-induced enterocolitis with a change in formula (101,102). Stools contain erythrocytes, neutrophils and eosinophils, and, not infrequently, reducing substances (101). Jejunal biopsy reveals partial villous atrophy, lymphocytosis (103), and plasma cells containing IgM and IgA (103,104). Skin-prick test results are characteristically negative, supporting the idea that the immunologic mechanism is not IgE mediated. However, some investigators propose a localized IgE mechanism with resultant mast cell degranulation (105,106). In addition, some children have a component of IgE sensitivity to milk or soy as well and there is increased atopy among family members. Resolution of symptoms occurs within 72 hours after elimination of the allergen, but diarrhea may persist longer due to the secondary development of disaccharidase deficiency. Rechallenge is hallmarked by a recurrence of symptoms within 1 to 8 hours, fecal leukocytes and erythrocytes, and an increase in peripheral blood leukocytes by 3,500 cells/m^3 (101).

Food-Induced Colitis

Food-induced colitis is similar to enterocolitis, with the same allergens being responsible–milk and soy (107–109). Involvement is limited to the colon (108–110). It is also seen in infants exclusively breast-fed for reasons described earlier (111). It appears in the same age group, but there is no diarrhea or marked dehydration, and children appear less ill (108,109). Hematochezia or occult blood in the stools is the most common clinical finding (109,110,112). Depending on the extent of involvement, sigmoidoscopy findings range from areas of patchy mucosal injection to severe friability with bleeding and aphthous ulcers (110,111). Colonic biopsies characteristi-

cally reveal eosinophilic infiltrate in the lamina propria and crypt epithelium with destruction of crypts; neutrophils are found in severe lesions (109,111). Blood loss usually resolves within 72 hours of discontinuing the allergen, but resolution of mucosal lesions may take up to 1 month.

Malabsorption Syndromes

Food hypersensitivity has been associated with malabsorption; cow's milk, soy, egg, and wheat are the most common offenders (113). Symptoms usually present in the first few months of life and are nonspecific with regard to the etiology. They range from steatorrhea to protracted diarrhea, poor weight gain, and failure to thrive (113). Stools have increased fecal fat and reducing substances. In the small intestine, there are frequently areas of villous atrophy interspersed with areas of normal mucosa, referred to as a "patchy enteropathy" (113,114). Severe, confluent, subtotal villous atrophy, as seen in gluten-sensitive enteropathy, is uncommon. The epithelium is hypercellular with a predominant mononuclear cell infiltrate and few eosinophils. Challenge with the allergen does not produce immediate symptoms but may take days to weeks (113). Likewise, resolution of symptoms after antigen elimination is slow, with resolution of lesions requiring 6 to 18 months (113).

Celiac Disease

Celiac disease, also known as gluten-sensitive enteropathy or celiac sprue, is characterized by malabsorption secondary to gluten ingestion (115,116). The allergen known to be the cause is gliadin, the alcohol-soluble portion of gluten found in wheat, oats, rye, and barley. The small intestine is involved with characteristic lesions (117), which resolve totally with elimination of gluten. The disease often presents in children 6 months to 2 years of age. Less severe disease may go unrecognized, not being diagnosed until adulthood (118). The small intestine is involved to varying degrees, with the proximal portion being involved most often (119). Clinical symptoms are those of malabsorption and are indistinguishable from other causes of malabsorption. The severity of symptoms correlates directly with the amount of intestine involved. Symptoms may be mild, such as ill-defined, vague symptoms of not feeling well, or patients may present with anemia secondary to vitamin B_{12} or folate malabsorption. Patients may have more classic symptoms of malabsorption, such as an increase in stool frequency or volume, foul smelling or rancid, frothy stools, weight loss, and weakness (120). In the most severe cases the total small intestine is involved, resulting in severe, life-threatening malnutrition, anemia, vitamin deficiencies, electrolyte imbalances, acidosis, failure to thrive, and dehydration (120). Extraintestinal manifestations, such as cheilosis, glossitis, and osteopenia reflecting severe malabsorption, also may be present (120).

Lesions of the small intestine are contiguous, not patchy, and most often involve the mucosa only, sparing the submucosa, muscularis, and serosa (118). There is shortening of the microvilli and flattening of the villi, frequently giving them a fused appearance (121). The crypts are hyperplastic with cytologically abnormal surface cells (121). The lamina propria is hypercellular, with a predominance of lymphocytes and plasma cells (118,121). These plasma cells are increased two- to sixfold and produce IgA, IgM, and IgG; there is a predominance of IgA-producing cells, as is normally found (122). Basophils, eosinophils, and mast cells are also present (123).

In addition to the classic intestinal lesions, serologic markers are often present in this disease. There are IgA antibodies found against reticulin and smooth muscle endomysium (124). Antiendomysial antibodies (AEAs) are highly sensitive and specific and therefore considered the gold standard in evaluating for celiac disease. Recently, this antibody has been identified as an antibody to tissue transglutaminase. IgA antitissue transglutaminase antibodies have been detected by enzyme-linked immunosorbent assay (ELISA) and were reported to be both sensitive and specific for the evaluation of celiac disease (125,126). Circulating IgG and IgA antibodies to gliadin are also found in most patients with celiac disease (127). Antigliadin antibodies are shown to be synthesized *in vitro* in cultured biopsy samples taken from the mucosa of pa-

tients with untreated celiac disease (128). Total IgA levels are frequently elevated, and total IgM levels decreased in many untreated patients. A recent study of healthy blood donors in the United States found the prevalence of AEAs to be 1:250, suggesting that celiac disease may not be rare, as defined by the presence of AEAs (129). Titers to IgA antigliadin, IgA antireticulin, and IgA AEAs decrease or disappear following gluten elimination and therefore can be used to follow response to treatment or to monitor compliance (130,131).

The clinical and pathophysiologic findings are consistent with an immunologic process in response to gluten ingestion: increased plasma cells and lymphocytes in the small intestine, destruction of the normal structure of the intestinal mucosa, specific antibodies to gliadin in the mucosa and the serum, and the reversal of mucosal lesions and serologic markers with the elimination of gluten with recurrence upon rechallenge. The exact mechanism, however, is as yet unknown. First thought to be immune complex mediated with the finding of specific antibodies, there is now evidence for T-cell–mediated mechanisms as well (132–134). Further support for T-cell involvement is the increased number of $\gamma\delta$-positive T cells noted in the peripheral blood of children with celiac disease, correlating with the density of $\gamma\delta$-positive T cells in the lamina propria (135).

Dermatitis Herpetiformis

Dermatitis herpetiformis is a food hypersensitivity manifested by a pruritic rash in association with gluten-sensitive enteropathy (136). It occurs most commonly in children 2 to 7 years of age. The rash is an erythematous, pleomorphic eruption involving predominantly the knees, elbows, shoulders, buttocks, and scalp. Lesions can be urticarial, papular, vesicular, or bullous (137). They may be hemorrhagic on the palms and soles, but mucous membranes are spared. Gluten-sensitive enteropathy is reported in 75% to 90% of cases. The remainder of patients usually have subclinical symptoms of celiac disease that are unmasked with aggressive gluten challenge.

The immunologic mechanism is unknown. In addition to its association with gluten sensitivity, there is other evidence for an immune-mediated process. IgA deposition in either a granular (85%–90%) or linear (10%–15%) pattern as well as C3 are found on immunofluorescent staining of dermal papillary tips both in normal and affected skin (136). Immune complexes are frequently found in the sera, although what role they play is uncertain (137). IgA antibodies against smooth muscle endomysium are found in approximately 70% of patients, and titers correlate with the severity of the intestinal disease. There is also an association with HLA-B8 (80%–90%) (137,138), and approximately 75% of patients are positive for HLA-DW3 (138). Both the cutaneous lesions and the enteropathy respond to gluten elimination. However, cutaneous lesions may respond more slowly to treatment and also may appear more slowly with rechallenge. Sulfones are the mainstay of therapy for the cutaneous lesions and may relieve pruritic symptoms within 24 hours (137).

Heiner's Syndrome

Heiner's syndrome is a form of primary pulmonary hemosiderosis associated with cow's milk sensitivity. It is rare, occurs in infants and young children, and is characterized by wheezing, chronic cough, recurrent pulmonary infiltrates, hypochromic microcytic anemia, and failure to thrive (139). Patients also may have rhinitis, hypertrophied nasopharyngeal tissue with resultant cor pulmonale (140), recurrent otitis media, GI symptoms, and growth retardation (141). Consistent with hemosiderosis, hemosiderin-laden macrophages may be seen in biopsy samples of the lung or in stomach aspirates (139). Patients have positive skin test results to cow's milk proteins and may have unusually high titers of precipitins to many cow's milk proteins as well as eosinophilia. The titers, however, do not correlate with disease severity, and their significance is as yet unknown (140). Symptoms improve when milk is eliminated from the diet and recur with rechallenge. With severe disease and acute GI symptoms, corticosteroids may be useful therapy.

Some patients with positive precipitins do not respond to milk elimination, whereas some with no titers do (142). In general, those patients who do have high titers of precipitins to cow's milk constituents respond to treatment and have a better prognosis than patients with other forms of pulmonary hemosiderosis (142). Although pulmonary hemosiderosis may have other causes, the presence of severe anemia should raise the suspicion of cow's milk–induced etiology.

IgE-MEDIATED ASTHMA FROM FOOD ALLERGEN INHALATION

IgE-mediated food reactions can result from inhalation of aerosolized antigens, usually in an occupational setting. The resultant symptoms are the same as respiratory symptoms seen with aeroallergens, rhinoconjunctivitis, and asthma. The asthma is often a more prominent symptom. Patients typically have IgE antibody to the food as demonstrated by skin tests, RAST, or enzyme assay. Baker's asthma, the first described occupational food allergy, was noted in 1705 by Bernadino Ramazzini in his treatise *De Moribus Artifucum Diatriba,* or *Disease of Workers* (143). This is the most common food-related lung disease, and affects workers who are regularly exposed to flour. Wheat is the most common allergen, and IgE antibody to wheat flour has been demonstrated in patients with Baker's asthma (144–146). Bronchial provocation has shown sensitivity to flour as well as to contaminants such as insects or molds (147–149). A study of crab processors reported that the IgE sensitization occurs through exposure to aerosolized proteins, in this case in the steam of cooking water, thus explaining the resultant respiratory symptoms (150). This also may explain some adverse reactions that food-sensitive individuals have experienced with smelling the food, or being in close vicinity while it is cooked. In a study of salmon processing workers, 24 of 291 employees developed occupational asthma. They worked in close proximity to machines that generated aerosolized salmon serum protein; IgE antibodies to salmon serum protein was demonstrated (151). Of interest, 12 of 54 snow crab workers who were sensitized by inhalation and developed asthma, experienced the same reaction with ingestion of the snow crab (150). This condition has been

TABLE 14.1. *Food causing occupational immunologic respiratory diseases*

Food	Associated occupation
Buckwheat flour	Food processors
Castor bean	Longshoremen, fertilizer workers, oil industry
Coffee bean	Longshoremen, food processors
Egg	Egg-processing workers
Garlic	Spice factory workers
Grain dust	Granary workers, farmers, millers, bakers
Guar gum	Carpet manufacturing
Gum acacia	Printers
Mushroom	Mushroom growers
Papain	Food processors
Salmon, crab	Food processors

described in a garlic worker as well (152). This, however, is not common because most patients with baker's asthma do not experience symptoms with wheat ingestion (145). Of note, there have been isolated reports of anaphylaxis from ingestion of food contaminated with an aeroallergen (153,154). Table 14.1 lists allergens implicated in food-related occupational lung disease.

FOOD-RELATED EXERCISE-INDUCED ANAPHYLAXIS

Exercise-induced anaphylaxis is a unique syndrome characterized by generalized body warmth, erythema, and pruritus, which can progress to fulminant anaphylaxis, including confluent urticaria, laryngeal edema, bronchospasm, GI symptoms, hypotension, and even vascular collapse (155). A subset of patients have these symptoms only if exercise is performed within 2 to 6 hours of food ingestion (156). With food alone or exercise alone, there is no anaphylaxis (156,157). For some patients, this postprandial exercise-induced anaphylaxis may occur with any food ingestion followed by exercise (156,157). Others have exercise-induced anaphylaxis only associated with the ingestion of specific foods, such as celery (156) or shellfish (158). These patients are skin test positive to the foods, yet they have no allergic reactions unless ingestion is followed by or preceded by rigorous exercise (156,158). Symptoms of exercise-induced anaphylaxis may be intermittent. For

all food-related exercise-induced anaphylaxis, episodes are prevented with avoidance of food ingestion 4 to 6 hours prior to or following exercise (157). Treatment also includes carrying self-injectable epinephrine, exercising with a "buddy," wearing medic alert identification, and exercising only if a medical facility is in reasonable proximity. If affordable, a cell phone should be carried. The mechanism of this type of anaphylaxis is not well understood, but it is thought to be mediated by mast cell degranulation (155).

FOOD RELATED REACTIONS OF UNCERTAIN ETIOLOGY

Food Additives

Allergic reactions to food additives are exceedingly rare. Many symptoms attributed to food additive intolerance such as mood changes and behavioral changes have not been substantiated by DBPCFC. In one study, 132 patients who responded to a survey stating they had an adverse reaction to food additives underwent different oral challenges with additives mixed in combination and with placebo capsules. Of these patients, only 3 had a consistent reaction: 2 to the natural yellow-orange annatto and one to the azo dye and the antioxidants, for an overall prevalence of 0.1% (159).

Metabisulfite reactions in asthmatic patients are both rare and variable (160). There were no positive oral challenges with metabisulfite in 12 patients with idiopathic anaphylaxis, and 1 patient with chronic urticaria, all of whom had reactions temporally related to restaurant meals (161). Two multicenter trials were conducted to evaluate claims of hypersensitivity to aspartame. These were double-blind, placebo-controlled crossover trials, one involving 40 patients presenting with headache after aspartame ingestion and the other involving 21 patients with urticaria or angioedema associated with aspartame ingestion. Both studies reported that aspartame was no more likely than placebo to cause the adverse reactions (162,163). In a multicenter double-blind placebo-controlled trial of 120 individuals who believed they had reactions to monosodium glutamate, none had reproducible reactions (164).

Other

Other diseases that appear to be exacerbated by certain foods have been reported in the literature. Some have been reported to be documented by DBPCFC, such as one case of arthritis (165) and 16 pediatric patients with migraine and epilepsy, 15 of whom had symptoms with exposure to several foods, 8 of whom had seizures (166). Although these DBPCFC show an association, they do not necessarily suggest an immunologic cause. Other symptoms such as fatigue, hyperreactivity, enuresis, and mood changes have not been substantiated by DBPCFC.

DIAGNOSIS

Diagnosis of food allergy requires a thorough history to differentiate between food intolerance and a true hypersensitivity reaction. Table 14.2 lists important data to obtain. Multiple food allergies are rare. Complaints of these as well as unusual clinical manifestations and excessive weight loss with elimination diets may all be manifestations of food aversion, possibly of a psychologic nature. Histories may more reliably implicate the offending agent in immediate-type reactions and may not be very helpful in chronic diseases such as atopic dermatitis (167). The physical examination may be helpful if a reaction is occurring and should also be used to rule out other disease processes.

In eliciting a history, one must be aware of "hidden" foods, and be aware that ingredients that comprise less than 2% of a new product may not be listed on the package. Hidden foods may

TABLE 14.2. *Data to gather in the evaluation of possible food allergy*

Implicated foods
Amount of food required to elicit a reaction
History of a reaction with each exposure
The amount of time between the exposure and the reaction (this is especially useful for an IgE-mediated reaction, which is usually immediate in onset but may occur up to 2 h following ingestion)
Clinical manifestations consistent with food allergy
Resolution of symptoms with elimination of the food
Duration of symptoms
Medications, if any, needed to treat reactions

TABLE 14.3. *Possible sources of hidden food allergy*

Cross-contamination
  At the manufacturing site
    Reworking[a]
    Shared machinery
  At the restaurant
Foods added for specific properties
  Inulin for health benefits such as increasing enteric bacteria
  Sodium caseinate added to tuna to promote its packing qualities
  Soy added to meat for bulk
Spices
  Not required to be labeled if not a primary ingredient
  May not be labeled individually

[a] Reworking is combining unacceptable pieces of candy to add to new production batches. This may combine chocolate that contains nuts with chocolate that doesn't.

be foods included in processing, such as egg-white used in meat processing (168), or contamination of a safe food, either in preparation of the food or from shared equipment at a factory. Inulin, a fructan and storage carbohydrate, has recently been reported to cause anaphylaxis (169). This carbohydrate is found in more than 36,000 plants, including chicory and artichokes. However inulin and oligofructose, a hydrolysate of inulin, are currently being added to many processed foods such as candy, ice cream, beverages, yogurt, butter, and cereals. This increased use is due to many postulated health benefits such as the ability to increase levels of enteric bacteria. This, added to foods, may be a new hidden food allergen. Table 14.3 lists some sources of hidden foods.

IgE-Mediated Reactions

A variety of *in vivo* and *in vitro* testing can be performed to corroborate a suspected food allergy. *In vivo* tests include skin-prick testing and elimination diets. Skin testing is recommended for histories suggestive of IgE-mediated food hypersensitivity. They are highly reliable (170) and give useful information in a short period of time (170,171). A drop of glycerinated food allergen extract (1:20 to 1:10 wt/vol dilution) is placed on the skin and the prick or puncture technique applied (171). Histamine and saline are used as positive and negative controls, respectively. Fruit and vegetable extracts are very labile, so fresh fruits and vegetables are recommended when testing for allergy to these foods (85). The food can be rubbed on the skin, which is then pricked, or the needle can first be introduced into the food with subsequent pricking of the skin. A wheal 3 mm greater than the negative control is considered a positive reaction (171). With reliable extracts, the incidence of false-negative results is low, rendering a negative predictive value of more than 95% (172). The positive predictive value, however, is significantly lower. It is approximately 60% in a patient population in which the likelihood of food allergies is fairly high (172), but may be as low as 3% in a patient population in which the prevalence is low and there is no suggestive history (172). In this same population, however, the negative predictive value of the prick test for foods approaches 100% (172,173). Intradermal food skin testing is not recommended because it has a higher chance of inducing systemic symptoms and a greater false-positive rate than skin-prick testing when compared with DBPCFC (171,173).

Elimination diets are 7- to 14-day diets in which all foods suspected of causing an allergic reaction are eliminated. When multiple foods are suspected, the elimination diet may be repeated, with only several foods eliminated each time. This may be helpful in chronic conditions such as atopic dermatitis or in children in whom specific foods may be difficult to implicate. If there is no resolution of symptoms, the foods are thought not to be responsible. Foods that are implicated may be reintroduced one at a time at 24- to 48-hour intervals to determine which foods are responsible. Elimination diets rarely diagnose food allergies and can be very tedious and time consuming. Foods thought to be implicated should generally be confirmed by skin testing and possibly DBPCFC because persistent elimination of foods can lead to nutritional inadequacies, especially in children (174). In adults who are nutritionally healthy, a diet of rice, lamb, and water for several days can be useful to exclude food allergy as a cause for variety of chronic conditions such as urticaria or rhinitis. Diet diaries are

occasionally useful when the cause-and-effect relationship are not initially perceived. Data of all foods ingested and any associated symptoms are recorded prospectively. Although there is no risk of nutritional inadequacies, these tend to yield little reward for the effort involved.

Occupational food-induced respiratory allergies (allergic rhinoconjunctivitis or asthma) may require spirometry to document asthma. Many patients will only have symptoms in the workplace initially and may benefit from serial peak flow monitoring or even spirometry at the workplace (175). Bronchial allergen challenges may be used, but patients can have severe life-threatening bronchospasm so this should be done only in a medical setting capable of treating such reactions, and only if necessary.

In vitro tests consist of measurement of specific serum IgE by RAST. This test is less specific (172) than skin-prick tests, considerably more expensive, and yields less immediate results. It may be considered, however, in cases of severe atopic dermatitis or dermographism where skin testing is more difficult. Recently, the CAP System FEIA, which quantifies allergen-specific IgE, was reported to have a positive predictive value similar to prick skin testing for milk, fish, egg, and peanut hypersensitivity (176). In addition, it identified patients with a high likelihood (>95%) of reacting clinically to these foods (176).

Double-blind placebo-controlled food challenge is considered the gold standard for the definitive diagnosis of food allergies (47). With foods that are not likely to cause an allergy or with negative skin test or RAST results, open or simple-blinded oral challenges may be used in the office setting and are much more practical. In the case of multiple positive results, however, DBPCFC may be used to confirm results, especially in children in whom elimination of multiple foods may lead to nutritional deficiencies (174). The choice of foods selected for the DBPCFC should be determined by history, skin test, or RAST results, or results of an elimination diet. Foods should be eliminated for 7 to 14 days and all medication that may interfere with interpretation of symptoms should be discontinued (i.e., antihistamines, corticosteroids). A standard scoring system (47) should be used, and there must be access to emergency medical treatment should anaphylaxis occur. Patients with a history consistent with an immediate reaction to food, especially those with a life-threatening reaction and positive skin test or RAST, should not be challenged.

The DBPCFC is administered in the fasting state. Lyophilized food is often used, and it is blinded to the patient and physician or nurse as either a capsule or liquid. The starting dose is usually 125 to 500 mg of lyophilized food, which is then doubled every 15 to 60 minutes. Symptoms are recorded using a standard scoring system, usually categorized by organs involved (47). A study is considered negative if 10 g of the substance has been tolerated. All blinded negative challenges must be confirmed by an open feeding under observation to rule out a false-negative reaction, which occurs in approximately 5% of patients. This may be secondary to the food processing such as the problems described previously with lyophilization of fish antigens. In summary, the DBPCFC may be especially useful in determining suspected food allergies, which are not apparent by history supplemented by skin testing or RAST testing or an elimination diet. It also may be helpful in interpreting positive skin tests that do not correlate with the patient's history.

Because children often develop tolerance to milk, soy, wheat, and eggs after several years of strict avoidance, it is recommended they be reevaluated with skin testing periodically (yearly or every 2 years). A negative skin test should be confirmed by oral challenge. Many patients, however, remain skin test positive despite losing clinical hypersensitivity. DBPCFC should then be performed. The CAP system FEIA quantifies allergen-specific IgE and can identify a subset of patients who have a greater than 95% chance of reacting to eggs, milk, peanuts, and fish. This can eliminate the need for DBPCFC in these patients (176).

Non–IgE-Mediated Reactions

Non–IgE-mediated food allergies involving the GI tract are diagnosed predominantly by response to elimination of the allergen from the diet, although some diseases require biopsies as well (Table 14.4). Food-induced enterocolitis and colitis resolve within 72 hours after elimination of the suspected antigen from the diet, although symptoms may persist if a secondary disaccharide deficiency has developed. Malabsorption syndromes may take days or weeks for symptoms to resolve. An oral food challenge can be used to confirm the diagnosis of

TABLE 14.4. *Diagnosis of non–IgE-mediated food allergy*

Manifestation	Diagnostic criteria
Food-induced enterocolitis	1. Resolution of symptoms within 72 h after elimination of the allergen (usually milk or soy). Symptoms may persist if a secondary disaccharidase deficiency develops.
	2. Open oral challenge, if elimination is inconclusive, consisting of 0.6 mg protein per kg body weight with simultaneous monitoring of the white blood cell count (WBC) and stools. Symptoms of vomiting and diarrhea appear in 1–6 h and can be severe. Peripheral WBC increases by 3,500 cells/m^3 and polymorphonuclear cells and eosinophils can be found in the stool.
Food-induced colitis	1 and 2. Same as above, but symptoms may take hours or days to appear and are not as severe.
	3. Biopsy.
Malabsorption syndromes	1,2, and 3. Same as above.
Celiac disease	Biopsy required for diagnosis with resolution of characteristic villous atrophy after 6–12 wk of a gluten-free diet.
	IgA levels useful for screening and monitoring the disease (i.e., compliance).
Allergic eosinophilic gastroenteritis	Biopsy-proven eosinophilic infiltration of the gastrointestinal wall.
	Multiple biopsies (as many as 10) may be needed because lesions are sporadic.
	Some patients have IgE to specific foods with improvement of symptoms and intestinal lesions after 6–12 wk of elimination.

enterocolitis. This consists of administering 0.6 g of the allergen/kg body weight with simultaneous monitoring of the peripheral white blood cell count. Vomiting and diarrhea will occur within 1 to 6 hours, and the absolute leukocyte count will increase by 3,500 cells/m^3 if the challenge is positive. Polymorphonuclear leukocytes and eosinophils can be found in the stool as well. Reactions to an oral challenge can be very severe, leading to dehydration and hypotension; therefore, such challenges need to be undertaken in a medical setting and should only be performed if the diagnosis is still in question after elimination of the allergen. In the case of food-induced colitis, symptoms may take hours to days to reappear with an oral challenge and are not as severe as those seen with enterocolitis. Both colitis and malabsorption syndromes can be confirmed by biopsy as well.

Celiac disease requires a biopsy showing characteristic villous atrophy with resolution after 6 to 12 weeks of a gluten-free diet. IgA against endomysium (124) or tissue transglutaminase (125,126) can be used for screening and following a patient's progress, but celiac disease can only be diagnosed by biopsy.

Allergic eosinophilic gastroenteritis is diagnosed with biopsy-proven eosinophilic infiltration of the GI wall. However, multiple biopsies, in some cases as many as 10, may be needed because the eosinophilic infiltrate is often sporadic and may be missed on a single biopsy. Some patients also may have positive skin test or RAST results to specific foods, with improvement in symptoms and normalization of intestinal lesions after 6 to 12 weeks of elimination of the food. Of note, many GI diseases, including inflammatory bowel disease and irritable bowel syndrome, may have somewhat increased eosinophilia on biopsy.

Other tests that have been reported in the evaluation of food allergies include basophil histamine release, IgG$_2$ and IgG$_4$ antibodies, antigen–antibody complexes, plasma histamine level, neutrophil chemotaxis, lymphocyte stimulation studies, and special intestinal biopsies. These tests are predominantly research tools, are not widely available, and, although appropriate for investigational purposes, are not sufficiently reliable to be used in clinical practice (177). Several tests including subcutaneous or sublingual provocation, the leukocytotoxicity assay, and intracutaneous or low-level modified RAST titration are widely promoted by some practitioners and laboratories for the diagnosis and treatment of food allergy. However, there is no generally accepted body of literature documenting the diagnostic utility of these methods (177,178).

TREATMENT

Once food hypersensitivity is diagnosed, the offending allergen must be strictly eliminated from the diet. This is the only proven treatment for food allergy. Patients and their families need to be properly educated in food avoidance, including hidden food sources. This may be particularly difficult with certain foods such as peanuts (5). Of 32 peanut-allergic patients studied by Bock et al., only 25% (8 patients) were able to successfully avoid peanut exposure for 5 years after their initial evaluation (51). In addition, some patients may be exquisitely sensitive, reportedly reacting to peanuts on airplanes without ingestion (179).

Patients with IgE-mediated reactions should be given injectable epinephrine (e.g., Epi-Pen or Ana-Kit) to be carried at all times, and its use should be demonstrated in the office. They should be instructed to use the epinephrine in case of accidental exposure and to go immediately to an emergency room for further evaluation as biphasic reactions can occur. Generally, these patients have immediate symptoms, appear to recover, then have a recurrence of severe anaphylactic symptoms. This was reported in one-third of fatal and near-fatal cases of anaphylaxis (12). For this reason, patients should be observed four additional hours after a reaction resolves because recurrence of symptoms may be fatal. School children should have their injectable epinephrine at school. The school administrators, nurse, and patient's teachers should be made aware of the allergy and what symptoms to look for in case of exposure. They should also be instructed in emergency treatment. These recommendations are extremely important because studies report that food anaphylaxis usually results from accidental exposure to a known allergen, and the risk for a fatal outcome is increased with a delay in treatment (12,13).

As previously mentioned, many food allergies diagnosed in childhood are not life-long, and an evaluation with skin test or RAST, and oral challenges should be considered every 1 to 3 years. This is not generally true for IgE-mediated allergy to peanuts, tree nuts, fish, or shellfish; nor is it useful in celiac disease, dermatitis herpetiformis, Heiner' syndrome, or allergic eosinophilic gastroenteritis. Thus, allergen avoidance for these is life-long. Pharmacologic agents are used to treat symptoms of anaphylaxis, but none have been shown reliably effective in preventing anaphylaxis (180). These include H_1 and H_2 antihistamines, oral cromolyn sodium, ketotifen, and antiprostaglandins. Immunotherapy was reported in one double-blind placebo-controlled study to be efficacious in three peanut-allergic patients (181). However, the rate of adverse systemic reactions was three times that of *aeroallergen rush* immunotherapy. This study had to be discontinued, so the long-term effect of immunotherapy was not evaluated.

Alternative immunotherapeutic strategies are being investigated, which may have future implications in humans. Roy et al. demonstrated reduction of allergen-induced anaphylaxis, specific IgE, plasma histamine, and vascular permeability in peanut-allergic mice using oral allergen-gene immunization (182). Horner et al. also reported decreased anaphylaxis in mice with DNA vaccination. In addition, they reported attenuation in the development of a type 2 helper T cell (T_H2)-based immune response after allergen exposure, which may have preventative implications as well (183).

Interest is growing in microbial antigens, particularly the gut microflora with their preferential expansion of the (T_H1) type 1 helper T cells and their role in the gut defense barriers. These microflora are termed probiotics. *Lactobacillus casei* GG is one such probiotic and has been reported to counteract increased gut permeability associated with prolonged cows milk exposure in rats (184). In a study of patients with atopic dermatitis and cow's milk hypersensitivity, the addition of lactobacillus with hydrolyzed whey formula resulted in decreased interstitial inflammation and improved clinical score of atopic dermatitis patients as compared with those treated with the hydrolyzed formula alone (185). *Lactobacillus* also has been shown to suppress lymphocyte proliferation *in vitro* (186), and thus may serve to promote tolerance and aid in the prevention of food allergy.

PREVENTION

The role of dietary manipulation in the prevention of atopic disease in infants of allergic parents has been under debate since 1936, when Grulee and Sanford noted a decreased incidence of atopy and food allergy among infants who were exclusively breast-fed (187). The mechanism by which breast-feeding may offer protection is unclear. It may be through the protective effects of secretory IgA or it may somehow induce gut maturity, aiding in the development of gut flora. In 1989, Zeiger et al. prospectively studied dietary manipulation in infants of atopic parents (188). With both maternal and infant avoidance of foods, the number of food-related symptoms (particularly atopic dermatitis, urticaria, and GI disease) was significantly reduced in the first 12 months of life while being less so at 2 years (188). The two groups became indistinguishable at 3, 4 (189), and 7 years of life (190). Of note, there was no difference in the incidence of asthma or rhinitis in the two groups at any time (188–190). Other studies have shown a persistent increased risk of food-related symptoms. A 10-year longitudinal study in New Zealand reported a risk of recurrent or chronic eczema that increased with the number of solid foods introduced before the age of 4 months. The highest risk was with four or more foods, and children in this group had a threefold higher risk of developing recurrent or chronic eczema as compared with those children fed no solid food before the age of 4 months (191). Because early introduction of foods, particularly those foods considered most allergenic, may increase the risk of developing food allergy, it is generally recommended that the introduction of eggs, fish, shellfish, tree nuts, and peanuts be delayed in children at high risk. Eggs should not be introduced before 2 years of age, and introduction of the others should be delayed until 4 years of age (191).

NATURAL HISTORY

Since the 1980s much has been learned about the natural history of food allergy. Children tend to lose their clinical reactivity to milk, soy, eggs, and wheat as they get older. In a prospective study of 501 children, only 2 of 15 patients with an allergy proved by DBPCFC during the first year of life remained reactive at 13 to 24 months of age (48). After 24 months of age, none retained their reactivity. In another study of patients who had severe reactions to eggs and milk, clinical reactivity lasted for years, but tolerance was eventually achieved (50). Of note, despite clinical tolerance, the presence of IgE as detected by skin test or RAST often still exists (48,50). Unlike the above foods, peanut, fish, tree nut, and shellfish hypersensitivity tends to persist. One long-term follow-up study of peanut-allergic patients reported that clinical reactions continue for a minimum of 14 years (51). Similar results were obtained from studies of patients with life-threatening anaphylaxis from fish (53), tree nuts, and crustacea (52). Recent evidence suggests that loss of clinical reactivity may be due to the structure of the allergenic epitopes. In children with cow's milk or egg IgE-mediated sensitivity, those who became tolerant had antibodies to conformational epitopes, whereas those with persistent hypersensitivity reacted primarily to linear epitopes (192). Immunodominant IgE epitopes of the major peanut allergens *Ara h 1* (recognized by >90% of peanut-allergic individuals) and *Ara h 2* are linear (193,194) and may explain the persistence of peanut allergy. Food allergies to peanuts, tree nuts, fish, and shellfish are considered lifelong, and patients must always carry emergency medicine.

REFERENCES

1. Anderson JA, Sogn DD, eds. *NIAID: adverse reactions to foods.* American Academy of Allergy and Immunology. NIH Publication. 1984:84–2442.
2. Eriksson NE. Food sensitivity reported by patients with asthma and hay fever. *Allergy* 1978;33:189–196.
3. Bock SA. Prospective appraisal of complaints of adverse reactions to foods in children during the first 3 years of life. *Pediatrics* 1987;79:683–688.
4. Høst A, Halken S. A prospective study of cow milk allergy in Danish infants during the first 3 years of life. *Allergy* 1990;45:587–596.
5. Sicherer SH, Munoz-Furlong A, Burks AW, et al. Prevalence of peanut and tree nut allergy in the US determined by a random digit dial telephone survey. *J Allergy Clin Immunol* 1999;103:559–562.
6. Buckley RH, Metcalfe DD. Food allergy. *JAMA* 1982;248:2627–2631.
7. Eigenmann PA, Sicherer SH, Borkowski TA, et al. Prevalence of IgE-mediated food allergy among children with atopic dermatitis. *Pediatrics* 1998;101:E8.
8. Roitt I, Brostoff J, Male D, eds. Hypersensitivity-type I. In: *Immunology,* 4th ed. Chicago: CV Mosby, 1996:22.
9. Smith PL, Kagey-Sobotka A, Bleeker ER, et al. Physiologic manifestations of human anaphylaxis. *J Clin Invest* 1980;66:1072–1080.
10. Kemp SF, Lockey RF, Wolf BL, et al. Anaphylaxis: a review of 266 cases. *Arch Intern Med* 1995;155:1749–1754.
11. Pumphrey RSH, Stanworth SJ. The clinical spectrum of anaphylaxis in north-west England. *Clin Exp Allergy* 1996;26:1364–1370.
12. Sampson HA, Mendelson L, Rosen JP. Fatal and near-fatal anaphylactic reactions to food in children and adolescents. *N Engl J Med* 1992;327:380–384.
13. Yunginger JW, Sweeney KG, Sturner WQ, et al. Fatal food-induced anaphylaxis. *JAMA* 1988;260:1450–1452.
14. Walker WA. Pathophysiology of intestinal uptake and absorption of antigens in food allergy. *Ann Allergy* 1987;59:7–16.
15. Walker WA. Antigen handling by the small intestine. *Clin Gastroenterol* 1986;15:1–20.
16. Walzer M. Allergy of the abdominal organs. *J Lab Clin Med* 1941;26:1867–1877.
17. Roitt I, Brostoff J, Male D, eds. The lymphoid system. In: *Immunology,* 4th ed. Chicago: CV Mosby, 1996:3.2.
18. Gearhart PJ, Cebra JJ. Differentiated B-lymphocytes: potential to express particular antibody variable and constant regions depends on site of lymphoid tissue and antigen load. *J Exp Med* 1979;149:216–227.
19. Mowat AM. The regulation of immune responses to dietary protein antigens. *Immunol Today* 1987;8:93–98.
20. Mowat AM, Strobel S, Drummond HE, et al. Immunological responses to fed protein antigens in mice. I. Reversal of oral tolerance to ovalbumin by cyclophosphamide. *Immunology* 1982;45:105–113.
21. Kleinman RE, Walker WA. The enteromammary immune system: an important new concept in breast milk host defense. *Dig Dis Sci* 1979;24:876–882.
22. Asherson GL, Zembala M, Perera MA, et al. Production of immunity and unresponsiveness in the mouse by feeding contact sensitizing agents and the role of suppressor cells in the Peyer's patches, mesenteric lymph nodes, and other tissues. *Cell Immunol* 1977;33:145–155.
23. Roitt I, Brostoff J, Male D, eds. Immunological tolerance. In: *Immunology,* 4th ed. Chicago: CV Mosby, 1996:12.
24. Bruce MG, Ferguson A. Oral tolerance to ovalbumin in mice: studies of chemically modified and "biologically filtered" antigen. *Immunology* 1986;57:627–630.
25. Bruce MG, Strobel S, Hanson DG, et al. Irradiated mice lose the capacity to "process" fed antigen for systemic

tolerance of delayed-type hypersensitivity. *Clin Exp Immunol* 1987;70:611–618.

26. Strobel S, Mowat AM, Ferguson A. Prevention of oral tolerance induction to ovalbumin and enhanced antigen presentation during a graft-versus-host reaction in mice. *Immunology* 1985;56:57–64.

27. Mowat AM, Ferguson A. Migration inhibition of lymph node lymphocytes as an assay for regional cell-mediated immunity in the intestinal lymph nodes of mice immunized orally with ovalbumin. *Immunology* 1982;47:365–370.

28. Natali PG, DeMartino C, Quaranta V, et al. Expression of Ia-like antigens in normal human nonlymphoid tissues. *Transplantation* 1981;31:75–78.

29. Mayer L, Shlien R. Evidence for function of Ia molecules on gut epithelial cells in man. *J Exp Med* 1987;166:1471–1483.

30. Heyman M, Grasset E, Ducroc R, et al. Antigen absorption by the jejunal epithelium of children with cow's milk allergy. *Pediatr Res* 1988;24:197–202.

31. Powell GK, McDonald PJ, Van Sickle GJ, et al. Absorption of food protein antigen in infants with food protein-induced enterocolitis. *Dig Dis Sci* 1989;34:781–788.

32. Selner JC, Merrill DA, Claman HN. Salivary immunoglobulin and albumin: development during the newborn period. *J Pediatr* 1968;72:685–689.

33. Kerner JA Jr. Formula allergy and intolerance. *Gastroenterol Clin North Am* 1995;24:1–25.

34. Ohsugi Y, Gershwin ME. The IgE response of New Zealand black mice to ovalbumin: an age-acquired increase in suppressor activity. *Clin Immunol* 1981;20:296–304.

35. Strobel S, Ferguson A. Immune responses to fed protein antigens in mice. 3. Systematic tolerance or priming is related to age at which antigen is first encountered. Pediatr Res 1984;18:588–594.

36. Businco L, Benincori N, Cantani A. Epidemiology, incidence and clinical aspects of food allergy. *Ann Allergy* 1984;53:615–622.

37. Hyman EPE, Clarke DD, Everett SL, et al. Gastric acid secretory function in pre-term infants. *J Pediatr* 1985;106:467–471.

38. Shub MD, Pang KY, Swann DA, et al. Age-related changes in chemical composition and physical properties of mucous glycoproteins from rat small intestine. *Biochem J* 1983;215:405–411.

39. Lebenthal E, Lee PC. Development of functional response in human exocrine pancreas. *Pediatrics* 1980;66:556–560.

40. Cummins AG, Munro GH, Miller HR, et al. Association of the maturation of the small intestine at weaning with mucosal mast cell activation in the rat. *Immunol Cell Biol* 1988;66:417–422.

41. Cummins AG, Labroy JT, Shearman DJ. The effect of cyclosporin A in delaying maturation of the small intestine during weaning in the rat. *Clin Exp Immunol* 1989;75:451–456.

42. Johansson SGO, Dannaeus A, Lilja G. The relevance of anti-food antibodies for the diagnosis of food allergy. *Ann Allergy* 1984;53:665–672.

43. May CD, Remigio L, Feldman J, et al. A study of serum antibodies to isolated milk proteins and ovalbumin in infants and children. *Clin Allergy* 1977;7:583–595.

44. Parrott DMV. The gut as a lymphoidal organ. *Clin Gastroenterol* 1976;5:211–228.

45. Marsh DG, Meyers DA, Bias WB. The epidemiology and genetics of atopic allergy. *N Engl J Med* 1981;305:1551–1559.

46. Lemanske RF Jr, Taylor SL. Standardized extracts, foods. *Clin Rev Allergy* 1987;5:23–36.

47. Bock SA, Sampson HA, Atkins FM, et al. Double-blind, placebo-controlled food challenge (DBPCFC) as an office procedure: a manual. *J Allergy Clin Immunol* 1988;82:986–997.

48. Bock SA. The natural history of adverse reaction to foods. *N Engl Regional Allergy Proc* 1986;7:504–510.

49. Foucard T. Developmental aspects of food sensitivity in childhood. *Nutr Rev* 1984;42:98–104.

50. Bock SA. Natural history of severe reactions to foods in young children. J Pediatr 1985;107:676–680.

51. Bock SA, Atkins F. The natural history of peanut allergy. *J Allergy Clin Immunol* 1989;83:900–904.

52. Atkins FM, Steinberg SS, Metcalfe DD. Evaluation of immediate adverse reactions to foods in adult patients. II. A detailed analysis of reaction patterns during oral food challenge. *J Allergy Clin Immunol* 1985;75:356–363.

53. Dannaeus A, Inganäs M. A follow-up study of children with food allergy. Clinical course in relation to serum IgE-and IgG-antibody levels to milk, egg and fish. *Clin Allergy* 1981;11;533–539.

54. Bleumink E, Young E. Identification of the atopic allergen in cow's milk. *Int Arch Allergy* 1968;34:521–543.

55. Bernhisel-Broadbent J, Strause D, Sampson HA. Fish hypersensitivity. II. Clinical relevance of altered fish allergenicity caused by various preparation methods. *J Allergy Clin Immunol* 1992;90:622–629.

56. Wertel SJ, Cooke SK, Sampson HA. Clinical reactivity to beef in children allergic to cow's milk. *J Allergy Clin Immunol* 1997;99:293–300.

57. Nordlee JA, Taylor SL, Jones RT, et al. Allergenicity of various peanut products as determined by RAST inhibition. *J Allergy Clin Immunol* 1981;68:376–382.

58. Taylor SL, Busse WW, Sachs MI, et al. Peanut oil is not allergenic to peanut-sensitive individuals. *J Allergy Clin Immunol* 1981;68:372–375.

59. Hoffman DR, Collins-Williams C. Cold-pressed peanut oils may contain peanut allergen. *J Allergy Clin Immunol* 1994;93:801–802.

60. Barnett D, Bonham B, Howden MEH. Allergenic cross-reactions among legume foods—an in vitro study. *J Allergy Clin Immunol* 1987;79:433–438.

61. Bernhisel-Broadbent J, Sampson HA. Cross-allergenicity in the legume botanical family in children with food hypersensitivity. *J Allergy Clin Immunol* 1989;83:435–440.

62. Bernhisel-Broadbent J, Taylor S, Sampson HA. Cross-allergenicity in the legume botanical family in children with food hypersensitivity. II. Laboratory correlates. *J Allergy Clin Immunol* 1989;84:701–709.

63. Bernhisel-Broadbent J, Scanlon SM, Sampson HA. Fish hypersensitivity. I. In vitro and oral challenge results in fish-allergic patients. *J Allergy Clin Immunol* 1992;89:730–737.

64. Jones SM, Magnolfi CF, Cooke SK, et al. Immunologic cross-reactivity among cereal grains and grasses in children with food hypersensitivity. *J Allergy Clin Immunol* 1995;96:341–351.

65. Waring NP, Daul CB, deShazo RD, et al. Hypersensitivity reactions to ingested crustacea: clinical evaluation

and diagnostic studies in shrimp-sensitive individuals. *J Allergy Clin Immunol* 1985;76:440–445.

66. Clein NW. Cow's milk allergy in infants and children. *Int Arch Allergy* 1958;13:245–256.

67. Langeland T. A clinical and immunological study of allergy to hen's egg white. VI. Occurrence of proteins cross-reacting with allergens in hen's egg white as studied in egg white from turkey, duck, goose, seagull, and in hen egg yolk, and hen and chicken sera and flesh. *Allergy* 1983;38:399–412.

68. Champion RH, Roberts SOB, Carpenter RG, et al. Urticaria and angio-oedema: a review of 554 patients. *Br J Dermatol* 1969;81:588–597.

69. Chan EF, Moward C. Contact dermatitis to food and spices. *Am J Contact Dermatitis* 1998;9:71–79.

70. Burks AW, Mallory SB, Williams LW, et al. MA. Atopic dermatitis: clinical relevance of food hypersensitivity reactions. *J Pediatr* 1988;113:447–451.

71. Sampson HA. Food hypersensitivity and atopic dermatitis. *Allergy Proc* 1991;12:327–331.

72. Sampson HA, Broadbent KR, Bernhisel-Broadbent J. Spontaneous release of histamine from basophils and histamine-releasing factor in patients with atopic dermatitis and food hypersensitivity. *N Engl J Med* 1989;321:228–232.

73. Stenton GR, Vliagoftis H, Befus AD. Role of intestinal mast cells in modulating gastrointestinal pathophysiology. *Ann Allergy Asthma Immunol* 1998;81:1–11.

74. Liu H-Y, Whitehouse WM, Giday Z. Proximal small bowel transit pattern in patients with malabsorption induced by bovine milk protein ingestion. *Radiology* 1975;115:415–420.

75. Fries JH, Zizmor J. Roentgen studies of children with alimentary disturbances due to food allergy. *Am J Dis Child* 1937;54:1239–1251.

76. Pollard HM, Stuart GJ. Experimental reproduction of gastric allergy in human beings with controlled observations on the mucosa. *J Allergy* 1942;13:467–473.

77. Gray I, Walzer M. Studies in mucous membrane hypersensitiveness. III. The allergic reaction of the passively sensitized rectal mucous membrane. *Am J Diff Dis* 1938;4:707.

78. Gray I, Harten M, Walzer M. Studies in mucous membrane hypersensitiveness. IV. The allergic reaction in the passively sensitized mucous membranes of the ileum and colon in humans. *Ann Intern Med* 1940;13:2050–2056.

79. Enberg RN, Leickly FE, McCullough J, et al. Watermelon and ragweed share allergens. *J Allergy Clin Immunol* 1987;79:867–875.

80. Lahti A, Bjørksten F, Hannuksela M. Allergy to birch pollen and apple, and cross-reactivity of allergens studied with the RAST. *Allergy* 1980;35:297–300.

81. Anderson KE, Lowenstein H. An investigation of the possible immunological relationship between allergen extracts from birch pollen, hazelnut, potato and apple. *Contact Dermatitis* 1978;4:73–79.

82. Halmepuro L, Lowenstein H. Immunological investigation of possible structural similarities between pollen antigens and antigens in apple, carrot, and celery tuber. *Allergy* 1985;40:264–272.

83. Ballmer-Weber BK, Vieths S, et al. Celery allergy confirmed by double-blind, placebo-controlled food challenge: a clinical study of 32 subjects with a history of adverse reactions to celery root. *J Allergy Clin Immunol* 2000;106;373–378.

84. Gall H, Kalveram KJ, Forck G, et al. Kiwi fruit allergy: a new birch pollen–associated food allergy. *J Allergy Clin Immunol* 1994;94:70–76.

85. Ortolani C, Ispano M, Pastorello EA, et al. Comparison of results of skin prick tests (with fresh foods and commercial food extracts) and RAST in 100 patients with oral allergy syndrome. *J Allergy Clin Immunol* 1989;83:683–690.

86. Jankiewicz A, Aulepp H, Baltes W, et al. Allergic sensitization to native and heated celery root in pollen-sensitive patients investigated by skin test and IgE binding. *Int Arch Allergy Immunol* 1996;111:268–278.

87. Steffen RM, Wyllie R, Petras RE, et al. The spectrum of eosinophilic gastroenteritis. *Clin Pediatr* 1991;30:404–411.

88. Talley NJ, Shorter RG, Phillips SF, et al. Eosinophilic gastroenteritis: a clinicopathological study of patients with disease of the mucosa, muscle layer and subserosal tissue. *Gut* 1990;31:54–58.

89. Goldman H, Ming S-C, eds. *Pathology of the gastrointestinal tract.* Philadelphia: WB Saunders, 1992:171–187.

90. Snyder JD, Rosenblum N, Wershil B, et al. Pyloric stenosis and eosinophilic gastroenteritis in infants. *J Pediatr Gastroenterol Nutr* 1987;6:543–547.

91. Kettlehut BV, Metcalfe DD. Adverse reactions to foods. In: Middleton E, Reed CE, Ellis EF, et al., eds. *Allergy: principles and practice,* 3rd ed. St. Louis, MO: CV Mosby, 1988:1481.

92. James JM, Sampson HA. An overview of food hypersensitivity. *Pediatr Allergy Immunol* 1991;3:67.

93. First year feeding problems. In: Nelson WE, Behrman RE, Kliegman RM, et al., eds. *Textbook of pediatrics,* 15th ed. Philadelphia: WB Saunders, 1996:165.

94. Forsyth BWC. Colic and the effect of changing formulas: a double-blind multiple-crossover study. *J Pediatr* 1989;115:521–526.

95. Lothe L, Lindberg T. Cow's milk whey protein elicits symptoms of infantile colic in colicky formula-fed infants: a double-blind crossover study. *Pediatrics* 1989;83:262–266.

96. Jakobsson I, Lindberg T. Cow's milk proteins cause infantile colic in breast-fed infants: a double-blind crossover study. *Pediatrics* 1983;71:268–271.

97. Infantile colic and food allergy: fact or fiction? *J Pediatr* 1989;115:583–584.

98. Gui X-Y. Mast cells: a possible link between psychological stress, enteric infection, food allergy and gut hypersensitivity in the irritable bowel syndrome. *J Gastroenterol Hepatol* 1998;13:980–989.

99. Weston AP, Biddle WL, Bhatia PS, et al. Terminal ileal mucosal mast cells in irritable bowel syndrome. *Dig Dis Sci* 1993;38:1590–1595.

100. Bock SA, Atkins FM. Patterns of food hypersensitivity during sixteen years of double-bind, placebo-controlled food challenges. *J Pediatr* 1990;117:561–567.

101. Powell GK. Milk-and soy-induced enterocolitis of infancy: clinical features and standardization of challenge. *J Pediatr* 1978;93:553–560.

102. Jakobsson I, Lindberg T. A prospective study of cow's milk protein intolerance in Swedish infants. *Acta Pediatr Scand* 1979;68:853–859.

103. Perkkio M, Savilahti E, Kuitunen P. Morphometric and immunohistochemical study of jejunal biopsies from children with intestinal soy allergy. *Eur J Pediatr* 1981;137:63–69.

104. Pearson JR, Kingston D, Shiner M. Antibody production to milk proteins in the jejunal mucosa of children with cow's milk protein intolerance. *Pediatr Res* 1983;17:406–412.

105. Selbekk BH. A comparison between in vitro jejunal mast cell degranulation and intragastric challenge in patients with suspected food intolerance. *Scand J Gastroenterol* 1985;20:299–303.

106. Nolte H, Schiotz PO, Kruse A, et al. Comparison of intestinal mast cell and basophil histamine release in children with food allergic reactions. *Allergy* 1989;44:554–565.

107. Jenkins HR, Pincott JR, Soothill JF, et al. Food allergy: the major cause of infantile colitis. *Arch Dis Child* 1984;59:326–329.

108. Berezin S, Schwarz SM, Glassman M, et al. Gastrointestinal milk intolerance of infancy. *Am J Dis Child* 1989;143:361–362.

109. Goldman H, Proujansky R. Allergic proctitis and gastroenteritis in children: clinical and mucosal features in 53 cases. *Am J Surg Pathol* 1986;10:75–86.

110. Gryboski JD. Gastrointestinal milk allergy in infants. *Pediatrics* 1967;40:354–362.

111. Lake AM, Whitington PF, Hamilton SR. Dietary protein-induced colitis in breast-fed infants. *J Pediatr* 1982;101:906–910.

112. Silber GH, Klish WJ. Hematochezia in infants less than 6 months of age. *Am J Dis Child* 1986;140:1097–1098.

113. Kuitunen P, Visakorpi JK, Savilahti E, et al. Malabsorption syndrome with cow's milk intolerance: clinical findings and course in 54 cases. *Arch Dis Child* 1975;50:351–356.

114. Manuel PD, Walker-Smith JA, France NE. Patchy enteropathy in childhood. *Gut* 1979;20:211–215.

115. Van de Kamer JH, Weyers HA, Dicke KW. Coeliac disease IV. An investigation into injurious constituents of wheat in connection with their action on patients with coeliac disease. *Acta Pediatr* 1953;42:223.

116. Anderson CM, Frazer AC, French JM, et al. Coeliac disease. Gastrointestinal studies and the effects of dietary wheat flour. *Lancet* 1952;1:836.

117. Paulley, LW. Observations on the aetiology of idiopathic steatorrhea. *BMJ* 1954;2:1328.

118. Rubin CE, Brandborg LL, Phelps PC, et al. Studies of celiac disease. I. The apparent identical and specific nature of the duodenal and proximal jejunal lesion in celiac disease and idiopathic sprue. *Gastroenterology* 1960;38:28–49.

119. MacDonald WC, Brandborg LL, Flick AL, et al. Studies of celiac sprue. IV. The response of the whole length of the small bowl to a gluten-free diet. *Gastroenterology* 1964;47:573–589.

120. Trier JS. Celiac sprue. In: Sleisenger MH, Fordtran JS, eds. *Gastrointestinal disease: pathophysiology, diagnosis, management,* 5th ed. Philadelphia: WB Saunders, 1993:1078.

121. Yardley JH, Bayless TM, Norton JH, et al. A study of the jejunal epithelium before and after a gluten-free diet. *N Engl J Med* 1962;267:1173–1179.

122. Baklien K, Brandtzaeg P, Fausa O. Immunoglobulins in jejunal mucosa and serum from patients with adult coeliac disease. *Scand J Gastroenterol* 1977;12:149–159.

123. Marsh MN, Hinde J. Inflammatory component of celiac sprue mucosa. I. Mast cells, basophils and eosinophils. *Gastroenterology* 1985;89:92–101.

124. Kumar V, Lerner A, Valeski JE, et al. Endomysial antibodies in the diagnosis of celiac disease and the effect of gluten on antibody titers. *Immunol Invest* 1989;18:533–544.

125. Levine A, Bujanover Y, Reif S, et al. Comparison of assays for anti-endomysial and anti-transglutaminase antibodies for the diagnosis of pediatric celiac disease. *Isr Med Assoc J* 2000;2:82–83.

126. Sugai E, Selvaggio G, Vazquez H. et al. Tissue transglutaminase antibodies in celiac disease; assessment of a commercial kit. *Am J Gastroenterol* 2000;95:2318–2322.

127. Levenson SD, Austin RK, Dietler MD, et al. Specificity of antigliadin antibody in celiac disease. *Gastroenterology* 1985;89:1–5.

128. Ciclitira PJ, Ellis HJ, Wood GM, et al. Secretion of gliadin antibody by coeliac jejunal mucosal biopsies cultured in vitro. *Clin Exp Immunol* 1986;64:119–124.

129. Not T, Horvath K, Hill ID, et al. Celiac disease risk in the USA: high prevalence of antiendomysium antibodies in healthy blood donors. *Scand J Gastroenterol* 1998;33:494–498.

130. O'Farrelly C, Feighery C, O'Brian DS, et al. Humoral response to wheat protein in patients with coeliac disease and enteropathy associated T cell lymphoma. *BMJ* 1986;293:908–910.

131. Walker-Smith JA, Guandalini S, Schmitz J, et al. Revised criteria for diagnosis of coeliac disease. *Arch Dis Child* 1990;65:909–911.

132. Howdle PD, Bullen AW, Losowsky MS. Cell mediated immunity to gluten within the small intestinal mucosa in coeliac disease. *Gut* 1982;23:115–122.

133. MacDonald TT, Spencer J. Evidence that activated mucosal T cells play a role in the pathogenesis of enteropathy in human small intestine. *J Exp Med* 1988;167:1341–1349.

134. Marsh MN. The immunopathology of the small intestinal reaction in gluten-sensitivity. *Immunol Invest* 1989;18:509–531

135. Klemola T, Tarkkanen J, Örmälä T, et al. Peripheral $\gamma\delta$ T cell receptor-bearing lymphocytes are increased in children with celiac disease. *J Pediatr Gastroenterol Nutr* 1994;18:435–439.

136. Hall RP. The pathogenesis of dermatitis herpetiformis: recent advances. *J Am Acad Dermatol* 1987;16:1129–1144.

137. Katz SI, Hall RP III, Lawley TJ, et al. Dermatitis herpetiformis: the skin and the gut. *Ann Intern Med* 1980;93:857–874.

138. Solheim BG, Ek J, Thune PO, et al. HLA antigens in dermatitis herpetiformis and coeliac disease. *Tissue Antigens* 1976;7:57–59.

139. Heiner DC, Sears JW. Chronic respiratory disease associated with multiple circulating precipitins to cow's milk. *Am J Dis Child* 1960;100:500–502.

140. Boat TF, Polmar SH, Whitman V, et al. Hyperreactivity to cow milk in young children with pulmonary hemosiderosis and cor pulmonale secondary to nasopharyngeal obstruction. *J Pediatr* 1975;87:23–29.

141. Heiner DC, Sears JW, Kniker WT. Multiple precipitins to cow's milk in chronic respiratory disease. A syndrome including poor growth, gastrointestinal symptoms, evidence of allergy, iron deficiency anemia and pulmonary hemosiderosis. *Am J Dis Child* 1962;103:634.

142. Lee SK, Kniker WT, Cook CD, et al. Cow's milk-induced pulmonary disease in children. *Adv Pediatr* 1978;25:39–57.

143. Cohen SG. Landmark commentary: Ramazzini on occupational disease. *Allergy Proc* 1990;11:49.

144. Blands J, Diamant B, Kallos P, et al. Flour allergy in bakers. I. Identification of allergenic fractions in flour and comparison of diagnostic methods. *Int Arch Allergy Appl Immunol* 1976;52:392–406.

145. Hendrick DJ, Davies RJ, Pepys J. Baker's asthma. *Clin Allergy* 1976;6:241.

146. Walker CL, Grammer LC, Shaughnessy MA, et al. Baker's asthma: report of an unusual case. *J Occup Med* 1989;31:439–442.

147. Frankland AW, Lunn JA. Asthma caused by the grain weevil. *Br J Indust Med* 1965;22:157.

148. Weiner A. Occupational bronchial asthma in a baker due to *Aspergillus. Ann Allergy* 1960;18:1004.

149. Stressman E. Results of bronchial testing in bakers. *Acta Allergol* 1967;22(suppl 8):99.

150. Cartier A, Malo J-L, Ghezzo H, et al. IgE sensitization in snow crab processing worker. J Allergy Clin Immunol 1986;78:344–348.

151. Douglas J, McSharry C, Blaikie L, et al. Occupational asthma caused by automated salmon processing. *Lancet* 1995;346:737–740.

152. Lybargar JA, Gallagher JS, Pulver DW, Litwin A, Brooks S, Bernstein IL. Occupational asthma induced by inhalation and ingestion of garlic. *J Allergy Clin Immunol* 1982;69:448–454.

153. Erben AM, Rodriguez JL, McCullough J, Ownby DR. Anaphylaxis after ingestion of beignets contaminated with *Dermatophagoides farinae. J Allergy Clin Immunol* 1993;92:846–849.

154. Matsumoto T, Hisano T, Hamaguchi M, et al. Systematic anaphylaxis after eating storage-mite–contaminated food. *Arch Allergy Immunol* 1996;109:197–200.

155. Sheffer AL, Tong AK, Murphy GF, et al. Exercise-induced anaphylaxis: a serious form of physical allergy associated with mast cell degranulation. *J Allergy Clin Immunol* 1985;75:479–484.

156. Kidd JM 3d, Cohen SH, Sosman AJ, et al. Food-dependent exercise-induced anaphylaxis. *J Allergy Clin Immunol* 1983;71:407–411.

157. Novey HS, Fairshter RD, Salness K, et al. Postprandial exercise- induced anaphylaxis. *J Allergy Clin Immunol* 1983;71:498–504.

158. Maulitz RM, Pratt DS, Schocket AL. Exercise-induced anaphylactic reaction to shellfish. *J Allergy Clin Immunol* 1979;63:433–434.

159. Young E, Patel S, Stoneham M, et al. The prevalence of reaction to food additives in a survey population. *J R Coll Physicians London* 1987;21:241–271.

160. Taylor SL, Bush RK, Selner JC, et al. Sensitivity to sulfited foods among sulfite-sensitive subjects with asthma. *J Allergy Clin Immunol* 1988;81:1159–1167.

161. Sonin L, Patterson R. Metabisulfite challenge in patients with idiopathic anaphylaxis. *J Allergy Clin Immunol* 1985;75;67–69.

162. Schiffman SS, Buckley CE III, Sampson HA, et al. Aspartame and susceptibility to headache. *N Engl J Med* 1987;317:1181–1185.

163. Geha R, Buckley CE, Greenberger P, et al. Aspartame is no more likely than placebo to cause urticaria/angioedema: results of a multicenter, randomized, double-blind, placebo-controlled, crossover study. *J Allergy Clin Immunol* 1993;92:513–520.

164. Geha RS, Beiser A, Ren C, et al. Multicenter, double-blind, placebo-controlled, multiple-challenge evaluation of reported reactions to monosodium glutamate. *J Allergy Clin Immunol* 2000;106:973–980.

165. Panush RS, Stroud RM, Webster EM. Food-induced (allergic) arthritis. Inflammatory arthritis exacerbated by milk. *Arthritis Rheumatol* 1986;29:220–226.

166. Egger J, Carter CM, Soothill JF, et al. Oligoantigenic diet treatment of children with epilepsy and migraine. *J Pediatr* 1989;114:51–58.

167. Sampson HA. Role of immediate food hypersensitivity in the pathogenesis of atopic dermatitis. *J Allergy Clin Immunol* 1983;71:473–480.

168. Leduc V, Demeulemester C, Polack B, et al. Immunochemical detection of egg-white antigens and allergens in meat products. *Allergy* 1999;54:464–472.

169. Gay-Crosier F, Schreiber G, Hauser C. Anaphylaxis from inulin in vegetables and processed food [Letter]. *N Engl J Med* 2000;342:1372–1373.

170. Bock SA, Lee W-Y, Remigio L, et al. Appraisal of skin tests with food extracts for diagnosis of food hypersensitivity. *Clin Allergy* 1978;8:559–564.

171. Bock SA, Buckley J, Holst A, et al. Proper use of skin tests with food extracts in diagnosis of hypersensitivity to food in children. *Clin Allergy* 1977;7:375–383.

172. Sampson HA, Albergo R. Comparison of results of skin tests, RAST, and double-blind placebo-controlled food challenges in children with atopic dermatitis. *J Allergy Clin Immunol* 1984;74:26.

173. May CD. Objective clinical and laboratory studies of immediate hypersensitivity reactions to foods in asthmatic children. *J Allergy Clin Immunol* 1976;58:500–515.

174. Roesler TA, Barry PC, Bock SA. Factitious food allergy and failure to thrive. *Arch Pediatr Adolesc Med* 1994;148:1150–1155.

175. Ditto AM, Grammer LC. Immunologic evaluation of environmental lung disease. *Clin Pulmon Med* 1995:2;276–285.

176. Sampson HA, Ho DG. Relationship between food-specific IgE concentrations and the risk of positive food challenges in children and adolescents. *J Allergy Clin Immunol* 1997;100:444–451.

177. Bahna SL. Diagnostic tests for food allergy. *Clin Rev Allergy* 1988;6:259–284.

178. Grieco MH. Controversial practices in allergy. *JAMA* 1982:247:3106–3111.

179. Sicherer SH, Furlong TJ, DeSimone J, et al. Self-reported reactions to peanut on commercial airliners. *J Allergy Clin Immunol* 1999;104:186–189.

180. Sogn DD. Medications and their use in the treatment of adverse reactions to foods. *J Allergy Clin Immunol* 1986;78:238.

181. Oppenheimer JJ, Nelson HS, Bock SA, et al. Treatment

of peanut allergy with rush immunotherapy. *J Allergy Clin Immunol* 1992;90:256–262.

182. Roy K, Mao H-Q, Huang S-K, et al. Oral gene delivery with chitosan-DNA nanoparticles generates immunologic protection in a murine model of peanut allergy. *Nature Med* 1999;4: 387–391.

183. Horner AA, Nguyen MD, Ronaghy A, et al. DNA-based vaccination reduces the risk of lethal anaphylactic hypersensitivity in mice. *J Allergy Clin Immunol* 2000;106:349–356.

184. Isolauri E, Majamaa H, Arvola T, et al. *Lactobacillus casei* strain GG reverses increased intestinal permeability induced by cow milk in suckling rats. *Gastroenterology* 1993;105:1643–1650.

185. Majamaa H, Isolauri E. Probiotics: a novel approach in the management of food allergy. *J Allergy Clin Immunol* 1997;99:179–185.

186. Sutas Y, Soppi E, Korhonen H, et al. Suppression of lymphocyte proliferation in vitro by bovine caseins hydrolyzed with *Lactobacillus casei* GG–derived enzymes. *J Allergy Clin Immunol* 1996;98:216–224.

187. Grulee EG, Sanford HN. The influence of breast and artificial feeding on infantile eczema. *J Pediatr* 1936;9:223.

188. Zeiger RS, Heller S, Mellon MH, et al. Effect of combinedmaternal and infant food-allergen avoidance on development of atopy in early infancy: a randomized study. *J Allergy Clin Immunol* 1989;84:72–89.

189. Zeiger RS, Heller S, Sampson HA. Genetic and environmental factors affecting the development of atopy from birth through age 4 in a prospective randomized controlled study of dietary avoidance [Abstract]. *J Allergy Clin Immunol* 1992;89:192.

190. Zeiger RS, Heller S. The development and prediction of atopy in high-risk children: follow-up at age seven years in a prospective randomized study of combined maternal and infant food allergen avoidance. *J Allergy Clin Immunol* 1995;95:1179–1190.

191. Fergusson DM, Horwood LJ, Shannon FT. Early solid feeding and recurrent childhood eczema: a 10-year longitudinal. *Pediatrics* 1990;86:541–546.

192. Sampson HA, Cooke SK, Huang SK. Variable response to ovomucoid in man. J Immunol 1997;159:2026–2032.

193. Burks AW, Shin D, Cockrell G, et al. Mapping and mutational analysis of the IgE-binding epitopes on Ara h 1, a legume vicilin protein and a major allergen in peanut hypersensitivity. *Eur J Biochem* 1997;245:334–339.

194. Stanley JS, King W, Burks AW, et al. Identification and mutational analysis of the immuno dominant IgE epitopes of the major peanut allergen Ara h 2. *Arch Biochem Biophys* 1997;347:244–253.

15

Atopic Dermatitis

Peck Y. Ong and Donald Y.M. Leung

Department of Pediatrics, University of Colorado Health Sciences Center,
Department of Pediatric Allergy-Immunology, National Jewish
Medical and Research Center, Denver Colorado

Atopic dermatitis (AD) is a chronic inflammatory skin disease that most commonly arises in childhood (1,2). It is frequently associated with a personal or family history of allergic rhinitis or asthma. Up to 85% of AD patients have elevated serum immunoglobulin E (IgE) and positive immediate skin test. A subgroup of AD patients, however, is nonatopic with no apparent sensitization to food or inhalant allergens (3).

EPIDEMIOLOGY

Between 5% and 20% of children worldwide are affected by AD (4). Sixty percent of affected children continue to have persistent AD after puberty (5), and nearly 80% of patients are at risk for developing respiratory allergies, including allergic rhinitis and asthma (6). The concordance rate for monozygotic twins with AD is 77% as compared with 15% for dizygotic twins with AD (7), indicating a genetic role in the pathogenesis of AD. However, the mode of inheritance for AD is not known. Various candidate genes for asthma and allergic diseases, including the region on chromosome 5q31 that contains the cytokine genes that regulate serum IgE levels and eosinophilia, have been studied for possible association with AD (8). It is likely that the expression of AD, as with other atopic diseases, involves the interaction of multiple genes, the environment, and the immune system.

PATHOGENESIS

The peripheral blood mononuclear cells (PBMCs) of AD patients produce increased levels of helper T cell type 2 (T_H2) cytokines, including interleukin-4 (IL-4) and IL-13 (9,10), which are crucial in the induction of IgE production (11). In addition, decreased expression of interferon-γ (IFN-γ) (12), which is a T_H1 cytokine that is known to mediate delayed-type hypersensitivity responses and inhibit IgE production (12), is another characteristic of PBMCs of AD patients. These peripheral blood abnormalities are consistent with the elevation of serum IgE in AD patients.

In the acute, erythematous skin lesions of AD patients, the majority of cellular infiltrate consists of $CD4^+$ T cells expressing the memory T-cell marker CD45RO (13) and the skin-homing receptor, cutaneous lymphocyte-associated antigen (CLA) (14). These T cells produce increased levels of IL-4, IL-5, and IL-13 (15,16). IL-4 and IL-13 play a critical role in the induction of endothelial adhesion molecules required for influx of allergic inflammatory cells (e.g., eosinophils) into the skin. IL-5 is also a T_H2 cytokine that promotes the development, activation, chemotaxis and survival of eosinophils, which in turn deposit extensive amounts of cytotoxic granule proteins in AD lesions (17). These proteins include major basic protein and eosinophil cationic protein. In addition to their cytotoxic properties, these proteins are also capable of inducing basophil and

TABLE 15.1. *Diagnostic criteria for atopic dermatitis*

The presence of itchy skin plus three or more of the following:
1. History of itchy skin involving flexural areas (elbows, behind the knees or fronts of ankles) or around the neck (add "or on the cheeks" for patients under 10 yr).
2. A personal history of asthma or allergic rhinitis (or family history of atopic disease in a first-degree relative for patients under 4 yr).
3. A history of generalized dry skin in the past year.
4. Visible dermatitis involving flexural areas (add "or on the cheeks/forehead and outer aspects of the limbs" for patients under 4 yr).
5. Onset of the skin condition under 2 yr (this criterion only applies to patients 4 yr or older).

Modified from Williams HC, Burney PG, Pembroke AC, et al. The U.K. Working Party's Diagnostic Criteria for Atopic Dermatitis. III. Independent hospital validation. *Br J Dermatol* 1994; 131:406–416.

mast cell degranulation to release inflammatory mediators (18). Increased IFN-γ expression has been found in chronic AD lesions (19). Thus, a biphasic model of inflammation in AD with a predominance of T_H2 cytokines (e.g., IL-4) in acute lesions and a predominance of T_H1 cytokines (e.g., IFN-γ and IL-12) in chronic lesions has been proposed (20).

The activation of T cells in AD skin is stimulated by antigen-presenting cells that consist mainly of epidermal Langerhans cells. These cells express high levels of the high-affinity receptor for IgE (FcRI), which bind to IgE molecules and facilitate the capture of allergens for processing and presentation to T cells (21). IgE-positive epidermal Langerhans cells from AD lesions have been found to be 100- to 1,000-fold more efficient in presenting house dust mite allergen to T cells than IgE–epidermal Langerhans cells (22).

In addition to allergens, superantigenic toxins also have been implicated in the pathogenesis of AD (23). These toxins are produced by *Staphylococcus aureus*, which are found in the skin lesions of 90% of AD patients (24). AD patients who have specific serum IgE to these superantigenic toxins have been found to have more severe disease than patients without specific IgE to these toxins (25). In addition, superantigenic toxins may contribute to the skin inflammation of nonatopic AD patients through the activation of T cells and production of inflammatory cytokines (26). The presence of IgE autoantibodies also has been demonstrated in AD patients, suggesting a role for IgE autoreactivity in the pathogenesis of AD (27).

CLINICAL MANIFESTATIONS AND DIAGNOSIS

Acute AD lesions are characterized by intense pruritus, erythematous papules, and excoriations with a serous exudate, whereas chronic lesions consist of nonerythematous thickened plaques of skin with accentuated skin markings (lichenification). Fibrotic papules (prurigo nodularis) may be present in long-standing chronic AD lesions.

There is currently no diagnostic laboratory test for AD. The diagnosis of AD is based on clinical features. The most frequently used clinical criteria are those proposed by Hanifin and Rajka (28). These criteria have been refined by the United Kingdom's Working Party (29). This refined set of criteria has a sensitivity of 85% and specificity of 96%. Its main features are shown in Table 15.1.

Eighty-seven percent of AD patients have onset of the disease before 5 years of age, and less than 2% of patients have disease onset after 20 years of age (30). Therefore, adult patients with suspected new-onset AD should raise a high index of suspicion for other skin conditions or diseases (Table 15.2). Of note, a significant number of adult patients who present with occupational hand eczema have a personal history of atopy (31).

EVALUATION

The grading of the severity of AD is based on the extent of affected areas, itch intensity, and appearance of the skin lesions (32,33). In general, patients with more than 20% skin involvement (or 10% skin involvement if affected areas

TABLE 15.2. *Differential diagnoses of atopic dermatitis*

Dermatologic diseases
  Seborrheic dermatitis, irritant or allergic contact dermatitis, psoriasis, nummular pilaris, keratosis pilaris, lichen simplex chronicus, pityriasis rosea, nonbullous congenital ichthyosiform erythroderma
Neoplastic diseases
  Cutaneous T-cell lymphoma (mycosis fungoides, Sézary syndrome), Letterer-Siwe disease (Langerhans cell histocytosis), necrolytic migratory erythema associated with pancreatic tumor.
Immunodeficiencies
  Hyper-IgE syndrome, Wiskott-Aldrich syndrome, severe combined immunodeficiency syndrome
Infectious diseases
  Human immunodeficiency virus–associated eczema, scabies, candidiasis, tinea versicolor
Congenital and metabolic disorders
  Netherton syndrome, phenylketonuria, zinc deficiency, essential fatty acid deficiency, histidine deficiency, infantile-onset multiple carboxylase deficiency

include the eyelids, hands, or intertriginous areas) who have not responded to first-line treatment (see section on Management) may be considered to have severe AD (34). Factors that contribute to severity of AD include the following:

- Patients who are erythrodermic and at risk for exfoliation
- Patients who require chronic high potency topical or systemic corticosteroids
- Patients who require hospitalization for management of AD or skin infection due to AD
- Patients with ocular complications such as keratoconus or keratoconjunctivitis
- Patients with significant sleep, psychological, or developmental disturbances due to AD

Food allergy is an important trigger of AD in infants and young children (35). The prevalence of food allergy in children with moderate to severe AD ranged from 33% to 39% in various studies (35). In addition, the severity of AD directly correlates with the presence of food allergy (36). A rational approach in evaluating children with AD and suspected food allergies is to screen them using skin-prick test for the most common offending foods, including eggs, milk, soy, wheat, fish, peanut, walnut (or cashew), and selected foods as suggested by history (35). Skin-prick tests are useful when they are negative because they have high negative predictive value of more than 95% (37,38). On the other hand, positive skin prick test have a positive predictive value of less than 50% (37,38). Sampson and Ho (39) evaluated the usefulness of quantitative serum IgE levels using the Pharmacia CAP System FEIA in predicting food-allergic reaction in AD patients and found that the IgE levels for the following four foods have positive predictive value of greater than 95%: eggs, 6 kU/L; milk, 32 kU/L; peanuts, 15 kU/L; and codfish, 20 kU/L. Thus, quantitative serum IgE levels using the CAP System FEIA for eggs, milk, peanuts, and codfish are useful in determining the need to perform oral challenge for these foods. Positive skin-prick tests should be followed by placebo-controlled oral food challenges unless the patient has a history of life-threatening reactions on ingestion of the suspected food or significant improvement of AD on dietary elimination. This approach can prevent unnecessary or harmful dietary limitations (40). Oral food challenges should be performed in a setting that is well prepared for managing severe allergic reactions. Double-blind, placebo-controlled oral food challenges are considered to be the gold standard for diagnosing food allergy (35).

Inhalant allergens, including house dust mite and animal danders, are potential triggers of AD (41). In a double-blind controlled study, Tan et al. showed that house dust mite avoidance could improve AD (42). It is therefore useful to obtain a skin-prick test or specific serum IgE to identify AD patients who are sensitive to these aeroallergens in order to implement appropriate avoidance measures.

Getting a bacterial culture with antibiotic sensitivity from skin wounds can direct antibiotic choice in patients with clinical evidence of staphylococcal skin infection (e.g., weeping or oozing lesions). Infected AD lesions that have not responded to appropriate systemic antibiotics in 48 hours (43) or the presence of vesicular rash should raise the suspicion for herpes simplex virus (HSV). A Tzanck smear and a viral culture can be obtained to establish the diagnosis. Fungi also have been implicated in the pathogenesis of AD (44), and a variant form of AD involving the head and neck has been associated with fungal colonization (45). These patients respond to antifungal therapy.

MANAGEMENT

First-line Treatment

First-line treatment of AD consists of avoidance of triggers, skin hydration, topical corticosteroids, and control of pruritus (Fig. 15.1). Irritants such as wool clothing, harsh soaps, extremes of temperatures, chemicals, and smoke should be avoided. For patients who are diagnosed with food allergy, the offending foods should be eliminated from the diet. A dietary consultation is often helpful in the elimination of food allergens, as well as in planning a nutritionally balanced diet. For AD patients who have house dust mite allergy, it is important to implement dust mite control such as the use of dust mite–proof bed and pillow covers, frequent carpet vacuuming, and minimizing the presence of soft furnishing and toys. For patients with indoor pet sensitivity, the animals should be removed from the home environment or kept outdoors (46).

Skin hydration therapy for patients with moderate to severe AD should include a soaking luke-warm bath for 15 to 20 minutes once to twice a day. The use of milder superfatted soaps for cleansing can help to prevent skin dryness. The bath should be followed immediately by the application of an emollient to uninvolved skin areas and topical corticosteroids to affected areas. Emollient creams (e.g., Vanicream) are better than ointments in humid conditions because creams are less occlusive and less likely to retain sweat, which may cause folliculitis. On the other hand, ointments (e.g., Aquaphor) are more effective in preventing evaporation and therefore more suitable for use in dry weather condition.

For patients with mild AD, low-potency topical corticosteroids such as 1% or 2.5% hydro-

cortisone (Table 15.3) may be used on affected skin areas once to twice a day after bathing. In patients who do not respond to low-potency topical corticosteroids, a medium-potency topical corticosteroids such as 0.1% triamcinolone ointment may be used on affected skin areas on the trunk and extremities. Hydrocortisone (2.5%) ointment may be used on affected areas on the face and intertriginous areas. Ointment preparations of corticosteroids used after baths generally have less drying effect due to their occlusive nature. Therefore, they are preferred over creams in dry weather conditions and in patients who do not sweat excessively. Potential side effects of topical corticosteroids include skin atrophy, striae, and adrenal suppression (47). These side effects are related to the potency of the corticosteroids, the body surface area covered, and the duration of use. High-potency topical corticosteroids (groups I and II in Table 15.3) should be reserved for severe AD patients only, and they should not be used for more than 1 week.

Localized superficial staphylococcal skin infection may be treated with topical antibiotic such as mupirocin (Bactroban). In AD patients who do not respond to topical treatment or who have widespread staphylococcal skin infection, systemic antibiotics such as azithromycin or cephalexin can be helpful (48). Because HSV infection in AD can lead to life-threatening dissemination (49), systemic acyclovir should be considered in infected AD patients, especially infants, immunocompromised individuals, and those with widespread AD.

The fingernails of AD patients should be kept short and clean to minimize skin trauma and infection from scratching. First-generation systemic antihistamines such as diphenhydramine and hydroxyzine may be helpful in relieving pruritus in some AD patients due to their sedating effects. Therefore, these medications are best used at bedtime. Studies on second-generation nonsedating antihistamines in the control of pruritus in AD patients have produced mixed results (50). Topical Doxepin cream in combination with topical corticosteroid has been found to be safe and effective in controlling pruritus in some AD patients, but there is an increased risk for developing contact sensitivity to doxepin with topical use (51). Tar shampoos or low-potency topical

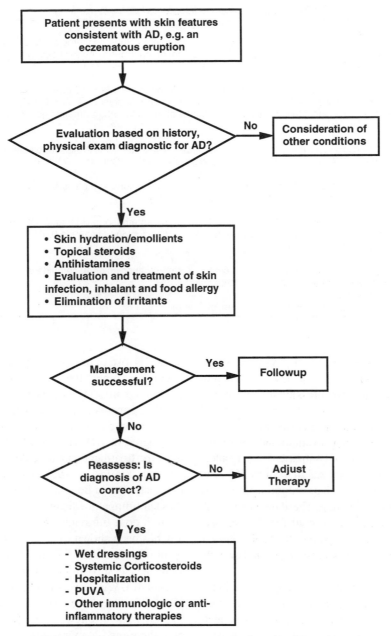

FIG. 15.1. Algorithm for management of atopic dermatitis.

corticosteroid lotions may be helpful in controlling scalp itching.

Treatment for Severe AD

For patients with severe AD, it is necessary for their skin to be clear before any definitive evaluations such as oral food challenges can be per- formed. In these patients, wet occlusive dressings are often helpful (52). This therapy increases hydration, penetration of topical corticosteroids, and pruritus control, and therefore allows rapid healing of excoriated lesions. However, overuse of wet dressings may lead to chilling, maceration of the skin, and secondary infection (34). Therefore, wet dressing therapy should be closely

TABLE 15.3. *Topical corticosteroid potency ranking*

Group I (most potent)
Betamethasone dipropionate 0.05% (Diprolene; cream, ointment), clobetasol propionate 0.05% (Temovate; cream, ointment), diflorasone diacetate 0.05% (Psorcon; ointment), halobetasol dipropionate 0.05% (Ultravate; cream, ointment)

Group II
Amcinonide 0.1% (Cyclocort; ointment), betamethasone dipropionate 0.05% (Diprosone; cream, ointment), desoximetasone (Topicort; 0.05% gel, 0.25% cream, ointment), fluocinonide 0.05% (Lidex; solution, gel, cream, ointment), halcinonide 0.1% (Halog; solution, cream, ointment), mometasone furoate 0.1% (Elocon; ointment)

Group III
Amcinonide 0.1% (Cyclocort; lotion, cream), betamethasone valerate 0.1% (Valisone; ointment), diflorasone diacetate 0.05% (Florone; cream), fluticasone propionate 0.005% (Cutivate; ointment)

Group IV
Triamcinolone acetonide 0.1% (Kenalog; cream, ointment), fluocinolone acetonide 0.025% (Synalar; ointment), mometasone furoate 0.1% (Elocon; lotion, cream)

Group V
Hydrocortisone valerate 0.2% (Westcort; cream, ointment), betamethasone valerate 0.1% (Valisone; lotion, cream), fluticasone propionate 0.05% (Cutivate; cream), fluocinolone acetonide 0.025% (Synalar; cream), Desonide 0.05% (Tridesilon; ointment)

Group VI
Alclometasone dipropionate 0.05% (Aclovate; cream, ointment), fluocinolone acetonide 0.01% (Synalar; solution, cream), desonide 0.05% (Tridesilon; cream).

Group VII (least potent)
Hydrocortisone 1%/2.5% (Hytone; lotion, cream, ointment)

monitored by an experienced physician, and is optimally administered in a day hospital program. In addition to wet dressing therapy, it may be necessary to implement temporary dietary and environmental limitations in order to prepare the patient for subsequent evaluations. Therefore, patients who have failed outpatient management will need to be hospitalized in a controlled environment. Sedatives such as chloral hydrate may be used to control itching. These medications allow antihistamines to be held for allergen skin testing. However, the adverse effects of sedatives, including respiratory depression, should be monitored closely.

Systemic corticosteroids may be required rarely in patients with severe AD who respond poorly to topical corticosteroids. AD patients who receive systemic corticosteroids often experience a rebound worsening of their dermatitis following the discontinuation of the medication (34). Therefore, a short course of systemic corticosteroids should be followed by implementation of intensified skin hydration and topical corticosteroid therapy during the tapering period to suppress the rebound flaring. Due to the potential side effects of systemic corticosteroids,

including osteoporosis and growth suppression in children, other alternative therapies should be considered in AD patients who have required multiple courses of systemic corticosteroids.

Systemic antifungal medications should be considered in AD patients who have failed the first-line treatment and are colonized with fungi on their skin lesions (53). However, liver function tests should be monitored in patients given these antifungal medications.

High-dose ultraviolet A1 (UVA1) phototherapy has been shown to be effective in the treatment of severe AD (54). Its efficacy in treating acute AD is also more superior than the conventional UVA-UVB combination therapy (54). However, it has been suggested that UVA-UVB therapy may have fewer side effects than UVA1 and therefore is more suitable for long-term treatment of chronic AD (54). UVB also has been shown to be effective in the treatment of AD (55). It has been suggested that UVB may be safer than the UVA-UVB combination in the treatment of AD (55). However, the long-term carcinogenic potential for skin cancer and other side effects of these different forms of UV phototherapy are unknown and need further evaluation.

Alternative Therapies

Recombinant Interferon-γ

Interferon-γ has been shown to suppress IL-4 and IgE production (12). The use of recombinant interferon-γ (rIFN-γ) in the treatment of AD is based on the rationale that this cytokine may restore the immunologic imbalance consisting of an aggravated T_H2 response. Several studies have shown the beneficial effects of rIFN-γ in AD, including one study that showed persistent long-term improvement in AD patients who were treated with rIFN-γ (56). However, the wide use of rIFN-γ in the treatment of AD has been limited by its high cost and difficulty in predicting responders (56).

Intravenous Immunoglobulin

There are few studies on the efficacy of IVIG in AD (57). The major disadvantage of this therapy is its high cost and transient efficacy. In addition, double-blind placebo-controlled studies will be needed to establish its efficacy in AD.

Phosphodiesterase Inhibitors

The antiinflammatory activity of a topical phosphodiesterase inhibitor, CP-80633, has been studied in AD (58). Currently, the mechanism of action for topical phosphodiesterase inhibitors is not fully understood but may be associated with their inhibitory effects on inflammatory cytokines (58). Other more potent topical phosphodiesterase inhibitors are also being studied for the treatment of AD (59).

Cyclosporine

Oral cyclosporine works primarily through the suppression of inflammatory cytokine production by T cells (60). This medication has been shown to improve severe AD significantly in both adults (61) and children (62) at a maximum dose of 5 mg/kg/day for about a year. After the discontinuation of cyclosporine, most patients experienced a relapse, but in some patients the improvement of AD was sustained for up to 3 months

(61). The major disadvantages of cyclosporine treatment consist of the need for frequent blood chemistry and cell count monitoring, renal toxicity, hypertension, and potential long-term risk for malignancy (61). Topical cyclosporine has been studied in AD, but no consistent beneficial effect has been found (63,64).

Tacrolimus

Tacrolimus (also known as FK506) is a potent immunosuppressive agent that behaves with a mechanism similar to that of cyclosporine by inhibiting the production of inflammatory cytokines by T cells (60). When administered systemically, tacrolimus is an effective immunosuppressant in organ transplantation but possesses systemic side effects similar to those of cyclosporine (65). Due to its smaller molecular size compared with cyclosporine and better skin penetration (65), a topical form of tacrolimus has been developed for the treatment of inflammatory skin diseases. Two well-controlled studies showed that a 3-week topical treatment with 0.03%, 0.1%, and 0.3% tacrolimus ointments resulted in significant improvement in both adults (67) and children (68) with moderate to severe AD. Signs and symptoms of AD, including erythema and pruritus, were decreased in the patients treated with tacrolimus ointment. There was no significant difference in efficacy between the three different concentrations of tacrolimus ointment in general. However, the 0.1% and the 0.3% ointments may be more effective in the treatment of AD on the face and neck than the 0.01% ointment (68). Importantly, no significant systemic side effect was noted in both studies. The only significant adverse effect was a local burning sensation at the site of tacrolimus application (67). Current studies on the long-term efficacy and safety of tacrolimus ointment in AD have been completed, and the medication has been found to be generally safe and efficacious.

Another topical medication with a mode of action similar to that of tacrolimus, SDZ ASM 981, also has been shown to be safe and effective in the treatment of AD (69). With their potent antiinflammatory effects and lack of significant side effects, topical tacrolimus and macrolactams such as SDZ ASM 981 are attractive nonsteroidal antiinflammatory medications for AD.

SUMMARY AND CONCLUSIONS

Atopic dermatitis is a common skin disease of childhood. Significant proportions of affected children have persistent AD after puberty and are at risk for developing respiratory allergies, including asthma and allergic rhinitis. The pathogenesis of AD is currently not fully understood but involves interactions between genetic factors, the immune system, and the environment. The majority of AD patients are atopic, with elevated total serum IgE and positive immediate skin test results to food or inhalant allergens. However, subgroups of AD patients are nonatopic, and their disease may involve nonallergic mechanisms of inflammation. In addition, superantigens produced by *S. aureus*, which are found on the skin lesions of 90% of AD patients, may contribute to the inflammation of AD through IgE- and non–IgE-mediated mechanisms.

There is currently no single diagnostic test or curative therapy for AD. The diagnosis of AD is based on a defined set of clinical criteria. The management of AD includes avoidance of potential triggers. Therefore, initial evaluation should include ruling out sensitivities to food (particularly in children) and inhalant allergens. Other first-line preventive and symptomatic treatments include adequate skin hydration, topical corticosteroids, and the use of first-generation antihistamine at bedtime. Secondary bacterial, viral, or fungal infection should be treated with appropriate antimicrobial agents. For patients with severe persistent AD, alternative therapies should be considered because chronic use of corticosteroids can cause significant local and systemic side effects. Currently, the most promising alternative antiinflammatory therapy for AD is topical macrolide immunomodulators, such as tacrolimus or SDZ ASM 981, which work by suppressing inflammatory cytokine production. These topical medications have been shown to have excellent clinical efficacy without significant side effects.

ACKNOWLEDGMENTS

This work was supported in part by National Institutes of Health Grants AR41256 and General Clinical and Research Center Grant MO1 RR00051 from the Division of Research Resources.

REFERENCES

1. Leung DYM, Rhodes AR, Geha RS, et al. Atopic dermatitis. In: Fitzpatrick TB, Eisen AZ, Wolff K, et al. *Dermatology in general medicine*, 4th ed. New York: McGraw-Hill, 1993:1543–1564.
2. Leung DYM. Atopic dermatitis: new insights and opportunities for therapeutic intervention. *J Allergy Clin Immunol* 2000;105:860–876.
3. Guillet G, Guillet MH. Natural history of sensitizations in atopic dermatitis. A 3-year follow-up in 250 children: food allergy and high risk of respiratory symptoms. *Arch Dermatol* 1992;128:187–192.
4. Williams H, Robertson C, Stewart A, et al. Worldwide variations in the prevalence of symptoms of atopic eczema in the International Study of Asthma and Allergies in Childhood. *J Allergy Clin Immunol* 1999;103:125–138.
5. Wuthrich B. Clinical aspects, epidemiology, and prognosis of atopic dermatitis. *Annals Allergy Asthma Immunol* 1999;83:464–470.
6. Linna O, Kokkonen J, Lahtela P, et al. Ten-year prognosis for generalized infantile eczema. *Acta Paediatr* 1992;81:1013–1016.
7. Schultz Larsen F. Atopic dermatitis: a genetic-epidemiologic study in a population-based twin sample. *J Am Acad Dermatol* 1993;28:719–723.
8. Forrest S, Dunn K, Elliott K, et al. Identifying genes predisposing to atopic eczema. *J Allergy Clin Immunol* 1999;104:1066–1070.
9. Renz H, Jujo K, Bradley KL, et al. Enhanced IL-4 production and IL-4 receptor expression in atopic dermatitis and their modulation by interferon-gamma. *J Invest Dermatol* 1992;99:403–408.
10. Takamatsu Y, Hasegawa M, Sato S, et al. IL-13 production by peripheral blood mononuclear cells from patients with atopic dermatitis. *Dermatology* 1998;196:377–381.
11. Vercelli D, Geha RS. Regulation of IgE synthesis: from the membrane to the genes. *Springer Semin Immunopathol* 1993;15:5–16.
12. Jujo K, Renz H, Abe J, et al. Decreased interferon gamma and increased interleukin-4 production in atopic dermatitis promotes IgE synthesis. *J Allergy Clin Immunol* 1992;90:323–331.
13. Leung DYM, Bhan AK, Schneeberger EE, et al. Characterization of the mononuclear cell infiltrate in atopic dermatitis using monoclonal antibodies. *J Allergy Clin Immunol* 1983;71:47–56.
14. Picker LJ, Michie SA, Rott LS, et al. A unique phenotype of skin-associated lymphocytes in humans. Preferential expression of the HECA-452 epitope by benign and malignant T cells at cutaneous sites. *Am J Pathol* 1990;136:1053–1068.

15. Hamid Q, Boguniewicz M, Leung DYM. Differential in situ cytokine gene expression in acute versus chronic atopic dermatitis. *J Clin Invest* 1994;94:870–876.

16. Hamid Q, Naseer T, Minshall EM, et al. In vivo expression of IL-12 and IL-13 in atopic dermatitis. *J Allergy Clin Immunol* 1996;98:225–231.

17. Leiferman KM. Eosinophils in atopic dermatitis. *J Allergy Clin Immunol* 1994;94:1310–1317.

18. Gleich GJ. Mechanisms of eosinophil-associated inflammation. *J Allergy Clin Immunol* 2000;105:651–663.

19. Grewe M, Gyufko K, Schopf E, et al. Lesional expression of interferon-gamma in atopic eczema. *Lancet* 1994;343:25–26.

20. Grewe M, Bruijnzeel-Koomen CA, Schopf E, et al. A role for Th1 and Th2 cells in the immunopathogenesis of atopic dermatitis. *Immunol Today* 1998;19:359–361.

21. Bieber T. Fc epsilon RI on human epidermal Langerhans cells: an old receptor with new structure and functions. *Int Arch Allergy Immunol* 1997;113:30–34.

22. Mudde GC, Van Reijsen FC, Boland GJ, et al. Allergen presentation by epidermal Langerhans' cells from patients with atopic dermatitis is mediated by IgE. *Immunology* 1990;69:335–341.

23. Leung DYM, Hauk P, Strickland I, et al. The role of superantigens in human diseases: therapeutic implications for the treatment of skin diseases, *Br J Dermatol* 1998;139(suppl 53):17–29.

24. Leung DYM, Harbeck R, Bina P, et al. Presence of IgE antibodies to staphylococcal exotoxins on the skin of patients with atopic dermatitis. Evidence for a new group of allergens. *J Clin Invest* 1993;92:1374–1380.

25. Bunikowski R, Mielke M, Skarabis H, et al. Prevalence and role of serum IgE antibodies to the *Staphylococcus aureus*–derived superantigens SEA and SEB in children with atopic dermatitis. *J Allergy Clin Immunol* 1999;103:119–124.

26. Akdis CA, Akdis M, Simon D, et al. T cells and T cell-derived cytokines as pathogenic factors in the nonallergic form of atopic dermatitis. *J Invest Dermatol* 1999;113:628–634.

27. Valenta R, Seiberler S, Natter S, et al. Autoallergy: a pathogenetic factor in atopic dermatitis? *J Allergy Clin Immunol* 2000;105:432–437.

28. Hanifin JM, Rajka G. Diagnostic features of atopic dermatitis. *Acta Dermatol Venereol (Stockh)* 1980;92:44–47.

29. Williams HC, Burney PG, Pembroke AC, et al. The U.K. Working Party's Diagnostic Criteria for Atopic Dermatitis. III. Independent hospital validation. *Br J Dermatol* 1994;131:406–416.

30. Rajka G. *Essential aspects of atopic dermatitis.* Berlin: Springer, 1989.

31. Rystedt I. Work-related hand eczema in atopics. *Contact Dermatitis* 1985;12:164–171.

32. Rajka G, Langeland T. Grading of the severity of atopic dermatitis. *Acta Dermatol Venereol Suppl* 1989;144:13–14.

33. Hanifin JM. Standardized grading of subjects for clinical research studies in atopic dermatitis: workshop report. *Acta Dermatol Venereol Suppl* 1989;144:28–30.

34. Leung DYM, Hanifin JM, Charlesworth EN, et al. Disease management of atopic dermatitis: a practice parameter. Joint Task Force on Practice Parameters, representing the American Academy of Allergy, Asthma and Immunology, the American College of Allergy, Asthma and Immunology, and the Joint Council of Allergy, Asthma and Immunology. Work Group on Atopic Dermatitis. *Ann Allergy Asthma Immunol* 1997;79:197–211.

35. Sicherer SH, Sampson HA. Food hypersensitivity and atopic dermatitis: pathophysiology, epidemiology, diagnosis, and management. *J Allergy Clin Immunol* 1999;104(suppl):114–122.

36. Guillet G, Guillet MH. Natural history of sensitizations in atopic dermatitis. A 3-year follow-up in 250 children: food allergy and high risk of respiratory symptoms. *Arch Dermatol* 1992;128:187–192.

37. Sampson HA, Albergo R. Comparison of results of skin tests, RAST, and double-blind, placebo-controlled food challenges in children with atopic dermatitis. *J Allergy Clin Immunol* 1984;74:26–33.

38. Bock SA, Lee WY, Remigio L, et al. Appraisal of skin tests with food extracts for diagnosis of food hypersensitivity. *Clin Allergy* 1978;8:559–564.

39. Sampson HA, Ho DG. Relationship between food-specific IgE concentrations and the risk of positive food challenges in children and adolescents. *J Allergy Clin Immunol* 1997;100:444–451.

40. Niggemann B, Sielaff B, Beyer K, et al. Outcome of double-blind, placebo-controlled food challenge tests in 107 children with atopic dermatitis. *Clin Exp Allergy* 1999;29:91–96.

41. Charlesworth EN. Practical approaches to the treatment of atopic dermatitis. *Allergy Proc* 1994;15:269–274.

42. Tan BB, Weald D, Strickland I, et al. Double-blind controlled trial of effect of housedust-mite allergen avoidance on atopic dermatitis. *Lancet* 1996;347:15–18.

43. David TJ, Longson M. Herpes simplex infections in atopic eczema. *Arch Dis Child* 1985;60:338–343.

44. Scalabrin DM, Bavbek S, Perzanowski MS, et al. Use of specific IgE in assessing the relevance of fungal and dust mite allergens to atopic dermatitis: a comparison with asthmatic and nonasthmatic control subjects. *J Allergy Clin Immunol* 1999;104:1273–1279.

45. Clemmensen O, Hjorth N. Treatment of dermatitis of the head and neck with ketoconazole in patients with type I sensitivity to *Pityrosporum orbiculare. Semin Dermatol* 1983;2:26–29.

46. Endo K, Hizawa T, Fukuzumi T, et al. Keeping dogs indoor aggravates infantile atopic dermatitis. *Arerugi* 1999;48:1309–1315.

47. Cornell RC, Stoughton RB. Six-month controlled study of effect of desoximetasone and betamethasone 17-valerate on the pituitary-adrenal axis. *Br J Dermatol* 1981;105:91–95.

48. Veien NK. The clinician's choice of antibiotics in the treatment of bacterial skin infection. *Br J Dermatol* 1998;139(suppl):30–36.

49. Sanderson IR, Brueton LA, Savage MO, et al. Eczema herpeticum: a potentially fatal disease. *BMJ* (Clin Res Ed), 1987;294:693–694.

50. Klein PA, Clark RA. An evidence-based review of the efficacy of antihistamines in relieving pruritus in atopic dermatitis. *Arch Dermatol* 1999;135:1522–1525.

51. Drake LA, Cohen L, Gillies R, et al. Pharmacokinetics of doxepin in subjects with pruritic atopic dermatitis. *J Am Acad Dermatol* 1999;41:209–214.

52. Nicol NH. Atopic dermatitis: the (wet) wrap-up. *Am J Nursing* 1987;87:1560–1563.

53. Kolmer HL, Taketomi EA, Hazen KC, et al. Effect of combined antibacterial and antifungal treatment in severe atopic dermatitis [see comments]. J Allergy Clin Immunol 1996;98:702–707.

54. Krutmann J, Diepgen TL, Luger TA, et al. High-dose UVA1 therapy for atopic dermatitis: results of a multicenter trial. *J Am Acad Dermatol* 1998;38:589–593.

55. Grundmann-Kollmann M, Behrens S, Podda M, et al. Phototherapy for atopic eczema with narrow-band UVB. *J Am Acad Dermatol* 1999;40:995–997.

56. Stevens SR, Hanifin JM, Hamilton T, et al. Long-term effectiveness and safety of recombinant human interferon gamma therapy for atopic dermatitis despite unchanged serum IgE levels [see comments]. *Arch Dermatol* 1998;134:799–804.

57. Jolles S, Hughes J, Rustin M. The treatment of atopic dermatitis with adjunctive high-dose intravenous immunoglobulin: a report of three patients and review of the literature. *Br J Dermatol* 2000;142:551–554.

58. Hanifin JM, Chan SC, Cheng JB, et al. Type 4 phosphodiesterase inhibitors have clinical and in vitro antiinflammatory effects in atopic dermatitis. *J Invest Dermatol* 1996;107:51–56.

59. Hanifin JM, Chan S. Biochemical and immunologic mechanisms in atopic dermatitis: new targets for emerging therapies. *J Am Acad Dermatol* 1999;41:72–77.

60. Schreiber SL, Crabtree GR. The mechanism of action of cyclosporin A and FK506. *Immunol Today* 1992;13:136–142.

61. Berth-Jones J, Graham-Brown RA, Marks R, et al. Longterm efficacy and safety of cyclosporin in severe adult atopic dermatitis. *Br J Dermatol* 1997;136:76–81.

62. Harper JI, Ahmed I, Barclay G, et al. Cyclosporin for severe childhood atopic dermatitis: short course versus continuous therapy. *Br J Dermatol* 2000;142:52–58.

63. de Prost Y, Bodemer C, Teillac D. Randomised doubleblind placebo-controlled trial of local cyclosporin in atopic dermatitis. *Acta Dermatol Venereol Suppl* 1989;144:136–138.

64. De Rie MA, Meinardi MM, Bos JD. Lack of efficacy of topical cyclosporin A in atopic dermatitis and allergic contact dermatitis. *Acta Dermatol Venereol* 1991;71:452–454.

65. Shimizu T, Tanabe K, Tokumoto T, et al. Clinical and histological analysis of acute tacrolimus (TAC) nephrotoxicity in renal allografts. *Clin Transplant* 1999;13:48–53.

66. Fleischer AB Jr. Treatment of atopic dermatitis: role of tacrolimus ointment as a topical noncorticosteroidal therapy. *J Allergy Clinical Immunol* 1999;104(suppl):126–130.

67. Ruzicka T, Bieber T, Schopf E, et al. A short-term trial of tacrolimus ointment for atopic dermatitis. European Tacrolimus Multicenter Atopic Dermatitis Study Group. *N Engl J Med* 1997;337:816–821.

68. Boguniewicz M, Fiedler VC, Raimer S, et al. A randomized, vehicle-controlled trial of tacrolimus ointment for treatment of atopic dermatitis in children. Pediatric Tacrolimus Study Group. *J Allergy Clin Immunol* 1998;102:637–644.

69. Van Leent EJ, Graber M, Thurston M, et al. Effectiveness of the ascomycin macrolactam SDZ ASM 981 in the topical treatment of atopic dermatitis. *Arch Dermatol* 1998;134:805–809.

16

Erythema Multiforme, Stevens-Johnson Syndrome, and Toxic Epidermal Necrolysis

Anju Tripathi, *Neill T. Peters, and †Roy Patterson

*Division of Allergy-Immunology, Department of Medicine, Northwestern University Medical School, Chicago, Illinois; *Department of Dermatology, Department of Medicine, Mercy Hospital and Medical Center, Chicago, Illinois; †Division of Allergy-Immunology, Department of Medicine, Northwestern University Medical School, Chicago, Illinois*

Erythema multiforme (EM), Stevens-Johnson syndrome (SJS), and toxic epidermal necrolysis (TEN) represent a spectrum of immunologically mediated diseases due to hypersensitivity to drugs or infections. There is no uniformly accepted definition or classification of these diseases, and understanding of their exact immunologic basis is lacking.

HISTORICAL BACKGROUND

Erythema multiforme is a term originally attributed to Ferdinand von Hebra. In 1866, he wrote about "erythema exudativum multiforme," a single cutaneous eruption with multiple evolving stages of lesions (1). Von Hebra described erythema multiforme as a mild cutaneous syndrome featuring symmetric acral lesions, which resolved without sequelae and had a tendency to recur. In 1922, Stevens and Johnson described a generalized eruption in two children characterized by fever, erosive stomatitis, and severe ocular involvement (2). This eruption became known as Stevens-Johnson syndrome. Thomas, in 1950, proposed that the milder von Hebra form of EM be called EM minor, and the more severe mucocutaneous eruption of SJS be called EM major (3). According to Thomas, fever and severe ocular involvement were the main points of distinction between the two types. The term

toxic epidermal necrolysis was first introduced in 1956 by Lyell to describe patients with extensive epidermal necrosis that resembled scalded skin (4).

In 1993, an international consensus conference attempted to classify severe EM, SJS, and TEN on the basis of skin lesions and the extent of epidermal detachment (5). Using an illustrated atlas to standardize the diagnosis of acute severe bullous disorders attributed to drugs and infectious agents, the researchers defined bullous EM, SJS, SJS-TEN overlap, and TEN (Table 16.1). Unfortunately, the ultimate classification of severe forms of EM remains a matter of debate and confusion for both primary care physicians and specialists. Given the rarity of SJS and TEN, it has been difficult to create a universally accepted standard of care for the management of these patients. Nonetheless, several concepts regarding EM, SJS, and TEN and their therapy have been proposed. It is well accepted that SJS and TEN represent varying severity of the same disease spectrum, with TEN being the most severe form.

ERYTHEMA MULTIFORME

Erythema multiforme, or the classic von Hebra type of erythema multiforme, is a symmetric eruption with a predilection for the extremities.

TABLE 16.1. *Classification of erythema multiforme, Stevens-Johnson syndrome (SJS) and toxic epidermal necrolysis (TEN)*

	Skin lesions	Extent of skin detachment
Bullous erythema multiforme	Typical targets or raised atypical targets	<10%
SJS	Erythematous or purpuric macules or flat atypical targets	<10%
Overlap SJS/TEN	Purpuric macules or flat atypical targets	10%–30%
TEN with spots	Purpuric macules or flat atypical targets	>30%
TEN without spots	Detachment of large epidermal sheets without any macules or targets	>10%

Adapted from Bastuji-Garin S, Rzany B, Stern RS, et al. Clinical classification of cases of toxic epidermal necrolysis, Stevens-Johnson syndrome, and erythema multiforme. *Arch Dermatol* 1993;129:92–96; with permission.

The characteristic primary lesion is a "target" comprised of three zones (6) (Figs. 16.1 and 16.2). Centrally there is a disk surrounded by an elevated, pale ring. This is concentrically bordered by a zone of erythema (5). Mucosal involvement occurs in a majority of cases of EM; however, it is usually limited to the oral mucosa and typically is not severe (7). EM is most often associated with herpes simplex virus (HSV) infections and follows an outbreak of HSV by 1 to 3 weeks (8,9). The eruption is self-limited, lasts 1 to 4 weeks, and requires symptomatic management. HSV-induced EM may be recurrent, and in such cases, recurrences can be prevented with suppressive antiherpetic therapy (10,11).

Drugs may cause a small proportion of EM cases (12,13). Discontinuation of the implicated medication and supportive therapy results in complete resolution of the skin eruption. Short courses of oral corticosteroids may hasten recovery. In some cases of EM, no obvious cause may be elicited (13).

STEVENS-JOHNSON SYNDROME

Stevens-Johnson syndrome is a diffuse, severe, mucocutaneous eruption involving two or more mucosal surfaces, with or without visceral involvement (Figs. 16.3 and 16.4). The majority of cases are attributed to drug exposures (13–20)

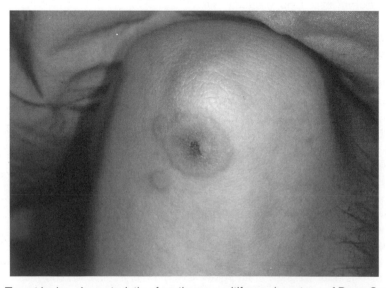

FIG. 16.1. Target lesion characteristic of erythema multiforme (courtesy of Dana Sachs, M.D.).

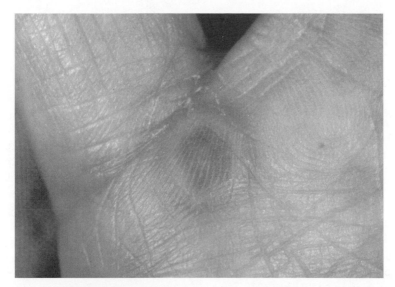

FIG. 16.2. Target lesion (courtesy of Dana Sachs, M.D.).

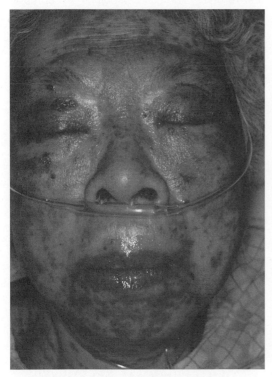

FIG. 16.3. Stevens-Johnson syndrome secondary to trimethoprim-sulfamethoxazole.

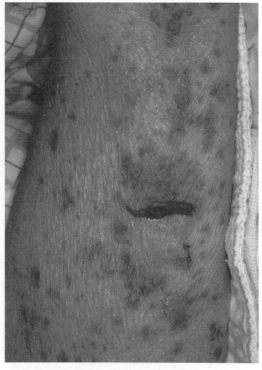

FIG. 16.4. Stevens-Johnson syndrome. Same patient as shown in Fig. 16.3.

TABLE 16.2. *Medications commonly implicated in Stevens-Johnson Syndrome and toxic epidermal necrolysis*

Sulfonamides	Allopurinol
Carbamazepine	Penicillins
Phenytoin	Nonsteroidal antiinflammatory agents
Phenobarbital	Fluoroquinolones
Chlormezanone[a]	Cephalosporins
Acetaminophen (Paracetamol)	Valproic acid

[a] muscle relaxant-sedative
Data from references 13–20.

(Table 16.2). The eruption classically starts 7 to 21 days after initiation of the drug. Reexposure of a sensitized individual to a drug that had previously induced SJS may result in an acute recurrence of the eruption in 1 to 2 days (21). Infections, especially with *Mycoplasma pneumoniae*, are also known to produce SJS (22,23).

Constitutional symptoms such as fever and malaise are often present in SJS. The eruption typically starts on the face and the upper torso and extends rapidly. Individual lesions include flat, atypical targets with dusky centers and purpuric macules (5). Flaccid blisters also may form. Oral, ocular, genitourinary, respiratory, and gastrointestinal mucosa all may be involved, and therefore require appropriate evaluation (21,24,25). Nearly 69% of patients have ocular manifestations ranging from mild conjunctivitis to corneal ulcerations (26).

Clinicians familiar with SJS usually have little difficulty recognizing a fully developed case. A skin biopsy, and in some cases a direct immunofluorescence study, can help confirm a diagnosis of SJS and exclude other diagnostic considerations.

Treatment

Hospital admission is necessary in most patients presenting with SJS. The extent of skin and mucosal involvement as well as laboratory findings need to be evaluated emergently. The extent of epidermal detachment is considered both a prognostic factor and a guide to therapy (27). If greater than 30% TBSA epidermal detachment is present, the patient has TEN and requires differ-

ent therapy (see discussion below on TEN). The laboratory investigation should include a complete blood cell count with differential, serum electrolytes, liver function tests, and urinalysis. The possible precipitating drug must be identified and discontinued. If a patient is on multiple medications, all nonessential drugs should be discontinued. Early discontinuation of the etiologic drug has been reported to improve survival in patients with SJS and TEN (20). Ophthalmologic consultation should be obtained early in all patients with ocular involvement. Further diagnostic evaluation is dictated by the patient's condition.

In addition to supportive care, we recommend early use of systemic corticosteroids. For mild cases, oral prednisone at doses of 1/mg/kg/day may be sufficient. Intravenous methylprednisolone, at doses of 1 to 4/mg/kg/day, may be necessary for severe SJS. The dose of corticosteroids should be gradually reduced as the eruption resolves. An exacerbation of the eruption may occur if corticosteroids are withdrawn too rapidly. Often patients receive systemic steroids on a daily basis for 2 weeks then are converted to alternate day prednisone for 3 to 4 weeks.

The use of systemic corticosteroids for SJS remains controversial (28–32). Some reports in the literature suggest an increased risk of complications with corticosteroids. We have observed complete recovery in all patients with SJS who are diagnosed early and in whom the precipitating cause is removed and corticosteroids are used promptly and in adequate doses. We have observed normalization of laboratory abnormalities, resolution of constitutional symptoms, and improvement of mucocutaneous lesions. In our series of 67 SJS patients treated with corticosteroids, no significant morbidity was observed (21,24,25,33,34). Three of the 67 patients in our series died; however, their deaths were not attributable to either SJS or corticosteroid therapy (21,24,25).

TOXIC EPIDERMAL NECROLYSIS

Toxic epidermal necrolysis is the most severe adverse drug reaction. A possible relationship with medications can be established in almost 90%

of patients with TEN (17,19) (Table 16.2). TEN, like SJS, features extensive mucosal involvement in over 90% of patients. Unlike SJS, however, the degree of epidermal detachment is over 30% of the TBSA (35). TEN has a significant morbidity, and a mortality rate of about 30% (17,19,27). Most deaths are attributed to sepsis (16,17,27).

Treatment

Therapy for TEN is supportive. Corticosteroid use therapy showed no benefit in the treatment of patients with TEN (36,37). Patients with TEN need aggressive fluid and electrolyte correction, local skin care, and fastidious infection precautions. This is best achieved in a burn unit (36,38).

Intravenous immune globulin, cyclosporine, and cyclophosphamide have been reported to improve outcomes in TEN (39–41). These results are based on small series of patients, and at the present time, the use of these agents in TEN is not universally accepted.

Pathogenesis

The exact immunologic basis for SJS and TEN is unknown. SJS is thought to occur through cell-mediated responses. CD8$^+$ T cells, the predominant cells found in the epidermis in bullous exanthems, SJS, and TEN, are thought to mediate keratinocyte destruction (40,42–44). One study has identified increased expression of adhesion molecules in the epidermis of patients with EM (45). Expression of these molecules, such as intracellular adhesion molecule type 1, on the surface of keratinocytes facilitates the cell trafficking of T lymphocytes into the epidermis. Perforin, a cytoplasmic peptide found in cytotoxic T cells, also has been detected in the dermis of SJS patients (46). Perforin can damage target cell membranes and therefore facilitate the entry of other granules such as granzymes into the target cell. These granules are known to trigger a series of reactions culminating in apoptosis (47). Histopathologic specimens from patients with SJS and TEN exhibit apoptosis (46,48).

Another mechanism involved in keratinocyte apoptosis in SJS and TEN may involve Fas-Fas ligand interactions. One study has identified high concentrations of soluble Fas ligand in the sera of TEN patients (41). Others have reported that cells of the monocyte-macrophage lineage also play a role in SJS. These cells act as antigen-presenting cells and may mediate keratinocyte destruction through the release of cytokines such as tumor necrosis factor α (49).

REFERENCES

1. von Hebra F. On diseases of the skin including the exanthemata. Vol. 1. Translated by CH Fogge. London: New Sydenham Society, 1866:285–289.
2. Stevens AM, Johnson FC. A new eruptive fever associated with stomatitis and ophthalmia. *Am J Dis Child* 1992;24:526–533.
3. Thomas BA. The so-called Stevens-Johnson syndrome. *BMJ* 1950;1:1393–1397.
4. Lyell A. Toxic epidermal necrolysis: an eruption resembling scalding of the skin. *Br J Dermatol* 1956;68:355–361.
5. Bastuji-Garin S, Rzany B, Stern RS, et al. Clinical classification of cases of toxic epidermal necrolysis, Stevens-Johnson syndrome, and erythema multiforme. *Arch Dermatol* 1993;129:92–96.
6. Huff JC, Weston WL, Tonnesen ME. Erythema multiforme: a critical review of characteristics, diagnostic criteria, and causes. *J Am Acad Dermatol* 1983;8:763–775.
7. Schofield JK, Tatnall FM, Leigh IM. Recurrent erythema multiforme: clinical features and treatment in a large series of patients. *Br J Dermatol* 1993;128:542–545.
8. Anderson NP. Erythema multiforme: its relationship to herpes simplex. *Arch Dermatol* 1945;5:10–16.
9. Shelley WB. Herpes simplex virus as a cause of erythema multiforme. *JAMA* 1967;201:153–156.
10. Kerob D, Assier-Bonnet H, Esnault-Gelly P, et al. Recurrent erythemata multiforme unresponsive to acyclovir prophylaxis and responsive to valacyclovir continuous therapy. *Arch Dermatol* 1998;134:876–877.
11. Lemak MA, Duric M, Bean SF. Oral acyclovir for the prevention of herpes associated erythema multiforme. *J Am Acad Dermatol* 1986;15:50–54.
12. Howland WW, Golitz LE, Weston WL, et al. Erythema multiforme, clinical, histopathologic and immunologic study. *J Am Acad Dermatol* 1984;10:438–446.
13. Assier M, Bastuji-Garin S, Revuz J, et al. Erythema multiforme with mucous membrane involvement and Stevens-Johnson syndrome are clinically different disorders with distinct causes. *Arch Dermatol* 1995;131:539–543.
14. Roujeau J-C, Kelly JP, Naldi L, et al. Medication use and the risk of Stevens-Johnson syndrome and toxic epidermal necrolysis. *N Engl J Med* 1995;333:1600–1607.
15. Roujeau J-C, Stern RS. Severe adverse reactions to drugs. *N Engl J Med* 1994;331:1272–1284.
16. Ruiz-Maldonado R. Acute disseminated epidermal necrosis types 1, 2, and 3. Study of sixty cases. *J Am Acad Dermatol* 1985;13:623–635.
17. Roujeau J-C, Guillaume J-C, Fabre J-P, et al. Toxic epidermal necrolysis (Lyell syndrome): incidence and

drug etiology in France, 1981–1985. *Arch Dermatol* 1990;127;839–842.

18. Guillaume J-C, Roujeau J-C, Revuz J, et al. The culprit drugs in 87 cases of toxic epidermal necrolysis (Lyell's syndrome). *Arch Dermatol* 1987;123:1166–1170.

19. Schöpf E, Stühmer A, Rzany B, et al. Toxic epidermal necrolysis and Stevens-Johnson syndrome: an epidemiologic study from West Germany. *Arch Dermatol* 1991;127:839–842.

20. Garcia DI, LeCleach L, Bocquet H, et al. Toxic epidermal necrolysis and Stevens-Johnson syndrome. Does early withdrawal of causative drugs decrease the risk of death? *Arch Dermatol* 2000;136:323–327.

21. Tripathi A, Ditto AM, Grammer LC, et al. Corticosteroid therapy in an additional 13 cases of Stevens-Johnson syndrome: a total series of 67 cases. *Allergy Asthma Proc* 2000;21:101–105.

22. Tay YK, Fluff JC, Weston WL. *Mycoplasma pneumoniae* infection is associated with Stevens-Johnson syndrome, not erythema multiforme (von Hebra). *J Am Acad Dermatol* 1996;35:757–760.

23. Leaute-Labreze C, Lamireau T, Chawki D, et al. Diagnosis, classification, and management of erythema multiforme and Stevens-Johnson syndrome. *Arch Dis Child* 2000;831:347–352.

24. Patterson R, Dykewicz MS, Gonzalzles A, et al. Erythema multiforme and Stevens-Johnson syndrome descriptive and therapeutic controversy. *Chest* 1990;98: 331–336.

25. Patterson R, Miller M, Kaplan M, et al. Effectiveness of early therapy with corticosteroids in Stevens-Johnson syndrome: experience with 41 cases and a hypothesis regarding pathogenesis. *Ann Allergy* 1994;73:27–34.

26. Power WJ, Ghoraishi M, Merayo-Lloves J, et al. Analysis of the acute ophthalmic manifestations of the erythema multiforme/Stevens-Johnson syndrome/toxic epidermal necrolysis disease spectrum. *Ophthalmology* 1995;102:1669–1676.

27. Ruiz J, Penso D, Roujeau J-C, et al. Toxic epidermal necrolysis. Clinical findings and prognosis factors in 87 patients. *Arch Dermatol* 1987;123:1160–1165.

28. Rasmussen JE. Erythema multiforme in children: response to treatment with systemic corticosteroids. *Br J Dermatol* 1976;95:181–186.

29. Shim S. Stevens-Johnson syndrome: a pediatric experience. *J Louisiana State Med Soc* 1976;128:331–333.

30. Ginsberg CM. Stevens-Johnson syndrome in children. *Pediatr Infect Dis* 1982;1:155–158.

31. Ting HC, Adam BA. Erythema multiforme: response to corticosteroids. *Dermatology* 1984;169:175–178.

32. Nethecott JR, Choi BCK. Erythema multiforme (Stevens-Johnson syndrome) chart review of 123 hospitalized patients. *Dermatology* 1985;171:383–396.

33. Patterson R, Grammer LC, Greenberger PA, et al. Stevens-Johnson Syndrome (SJS): effectiveness of corticosteroids in management and recurrent SJS. *Allergy Proc* 1992;2:89–95.

34. Cheriyan S, Patterson R, Greenberger PA, et al. The outcome of Stevens-Johnson syndrome treated with corticosteroids. *Allergy Proc* 1995;16:151–155.

35. Roujeau J-C. The spectrum of Stevens-Johnson syndrome and toxic epidermal necrolysis: a clinical classification. *J Invest Dermatol* 1994;102:285–305.

36. Helebran PH, Corder VJ, Madden MR, et al. Improved burn center survival of patients with toxic epidermal necrolysis managed without corticosteroids. *Ann Surg* 1986;204:503–511.

37. Kim PS, Goldfard IW, Gaisford JC, et al. Stevens-Johnson syndrome and toxic epidermal necrolysis: a physiologic review with recommendations for a treatment protocol. *J Burn Care Rehabil* 1983;4:91–100.

38. Heimbach DM, Engrau LH, Marvin JA, et al. Toxic epidermal necrolysis: a step forward in treatment. *JAMA* 1987;257:2171–2175.

39. Hewitt J, Onerod AP. Toxic epidermal necrolysis treated with cyclosporin. *Clin Exp Dermatol* 1992;19:264–265.

40. Heng MCY, Allen SG. Efficacy of cyclophosphamide in toxic epidermal necrolysis. Clinical and pathophysiologic aspects. *J Am Acad Dermatol* 1991;25:773–786.

41. Viard I, Wehrli P, Bullani R, et al. Inhibition of toxic epidermal necrolysis by blockade of CD95 with human intravenous immunoglobulin. *Science* 1998;282:490–493.

42. Margolis RJ, Tonneson MG, Harrist TJ, et al. Lymphocyte subsets and Langerhans cells/indeterminate cells in erythema multiforme. *J Invest Dermatol* 1983;81:403–406.

43. Miyauchi H, Losokawa H, Akaeda T, et al. Cell subsets in drug induced toxic epidermal necrolysis. *Arch Dermatol* 1991;127:851–855.

44. Hertl M, Bohlem H, Jugert F, et al. Predominance of epidermal CD8$^+$ T lymphocytes in bullous cutaneous reactions caused by β-lactam antibiotics. *J Invest Dermatol* 1993;101:794–799.

45. Shiohara T, Chiba M, Tanaka Y, et al. Drug induced photosensitive erythema multiforme–like eruptions: possible role for cell adhesion molecules in a flare induced by rhus dermatitis. *J Am Acad Dermatol* 1990;22:647–650.

46. Inachi S, Mizutani H, Shimizu M. Epidermal apoptotic cell death in erythema multiforme and Stevens Johnson syndrome. *Arch Dermatol* 1997;133:845–849.

47. Cohen JJ, Duke RC. Apoptosis and programmed cell death in immunity. *Annu Rev Immunol* 1992;10:167–193.

48. Paul C, Wolkenstein P, Adle H, et al. Apoptosis as a mechanism of keratinocyte death in toxic epidermal necrolysis. *Br J Dermatol* 1996;134:710–714.

49. Pacquet P, Nikkels A, Arrese J, et al. Macrophages and tumor factor in toxic epidermal necrolysis. *Arch Dermatol* 1994;130:605–608.

17

Drug Allergy

Part A: Introduction, Epidemiology, Classification of Adverse Reactions, Immunochemical Basis, Risk Factors, Evaluation of Patients with Suspected Drug Allergy, Patient Management Considerations

Anne Marie Ditto

Division of Allergy-Immunology, Department of Medicine, Northwestern University Medical School, Chicago, Illinois

In the last edition of this text, the subject of drug allergy was extensively reviewed (1). Although a reasonably comprehensive overview of this important topic is addressed in this edition, an effort has been made to focus more sharply on clinically applicable information. An even more concise, practical review is published elsewhere (2). Other reviews of drug allergy are also recommended (3,4). Further, although specific recommendations are suggested regarding drug challenges and desensitization protocols, it is advisable, if possible, for those inexperienced in such matters to consult with physicians who regularly evaluate and manage hypersensitivity phenomena.

EPIDEMIOLOGY

A consequence of the rapid development of new drugs to diagnose and treat human illness has been the increased incidence of adverse reactions to these agents, which may produce additional morbidity and, on occasion, mortality. Their occurrence violates a basic principle of medical practice, *primum non nocere* (above all, do no harm). It is a sobering fact that adverse drug reactions are responsible for most iatrogenic illnesses. This should serve to remind physicians not to select potent and often unnecessary drugs to treat inconsequential illnesses. Many patients have come to expect drug treatments for the most trivial of symptoms. On the other hand, a physician should not deprive a patient of necessary medication for fear of a reaction. Fortunately, most adverse reactions are not severe, but the predictability of seriousness is usually not possible in the individual case or with the individual drug.

An *adverse drug reaction* may be defined as any undesired and unintended response that occurs at doses of an appropriate drug given for the therapeutic, diagnostic, or prophylactic benefit of the patient. The reaction should appear within a reasonable time after administration of the drug. This definition excludes therapeutic failure, which the patient may perceive as an adverse drug reaction. A *drug* may be defined as any substance used in diagnosis, therapy, and prophylaxis of disease.

Although the exact incidence of adverse drug reactions is unknown, some estimates of their magnitude are available. Reported estimates of the incidence of adverse drug reactions leading to hospitalization vary, but one study based on a computerized surveillance system determined that 2% of hospital admissions were a result of adverse drug reactions (5). As many as 15% to 30% of medical inpatients experience an adverse drug reaction (6). Drug-attributed deaths occur in 0.01% of surgical inpatients and in 0.17% of medical inpatients (7,8). Most of these fatalities occurred among patients who were terminally ill (9). Most deaths were due to a small number of drugs that, by their nature, are known to be quite toxic.

Information regarding outpatient adverse drug events is scant by comparison because most are not reported to pharmaceutical companies and appropriate national registries. Such surveys are complicated by the problem of differentiating between signs and symptoms attributable to the natural disease and those related to its treatment. Adverse drug reactions may mimic virtually every disease, including the disease being treated. The challenge of monitoring adverse drug reactions is further complicated by multiple drug prescribing and the frequent use of non prescription medications. Despite these limitations, such monitoring did identify the drug-induced skin rash that often follows ampicillin therapy.

Although most drug safety information is obtained from clinical trials before drug approval, premarketing studies are narrow in scope and thus cannot uncover adverse drug reactions in all patient populations. Adverse effects that occur over time or that are less frequent than 1 in 1,000, such as drug hypersensitivity, will not be detected until used by large numbers of patients after drug approval (10).

Thus, postmarketing surveillance is essential to the discovery of unexpected adverse drug effects. However, one estimate is that only 1% of adverse drug reactions are voluntarily reported to pharmaceutical companies and the U.S. Food and Drug Administration (FDA) (11). In an attempt to ensure the timely collection of adverse drug reactions, the FDA introduced a simplified medical products reporting program in 1993, MedWatch (12). Although the FDA had an adverse drug reaction reporting system in place before MedWatch, it was awkward to use and

TABLE 17.1. *Reporting adverse reactions to MedWatch*

By mail:
- Use postage-paid MedWatch form 3500

By phone:
- 1-800-FDA-1088 to report by phone, to receive copies of form 3500 or a copy of *FDA Desk Guide for Adverse Event and Product Problem Reporting*
- 1-800-FDA-0178 to FAX report
- 1-800-FDA-7967 for a Vaccine Adverse Event Reporting System (VAERS) form for vaccines

By internet:
- http://www.fda.gov/medwatch

understandably discouraged health professionals' participation. Using MedWatch, the reporting individual does not have to prove absolutely an association between the drug and the adverse reaction. When reported, the information becomes part of a large database and can be investigated further. A simple, self-addressed, one-page form is available and can be sent by mail, fax, or computer modem. This form may be obtained directly from the FDA and is also available in hospital pharmacies, the *Physicians' Desk Reference*, and the *FDA Medical Bulletin*. The FDA can also provide a copy of their new *FDA Desk Guide to Adverse Event and Product Problem Reporting*. Table 17.1 summarizes how to report adverse drug reactions to MedWatch. Voluntary reporting led to the observation that ventricular arrhythmias, such as torsades de pointes, may occur when terfenadine is administered with erythromycin or ketoconazole (13).

Most adverse drug reactions do not have an allergic basis. What follows is a discussion that primarily focuses on those reactions that are, or possibly could be, mediated by immunologic mechanisms.

Allergic drug reactions account for 6% to 10% of all observed adverse drug reactions. It has been suggested that the risk for an allergic reaction is about 1% to 3% for most drugs. It is estimated that about 5% of adults may be allergic to one or more drugs. However, as many as 15% believe themselves to be or have been incorrectly labeled as being allergic to one or more drugs and, therefore, may be denied treatment with an essential medication. At times, it may be imperative to establish the presence or absence of allergy to a drug when its use is necessary and there are no safe alternatives. Although many patients with a history of reacting to a drug could safely receive that drug again, the outcome could be serious if that patient is truly allergic. Hence, a suspicion of drug hypersensitivity must be evaluated carefully.

CLASSIFICATION OF ADVERSE DRUG REACTIONS

Before proceeding with a detailed analysis of drug hypersensitivity, it is appropriate to attempt to place it in perspective with other adverse drug reactions. Physicians should carefully analyze adverse drug reactions to determine their nature because this will influence future use. For example, a drug-induced side effect may be corrected by simply reducing the dose. On the other hand, an allergic reaction to a drug may mean that drug cannot be used or may require special considerations before future administration.

Adverse drug reactions may be divided into two major groups: (a) *predictable adverse reactions,* which are (i) often dose dependent, (ii) related to the known pharmacologic actions of the drug, (iii) occur in otherwise normal patients, and (iv) account for 80% or more of adverse drug effects; and (b) *unpredictable adverse reactions,* which are (i) usually dose-independent, (ii) usually unrelated to the drug's pharmacologic actions, and (iii) often related to the individual's immunologic responsiveness or, on occasion, to genetic differences in susceptible patients.

Not included in this classification are those reactions that are unrelated to the drug itself but are attributable to events associated with and during its administration. Such events are often mistakenly ascribed to the drug, and the patient is inappropriately denied that agent in the future. Particularly after parenteral administration of a drug, *psychophysiologic reactions* in the form of hysteria, hyperventilation, or vasovagal response may ensue. Some of these reactions may be manifestations of underlying psychiatric disorders (15). Even anaphylactoid symptoms have been observed in placebo-treated patients (16). Another group of signs and symptoms is considered a *coincidental reaction.* They are a result

TABLE 17.2. *Classification of adverse drug reactions*

Predictable adverse reactions occurring in normal patients
Overdosage: toxicity
Side effects
- Immediate expression
- Delayed expression
Secondary or indirect effects
- Drug related
- Disease associated
Drug–drug interactions

Unpredictable adverse reactions occurring in susceptible patients
Intolerance
Idiosyncratic reactions
Allergic (hypersensitivity) reactions
Pseudoallergic reactions

of the disease under treatment and may be incorrectly attributed to the drug, for example, the appearance of viral exanthems and even urticaria during the course of a treatment with an antibiotic. Although it may be difficult to characterize a particular drug reaction, a helpful classification is shown in Table 17.2, followed by a brief description of each.

Overdosage: Toxicity

The toxic effects of a drug are directly related to the systemic or local concentration of the drug in the body. Such effects are usually predictable on the basis of animal experimentation and may be expected in any patient provided a threshold level has been exceeded. Each drug tends to have its own characteristic toxic effects. Overdosage may result from an excess dose taken accidentally or deliberately. It may be due to accumulation as a result of some abnormality in the patient that interferes with normal metabolism and excretion of the drug. The toxicity of morphine is enhanced in the presence of liver disease (inability to detoxify the drug) or myxedema (depression of metabolic rate). The toxicity of chloramphenicol in infants is due to immaturity of the glucuronide conjugating system, allowing a toxic concentration to accumulate. In the presence of renal failure, drugs such as the aminoglycosides, normally excreted by this route, may accumulate and produce toxic reactions.

Side Effects

Side effects are the most frequent adverse drug reactions. They are therapeutically undesirable, but often unavoidable, pharmacologic actions occurring at usual prescribed drug dosages. A drug frequently has several pharmacologic actions, and only one of those may be the desired therapeutic effect. The others may be considered side effects. The first-generation antihistamines commonly cause adverse central nervous system effects, such as sedation. Their anticholinergic side effects include dry mouth, blurred vision, and urinary retention.

Other side effects may be delayed in expression and include teratogenicity and carcinogenicity. Methotrexate, which has been used in some steroid-dependent asthmatic patients, is teratogenic and should not be used during pregnancy. Immunosuppressive agents can alter host immunity and may predispose the patient to malignancy (17).

Secondary or Indirect Effects

Secondary effects are indirect, but not inevitable, consequences of the drug's primary pharmacologic action. They may be interpreted as the appearance of another naturally occurring disease rather than being associated with administration of the drug. Some appear to be due to the drug itself, creating an ecologic disturbance and permitting the overgrowth of microorganisms. In the presence of antimicrobial (notably ampicillin, clindamycin, or cephalosporins) exposure, *Clostridium difficile* can flourish in the gastrointestinal tract in an environment in which there is reduced bacterial competition. Toxins produced by this organism may result in the development of pseudomembranous colitis (18).

Antimicrobial agents may be associated with another group of reactions that may mimic hypersensitivity, but appear to be disease associated. The *Jarisch-Herxheimer* phenomenon involves the development of fever, chills, headaches, skin rash, edema, lymphadenopathy, and often an exacerbation of preexisting skin lesions. The reaction is believed to result from the release of microbial antigens, endotoxins, or both

(19). This has usually followed penicillin treatment of syphilis and leptospirosis, but also has been observed during treatment of parasitic and fungal infections. With continued treatment, the reaction subsides, thus confirming it is not an allergic response. Unfortunately, treatment is often discontinued and the drug blamed for the reaction. Another example would include the high incidence of skin rash in patients with the Epstein-Barr virus treated with ampicillin.

Drug–Drug Interactions

A drug–drug interaction is generally regarded as the modification of the effect of one drug by prior or concomitant administration of another. Fortunately, drug–drug interactions of major clinical consequence are relatively infrequent (20). It is also important to recall that not all drug interactions are harmful, and some may be used to clinical advantage.

As the number of drugs taken concurrently increases, the greater the likelihood of an adverse drug interaction. When an interaction is reported, an average of between four and eight drugs are being taken by the patient. Therefore, the largest risk group are elderly patients, who often receive polypharmacy. The danger of an interaction also escalates when several physicians are treating a patient, each for a separate condition. It is the physician's responsibility to determine what other medications the patient is taking, even nonprescription drugs.

Several widely prescribed agents used to treat allergic rhinitis and asthma interacted significantly with other drugs. The second-generation antihistamines, terfenadine and astemizole, were metabolized by cytochrome P-450 mixed-function oxidase enzymes. These antihistamines, in combination with drugs that inhibited the P-450 enzyme system, such as the imidazole antifungals ketoconazole and itraconazole or the macrolide antibiotics erythromycin and clarithromycin, resulted in increased concentrations of the antihistamines. This caused potential for prolongation of the QT interval, sometimes producing torsades de pointes or other serious cardiac arrhythmias (13). These antihistamines are no longer available in the United States.

Although plasma concentrations of loratadine increased with concomitant administration of ketoconazole, this did not cause prolongation of the QT interval and the risk for torsades de pointes (21).

An excellent review of other adverse drug interactions may be found in a looseleaf publication authored by Hansten and Horn (22).

Intolerance

Intolerance is a characteristic pharmacologic effect of a drug which is quantitatively increased, and often is produced, by an unusually small dose of medication. Most patients develop tinnitus after large doses of salicylates and quinine, but few experience it after a single average dose or a smaller dose than usual. This untoward effect may be genetically determined and appears to be a function of the recipient, or it may occur in individuals lying at the extremes of dose-response curves for pharmacologic effects.

In contrast to intolerance, which implies a quantitatively increased pharmacologic effect occurring among susceptible individuals, *idiosyncratic and allergic reactions* are qualitatively aberrant and inexplicable in terms of the normal pharmacology of the drug given in usual therapeutic doses.

Idiosyncratic Reactions

Idiosyncrasy is a term used to describe a qualitatively abnormal, unexpected response to a drug, differing from its pharmacologic actions and thus resembling hypersensitivity. However, this reaction does not involve a proven, or even suspected, allergic mechanism.

A familiar example of an idiosyncratic reaction is the hemolytic anemia occurring commonly in African and Mediterranean populations and in 10% to 13% of African American males (sex-linked) exposed to oxidant drugs or their metabolites. About 25% of African American females are carriers, and of these, only one fifth have a sufficiently severe expression of the deficiency to be clinically important. A more severe form of the deficiency occurs in Caucasian Americans, primarily among people of Mediterranean origin. The erythrocytes of such individuals lack the enzyme glucose-6-phosphate dehydrogenase (G6PD) that is essential for aerobic metabolism of glucose and, consequently, cellular integrity (23). Although the original observations of this phenomenon were among susceptible individuals receiving primaquine, more than 50 drugs are known that induce hemolysis in G6PD-deficient patients. Clinically, the three classes of drugs most important in terms of their hemolytic potential are sulfonamides, nitrofurans, and water-soluble vitamin K analogues. If G6PD deficiency is suspected, simple screening tests dependent on hemoglobin oxidation, dye reduction, or fluorescence generation provide supporting evidence. The study of genetic G6PD deficiency and other genetic defects leading to adverse drug reactions has been termed *pharmacogenetics* (24).

Allergic Reactions

Allergic drug reactions occur in only a small number of individuals, are unpredictable and quantitatively abnormal, and are unrelated to the pharmacologic action of the drug. Unlike idiosyncrasy, allergic drug reactions are the result of an immune response to a drug following previous exposure to the same drug or to an immunochemically related substance that had resulted in the formation of specific antibodies, of sensitized T lymphocytes, or of both. Ideally, the term *drug allergy* or *hypersensitivity* should be restricted to those reactions proved, or more often presumed, to be the result of an immunologic mechanism.

The establishment of an allergic mechanism should be based on the demonstration of specific antibodies, sensitized lymphocytes, or both. This is not often possible for many reactions ascribed to drug allergy. The diagnosis is usually based on clinical observations and, in selected instances, reexposure to the suspected agent under controlled circumstances. Even in the absence of direct immunologic evidence, an allergic drug reaction often is suspected when certain clinical and laboratory criteria are present, as suggested in Table 17.3. Obviously, none of these is absolutely reliable (25).

Immediate reactions occurring within minutes often include manifestations of anaphylaxis.

TABLE 17.3. *Clinical criteria of allergic drug reactions*

1. Allergic reactions occur in only a small percentage of patients receiving the drug and cannot be predicted from animal studies.
2. The observed clinical manifestations do not resemble known pharmacologic actions of the drug.
3. In the absence of prior exposure to the drug, allergic symptoms rarely appear before 1 week of continuous treatment. After sensitization, even years previously, the reaction may develop rapidly upon reexposure to the drug. As a rule, drugs used with impunity for several months or longer are rarely the culprits. This temporal relationship is often the most vital information in determining which of many drugs being taken needs to be considered most seriously as the cause of a suspected drug hypersensitivity reaction.
4. The reaction may resemble other established allergic reactions, such as anaphylaxis, urticaria, asthma, and serum sickness–like reactions. However, a variety of skin rashes (particularly exanthems), fever, pulmonary infiltrates with eosinophilia, hepatitis, acute interstitial nephritis, and lupus syndrome have been attributed to drug hypersensitivity.
5. The reaction may be reproduced by small doses of the suspected drug or other agents possessing similar or cross-reacting chemical structures.
6. Eosinophilia may be suggestive if present.
7. Rarely, drug-specific antibodies or T lymphocytes have been identified that react with the suspected drug or relevant drug metabolite.
8. As with adverse drug reactions in general, the reaction usually subsides within several days after discontinuation of the drug.

Accelerated reactions taking place after 1 hour to 3 days frequently are manifested as urticaria and angioedema and occasionally as other rashes, especially exanthems, and fever. Delayed or late reactions do not appear until 3 days or longer after drug therapy is initiated and commonly include a diverse group of skin rashes, drug fever, and serum sickness–like reactions and, less commonly, hematologic, pulmonary, hepatic, and renal reactions, vasculitis, and a condition resembling lupus erythematosus.

Because clinical criteria are often inadequate, specific immunologic testing is desirable. Until this is accomplished, at best the relationship can be considered only presumptive. With few exceptions, safe, reliable *in vivo* tests and simple, rapid, predictable *in vitro* tests for the absolute diagnosis of drug allergy are unavailable. The most conclusive test is cautious readministration of the suspected drug, but usually the risk is not justified.

Pseudoallergic Reactions

Pseudoallergy refers to an immediate generalized reaction involving mast cell mediator release by an immunoglobulin E (IgE)-independent mechanism (26). Although the clinical manifestations often mimic or resemble IgE-mediated events (anaphylaxis), the initiating event does not involve an interaction between the drug or drug metabolites and drug-specific IgE antibodies.

A differential point is that these reactions may occur in patients without a previous exposure to these substances.

Such reactions appear to result from non-immunologic activation of effector pathways. Certain drugs, such as opiates, vancomycin, polymyxin B, and D-tubocurarine, may directly release mediators from mast cells, resulting in urticaria, angioedema, or even a clinical picture resembling anaphylaxis. In general, these reactions can be prevented by pretreatment with corticosteroids and antihistamines, as outlined for radiographic contrast media (RCM) (27). IgE-mediated allergic reactions, however, cannot.

Overview

The classification of adverse drug reactions presented here must be considered tentative. At times, it may be impossible to place a particular drug reaction under one of these headings. However, the common practice of labeling any drug reaction as "allergic" should be discouraged.

IMMUNOCHEMICAL BASIS OF DRUG ALLERGY

Drugs as Immunogens

The allergenic potential of drugs is largely dependent on their chemical properties. Increases in molecular size and complexity are associated with an increased ability to elicit an immune response. Hence, large-molecular-weight drugs, such as heterologous antisera, chymopapain, streptokinase, L-asparaginase, and insulin, are complete antigens that can induce immune responses and elicit hypersensitivity reactions. Immunogenicity is weak or absent when substances have a molecular weight of less than 4,000 daltons (28).

Most drugs are simple organic chemicals of low molecular weight, usually less than 1,000 daltons. For such low-molecular-weight drugs to become immunogenic, the drug or a drug metabolite must be bound to a macromolecular carrier, often by covalent bonds, for effective antigen processing. The simple chemical (hapten), nonimmunogenic by itself, becomes immunogenic in the presence of the carrier macromolecule and now directs the specificity of the response.

β-Lactam antibiotics are highly reactive with proteins and can directly haptenate carrier macromolecules. However, most drugs are not sufficiently reactive to form a stable immunogenic complex. It is likely that haptens derived from most drugs are *reactive metabolites* of the parent compound, which then bind to carrier macromolecules to become immunogenic. This requirement for metabolic processing may help to explain the low incidence of drug allergy; the predisposition of certain drugs to cause sensitization as they are prone to form highly reactive metabolites; and the inability of skin testing and other immunologic tests with the unaltered drug to predict or identify the reaction as being allergic in nature.

Penicillin allergy has received most attention as a model of drug haptenization (29). Unfortunately, relevant drug haptens have not been identified for most allergic drug reactions. Recent studies of human IgE and IgG to sulfonamides have established the N^4-sulfonamidoyl determinant to be the major sulfonamide haptenic determinant (30).

It should be noted that an antigen must have multiple combining sites (multivalent) to elicit hypersensitivity reactions. This requirement permits bridging of IgE and IgG antibody molecules or antigen receptors on lymphocytes.

Conjugation of the free drug or metabolite (hapten) with a macromolecular carrier to form a multivalent hapten-carrier conjugate is necessary to initiate an immune response and elicit a hypersensitivity reaction. The univalent ligand (free drug or metabolite), in large excess, may inhibit the response by competing with the multivalent conjugates for the same receptors. Therefore, the relative concentration of each will determine the frequency, severity, and rate of allergic drug reactions. Also, removal of haptens from carrier molecules by plasma enzymes (dehaptenation) will influence the likelihood of such reactions (31).

Finally, some low-molecular-weight drugs, such as quaternary ammonium muscle relaxants and aminoglycosides, have enough distance between determinants to act as bivalent antigens without requiring conjugation to a carrier (32).

Immunologic Response to Drugs

Drugs often induce an immune response, but only a small number of patients actually experience clinical hypersensitivity reactions. For example, most patients exposed to penicillin and insulin develop demonstrable antibodies; however, in most instances, these do not result in allergic reactions or reduced effectiveness of the drug.

Mechanisms of Drug-Induced Immunopathology

An immunologic response to any antigen may be quite diverse and the attendant reactions quite complex. Drugs are no exception and have been associated with all of the immunologic reactions proposed by Gell and Coombs (33) subsequently modified by Kay (34) and Janeway (35). It is likely that more than one mechanism may contribute to a particular reaction, but often one will predominate. Table 17.4 is an attempt to provide an overview of the immunopathology of allergic drug reactions based on the original Gell and Coombs classification.

Penicillin alone has been associated with many of these reactions. Anaphylaxis and urticaria following penicillin administration are examples of type I reactions. The hemolytic anemia

TABLE 17.4. *Immunopathology of allergic reactions to drugs*

Classification	Immunoreactants	Clinical presentation
Type I	Mast cell–mediated IGR • IgE-dependent (anaphylactic) • IgE-independent (pseudo allergic or anaphylactoid)	Anaphylaxis, urticaria, angioedema, asthma, rhinitis
Type IIa	Antibody-mediated cytotoxic reactions—IgG and IgM antibodies Complement often involved	Immune cytopenias Some organ inflammation
Type III	Immune complex–mediated reactions Complement involved	Serum sickness, vasculitis
Type IVa$_1$	T-lymphocyte–mediated reactions (CD4 and T$_H$1) type 1 cytokines	Contact dermatitis Some exanthems

IGR, immediate generalized reactions; IgE, immunoglobulin E; IgM, immunoglobulin M.
Adapted from Kay AB. Concepts of allergy and hypersensitivity. In: Kay AB, ed. *Allergy and allergic diseases.* Oxford, UK: Blackwell Science, 1997:23, with permission.

associated with high-dose penicillin therapy is a type II reaction. A serum sickness–like reaction, now most commonly associated with penicillin treatment, is a type III reaction. Finally, the contact dermatitis that occurred when penicillin was used topically in the past is an example of a type IV reaction.

RISK FACTORS FOR DRUG ALLERGY

Several factors have been identified that may influence the induction of drug-specific immune responses and the elicitation of clinical reactions to these agents (36,37) (Table 17.5).

Drug- and Treatment-related Factors

Nature of the Drug

Macromolecular drugs, such as heterologous antisera and insulin, are complex antigens and have the potential to sensitize any patient. As noted earlier, most drugs have molecular weights of less than 1,000 daltons and are not immunogenic by themselves. Immunogenicity is determined by the potential of the drug or, more often, a drug metabolite to form conjugates with carrier proteins.

β-Lactam antibiotics, aspirin and nonsteroidal antiinflammatory drugs (NSAIDs), and sulfonamides account for 80% for allergic or pseudoallergic reactions.

Drug Exposure

Cutaneous application of a drug is generally considered to be associated with the greatest risk for sensitizing patients (37). In fact, penicillin, sulfonamides, and antihistamines are no longer used topically because of this potential. The adjuvant effect of some intramuscular preparations may increase the risk for sensitization; for example, the incidence of reactions to benzathine penicillin is higher than other penicillin preparations.

TABLE 17.5. *Risk factors for drug allergy*

Drug- and treatment-related factors
  Nature of the drug
    Immunologic reactivity
    Nonimmunologic activity
  Drug exposure
    Route of administration
    Dose, duration, and frequency of treatment
Patient-related factors
  Age and gender
  Genetic factors
    Role of atopy
    Acetylator status
    Human leukocyte antigen type
    Familial drug allergy
  Prior drug reactions
    Persistence of drug-immune response
    Cross-sensitization
    Multiple drug allergy syndrome
  Concurrent medical illness
    Asthma
    Cystic fibrosis
    Epstein-Barr viral infection
    Human immunodeficiency virus–infected patients
  Concurrent medical therapy
    β-Adrenergic receptor blocking agents

The intravenous route may be the least likely to sensitize patients.

Once a patient is sensitized, the difference in reaction rates between oral and parenteral drug administration is likely related to the rate of drug administration. Anaphylaxis is less common after oral administration of a drug, although severe reactions have occurred. For other allergic drug reactions, the evidence supporting oral administration is less clear.

The dose and duration of treatment appear to affect the development of a drug-specific immunologic response. In drug-induced lupus erythematosus (DIL), the dose and duration of hydralazine therapy are important factors. Penicillin-induced hemolytic anemia follows high, sustained levels of drug therapy.

There is currently little evidence that the frequency of drug administration affects the likelihood of sensitization (37). However, frequent courses of treatment are more likely to elicit an allergic reaction as is interrupted therapy. The longer the intervals between therapy, the less likely an allergic reaction.

Patient-related Factors

Age and Gender

There is a general impression that children are less likely to become sensitized to drugs than adults. However, serious allergic drug reactions do occur in children. Some confusion may arise in that the rash associated with a viral illness in children may incorrectly be ascribed to an antibiotic being administered as treatment.

Genetic Factors

Allergic drug reactions occur in only a small percentage of individuals treated with a given drug. It is likely that many factors, both genetic and environmental, are involved in determining which individuals in a large random population will develop an allergic reaction to a given drug.

Patients with a history of allergic rhinitis, asthma, or atopic dermatitis (*the atopic constitution*) are not at increased risk for being sensitized to drugs compared with the general population (37). However, it does appear that atopic patients are more likely to develop pseudoallergic reactions, especially to RCM (38).

The rate of metabolism of a drug may influence the prevalence of sensitization. Individuals who are genetically *slow acetylators* are more likely to develop DIL associated with the administration of hydralazine and procainamide (39,40). Adverse reactions to sulfonamides may be more severe among slow acetylators (41).

Specific *human leukocyte antigen (HLA)* genes have been associated with the risk for drug allergy. The susceptibility for drug-induced nephropathy in patients with rheumatoid arthritis treated with gold salts or penicillamine is associated with the HLA-DRw3 and HLA-B8 phenotypes (42). In addition, specific HLA genes have been associated with hydralazine-induced lupus erythematosus, levamisole-induced agranulocytosis, and sulfonamide-induced toxic epidermal necrolysis (TEN) (43).

The possibility of *familial drug allergy* has been reported recently (44). Among adolescents whose parents had sustained an allergic reaction to antibiotics, 25.6% experienced an allergic reaction to an antimicrobial agent, whereas only 1.7% reacted when their parents tolerated antibiotics without an allergic reaction.

Prior Drug Reactions

Undoubtedly, the most important risk factor is a history of a prior hypersensitivity reaction to a drug being considered for treatment or one that may be immunochemically similar. However, drug hypersensitivity may not persist indefinitely. It is well established that, after an allergic reaction to penicillin, the half-life of antipenicilloyl IgE antibodies in serum ranges from 55 days to an indeterminate, long interval in excess of 2,000 days (37). Ten years after an immediate-type reaction to penicillin, only about 20% of individuals are still skin test positive.

There may be *cross-sensitization* between drugs. The likelihood of cross-reactivity among the various sulfonamide groups (antibacterials, sulfonylureas, diuretics) is an issue that has not been resolved. There is little supporting evidence in the medical literature that cross-sensitization is a significant problem. Patients who have demonstrated drug hypersensitivity in the past appear to have an increased tendency to develop sensitivity to new drugs. Penicillin-allergic patients have about a 10-fold increased risk for an allergic reaction to non–β-lactam antimicrobial drugs (45,46). The reactions were not restricted to immediate-type hypersensitivity. Fifty-seven percent reacted to a sulfonamide. With the exception of the aminoglycosides, reaction rates were much higher than expected in all other antibiotic classes, including erythromycin. Among children with multiple antibiotic sensitivities by history, 26% had positive penicillin skin tests (47). These observations suggest that such patients are prone to react to haptenating drugs during an infection (48). Obviously, such patients present difficult clinical management problems.

Concurrent Medical Illness

Although atopy does not predispose to the development of IgE-mediated drug hypersensitivity, it appears to be a risk factor for more severe reactions once sensitivity has occurred, especially in asthmatic patients (36,37). Children with cystic fibrosis are more likely to experience allergic drug reactions, especially during drug desensitization (49).

Maculopapular rashes following the administration of ampicillin occur more frequently during Epstein-Barr viral infections and among patients with lymphatic leukemia (50).

Immune deficiency is associated with an increased frequency of adverse drug reactions, many of which appear to be allergic in nature. Patients who are immunosuppressed may become deficient in suppressor T lymphocytes that regulate IgE antibody synthesis.

In recent years, much attention has been given to adverse drug reactions, in particular hypersensitivity, which occur with a much higher frequency among human immunodeficiency virus (HIV)-infected patients than among patients who are HIV seronegative (51,52). A retrospective study comparing *Pneumocystis carinii* pneumonia (PCP) in patients with acquired immunodefi-

ciency syndrome (AIDS) to a similar pneumonia in patients with other underlying immunosuppressive conditions reported adverse reactions to trimethoprim-sulfamethoxazole (TMP-SMX) in 65% of AIDS patients compared with 12% of patients with other immunosuppressive diseases, suggesting the abnormality may be due to the HIV infection (53). TMP-SMX has been associated with rash, fever, and hematologic disturbances and, less frequently, with more severe reactions such as Stevens-Johnson syndrome, toxic epidermal necrolysis, and anaphylactic reactions. Also, pentamidine, antituberculosis regimens containing isoniazid and rifampin, amoxicillin-clavulanate, and clindamycin have been associated with an increased incidence of adverse drug reactions, some of which may involve an allergic mechanism. It also appears that progression of HIV disease to a more advanced stage confers an increased risk for hypersensitivity reactions (51).

Concurrent Medical Therapy

Some medications may alter the risk and severity of reactions to drugs. Patients treated with β-adrenergic blocking agents, even timolol maleate ophthalmic solution, may be more susceptible to, and prove to be more refractory to, treatment of drug-induced anaphylaxis (54).

CLINICAL CLASSIFICATION OF ALLERGIC REACTIONS TO DRUGS

A useful classification is based primarily on the clinical presentation or manifestations of such reactions. The presumption of allergy is based on clinical criteria cited earlier (Table 17.3). Table 17.6 provides an overview of a clinical classification based on organ systems involved; namely, generalized multisystem involvement and predominantly organ-specific responses.

What follows is a brief discussion of each of these clinical entities, including a list of most commonly implicated drugs. Detailed lists of implicated drugs appear in periodic literature reviews (55,56).

TABLE 17.6. *Clinical classification of allergic reactions to drugs*

Generalized or multisystem involvement
  Immediate generalized reactions
    Anaphylaxis (IgE-mediated reactions)
    Anaphylactoid reactions (IgE-independent)
  Serum sickness and serum sickness–like reactions
  Drug fever
  Drug-induced autoimmunity
    Reactions simulating systemic lupus
      erythematosus
    Other reactions
  Hypersensitivity vasculitis
Reactions predominantly organ specific
  Dermatologic manifestations[a]
  Pulmonary manifestations
    Asthma
    Pulmonary infiltrates with eosinophilia
    Pneumonitis and fibrosis
    Noncardiogenic pulmonary edema
  Hematologic manifestations
    Eosinophilia
    Drug-induced immune cytopenias
      Thrombocytopenia
      Hemolytic anemia
      Agranulocytosis
  Hepatic manifestations
    Cholestasis
    Hepatocellular damage
    Mixed pattern
  Renal manifestations
    Glomerulonephritis
    Nephrotic syndrome
    Acute interstitial nephritis
  Lymphoid system manifestations
    Pseudolymphoma
    Infectious mononucleosis–like syndrome
  Cardiac manifestations
  Neurologic manifestations

[a]A separate listing of dermatologic manifestations is included in that section (Table 17.8).
IgE, immunoglobulin E.

Generalized or Multisystem Involvement

Immediate Generalized Reactions

The acute systemic reactions are among the most urgent of drug-related events. Greenberger has used the term *immediate generalized reactions* to underscore the fact that many are not IgE mediated (57). Drug-induced *anaphylaxis* should be reserved for a systemic reaction proved to be IgE mediated. Drug-induced *anaphylactoid reactions* are clinically indistinguishable from anaphylaxis but occur through IgE-independent mechanisms. Both ultimately result in the release of potent vasoactive and inflammatory mediators from mast cells and basophils.

In a series of 32,812 continuously monitored patients, such reactions occurred in 12 patients (0.04%), and there were 2 deaths (58). Because anaphylaxis is more likely to be reported when a fatality occurs, its prevalence may be underestimated. Drug-induced anaphylaxis does not appear to confer increased risk for such generalized reactions to allergens from other sources (59).

Most reactions occur within 30 minutes, and death may ensue within minutes. Anaphylaxis occurs most commonly after parenteral administration, but it has also followed oral, percutaneous, and respiratory exposure. Symptoms usually subside rapidly with appropriate treatment, but may last 24 hours or longer, and recurrent symptoms may appear several hours after apparent resolution of the reaction. As a rule, the severity of the reaction decreases with increasing time between exposure to the drug and onset of symptoms. Death is usually due to cardiovascular collapse or respiratory obstruction, especially laryngeal or upper airway edema. Although most reactions do not terminate fatally, the potential for such must be borne in mind, and the attending physician must respond immediately with appropriate treatment.

Table 17.7 summarizes most agents frequently associated with immediate generalized reactions. In some situations, drugs, such as general anesthetic agents and vancomycin, which are primarily direct mast cell mediator releasers, can produce an IgE-mediated reaction (32,60). This distinction has clinical relevance in that IgE-independent reactions may be prevented or modified by pretreatment with corticosteroids and antihistamines, whereas such protection from drug-induced IgE-mediated reactions is less likely. In the latter situation, when the drug is medically necessary, desensitization is an option.

The *β*-lactam antibiotics, notably penicillin, are by far the most common causes of drug-induced anaphylaxis. Essentially all *β*-lactam anaphylactic reactions are IgE mediated. Immediate generalized reactions to other antibiotics occur but are relatively uncommon. Recently,

TABLE 17.7. *Drugs implicated in immediate generalized reactions*

Anaphylaxis (IgE mediated)
β-Lactam antibiotics
Allergen extracts
Heterologous antisera
Insulin
Vaccines (egg based)
Streptokinase
Chymopapain
L-Asparaginase
Cisplatin
Carboplatin
Latex[a]

Anaphylactoid (IgE independent)
Radiocontrast material
Aspirin
Nonsteroidal antiinflammatory drugs
Dextran and iron dextran
Anesthetic drugs
   Induction agents[b]
   Muscle relaxants[b]
Protamine[b]
Vancomycin[b]
Ciprofloxacin
Paclitaxel (Taxol)

[a]Not a drug per se, but often an important consideration in a medical setting.
[b]Some reactions may be mediated by IgE antibodies.
IgE, immunoglobulin E.

anaphylactoid reactions have been reported after the administration of ciprofloxacin and norfloxacin (61).

Cancer chemotherapeutic agents have been associated with hypersensitivity reactions, most commonly type I immediate generalized reactions (62). L-Asparaginase has the highest risk for such reactions. Serious anaphylactic reactions with respiratory distress and hypotension occur in about 10% of patients treated. It is likely that most of these reactions are IgE mediated. However, skin testing appears to be of no value in predicting a reaction because there are both false-positive and false-negative results. Therefore, one must be prepared to treat anaphylaxis with each dose. For those reacting to L-asparaginase derived from *Escherichia coli*, one derived from *Erwinia chyoanthermia* (a plant pathogen) or a modified asparaginase (pegaspargase) may be a clinically effective substitute. Cisplatin and carboplatin are second only to L-asparaginase in producing such reactions. Skin testing with these agents appears to have pre-

dictive value, and desensitization has been successful when these drugs are medically necessary (63). The initial use of paclitaxel (Taxol) to treat ovarian and breast cancer was associated with a 10% risk for anaphylactoid reactions. However, with premedication and lengthening of the infusion time, the risk is significantly reduced (64). All other antitumor drugs, except altretamine, the nitrosoureas, and dactinomycin, have occasionally been associated with hypersensitivity reactions (62). Some appear to be IgE mediated, but most are probably IgE independent.

Anaphylactic and anaphylactoid reactions occurring during the perioperative period have received increased attention. The evaluation and detection of these reactions is complicated by the use of multiple medications and the fact that patients are often unconscious and draped, which may mask the early signs and symptoms of an immediate generalized reaction (65). During anesthesia, the only feature observed may be cardiovascular collapse or airway obstruction. Cyanosis due to oxygen desaturation may be noted. One large multicenter study indicated that 70% of cases were due to muscle relaxants, while 12% were due to latex (66). Other agents, such as intravenous induction drugs, plasma volume expanders (dextran), opioid analgesics and antibiotics, also require consideration. With the increased use of cardiopulmonary bypass surgery, the incidence of protamine-induced immediate life-threatening reactions has risen (67). Anaphylaxis to ethylene oxide–sterilized devices has been described; hence, such devices used during anesthesia could potentially cause anaphylaxis (68).

Psyllium seed is an active ingredient of several bulk laxatives, and has been responsible for asthma following inhalation and anaphylaxis after ingestion, particularly in atopic subjects (69). Anaphylactoid reactions following intravenous fluorescein may be modified by pretreatment with corticosteroids and antihistamines (70). Of patients reacting to iron-dextran, 0.6% had a life-threatening anaphylactoid reaction (71). Anaphylactoid reactions may also be caused by blood and blood products through the activation of complement and the production of anaphylatoxins. Adverse reactions to monoclonal antibodies include immediate generalized reactions, but the mechanism for such remains unclear (72).

If one surveys the medical literature, one will find that virtually all drugs, including corticosteroids, tetracycline, cromolyn, erythromycin, and cimetidine, have been implicated in such immediate generalized reactions. However, these infrequent reports should not be a reason to withhold essential medication.

Serum Sickness and Serum Sickness–like Reactions

Serum sickness results from the administration of heterologous (often equine) antisera and is the human equivalent of immune complex–mediated serum sickness observed in experimental animals (73). A serum sickness–like illness has been attributed to a number of nonprotein drugs, notably the β-lactam antibiotics. These reactions are usually self-limited and the outcome favorable, but H₁ blockers and prednisone may be needed.

With effective immunization procedures, antimicrobial therapy, and the availability of human antitoxins, the incidence of serum sickness has declined. Currently, heterologous antisera are still used to counteract potent toxins such as snake venoms, black widow and brown recluse spider venom, botulism, and gas gangrene toxins as well as to treat diphtheria and rabies. Equine and murine antisera, used as antilymphocyte or antithymocyte globulins and as monoclonal antibodies for immunomodulation and cancer treatment, may cause serum sickness (74). Serum sickness has also been reported in patients receiving streptokinase (75).

β-Lactam antibiotics are considered to be the most common nonserum causes of serum sickness–like reactions. One literature review did not support this assertion (76). In fact, such reactions appear to be quite infrequent, with an incidence of 1.8 per 100,000 prescriptions of cefaclor and 1 per 10 million for amoxicillin and cephalexin (77). Other drugs occasionally incriminated include ciprofloxacin, metronidazole, streptomycin, sulfonamides, allopurinol, carbamazepine, hydantoins, methimazole, phenylbu-

tazone, propanolol, and thiouracil. It should be noted that the criteria for diagnosis might not be uniform for each drug.

The onset of serum sickness typically begins 6 to 21 days after administration of the causative agent. The latent period reflects the time required for the production of antibodies. The onset of symptoms coincides with the development of immune complexes. Among previously immunized individuals, the reaction may begin within 2 to 4 days following administration of the inciting agent. The manifestations include fever and malaise, skin eruptions, joint symptoms, and lymphadenopathy.

There is no laboratory finding specific for the diagnosis of serum sickness or serum sickness–like reactions. Laboratory abnormalities may be helpful, if present. The erythrocyte sedimentation rate may be elevated, although it has been noted to be normal or low (78). There may be a transient leukopenia or leukocytosis during the acute phase (79,80). Plasmacytosis may occasionally be present; in fact, serum sickness is one of the few illnesses in which plasma cells may be seen in the peripheral blood (81). The urinalysis may reveal slight proteinuria, hyaline casts, hemoglobinuria, and microscopic hematuria. However, nitrogen retention is rare. Transaminases and serum creatinine may be transiently elevated (82).

Serum concentrations of C3, C4, and total hemolytic complement are depressed, providing some evidence that an immune complex mechanism is operative. These may rapidly return to normal. Immune complex and elevated plasma concentrations of C3a and C5a anaphylatoxins have been documented (83).

The prognosis for complete recovery is excellent. The symptoms may be mild, lasting only a few days, or quite severe, persisting for several weeks or longer.

Antihistamines control urticaria. If symptoms are severe, corticosteroids (e.g., prednisone, 40 mg/day for 1 week and then taper) are indicated. However, corticosteroids do not prevent serum sickness, as noted in patients receiving antithymocyte globulin (74). Skin testing with foreign antisera is routinely performed to avoid anaphylaxis with future use of foreign serum.

Drug Fever

Fever is a well-known drug hypersensitivity reaction. An immunologic mechanism is often suspected. Fever may be the sole manifestation of drug hypersensitivity and is particularly perplexing in a clinical situation in which a patient is being treated for an infection.

The height of the temperature does not distinguish drug fever, and there does not appear to be any fever pattern typical of this entity. Although a distinct disparity between the recorded febrile response and the relative well-being of the patient has been emphasized, clearly such individuals may be quite ill with high fever and shaking chills. A skin rash is occasionally present and tends to support the diagnosis of a drug reaction.

Laboratory studies usually reveal leukocytosis with a shift to the left, thus mimicking an infectious process. Mild eosinophilia may be present. An elevated erythrocyte sedimentation rate and abnormal liver function tests are present in most cases.

The most consistent feature of drug fever is prompt defervescence, usually within 48 to 72 hours after withdrawal of the offending agent. Subsequent readministration of the drug produces fever, and occasionally chills, within a matter of hours.

In general, the diagnosis of drug fever is usually one of exclusion after eliminating other potential causes of the febrile reaction. Prompt recognition of drug fever is essential. If not appreciated, patients may be subjected to multiple diagnostic procedures and inappropriate treatment. Of greater concern is the possibility that the reaction may become more generalized with resultant tissue damage. Autopsies on patients who died during drug fever show arteritis and focal necrosis in many organs, such as myocardium, lung, and liver.

Drug-induced Autoimmunity

Drug-induced Lupus Erythematosus

DIL is the most familiar drug-induced autoimmune disease, in part because systemic lupus erythematosus (SLE) remains the prototype of autoimmunity. DIL is termed autoimmune because of its association with the development of antinuclear antibodies (ANAs). However, these same autoantibodies are found frequently in the absence of frank disease. An excellent review of drug-induced autoimmunity appears elsewhere (84).

Convincing evidence for DIL first appeared in 1953 after the introduction of hydralazine for treatment of hypertension (85). Procainamide-induced lupus was first reported in 1962 and is now the most common cause of DIL in the United States (86). These drugs have also been the best studied. Other agents for which there has been definite proof of an association include isoniazid, chlorpromazine, methyldopa, and quinidine. Another group of drugs probably associated with the syndrome includes many anticonvulsants, β blockers, antithyroid drugs, penicillamine, sulfasalazine, and lithium.

The incidence of DIL is not precisely known. In a recent survey of patients with lupus erythematosus seen in a private practice, 3% had DIL (87). Patients with idiopathic SLE do not appear to be at increased risk from drugs implicated in DIL (88).

Fever, malaise, arthralgias, myalgias, pleurisy, and slight weight loss may appear acutely in a patient receiving an implicated drug. Pleuropericardial manifestations, such as pleurisy, pleural effusions, pulmonary infiltrates, pericarditis, and pericardial effusions, are more often seen in patients taking procainamide. Unlike idiopathic SLE, the classic butterfly malar rash, discoid lesions, oral mucosal ulcers, Raynaud's phenomenon, alopecia, and renal and central nervous system disease are unusual in DIL. Glomerulonephritis has occasionally been reported in hydralazine-induced lupus. As a rule, DIL is a milder disease than idiopathic SLE. Because many clinical features are nonspecific, the presence of ANAs is essential in the diagnosis of drug-induced disease.

Clinical symptoms usually do not appear for many months after institution of drug treatment. Clinical features of DIL usually subside within days to weeks after the offending drug is discontinued. In an occasional patient, the symptoms may persist or recur over several months before disappearing. ANAs often disappear in a few weeks to months but may persist for a year or longer. Mild symptoms may be managed with NSAIDs; more severe disease may require corticosteroid treatment.

If no satisfactory alternative drug is available and treatment is essential, the minimum effective dose of the drug and corticosteroids may be given simultaneously with caution and careful observation. With respect to procainamide, DIL can be prevented by giving *N*-acetylprocainamide, the major acetylated metabolite of procainamide. In fact, remission of procainamide-induced lupus has occurred when patients were switched to *N*-acetylprocainamide therapy (89,90).

Finally, there are no data to suggest that the presence of ANAs necessitates discontinuance of the drug in asymptomatic patients. The low probability of clinical symptoms in seroreactors and the fact that major organs are usually spared in DIL support this recommendation (91).

Other Drug-induced Autoimmune Disorders

In addition to DIL, D-penicillamine has been associated with several other autoimmune syndromes, such as myasthenia gravis, polymyositis and dermatomyositis, pemphigus and pemphigoid, membranous glomerulonephritis, Goodpasture's syndrome, and immune cytopenias (84). It has been suggested that by binding to cell membranes as a hapten, penicillamine could induce an autologous T-cell reaction, B-cell proliferation, autoantibodies, and autoimmune disorders (92).

Hypersensitivity Vasculitis

Vasculitis is a condition that is characterized by inflammation and necrosis of blood vessels. Organs or systems with a rich supply of blood vessels are most often involved. Thus, the skin is often involved in vasculitic syndromes. In the systemic necrotizing vasculitis group (polyarteritis nodosa, allergic granulomatosis of Churg-Strauss) and granulomatous vasculitides (Wegener granulomatosis, lymphomatoid granulomatosis, giant cell arteritides), cutaneous involvement is not as common a presenting feature as seen in the hypersensitivity vasculitides

(HSV). Also, drugs do not appear to be implicated in the systemic necrotizing and granulomatous vasculitic syndromes.

Drugs do appear to be responsible for or associated with a significant number of cases of HSV (93). These may occur at any age, but the average age of onset is in the fifth decade (94). The older patient is more likely to be taking medications that have been associated with this syndrome, for example, diuretics and cardiac drugs. Other frequently implicated agents include penicillin, sulfonamides, thiouracils, hydantoins, iodides, and allopurinol. Allopurinol administration, particularly in association with renal compromise and concomitant thiazide therapy, has produced a vasculitic syndrome manifested by fever, malaise, rash, hepatocellular injury, renal failure, leukocytosis, and eosinophilia. The mortality rate approaches 25% (95). However, in many cases of HSV, no cause is ever identified. Fortunately, idiopathic cases tend to be self-limited.

The most common clinical feature of HSV is palpable purpura, and the skin may be the only site where vasculitis is recognized. The lesions occur in recurrent crops of varying size and number and are usually distributed in a symmetric pattern on the lower extremities and sacral area. Fever, malaise, myalgia, and anorexia may accompany the appearance of skin lesions. Usually, only cutaneous involvement occurs in drug-induced HSV, but glomerulonephritis, arthralgias or arthritis, abdominal pain and gastrointestinal bleeding, pulmonary infiltrates, and peripheral neuropathy are occasionally present.

The diagnosis of HSV is established by skin biopsy of a lesion demonstrating characteristic neutrophilic infiltrate of the blood vessel wall terminating in necrosis, leukocytoclasis (nuclear dust or fragmentation of nuclei), fibrinoid changes, and extravasation of erythrocytes. This inflammation involves small blood vessels, predominantly postcapillary venules.

When a patient presents with palpable purpura and has started a drug within the previous few months, consideration should be given to stopping that agent. Generally, the prognosis for HSV is excellent, and elimination of the offending agent, if one exists, usually suffices for therapy. For a minority of patients who have persistent lesions or significant involvement of other organ systems, corticosteroids are indicated.

Predominantly Organ-specific Reactions

Dermatologic Manifestations

Cutaneous eruptions are the most frequent manifestations of adverse drug reactions and occur in 2% to 3% of hospitalized inpatients (96). The offending drug could be easily identified in most cases and in one study was confirmed by drug challenges in 62% of patients (97). Frequently implicated agents include β-lactam antibiotics (especially ampicillin and amoxicillin), sulfonamides (especially TMP-SMX), NSAIDs, anticonvulsants, and central nervous system depressants (98).

Drug eruptions are most often exanthematous or morbilliform in nature. Most are of mild or moderate severity, often fade within a few days, and pose no threat to life or subsequent health. On rare occasions, such drug eruptions may be severe or even life threatening, for example, Stevens-Johnson syndrome and toxic epidermal necrolysis. Some more typical features of a drug-induced eruption include an acute onset within 1 to 2 weeks after drug exposure, symmetric distribution, predominant truncal involvement, brilliant coloration, and pruritus. Features that suggest that a reaction is serious include the presence of urticaria, blisters, mucosal involvement, facial edema, ulcerations, palpable purpura, fever, lymphadenopathy, and eosinophilia (99). The presence of these usually necessitates prompt withdrawal of the offending drug.

Table 17.8 provides a list of recognizable cutaneous eruptions frequently induced by drugs and presumably on an immunologic basis.

Exanthematous or Morbilliform Eruptions

Exanthematous or morbilliform eruptions are the most common drug-induced eruptions and may be difficult to distinguish from viral exanthems. The rash may be predominantly erythematous, maculopapular, or morbilliform (measles-like), and often begins on the trunk or in areas of pressure, for example, the backs of bedridden

TABLE 17.8. *Drug-induced cutaneous manifestations*

Most frequent
Exanthematous or morbilliform eruptions
Urticaria and angioedema
Contact dermatitis[a]
   Allergic eczematous contact dermatitis
   Systemic eczematous "contact-type" dermatitis

Less frequent
Fixed drug eruptions
Erythema multiforme–like eruptions
   Stevens-Johnson syndrome
Generalized exfoliative dermatitis
Photosensitivity

Uncommon
Purpuric eruptions
Toxic epidermal necrolysis (Lyell's syndrome)
Erythema nodosum

[a]Contact dermatitis is still listed among the top three, but there is evidence that this problem may be decreasing with the purposeful avoidance of topical sensitizers.

patients. Pruritus is variable or minimal. Occasionally, pruritus may be an early symptom, preceding the development of cutaneous manifestations. Gold salts and sulfonamides have been associated with pruritus as an isolated feature. This rarely progresses to overt exfoliation, although this is possible (100). Usually, this drug-induced eruption appears within a week or so after institution of treatment. Unlike the generally benign nature of this adverse drug reaction, a syndrome with a similar rash and fever, often with hepatitis, arthralgias, lymphadenopathy, and eosinophilia, has been termed *hypersensitivity syndrome* (99). It has a relatively later onset (2 to 6 weeks after initiation of treatment), evolves slowly, and may be difficult to distinguish from drug-induced vasculitis. Anticonvulsants, sulfonamides, and allopurinol are the most frequent causes of hypersensitivity syndrome. Recovery is usually complete, but the rash and hepatitis may persist for weeks.

Urticaria and Angioedema

Urticaria with or without angioedema is the second most frequent drug-induced eruption. It may occur alone or may be part of an immediate generalized reaction, such as anaphylaxis, or serum sickness. An allergic IgE-mediated mechanism is often suspected, but it may be the result of a pseudoallergic reaction. A recent study reported that β-lactam antibiotics (through an allergic mechanism) accounted for one third, and NSAIDs (through a pseudoallergic mechanism) accounted for another third, of drug-induced urticarial reactions (101).

Often, urticaria appears shortly after drug therapy is initiated, but its appearance may be delayed for days to weeks. Usually, individual urticarial lesions do not persist much longer than 24 hours, but new lesions may continue to appear in different areas of the body for 1 to 2 weeks. If the individual lesions last longer than 24 hours, or if the rash persists for much longer than 2 weeks, the possibility of another diagnosis such as urticarial vasculitis should be considered. A drug etiology should be considered in any patient with chronic urticaria, which is defined as lasting more than 6 weeks.

Angioedema is most often associated with urticaria, but it may occur alone. Angiotensin-converting enzyme (ACE) inhibitors are responsible for most cases of angioedema requiring hospitalization (102). The risk for angioedema is estimated to be between 0.1% and 0.2% in patients receiving such therapy (103). The angioedema commonly involves the face and oropharyngeal tissues and may result in acute airway obstruction necessitating emergency intervention. Most episodes occur within the first week or so of therapy, but there are occasional reports of angioedema as long as 2 years after initiation of treatment (104). The mechanism of angioedema is probably ACE inhibitor potentiation of bradykinin production (105). Because treatment with epinephrine, antihistamines, and corticosteroids may be ineffective, the physician must be aware of the potential for airway compromise and the possible need for early surgical intervention. When angioedema follows the use of any one of these agents, treatment with any ACE inhibitor should be avoided. Angiotensin II receptor inhibitors may be a good alternative, although angioedema has been reported with these (106,107).

Allergic Contact Dermatitis

Allergic contact dermatitis is produced by medications or by components of the drug delivery system applied topically to the skin and is an example of a type IV cell-mediated immune reaction (Table 17.4). Following topical sensitization, the contact dermatitis may be elicited by subsequent topical application. The appearance of the skin reaction and diagnosis by patch testing is similar to allergic contact dermatitis from other causes. The diagnosis should be suspected when the condition for which the topical preparation is being applied fails to improve, or worsens. Patients at increased risk for allergic contact dermatitis include those with stasis dermatitis, leg ulcers, perianal dermatitis, and hand eczema (108). Common offenders include neomycin, benzocaine, and ethylenediamine. Less common sensitizers include paraben esters, thimerosal, antihistamines, bacitracin, and, rarely, sunscreens and topical corticosteroids (109).

Neomycin is the most widely used topical antibiotic and has become the most sensitizing of all antibacterial preparations. Other aminoglycosides (e.g., streptomycin, kanamycin, gentamicin, tobramycin, amikacin, and netilmicin) may cross-react with neomycin, but this is variable (110). Neomycin-allergic patients may develop a systemic "contact-type" dermatitis when exposed to some of these drugs systemically. Many neomycin-allergic patients also react to bacitracin. In addition to neomycin, other topical antibiotics that are frequent sensitizers include penicillin, sulfonamides, chloramphenicol, and hydroxyquinolones. For this reason, they are seldom prescribed in the United States.

Benzocaine, a paraaminobenzoic acid (PABA) derivative, is the most common topical anesthetic associated with allergic contact dermatitis. It is found in many nonprescription preparations, such as sunburn and poison ivy remedies, topical analgesics, throat lozenges, and hemorrhoid preparations. In some benzocaine-sensitive patients, there may be cross-reactivity with other local anesthetics that are based on PABA esters, such as procaine, butacaine, and tetracaine. Suitable alternatives are the local anesthetics based on an amide structure, such as lidocaine, mepivacaine, and bupivacaine. Such individuals may also react to other paraamino compounds, such as some hair dyes (paraphenylenediamine),

PABA-containing sunscreens, aniline dyes, and sulfonamides.

Ethylenediamine, a stabilizer used in some antibiotics, corticosteroids, and nystatin-containing combination creams, is a common sensitizer. Once sensitized to ethylenediamine topically, a patient may experience widespread dermatitis following the systemic administration of medicaments that contain ethylenediamine, such as aminophylline, hydroxyzine, and tripelennamine (111).

Among the less frequent topical sensitizers, paraben esters, used as preservatives in topical corticosteroid creams, were thought to be important; however, a recent study failed to support this assertion (112). Thimerosal (Merthiolate) is used topically as an antiseptic and also as a preservative. In one study, 7.5% of patients had a positive patch test with this material. Not all such patients are mercury allergic; many react to the thiosalicylic moiety. Local and even systemic reactions have been ascribed to thimerosal used as a preservative in some vaccines (113). Systemic administration of antihistamines is rarely, if ever, associated with an allergic reaction; however, topical antihistamines are potential sensitizers, and their use should be avoided. Most instances of allergic contact dermatitis attributed to topical corticosteroids are due to the vehicle, not to the steroid itself. Patch testing with the highest concentration of the steroid ointment may help identify whether the steroid itself or the vehicle constituent is responsible. Some attention has already been focused on systemic eczematous contact-type dermatitis.

In summary, physicians should attempt to avoid or minimize the use of common sensitizers, such as neomycin and benzocaine, in the treatment of patients with chronic dermatoses such as stasis dermatitis and hand eczema. A more comprehensive review of drug-induced allergic contact dermatitis is found elsewhere (114).

Fixed Drug Eruptions

Fixed drug eruptions, in contrast to most other drug-induced dermatoses, are considered to be pathognomonic of drug hypersensitivity. Men are more frequently affected then women, but children may also be affected (115,116). The term *fixed* relates to the fact that these lesions tend to recur in the same sites each time the specific drug is administered. On occasion, the dermatitis may flare with antigenically related and even unrelated substances.

The characteristic lesion is well delineated and round or oval; it varies in size from a few millimeters to 25 to 30 cm. Edema appears initially, followed by erythema, which then darkens to become a deeply colored, reddish purple, dense raised lesion. On occasion, the lesions may be eczematous, urticarial, vesiculobullous, hemorrhagic, or nodular. Lesions are most common on the lips and genitals but may occur anywhere on the skin or mucous membranes (117,118). Usually, a solitary lesion is present, but the lesions may be more numerous, and additional ones may develop with subsequent administration of the drug. The length of time from reexposure to the drug to the onset of symptoms is 30 minutes to 8 hours (mean, 2.1 hours). The lesions usually resolve within 2 to 3 weeks after drug withdrawal, leaving transient desquamation and residual hyperpigmentation.

The mechanism is unknown, but the histopathology is consistent with T-cell–mediated destruction of epidermal cells, resulting in keratinocyte damage (119). Commonly implicated drugs include phenolphthalein, barbiturates, sulfonamides, tetracycline, and NSAIDs. Drugs most commonly implicated vary depending on the country, the availability of drugs, and their pattern of use (120,121). In addition, some authors believe the location of lesions may be specific to the drug (122).

Treatment is usually not required after the offending drug has been withdrawn because most fixed drug eruptions are mild and not associated with significant symptoms. Corticosteroids may decrease the severity of the reaction without changing the course of the dermatitis (115).

Erythema Multiforme–like Eruptions

A useful classification for the heterogeneous syndrome of erythema multiforme has been suggested (123). It is often a benign cutaneous illness with or without minimal mucous membrane involvement and has been designated *erythema multiforme minor* (EM minor). A more severe cutaneous reaction with marked mucous membrane (at least two mucosal surfaces) involvement and constitutional symptoms has been termed *erythema multiforme major* (EM major). The eponym Stevens-Johnson syndrome has become synonymous with EM major. In addition, some have considered TEN to represent the most severe form of this disease process, but others believe it should be considered as a separate entity.

EM minor is a mild, self-limited cutaneous illness characterized by the sudden onset of symmetric erythematous eruptions on the dorsum of the hands and feet and on the extensor surfaces of the forearms and legs; palms and soles are commonly involved. Lesions rarely involve the scalp or face. Truncal involvement is usually sparse. The rash is minimally painful or pruritic. It is a relatively common condition in young adults 20 to 40 years of age and is often recurrent in nature. Mucous membrane involvement is usually limited to the oral cavity. Typically, the lesions begin as red, edematous papules that may resemble urticaria. Some lesions may develop concentric zones of color change, producing the pathognomonic "target" or "iris" lesions. The rash usually resolves in 2 to 4 weeks, leaving some residual postinflammatory hyperpigmentation but no scarring or atrophy. Constitutional symptoms are minimal or absent. The most common cause is believed to be herpes simplex infection, and oral acyclovir has been used to prevent recurrence of EM minor (124).

Most instances of drug-induced erythema multiforme result in more severe manifestations, classified as EM major or Stevens-Johnson syndrome. This bullous-erosive form is often preceded by constitutional symptoms of high fever, headache, and malaise. Involvement of mucosal surfaces is a prominent and consistent feature. The cutaneous involvement is more extensive than in EM minor, and there is often more pronounced truncal involvement. Painful oropharyngeal mucous membrane lesions may interfere with nutrition. The vermilion border of the lips becomes denuded and develops serosanguinous crusts, a typical feature of this syndrome. Eighty-five percent of patients develop conjunc-

tival lesions, ranging from hyperemia to extensive pseudomembrane formation. Serious ocular complications include the development of keratitis sicca, corneal erosions, uveitis, and even bulbar perforation. Permanent visual impairment occurs in about 10% of patients. Mucous membrane involvement of the nares, anorectal junction, vulvovaginal region, and urethral meatus is less common. The epithelium of the tracheobronchial tree and esophagus may be involved, leading to stricture formation. EM major has a more protracted course, but most cases heal within 6 weeks (123). The mortality rate approaches 10% among patients with extensive disease. Sepsis is a major cause of death. Visceral involvement may include liver, kidney, or pulmonary disease.

The pathogenesis of this disorder is uncertain, however, the histopathologic features are similar to graft-versus-host disease and suggest an immune mechanism. Deposition of C3, IgM, and fibrin can be found in the upper dermal blood vessels (125). Upregulation of intercellular adhesion molecule 1, an adhesion molecule that facilitates recruitment of inflammatory cells, has been found in the epidermis of patients with erythema multiforme (126). However, unlike immune complex–mediated cutaneous vasculitis in which the cell infiltrate is mostly polymorphonuclear leukocytes, a mononuclear cell infiltrate (mostly lymphocytes) is present around the upper dermal blood vessels (127,128). Activated lymphocytes, mainly $CD8^+$ cells, are present, and there is increasing evidence that they are responsible for keratinocyte destruction (128–131). Epidermal apoptosis has also been reported in patients with Stevens-Johnson syndrome and TEN (128–132), and the role of the T cell in apoptosis is well established. It is possible that a drug or drug metabolite may bind to the cell surface, after which the patient then develops lymphocyte reactivity directed against the drug–cell complex.

Drugs are the most common cause of Stevens-Johnson syndrome, accounting for at least half of cases (99). Drugs most frequently associated with this syndrome and also TEN include sulfonamides (especially TMP-SMX), anticonvulsants (notably carbamazepine), barbiturates, phenylbutazone, piroxicam, allopurinol, and the aminopenicillins. Occasional reactions have followed the use of cephalosporins, fluoroquinolones, vancomycin, antituberculous drugs, and NSAIDs. Typically, symptoms begin 1 to 3 weeks after initiation of therapy.

Although there is some disagreement, based on a series of 67 patients, early management of Stevens-Johnson syndrome with high-dose corticosteroids (160 to 240 mg methylprednisolone a day initially) should be implemented (133,134). Corticosteroids hastened recovery, produced no major side effects, and were associated with 100% survival and full recovery with no significant residual complications. This recommendation does not apply to the management of TEN. Drug challenges to establish whether a patient can safely tolerate a drug following a suspected reaction should not be considered with serious adverse reactions such as Stevens-Johnson syndrome, TEN, and exfoliative dermatitis.

Generalized Exfoliative Dermatitis

Exfoliative dermatitis is a serious and potentially life-threatening skin disease characterized by erythema and extensive scaling in which the superficial skin is shed over virtually the entire body. Even hair and nails are lost. Fever, chills, and malaise are often prominent, and there is a large extrarenal fluid loss. Secondary infection frequently develops, and on occasion, a glomerulonephritis has developed. Fatalities occur most often in elderly or debilitated patients. Laboratory tests and skin biopsy are helpful only to exclude other causes, such as psoriasis or cutaneous lymphoma. High-dose systemic corticosteroids and careful attention to fluid and electrolyte replacement are essential.

Exfoliative dermatitis may occur as a complication of preexisting skin disorders (e.g., psoriasis, seborrheic dermatitis, atopic dermatitis, and contact dermatitis); in association with lymphomas, leukemias, and other internal malignancies; or as a reaction to drugs. At times, a predisposing cause is not evident. The drug-induced eruption may appear abruptly or may follow an apparently benign, drug-induced exanthematous eruption. The process may continue for weeks or months after withdrawal of the offending drug.

Many drugs have been implicated in the development of exfoliative dermatitis, but the most frequently encountered are sulfonamides, penicillins, barbiturates, carbamazepine, phenytoin, phenylbutazone, allopurinol, and gold salts (135). No immunologic mechanism has been identified. The diagnosis is based on clinical grounds, the presence of erythema followed by scaling, and drug use compatible with this cutaneous reaction. The outcome is usually favorable if the causative agent is identified and then discontinued and corticosteroids are initiated. However, an older study reported a 40% mortality rate, reminding us of the potential seriousness of this disorder (136).

Photosensitivity

Photosensitivity reactions are produced by the interaction of a drug present in the skin and light energy. The drug may be administered topically, orally, or parenterally. Although direct sunlight (ultraviolet spectrum 2,800 to 4,500 nm or 280 to 450 mm) is usually required, filtered or artificial light may produce reactions. African Americans have a lower incidence of drug photosensitivity, presumably because of greater melanin protection. The eruption is limited to light-exposed areas, such as the face, the V area of the neck, the forearms, and the dorsa of the hands. Often, a triangular area on the neck is spared because of shielding by the mandible. The intranasal areas and the groove of the chin are also spared. Although symmetric involvement is usual, unilateral distribution may result from activities such as keeping an arm out of the window while driving a car.

Photosensitivity may occur as a phototoxic nonimmunologic phenomenon and, less frequently, as a photoallergic immunologic reaction. Differential features are shown in Table 17.9. Phototoxic reactions are nonimmunologic, occurring in a significant number of patients upon first exposure when adequate light and drug concentrations are present. The drug

TABLE 17.9. *Differential features of photosensitivity*

Feature	Phototoxic	Photoallergic
Incidence	Common	Uncommon
Clinical picture	Sunburn-like	Eczematous
Reaction possible with first drug exposure	Yes	Requires sensitization period of days to months
Onset	4–8 hr after exposure	12–24 hr after exposure once sensitized
Chemical alteration of drug	No	Yes
Ultraviolet range	2800–3100 nm	3200–4500 nm
Drug dosages	Dose related	Dose-independent once sensitized
Immunologic mechanism	None	T-cell mediated
Flares at distant previously involved sites	No	May occur
Recurrence from exposure to ultraviolet light alone	No	May occur in persistent eruptions

absorbs light, and this oxidative energy is transferred to tissues, resulting in damage. The light absorption spectrum is specific for each drug. Clinically, the reaction resembles an exaggerated sunburn developing within a few hours after exposure. On occasion, vesiculation occurs, and hyperpigmentation remains in the area. Most phototoxic reactions are prevented if the light is filtered through ordinary window glass. Tetracycline and amiodarone are two of the many agents implicated in phototoxic reactions (137).

Photoallergic reactions, in contrast, generally start with an eczematous phase and more closely resemble contact dermatitis. Here, the radiant energy presumably alters the drug to form reactive metabolites that combine with cutaneous proteins to form a complete antigen, to which a T-cell–mediated immunologic response is directed. Such reactions occur in only a small number of patients exposed to the drug and light. The sensitization period may be days or months. The concentration of drug required to elicit the reaction can be very small, and there is cross-reactivity with immunochemically related substances. Flare-ups may occur at lightly covered or unexposed areas and at distant, previously exposed sites. The reaction may recur over a period of days or months after light exposure, even without further drug administration. As a rule, longer ultraviolet light waves are involved, and window glass does not protect against a reaction. The photoallergic reaction may be detected by a positive photo patch test, which involves application of the suspected drug as an ordinary patch test for 24 hours, followed by exposure to a light source. Drugs implicated include the sulfonamides (antibacterials, hypoglycemics, diuretics), phenothiazines, NSAIDs, and griseofulvin (138).

Purpuric Eruptions

Purpuric eruptions may occur as the sole expression of drug allergy, or they may be associated with other severe eruptions, notably erythema multiforme. Purpura caused by drug hypersensitivity may be due to thrombocytopenia.

Simple, nonthrombocytopenic purpura has been described with sulfonamides, barbiturates, gold salts, carbromal, iodides, antihistamines, and meprobamate. Phenylbutazone has produced both thrombocytopenic and nonthrombocytopenic purpura. The typical eruption is symmetric and appears around the feet and ankles or on the lower part of the legs, with subsequent spread upward. The face and neck usually are not involved. The eruption is composed of small, well-defined macules or patches of a reddish brown color. The lesions do not blanch on pressure and often are quite pruritic. With time, the dermatitis turns brown or grayish brown, and pigmentation may persist for a relatively long period. The mechanism of simple purpura is unknown.

A very severe purpuric eruption, often associated with hemorrhagic infection and necrosis with large sloughs, has been associated with coumarin anticoagulants. Although originally thought to be an immune-mediated process, it is now believed to be the result of an imbalance between procoagulant and fibrinolytic factors (139,140).

Toxic Epidermal Necrolysis

TEN (Lyell syndrome) induced by drugs is a rare, fulminating, potentially lethal syndrome characterized by the sudden onset of widespread blistering of the skin, extensive epidermal necrosis, and exfoliation of the skin associated with severe constitutional symptoms. It has been suggested that TEN may represent the extreme manifestation of EM major, but this position has been contested by others who cite the explosive onset of widespread blistering, the absence of target lesions, the peridermal necrosis without dermal infiltrates, and the paucity of immunologic deposits in the skin in TEN (141).

However, it has generally been assumed that TEN is an immunologically mediated disease because of its association with graft-versus-host disease, reports of immunoreactants in the skin, drug-dependent antiepidermal antibodies in some cases, and altered lymphocyte subsets in peripheral blood and the inflammatory infiltrate (141). An increased expression of HLA-B12 has been reported in TEN cases (142), and high concentrations of soluble fas ligand have been found in the sera of patients with TEN (143).

TEN usually affects adults and is not to be confused with the staphylococcal scalded-skin syndrome seen in children. The latter is characterized by a staphylococcal elaborated epidermolytic toxin, a cleavage plane high in the epidermis, and response to appropriate antimicrobial therapy. Features of TEN include keratinocyte necrosis and cleavage at the basal layer with loss of the entire epidermis (144). In addition, the mucosa of the respiratory and gastrointestinal tracts may be affected.

These patients are seriously ill with high fever, asthenia, skin pain, and anxiety. Marked skin erythema progresses over 1 to 3 days to the formation of huge bullae, which peel off in sheets, leaving painful denuded areas. Detachment of more than 30% of the epidermis is expected,

whereas detachment of less than 10% is compatible with Stevens-Johnson syndrome (145). A positive Nikolsky sign (i.e., dislodgment of the epidermis by lateral pressure) is present on erythematous areas. Mucosal lesions, including painful erosions and crusting, may be present on any surface. The complications of TEN and extensive thermal burns are similar. Unlike Stevens-Johnson syndrome, high-dose corticosteroids are of no benefit (133,134). Mortality may be reduced from an overall rate of 50% to less than 30% by early transfer to a burn center (146).

The drugs most frequently implicated in TEN include sulfonamides (20% to 28%; especially TMP-SMX), allopurinol (6% to 20%), barbiturates (6%), carbamazepine (5%), phenytoin (18%), and NSAIDs (especially oxyphenbutazone, 18%; piroxicam, isoxicam, and phenylbutazone, 8% each) (147,148).

Erythema Nodosum

Erythema nodosum–like lesions are usually bilateral, symmetric, ill-defined, warm and tender, subcutaneous nodules involving the anterior aspects (shins) of the legs. The lesions are usually red or sometimes resemble a hematoma and may persist for a few days to several weeks. They do not ulcerate or suppurate, and usually resemble contusions as they involute. Mild constitutional symptoms of low-grade fever, malaise, myalgia, and arthralgia may be present. The lesions occur in association with streptococcal infections, tuberculosis, leprosy, deep fungal infections, cat scratch fever, lymphogranuloma venereum, sarcoidosis, ulcerative colitis, and other illnesses.

There is some disagreement whether drugs may cause erythema nodosum. Because the etiology of this disorder is unclear, its occurrence simultaneously with drug administration may be more coincidental than causative. Drugs most commonly implicated include sulfonamides, bromides, and oral contraceptives. Several other drugs, such as penicillin, barbiturates, and salicylates, are often suspected but seldom proved as causes of erythema nodosum. Treatment with corticosteroids is effective but is seldom necessary after withdrawal of the offending drug.

Pulmonary Manifestations

Bronchial Asthma

Pharmacologic agents are a common cause of acute exacerbations of asthma, which, on occasion, may be severe or even fatal. Drug-induced bronchospasm most often occurs in patients with known asthma but may unmask subclinical reactive airways disease. It may occur as a result of inhalation, ingestion, or parenteral administration of a drug. Although asthma may occur in drug-induced anaphylaxis or anaphylactoid reactions, bronchospasm is usually not a prominent feature; laryngeal edema is far more common and is a potentially more serious consideration.

Airborne exposure to drugs during manufacture or during final preparation in the hospital or at home has resulted in asthma. Parents of children with cystic fibrosis have developed asthma following inhalation of pancreatic extract powder in the process of preparing their children's meals (149). Occupational exposure to some of these agents has caused asthma in nurses, for example, psyllium in bulk laxatives (150), and in pharmaceutical workers following exposure to various antibiotics (151). Spiramycin used in animal feeds has resulted in asthma among farmers, pet shop owners, and laboratory animal workers who inhale dusts from these products. NSAIDs account for more than two thirds of drug-induced asthmatic reactions, with aspirin being responsible for more than half of these (152).

Both oral and ophthalmic preparations that block β-adrenergic receptors may induce bronchospasm among individuals with asthma or subclinical bronchial hyperreactivity. This may occur immediately after initiation of treatment, or rarely after several months or years of therapy. Metoprolol, atenolol, and labetalol are less likely to cause bronchospasm than are propranolol, nadolol, and timolol (153). Timolol has been associated with fatal bronchospasm in patients using this ophthalmic preparation for glaucoma. Occasional subjects without asthma have developed bronchoconstriction after treatment with β-blocking drugs (154). One should also recall that β blockers may increase the occurrence and magnitude of immediate generalized reactions to other agents (54).

Cholinesterase inhibitors, such as echothiophate ophthalmic solution used to treat glaucoma, and neostigmine or pyridostigmine used for myasthenia gravis, have produced bronchospasm. For obvious reasons, methacholine is no longer used in the treatment of glaucoma.

Although ACE inhibitors have been reported to cause acute bronchospasm or aggravate chronic asthma (155), a harsh, at times disabling, cough is a more likely side effect that may be confused with asthma. This occurs in 10% to 25% of patients taking these drugs, usually within the first 8 weeks of treatment, although it may develop within days or may not appear for up to 1 year (156). Switching from one agent to another is of no benefit. The cough typically resolves within 1 to 2 weeks after discontinuing the medication; persistence longer than 4 weeks should trigger a more comprehensive diagnostic evaluation. The mechanism of ACE inhibitor–induced cough is unclear. Cough may be avoided with the use of an ACE II receptor antagonist (157,158). As stated previously, ACE inhibitors may cause angioedema and may be a source of cough and dyspnea (159).

Sulfites and metabisulfites can provoke bronchospasm in a subset of asthmatic patients. The incidence is probably low but may be higher among those who are steroid dependent (160). These agents are used as preservatives to reduce microbial spoilage of foods, as inhibitors of enzymatic and nonenzymatic discoloration of foods, and as antioxidants that are often found in bronchodilator solutions. The mechanism responsible for sulfite-induced asthmatic reactions may be the result of the generation of sulfur dioxide, which is then inhaled. However, sulfite-sensitive asthmatic patients are not more sensitive to inhaled sulfur dioxide than are other asthmatic patients (161). The diagnosis of sulfite sensitivity may be established on the basis of sulfite challenge. There is no cross-reactivity between sulfites and aspirin (162). Bronchospasm in these patients may be treated with metered-dose inhalers or nebulized bronchodilator solutions containing negligible amounts of metabisulfites. Although epinephrine does contain sulfites, its use in an emergency situation even among sulfite-sensitive asthmatic patients should not be discouraged (161).

Pulmonary Infiltrates with Eosinophilia

An immunologic mechanism is probably operative in two forms of drug-induced acute lung injury, namely hypersensitivity pneumonitis and pulmonary infiltrates associated with peripheral eosinophilia. Pulmonary infiltrates with peripheral eosinophilia syndrome has been associated with the use of a number of drugs, including sulfonamides, penicillin, NSAIDs, methotrexate, carbamazepine, nitrofurantoin, phenytoin, cromolyn sodium, imipramine, and L-tryptophan (163). Although a nonproductive cough is the main symptom, headache, malaise, fever, nasal symptoms, dyspnea, and chest discomfort may occur. The chest radiograph may show diffuse or migratory focal infiltrates. Peripheral blood eosinophilia is usually present. Pulmonary function testing reveals restriction with decreased carbon dioxide diffusing capacity (DLCO). A lung biopsy demonstrates interstitial and alveolar inflammation consisting of eosinophils and mononuclear cells. The outcome is usually excellent, with rapid clinical improvement upon drug cessation and corticosteroid therapy. Usually, the patient's pulmonary function is restored with little residual damage.

Nitrofurantoin may also induce an acute syndrome, in which peripheral eosinophilia is present in about one third of patients. However, this reaction differs from the drug-induced pulmonary infiltrates with peripheral eosinophilia syndrome just described because tissue eosinophilia is not present, and the clinical picture frequently includes the presence of a pleural effusion (164). Adverse pulmonary reactions occur in less than 1% of those taking the drug. Typically, the onset of the acute pulmonary reaction begins a few hours to 7 to 10 days after commencement of treatment. Typical symptoms include fever, dry cough, dyspnea (occa-

sional wheezing), and, less commonly, pleuritic chest pain. A chest radiograph may show diffuse or unilateral involvement, with an alveolar or interstitial process that tends to involve lung bases. A small pleural effusion, usually unilateral, is seen in about one third of patients. With the exception of DIL, nitrofurantoin is one of the only drugs producing an acute drug-induced pleural effusion. Knowledge of this reaction can prevent unnecessary hospitalization for suspected pneumonia. Acute reactions have a mortality rate of less than 1%. Upon withdrawal of the drug, resolution of the chest radiograph findings occurs within 24 to 48 hours.

Although the acute nitrofurantoin-induced pulmonary reaction is rarely fatal, a chronic reaction that is uncommon has a higher mortality rate of 8%. Cough and dyspnea develop insidiously after 1 month or often longer of treatment. The chronic reaction mimics idiopathic pulmonary fibrosis clinically, radiologically, and histologically. Although somewhat controversial, if no improvement occurs after the drug has been withdrawn for 6 weeks, prednisone, 40 mg/day, should be given and continued for 3 to 6 months (163,164).

Of the cytotoxic chemotherapeutic agents, methotrexate is the most common cause of a noncytotoxic pulmonary reaction in which peripheral blood, but not tissue, eosinophilia may be present (165). In recent years, this drug has also been used to treat nonmalignant conditions, such as psoriasis, rheumatoid arthritis, and asthma. Symptoms usually begin within 6 weeks after initiation of treatment. Fever, malaise, headache, and chills may overshadow the presence of a nonproductive cough and dyspnea. Eosinophilia is present in 40% of cases. The chest radiograph demonstrates a diffuse interstitial process, and 10% to 15% of patients develop hilar adenopathy or pleural effusions. Recovery is usually prompt upon withdrawal of methotrexate, but it can occasionally be fatal. The addition of corticosteroid therapy may hasten recovery time. Although an immunologic mechanism has been suggested, some patients who have recovered may be able to resume methotrexate without adverse sequelae. Bleomycin and procarbazine, chemotherapeutic agents usually associated with cytotoxic pulmonary reactions, have occasionally produced a reaction similar to that of methotrexate.

Pneumonitis and Fibrosis

Slowly progressive pneumonitis or fibrosis is usually associated with cytotoxic chemotherapeutic drugs, such as bleomycin. However, some drugs, such as amiodarone, may produce a clinical picture similar to hypersensitivity pneumonitis without the presence of eosinophilia. In many cases, this category of drug-induced lung disease is often dose dependent.

Amiodarone, an important therapeutic agent in the treatment of many life-threatening arrhythmias, has produced an adverse pulmonary reaction in about 6% of patients, with 5% to 10% of these reactions being fatal (166). Symptoms rarely develop in a patient receiving less than 400 mg/day for less than 2 months. The clinical presentation is usually subacute with initial symptoms of nonproductive cough, dyspnea, and occasionally low-grade fever. The chest radiograph reveals an interstitial or alveolar process. Pulmonary function studies demonstrate a restrictive pattern with a diffusion defect. The sedimentation rate is elevated, but there is no eosinophilia. Histologic findings include the intraalveolar accumulation of foamy macrophages, alveolar septal thickening, and occasional diffuse alveolar damage (167). Amiodarone has the unique ability to stimulate the accumulation of phospholipids in many cells, including type II pneumocytes and alveolar macrophages. It is unclear whether these changes cause interstitial pneumonitis, as these findings are seen in most patients receiving this drug without any adverse pulmonary reactions. Although an immunologic mechanism has been suggested, the role of hypersensitivity in amiodarone-induced pneumonitis remains speculative (168). Most patients recover completely after cessation of therapy, although the addition of corticosteroids may be required. Further, when the drug is absolutely required to control a potentially fatal cardiac arrhythmia, patients may be able to continue treatment at the lowest dose possible when corticosteroids are given concomitantly (169).

Gold-induced pneumonitis is subacute in onset, occurring after a mean duration of therapy of 15 weeks and a mean cumulative dose of 582 mg (170). Exertional dyspnea is the predominant symptom, although a nonproductive cough and fever may be present. Radiographic findings include interstitial or alveolar infiltrates, whereas pulmonary function testing reveals findings compatible with a restrictive lung disorder. Peripheral blood eosinophilia is rare. Intense lymphocytosis is the most common finding in bronchoalveolar lavage. The condition is usually reversible after discontinuation of the gold injections, but corticosteroids may be required to reverse the process. Although this pulmonary reaction is rare, it must not be confused with rheumatoid lung disease.

Drug-induced chronic fibrotic reactions are probably nonimmunologic in nature, but their exact mechanism is unknown. Cytotoxic chemotherapeutic agents (azathioprine, bleomycin sulfate, busulfan, chlorambucil, cyclophosphamide, hydroxyurea, melphalan, mitomycin, nitrosoureas, and procarbazine hydrochloride) may induce pulmonary disease that is manifested clinically by the development of fever, nonproductive cough, and progressive dyspnea of gradual onset after treatment for 2 to 6 months or, rarely, years (171). It is essential to recognize this complication because such reactions may be fatal and could mimic other diseases, such as opportunistic infections. The chest radiograph reveals an interstitial or intraalveolar pattern, especially at the lung bases. A decline in carbon monoxide diffusing capacity may even precede chest radiograph changes. Frequent early etiologic findings include damage to type I pneumocytes, which are the major alveolar lining cells, and atypia and proliferation of type II pneumocytes. Mononuclear cell infiltration of the interstitium may be seen early, followed by interstitial and alveolar fibrosis, which may progress to honeycombing. The prognosis is often poor, and the response to corticosteroids is variable. Even those who respond to treatment may be left with clinically significant pulmonary function abnormalities. Although an immunologic mechanism has been suspected in some cases (172), it is now generally believed that these drugs induce the formation of toxic oxygen radicals that produce lung injury.

Noncardiogenic Pulmonary Edema

Another acute pulmonary reaction without eosinophilia is drug-induced noncardiogenic pulmonary edema. This develops very rapidly and may even begin with the first dose of the drug. The chest radiograph is similar to that caused by congestive heart failure. Hydrochlorothiazide is the only thiazide associated with this reaction (173). Most of the drugs associated with this reaction are illegal, including cocaine, heroin, and methadone (174,175). Salicylate-induced noncardiogenic pulmonary edema may occur when the blood salicylate level is over 40 mg/dL (176). In most cases, the reaction resolves rapidly after the drug is stopped. However, some cases may follow the clinical course of acute respiratory distress syndrome, notably with chemotherapeutic agents, such as mitomycin C or cytosine arabinoside (177), and rarely 2 hours after administration of RCM (178). The mechanism is unknown.

Hematologic Manifestations

Many instances of drug-induced thrombocytopenia and hemolytic anemia have been unequivocally shown by *in vitro* methods to be mediated by immunologic mechanisms. There is less certainty regarding drug-induced agranulocytosis. These reactions usually appear alone, without other organ involvement. The onset is usually abrupt, and recovery is expected within 1 to 2 weeks after drug withdrawal.

Eosinophilia

Eosinophilia may be present as the sole manifestation of drug hypersensitivity (179). More commonly, it is associated with other manifestations of drug allergy. Its recognition is useful because it may give early warning of hypersensitivity reactions that could produce permanent tissue damage or even death. However, most would agree that eosinophilia alone is not sufficient reason to discontinue treatment. In fact, some drugs, such as digitalis, may regularly produce eosinophilia, yet hypersensitivity reactions to this drug are rare.

Drugs that may be associated with eosinophilia in the absence of clinical disease include gold salts, allopurinol, aminosalicylic acid, ampicillin, tricyclic antidepressants, capreomycin sulfate, carbamazepine, digitalis, phenytoin, sulfonamides, vancomycin, and streptomycin. There does not appear to be a common chemical or pharmacologic feature of these agents to account for the development of eosinophilia. Although the incidence of eosinophilia is probably less than 0.1% for most drugs, gold salts have been associated with marked eosinophilia in up to 47% of patients with rheumatoid arthritis and may be an early sign of an adverse reaction (180). Drug-induced eosinophilia does not appear to progress to a chronic eosinophilia or hypereosinophilic syndrome. However, in the face of a rising eosinophil count, discontinuing the drug may prevent further problems.

Thrombocytopenia

Thrombocytopenia is a well-recognized complication of drug therapy. The usual clinical manifestations are widespread petechiae and ecchymoses and occasionally gastrointestinal bleeding, hemoptysis, hematuria, and vaginal bleeding. Fortunately, intracranial hemorrhage is rare. On occasion, there may be associated fever, chills, and arthralgia. Bone marrow examination shows normal or increased numbers of normal-appearing megakaryocytes. With the exception of gold-induced immune thrombocytopenia, which may continue for months because of the persistence of the antigen in the reticuloendothelial system, prompt recovery within 2 weeks is expected upon withdrawal of the drug (181). Fatalities are relatively infrequent. Readministration of the drug, even in minute doses, may produce an abrupt recrudescence of severe thrombocytopenia, often within a few hours.

Although many drugs have been reported to cause immune thrombocytopenia, the most common offenders in clinical practice today are quinidine, the sulfonamides (antibacterials, sulfonylureas, thiazide diuretics), gold salts, and heparin.

The mechanism of drug-induced immune thrombocytopenia is thought to be the "innocent bystander" type. Shulman suggested the formation of an immunogenic drug–plasma protein complex to which antibodies are formed; this antibody drug complex then reacts with the platelet (the innocent bystander), thereby initiating complement activation with subsequent platelet destruction (182). Some studies indicate that quinidine antibodies react with a platelet membrane glycoprotein in association with the drug (183). Patients with HLA-DR3 appear to be at increased risk for gold-induced thrombocytopenia.

Because heparin has had more widespread clinical use, the incidence of heparin-induced thrombocytopenia is about 5% (184). Some of these patients simultaneously develop acute thromboembolic complications. A heparin-dependent IgG antibody has been demonstrated in the serum of these patients. A low-molecular-weight heparinoid can be substituted for heparin in patients who previously developed heparin-induced thrombocytopenia (185).

The diagnosis is often presumptive because the platelet count usually returns to normal within 2 weeks (longer if the drug is slowly excreted) after the drug is discontinued. Many *in vitro* tests are available at some centers to demonstrate drug-related platelet antibodies. A test dose of the offending drug is probably the most reliable means of diagnosis, but this involves significant risk and is seldom justified. Treatment involves stopping the suspected drug and observing the patient carefully over the next few weeks. Corticosteroids do not shorten the duration of thrombocytopenia but may hasten recovery because of their capillary protective effect. Platelet transfusions should not be given because transfused platelets are destroyed rapidly and may produce additional symptoms.

Hemolytic Anemia

Drug-induced immune hemolytic anemia may develop through three mechanisms: (a) immune complex type; (b) hapten or drug adsorption type; and (c) autoimmune induction (84). Another mechanism involves nonimmunologic adsorption of protein to the red blood cell membrane, which results in a positive Coombs test but seldom causes a hemolytic anemia. Hemolytic anemia after drug administration accounts for about 16% to 18% of acquired hemolytic anemias.

The *immune complex mechanism* accounts for most cases of drug-induced immune hemolysis. The antidrug antibody binds to a complex of drug and a specific blood group antigen, for example, Kidd, Kell, Rh, or Ii, on the red blood cell membrane (186). Drugs implicated include quinidine, chlorpropamide, nitrofurantoin, probenecid, rifampin, and streptomycin. Of note is that many of these drugs have also been associated with immune complex-mediated thrombocytopenia. The serum antidrug antibody is often IgM, and the direct Coombs test is usually positive.

Penicillin is the prototype of a drug that induces a hemolytic anemia by the *hapten or drug absorption mechanism* (187). Penicillin normally binds to proteins on the red blood cell membrane, and among patients who develop antibodies to the drug hapten on the red blood cell, a hemolytic anemia may occur. In sharp contrast to immune complex–mediated hemolysis, penicillin-induced hemolytic anemia occurs only with large doses of penicillin, at least 10 million units daily intravenously. Anemia usually develops after 1 week of therapy, more rapidly in patients with preexisting penicillin antibodies. The antidrug antibody is IgG, and the red blood cells are removed by splenic sequestration independent of complement. About 3% of patients receiving high-dose penicillin therapy develop positive Coombs test results, but only some of these patients actually develop hemolytic anemia. The anemia usually abates promptly, but mild hemolysis may persist for several weeks. Other drugs occasionally associated with hemolysis by this mechanism include cisplatin and tetracycline.

Methyldopa is the most common cause of an *autoimmune* drug-induced hemolysis. A positive Coombs test develops in 11% to 36% of patients, depending on drug dosage, after 3 to 6 months of treatment (188). However, less than 1% of patients develop hemolytic anemia. The IgG autoantibody has specificity for antigens related to the Rh complex. The mechanism of autoantibody production is not clear. Hemolysis usually subsides within 1 to 2 weeks after the drug is stopped, but the Coombs test may remain positive for up to 2 years. These drug-induced antibodies will react with normal red blood cells. Because only a small number of patients actually develop hemolysis, a positive Coombs test alone is not sufficient reason to discontinue the medication. Several other drugs have induced autoimmune hemolytic disease, including levodopa, mefenamic acid, procainamide, and tolmetin.

A small number of patients treated with cephalothin develop a positive Coombs test as a result of *nonspecific adsorption of plasma proteins* onto red blood cell membranes. This does not result in a hemolytic anemia but may provide confusion in blood bank serology. Finally, several other drugs have been associated with hemolytic disease, but the mechanism is unclear. Such agents include chlorpromazine, erythromycin, ibuprofen, isoniazid, mesantoin, paraaminosalicylic acid, phenacetin, thiazides, and triamterene.

Agranulocytosis

Most instances of drug-induced neutropenia are due to bone marrow suppression, but they can also be mediated by immunologic mechanisms (189). The process usually develops 6 to 10 days after initial drug therapy; readministration of the drug after recovery may result in a hyperacute fall in granulocytes within 24 to 48 hours. Patients frequently develop high fever, chills, arthralgias, and severe prostration. The granulocytes disappear within a matter of hours, and this may persist 5 to 10 days after the offending drug is stopped. The role of drug-induced leukoagglutinins in producing the neutropenia has been questioned because such antibodies have also been found in patients who are not neutropenic. The exact immunologic mechanism by which some drugs induce neutropenia is unknown (190). Although many drugs have been occasionally incriminated, sulfonamides, sulfasalazine, propylthiouracil, quinidine, procainamide, phenytoin, phenothiazines, semisynthetic penicillins, cephalosporins, and gold are more commonly reported offenders. After withdrawal of the offending agent, recovery is usual within 1 to 2 weeks, although it may require many weeks or months. Treatment includes the use of antibiotics and other supportive measures. The value of leukocyte transfusions is unclear.

Hepatic Manifestations

The liver is especially vulnerable to drug-induced injury because high concentrations of drugs are presented to it after ingestion and also because it plays a prominent role in the biotransformation of drugs to potentially toxic reactive metabolites. These reactive metabolites may induce tissue injury through inherent toxicity, or possibly on an immunologic basis (191). Drug-induced hepatic injury may mimic any form of acute or chronic hepatobiliary disease; however, these hepatic reactions are more commonly associated with acute injury.

Some estimates of the frequency of liver injury due to drugs follow (192):

- >2%: Aminosalicylic acid, troleandomycin, dapsone, chenodeoxycholate
- 1% to 2%: Lovastatin, cyclosporine, dantrolene
- 1%: Isoniazid, amiodarone
- 0.5% to 1%: Phenytoin, sulfonamides, chlorpromazine
- 0.1% to 0.5%: Gold salts, salicylates, methyldopa, chlorpropamide, erythromycin estolate
- <0.01%: Ketoconazole, contraceptive steroids
- <0.001%: Hydralazine, halothane
- <0.0001%: Penicillin, enflurane, cimetidine

Drug-induced liver injury due to intrinsic toxicity of the drug or one of its metabolites is becoming less common. Such toxicity is often predictable because it is frequently detected in animal studies and during the early phases of clinical trials. A typical example of a drug producing such hepatotoxicity follows massive doses of acetaminophen (193). The excess acetaminophen is shunted into the cytochrome P-450 system pathway, resulting in excess formation of the reactive metabolite that binds to subcellular proteins, which in turn leads to cellular necrosis.

Although there is little direct evidence that an immunologic mechanism (hepatocyte-specific antibodies or sensitized T lymphocytes) is operative in drug-induced hepatic injury, such reactions are often associated with other hypersensitivity features. Injury attributed to hypersensitivity is suspected when there is a variable sensitization period of 1 to 5 weeks; when the hepatic injury is associated with clinical features of hypersensitivity (fever, skin rash, eosinophilia, arthralgias, and lymphadenopathy); when histologic features reveal an eosinophil-rich inflammatory exudate or granulomas in the liver; when hepatitis-associated antigen is absent; and when there is prompt recurrence of hepatic dysfunction following the readministration of small doses of the suspected drug (not usually recommended). After withdrawal of the offending drug, recovery is expected unless irreversible cell damage has occurred. Such liver injury may take the form of cholestatic disease, hepatocellular injury or necrosis, or a mixed pattern.

Drug-induced cholestasis is most often manifested by icterus, but fever, skin rash, and eosinophilia may also be present. The serum alkaline phosphatase levels are often elevated 2 to 10 times normal, whereas the serum aminotransferases are only minimally increased. Occasionally, antimitochondrial antibodies are present. Liver biopsy reveals cholestasis, slight periportal mononuclear and eosinophilic infiltration, and minimal hepatocellular necrosis. After withdrawal of the offending drug, recovery may take several weeks. Persistent reactions may mimic primary biliary cirrhosis; however, antimitochondrial antibodies are usually not present. The most frequently implicated agents are the phenothiazines (particularly chlorpromazine), the estolate salt of erythromycin, and less frequently, nitrofurantoin and sulfonamides (194).

Drug-induced hepatocellular injury mimics viral hepatitis but has a higher morbidity rate. In fact, 10% to 20% of patients with fulminant hepatic failure have drug-induced injury. The serum aminotransferases are increased, and icterus may develop, the latter associated with a higher mortality rate. The histologic appearance of the liver is not specific for drug-induced injury. Drugs commonly associated with hepatocellular damage are halothane, isoniazid, phenytoin, methyldopa, nitrofurantoin, allopurinol, and sulfonamides. It is now clear that damage from isoniazid is due to metabolism of the drug to a toxic metabolite, acetylhydrazine (195).

Only halothane-induced liver injury has reasonably good support for an immune-mediated process, primarily on the basis of finding circulating antibodies that react with halothane-induced hepatic neoantigen in a significant number of patients with halothane-induced hepatitis (196). In the United States, enflurane and isoflurane have largely replaced halothane (except in children) because the incidence of hepatic injury appears to be less. However, cross-reacting antibodies have been identified in some patients (197).

Mixed pattern disease denotes instances of drug-induced liver disease that do not fit exactly into acute cholestasis or hepatocellular injury. There may be moderate abnormalities of serum aminotransferases and alkaline phosphatase levels with variable icterus. Among patients with phenytoin-induced hepatic injury, the pattern may resemble infectious mononucleosis with fever, lymphadenopathy, lymphoid hyperplasia, and spotty necrosis. Granulomas in the liver with variable hepatocellular necrosis are a hallmark of quinidine-induced hepatitis (198). Other drugs associated with hepatic granulomas are sulfonamides, allopurinol, carbamazepine, methyldopa, and phenothiazines.

Drug-induced chronic liver disease is rare but may also mimic any chronic hepatobiliary disease. Drug-induced chronic active hepatitis has been associated with methyldopa, isoniazid, and nitrofurantoin (199). Some of these patients may develop antinuclear and smooth muscle antibodies. Also, the chronic liver injury may not improve after withdrawal of the offending drug.

Renal Manifestations

The kidney is especially vulnerable to drug-induced toxicity because it receives, transports, and concentrates within its parenchyma a variety of potentially toxic substances. Tubular necrosis may follow drug-induced anaphylactic shock or drug-induced immunohemolysis. Immune drug-induced renal disease is rare, but glomerulonephritis, nephrotic syndrome, and acute interstitial nephritis (AIN) occasionally have been ascribed to drug hypersensitivity.

Glomerulitis is a prominent feature of experimental serum sickness but is rarely of clinical significance in drug-induced, serum sickness–like reactions in humans. In all probability, it is a transient, completely reversible phenomenon that completely subsides once the offending drug has been discontinued. Although spontaneously occurring SLE is frequently associated with glomerulonephritis, drug-induced SLE rarely manifests significant renal involvement. As a rule, cutaneous involvement is the prominent feature of drug-induced vasculitis, but occasionally glomerulonephritis may be present. Chronic glomerulonephritis was described in a patient with Munchausen syndrome who repeatedly injected herself with DPT vaccine (200). Among heroin addicts, there is a 10% incidence of chronic glomerulonephritis at autopsy. It is suggested that this may be due to immune complexes developing as a result of an immune response to contaminants acquired in the "street" processing of the drug (201). A case of Goodpasture syndrome (pulmonary hemorrhage and progressive glomerulonephritis) was associated with D-penicillamine treatment of Wilson disease—the first case report of a drug being implicated in the etiology of this syndrome (202).

Nephrotic syndrome induced by drugs occurs primarily from immunologic processes that result in membranous glomerulonephritis. This has been more commonly associated with heavy metals (especially gold salts), captopril, heroin, NSAIDs, penicillamine, and probenecid, and less commonly with anticonvulsants (mesantoin, trimethadione, paramethadione), sulfonylureas, lithium, ampicillin, rifampin, and methimazole. An immune complex mechanism is probably responsible for this drug-induced nephropathy (203,204). Proteinuria usually resolves when these agents are discontinued.

AIN, thought to be due to drug hypersensitivity, has been recognized with many agents (205). More frequently reported drugs include the β-lactam antibiotics (especially methicillin), NSAIDs, rifampin, sulfonamide derivatives, captopril, allopurinol, methyldopa, anticonvulsants, cimetidine, and ciprofloxacin. Drug-induced AIN should be suspected when acute renal insufficiency is associated with fever, skin rash, arthralgias, eosinophilia, mild proteinuria, microhematuria, and eosinophiluria beginning days to weeks after initiation of therapy. NSAID-induced AIN usually develops in elderly patients on long-term therapy and is often associated with massive proteinuria and rapidly progressive renal failure (206). Although the pathogenesis of this drug-induced nephropathy is uncertain, a number of immunologic findings have been documented in methicillin-induced AIN (207). These include the detection of penicilloyl haptenic groups and immunoglobulin deposition along glomerular and tubular basement membranes, circulating antitubular basement-membrane antibodies, a positive delayed skin test reaction to methicillin, and a positive lymphocyte transformation test to methicillin. Also, the lymphocytes infiltrating the renal interstitium are cytotoxic T cells. The prognosis is excellent following discontinuation of the drug, with full recovery expected within 12 months. After recovery, the offending drug or a chemically related one should be avoided because there have been several cases of cross-reactivity between methicillin and another β-lactam drug, or among various NSAIDs.

Lymphoid System Manifestations

Lymphadenopathy is a common feature of the serum sickness syndrome and may be present in drug-induced SLE. Lymphadenopathy associated with prolonged treatment with anticonvulsants, notably phenytoin, is a rare but well-established disorder that may mimic clinically and pathologically a malignant lymphoma (208). Cervical lymphadenopathy is most frequent, but may be generalized; hepatomegaly and splenomegaly are uncommon. Other features may include fever, a morbilliform or erythematous skin rash, and eosinophilia. Rarely, arthritis and jaundice may be present. The pathogenesis of this syndrome is unknown. However, phenytoin may induce immunosuppression, which then leads to lymphoreticular malignancies. The reaction usually subsides within several weeks after the drug is stopped and reappears promptly upon readministration of the offending drug. However, not all patients recover after drug withdrawal, and some develop Hodgkin's disease and lymphoma (209). An infectious mononucleosis-like syndrome has been described with phenytoin, aminosalicylic acid, and dapsone (210).

Cardiac Manifestations

Hypersensitivity myocarditis is rarely identified as a clinical entity. Although endomyocardial biopsy has, on occasion, suggested hypersensitivity myocarditis, reported cases are usually diagnosed at autopsy (211). Many drugs have been implicated, but the main offenders are the sulfonamides, methyldopa, penicillin, and its derivatives. Many of these drugs have also been associated with hypersensitivity vasculitis. In most cases diagnosed at autopsy, the patients died suddenly and unexpectedly while being treated for an unrelated and nonlethal illness (212).

The diagnosis should be considered when new electrocardiographic changes appear in association with unexpected tachycardia, mildly elevated cardiac enzymes, and cardiomegaly in a patient with an allergic drug reaction, usually with evidence of eosinophilia (213). Confirmation is usually obtained by a biopsy of the endomyocardium that demonstrates diffuse interstitial infiltrates rich with eosinophils.

Because cellular necrosis is less prominent than in other forms of myocarditis, permanent cardiac damage is less if the entity is recognized and the offending drug eliminated. Most patients recover in a few days to a few weeks. Aggressive treatment with corticosteroids or immunosuppressives may be necessary if myocarditis is severe and persistent. The diagnosed cases probably represent only the tip of the iceberg, with many cases presumably self-limited and unrecognized. This reaction should not be confused with other types of chronic eosinophilic myocardiopathy, which often lead to permanent cardiac damage and impairment of function.

Neurologic Manifestations

An allergic etiology for drug-induced damage to the central and peripheral nervous system is unusual. Postvaccinal encephalomyelitis does resemble experimental encephalomyelitis in animals. A peripheral neuritis has been reported in patients receiving gold salts, colchicine, nitrofurantoin, and sulfonamides; although such reactions have not been analyzed sufficiently to implicate an immunologic mechanism, this has been suggested.

EVALUATION OF PATIENTS WITH SUSPECTED DRUG HYPERSENSITIVITY

The investigation and identification of a drug responsible for a suspected allergic reaction still depends largely on circumstantial evidence and clinical skills of the physician. Absolute proof that a drug is the actual offender is usually lacking because, with few exceptions, conventional methods to diagnose allergic disorders are either unavailable or unreliable.

Knowledge of the clinical criteria (Table 17.3) and clinical manifestations ascribed to drug hypersensitivity is helpful in evaluation. None of these clinical manifestations is unique for drug allergy, but physicians should consider this very treatable condition along with other diagnostic possibilities.

The complexity and heterogeneity of immune responses induced by drugs, the variety of immunologic tests needed for their detection, and the fact that the relevant drug antigens are in most cases not able to be prepared *in vitro*, but rather are the result of complex metabolic interactions occurring *in vivo*, have largely prevented the development of clinically applicable *in vivo* and *in vitro* diagnostic tests. Table 17.10 provides an overview of useful approaches available to evaluate and diagnose allergic drug reactions.

Detailed History

The most important consideration in the evaluation of patients for possible drug allergy is a suspicion by the physician that an unexplained symptom or sign may be due to a drug currently being administered. Next in importance is obtaining a complete history of *all* drugs taken currently, and within the past month or so, as well as a history of any drug reactions in the past. It is helpful to be aware of those drugs most frequently implicated in allergic reactions (Table 17.11).

The clinical features of the reaction may suggest drug hypersensitivity, although morphologic changes associated with drug allergy are often protean in nature and usually not agent specific. It is obviously helpful to know whether the presenting manifestations have been reported

TABLE 17.10. *Overview of methods used to evaluate patents with suspected drug hypersensitivity*

Detailed history[a]—basis for diagnosis in most cases
- Consider the possibility
- Complete history of *all* drugs taken and any prior reactions
- Compatible clinical manifestations
- Temporal eligibility

***In vivo* testing**—clinically indicated in some cases
- Cutaneous tests for IgE-mediated reactions[a]
- Patch tests[a]
- Incremental provocative test dosing[a]

***In vitro* testing**—rarely helpful clinically
- Drug-specific IgE antibodies (RAST)
- Drug-specific IgG and IgM antibodies
- Lymphocyte blast transformation
- Others: mediator release, complement activation, immune complex detection

Withdrawal of the suspected drug—presumptive evidence if symptoms clear
- Eliminate any drug not clearly indicated
- Use alternate agents if possible

[a] These methods are clinically most available and useful in evaluating allergic drug reactions.
　IgE, immunoglobulin E; IgM, immunoglobulin M; RAST, radioallergosorbent test.

TABLE 17.11. *Drugs frequently implicated in allergic drug reactions*

Aspirin and nonsteroidal antiinflammatory drugs	Radiocontrast media
β-Lactam antibiotics	Antihypertensive agents (angiotensin-converting enzyme inhibitors, methyldopa)
Sulfonamides (antibacterial, hypoglycemics, diuretics)	Antiarrhythmia drugs (procainamide, quinidine)
Antituberculous drugs (isoniazid, rifampicin)	Heavy metals (gold salts)
Nitrofurans	Organ extracts (insulin, other hormones)[a]
Anticonvulsants (hydantoin, carbamazepine)	Antisera (antitoxins, monoclonal antibodies)[a]
Anesthetic agents (muscle relaxants, thiopental)	Enzymes (L-asparaginase, streptokinase, chymopapain)[a]
Allopurinol	Vaccines (egg-based)[a]
Antipsychotic tranquilizers	Latex[a,b]
Cisplatin	

[a] Complete antigens.
[b] Not a drug per se, but frequently present in a medical setting.

previously as features of a reaction to the drug being taken.

The history should establish temporal eligibility of the suspected drug. Unless the patient has been sensitized previously to the same or a cross-reacting drug, there should be an interval between initiation of treatment and the subsequent reaction. For most medications, this interval is rarely less than 1 week, and reactions generally appear within a month or so following initiation of therapy. It is unusual for a drug taken for long periods of time to be incriminated. This information has proved especially useful in deciding which drug is the likely offender when patients are receiving multiple medications. It is helpful to construct a graph denoting times when drugs were added and discontinued, along with the time of onset of clinical manifestations. For patients previously sensitized to a drug, allergic reactions may occur within minutes or hours after institution of therapy.

In Vivo Testing

In vivo testing for drug hypersensitivity involves skin testing or cautious readministration of the suspected provocative agent, test dosing. Such an approach may be clinically indicated in selected cases.

Immediate Wheal-and-Flare Skin Tests

Prick (puncture) and intradermal cutaneous tests for IgE-mediated drug reactions may be quite helpful in some clinical situations. Tests must be performed in the absence of medications that interfere with the wheal-and-flare response, such as antihistamines and tricyclic antidepressants. Positive (histamine) and negative (diluent) control skin tests should be performed. For safety, prick tests must be negative before proceeding with intradermal tests. A wheal without surrounding erythema is clinically insignificant (214).

For large-molecular-weight agents that have multiple antigenic determinants, such as foreign antisera, hormones (e.g., insulin), enzymes, egg-containing vaccines, and latex, positive immediate wheal-and-flare skin test reactions identify patients at risk for anaphylaxis. With low-molecular-weight drugs, skin testing has a role in the evaluation of IgE-mediated reactions to β-lactam antibiotics and at times has been helpful in the detection of IgE antibodies to muscle relaxants, aminoglycosides, and sulfamethoxazole.

There are occasional reports of immediate wheal-and-flare skin tests to other drugs implicated in immediate generalized reactions, but their significance is uncertain. However, this should not deter one from attempting such with dilute solutions of the suspected drug (215). It is theoretically possible that a drug may bind to high-molecular-weight carriers at the skin test site, thus permitting the required IgE antibody cross-linking for mast cell mediator release and the attendant wheal-and-flare response. When such testing is attempted with drugs that have not been previously validated, normal controls must also be tested to eliminate the possibility of false-positive responses. A positive skin test suggests that the patient may be at risk for an IgE-mediated reaction; however, a negative skin test reaction does not eliminate that possibility.

Patch Tests

Patch and photo patch tests are of value in cases of contact dermatitis to topically applied medicaments, even if the eruption was provoked by systemic administration of the drug. In photoallergic reactions, the patch test may become positive only after subsequent exposure to an erythemic dose of ultraviolet light (photo patch testing). The value of the patch test as a diagnostic tool in systemic drug reactions is unclear. However, some patients who have developed maculopapular or eczematous rashes after the administration of carbamazepine, practolol, and diazepam have consistently demonstrated positive patch tests to these drugs (216).

Incremental Provocative Test Dosing

Direct challenge of the patient with a test dose of the drug (provocative test dosing) remains the only absolute method to establish or exclude an etiologic relationship between most suspected drugs and the clinical manifestations produced. In certain situations, it is essential to determine whether a patient reacts to the drug, especially if there are no acceptable substitutes. Provocative testing only to satisfy the patient's curiosity or physician's academic interest is not justified. The procedure is potentially dangerous and is inadvisable without appropriate consultation and considerable experience in management of hypersensitivity phenomena. In fact, in one large series, patients were rechallenged with a drug suspected of producing a cutaneous reaction; 86% recurred, 11% of which were severe reactions (97).

The principle of incremental test dosing, also known as *graded challenge*, is to administer sufficiently small doses that would not cause a serious reaction initially, and to increase the dose by safe increments (usually 2- to 10-fold) over a matter of hours or days until a therapeutic dose is achieved (2). Generally, the initial starting dose is 1% of the therapeutic dose; it is 100- to 1,000-fold less if the previous reaction was severe. If the prior reaction was acute (e.g., anaphylaxis), the increased doses may be given at 15- to 30-minute intervals, with the entire procedure completed in 4 hours or less. When the previous reaction was delayed (e.g., morbilliform dermatitis), the interval between doses may be 24 to 48 hours and requires several weeks or longer for completion. Such slow test dosing may not be feasible in urgent situations, such as the need for TMP-SMX in AIDS patients with life-threatening *Pneumocystis carinii* pneumonia. If a reaction occurs during test dosing, a decision must be made as to whether the drug should be terminated or desensitization attempted.

Provocative test dosing should not be confused with desensitization (217). With respect to test dosing, the probability of a true allergic reaction is low, but the clinician is concerned about the possibility of such a reaction. It is likely that many of these patients could have tolerated the drug without significant risk, but for safety, reassurance, and medicolegal concerns, this cautious administration has merit. Desensitization is the procedure employed to administer a drug to a patient in whom true allergy has been reasonably well established, specifically IgE-mediated, immediate hypersensitivity.

Before proceeding with drug challenges, informed consent must be obtained and the information recorded in the medical record. It is advisable to explain the risks of giving as well as withholding the drug. Appropriate specialty consultation to underscore the need for the drug is desirable, if available. Hospitalization is usually required, and emergency equipment to treat anaphylaxis must be available. The drug challenge is performed immediately before treatment, not weeks or months in advance of therapy. Also, prophylactic treatment with antihistamines and corticosteroids before drug challenges is not recommended because these mask more mild reactions that may occur at low doses, risking a more serious reaction at higher doses. Drug rechallenges should not be considered when the previous reaction resulted in erythema multiforme major (Stevens-Johnson syndrome), TEN, exfoliative dermatitis, and drug-induced immune cytopenias.

In Vitro Testing

Testing *in vitro* to detect drug hypersensitivity has the obvious advantage of avoiding the inherent dangers in challenging patients with the drug. Although the demonstration of the drug-specific IgE is usually considered significant, the presence of other drug-specific immunoglobulin classes or cell-mediated allergy correlates poorly with a clinical adverse reaction. Drug-specific immune responses occur more frequently than clinical allergic drug reactions.

Drug-specific Immunoglobulin E Antibodies

The *in vitro* detection of drug-specific IgE antibodies is generally less sensitive than skin testing with the suspected agent. Further, this approach, as was true for skin testing with drugs, is hampered by the lack of information regarding relevant drug metabolites that are immunogenic.

A solid-phase radioimmunoassay, the radioallergosorbent test (RAST) has been validated mainly for the detection of IgE antibodies to the major (penicilloyl) determinant of penicillin and correlates reasonably well with skin tests using penicilloyl-polylysine. A RAST test for penicillin minor determinant sensitivity remains elu-

sive. In addition to penicillin, specific IgE antibodies have been detected in the sera of patients who sustained generalized immediate reactions to other β-lactam antibiotics, sulfamethoxazole, trimethoprim, sodium aurothiomalate, muscle relaxants, insulin, chymopapain, and latex (218). If positive, these tests may be helpful in identifying patients at risk; if negative, they do not exclude the possibility.

Drug-specific Immunoglobulin G and Immunoglobulin M Antibodies

With the exception of drug-induced immune cytopenias, there is often little correlation between the presence of drug-specific IgG and IgM antibodies and other drug-induced immunopathologic reactions. It has been reported that the presence of IgG antibodies to protamine in diabetic patients treated with NPH insulin increased the risk for immediate generalized reactions to protamine sulfate (219).

Drug-induced immune cytopenias afford an opportunity to test affected cells *in vitro*. Such testing should be performed as soon as the suspicion arises because the antibodies may disappear rapidly after withdrawal of the drug. For drug-induced immune hemolysis, a positive Coombs test is a useful screening procedure and may be followed by tests for drug-specific antibodies if available. Antiplatelet antibodies are best detected by the complement fixation test and the liberation of platelet factor 3. *In vitro* tests for drug-induced immune agranulocytosis are often disappointing because leukoagglutinins disappear very rapidly and are occasionally present in neutropenic conditions where no drug is involved.

Lymphocyte Blast Transformation

T-lymphocyte—mediated reactions (delayed hypersensitivity) have been suspected in some patients with drug allergy. Lymphocyte blastogenesis (lymphocyte transformation test) has been suggested as an *in vitro* diagnostic test for such reactions. This test detects *in vitro* proliferation of the patient's lymphocytes in response to drugs

(220). A variation on this assay measures the T-lymphocyte cytokine production rather than proliferation (221). There is disagreement regarding the value of this procedure in the diagnosis of drug allergy. However, because there appears to be a high incidence of false-negative and false-positive results, these tests have little clinical relevance (222).

Other Tests

The measurement of mast cell mediator release during drug-induced anaphylaxis or anaphylactoid reactions appears to be promising. Tryptase is a neutral protease that is specifically released by mast cells and remains in the serum for at least 3 hours after the reaction (223). It is a relatively stable protein that may be measured in stored serum samples. After a reaction, several serum samples should be obtained during the first 8 to 12 hours. A positive test for tryptase is helpful, but a negative result does not rule out an immediate generalized reaction.

Complement activation and immune complex assays are other tests that may be helpful in the evaluation of drug-induced serum sickness–like reactions. Immunoglobulins and complement have been demonstrated in drug-induced immunologic nephritis, but it is often unclear whether the drugs themselves are present in the immune complexes (224).

Withdrawal of the Suspected Drug

With a reasonable history suggesting drug allergy and the usual lack of objective tests to support the diagnosis, further clinical evaluation involves withdrawal of the suspected drugs, followed by prompt resolution of the reaction, often within a few days or weeks. This is presumptive evidence of drug allergy and usually suffices for most clinical purposes.

Typically, patients are taking several medications. Those drugs that are not clearly indicated should be stopped. For drugs that are necessary, an attempt should be made to switch to alternative, non–cross-reacting agents. After the reaction subsides, resumption of treatment with the drug least likely to have caused the problem may be considered, if that drug is sufficiently important. However, there may be risk for anaphylaxis if the causative agent is resumed after interruption of therapy. Therefore, this should be considered before any therapy is discontinued.

There may be circumstances in which it would be detrimental to discontinue a drug when there is no suitable alternative available. The physician must then consider whether the drug reaction or the disease poses a greater risk. If the reaction is mild and does not appear to be progressive, it may be desirable to treat the reaction symptomatically and continue therapy. For example, in patients being treated with a β-lactam antibiotic, the appearance of urticaria may be managed with antihistamines or low-dose prednisone. Anaphylaxis has not developed in this setting (3). However, interruption of therapy for 24 to 48 hours may result in anaphylaxis if treatment is resumed.

PATIENT MANAGEMENT CONSIDERATIONS: TREATMENT, PREVENTION, AND REINTRODUCTION OF DRUGS

Treatment of Allergic Drug Reactions

General Principles

Withdrawal of the suspected drug is the most helpful diagnostic maneuver. At the same time, it is also the treatment of choice. Frequently, no additional treatment is necessary, and the clinical manifestations often subside within a few days or weeks without significant morbidity. If the reaction is not severe, and more than one drug is a candidate, withdrawal of one drug at a time may clarify the situation.

There may be clinical situations in which continued use of the suspected drug is essential. Here, the risk of continuing the drug may be less than the risk of not treating the underlying disease, particularly if no suitable alternative drug is available. Careful observation of the patient to detect any progression of the reaction, for example, a morbilliform rash becoming exfoliative in nature, and use of antihistamines and prednisone, may permit completion of the recommended course of therapy. Some physicians may elect to "treat through" milder reactions, but this is not without risk and should be supervised by physicians with experience. There are also situations in which a manifestation, often cutaneous, appears during the treatment but is due to the basic illness and not the drug.

Symptomatic Treatment

Pharmacologic management of allergic drug reactions is aimed at alleviating the manifestations until the reaction subsides. For mild reactions, therapy is usually not required. Treatment of more severe reactions depends on the nature of the skin eruption and the degree of systemic involvement.

Drug-induced anaphylaxis and anaphylactoid reactions, urticaria, angioedema, and asthma are treated in a manner described in other chapters in this text dealing with these entities.

For most patients with drug-induced serum sickness or serum sickness-like reactions, treatment with antihistamines and NSAIDs is all that is required. More severe manifestations require treatment with prednisone, 40 to 60 mg daily to start, with tapering over 7 to 10 days. Occasionally, plasmapheresis has been used to remove immune reactants.

The treatment of Stevens-Johnson syndrome includes high-dose corticosteroid therapy (133,134). For milder ambulatory cases, a minimum of 80 mg of prednisone daily is advised. Severe cases require hospitalization and administration of 60 mg of intravenous methylprednisolone every 4 to 6 hours until the lesions show improvement. Corticosteroids should then be tapered slowly over 2 to 3 weeks because tapering prematurely may result in recurrence of the lesions (133,134). For TEN, corticosteroids will not suppress the severe cutaneous involvement, and such patients are most efficiently managed in a burn unit. Sepsis is the principal cause of death in affected patients.

For other drug-induced immune reactions, such as drug fever, DIL, and vasculitis, and for reactions involving circulating blood elements and solid organs, corticosteroids accelerate resolution of these adverse drug effects.

Prevention of Allergic Drug Reactions

Drug Considerations

The best way to reduce the incidence of allergic drug reactions is to prescribe only those medications that are clinically essential. Of 30 penicillin anaphylactic deaths, only 12 patients had clear indication for penicillin administration (225). A survey of patients with allopurinol hypersensitivity syndrome reported that the drug was given correctly in only 14 of 72 cases, and there were 17 deaths (226). Also, using many drugs when fewer would be adequate will complicate identification of the offending drug should a reaction occur. The use of drugs in Scotland is about half that in the United States, and not surprisingly, the incidence of adverse drug reactions is considerably less (227). Interruption of therapy increases risk for allergy and should be avoided. The physician must be well informed regarding adverse reactions to drugs being prescribed.

Patient Considerations

The patient or a responsible person must be questioned carefully about a previous reaction to any drug about to be prescribed, and information should also be obtained about all other drugs previously taken. If available, a review of the patient's medical records may uncover essential information regarding prior drug reactions. Unfortunately, studies have demonstrated that many health care professionals do not obtain adequate drug histories and document them in the medical record. This incomplete documentation did not appear to be related to the patients' inability to provide accurate information (228). Failure to follow these simple procedures not only may harm patients but also may result in significant malpractice claims (229).

Although overdiagnosis may be a problem, it is generally advisable to accept what the patient believes or has been advised without the need for further documentation. Fortunately, there are alternative, non–cross-reacting agents available for most clinical situations. However, there may be situations in which one might choose an alternative drug when there is a chance of cross-reactivity; for example, selecting a cephalosporin in a penicillin-allergic patient to avoid using a more toxic drug, such as an aminoglycoside. In this situation, the patient should be skin tested for penicillin, and if test results are positive, the cross-reacting drug should be administered with a desensitization protocol in a monitored setting. Although cross-reactivity risk may be low, reactions may be severe (230).

Available Screening Tests

For acute generalized reactions, immediate wheal-and-flare skin tests are sensitive indicators for the detection of specific IgE antibodies to proteins. Skin testing is mandatory before administration of foreign antisera to reduce the likelihood of anaphylaxis.

Immediate wheal-and-flare skin tests with nonprotein, haptenic drugs have been validated for penicillin, thus permitting identification of patients with a history of penicillin allergy who are no longer at significant risk for readministration of this agent. For other haptenic drugs, such testing may detect drug-specific IgE antibodies when positive at concentrations that do not result in false-positive reactions in normal subjects. However, negative skin tests do not eliminate the possibility of clinically significant allergic sensitivity. None of the available *in vitro* tests for assessment of drug hypersensitivity qualify as screening procedures. Obviously, the simplicity, rapidity, and sensitivity of skin testing make it a logical choice for clinical purposes.

Methods of Drug Administration

Although there is some disagreement (37), the oral route of drug administration is perhaps preferable to parenteral administration because allergic reactions are less frequent and generally less severe. Clearly, topical use of drugs carries the highest risk for sensitization. For drugs given parenterally, an extremity should be used if possible to permit placement of a tourniquet if a reaction occurs. In addition, patients should be kept under observation for 30 minutes after parenteral administration of a drug. If the patient is likely to

develop a vasovagal reaction after an injection, the drug may be given while the patient is sitting or in a recumbent position.

Prolonged exposure to a drug increases the likelihood of sensitization. The frequency of drug usage increases the chance of eliciting an allergic response. The risk for a reaction appears to be greater during the first few months after a preceding course of treatment.

Follow-up after an Allergic Drug Reaction

The responsibility to a patient who has sustained an adverse drug reaction does not end with discontinuation of the agent and subsequent management of the reaction. The patient or responsible people must be informed of the reaction and advised how to avoid future exposure to the suspected agent and any agents that may cross-react with the offending drug. It is also helpful to mention alternative drugs that may be useful in the future. The patient should be educated regarding the importance of alerting other treating physicians about drugs being taken and any past adverse drug reactions.

All medical records must prominently display this information in a conspicuous location. The patient could carry a card (231) or wear an identification tag or bracelet (MedicAlert Emblems, Turlock, California) noting those drugs to be avoided if possible.

Reintroduction of Drugs to Patients with a History of a Previous Reaction

If the patient has had a previous documented or suspected allergic reaction to a medication, and now requires its use again, the physician must consider the risks and benefits of readministration of that drug. Cautious reintroduction of that medication may be considered when there are no acceptable alternatives available or when the alternative drug produces unacceptable side effects, is clearly less effective, or requires limited use because of resistance (e.g., increased vancomycin use leading to vancomycin-resistant enterococci). Physicians specializing in hypersensitivity reactions have developed a number of management strategies that permit many patients

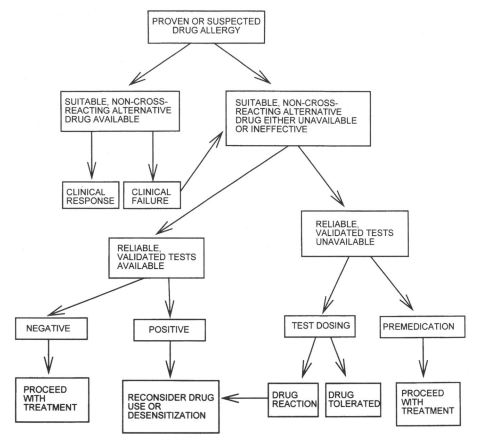

FIG. 17.1. This algorithm provides guidelines for the reintroduction of drugs to patients with a history of a previous drug reaction.

to receive appropriate drug therapy safely or to undergo an essential diagnostic evaluation (2). These procedures include premedication protocols, desensitization schedules, and test dosing regimens (Fig. 17.1).

Because these approaches constitute reintroduction of an agent previously implicated in an allergic reaction and thereby carry a risk for a potentially severe, even fatal, reaction, consultation should be obtained from the appropriate specialist (e.g., infectious disease specialist) to underscore the essentiality of the drug and its subsequent readministration. The medical record must contain this information in writing as well as informed consent from the patient or other responsible individuals. Informed consent must include a statement of potential risks of the pro-

cedure as well as risks that may develop without the treatment. Further, the medical setting should provide arrangements for emergency treatment of an acute reaction. Ideally, patients should not be receiving β-blocking drugs (even timolol ophthalmic solution); and asthma, if present, must be under optimal control.

Desensitization is best performed by an experienced allergist. Medical supervision is required throughout the procedure. Patients are often frightened by the risks of these procedures, and symptoms of anxiety may make evaluation difficult. The physicians must quickly decide whether to continue or abandon the procedure. In general, the presence of symptoms without objective findings suggests that the reaction may be hysterical in nature, and treatment should be continued.

Premedication

The prophylactic administration of antihistamines and corticosteroids alone or in combination with β-adrenergic agonists has been effective in reducing the incidence and severity of anaphylactoid reactions to RCM among patients with a previous history of such reactions. A similar approach has been used to minimize the likelihood of an anaphylactoid reaction following the administration of intravenous muscle relaxants, opiates, iron dextran, and protamine (2,232). It appears likely that drug-induced anaphylactoid events and possibly other situations in which the mechanisms of the reactions are unknown may be amenable to medication by such pretreatment regimens. Such premedication protocols are ineffective in blocking drug-induced IgE-mediated anaphylaxis. For this reason, prophylactic therapy before desensitization or test dosing to drugs is not recommended (2). Pretreatment may mask a mild reaction occurring at low doses of the drug and risk a more serious reaction at higher doses, which may be more difficult to manage.

Desensitization

Desensitization involves the conversion from a highly sensitive state to one in which the drug is now tolerated. This is reserved for patients with a history of an IgE-mediated immediate generalized reaction to a drug, confirmed by skin testing if available (e.g., PCN skin testing). Ideally, the term *desensitization* should be reserved for those reactions that have an established immunologic basis, and the cautious reaction with, and elimination of, IgE antibody is the goal. This produces a temporary, nonresponsive state lasting as long as therapy is uninterrupted. If therapy is interrupted, anaphylactic sensitivity may return within 48 hours of stopping the drug. Thus, continuation of an agent, such as insulin, after desensitization, is appropriate.

Acute desensitization with agents causing IgE-mediated reactions involves the administration of gradually increasing doses of the drug over several hours (e.g., penicillin) or days (e.g., insulin),

often starting with amounts as low as $\frac{1}{1,000,000}$ to $\frac{1}{100,000}$ of the therapeutic dose. The initial desensitizing dose may be based on the results of skin testing or test dosing. This process is accomplished with the agent that is required for treatment. Both oral and parenteral routes have been used for desensitization. The choice of route depends on the clinical condition, the drug being given, and the experience or preference of the attending physician. The intravenous dose is then doubled every 15 minutes while carefully monitoring the patient. Using such a protocol, anaphylaxis has not been reported during desensitization, or with continued uninterrupted treatment using a reduced dose. However, mild systemic reactions, notably urticaria and pruritus, occur in about one third of patients during desensitization. These mild reactions may subside spontaneously; they usually respond to symptomatic treatment, dosage adjustment, or both.

This approach has been used successfully to permit treatment with β-lactam antibiotics among patients with a history of penicillin allergy and positive tests for the major and minor haptenic determinants of penicillin; among diabetic patients with systemic insulin allergy; and among patients with positive skin tests for heterologous antisera. Desensitization to these IgE-mediated reactions renders mast cells specifically unresponsive to only the drug antigen used for desensitization. In many patients, successful desensitization is accompanied by a marked decrease or disappearance of the cutaneous wheal-and-flare response. Similar changes in skin test responses have been reported after successful desensitization to aminoglycosides and vancomycin (233,234). This is temporary; within 48 hours of discontinuing the drug, the skin tests are again positive. The patient is then at risk for anaphylaxis if the drug is resumed.

Although desensitization, as described, is limited to IgE-mediated reactions, the term has also been used in its broadest sense to describe a state of unresponsiveness to a drug that is accomplished by repeated and increasing exposure to that agent. This may include delayed, not IgE-mediated, reactions. This also is applied to patients who have had undeniable reactions to these drugs in the past. However, this does not involve elimination of available IgE antibodies through "controlled anaphylaxis" and may best be described as cautious readministration of the offending agent. Protocols have been described for the cautious administration of aspirin, sulfonamides (especially TMP-SMX and sulfasalazine), allopurinol (235), and others (2). Unlike desensitization to IgE-mediated reactions, these protocols are often more cumbersome and may require days or even weeks to complete. It should be emphasized that desensitization is a potentially hazardous procedure best left to physicians experienced in managing hypersensitivity reactions.

Test Dosing

In situations in which a drug is needed and the history of a previous reaction to that agent is vague, the possibility of true allergy is low, or the drug itself is an unlikely cause of such a reaction, test dosing or graded challenge is a method used to clarify the situation and safely determine whether it may be administered. A common example is a patient who has been advised to avoid all "caines," and now requires the use of a local anesthetic agent. True systemic allergy to local anesthetics is very rare. Test dosing provides

reassurance to the patient, physician, or dentist that this agent can be given safely.

The principle of test dosing is to select a dose of the drug below that which would potentially cause a serious reaction, and then proceed with relatively large incremental increases to full therapeutic doses. Using this technique, one can determine whether a reaction occurs before proceeding to the next dose. If a reaction occurs, it can be easily treated. If the drug is necessary, a desensitization protocol may then be considered.

The starting dose, incremental increase, and interval between challenges depend on the drug and the urgency of reaching therapeutic doses. For oral drugs, a usual starting dose is 0.1 mg or 1.0 mg, and then proceeds to 10 mg, 50 mg, 100 mg, and 200 mg. For parenteral drugs, the initial dose is less, for example, 0.01 mg or 0.001 mg. If the suspected reaction was immediate, a 30-minute interval between doses is appropriate, and the procedure is usually completed in 3 to 5 hours or less. For late-onset reactions, such as dermatitis, the dosing interval may be as long as 24 to 48 hours, with the procedure requiring 1 to 2 weeks or longer to complete. Although there is always the possibility of a severe reaction, the risk of test dosing appears to be very low (217).

Part B: Allergic Reactions to Individual Drugs: Low Molecular Weight

Paul A. Greenberger

Division of Allergy-Immunology, Department of Medicine, Northwestern University Medical School, Chicago, Illinois

The approach described in this part has been used successfully to permit treatment with β-lactam antibiotics among patients with a history of penicillin allergy and positive tests for the major and minor haptenic determinants of penicillin; among diabetic patients with systemic insulin allergy; and among patients with positive skin tests for heterologous antisera. Desensitization to these IgE-mediated reactions renders mast cells specifically unresponsive to only the drug antigen used for desensitization. In many patients, successful desensitization is accompanied by a marked decrease or disappearance of the cutaneous wheal-and-flare response. Similar changes in skin test responses have been reported following successful desensitization to aminoglycosides and vancomycin (1,2).

As noted earlier, the term desensitization also has been used in its broadest sense to describe a state of unresponsiveness to a drug that is accomplished by repeated and increasing exposure to that agent (3). Similar to acute desensitization for IgE-mediated reactions, these patients have had undeniable reactions to these drugs in the past. Protocols have been described for the cautious administration of aspirin (4,5), sulfonamides (especially TMP-SMX and sulfasalazine) (3,5,6), allopurinol (7), and others. Unlike desensitization to IgE-mediated reactions, these protocols are often more cumbersome and may require days or even weeks to complete. Finally, one should be reminded that desensitization is a potentially hazardous procedure best left to physicians experienced in managing hypersensitivity reactions.

TEST DOSING

In situations in which a drug is needed and the history of a previous reaction to that agent is vague, and the possibility of true allergy is low, or the drug itself is an unlikely cause of such a reaction, test dosing or graded challenge is a method used to clarify the situation and safely determine whether it may be administered. A common example is a patient who has been advised to avoid all "caines," and now requires the use of a local anesthetic agent. True systemic allergy to local anesthetics is almost unheard of. Test dosing provides reassurance to the patient, physician, or dentist that this agent can be safely given.

The principle of test dosing is to select a dose of the drug below that which would potentially cause a serious reaction, and then proceed with relatively large incremental increases to full therapeutic doses. Using this technique, one can determine whether a reaction has occurred before proceeding to the next dose. If a reaction occurs, it can be easily treated. If the drug is necessary, a desensitization protocol may then be considered.

The starting dose, incremental increase, and interval between challenges depend on the drug and the urgency of reaching therapeutic doses. For oral drugs, a usual starting dose is 0.1 mg or 1.0 mg, and then proceeds to 10 mg, 50 mg, 100 mg, and 200 mg. For parenteral drugs, the initial dose is less, for example, 0.01 mg or 0.001 mg. When the suspected reaction was immediate, a 20 to 30-minute interval between doses is appropriate, and the procedure is usually completed in 3 to 5 hours or less. For late-onset reactions, such as a dermatitis, the dosing interval may be as long as 24 to 48 hours, with the same protocols requiring 1 to 2 weeks or longer. Although there is always the possibility of a severe reaction, the risk of test dosing appears to be very low (8).

SPECIAL CONSIDERATIONS FOR PROVEN OR SUSPECTED ALLERGIC REACTIONS TO INDIVIDUAL DRUGS

In this section, specific recommendations as they pertain to important drugs commonly used in clinical practice are reviewed. For each agent, relevant background information is provided. Additional information about those drugs may be found in the last edition of this text (9) and elsewhere (6,10–12). Table 17.12 summarizes useful strategies for administering agents, once indication for the agent to be administered has been verified.

Penicillins and Other β-Lactam Antibiotics

Background

β-Lactam antibiotic hypersensitivity deserves special consideration because of its medical importance. Penicillin has been studied extensively and has become a prototype for the study of allergic drug reactions. As many as 10% of hospitalized patients report a history of penicillin allergy. In a study of 1,893 consecutive adult patients who had an order written for an antimicrobial agent while hospitalized, 470 (25%) patients reported an allergy to at least one drug (13). Two hundred and ninety-five (15.6%) patients listed penicillin. A manual review of the charts revealed that just 32% of records specified the details of the allergic reaction. Some patients have been labeled falsely as penicillin allergic and are denied this useful, remarkably nontoxic agent. The reasons for this discrepancy are either a previously incorrect diagnosis or the frequently evanescent nature of penicillin allergy. Following an acute allergic reaction, there is a time-dependent decline in the rate of positive skin tests to penicillin. In the first year, 90% to 100% retain sensitivity after a convincing allergic reaction, but that percentage drops to about 30% at 10 years (14). Some patients, however, maintain penicillin-specific IgE antibody for 30 to 40 years. It is therefore highly desirable to predict which patients are at risk for a penicillin reaction. Alternatively, a literature review reported that 347 of 1,063 (33%) patients who tested positive on penicillin skin test had vague histories of penicillin allergy (15).

The overall prevalence of β-lactam allergy is estimated to be about 2% per course of treatment (16). The most frequent manifestations are cutaneous, notably morbilliform, and urticarial eruptions; the most serious is anaphylaxis. In an older, often quoted study, penicillin-induced anaphylaxis occurred in about 0.01% to 0.05% (1 per 5,000 to 10,000) of patient treatment courses, with a fatal outcome in 0.0015% to 0.002% (1 death per 50,000 to 100,000 treatment courses) (17). This would translate to 500 to 1,000 deaths per year in the United States (18).

An atopic background (allergic rhinitis, asthma, atopic dermatitis) does not predispose an individual to the development of penicillin hypersensitivity, but once sensitized, such individuals are at increased risk for severe or fatal anaphylactic reactions (19). Anaphylaxis occurring in patients with asthma may result in acute severe respiratory failure. Also, atopic patients with *Penicillium* species "mold" allergy can receive penicillin unless specifically allergic to penicillin.

Patients with a history of prior penicillin reaction have a fourfold to sixfold increased risk for subsequent reactions to β-lactam antibiotics, including imipenem and meropenem. Among penicillin-allergic individuals, the unmodified administration of these drugs causes acute reactions in about two thirds of patients. If desensitization is performed, the incidence of reactions is much lower.

Although this discussion focuses primarily on the evaluation of and strategies to deal with IgE-mediated reactions, this group of agents has also been associated with other adverse, IgE-independent immunologic events that are briefly noted here and have been extensively reviewed elsewhere (16). *Immediate reactions* occur within the first hour following administration of the β-lactam drug, are IgE mediated, and may present an immediate threat to life. *Accelerated reactions* develop 1 to 72 hours after drug administration, are usually IgE mediated, usually present as urticaria and angioedema, and are

TABLE 17.12. *Examples of useful evaluation techniques and management strategies for selected drugs and agents*

Drugs or agents	Skin tests of value	Premedication useful	Test dosing indicated	Desensitization if essential	Additional comments
Immediate generalized reactions (IgE mediated)					
β-Lactam antibiotics	✓		See comments	✓	Test dose in absence of penicillin. MDM or validated cephalosporin skin tests.
Insulin	✓			✓	Use least reactive insulin by skin test for desensitization.
Immune sera	✓			✓	Risky in atopic patients allergic to horse dander.
Egg-containing vaccines	✓			✓	May be unnecessary for MMR vaccine.
Tetanus toxoid	✓			✓	If serum antitoxin levels adequate, desensitization not required.
Latex	See comments				No standardized skin test available. Avoidance only effective treatment.
Protamine		See comments			No studies to validate premedication.
Streptokinase	✓				Substitute urokinase or tissue plasminogen activator.
Chymopapain	✓				Consider laminectomy.
Immediate generalized reactions (IgE independent)					
Aspirin and nonsteroidal antiinflammatory drugs			✓	See comments	Term *desensitization* used, although reaction is not IgE mediated. Also useful for nonvascular studies.
Contrast media		✓			Lower osmolality media a better choice.
Opioid analgesics			✓		Pentazocaine or fentanyl are less active histamine releasers.
Cancer chemotherapy		✓			Slow infusion and premedication has been useful.
Allergy presumed mechanism unclear					
Sulfonamides			✓	See comments	Term *desensitization* often used, but reaction is usually IgE independent.
Local anesthetics			✓		True systemic reactions are rare. Reassurance is primary goal.
Anticonvulsants			✓		A potentially dangerous procedure.
Other rarely incriminated drugs or agents			✓		Seek consultation with experienced allergist

MDM, minor determinant mixture; MMR, measles, mumps, and rubella.
Adapted from Reference 5.

rarely life endangering. *Delayed or late reactions* occur after 3 days, are IgE independent, and usually present as benign morbilliform skin eruptions. Exfoliative dermatitis and Stevens-Johnson syndrome may occur. Late noncutaneous reactions include serum sickness–like reactions (20) and drug fever (21). Unusual late reactions are immune cytopenias, AIN, pulmonary infiltrates with eosinophilia, and hypersensitivity vasculitis.

In general, the previously described adverse events are common to all β-lactam antibiotics, such as the natural penicillins (penicillin G, penicillin V), the penicillinase-resistant penicillins (methicillin, nafcillin, dicloxacillin, imipenem, and meropenem), the aminopenicillins (ampicillin, amoxicillin), and the extended spectrum penicillins (carbenicillin, ticarcillin, mezlocillin, azlocillin, piperacillin). Hypersensitivity is usually less with the cephalosporins.

Individual β-lactam antibiotics have been associated more commonly with certain types of reactions. For instance, ampicillin and amoxicillin therapy is associated with a higher incidence (about 10%) of nonpruritic maculopapular rash than are other penicillins (about 2%) (21). The rash usually appears after at least 1 week of therapy, initially develops on the knees and elbows, and then spreads symmetrically to cover the entire body (22). If the patient has infectious mononucleosis, the incidence approaches 90%. The incidence of this cutaneous reaction is increased in patients with HIV and cytomegalovirus (CMV) infection, chronic lymphatic leukemia, and hyperuricemia (23). This eruption does not appear to be allergic in nature, but if there is an urticarial component, it may represent true IgE-mediated penicillin allergy, and rechallenge could result in a severe immediate generalized allergic reaction.

Cephalosporins produce reactions similar to those described for penicillins. The more common reactions include maculopapular or morbilliform skin eruption, drug fever, and a positive Coombs test (clinical hemolysis unusual). Less common reactions are urticaria, serum sickness–like reactions (especially with cefaclor in children) (24,25), and anaphylaxis (26,27). Drug-induced cytopenias and AIN are rare. Compared with the first-generation (e.g., cephalothin, cefazolin, cephalexin,* cefadroxil,* cefaclor*) and second-generation (e.g., cefamandole, cefuroxime, cefuroxime axetil*) cephalosporins, the third-generation (e.g., cefotaxime, ceftizoxime, ceftriaxone, ceftazidime, cefixime*) cephalosporins have a lower incidence of immediate, presumably IgE-mediated, generalized allergic reactions (28).

Some degree of cross-reactivity among the different classes of β-lactam antibiotics is well established (29). Because the semisynthetic penicillins contain the same 6-aminopenicillanic acid nucleus as natural penicillin G, it is not surprising that cross-allergenicity among these agents exists, albeit to various degrees. Individuals have been identified who have reacted to ampicillin and amoxicillin but not to penicillin (30,31). It is presumed that this is related to hypersensitivity to the side chains that differentiate the antibiotic from the parent compound. The incidence and clinical significance of these side-chain–specific reactions remains unknown. However, at this time, if a patient reports a history of penicillin allergy, it is prudent to assume that the individual is allergic to all penicillins (5,9,29). Because 9% to 15% of patients receiving antibiotics report a penicillin allergy (13,32–34), the impact of penicillin allergy in hospitalized patients remains significant.

Cephalosporins share a common β-lactam ring with penicillin but have a six-member dihydrothiazine ring instead of the five-membered thiazolidine ring of the penicillin molecule. Shortly after the introduction of the cephalosporins into clinical use, allergic reactions, including anaphylaxis, were reported, and the question of cross-reactivity between cephalosporins and penicillins was raised (35). To date, the issue has not been completely resolved. Significant *in vitro* and *in vivo* cross-reactivity has been demonstrated with first-generation cephalosporins (5% to 16.5%) (36). Fortunately, clinically relevant cross-reactivity between penicillin and the cephalosporins (especially second and third generation) is about 10% (37) and 2% to 3% (38,39), respectively. A

---

*Oral agents.

literature review of patients with a history of penicillin allergy challenged with cephalosporins revealed allergic reactions in 5.6% of patients with positive penicillin skin tests, compared with 1.7% among those with negative penicillin skin tests (16). A more recent but controversial review suggests that penicillin-allergic patients who are identified by either history or positive penicillin skin tests are not at increased risk compared with the general population, and they may be safely treated with cephalosporin antibiotics (38). However, cautious administration of cephalosporins to penicillin-allergic patients is advisable, especially when the history is that of acute urticaria or other anaphylactic reaction. Regrettably, in a report of six penicillin-allergic patients, three experienced fatal anaphylactic reactions from a first dose of a cephalosporin (27).

Primary cephalosporin allergy, including anaphylaxis, has occasionally been reported in both penicillin-allergic and penicillin-nonallergic patients and may be fatal (27). Most investigators have studied tolerance to the cephalosporins in penicillin-allergic patients, but little information is available regarding tolerance to other β-lactam antibiotics in patients with primary cephalosporin allergy. Such studies are limited by the lack of reliable cephalosporin haptenic determinants for skin testing. It appears that antibodies directed against unique side chains rather than against the common ring structure are more important in the immune response to cephalosporins (40). This would explain the low cross-reactivity among different cephalosporins, which share the same nucleus but have different side chains (41). Also, it may help to explain the low cross-reactivity between cephalosporins and penicillins, which share the same β-lactam ring in the nucleus but have different side chains. Until better information is available, it is best to avoid the use of β-lactam antibiotics in cephalosporin-allergic patients; if absolutely indicated, cautious administration is advisable with a third- or fourth-generation cephalosporin.

The carbapenems (imipenem, meropenem), monobactams (aztreonam), and carbacephems (loracarbef) are three classes of antibiotics that possess β-lactam ring structures. There is significant cross-reactivity between penicillin and imipenem (42) and meropenem based on structure. Immediate skin reactivity to imipenem (1 mg/mL) by prick test was demonstrated in a patient who experienced shock and cardiac arrest from imipenem (43). Aztreonam is the prototypical monobactam antibiotic. It is weakly cross-reactive in the penicillin-allergic patient and may be administered safely to most, if not all, patients allergic to other β-lactam antibiotics (44). The antibodies generated are specific to the side chain rather than the β-lactam ring. It should be noted, however, that ceftazidime, a third-generation cephalosporin, shares an identical side chain with aztreonam. It may be prudent not to use ceftazidime in rare subjects allergic to aztreonam. Loracarbef, a carbacephem, structurally resembles cefaclor, but the degree of cross-reactivity with penicillins and cephalosporins is unknown. For now, it is best to avoid its use among patients allergic to β-lactam antibiotics. Finally, clavulanic acid is also a β-lactam antibiotic with weak antibacterial activity but is a potent inhibitor of β-lactamase. It is often combined with amoxicillin to enhance antimicrobial activity. There is a recent report of two immediate generalized allergic reactions attributed to clavulanic acid (45).

Diagnostic Testing

Although obtaining a past history of penicillin allergy is essential, one cannot completely rely on that information to predict who is allergic. The history may be inaccurate, and many patients do lose their sensitivity over time. The failure to elicit this information has resulted in several fatalities following the administration of these drugs to patients with a good history of β-lactam hypersensitivity (46). To help clarify this situation, when the drug is essential, skin testing with penicillin has been useful to identify those patients at risk for anaphylaxis and other, milder IgE-mediated reactions. When appropriate skin testing reagents are either unavailable or have not been validated, test dosing with the desired β-lactam antibiotic is recommended.

Benzylpenicillin (BP) has a molecular weight of 300 and is metabolized in large part (about 95%) into a penicilloyl hapten moiety. This metabolite is referred to as the major determinant and has been conjugated to poly-D-lysine to form penicilloyl-polylysine (PPL), which has been commercially available as Pre-Pen (Hollister-Stier, Spokane, WA) for skin testing. Other penicillin metabolites, including BP itself, constitute 5% or less of administered penicillin and are collectively referred to as the *minor determinant mixture* (MDM). They are minor in name only but are responsible for some penicillin anaphylactic reactions. A standardized MDM is not available commercially for skin testing. Therefore, a fresh solution of BP (10,000 units/mL) has been used for skin testing purposes. Skin testing with both PPL and freshly prepared BP (as the sole minor determinant) should detect 85% to 88% of potential reactors (14,17). Almost all patients (99%) with negative skin tests to PPL and MDM reagents can be treated safely with penicillin (47). If PPL is not used but MDM is, from 34% to 60% of skin test–positive patients would be missed (14,48). Thus, the major determinant identified a significant proportion of skin test–positive patients, and its use improves safety during testing and desensitization.

In general, skin testing with BP-derived reagents, PPL and MDM, is also predictive of reactions to other β-lactam antibiotics (14,49); however, there are patients with reactions to ampicillin, amoxicillin, and cephalosporin side chains who may not be detected by skin testing (30,31). Although skin testing with the β-lactam antibiotic of therapeutic choice has been advocated to detect additional potential reactors, skin test reagents prepared from other penicillins, cephalosporins, imipenem, and aztreonam have not been standardized, and the results are not validated (16,50). A positive skin test using these materials suggests the potential for an IgE-mediated reaction, but a negative test does not eliminate this concern. The incidence of such reactions to other β-lactam antibiotics when skin tests are negative to standard penicillin reagents is unknown but is probably small (51). Some minor determinant mixtures are not as sensitive as others and have led to confusion about the need to detect side-chain–specific IgE.

In practice, penicillin skin testing to evaluate the potential or risk for an IgE-mediated reac-

tion should be reserved for patients with a history suggesting penicillin allergy when administration of the drug is essential or when confusion about penicillin interferes with optimal antibiotic selection. Such testing is of no value in predicting the occurrence of non–IgE-mediated reactions and is contraindicated when the previous reaction was Stevens-Johnson syndrome, TEN, or exfoliative dermatitis. Elective penicillin skin testing followed by an oral challenge and subsequent 10-day course of treatment with penicillin or amoxicillin in skin test–negative subjects has been recommended, particularly in children with a history suggesting penicillin allergy (52). It was hoped that this procedure would "clear the air" and eliminate the need to carry out such testing when the child is ill and in need of penicillin therapy. Using this approach, the risk for resensitization was about 1%. In one small study of 19 patients, 16% of penicillin history–positive, but skin test–negative adults receiving intravenous penicillin therapy became skin test positive 1 to 12 months after completion of treatment (53). In another study, none of 33 penicillin history–positive, skin test–negative patients had evidence of IgE-mediated reactions, suggesting loss of antipenicillin IgE antibodies (54). The overall data support the use of penicillin skin tests in managing patients with a history of penicillin allergy, regardless of the severity of the previous reaction. Penicillin skin testing is rapid, and the risk for a serious reaction is minimal when performed by trained personnel, using recommended drug concentrations, and completing skin-prick tests before attempting intradermal skin tests. Testing should be completed shortly before administration of the drug.

Table 17.13 summarizes the reagents used for β-lactam antibiotic skin tests and the recommended starting concentrations of these reagents, which are adequately sensitive but have a low risk for provoking a systemic or nonspecific irritant reaction. In patients with a history of a life-threatening reaction to penicillin, it is advisable to dilute the skin test reagents 100-fold for initial testing. Skin-prick testing is accomplished by pricking through a drop of the reagent placed on the volar surface of the forearm and observing for

TABLE 17.13. β-*Lactam antibiotic skin tests*

Skin test reagents	Route	Drug test concentration	Skin test volume	Dose
Penicilloyl-polylysine[a] (Pre-Pen) (6×10^{-5} M)	Prick Intradermal	Full strength Full strength	1 drop 0.02 mL	
Penicillin G[a] potassium (freshly prepared)	Prick Intradermal (serial 10-fold dilutions optional)[d]	10,000 U/mL 10,000 U/mL	1 drop 0.02 mL	200 units
Penicillin minor determinant mixture[b] (10^{-2} M)	Prick Intradermal (serial 10-fold dilutions optional)[d]	Full strength Full strength	1 drop 0.01–0.02 mL	
Cephalosporins and other penicillins[c]	Prick Intradermal (serial 10-fold dilutions optional)[d]	3 mg/mL 3 mg/mL	1 drop 0.02 mL	60 μg
Aztreonam[c]	Prick Intradermal (serial 10-fold dilutions optional)[d]	3 mg/mL 3 mg/mL	1 drop 0.02 mL	60 μg
Imipenem[c]	Prick Intradermal (serial 10-fold dilutions optional)[d]	1 mg/mL 1 mg/mL	1 drop 0.02 mL	20 μg
Histamine (Histatrol)— positive control	Prick Intradermal	1 mg/mL 0.1 mg/mL	1 drop 0.02 mL	
Saline or diluent— negative control	Prick Intradermal	NA NA	1 drop 0.02 mL	

[a]Testing validated.
[b]Testing validated; reagents not available (except at some medical centers).
[c]Testing not validated. Negative tests do not rule out possibility of a reaction.
[d]Serial skin tests may be prudent when previous reaction was anaphylactic in nature.

15 to 20 minutes. A significant reaction is a wheal 3 mm or larger than the control with surrounding erythema. If negative, proceed with intradermal skin tests. Using a tuberculin or allergy syringe, inject 0.01 to 0.02 mL of the reagent, sufficient to raise a 2- to 3-mm bleb on the volar surface of the forearm. After 15 to 20 minutes, a positive test produces a wheal of 4 mm or larger with surrounding erythema. If the results are equivocal or difficult to interpret, the tests should be repeated. It should be noted that there is some disagreement among investigators as to what constitutes an acceptable positive skin test (50). A 4-mm wheal with surrounding erythema is positive; a 4-mm or greater wheal without erythema is "indeterminate" and usually not representative of antipenicillin IgE antibodies. Caution is required on test dose challenging though.

Because penicillin MDM is not commercially available and skin testing with other β-lactam antibiotics has not been standardized, nor have

the results been validated, test dosing is recommended in patients with a past history of penicillin allergy and negative skin tests to Pre-Pen and penicillin G (5). How one approaches this procedure depends on the severity of the previous reaction and the experience of the managing physician. After documenting the need for the drug, obtaining informed consent, and being prepared to treat anaphylaxis, a test dose protocol may be initiated with a physician in constant attendance; 0.001 mg (1 unit) of the therapeutic β-lactam antibiotic is administered by the desired (oral, intravenous) route. The patient is observed for signs of pruritus, flushing, urticaria, dyspnea, and hypotension. In the absence of these signs, at 15-minute intervals, subsequent doses are given as outlined in Table 17.14. If a reaction occurs during this procedure, it is treated with epinephrine and antihistamines; the need for the drug should be reevaluated and desensitization considered if this agent is essential. This is a

TABLE 17.14. *Suggested test dosing schedule for β-lactam antibiotics*

Dose (mg)[a]	Dose (units)[a]
0.001	1
0.005	10
0.01	20
0.05	100
0.10	200
0.50	800
1.00	1,600
10.00	16,000
50.00	80,000
100.00	160,000
200.00	320,000
Full dose may be administered	

[a]400,000 units penicillin G potassium is roughly equivalent to 250 mg of other β-lactam antibiotics (1 μg = 1.8 units).

rather conservative test dosing schedule and may even be useful in situations in which skin testing with Pre-Pen and penicillin G potassium has not been successfully completed. More experienced physicians may elect to shorten this procedure; one suggestion has been to test dose with $\frac{1}{100}$ of the therapeutic dose ($\frac{1}{1,000}$ of the therapeutic dose if the previous reaction was severe), and then move quickly to the full therapeutic dose if there is no reaction (16).

Because there is a small risk associated with skin testing and test dosing, *in vitro* tests have obvious appeal. Solid-phase immunoassays, such as the RAST and the enzyme-linked immunosorbent assay (ELISA), have been developed to detect serum IgE antibodies against the major penicilloyl determinant. The RAST or fluorescent immunoassay generally correlates with skin testing to PPL. RAST and fluorescent immunoassays for cephalosporins and other antimicrobial drugs have been reported but are only available for research. At present, RAST and other *in vitro* tests have limited clinical usefulness because there are many unidentified metabolites that may become haptens.

Management of Patients with a History of Penicillin Allergy

Preferable management of patients with a history of penicillin or other β-lactam antibiotic allergy is the use of an equally effective, non–cross-reacting antibiotic. In most situations, adequate substitutes are available (55), and consultation with infectious disease experts is valuable. Aztreonam, a monocyclic β-lactam antibiotic, has little if any cross-reactivity with penicillins or cephalosporins and can be administered to patients with prior anaphylactic reactions to penicillin. Unfortunately, this antibiotic's activity is limited to aerobic gram-negative bacilli, such as *Pseudomonas aeruginosa*.

If alternative drugs fail, or if there is known antibiotic resistance by suspected pathogens, skin testing and test dosing with the β-lactam antibiotic of choice should be performed. If skin tests are positive, if the patient reacts to test doses, or if such testing is not done, administration of the β-lactam antibiotic, using a desensitization protocol, is advised. One begins with a subanaphylactic dose so that if anaphylaxis occurs, it can be controlled.

Some infections in which this approach becomes necessary include enterococcal infections, brain abscess, bacterial meningitis, sepsis with staphylococci, *Neisseria* or *Pseudomonas* species organisms, *Listeria* infections, neurosyphilis, and syphilis in pregnant women. In fact, penicillin desensitization is indicated for pregnant women with syphilis who demonstrate immediate hypersensitivity to that drug (56). Also, at present, there are no data to support the use of alternatives to penicillin for treatment of neurosyphilis and all stages of syphilis among HIV-infected patients (55).

The usual scenario involves a patient who presents with a convincing history of penicillin allergy and, if available and performed, negative skin tests for Pre-Pen and penicillin G. Many physicians do not have access to important minor determinants for skin testing; therefore, test dosing as previously outlined is recommended because 12% to 15% of patients may not have been identified as skin test positive (14,47). If a reaction occurs at any test dose, the need for the drug should be reevaluated. If essential, a desensitization protocol should be considered. A more unusual scenario is a patient with a positive history and positive skin tests for available penicillin reagents. Such patients are at significant risk for anaphylaxis. Desensitization protocols significantly reduce the risk for anaphylaxis in skin test–positive patients, whereas deliberate infusion of a β-lactam antibiotic at the usual rate could cause a severe or fatal anaphylactic reaction.

Acute β-lactam antibiotic desensitization should be performed in an intensive care setting. Informed consent (verbal or written) is advised. Patients with asthma or congestive heart failure should be under optimal control. Premedication with antihistamines and corticosteroids is not recommended because these drugs have not proved effective in suppressing anaphylaxis and could mask mild allergic manifestations that may have resulted in a modification of the desensitization protocol (19).

Before initiation of desensitization, two intravenous lines are established, and baseline vital signs are recorded. The clinical state of the patient is recorded. A baseline electrocardiogram and spirometry have been advocated by some as well as continuous electrocardiographic monitoring. During desensitization, vital signs and the clinical state of the patient are noted before each dose, and at 10- to 20-minute intervals following each dose. A physician must be in close attendance during the entire procedure so that unexpected reactions such as hypotension can be reversed quickly.

Desensitization has been accomplished successfully using either the oral or intravenous routes of administration (57,58). Oral desensitization is favored by some who believe that the risk for a serious reaction is less. The intravenous route is chosen by others, including myself, who prefer absolute control of the drug concentration used and its rate of administration. Unfortunately, there is no completely standardized regimen, and there have been no direct comparative studies between oral and intravenous desensitizing protocols.

Regardless of the method chosen for desensitization, the basic principles are similar. The initial dose is typically $\frac{1}{10,000}$ of the therapeutic dose. Oral desensitization may begin with the dose that is tolerated during oral test dosing. Intravenous desensitization should begin with $\frac{1}{10}$ or $\frac{1}{100}$ (if the previous reaction was severe) of the dose producing a positive skin test or intravenous test dose response. The dose is then usually doubled at 7- to 15-minute intervals until full therapeutic doses are achieved, typically within 4 to 5 hours. Representative protocols for intravenous (Table 17.15) and oral (Table 17.16) desensitization are presented.

Table 17.15 outlines an intravenous desensitization protocol for penicillin G potassium or any other β-lactam antibiotic (10). The dose to be administered is placed in a small volume of 5% dextrose in water for piggyback delivery into the already established intravenous line. It is administered slowly at first, then more rapidly if no warning signs, such as pruritus or flushing, appear. If symptoms develop during the procedure, the flow rate is slowed or stopped and the patient treated appropriately, using the other intravenous site if necessary. After symptoms subside, the flow rate is slowly increased once again. Once the patient has received and tolerated 800,000 units of penicillin G or 800 mg of any other β-lactam antibiotic, the full therapeutic dose may be given and therapy continued without interruption.

Table 17.16 provides a protocol for oral desensitization with β-lactam antibiotics. If the patient is unable to take oral medication, it may be administered through a feeding tube. Mild reactions during desensitization, such as pruritus, fleeting urticaria, mild rhinitis, or wheezing, require the dose to be repeated until tolerated. If a more serious reaction occurs, such as hypotension, laryngeal edema, or severe asthma, the next dose should be decreased to at least one third of the provoking dose and withheld until the patient is stable. If an oral form of the desired β-lactam agent is unavailable, intravenous desensitization should be considered. Once desensitized, treatment must not lapse. Regardless of the route selected for desensitization, mild reactions, usually pruritic rashes, may be expected in about 30% of patients during and after the procedure. These reactions usually subside with continued treatment, but symptomatic therapy may be necessary.

After successful desensitization, some individuals may have predictable needs for future exposures to β-lactam antibiotics. Patients with

TABLE 17.15. *Protocol for intravenous desensitization with β-lactam antibiotics*

β-Lactam concentration (mg/mL)	Penicillin G concentration (U/mL)	Dose No.[a]	Amount given (mL)	Dose given (mg/units)
0.1	160	1	0.10	0.01/16
		2	0.20	0.02/32
		3	0.40	0.04/64
		4	0.80	0.08/128
1.0	1,600	5	0.15	0.15/240
		6	0.30	0.30/480
		7	0.60	0.06/960
		8	1.00	1.0/1600
10.0	16,000	9	0.20	2.0/3200
		10	0.40	4.0/6400
		11	0.80	8.0/12,800
100.0	160,000	12	0.15	15.0/24,000
		13	0.30	30.0/48,000
		14	0.60	60.0/96,000
		15	1.00	100.0/160,000
1000.0	1,600,000	16	0.20	200.0/320,000
		17	0.40	400.0/640,000
		18	0.80	800.0/1,280,000

Observe patient for 30 minutes; administer full therapeutic dose intravenously.

[a]Dose approximately doubled every 7–15 min.

Adapted from Adkinson NF Jr. Drug allergy. In: Middleton EJ, Reed CE, Ellis EF, et al, eds. *Allergy: principles and practice.* 5th ed. St. Louis: CV Mosby, 1998:1212–1224, with permission.

TABLE 17.16. *Protocol for oral desensitization with β-lactam antibiotics*

β-Lactam concentration (mg/mL)[a]	Dose no.[b]	Amount given[c] (mL)	Dose given (mg)
0.5	1	0.10	0.05
	2	0.20	0.10
	3	0.40	0.20
	4	0.80	0.40
	5	1.60	0.80
	6	3.20	1.60
	7	6.40	3.20
5.0	8	1.20	6.00
	9	2.40	12.00
	10	4.80	24.00
50.0	11	1.00	50.00
	12	2.00	100.00
	13	4.00	200.00
	14	8.00	400.00

Observe patient for 30 minutes; give full therapeutic dose by route of choice.

[a]Dilutions prepared from antibiotic syrup, 250 mg/5 mL.
[b]Dose approximately doubled every 15 min.
[c]Drug amount given in 30 mL water or flavored beverage.

Adapted from Sullivan TJ. Drug Allergy. In: Middleton EJ, Reed CE, Ellis EF, et al., eds. *Allergy: principles and practice.* 4th ed. St. Louis: CV Mosby, 1993:1726, with permission.

cystic fibrosis, chronic neutropenia, or occupational exposure to these agents may benefit from chronic twice-daily oral penicillin therapy to sustain a desensitized state between courses of high-dose parenteral therapy (59,60). However, some investigators are concerned about the ability to maintain 100% compliance among cystic fibrosis patients in an outpatient setting and therefore prefer to perform intravenous desensitization each time β-lactam antibiotic therapy is required (61).

In summary, β-lactam antibiotics can be administered by desensitization with relatively little risk in patients with a history of allergy to these drugs and a positive reaction to skin testing. Once successfully desensitized, the need for uninterrupted therapy until treatment has been completed is advisable. Any lapse in therapy greater than 12 hours may permit such sensitivity to return. Mild reactions during and after desensitization are not an indication to discontinue treatment. Many resolve spontaneously or may require symptomatic therapy.

Among successfully desensitized patients with a positive history of β-lactam allergy and a positive response to skin testing or test dosing, this same approach may be repeated before a future course of therapy. There appears to be little risk for resensitization following an uneventful course of therapy among patients with positive histories and negative skin tests or after uneventful test dosing (52,54).

Non–β-Lactam Antimicrobial Agents

Allergic reactions to non–β-lactam antimicrobial drugs, most commonly cutaneous eruptions, are common causes of morbidity and, rarely, mortality. Anaphylaxis to these agents is a rare event. The estimated overall incidence of a hypersensitivity-type reaction to non–β-lactam drugs is about 1% to 3%. Some antimicrobial agents, however, such as TMP-SMX, produce reactions more commonly; in contrast, others, such as tetracycline, are much less likely to do so.

Unlike the β-lactam antimicrobials, other antibiotics have been less well studied and also include a wide variety of chemical agents. Research has been hampered by the lack of information regarding the immunochemistry of most of these drugs and, therefore, the unavailability of proven immunodiagnostic tests to assist the physician. Although skin testing with the free drug and some *in vitro* tests have been described for sulfonamides, aminoglycosides, and vancomycin, there are no large series reported to validate their clinical usefulness.

Despite these shortcomings, when such agents, notably TMP-SMX, are medically necessary, protocols have been developed to administer these drugs. With the exception of sulfonamides and occasionally other non–β-lactam drugs, urgent administration is usually not required. Slow, cautious test dosing is generally a safe and effective method to determine whether the drug is now tolerated. An example with TMP-SMX is to begin with 0.1 mg orally and, at 30- to 60-minute intervals, administer 1 mg, 10 mg, and 50 mg. If there is no reaction, on the following day, 100 mg and 200 mg may be given. On occasion, particularly in life-threatening pneumocystis or toxoplasma infections in AIDS patients, an every-4-hour dosing schedule may be required. Because most reactions to non–β-lactam antimicrobial agents are nonanaphylactic (IgE independent), desensitization is indicated rarely and may be quite dangerous, as described later.

Sulfonamides

Background

The stimulus for continued attention to sulfonamide and trimethoprim hypersensitivity is due to their utility in treatment of a wide variety of gram-positive and gram-negative bacterial infections and to their importance in the treatment of infectious complications in patients with AIDS. In patients infected with HIV, TMP-SMX is effective as prophylaxis and primary therapy for PCP, as prophylaxis for *Toxoplasma gondii* infections, and as treatment for *Isospora belli* gastroenteritis. The combination of sulfadiazine and pyrimethamine is most effective to treat chorioretinitis and encephalitis due to toxoplasmosis in HIV-positive patients. Another sulfonamide, sulfasalazine, may be used in the management of inflammatory bowel disease.

The most common reaction ascribed to sulfonamide hypersensitivity is a generalized rash, usually maculopapular in nature, developing 7 to 12 days after initiation of treatment. Fever may be associated with the rash. Urticaria is occasionally present, but anaphylaxis is a rare event. In addition, severe cutaneous reactions, such as Stevens-Johnson syndrome and toxic-epidermal necrolysis, may occur. Hematologic reactions, notably thrombocytopenia and neutropenia, serum sickness–like reactions, as well as hepatic and renal complications may occur occasionally.

Diagnostic Testing

There are no *in vivo* or *in vitro* tests available to evaluate the presence of sulfonamide allergy. However, there is evidence that some of these reactions are mediated by an IgE antibody directed against its immunogenic metabolite, N^4-sulfonamidoyl (61). Further, studies using multiple N^4-sulfonamidoyl residues attached to polytyrosine carrier as a skin test reagent have been reported (62), but additional studies are necessary to evaluate its clinical usefulness. Also, it appears that most sulfonamide reactions are not IgE mediated. It is likely that most adverse reactions are due to hydroxylamine metabolites, which induce *in vitro* cytotoxic reactions in peripheral blood lymphocytes of patients with sulfonamide hypersensitivity (63–65).

Clinical confirmation of sulfonamide reaction is accomplished by test dosing. This is of concern, particularly when treating HIV-positive patients with TMP-SMX, and also with the use of sulfasalazine in the management of inflammatory bowel disease.

Management of Sulfonamide Reactions in Patients with Acquired Immunodeficiency Syndrome

Patients infected with HIV are at increased risk for hypersensitivity reactions to certain drugs (66,67). The best-known example of a drug that produces hypersensitivity reactions in such patients is TMP-SMX. Cutaneous eruptions from TMP-SMX occur in 3.4% of medical inpatients (68) and in 29% to 65% of patients with AIDS being treated for PCP with this drug (69). A retrospective study comparing PCP in patients with AIDS to PCP in patients with other underlying immunosuppressive disorders reported adverse reactions to TMP-SMX in 65% of AIDS patients compared with 12% of patients with other immunosuppressive diseases, suggesting that the abnormality may result from the HIV infection rather than from PCP (70). Such reactions are less frequent among HIV-infected African American patients (71). The exact pathogenesis of these reactions remains unknown. It is generally accepted that it is the sulfamethoxazole moiety that is responsible for these reactions; trimethoprim may be a cause of acute urticaria or anaphylaxis (72–74).

With a reasonable or definite history of a previous reaction, the preferred approach is to use alternative drugs with similar efficacy. However, TMP-SMX remains the drug of choice for prophylactic treatment of PCP in AIDS patients. Pentamidine is an alternative to TMP-SMX but is also associated with serious adverse reactions (75,76). Cautious readministration of these agents becomes an important consideration. However, this can be risky because reactions may be severe or delayed in appearance, the disease may progress during the attempt, and the reaction may not be completely reversible.

Conversely, these may be insignificant concerns when compared with expected fatal outcome from untreated PCP.

One recommended test dosing schedule (sometimes referred to as desensitization) for TMP-SMX begins with administration of 1% of the full dose on day 1, 10% on day 2, 30% on day 3, and the full dose on day 4 (5). By taking several days to complete, delayed reactions may become evident. When more urgent administration is necessary, TMP-SMX has been given intravenously in doses of 0.8, 7.2, 40, 80, 400, and 680 mg (based on the SMX component) at 20-minute intervals (77). Desensitization may be performed with the pediatric suspension of TMP-SMX (5 mL contains 40 mg TMP and 200 mg of SMX) (3). The first dose is 0.05 mL ($\frac{1}{100}$ of a reduced adult dose). More prolonged courses of oral test dosing, such as 10 and 26 days, have been described (78,79). Delayed reactions may be treated with 30 to 50 mg prednisone daily and antihistamines to permit completion of the course of therapy for PCP. In one study, when the history was rash or rash and fever, a 5-day oral course was successful in 14 of 17 patients (80).

Test dosing with intravenous pentamidine has been successfully performed in the face of a previous reaction to this agent. A stock solution containing 200 mg pentamidine in 250 mL dextrose in water (0.8 mg/mL) is prepared. Starting with a 1:10,000 dilution of this solution, 2 mL is given intravenously over 2 minutes. At 15-minute intervals, 2 mL of 1:1,000, 2 mL of 1:100, and 2 mL of 1:10 dilution are administered. After this, 250 mL full-strength solution is given over 2 hours. Successful treatment with aerosolized pentamidine in patients with adverse reactions to systemic pentamidine has been reported using a rapid test dosing schedule (81).

There are reports of anaphylactic-like reactions in patients with previous TMP-SMX–induced cutaneous reactions (72–74,82). Several investigators have reported an association between the progression of HIV disease and serum IgE levels (83). Oral desensitization with TMP-SMX in one such patient has been described, beginning with 0.00001 mg (SMX component) and progressing to full-dose treatment in 7 hours

(84). This procedure is rarely indicated and is dangerous.

Prophylaxis against PCP has been suggested for AIDS patients with CD4 cell counts below 200 cells/mm^3, for patients with unexplained persistent fever (> 37.8°C or 100°F) for 2 weeks, for oropharyngeal candidiasis regardless of CD4 cell count, and for patients who have recovered from an episode of PCP. TMP-SMX is the drug of choice; if there has been a previous reaction to this agent, oral test dosing followed by daily administration has been effective (85). If this is not tolerated, aerosolized pentamidine administered by nebulizer once a month has been recommended. For patients who are unable to tolerate both drugs, dapsone may be a reasonable alternative. However, TMP-SMX is more effective than aerosolized pentamidine or oral dapsone (86).

Sulfadiazine, together with pyrimethamine, is the treatment of choice of toxoplasmosis in HIV-infected patients. Among patients who react to sulfadiazine, clindamycin and pyrimethamine are less satisfactory alternatives for treatment of *T. gondii* encephalitis or chorioretinitis. Should this fail, rapid test dosing with sulfadiazine can be accomplished by using 1 mg, 10 mg, 100 mg, 500 mg, 1,000 mg, and 1,500 mg at 4-hour intervals (87). Delayed cutaneous reactions can be treated with prednisone in an effort to complete the recommended course of therapy.

Various protocols have been published for test dosing in patients with AIDS (78–80,84,87–93). All share the same principles with the doses recommended, method of delivery, increment in doses, and interval between dosing based on the severity and type of the previous reaction and the urgency for treatment. Such strategies have generally been successful and could be applied to other drugs, for example, antituberculous regimens or zidovudine (94) for treatment of hypersensitivity reactions in AIDS patients.

A history of Stevens-Johnson syndrome is nearly always an absolute contraindication to test dosing or desensitization with TMP-SMX (5). Two patients with previous Stevens-Johnson syndrome were successfully treated with TMP-SMX after an 8-day protocol beginning with 1 mL of 1:1,000,000 dilution of TMP-SMX suspension (95). Only in extreme circumstances should such a procedure be performed.

Management of Sulfasalazine Reactions in Patients with Inflammatory Bowel Disease

The active therapeutic component in sulfasalazine is 5-aminosalicylic acid (5-ASA), which is linked by an azobond to sulfapyridine. After oral ingestion, sulfasalazine is delivered intact to the colon, where bacteria split the azobond to release 5-ASA, which acts topically on inflamed colonic mucosa. (5-ASA may be administered as a suppository for ulcerative proctitis). The sulfapyridine component is absorbed systemically and accounts for most of the adverse effects attributed to sulfasalazine. The drug has been used for mildly or moderately active ulcerative colitis and for maintaining remission of inactive ulcerative colitis. Its role in the management of Crohn's disease is less clear. An estimated 2% of patients develop what is assumed to be a hypersensitivity reaction, usually a maculopapular rash, fever, or both. Oral 5-ASA preparations (e.g., olsalazine, mesalamine, or its prodrug balsalazide) are preferred as first-line agents because of their superior side-effect profile and equivalent therapeutic efficacy compared with sulfasalazine (96).

For the occasional patient with possible drug allergy who requires sulfasalzine, test dosing has been recommended. One approach starts with a dilute suspension of the drug (liquid sulfasalazine suspension diluted with simple syrup) and advancing the dose slowly, as shown in Table 17.17 (97). If a rash or fever develops, the dose may be reduced and then advanced more slowly. This approach is ineffective for nonallergic toxicity (headache, nausea, vomiting, abdominal pain) and should not be considered in patients who have had severe reactions, such as Stevens-Johnson syndrome, TEN, agranulocytosis, or fibrosing alveolitis. Most patients were able to achieve therapeutic doses, although some patients did require several trials.

With the newer aminosalicylate preparations, newer corticosteroid enemas (budesonide), and the use of other immunosuppressive drugs, the medical management of inflammatory bowel

TABLE 17.17. *Test dosing with sulfasalazine*[a]

Day	Dose (mg)
1	1
2	2
3	4
4	8
5–11	10
12	20
13	40
14	80
15–21	100
22	200
23	400
24	800
25–31	1000
32 on	2000

[a]Patients should have failed newer antiinflammatory agents.
Adapted from Purdy BH, Philips DM, Summers RW. Desensitization for sulfasalazine rash. *Ann Intern Med* 1984;100:512, with permission.

disease will continue to improve, and, consequently, the need for sulfasalazine should decrease.

Other Antimicrobial Agents

Aminoglycosides

Despite the introduction of newer, less toxic antimicrobial agents, the aminoglycosides continue to be useful in the treatment of serious enterococcal and aerobic gram-negative bacillary infections. These agents have considerable intrinsic toxicity, namely nephrotoxicity and ototoxicity.

Hypersensitivity-type reactions to aminoglycosides are infrequent and minor, usually taking the form of benign skin rashes or drug-induced fever. Anaphylactic reactions are rare but have been reported after tobramycin and streptomycin administration. Intravenous tobramycin has caused acute respiratory failure requiring intubation. Successful desensitization to tobramycin (98) and streptomycin (99) has been accomplished.

Vancomycin

Vancomycin is an alternative treatment for serious infections in patients with hypersensitivity reactions or in whom there is bacterial resistance to β-lactam antibiotics.

Except for the "red-man" or "red-neck" syndrome, adverse reactions to vancomycin are relatively rare. Red-man syndrome is characterized by pruritus and erythema or flushing involving the face, neck and upper torso, occasionally accompanied by hypotension. This has been attributed to the nonimmunologic release of histamine (100). This complication may be minimized by administering vancomycin over at least a 1- to 2-hour period. Otherwise 1,000 mg of vancomycin administered over 30 minutes or less will cause mast cell histamine release (100). A rare patient may require a slower infusion (over 5 hours) of 500 mg or 1 g (101). Pretreatment with antihistamines (e.g., hydroxyzine) may be protective. Vasopressors may be required if severe hypotension occurs.

Vancomycin has been reported to cause Stevens-Johnson syndrome (102) and exfoliative dermatitis (103). Test dosing or desensitization should be avoided in such patients except in the most demanding circumstances.

Fluoroquinolones

Fluoroquinolones are antimicrobial agents with a broad range of activity against both gram-negative and gram-positive organisms. Skin rashes and pruritus have been reported in less than 1% of patients receiving these drugs. Phototoxicity may occur. Rarely, Achilles tendon inflammation or rupture occurs. Anaphylactoid reactions, following the initial dose of ciprofloxacin, have been described (104), as has severe respiratory distress necessitating intubation (105).

Tetracyclines

Tetracyclines are bacteriostatic agents with broad-spectrum antimicrobial activity. Hypersensitivity-type reactions, including morbilliform rashes, urticaria, and anaphylaxis, occur very rarely with tetracycline drugs. Doxycycline and demeclocycline may produce a mild to severe phototoxic dermatitis; minocycline does not. Photosensitivity may occur with all tetracycline drugs.

Chloramphenicol

With the availability of numerous alternative agents and the concern about toxicity, this drug is used infrequently. In patients with bacterial meningitis and a history of severe β-lactam hypersensitivity, chloramphenicol is a reasonable first choice, or ceftriaxone after testing. For treatment of rickettsial infections in young children or pregnant women, when tetracycline is contraindicated, this agent is useful.

Bone marrow aplasia is the most serious toxic effect. Believed to be idiosyncratic, occurring in 1 in 40,000 cases of therapy, it tends to occur in patients who undergo prolonged treatment, particularly if the drug has been administered on multiple occasions. This might suggest an immunologic mechanism, but this has not been established. Skin rash, fever, and eosinophilia are observed rarely. Anaphylaxis has been reported (106).

Macrolides

Erythromycin is one of the safest antibiotics even though it causes nausea or vomiting. Hypersensitivity-type reactions are uncommon, and they consist of usually benign skin rashes, fever, eosinophilia or acute urticaria and angioedema (107). Anaphylaxis to oral erythromycin, 500 mg, has been reported (108). Cholestatic hepatitis occurs infrequently, most often in association with erythromycin estolate. Recovery is expected upon withdrawal of the drug, although it may require a month or so to resolve.

The newer macrolides, azithromycin and clarithromycin, are even better tolerated and less toxic. Cholestatic hepatitis has been reported with clarithromycin (109).

Clindamycin

This drug is active against most anaerobes, most gram-positive cocci, and certain protozoa. The main concern with clindamycin use is *Clostridium difficile* pseudomembranous colitis.

Adverse drug reactions to clindamycin occurred in less than 1% of hospitalized patients (110). Urticaria, drug fever, eosinophilia, and erythema multiforme have been reported occasionally.

Metronidazole

Metronidazole is useful against most anaerobes, certain protozoa, and *Helicobacter pylori*. The most common adverse reactions are gastrointestinal. Hypersensitivity reactions, including urticaria, pruritus, and erythematous rash have been reported. There is a case report of successful oral desensitization in a patient after what appeared to be an anaphylactic event (111).

Antifungal Agents

Allergic reactions to amphotericin B are quite rare. A report described a patient with amphotericin B–induced anaphylaxis (112). The patient was successfully challenged intravenously with amphotericin, using a desensitization-type protocol. Acute stridor during testing with amphotericin B may occur and require racemic epinephrine. Liposomal amphotericin is not necessarily safer than amphotericin B in terms of nephrotoxic effects. Anaphylactic reactions have been reported in patients receiving liposomal preparations (113), including one fatality (114).

Hypersensitivity-type reactions, notably rash and pruritus, occur in 4% to 10% of patients receiving ketoconazole. Itraconazole has been associated with a generalized maculopapular rash. There is a report of successful oral desensitization to itraconazole in a patient with localized coccidioidomycosis (115).

Antiviral Agents

Hypersensitivity reactions to antimicrobial and antiretroviral agents are common among HIV-infected patients. There is a report of a patient who was successfully desensitized to zidovudine using a protocol requiring 37 days (116) and a shorter, 10-day protocol (94). Because there is a limited number of drugs available to treat individuals with HIV, such protocols may become increasingly necessary to provide treatment when alternatives are unavailable.

Acute tongue and pharyngeal swelling with urticaria, stridor, and hypotension has been reported with another antiviral agent, lamivudine (117).

Antituberculous Agents

Many manifestations of hypersensitivity resulting from antituberculous drugs usually appear within 3 to 7 weeks after initiation of treatment. The most common signs are fever and rash, and the fever may be present alone for a week or more before other manifestations develop. The skin rash is usually morbilliform but may be urticarial, purpuric, or rarely exfoliative. Less common manifestations include a lupus-like syndrome (especially with isoniazid). Anaphylaxis rarely has been associated with streptomycin and ethambutol.

A common approach is to discontinue all drugs (usually isoniazid, rifampin, pyrazinamide) and allow the reaction (usually a rash) to subside. Subsequently, each drug is reintroduced by test dosing to identify the responsible agent. Another drug then may be substituted for the causative agent. Another approach has been to suppress the reaction with an initial dose of 40 to 80 mg prednisone daily while antituberculous therapy is maintained. This has resulted in prompt clearing of the hypersensitivity reaction, and with adequate chemotherapy, steroids do not appear to affect the course of tuberculosis unfavorably. After taking prednisone for several months, the corticosteroid preparation may be discontinued, and the reaction may not reappear.

Adverse drug reactions occurred in 23 of 132 (18%) patients with AIDS (118). Cutaneous eruptions were reported in 13 patients with a life-threatening anaphylactic reaction in another patient (119).

Multiple Antibiotic Sensitivity Syndrome

Patients who have reacted to any antimicrobial drug in the past have as high as a 10-fold increased risk for an allergic reaction to another antimicrobial agent (120). The physician should be aware of this possibility and be prepared for such and institute prompt treatment.

Aspirin and other Nonsteroidal Antiinflammatory Drugs

Background

Aspirin (ASA) and nonselective NSAIDs rank second or third to the β-lactam antibiotics in producing "allergic-type" drug reactions. Unpredictable reactions to these agents include (a) acute bronchoconstriction in some patients with nasal polyps and persistent asthma; (b) an exacerbation of urticaria in 21% to 30% of patients with idiopathic urticaria or angioedema; and (c) anaphylactic reactions with a threat to life. The occurrence of both asthma and urticaria triggered by ASA administration in the same individual is a rare event (121). In addition, among otherwise normal individuals, anaphylactoid and urticarial reactions have occurred within minutes after the ingestion of ASA or a nonselective NSAID. Although ASA has been recommended to treat systemic mast cell disease, there is a subset of patients with this disorder who experience anaphylactoid reactions after the ingestion of ASA and NSAIDs (122).

The prevalence of *ASA-induced respiratory reactions* based on the patient's history alone is thought to be less than 10% among asthmatic patients older than 10 years of age (123); based upon oral challenge, it is 10% to 20% (124). In the subpopulation of asthmatic patients with associated rhinosinusitis or nasal polyps, even without a history of ASA-induced respiratory reactions, the prevalence by oral challenge increases to 30% to 40% (125). Among adult asthmatics with a prior history of ASA sensitivity, the prevalence of ASA-induced respiratory reactions following oral ASA challenges has been confirmed in 66% to 97% of cases (126,127). Among asthmatic children less than 10 years of age, the prevalence of ASA sensitivity appears to be less but increases in frequency to that reported in adults during the teenage years. If adequate doses of certain other nonselective NSAIDs are used, they induce reactions in a significant number of patients reacting to ASA.

The typical patient is an adult with chronic nonallergic rhinosinusitis, often with nasal polyps, and persistent asthma. Most commonly, such patients have had established respiratory manifestations for months or years before the first clear episode of an ASA-induced respiratory reaction. Such reactions usually occur within 2 hours after the ingestion of ASA or NSAIDs, and may be quite severe and, rarely, are fatal. The reaction may be associated with profound nasal congestion, rhinorrhea, and ocular injection (125).

Currently, one of the more attractive hypotheses to explain these ASA- and NSAID-induced respiratory reactions stems from the observation that these drugs share the property of inhibiting the generation of cyclooxygenase-1 products, thereby permitting the synthesis of lipoxygenase products, most notably leukotriene-D_4, which is capable of inducing acute bronchoconstriction and increasing vascular permeability. To support this assertion, the 5-lipoxygenase inhibitor, zileuton, has been shown to block the decline in forced expiratory volume at 1 second (FEV_1) after ASA ingestion among ASA-sensitive asthmatic patients (128). Also, after aspirin challenge, there is a 10-fold increase in urine LTE-4 concentration, reflecting heightened synthesis of LTD-4 (129). Furthermore, patients with ASA-sensitive asthma are hyperresponsive to LTE-4 given during bronchoprovocation; indeed, they are hypersensitive by a factor of 13 compared with ASA-tolerant patients with asthma (127).

The selective cyclooxygenase-2 antagonists, celecoxib and refecoxib, have been tolerated uneventfully in 42 aspirin-intolerant patients with asthma to date (130,131).

A subpopulation of patients with *chronic urticaria or angioedema* experience an exacerbation of urticaria after ingesting ASA or NSAIDs (132). Using appropriate challenge techniques, the prevalence is between 21% and 30%. A reaction is much more likely to occur when the urticaria is active at the time of challenge (133). Avoidance of these agents eliminates acute exacerbations of urticaria following their ingestion but appears to have little effect on the ongoing chronic urticaria.

The prevalence of *anaphylactoid reactions* after the ingestion of both ASA or specific NSAIDs is unknown. Characteristically, such patients appear to be normal and react to only one NSAID or to ASA. Cross-reactivity within the entire class of cyclooxygenase inhibitors is rare. Further, some such reactions occur after two or more exposures to the same NSAID. These features suggest the possibility of an IgE-mediated response, but specific IgE against ASA or any NSAID has not been demonstrated. On occasion, urticaria or angioedema alone may occur after the ingestion of ASA or a nonselective NSAID in patients without ongoing chronic urticaria.

Diagnostic Tests

The diagnosis can usually be established by history and does not require confirmatory testing. On occasion, there may be circumstances in which the diagnosis is unclear or a specific diagnosis is required. Skin tests are of no value in the diagnosis of ASA or NSAID sensitivity. Also, there are currently no reliable *in vitro* tests available for the detection of ASA sensitivity. The only definitive diagnostic test is oral test dosing (5,127).

Among asthmatic patients, test dosing with ASA or nonselective NSAIDs can provoke a severe acute respiratory reaction and should be attempted only by experienced physicians capable of managing acute, severe asthma in an appropriate medical setting. The asthma should be under optimal control before test dosing is begun. The high risk for this procedure must be considered in relation to its potential benefit. A detailed description of a 3-day test dosing protocol may be found elsewhere (127,132). A typical starting dose of ASA is 3 mg, and progresses to 30 mg, 60 mg, 100 mg, 150 mg, 325 mg, and 650 mg at 3-hour intervals if there is no reaction. If a reaction occurs, subsequent ASA challenges are suspended, and the reaction is treated vigorously. After an ASA-induced respiratory reaction, there is a 2- to 5-day refractory period during which the patient may tolerate ASA and all other NSAIDs (134). Although not currently available in the United States, ASA-lysine has been used for inhalation challenge to verify ASA-sensitive asthmatic patients in Europe (135). Considering the potential difficulties with test dosing and the fact that ASA and other NSAIDs can usually be avoided, such diagnostic challenges should be reserved for research purposes or for patients with suspected sensitivity to ASA or NSAIDs who now require those agents for management of chronic conditions.

For patients with chronic urticaria, test dosing may be performed in an outpatient setting. For those with ongoing urticaria, treatment of the condition should be continued to avoid false-positive results (133). If the urticaria is intermittent, test dosing can be accomplished during a remission. A typical ASA test dosing protocol is to give 100 mg and 200 mg twice in the morning at 2-hour intervals on day 1, and 325 mg and 650 mg on day 2 (127). Most patients react at doses of 325 mg or 650 mg, and the elapsed time before the reaction appears is 3 to 6 hours after ingestion of the drug. This protocol may be modified by including placebo capsules between ASA dosing.

Test dosing for anaphylactoid reactions is seldom indicated and can be dangerous. However, as previously noted, anaphylactoid reactions are limited usually to either ASA or a single nonselective NSAID. Therefore, test dosing with another NSAID may demonstrate its safety for use in treating a medical condition. Unfortunately, if ASA sensitivity is the culprit, other NSAIDs are unacceptable alternatives as platelet inhibitors. For this reason, an oral ASA test protocol in a monitored setting to reach a final dose of 80 mg has been reported (136).

Management of Aspirin- and other Nonsteroidal Antiinflammatory Drug–Sensitive Patients

Once ASA and other NSAID sensitivity develops, it may last for years. Therefore, strict avoidance of these drugs is critical. Patients should be attentive to the variety of commonly available nonprescription preparations that contain ASA or NSAIDs, such as "cold," headache, and analgesic remedies. All nonselective NSAIDs that inhibit the cyclooxygenase pathway cross-react to varying degrees with ASA in causing respiratory reactions among ASA-sensitive asthmatic patients and in triggering urticarial reactions among patients with chronic urticaria who react to ASA. A current list of NSAIDs that cross-react with ASA is provided in Table 17.18.

TABLE 17.18. *Strong inhibitors, weak inhibitors, and noninhibitors of cyclooxygenase-1*

Strong inhibitors of cyclooxygenase-1
Diclofenac (Voltaren, Arthrotec, Cataflam)
Diflunisal (Dolobid)
Etodolac (Lodine)
Fenoprofen (Nalfon)
Flubiprofen (Ansaid)
Ibuprofen (Motrin, Advil, Nuprin, Haltran, Medipren)
Indomethacin (Indocin)
Ketoprofen (Orudis, Oruvail)
Ketorolac (Toradol)
Meclofenamate (Meclomen)
Mefanamic acid (Ponstel)
Meloxicam (Mobic)
Nabumetone (Relafen)
Naproxen (Naprosyn, Anaprox, Aleve, Naprelan)
Oxaprozin (Daypro)
Piroxicam (Feldene)
Sulindac (Clinoril)
Tolmetin (Tolectin)

**Weak inhibitors of cyclooxygenase-1
(suitable, initial alternatives)**
Acetaminophen (Tylenol, Datril, Excedrin, Midol, Percogesic)
Salsalate (Disalcid)

Noninhibitors of cyclooxygenase-1
Choline magnesium trisalicylate (Trilisate)
Celebrex (Celebrex)
Hydroxychloroquine (Plaquenil)
Refecoxib (Vioxx)

Among ASA-sensitive patients, acetaminophen is most commonly recommended as an alternative and is almost always tolerated uneventfully. However, in one study, high doses of acetaminophen, such as 1,000 mg, were reported to provoke acute bronchoconstriction (decreases in FEV_1) in about one third of ASA-sensitive asthmatic patients (137). In general, acetaminophen-induced respiratory reactions are much milder and of shorter duration than those induced by ASA. When asthma is stable, if necessary, test dosing with acetaminophen may be attempted starting with 325 mg. If there is no reaction after 2 to 3 hours, 650 mg is given. After 3 more hours, if there has been no adverse reaction, 1,000 mg of acetaminophen may be given (138). Salsalate is also a weak cyclooxygenase inhibitor, which has caused a decrease in FEV_1 in up to 20% of ASA-sensitive asthmatic patients when 2,000 mg is given (139). Salsalate and choline magnesium trisalicylate have no effect on cyclooxygenase *in vitro* and do not cause acute bronchoconstriction in ASA-sensitive asthmatic patients in recommended doses. Although there was a report of a bronchoconstrictive reaction to hydrocortisone sodium succinate (Solu-Cortef) in 1 of 45 ASA-sensitive asthmatic patients (140), this occurrence seems exceedingly rare. Also, tartrazine (FD& C yellow dye) does not cross-react with ASA in ASA-sensitive patients or induce acute respiratory reactions, as was thought at one time (127,141).

A practical problem is what advice to give to historically non–ASA-sensitive asthmatic patients regarding the use of ASA and other NSAIDs. One approach is to caution such patients about the potential for such a reaction, particularly if they have nasal polyps and are steroid dependent (142). There is a low incidence of ASA sensitivity in patients with asthma with normal computed tomography scans of the sinuses and in patients with clear evidence of IgE-mediated asthma (143). Treatment with ASA or other NSAIDs may be medically necessary in some patients with ASA-sensitive asthma, such as the management of a rheumatoid or osteoarthritis or to inhibit platelet aggregation for coronary artery or carotid disease. The term desensitization has been applied to this procedure, although many would prefer that this term be reserved for IgE-mediated reactions. The process is identical to oral test dosing with ASA for diagnostic purposes, except that the challenge continues following a positive respiratory reaction (127,134). The dose of ASA that caused the reaction is reintroduced after the patient has recovered. If no further reaction occurs, at 3-hour intervals, the dose is gradually increased until either another reaction occurs or the patient can tolerate 650 mg of ASA without a reaction. Once successfully "desensitized," cross-desensitization between ASA and all other nonselective NSAIDs is complete. This state can be maintained indefinitely if the patient takes at least one ASA daily; if ASA is stopped, it persists for only 2 to 5 days.

ASA desensitization followed by long-term ASA treatment has been advocated for treatment of ASA-sensitive asthma (127,144). Such treatment has resulted in improvement in rhinosinusitis with prevention of nasal polyp reformation and improved sense of smell, as well as allowing a significant reduction in the need for systemic and inhaled corticosteroids. Nevertheless, as with other antiasthma treatments, ASA desensitization does not induce a remission of asthma.

Unlike ASA-sensitive asthma, ASA-sensitive urticaria and angioedema do not appear to respond to ASA desensitization (145). Aspirin desensitization has been employed to prevent synthesis of mast cell–derived prostaglandin D_2, a cyclooxygenase product thought to be largely responsible for systemic reactions, among patients with systemic mastocytosis disease who also have experienced anaphylactoid reactions after the ingestion of ASA or NSAIDs (122).

Acetaminophen

In contrast to the rare ASA-sensitive patient with asthma who develops a 25–33% decrease in FEV_1 with 1,000 mg challenge with acetaminophen (146), true anaphylactoid reactions to acetaminophen have been reported (147–149). The provoking doses necessary to induce shock were 125 mg, 191 mg, and 300 mg (147–149). Elevated plasma or urine histamine concentrations were demonstrated (147,149). These patients were not ASA-sensitive and had anaphylactoid reactions, as compared with the rare ASA-sensitive patient with asthma who has a moderate bronchoconstrictive response to 1,000 mg of acetaminophen.

Concurrent acetaminophen and aspirin sensitivity was reported in a 13-year-old girl with asthma (150). She experienced acute urticaria, angioedema, and dyspnea within 10 minutes of ingesting 650 mg of acetaminophen. Aspirin, 325 mg, and indomethacin, 300 mg, caused acute urticaria (150). Such sensitivity must be exceedingly rare.

For practical purposes, ASA-sensitive patients can use acetaminophen without initial test dosing.

Radiographic Contrast Media

Background

RCM are clear solutions and should not be called "dyes." Nonfatal immediate generalized reactions (most commonly urticaria) occur in 2% to 3% of patients receiving conventional ionic high-osmolality RCM and in less than 0.5% of patients receiving the lower-osmolality agents. A large prospective study reported severe life-threatening (often anaphylactoid) reactions occurring in 0.22% of those receiving the high-osmolality media compared with only 0.04% of those receiving lower-osmolality preparations (151). It is clear that the lower-osmolality RCM causes significantly fewer adverse reactions (152,153), but severe reactions may occur (154,155). In fact, the risk for a fatal reaction may be the same with either class of RCM and is estimated to be 0.9 cases per 100,000 infusions (156). Deaths have occurred with all types of RCM (155). The volume infused in fatal reactions may be less than 10 mL in some cases (157).

The overall prevalence of reactions to the non-iodinated, gadolinium-based contrast agents for magnetic resonance imaging (MRI) is about 1% to 2%. Severe systemic anaphylactoid reactions to these agents can occur rarely, in the order of 1:350,000 injections (158).

Clearly, there are patients at increased risk for an immediate generalized reaction to RCM. The most obvious and important risk factor is a history of a previous reaction to these agents. The exact reaction rate is unknown, but with ionic hyperosmolality RCM, it ranges between 17% and 60% (159). The administration of nonionic lower-osmolality agents to such patients reduces the risk to 4% to 5.5% (160,161). Severe coronary artery disease, unstable angina, advanced age, female sex, and receipt of large volumes of contrast media are also risk factors (154,155). Atopic individuals and asthmatic patients appear to be more susceptible to anaphylactoid reactions to RCM (151,155,162). There is some disagreement about the risk for an immediate generalized reaction to RCM among patients receiving β-adrenergic blocking agents (163,164). The risk was not found to be increased in a prospective study (163); however, reactions may be more severe and less responsive to treatment in patients with cardiac impairment. Among such patients, the use of lower-osmolality RCM and possibly pretreatment with antihistamines and corticosteroids (discussed later) may be advisable. The data that patients who have reacted to topical iodine cleansing solutions and iodides and those allergic to shellfish are at slightly increased risk for RCM reactions was based on use of older RCM (165) and does not justify use of lower-osmolality RCM in the absence of a previous anaphylactoid reaction to RCM or very high anxiety about the procedure.

Typically, most reactions begin within 1 to 3 minutes after intravascular RCM administration, rarely after 20 minutes. Nausea, emesis, and flushing are most common and may be due to vagal stimulation. Such reactions are to be distinguished from immediate generalized reactions, which include pruritus, urticaria, angioedema, bronchospasm, hypotension, and syncope. Urticaria is the most common reaction. Most of these reactions are self-limited and respond promptly to the administration of epinephrine and antihistamines. However, the potential for a fatal outcome must not be ignored, and trained personnel must be available to recognize and treat hypotension and cardiac or respiratory arrest. Sudden-onset grand mal seizure likely reflects cerebral hypoperfusion and not epilepsy.

The mechanism of RCM-induced immediate generalized reactions is not fully understood. These reactions are not IgE mediated but involve mast cell activation with release of histamine and other mediators (155,166).

Diagnostic Testing

There are no *in vivo* or *in vitro* tests to identify potential reactors to RCM. Severe and fatal reactions have occurred after an intravenous test dose of 1 to 2 mL. Also, severe reactions have followed a negative test dose. Graded test dosing has been abandoned.

As noted previously, a history of a previous reaction to RCM is the most essential information necessary to assess the risk for a repeat reaction (155,166).

Management of Patients at Increased Risk for a Repeat Radiographic Contrast Media Reaction

Among patients with a previous reaction to RCM, the incidence and severity of subsequent reactions has been reduced using pretreatment regimens of corticosteroids, antihistamines, and adrenergic agents. Using older higher-osmolality RCM, pretreatment with prednisone and diphenhydramine reduced the prevalence of repeat reactions to about 10%, whereas the addition of ephedrine to this protocol reduced it further to 5% (167). The addition of lower-osmolality RCM to the prednisone-diphenhydramine regimen decreased the incidence of repeat reactions even further to 0.5% (159,168). Most repeated reactions tended to be quite mild. Unfortunately, the higher cost of these lower-osmolality RCM remains an issue for some hospitals and physicians.

The following summarizes a useful approach that can be recommended when patients with a history of a RCM-associated immediate generalized reaction require a repeated study (5,9):

1. Document in the medical record the need for the procedure and that alternative procedures are unsatisfactory.
2. Document in the record that the patient or responsible person understands the need for the test and that the pretreatment regimen may not prevent all adverse reactions.
3. Recommend the use of lower-osmolality RCM if available.
4. Pretreatment medications are as follows:
   A. Prednisone, 50 mg orally, 13 hours, 7 hours, and 1 hour before the RCM procedure
   B. Diphenhydramine, 50 mg intramuscularly or orally, 1 hour before the RCM procedure
   C. Albuterol, 4 mg orally, 1 hour before the RCM procedure (withhold if the patient has unstable angina, cardiac arrhythmia, or other cardiac risks)
5. Proceed with the RCM study and have emergency therapy available.

There may be situations in which high-risk patients require an emergency RCM study. The following emergency protocol is recommended (5):

1. Administer hydrocortisone, 200 mg intravenously, immediately and every 4 hours until the study is completed.
2. Administer diphenhydramine, 50 mg intramuscularly, immediately before or 1 hour before the procedure.
3. Administer albuterol, 4 mg orally, immediately before or 1 hour before the procedure (optional).
4. Recommend the use of lower-osmolality RCM if available.

Because several hours are required for corticosteroids to be effective, it is best to avoid the emergency administration of RCM unless absolutely necessary. The medical record should note that there has not been time for conventional pretreatment and that there is limited experience with such abbreviated programs.

It is also important to be aware that anaphylactoid reactions to RCM may occur when these agents are administered by nonvascular routes, for example, retrograde pyelograms, hysterosalpingograms, myelograms, and arthrograms. Previous reactors undergoing those procedures should receive pretreatment as described previously.

Finally, it should be noted that the pretreatment protocols are useful only for the prevention of anaphylactoid reactions, but not for other types of life-threatening reactions, such as the adult respiratory tract distress syndrome or noncardiogenic pulmonary edema (169).

Patients with asthma should have their respiratory status stable under ideal circumstances. Similarly, hydration and perhaps acetylcysteine should be employed to prevent acute renal failure (170).

Local Anesthetics

Background

Patients who experience adverse reactions of virtually any type following the injection of a local anesthetic may be advised erroneously that they are allergic to these agents and should never receive "caines" in the future. Such patients may be denied the benefit of dental care or a surgical procedure.

Most commonly, these adverse effects are vasovagal reactions, toxic reactions, hysterical reactions, or epinephrine side effects. Allergic

TABLE 17.19. *Classification of local anesthetics*

Benzoic acid esters (group I)
  Benzocaine[a]
  Butamben picrate (Butesin)[a]
  Chloroprocaine (Nesacaine)
  Cocaine[a]
  Procaine (Novocain)
  Proparacaine[a]
  Tetracaine (Pontocaine)
Amide or miscellaneous structures (group II)
  Bupivacaine (Marcaine, Sensorcaine)[b]
  Dibucane (Nupercaine)[b]
  Dyclonine (Dyclone)[a]
  Etiodocaine (Duranest)[b]
  Levobupivacaine (Chirocaine)[b]
  Lidocaine (Xylocaine)[b]
  Mepivacaine (Carbocaine, Polocaine)[b]
  Pramoxine (Tronothane)[a]
  Prilocaine (Citanest)[b]
  Roprivacaine (Naropin)[b]

[a] Primarily topical agents.
[b] Contain amide structure.

contact dermatitis is the most common immunologic reaction to local anesthetics. On occasion, clinical manifestations suggestive of immediate-type reactions are described, but most reported series have shown that such reactions occur rarely, if ever (171–174).

As shown in Table 17.19, local anesthetics may be classified as benzoic acid esters (group I) or others (group II). On the basis of local anesthetic contact dermatitis and patch testing studies, the benzoic acid esters often cross-react with each other but do not cross-react with those agents in group II. Also, drugs in group II do not cross-react with each other and appear to be less sensitizing.

It has been suggested that sulfites and parabens, which are used as preservatives in local anesthetics, may be responsible for allergic-like reactions. However, such reactions are so rare as to be reportable (175). When confronted with this remote possibility, the pragmatic approach is to avoid preparations containing them. On the other hand, latex-containing products, such as gloves and rubber dams, are often used in dental and surgical practices. Local or systemic reactions may occur in latex-sensitive patients, and this possibility should be considered in the differential diagnosis of adverse reactions attributed to local anesthetic agents.

Diagnostic Testing

Initial skin testing as a part of a test dosing protocol is the preferred approach. Prick tests are usually negative. Positive intradermal skin tests are often found in otherwise healthy controls and do not correlate with the outcome of test dosing (171,173). *In vitro* testing is not applicable.

Management of Patients with a History of Reactions to Local Anesthetics

If the local anesthetic agent causing the previous reaction is known, a different local anesthetic agent should be selected for administration for reassurance. For example, if the drug is an ester, an amide may be chosen. If the drug is an amide, another amide may be used.

The use of diphenhydramine may provide reasonable anesthesia required for suturing, but clearly this is inadequate for dental anesthesia.

Unfortunately, the local anesthetic agent is often unknown, and the clinical details of the previous reaction are often vague, unavailable, or of uncertain significance. For this reason, the following protocol has been effective in identifying a local anesthetic agent that the patient will tolerate (5):

1. Obtain consent.
2. Determine the local anesthetic agent to be used by the dentist or physician. It must not contain epinephrine. These are usually available as ampules.
3. At 15-minute intervals:
   A. Perform a skin-prick test using the undiluted local anesthetic.
   B. If negative, inject 0.1 mL of a 1:100 dilution subcutaneously in an extremity.
   C. If there is no local reaction, inject 0.1 mL of a 1:10 dilution of local anesthetic subcutaneously.
   D. If there is no local reaction, inject 0.1 mL of undiluted local anesthetic agent.
   E. If there is no local reaction, inject 1 mL and then 2 mL of the undiluted local anesthetic agent.
4. Following this procedure, a letter is given to the patient indicating that the patient has received 3 mL of the respective local anesthetic

with no reaction and is at no greater risk for a subsequent allergic reaction than the general population.

5. Such test dosing should be undertaken by individuals with training and experience in such tests, and also in treatment of anaphylactic reactions.

This regimen should be completed before the anticipated procedure, and in some cases, it can be done to help exclude local anesthetic "allergy." To date, we are not aware of any patient with negative test dosing who reacted later when the local anesthetic agent was used for a procedure, with the exception of hysterical reactions. The success of this approach is undoubtedly related to the extreme rarity of true allergic reactions to local anesthetic agents. However, at the least, the protocol serves to allay some or all of the anxiety of patients and referring dentists and physicians, and at the most, it may permit one to identify safely that rare patient truly at risk for an allergic reaction to subsequent local anesthetic administration.

Angiotensin-converting Enzyme Inhibitors and Angiotensin II Receptor Antagonists

ACE inhibitors have efficacy in treatment of patients with left ventricular systolic dysfunction or congestive heart failure, as secondary prevention in patients who have experienced a myocardial infarction, in diabetic patients, and as antihypertensive agents. ACE inhibitors have been reported to cause a nonproductive cough in 1% to 39% of patients; this cough subsides in a few days or in less than 4 weeks in exceptional cases (176). Angioedema has been recognized in other patients, perhaps with an incidence of 0.1% to 0.2% (177,178). The angioedema may cause marked tongue or pharyngeal swelling such that intubation is required. It has a predilection for the tongue, pharynx, and face as opposed to gastrointestinal tract or as isolated dysphagia (177). It has been reported that first episodes occurred in the first 4 weeks of ACE inhibitor use in 22% of patients, and 77% occurred after that time, with an overall mean duration until presentation of 11 months (178,179). In another study, the mean

time was 19 months, with a range of 3 days to 6.3 years (180). African Americans appear to be at increased risk for experiencing angioedema from ACE inhibitors (179,180). Because 7 of 9 patients in one series were using aspirin, it has been hypothesized that aspirin could be a cofactor in ACE inhibitor angioedema (180). Complement is not consumed during these reactions.

ACE inhibitors have been reported to induce anaphylactoid reactions during hemodialysis, especially when the dialysis membrane is polyacrilonitrile but not cuprophane or polysulfone (181–183).

The mechanism of acute angioedema is thought to be attributable to production of excessive bradykinin in that ACE inhibitors, which block generation of angiotensin II from angiotensin I, also inhibit inactivation of bradykinin. Accumulation of bradykinin is thought to cause cough and angioedema and contribute to anaphylactoid reactions by causing vasodilation. It remains to be determined whether this hypothesis is the correct explanation because reports of acute angioedema from angiotensin II receptor antagonists have appeared (184,185). These drugs do not inhibit ACE so that buildup of bradykinin because of inhibition of the bradykinase enzyme does not occur. Reactions to losartan have occurred within 1 day to 16 months after beginning therapy (185). Some patients have never received an ACE inhibitor. Angiotensin II receptor antagonists are not contraindicated in patients who have experienced angioedema from an ACE inhibitor, but physician awareness of potential future episodes is warranted.

In patients with idiopathic anaphylaxis, ACE inhibitors (and β-adrenergic antagonists) are contraindicated at least on a relative basis until our understanding of these reactions improves.

Opiates

Opiates have their historical basis traced back 1800 years ago related to opium (186). Opioid receptors have been identified as μ, δ, κ, and nociceptin/orphanin FQ (186). The classic opioid actions are mediated by μ-receptor stimulation which results in analgesia, decreased gastrointestinal transit time, contraction of the sphincter of Oddi, respiratory depression, decreased cough, and pupillary constriction. Analgesia is caused by activation of μ, δ, and κ receptors. However, μ receptors are present in ascending nerves in the spinal tract and in the brain, whereas κ receptors are present only in spinal nerves. Morphine activates μ and κ receptors while fentanyl acts on μ, δ, and κ receptors.

Morphine and codeine are most likely to activate mast cells and cause flushing or acute urticaria. Meperidine, tramadol, and fentanyl are ineffective triggers of mast cells. Meperidine is out of favor because of sharp rises and falls in serum concentrations, but although it can cause diaphoresis, it is an unlikely cause of urticaria.

Patients may have confused opioid effects for hypersensitivity, but when there is a history of codeine- or morphine-induced urticaria, alternative agents may be selected if narcotics are required. For example, fentanyl can be administered intravenously or transdermally. Lower doses of long-acting formulations of morphine may be tried as well.

Chemotherapy For Neoplastic Diseases

Many chemotherapeutic agents result in bone marrow suppression or other particular adverse effects including serious cutaneous eruptions. Interstitial lung disease or infiltrates can occur with use of bleomycin, methotrexate, cyclophosphamide, busulfan, carmustine (BCNU), and all trans-retinoic acid as examples (187,188). The latter has been associated with basophil-derived histamine release causing acute bronchoconstriction when administered to patients with acute promyelocytic leukemia. The promyelocytes resemble basophils! Capillary leak syndromes occur with IL-2, cytosine arabinoside, the combination of mitomycin and vinca alkaloids and other agents.

Anaphylaxis has occurred with various chemotherapeutic agents but fortunately is rare. Cisplatin and carboplatin can cross-react and are potent sensitizers (189,190). Because some of these reactions are IgE mediated, prednisone-diphenhydramine pretreatment is not expected to be successful. If either of these agents is truly essential and the patient agrees, skin testing can be carried out with prick tests of 0.1 mg/ml concentration with intradermals of 0.001 mg/ml, 0.01 mg/ml, and 0.1 mg/ml (190). Desensitization should begin with 0.01 mg or less depending on the skin test results. In some cases, desensitization will be successfully carried out, but not in all cases. Indeed, as little as 3.5 mg of cisplatin has caused anaphylaxis (190). The physician must be in attendance with epinephrine available.

Anticonvulsants

Phenytoin hypersensitivity syndrome is rare but typically begins within 2 months of initiation of phenytoin. In a few cases, the onset is in the third month of therapy. Reactions consist of fever; marked erythematous papules that may blister, demonstrate necrosis from vasculitis, and desquamate; and other findings such as tender lymphadenopathy, liver enlargement, and oral ulcerations (191,192). This author believes that such patients have sufficient criteria for the diagnosis of Stevens-Johnson syndrome. In fact, in a series of patients with Stevens-Johnson syndrome, phenytoin, carbamazepine, valproic acid, and phenobarbital all were identified (193). Associated laboratory findings may include atypical lymphocytes, eosinophilia, elevation of serum creatinine, and liver function test abnormalities. Leukopenia may occur in some patients. Pulmonary eosinophilia with respiratory failure has been reported (194). The name of *anticonvulsant hypersensitivity syndrome* has been suggested because of the combination of fever, severe pruritic rash, and lymphadenopathy associated with multisystem involvement (191). Some cases are familial (195). Carbamazepine can cause a similar reaction and is contraindicated on a relative basis. Because of shared structures and metabolism, it is thought that when a patient develops the anticonvulsant hypersensitivity syndrome to either phenytoin or carbamazepine, that neither of these medications or phenobarbital should be re-administered. However, phenobarbital is not automatically contraindicated in patients allergic to phenytoin or carbamazepine (195). When the diagnosis has not been clear or an error occurs, even 1 dose of phenytoin or carbamazepine may elicit the syndrome in a susceptible patient. Thus, challenges must be carried out in exceptional cases and with very small doses.

The mechanism may relate to inadequate detoxification by epoxide hydrolase of hepatic microsome-generated metabolites of phenytoin and carbamazepine (192,195). The relatives of affected patients who are themselves non-epileptic and non-exposed to phenytoin may have findings of delayed metabolism (195). The metabolites are thought to cause either apoptosis or neoantigen formation with the clinical hypersensitivity syndrome (195). Sensitized T_{H2} lymphocytes and presence of the skin-homing receptor, CLA, have been reported in a patient with erythema multiforme attributable to phenobarbital (196). Whatever the mechanism, systemic corticosteroids should be administered and anticonvulsants discontinued (3,5,197) (See Chapter 16).

Alternative anticonvulsants, if necessary, should be selected, such as valproic acid, divalproex, phenobarbital, benzodiazepines, or gabapentin. Valproic acid and divalproex are hepatotoxic, so caution is advised in patients with the liver involvement. Felbamate can cause aplastic anemia and hepatic failure and is contraindicated in patients with liver disease. Appropriate neurologic consultation is advisable.

Muscle Relaxants

The neuromuscular blocking agents are divided into depolarizing (succinylcholine) and non-depolarizing (vecuronium, pancuronium) categories. Acute anaphylactic reactions present as sudden onset hypotension, shock, or acute bronchoconstriction with difficulty in ventilation by the anesthesiologist. Emergent intubation and cardiopulmonary resuscitation may be necessary. Generalized urticaria may or may not be reported but flushing or angioedema may be observed on the face. The neuromuscular blocking agents may cause an IgE mediated reaction or induce mast cell activation independent of IgE antibodies. Improvements in synthesis have resulted in agents with little ability to activate mast cells. In some cases, very rapid infusion of the agent causes an immediate reaction, whereas administration over 30–60 seconds does not. The incidence of immediate generalized reactions during general anesthesia ranges from about 1:5000 to 1:20,000 (198). Up to 25% of reactions occur on the initial anesthetic exposure (198), which might be explained by the presence of quaternary and tertiary ammonium ions being present in cosmetics, disinfectants, foods, and other medications.

The non-depolarizing neuromuscular blocking agents have tertiary and quaternary ammonium groups that are considered to be the antigenic sites for IgE. Cross-reactivity exists based on skin test results. The neuromuscular blocking agents can be diluted from 10^{-1} to 10^{-4}. For prick (epicutaneous) testing, use the 10^{-1} dilution (199). The lowest dilution (10^{-4}) is used for intradermal testing if the prick test is positive. If the prick test is negative, begin with the 10^{-3} dilution (199). If the first intradermal skin test is negative, continue with step-wise skin testing until the 10^{-1} dilution is used. If it also is negative, the agent can be considered for administration. Incriminated agents include vecuronium, pancuronium, atracurium, cisatracurium, rocuronium, d-tubocurarine, and succinylcholine. Skin testing will identify cross-reactive agents, but some patients have immediate cutaneous reactivity to a single agent. Negative skin tests help identify the agents that can be administered safely.

Anesthetic agents such as benzodiazepines, thiopental, and propofol rarely are proven to be causative, but adverse reactions have been reported to all of them. The hypnotic agent ketamine, which has sympathetic stimulating actions, caused acute severe pulmonary edema in an 8-year-old child (200). Latex allergy, antibiotics, and protamine are in the differential diagnosis of allergic reactions.

Part C: Immunologic Reactions to High-Molecular-Weight Therapeutic Agents

Leslie C. Grammer

Division of Allergy-Immunology, Department of Medicine, Northwestern University Medical School, Chicago, Illinois

Most therapeutic agents are small haptens, less than 1 kDa, which require conjugation to a large molecule, usually a protein, in order to be recognized by the human immunologic system. This recognition can result in sensitization and hypersensitivity reactions on subsequent exposure. Therapeutic agents that are proteins, either of human or nonhuman origin, greater than 3 to 5 kDa, can be recognized by the human immunologic system and can cause sensitization and hypersensitivity reactions. Because these proteins are complete antigens, they can be used as skin testing reagents or as antigens in *in vitro* assays. Nonhuman proteins like porcine insulin and adrenocorticotropic hormone (ACTH) are well-recognized causes of hypersensitivity reactions (1,2). Nonhuman protein enzymes like chymopapain and streptokinase have been reported to cause anaphylaxis and other milder hypersensitivity reactions (3). Antithymocyte globulin (ATG), derived from rabbit or equine sources, has been reported to cause immediate type I hypersensitivity as well as type III immune complex–mediated hypersensitivity (4).

Human recombinant proteins are less likely than nonhuman proteins to result in hypersensitivity reactions, but they do occur (5). A likely explanation for this somewhat unexpected occurrence is that they are caused by B-cell recognition of alteration in tertiary or quaternary structure because the primary amino acid sequence, recognized by T cells, is an exact copy of the endogenously produced human protein (6). Insulin was the first recombinant human protein to which hypersensitivity reactions were reported (1). Initially, most of the patients who were reported to be allergic to human recombinant insulin had actually been sensitized to porcine or bovine insulin. Subsequently, however, there were reports of human recombinant proteins, including insulin, granulocyte-macrophage colony-stimulating factor (GM-CSF), and soluble type I interleukin-1 (IL-1) receptor, causing hypersensitivity reactions with no prior sensitization to nonhuman analogue proteins (7–9).

INSULIN

Background

The exact incidence of insulin allergy is unknown; however, the incidence appears to be declining (1). The increasing use of human recombinant DNA (rDNA) insulin may in part be responsible. However, it should be noted that human rDNA insulin has been associated with severe allergic reactions. Patients with systemic allergy to animal source insulins have demonstrated cutaneous reactivity to human rDNA insulin (10). In addition, IgE and IgG antibody directed against human rDNA insulin was detected in the sera of these patients (11). In most patients, the antiinsulin antibody appears to be directed against a determinant present in all commercially available insulins (12). There has even been a report of systemic allergy to endogenous insulin during therapy with recombinant insulin (13).

About 40% of patients receiving porcine insulin develop clinically insignificant immediate wheal-and-flare skin test reactivity to insulin. The prevalence of cutaneous reactivity in patients receiving human rDNA insulin is unknown. It has been suggested that the presence of antiinsulin IgG antibodies may serve as "blocking" antibodies and prevent allergic reactions in patients with antiinsulin IgE antibodies. Immunologic insulin resistance that is due to antiinsulin IgG antibodies may follow or occur simultaneously with IgE-mediated insulin allergy (10). The most common, clinically important, immunologic reactions to insulin are local and systemic allergic reactions and insulin resistance.

Local allergic reactions are not uncommon and usually appear within the first 1 to 4 weeks of treatment. They are usually mild and consist of erythema, induration, burning, and pruritus at the injection site. They may occur immediately (15 to 30 minutes) after the injection or may be delayed for 4 hours or more. Some patients have a biphasic IgE reaction in which the initial local reaction resolves within an hour or so and is followed by a delayed indurated lesion 4 to 6 hours later that persists for 24 hours (14). These local allergic reactions almost always disappear in 3 to 4 weeks with continued insulin administration. Occasionally, they may persist and may precede a systemic reaction. In fact, stopping treatment because of local reactions may increase the risk for a systemic allergic reaction when insulin therapy is resumed. Treatment of local reactions, if necessary at all, involves the administration of antihistamines for several weeks for symptomatic relief until the reaction disappears. On occasion, it may be necessary to switch to a different preparation.

Systemic allergic reactions to insulin are IgE mediated and are characterized by urticaria, angioedema, bronchospasm, and hypotension. Such reactions are rare. Most commonly, these patients have a history of interruption in insulin treatment. Systemic reactions occur most frequently within 12 days of resumption of insulin therapy and are often preceded by the development of progressively larger local reactions. It is most common to have a large urticarial lesion at the site of insulin injection.

Immunologic insulin resistance is even more rare than insulin allergy and is related to the development of anti-insulin IgG antibodies of sufficient titer and affinity to inactivate large amounts of exogenously administered insulin (in excess of 200 units daily). It occurs most commonly in patients older than 40 years of age and usually appears during the first year of insulin treat-

ment. When nonimmune causes of insulin resistance (obesity, infection, endocrinopathies) have been excluded, treatment involves the use of corticosteroids, for example, 60 to 100 mg prednisone daily. This is effective in about 75% of patients, and improvement is expected during the first 2 weeks of treatment. The dose of prednisone is decreased gradually once a response has occurred, but many patients may require small doses, such as 20 mg on alternate days, for up to 6 to 12 months (5).

Diagnostic Testing

About half of patients receiving porcine insulin have positive skin tests to insulin. Therefore, such testing has limited value in the diagnostic evaluation. However, skin testing is of value in selection of the least allergenic insulin (porcine, human) to be used for desensitization. Also, the presence of a negative skin test makes insulin allergy unlikely.

Management of Patients with Systemic Insulin Allergy

After a systemic allergic reaction to insulin, and presuming insulin treatment is necessary, insulin should not be discontinued if the last dose of insulin has been given within 24 hours. The next dose should be reduced to about one third to one tenth of the dose that produced the reaction, depending on the severity of the initial reaction. Subsequently, insulin can be increased slowly by 2 to 5 units per injection until a therapeutic dose is achieved (15).

If more than 24 hours has elapsed since the systemic allergic reaction to insulin, desensitization may be attempted cautiously if insulin is absolutely indicated. The least allergenic insulin may be selected by skin testing with commercially available insulins: porcine, insulin lispro, or human rDNA (16). Table 17.20 provides a representative insulin desensitization schedule (5).

When no emergency exists, slow desensitization over several days is appropriate. The schedule may require modifications if large local or systemic reactions occur. In addition to being prepared to treat anaphylaxis, the physician must

TABLE 17.20. *Insulin desensitization schedule*

Day	Time[a]	Insulin (units)	Route[b]
1	7:30 AM	0.00001[c]	Intradermal
	12:00 noon	0.0001	Intradermal
	4:30 PM	0.001	Intradermal
2	7:30 AM	0.01	Intradermal
	12:00 noon	0.1	Intradermal
	4:30 PM	1.0	Intradermal
3	7:30 AM	2.0	Subcutaneous
	12:00 noon	4.0	Subcutaneous
	4:30 PM	8.0	Subcutaneous
4	7:30 AM	12.0	Subcutaneous
	12:00 noon	16.0	Subcutaneous
5	7:30 AM	20.0[d]	Subcutaneous
6	7:30 AM	25.0[d]	Subcutaneous

Increase by 5 units per day until therapeutic levels are achieved.

[a]In ketoacidosis, the doses may be given every 15 to 30 minutes.
[b]Some physicians prefer to give all doses subcutaneously.
[c]Days 1 through 4: regular insulin.
[d]Days 5 and 6: NPH or Lente insulin.

also be prepared to treat hypoglycemia, which may complicate the frequent doses of insulin required for desensitization. More rapid desensitization may be required if ketoacidosis is present. The schedule suggested in Table 17.20 may be used, but the doses are administered at 15- to 30-minute intervals. Desensitization is usually successful and is associated with a decline in both specific IgE insulin-binding levels, and skin tests may actually become negative (17). This is clearly an example of true desensitization.

PROTAMINE SULFATE

Protamine is a small polycationic polypeptide (4.5 kDa). It is derived from salmon sperm, and it is used to retard the absorption of insulins, such as neutral protamine Hagedorn (NPH), and to reverse heparin anticoagulation. This latter application has increased significantly with the increased use of cardiopulmonary bypass procedures, cardiac catheterization, hemodialysis, and leukopheresis. Increased reports of life-threatening adverse reactions have coincided with increased use.

Acute reactions to intravenous protamine may be mild and consist of rash, urticaria, and tran-

sient elevations in pulmonary artery pressure. Other reactions are more severe and include bronchospasm, hypotension, and at times, cardiovascular collapse and death (18). The exact incidence of these reactions is unknown. However, a prospective study of patients undergoing cardiopulmonary bypass surgery reported a reaction rate of 10.7%, although severe reactions were 1.6% (19).

Diabetic patients treated with protamine-containing insulins have a 40-fold increased risk (2.9% versus 0.07%) for sensitization to protamine (20). Initially, it was believed that men who have had vasectomies were at increased risk; however, the incidence of protamine reactions is not significantly increased in that population (21). A history of fish allergy is not a significant risk factor (20). Previous exposure to protamine intravenously may increase the risk for a reaction on subsequent administration (18).

The exact mechanisms by which protamine produces adverse reactions are not completely understood (22). Some appear to be IgE-mediated anaphylaxis, whereas others may be complement-mediated anaphylactoid reactions due to heparin–protamine complexes or protamine–antiprotamine complexes.

Although skin-prick tests have been recommended using 1 mg/mL of protamine, in normal volunteers, there was an unacceptable rate of false-positive reactions (19). Using more dilute solutions did not appear to be predictive of an adverse reaction to protamine. Although serum antiprotamine IgE and IgG antibodies have been demonstrated *in vitro*, this has not been reported to be helpful in evaluating potential reactors.

There are no widely accepted alternatives to the use of protamine to reverse heparin anticoagulation. Allowing heparin anticoagulation to reverse spontaneously has been advocated, but at the risk of significant hemorrhage. Pretreatment with corticosteroids and antihistamines may be considered, but there are no studies to support this approach. Hexadimethrine (Polybrene) has been used in the past to reverse heparin anticoagulation, but the potential for renal toxicity has led to its removal from general use. However, it may be available as a compassionate-use drug for patients who previously had a life-threatening reaction to protamine used as a heparinase. Test dosing may be valuable, but it is unproved. Emergency treatment for anaphylaxis should be immediately available.

STREPTOKINASE

A nonenzymatic protein produced by group C β-hemolytic streptococci, streptokinase has been used for thrombolytic therapy but is associated with allergic reactions. The reported reaction rate ranges from 1.7% to 18% (23). The descriptions of allergic reactions have not been well characterized but have included urticaria, serum sickness, bronchospasm, and hypotension. Both *in vivo* and *in vitro* evidence for an IgE-mediated mechanism have been reported (24).

Because there is a need to institute therapy immediately, there is not sufficient time for an *in vitro* immunoassay. Intradermal skin tests with 100 IU of streptokinase are recommended (25). Using this approach, patients who are at risk for anaphylaxis can be identified. If there is a negative skin test, streptokinase may be administered. However, such testing does not eliminate the possibility of a late reaction, such as serum sickness (26). If the skin test is positive, urokinase or recombinant tissue plasminogen activator (rt-PA) may be used. In fact, current regimens of rt-PA and streptokinase are equally effective in salvaging myocardium during an evolving infarction (27). In two recent studies, one including 20,201 patients, it was reported that allergic reactions still occur to streptokinase (28,29).

CHYMOPAPAIN

Chymopapain is occasionally used for intradiskal injection for chemonucleolysis of herniated lumbar intervertebral disks (30). Women are more likely than men to experience anaphylaxis. Because anaphylaxis in patients treated with chymopapain has occurred on the initial injection, prior sensitization obviously has been present. Chymopapain is obtained from a crude fraction from the papaya tree, papain, which has enzymatic properties. Consequently, it is used for such purposes as tenderizing meat and clarifying beer or in solutions for use with soft contact lenses.

It is likely that exposure to crude papain, a component of which is chymopapain, may sensitize patients to chymopapain.

Because anaphylaxis may occur after the first injection, it is desirable to have a method to identify patients at risk. Both *in vivo* skin tests and *in vitro* immunoassays have been used to detect antichymopapain IgE antibody (31).

Skin testing with chymopapain has been useful in screening patients. Dilutions of chymopapain are made in saline with 0.1% human serum albumin as a stabilizer. If a histamine control is positive and a saline control is negative, skin-prick tests are performed using 1 mg/mL and 10 μg/mL of chymopapain. If the skin-prick tests are negative, proceed with an intradermal skin test using 0.02 mL of 100 μg/mL chymopapain. A positive reaction produces a wheal and erythema. If skin tests are negative, one may proceed with the intradiskal injection. If skin tests are positive, laminectomy should be considered. At present, the number of reactions to chymopapain is decreasing, largely because of the decreased use of chemonucleolysis in the United States. In other countries, it is still used (32).

LATEX

Latex is covered extensively in Chapter 31. It is mentioned here only because it is a high-molecular-weight agent that has some therapeutic uses, such as a urethral catheter to treat urinary tract obstruction. Latex is the natural milky rubber sap that is harvested from the rubber tree, *Hevea brasiliensis.* Latex allergy has been reported to cause contact dermatitis and IgE-mediated reactions during procedures involving latex exposure.

During the manufacturing process, various accelerators, antioxidants, and preservatives are added to ammoniated latex. These agents are responsible for the type IV contact dermatitis. Latex gloves are then formed by dipping porcelain molds into the compounded latex. Subsequent steps include oven heating, leaching to remove water-soluble proteins and excess additives, curing by vulcanization, and finally powdering the gloves with cornstarch to decrease friction and provide comfort. Powder-free gloves are passed through a chlorination wash, which may also reduce the amount of water-soluble antigen. The natural rubber latex allergens are proteins present in raw latex and are not a result of the manufacturing process (33).

In 1979, the first case of rubber-induced contact urticaria was reported (34). Since then, many reports of IgE-mediated hypersensitivity reactions have been reported, including contact urticaria, rhinitis, asthma, and anaphylaxis. Contact urticaria is the most common early manifestation of IgE-mediated rubber allergy, particularly in latex-sensitive health care workers, who report contact urticaria involving their hands. These symptoms are often incorrectly attributed to the powder in the gloves or frequent handwashing. Inhalation of latex-coated cornstarch particles from powdered gloves has evoked rhinitis and asthma in latex-sensitive people. Many of these individuals are atopic with a history of rhinitis due to pollens and asthma due to dust mites and animal dander (33). These reactions have been noted in both health care workers and people employed in a rubber glove factory.

Anaphylaxis is usually associated with parenteral or mucosal exposure. Reactions have occurred after contact with rubber bladder catheters or condoms and during surgery, childbirth, and dental procedures. Patients with latex-induced anaphylaxis during anesthesia often have a prior history of contact urticaria or angioedema from rubber products, such as gloves or balloons. Also, anaphylaxis has followed the blowing up of toy balloons. Fatal anaphylactic reactions have been reported with rubber balloon catheters used for barium enemas (35). This device is no longer available in the United States.

At the present time, the diagnosis of latex allergy is primarily based on the clinical history. Patients should be questioned if they have ever noted erythema, pruritus, urticaria, or angioedema after contact with rubber products. Unexplained episodes of urticaria and anaphylaxis should be scrutinized. Also, the work history may uncover potential occupational exposure to latex. In some patients, contact dermatitis may precede IgE-mediated reactions.

In vivo and in vitro testing for the presence of latex-induced IgE antibodies has limited value.

Skin-prick tests using commercial latex reagents have been widely used in Europe and Canada. In the United States, there are no standardized, licensed latex extracts for diagnostic use. Some investigators have used their own extracts prepared from latex gloves. However, latex gloves vary significantly in their allergen content (36), and systemic reactions have occurred with these unstandardized preparations (37). Intradermal skin testing for latex allergy is generally not recommended. However, experienced allergists may prepare latex allergens for cautious prick and then intradermal tests beginning with low and then increasing concentrations.

"Use" tests have been advocated wherein the patient's wet hands are exposed to latex gloves. Initially, one finger is exposed for 15 minutes; if there is no reaction, the entire hand is exposed for an additional 15 minutes. In one series, 92% of patients with latex allergy had a positive provocative test (38).

In summary, there is no reliable test for latex allergy currently available in the United States. A standardized reagent for skin-prick tests is the diagnostic method of choice offering the best combination of speed and sensitivity. Hopefully, unlike the delay in the availability of a standardized reagent for the detection of penicillin minor determinant sensitivity, a reliable skin test material for the diagnosis of latex allergy will soon be commercially available.

Once the diagnosis of latex allergy is established, avoidance is the only effective therapy. Natural rubber latex is ubiquitous, and avoidance is often difficult. Additional protective measures for individuals with known latex allergy include wearing a MedicAlert bracelet, having autoinjectable epinephrine (EpiPen) available, and keeping a supply of nonlatex gloves for emergencies. Because there has been association between latex allergy and certain foods, latex-sensitive patients should be queried about reactions to bananas, avocado, kiwi fruit, chestnuts, and passion fruit, and advised to be cautious when ingesting them.

Prevention of latex allergy is the goal. When the Mayo Clinic changed to low-latex nonpowdered gloves, the incidence of latex sensitization decreased significantly (39,40). Dr. Baur and his colleagues reported reduction of latex aeroallergens after removal of powdered latex gloves from their hospital (41). Other studies to address this strategy are ongoing.

ADRENOCORTICOTROPIC HORMONE

Historically, patients with multiple sclerosis were treated with ACTH derived from porcine sources. There have been case reports of patients having anaphylaxis after being so treated. In one patient with anaphylaxis to porcine ACTH, positive cutaneous tests and serologic evidence of IgE against porcine ACTH was described (2). Cosyntropin, synthetic ACTH, has not been described to cause anaphylaxis.

BLOOD PRODUCTS

Blood transfusions or plasma transfusions may elicit immediate generalized reactions in 0.1% to 0.2% of these administration procedures. Anaphylactic shock occurs in 1:20,000 to 1:50,000. Patients with IgA deficiency should receive preparations from IgA-deficient donors because they may have preexisting serum IgE or IgG antibodies to IgA. Alternatively, thoroughly washed red blood cells may be administered. It has been suggested that pretreatment with corticosteroids and antihistamines may be helpful in some cases, but severe reactions may occur, and epinephrine must be readily available for treatment.

Other immunologically mediated reactions may occur with blood transfusions. If the antigens are leukocyte cell surface proteins, a reaction consisting of fever, chills, myalgias, and dyspnea, with or without hypotension, can occur (42). The treatment for this is supportive care. Fewer reactions are reported when reduced-reduced components are used.

Treatment and prevention of disease through manipulation of the immune system is a major achievement of modern medicine that has eliminated smallpox and has nearly eradicated polio, tetanus, diphtheria, pertussis, measles, mumps, and rubella in the United States. Extensive serum therapy began in the 1890s with the use of horse antisera to diphtheria and tetanus toxins. Until the use of antibiotics in the 1940s, treatment of infectious disease often involved the use of type-specific antisera to bacteria or their toxins. Today, active immunizations to prevent infectious diseases has limited the use of passively transferred, immunologically active serum products; however, passive immunization with serum immunoglobulin concentrates still have an important role in well-defined clinical situations.

IMMUNE SERA THERAPY: HETEROLOGOUS AND HUMAN

Background

The two major allergic reactions that may follow an injection of heterologous antisera are anaphylaxis and serum sickness. Anaphylaxis is less common but is very likely to occur among patients who are atopic and have IgE antibodies directed against the corresponding animal dander, most commonly horse. For this reason, such individuals may react after the first injection of antisera. Serum sickness is more common and is dose related.

Current immunization procedures and the availability of human immune serum globulin (ISG) and specific human immune serum globulin (SIG) preparations have reduced the need for heterologous antisera. However, equine antitoxins may still be required in the management of snakebite (pit vipers and coral snake), black widow spider bite, diphtheria, and botulism (43,44). Antilymphocyte and antithymocyte globulins, prepared in horses and rabbits, have been used to provide immunosuppression for transplants and to treat aplastic anemia. Murine monoclonal antilymphocyte antibodies to treat lymphocytic malignancies have also produced immediate generalized reactions but such reactions do not appear to be IgE dependent (45).

Where available and appropriate, human ISG preparations should be used in preference to animal antisera. Although infrequent, immediate generalized reactions have followed the administration of human ISG preparations. Intramuscular ISG preparations contain high-molecular-weight IgG aggregates that are biologically active and may activate serum complement to produce anaphylactoid reactions. Anaphylaxis has also followed the administration of both intramuscular and intravenous human ISG among IgA-deficient patients who may produce IgE and IgG antibodies directed against IgA (46). Such patients are at risk for anaphylaxis upon infusion of IgA-containing blood products. Only one preparation of intravenous ISG (Gammagard) is sufficiently IgA poor to be considered in the treatment of IgA-deficient patients.

Tests before Heterologous Antisera Administration

Before administering heterologous antisera to any patient, regardless of history, skin testing *must* be performed on the volar surface of the forearm to determine whether there is the presence of IgE antibodies and thereby predict the likelihood of anaphylaxis. Many package inserts have suggested procedures. If not, skin-prick tests using antisera diluted 1:10 with normal saline and a saline control are performed. If negative after 15 minutes, intradermal skin tests using 0.02 mL of a 1:100 dilution of antisera and a saline control are completed. If the history suggests a previous reaction, or if the patient has atopic symptoms after exposure to the corresponding animal (usually horse), begin intradermal testing using 0.02 mL of a 1:1,000 dilution. A negative skin test virtually excludes significant anaphylactic sensitivity, but some would recommend giving a test dose of 0.5 mL of undiluted antisera intravenously before proceeding with recommended doses. It should be remembered that this approach does not exclude the possibility of a late reaction, notably serum sickness 8 to 12 days later.

Desensitization

When there is no alternative to the use of heterologous antisera, desensitization has occasionally been successful despite a positive skin test to the material. The procedure is dangerous and may be more difficult to accomplish in patients who are allergic to the corresponding animal dander.

There are several protocols recommended for desensitization. The package insert often recommends at least one such schedule. An intravenous infusion should be established in both arms. A conservative schedule begins with the subcutaneous administration of 0.1 mL of a 1:100 dilution in an extremity, where a tourniquet may be placed proximally if required. The dose is doubled every 15 minutes. If a reaction occurs, it is treated, and desensitization is resumed using half the dose provoking the reaction. After reaching 1 mL of the undiluted antiserum, the remainder may be given by slow intravenous infusion.

At times, more rapid delivery of the antisera may be required (47). Here, intravenous infusions are also established in both arms; one to administer the antisera, and the other for treatment of complications. Initiate a slow infusion of the antisera through one of the intravenous lines. If there is no reaction after 15 minutes, the infusion rate may be increased. If a reaction occurs, the antisera infusion is stopped and the reaction treated appropriately. After the reaction has been controlled, the slow infusion is reestablished. Most patients can be given 80 to 100 mL over 4 hours. If there is no reaction, it is possible to give that amount in the first hour. However, some patients do not tolerate desensitization despite adherence to the above procedure (48).

After successful desensitization, it is possible that serum sickness will develop in 8 to 12 days. If the dose of antisera is in excess of 100 mL, virtually all patients will experience some degree of serum sickness. Treatment with corticosteroids is effective, the prognosis is excellent, and long-term complications are rare.

RECOMBINANT HUMAN PROTEINS

Monoclonal Antibodies

Clinical trials with monoclonal antibodies have reported their potential uses as diagnostic and therapeutic agents for malignant disease, inflammatory bowel disease, and various autoimmune diseases. However, various immunologic mechanisms can make their administration difficult. With the human monoclonal antibodies that are chimerized with some murine proteins, hypersensitivity may occur. Hypersensitivity reactions may include fever, chills, rigors, diaphoresis, malaise, pruritus, urticaria, nausea, dyspnea, and hypotension. Although rare, anaphylaxis has also been reported (49). Monoclonal antibodies may also cross-react with normal tissue, resulting in various adverse effects depending on the affected tissue (50). For example, both neuropathy and encephalopathy have been reported.

In patients with colorectal carcinoma treated with monoclonal antibody 17-1A, allergic reactions were reported that necessitated reducing the dose of the antibody (51). In one study, rituximab, an anti-CD20, was well tolerated by patients with non-Hodgkin lymphoma (52). However, in a study of patients with chronic lymphocytic leukemia, cytokine release syndrome was reported to occur in several patients after receiving rituximab (53). The elevated cytokine levels were associated with clinical symptoms, including fever, chills, nausea, vomiting, dyspnea, and hypotension. The severity and frequency of these events were associated with the number of circulating tumor cells at baseline.

Abciximab, a monoclonal antibody (7E3) that prevents platelet aggregation by binding glycoprotein IIb/IIIa, generally does not cause hypersensitivity reactions. However, a case of probable anaphylaxis has been reported (54). A monoclonal peptide inhibitor of glycoprotein IIb/IIIa, eptifibatide, has been reported to be nonimmunogenic in a study of 441 patients (55).

Tumor necrosis factor (TNF) is a key cytokine in the inflammation of inflammatory bowel disease and in rheumatoid arthritis. Two monoclonal antibodies against TNF, infliximab and etanercept, were approved by the FDA in 1998. Infliximab is approved for Crohn disease and etanercept for rheumatoid arthritis (56,57). No reports of significant adverse immunologic events have been published with these agents. Similarly, basiliximab, an anti–IL-2 receptor monoclonal antibody (58), and SB 209763, a monoclonal antibody against respiratory syncytial virus (59), have not been associated with hypersensitivity or other adverse immunologic events.

Polyclonal sheep antidigoxin antibodies have proved useful when administered to patients with digoxin overdose. Unfortunately, significant hypersensitivity reactions, including severe anaphylaxis, have been described. Human monoclonal antidigoxin antibodies are currently under development (60). OKT3, a monoclonal antibody against CD3, has not been reported to cause hypersensitivity reactions, but patients may become resistant to treatment as a result of development of antiidiotypic antibody (61).

Colony-Stimulating Factors

Recombinant human GM-CSF is used to accelerate myeloid recovery after bone marrow transplantation or high-dose chemotherapy. In a patient with pruritus, urticaria, and angioedema after GM-CSF administration, positive prick tests were reported with 100 and 250 μg/mL (8). There are other reports of anaphylaxis in the literature (62,63). There are also reports of localized reactions and generalized maculopapular eruptions. The immunopathogenesis of the latter reactions has not been well characterized (64). GM-CSF has also been reported to induce antibodies that neutralize the biologic activity of GM-CSF, thus compromising its therapeutic efficacy (65). Recombinant G-CSF has not yet been reported to cause hypersensitivity reactions, nor are there reports of neutralizing antibody induction.

Soluble Type 1 Interleukin-1 Receptor

Interleukin-1 is a cytokine important in many types of inflammation. The receptor for IL-1 exists both in a cell-bound form and in a soluble form. Recombinant IL-1 receptor has the potential to downregulate inflammation that is IL-1 dependent. A patient has been reported with large local reactions to soluble IL-1 receptor and a positive intradermal skin test with 125 μg/mL (9). She also had IgE against IL-1 receptor in her serum.

Erythropoietin

Although hypersensitivity reactions have not yet been reported with erythropoietin, antibodies, including neutralizing antibodies, have been reported. In one patient, antibody development was actually associated with red blood cell aplasia that resolved when erythropoietin was discontinued and the antibody titers declined (66). A rapid serologic method for detecting antirecombinant human erythropoietin antibodies has been published as a tool for the diagnosis of erythropoietin resistance (67). Antibody production against erythropoietin should be considered in the evaluation of patients whose anemia becomes refractory to erythropoietin therapy.

Interferons

Recombinant interferon-α (rIFN-α) has been reported to be a useful therapy in a subpopulation of patients with chronic hepatitis C. In some of these patients, development of antibody against rIFN-α has been reported (68). The prevalence varies from 1.2% to 20.2%, depending on the preparation. In one study, the development of antibodies was associated with a relapse of their disease (69). It is presumed that the antibody was inactivating the rIFN-α. In the treatment of patients with CML, neutralizing antibody has also been associated with relapse (70). It has been reported that the epitopes, which are recognized by neutralizing antibody, are located in the N-terminal function domain of rife-a (71).

Chronic granulomatous disease has been reported to be treated safely and effectively with rife-a (72). However, high-avidity IFN-neutralizing antibodies have been reported in pharmacologically prepared human immunoglobulin (73). In a patient receiving rife-a for systemic mastocytosis, anti-IFN antibodies were reported. Cessation of the IFN therapy resulted in a decline of antibody titer (74).

Follicle-stimulating Hormone

With the increasing number of infertile couples deciding to pursue *in vitro* fertilization, the use of a variety of hormones has increased. Follicle-stimulating hormone (FSH) is one such hormone. Before the advent of recombinant FSH, it was recovered from human urine, purified, sterilized, and administered. One patient was reported who developed a severe anaphylactic reaction to urine-derived FSH (75). She had a positive intradermal test as corroborative evidence. She tolerated the administration of recombinant FSH and had establishment of a clinical pregnancy. There

are other documented hypersensitivity reactions to urine-derived preparations while subsequently tolerating the recombinant protein (76). Whether these phenomena are explained by immunologic reactions to proteins other than FSH in the urine has not been studied.

Factor VIII

Until recombinant factor VIII was available, patients with hemophilia were treated with factor VIII concentrates derived from human plasma. Because factor VIII is a "foreign protein" to patients with hemophilia, the development of an immunologic response is expected. There is one report of anaphylaxis to factor VIII concentrate (77). When that patient suffered another episode of hemorrhage, desensitization with pretreatment was attempted, but a moderately severe reaction occurred. No anaphylactic reactions definitely due to recombinant factor VIII have been reported (78). The major immunologic problem in hemophilia is not hypersensitivity to factor VIII, but developing inhibitors of factor VIII, namely neutralizing antibody (79–81). Several investigators predicted that the incidence of inhibitors in patients treated only with the recombinant product would be higher (82,83). However, the studies suggest that the prevalence is about the same, with most patients having a low level of inhibitor that does not significantly affect the efficacy (84).

Other Recombinant Proteins

Hirudin is a thrombin inhibitor found in the salivary glands of leeches. In a trial of use of recombinant hirudin as an anticoagulant, an IgE-mediated hypersensitivity reaction was reported (85). Although tissue plasminogen activator (tPA) is generally not a cause of hypersensitivity reactions, a case of anaphylaxis temporally related to its administration has been reported (86). That patient also had IgE directed against tPA detected in the serum. In patients with cystic fibrosis treated with recombinant DNAase, a few patients developed antibody, but there have been no reports of anaphylaxis or other significant hypersensitivity reactions (87). In patients treated with humanized monoclonal antibody against IgE (rhuMAb-E25), no patients developed antibody or evidence of hypersensitivity reactions (88).

VACCINES

A variety of adverse effects can result from vaccine administration: arthralgias from rubella vaccines, significant fever from pertussis vaccines, and fever with rash from live measles vaccine. A second risk of immunization is the possibility of reactions to vaccine components, such as eggs, gelatin, and neomycin. Another risk that occurs, for example, with frequent tetanus toxoid exposure, is development of IgE antibodies with resultant anaphylaxis or urticaria (89,90). Finally, as happened with killed rubeola and respiratory syncytial virus vaccines, the protective immunity declined with time. When natural exposure resulted in infection, it was often atypical and actually more severe than in individuals who had never been immunized (91–94).

Tetanus Toxoid

Although minor reactions, such as local swelling, are common after tetanus toxoid or diphtheria-tetanus (dT) toxoid vaccinations, true IgE-mediated reactions are rare. However, the *Institute of Medicine Report 1994* concluded that there was a causative relationship between anaphylaxis and administration of tetanus toxoid with or without diphtheria (95). A number of case reports have been published (96–98), but surveys estimate the risk for a systemic reaction to be very small, 0.00001% (99). Because diphtheria toxoid is not available as a single agent, it is impossible to separate the true incidence of diphtheria-associated reactions from those due to tetanus toxoid.

When it appears necessary to administer tetanus toxoid to a patient with a history of a previous adverse reaction, a skin test–graded challenge may be performed (100,101). One recommended approach is to begin with a skin-prick test using undiluted toxoid. If negative, at 15-minute intervals, 0.02 mL of successive dilutions of toxoid 1:1,000 and 1:100 are injected intradermally. If the prick test was positive, begin with a 1:10,000 dilution. Subsequently,

0.02 mL and 0.20 mL of a 1:10 dilution are given subcutaneously. This may be followed by 0.05 mL, 0.10 mL, 0.15 mL, and 0.20 mL of full-strength toxoid given subcutaneously. Some would prefer to wait for 24 hours after 0.10 mL is given to detect delayed reactivity. After that, the balance of full-strength material may be given for a final total dose of 0.50 mL.

Pertussis and Rubella

The Institute of Medicine analyzed adverse effects of pertussis and rubella vaccines (102). With pertussis vaccines, reactions at the site are common, as is fever. Seizures occur in 1 in every 1,750 injections, as does the "collapse syndrome," hypotonic, hyporesponsive episodes. Encephalitis and other neurologic sequelae were once thought to be a consequence of pertussis vaccine, but the evidence does not report a causal association.

Rubella vaccination results in arthritis and arthralgia in a significant percentage of adult and adolescent females. The incidence of arthralgia among children is very low (101).

Measles, Mumps, Rubella

Because the live attenuated virus used in the measles, mumps, rubella (MMR) vaccine is grown in cultured chick-embryo fibroblasts, concern has been raised regarding its administration to egg-allergic children. The fibroblast cultures used to produce MMR vaccine contain no or trivial amounts of egg allergen. For this reason, and also based on extensive clinical experience, it has been suggested that egg-allergic children be given MMR vaccine without preliminary skin testing with the vaccine (102). The Advisory Committee on Immunization Practices no longer recommends skin testing or test dosing in egg-allergic subjects who are to receive MMR (103). It should be noted that hypersensitivity reactions to MMR vaccine have been described in children who tolerate eggs. There are several reports that indicate that those reactions are due to another component, gelatin (104–106). In addition to causing anaphylaxis in patients receiving MMR, anaphylaxis due to gelatin has been reported in patients receiving Japanese encephalitis vaccine (107).

If it is deemed necessary to test an egg-allergic patient for MMR vaccine, a prick test is performed with a 1:10 dilution of MMR vaccine in normal saline, and a normal saline control. Intradermal skin tests, following a negative prick skin test, are probably unnecessary and may be misleading. After a negative prick test, the vaccine may be administered in the routine fashion.

After a positive skin-prick test for MMR vaccine, at 15-minute intervals, the following dilutions of vaccine are administered subcutaneously: 0.05 mL of a 1:100 dilution, 0.05 mL of a 1:10 dilution, and 0.05 mL of the undiluted vaccine. Subsequently, at 15-minute intervals, increasing amounts of the undiluted vaccine (0.10 mL, 0.15 mL, and 0.20 mL) are given until the total immunizing dose of 0.50 mL is received. Using this protocol, systemic reactions have been reported; hence, a physician must be prepared to treat anaphylaxis (108). After completion of the procedure, it is advisable to keep the patient under observation for an additional 30 minutes.

Influenza and Yellow Fever Vaccine in Egg-Allergic Patients

Allergic reactions to influenza vaccine are rare, and the vaccine may be given safely to people who are able to tolerate eggs by ingestion, even if they demonstrate a positive skin test to egg protein (109). There is a report of 83 egg-allergic patients who received the influenza vaccine uneventfully, even though 4 had a positive prick test for the vaccine (110). Anaphylaxis has been reported at a rate of 0.024:100,000. The Advisory Committee on Immunization Practices does state that influenza vaccine should not be administered to people known to have anaphylactic hypersensitivity to eggs or other components of the vaccine without first consulting a physician (111). Among asthmatic patients, there was some concern about inducing bronchospasm after administration; however, there appears to be no evidence of asthmagenicity after influenza vaccine (112). Clearly, the patient with moderate-to-severe asthma is at risk from natural infection and will benefit from influenza vaccination.

Although yellow fever vaccine is not required in the United States, travelers to endemic areas may require immunization. Of the egg-based vaccines, yellow fever vaccine contains the most egg protein. Yellow fever vaccine also contains gelatin. In a review of 5,236,820 vaccinations, it was estimated that the risk for anaphylaxis was about 1 in 131,000 (113). In another study, two of 493 individuals with a positive history of egg allergy had anaphylaxis following yellow fever immunization; both of these patents had positive skin tests to both egg and the vaccine (114). The Centers for Disease Control and Prevention lists egg hypersensitivity as one of the reasons that an individual should not receive yellow fever vaccine. It is suggested that the individual obtain a waiver letter from a consular or embassy official (115). For patients with a clear history of egg allergy or when in doubt, skin testing with the appropriate vaccine is a reliable method to identify the patients at risk (111). A prick test is performed with a 1:10 dilution of the vaccine in normal saline, and a normal saline control. If negative or equivocal, an intradermal skin test using 0.02 mL of a 1:100 dilution of the vaccine is performed, and a saline control. If negative, the vaccine may be administered in a routine fashion.

After a positive skin test to the vaccine, if it is considered essential, administer 0.05 mL of a 1:100 dilution intramuscularly and, at 15- to 20-minute intervals, give 0.05 mL of a 1:10 dilution, 0.05 mL of undiluted vaccine, followed by 0.10 mL, 0.15 mL, and 0.20 mL of undiluted vaccine for a total dose of 0.50 mL. Using this format, patients develop adequate protective antibody titers (116).

Other Vaccines

Both typhoid and paratyphoid vaccines have been reported to cause anaphylaxis (117,118). In a study of 14,249 marines who received Japanese encephalitis vaccine, the reaction rate was 0.00267% (119). The reactions were primarily urticaria, angioedema, and pruritus. In a study of 1,198,751 individuals who received meningococcal vaccine, the rate of anaphylaxis was reported as 0.1 in 100,000, a very rare event (120). Because varicella vaccine contains neomycin, individuals with neomycin hypersensitivity would be at potential risk for an allergic reaction (121). There are several case reports of anaphylactic episodes after hepatitis B vaccine (122,123). Until 1999, the only hepatitis B vaccines available contained thimerosal, making them difficult to administer to individuals with thimerosal allergy (124).

REFERENCES

Part A: Introduction, Epidemiology, Classification of Adverse Reactions, Immunochemical Basis, Risk Factors, Evaluation of Patients with Suspected Drug Allergy, Patient Management Considerations

1. DeSwarte RD. Drug allergy. In: Patterson R, Grammer LC, Greenberger PA, et al, eds. *Allergic diseases: diagnosis and management.* 4th ed. Philadelphia: JB Lippincott, 1993:395.
2. Patterson R, DeSwarte RD, Greenberger PA, et al. Drug allergy and protocols for management of drug allergies. *Allergy Proc* 1994;15:239.
3. Sullivan TJ. Drug allergy. In: Middleton E, Reed CE, Ellis EF, et al, eds. *Allergy: principles and Practice.* 4th ed. St Louis: CV Mosby, 1993:1726.
4. Anderson JA. Allergic reactions to drugs and biological agents. *JAMA* 1992;268:2845.
5. Classen DC, Pestotnik SL, Evans RS, et al. Computerized surveillance of adverse drug events in hospitalized patients. *JAMA* 1991;266:2847.
6. Jick H. Adverse drug reactions: the magnitude of the problem. *J Allergy Clin Immunol* 1985;74:555.
7. Armstrong B, Dinan B, Jick H. Fatal drug reactions in patients admitted to surgical services. *Am J Surg* 1976;132:643.
8. Porter J, Jick H. Drug-related deaths among medical inpatients. *JAMA* 1977;237:879.
9. Jick H. Drugs: remarkably nontoxic. *N Engl J Med* 1974;291:284.
10. Spilker B. *Guide to clinical trials.* New York: Raven, 1991:565.
11. Scott HD, Rosenbaum SE, Waters WJ. Rhode Island physicians' recognition and reporting of adverse drug reactions. *Rhode Island Med J* 1987;70:311.
12. Kessler DA. Introducing MedWatch: a new approach to reporting and device adverse effects and product problems. *JAMA* 1993;269:2765.
13. Honig PK, Wortham DC, Zamani K, et al. Terfenadine-ketoconazole interaction: pharmacokinetic and electro-cardiographic consequences. *JAMA* 1993;269:1513.
14. DeSwarte RD. Drug allergy: problems and strategies. *J Allergy Clin Immunol* 1984;74:209.
15. Schatz M, Patterson R, DeSwarte RD. Non-organic adverse reactions to aeroallergen immunotherapy. *J Allergy Clin Immunol* 1976;58:198.
16. Wolf S. The pharmacology of placebos. *Pharmacol Rev* 1959;11:689.
17. Penn I. Cancers following cyclosporine therapy. *Transplantation* 1987;43:32.
18. Kelly CP, Pothoulakis C, LaMont JT. Clostridium difficile colitis. *N Engl J Med* 1994;330:257.
19. Gelfand JA, Elin RJ, Berry FW, et al. Endotoxemia associated with the Jarisch-Herxheimer reactions. *N Engl J Med* 1976;295:211.
20. McInnes GT, Brodie MJ. Drug interactions that matter: a critical appraisal. *Drugs* 1988;36:83.
21. Affrime MB, Lorber R, Danzig M, et al. Three month evaluation of electrocardiographic effects of loratidine in humans. *J Allergy Clin Immunol* 1993;91:259.
22. Hansten PD, Horn JR. *Drug interactions.* 6th ed. Philadelphia and London: Lea & Febiger, 1989.
23. Beutler E. Glucose-6-phosphate dehydrogenase deficiency. *N Engl J Med* 1991;324:169.
24. Landu BM. Pharmacogenetics. *Med Clin North Am* 1969;53:839.
25. DeSwarte RD. Drug allergy: an overview. *Clin Rev Allergy* 1986;4:143.
26. Ring J. Pseudoallergic drug reactions. In: Korenblat PE, Wedner HJ, eds. *Allergy: theory and practice.* 2nd ed. Philadelphia: WB Saunders, 1992:243.
27. Greenberger PA, Patterson R. The prevention of immediate generalized reactions to radiocontrast media in high risk patients. *J Allergy Clin Immunol* 1991;87:867–872.
28. deWeck AL. Pharmacologic and immunochemical mechanisms of drug hypersensitivity. *Immunol Allergy Clin North Am* 1991;11:461.
29. Levine BB. Immunologic mechanisms of penicillin allergy: a haptenic model system for the study of allergic diseases in man. *N Engl J Med* 1966;275:1115.
30. Carrington DM, Earl HS, Sullivan TJ. Studies of human IgE to a sulfonamide determinant. *J Allergy Clin Immunol* 1987;79:442.
31. Sullivan TJ. Dehaptenation of albumin substituted with benzylpenicillin G determinants. *J Allergy Clin Immunol* 1988;81:222.
32. Didier A, Cador D, Bongrand P, et al. Role of quaternary ammonium ion determinants in allergy to muscle relaxants. *J Allergy Clin Immunol* 1987;79:578.
33. Coombs RRA, Gell PGH. Classification of allergic reactions responsible for clinical hypersensitivity and disease. In: Gell PGH, Coombs RRA, Lachman PJ, eds. *Clinical aspects of immunology.* 3rd ed. Oxford: Blackwell Scientific Publications, 1975:761.
34. Kay, AB. Concepts of allergy and hypersensitivity. In: Kay, AB, ed. *Allergy and allergic diseases.* Malden, MA: Blackwell Science, 1997:23–35.
35. Janeway CA Jr, Travers P. Immune responses in the absence of infection, Chapter 11. In: *Immunobiology: the immune system in health and disease.* 2nd ed. London: Garland Press, 1995.
36. VanArsdel PP Jr. Classification and risk factors for drug allergy. *Immunol Allergy Clin North Am* 1991;11:475.
37. Adkinson NF Jr. Risk factors for drug allergy. *J Allergy Clin Immunol* 1984;74:567.
38. Enright T, Chua-Lim A, Duda E. The role of a documented allergic profile as a risk factor for radiographic contrast media reactions. *Ann Allergy* 1989;62:302.
39. Perry HM, Tan EM, Carmody S, et al. Relationship of acetyltransferase activity to antinuclear antibodies and toxic symptoms in hypertensive patients treated with hydralazine. *J Lab Clin Med* 1970;76:114.

40. Woosley RL, Drayer DE, Reidenberg MM, et al. Effect of acetylator phenotype on the rate at which procainamide induces antinuclear antibodies and the lupus syndrome. *N Engl J Med* 1978;298:1157.
41. Reider MJ, Vetrecht J, Shear NH, et al. Diagnosis of sulfonamide hypersensitivity reactions by in vitro "rechallenge" with hydroxylamine metabolites. *Ann Intern Med* 1989;110:286.
42. Wooley PH, Griffin J, Panayi GS, et al. HLA-DR antigens and toxic reactions to sodium aurothiomalate and D-penicillamine in patients with rheumatoid arthritis. *N Engl J Med* 1980;303:300.
43. Roujeau JC, Huynh TN, Bracq C, et al. Genetic susceptibility to toxic epidermal necrolysis. *Arch Dermatol* 1987;123:171.
44. Attaway NJ, Jasin HM, Sullivan TJ. Familial drug allergy. *J Allergy Clin Immunol* 1991;87:227.
45. Sullivan TJ, Ong RC, Gilliam LK. Studies of the multiple drug allergy syndrome. *J Allergy Clin Immunol* 1989;83:270.
46. Moseley EK, Sullivan TJ. Allergic reactions to antimicrobial drugs in patients with a history of prior drug allergy. *J Allergy Clin Immunol* 1991;87:226.
47. Kamada MM, Twarog F, Leung DYM. Multiple antibiotic sensitivity in a pediatric population. *Allergy Proc* 1991;12:347.
48. Sullivan TJ. Management of patients allergic to antimicrobial drugs. *Allergy Proceed* 1992;12:361.
49. Moss RB. Sensitization to aztreonam and cross-reactivity with other beta-lactam antibiotics in high-risk patients with cystic fibrosis. *J Allergy Clin Immunol* 1991;87:78.
50. Bierman CW, Pierson WE, Zeitz SJ, et al. Reactions associated with ampicillin therapy. *JAMA* 1972;220:1098.
51. Harb GE, Jacobson MA. Human immunodeficiency virus (HIV) infection: does it increase susceptibility to adverse drug reactions? *Drug Safety*, 1993;9:1.
52. Bayard PJ, Berger TG, Jacobson MA. Drug hypersensitivity reactions and human immunodeficiency virus disease. *J Acquir Immune Defic Syndr* 1992;5:1237.
53. Kovacs JA, Hiemenz JW, Macher AM, et al. Pneumocystis carinii pneumonia: a comparison between patients with the acquired immunodeficiency syndrome and patients with other immunodeficiencies. *Ann Intern Med* 1984;100:663.
54. Toogood JH. Risk of anaphylaxis in patients receiving beta-blocker drugs. *J Allergy Clin Immunol* 1988;81:1.
55. Dukes MNG, ed. *Meyler's side effects of drugs: an encyclopedia of adverse reactions and interactions*. 13th ed. Amsterdam-New York-Oxford: Elsevier, 1992.
56. Dukes MNG, ed. *Side effects of drugs, annual 22*. Amsterdam-New York-Oxford: Elsevier, 1999.
57. Greenberger PA. Drug allergies. In: Rich RR, Fleisher TA, Schwartz BD, et al, eds. *Clinical immunology: principles and practice*. St. Louis: Mosby-Year Book, 1996:988.
58. Porter J, Jick H. Boston Collaborative Drug Surveillance Programs: drug induced anaphylaxis, convulsions, deafness, and extrapyramidal symptoms. *Lancet* 1977;1:587.
59. Herrera AM, deShazo RD. Current concepts in anaphylaxis. *Immunol Allergy Clin North Am* 1992;12:517.
60. Weiss ME, Adkinson NF, Hirshman CA. Evaluation of allergic drug reactions in the perioperative period. *Anesthesiology* 1989;71:483.
61. Davis H, McGoodwin E, Reed TG. Anaphylactoid reactions reported after treatment with ciprofloxacin. *Ann Intern Med* 1989;111:1041.
62. Weiss RB. Hypersensitivity reactions. *Semin Oncol* 1992;19:458.
63. Windom HH, McGuire WP III, Hamilton RG, et al. Anaphylaxis to carboplatin: a new platinum chemotherapeutic agent. *J Allergy Clin Immunol* 1992;90:681.
64. Weiss RB, Donehower RC, Wiernik PH, et al. Hypersensitivity reactions from taxol. *J Clin Oncol* 1990; 8:1263.
65. Weiss ME. Drug allergy. *Med Clin North Am* 1992; 76:857.
66. Laxenaire MC, Monneret-Vautrin DA, Guaént JL. Drugs and other agents involved in anaphylactic shock occuring during anesthesia: a French multicenter epidemiological inquiry. *Ann Fr Anesth Reanim* 1993;12:91.
67. Weiler JM, Gellhaus AA, Carter JG, et al. A prospective study of the risk of an immediate adverse reaction to protamine sulfate during cardiopulmonary bypass surgery. *J Allergy Clin Immunol* 1990;85:713.
68. Grammer LC, Paterson BF, Roxe D, et al. IgE against ethylene oxide-altered human serum albumin in patients with anaphylactic reactions to dialysis. *J Allergy Clin Immunol* 1985;76:511.
69. Seggev JS, Ohta K, Tipton WR. IgE mediated anaphylaxis due to a psyllium-containing drug. *Ann Allergy* 1984;53:325.
70. Rohr AS, Pappano JE. Prophylaxis against fluorescein-induced anaphylactoid reactions. *J Allergy Clin Immunol* 1992;90:407.
71. Hamstra RD, Block MH, Schocket AL. Intravenous iron dextran in clinical medicine. *JAMA* 1980;243:1726.
72. Dykewicz MS, Rosen ST, O'Connell MM, et al. Plasma histamine but not anaphylatoxin levels correlate with generalized urticaria from infusions of antilymphocyte monoclonal antibodies. *J Lab Clin Med* 1992;120:290.
73. Dixon FJ, Vasquez JJ, Weigle WO, et al. Pathogenesis of serum sickness. *Arch Pathol* 1968;63:18.
74. Bielory L, Gascon P, Lawley TJ, et al. Human serum sickness: a prospective analysis of 35 patients treated with equine anti-thymocyte globulin for bone marrow failure. *Medicine* 1988;67:40.
75. Davidson JR, Bush RK, Grogan EW, et al. Immunology of a serum sickness/vasculitis reaction secondary to streptokinase used for acute myocardial infarction. *Clin Exp Rheumatol* 1988;6:381.
76. Erffmeyer JE. Serum sickness. *Ann Allergy* 1986;56: 105.
77. Platt R, Dreis MW, Kennedy DL, et al. Serum sickness-like reactions to amoxicillin, cefaclor, cephalexin, and trimethoprim-sulfamethoxazole. *J Infect Dis* 1988;158:474.
78. Tatum AJ, Ditto AM, Patterson R. Severe serum sickness-like reaction to oral penicillin drugs: three case reports. *Ann Allergy Asthma Immunol* 2001;36:330–334.
79. Fauci AS. Vasculitis. In: Parker CW, ed. *Clinical immunology*. Philadelphia: WB Saunders, 1980:473–519.
80. Naguwa SM, Nelson BL. Human serum sickness. *Clin Rev Allergy* 1985;3:117–126.
81. Barnett EV, Stone G, Swisher SN, et al. Serum sickness and plasmacytosis: clinical, immunologic, and hematologic analysis. *Am J Med* 1963;35:113.

82. Bielory L, Gascon P, Lawley TJ, et al. Human serum sickness: a prospective analysis of 35 patients treated with equine and thymocyte globulin for bone marrow failure. *Medicine* 1988;67:40–57.

83. Lawley TJ, Bielory L, Gascon R, et al. A prospective clinical and immunologic analysis of patients with serum sickness. *N Engl J Med* 1984;311:1407.

84. Gilliland BC. Drug-induced autoimmune and hematologic disorders. *Immunol Allergy Clin North Am* 1991;11:525.

85. Morrow JD, Schroeder HA, Perry Jr HM. Studies on the control of hypertension by hyphex. II. Toxic reactions and side effects. *Circulation* 1953;8:829.

86. Ladd AT. Procainamide-induced lupus erythematosus. *N Engl J Med* 1962;267:1357.

87. Pistiner M, Wallace DJ, Nessim S, et al. Lupus erythematosus in the 1980's: a survey of 570 patients. *Semin Arthritis Rheum* 1991;21:55.

88. Steinberg AD, Gourley MF, Klinman DM, et al. Systemic lupus erythematosus. *Ann Intern Med* 1991;115:548.

89. Lahita R, Kluger J, Drayer DE, et al. Antibodies to nuclear antigens in patients treated with procainamide or acetylprocainamide. *N Engl J Med* 1979;301:1382.

90. Stec GP, Lertora JJL, Atkinson AJ Jr, et al. Remission of procainamide-induced lupus erythematosus with N-acetylprocainamide therapy. *Ann Intern Med* 1979;90:799.

91. Blomgren SE, Condemi JJ, Bignall MC, et al. Antinuclear antibody induced by procainamide. A prospective study. *N Engl J Med* 1969;281:64.

92. Gleichmann E, Pals ST, Rolink AG, et al. Graft-versus-host reactions: clues to the etiopathology of a spectrum of immunological disease. *Immunol Today* 1984;5: 324.

93. Fauci AS. Vasculitis. *J Allergy Clin Immunol* 1983;72:211.

94. Hunder GG, Arend WP, Bloch DA, et al. The American College of Rheumatology 1990 criteria for the classification of vasculitis: introduction. *Arthritis Rheum* 1990;33:1065.

95. Arellano F, Sacristán JA. Allopurinol hypersensitivity syndrome: a review. *Ann Pharmacother* 1993;27:337.

96. Bigby M, Jick S, Jick H, et al. Drug-induced cutaneous reactions: a report from the Boston Collaborative Drug Surveillance Program on 15,438 consecutive inpatients, 1975 to 1983. *JAMA* 1986;256:3358.

97. Kauppinen K. Rational performance of drug challenge in cutaneous hypersensitivity. *Semin Dermatol* 1983;2:227.

98. Kauppinen K, Stubb S. Drug eruptions: causative agents and clinical types: a series of in-patients during a 10-year period. *Acta Derm Venereol* 1984;64:320.

99. Roujeau JC, Stern RS. Severe adverse cutaneous reactions to drugs. *N Engl J Med* 1994;331:1272.

100. Levenson DE, Arndt KA, Stern RS. Cutaneous manifestations of adverse drug reactions. *Immunol Allergy Clin North Am* 1991;11:493.

101. Alanko K, Stubb S, Kauppinen K. Cutaneous drug reactions: clinical types and causative agents. A five-year survey of in-patients (1982–1985). *Acta Derm Venereol* 1989;69:223.

102. Hedner T, Samuelsson O, Lunde H, et al. Angio-oedema in relation to treatment with angiotensin converting enzyme inhibitors. *Br Med J* 1992;304:941.

103. Orfan N, Patterson R, Dykewicz MS. Severe angioedema related to ACE inhibitors in patients with a history of idiopathic angioedema. *JAMA* 1990;264:1287.

104. Chin HL, Buchan DA. Severe angioedema after long term use of an angiotensin-converting-enzyme inhibitor. *Ann Intern Med* 1990;112:312.

105. Anderson MW, deShazo RD. Studies of the mechanism of angiotensin-converting enzyme (ACE) inhibitor-associated angioedema: the effect of an ACE inhibitor on cutaneous responses to bradykinin, codeine, and histamine. *J Allergy Clin Immunol* 1990;85:856.

106. Sharma PK, Yium JJ. Angioedema associated with angiotensin II receptor antagonist losartan. *South Med J* 1997;90:525–553.

107. Rupprecht R, Vente C, Grafe A, et al. Angiodema due to losartan. *Allergy* 1999;54:81–82.

108. Angelini G, Vena GA, Meneghini CL. Allergic contact dermatitis to some medicaments. *Contact Dermatitis* 1985;12:263.

109. Storrs FJ. Contact dermatitis caused by drugs. *Immunol Allergy Clin North Am* 1991;11:509.

110. Rudzki E, Zakrzewski Z, Rebandel P, et al. Cross reactions between aminoglycoside antibiotics. *Contact Dermatitis* 1988;18:314.

111. Elias J, Levinson A. Hypersensitivity reactions to ethylenediamine in aminophylline. *Am Rev Respir Dis* 1981;123:550.

112. Storrs FJ, Rosenthal LE, Adams RM, et al. Prevalence and relevance of allergic reactions in patients patch tested in North America—1984 to 1985. *J Am Acad Dermatol* 1989;20:1038.

113. Rietschal RL, Adams RM. Reactions to thimerosal in hepatitis B vaccines. *Dermatol Clin* 1990;8:161.

114. Fisher AA. Contact dermatitis from topical medicaments. *Semin Dermatol* 1982;1:49.

115. Stubb S, Heikkila H, Kauppinen K. Cutaneous reactions to drugs: a series of in-patients during a five-year period. *Acta Dermatol Venerol* 1994;74:289–291.

116. Sharma VK, Dhar S. Clinical pattern of cutaneous eruption among children and adolescents in North India. *Pediatr Dermatol* 1995;12:178–183.

117. Cohen HA, Barzilai A, Matalon A, et al. Fixed drug eruption of the penis due to hydroxyzine, hydrochloride. *Ann Pharmacother* 1997;31:327–329.

118. Gruber F, Stasic A, Lenkovic M, et al. Postcoital fixed drug eruption in a man sensitive to trimethoprim-sulfamethoxazole. *Clin Exp Dermatol* 1997;22:144–145.

119. Shiohara T. The interaction between keratinocytes and T cells-and overview of the role of adhesion molecules and the characterization of epidermal T cells. *J Dermatol* 1992;19:726–730.

120. Mahoob A, Haroon TS. Drugs causing fixed drug eruptions: a study of 450 cases. *Int J Dermatol* 1998;37:833–838.

121. Lee AY. Topical provocation in 31 cases of fixed drug eruptions: change of causative drugs in 10 years. *Contact Dermatitis* 1998;38:258–260.

122. Thankappan TP, Zachariah J. Drug-specific clinical pattern in fixed drug eruptions. *Int J Dermatol* 1991;30:867–870.

123. Huff JC, Weston WL, Tonnesen MG. Erythema multiforme: a critical review of characteristics, diagnostic criteria, and causes. *J Am Acad Dermatol* 1983;8:763.

124. Brice DL, Krzemien BS, Weston WL, et al. Detection of herpes simplex virus DNA in cutaneous lesions of erythema multiforme. *J Invest Dermatol* 1989;93:183.

125. Finan MC, Schroeter AL. Cutaneous immunofluorescence study of erythema multiforme: correlation with light microscopic patterns and etiologic agents. *J Am Acad Dermatol* 1984;10:497.

126. Shiohara T, Chiba M, Tanaka Y, et al. Drug-induced, photosensitive, erythema multiforme-like eruption: possible role for cell adhesion molecules in a flare induced by rhus dermatitis. *J Am Acad Dermatol* 1990;22:647–650.

127. Tonnesen MG, Harrist TJ, Wintroub BV, et al. Erythema multiforme: microvascular damage and infiltration of lymphocytes and basophils. *J Invest Dermatol* 1983;80:282.

128. Margolis RJ, Tonneson MG, Harrist TJ, et al. Lymphocyte subsets and langerhans cells/indeterminate cells in erythema multiforme. *J Invest Dermatol*1983;81:403–406.

129. Heng MCY, Allen SG. Efficacy of cyclophosphamide in toxic epidermal necrolyses. *J Am Acad Dermatol* 1991;25:778–786.

130. Miyauchi H, Losokawa H, Akaeda T, et al. T-cell subsets in drug induced toxic epidermal necrolysis. *Arch Dermatol* 1991;127:851–855.

131. Hertl M, Bohlen H, Jugert F, et al. Predominance of epidermal CD8+ T lymphocytes in bullous cutaneous reactions caused by β-lactam antibiotics. *J Invest Dermatol* 1993;101:794–799.

132. Correia O, Delgado L, Ramos JP, et al. Cutaneous T-cell recruitment in toxic epidermal necrolysis: further evidence of CD8⁺ lymphocyte involvement. *Arch Dermatol* 1993;129:466.

133. Cheriyan S, Patterson R, Greenberger PA, et al. The outcome of Stevens-Johnson syndrome treated with corticosteroids. *Allergy Proc* 1995;16:151–155.

134. Tripathi A, Ditto AM, Grammar LC, et al. Corticosteroid therapy in an additional 13 cases of Stevens-Johnson syndrome: a total series of 67 cases. *Allergy Asthma Proc* 2000;21:101–105

135. Adam JE. Exfoliative dermatitis. *Can Med Assoc J* 1968;99:661.

136. Nicolis GD, Helwig EB. Exfoliative dermatitis: a clinicopathologic study of 135 cases. *Arch Dermatol* 1973;109:682.

137. Bigby M, Stern RS, Arndt KA. Allergic cutaneous reactions to drugs. *Primary Care* 1989;16:713.

138. Epstein JH, Wintroub BV. Photosensitivity due to drugs. *Drugs* 1985;30:42.

139. Nalbandian RM, Mader IJ, Barret JL, et al. Petechiae, ecchymoses, and necrosis of skin induced by coumarin congeners. *JAMA* 1965;192:603.

140. Bauer KA. Coumarin-induced skin necrosis. *Arch Dermatol* 1993;129:766.

141. Goldstein SM, Wintroub BW, Elias PM, et al. Toxic epidermal necrolysis: unmuddying the waters. *Arch Dermatol* 1987;123:1153.

142. Roujeau JC, Huynh TN, Bracq C, et al. Genetic susceptibility to toxic epidermal necrolysis. *Arch Dermatol* 1987;123:1171.

143. Viard I, Wehrli P, Bullani R, et al. Inhibition of toxic epidermal necrolysis by blockade of CD95 with human intravenous immunoglobulin. *Science* 1998;282:490–493.

144. Amon RB, Dimond RL. Toxic epidermal necrolysis: rapid differentiation between staphylococcal-induced disease and drug-induced disease. *Arch Dermatol* 1975;111:1433.

145. Bastuji-Garin S, Rzany B, Stern RS, et al. Clinical classification of cases of toxic epidermal necrolysis, Stevens-Johnson syndrome, and erythema multiforme. *Arch Dermatol* 1993;129:92.

146. Heinbach DM, Engrav LH, Marvin JA, et al. Toxic epidermal necrolysis: a step forward in treatment. *JAMA* 1987;257:2171.

147. Guillaume J-C, Ronjeau J-C, Revoz J, et al. The culprit drugs in 87 cases of toxic epidermal necrolysis (Lyell's syndrome). *Arch Dermatol* 1987;123:1166.

148. Stern RS, Chan HL. Usefulness of case report literature in determining drugs responsible for toxic epidermal necrolysis. *J Am Dermatol* 1989;21:317.

149. Twarog FG. Hypersensitivity to pancreatic extracts in parents of patients with cystic fibrosis. *J Allergy Clin Immunol* 1977;59:35.

150. Pozner LH, Mandarano C, Zitt MJ, et al. Recurrent bronchospasm in a nurse. *Ann Allergy* 1986;56:14.

151. Coutts II, Dally MB, Newman Taylor AJ, et al. Asthma in workers manufacturing cephalosporins. *Br Med J* 1981;283:95.

152. Hunt LW, Rosenow EC III. Asthma-producing drugs. *Ann Allergy* 1992;68:453.

153. Mecker DP, Wiedemann HP. Drug-induced bronchospasm. *Clin Chest Med* 1990;11:163.

154. Fraley DS, Bruns FJ, Segel DP, et al. Propanolol-related bronchospasm in patients without a history of asthma. *South Med J* 1980;73:238.

155. Lunde H, Herdner T, Samuelson O, et al. Dyspnea, asthma, and bronchoconstriction in relation to treatment with angiotensin converting enzyme inhibitors. *Br Med J* 1994;308:18.

156. Simon SR, Black HR, Moser M, et al. Cough and ACE inhibitors. *Arch Intern Med* 1992;152:1698.

157. Pylypchuk GB. ACE inhibitor versus angiotensin II blocker-induced cough and angioedema. *Ann Pharmacother* 1998;32:1060–1066.

158. Lacourciere Y, Lefebvre J, Nakhle G, et al. Association between cough and angiotensin converting enzyme inhibitors versus angiotensin II antagonists: the design of a prospective, controlled study. *J Hypertens* 1994;12:S49.

159. Israili ZH, Hall WD. Cough and angioneurotic edema associated with angiotensin-converting enzyme inhibitor therapy: a review of the literature and pathophysiology. *Ann Intern Med* 1992;117:234.

160. Bush RK, Taylor SL, Holden K, et al. Prevalence of sensitivity to sulfiting agents in asthmatic patients. *Am J Med* 1986;81:816.

161. Goldfarb G, Simon RA. Provocation of sulfite sensitive asthma. *J Allergy Clin Immunol* 1984;73:135.

162. Simon RA, Stevenson DD. Lack of cross sensitivity between aspirin and sulfite in sensitive asthmatics. *J Allergy Clin Immunol* 1987;79:257.

163. Pisani RJ, Rosenow EC III. Drug-induced pulmonary disease. In: Simmons DH, Tierney DF, eds. *Current pulmonology.* Vol. 13. St. Louis: Mosby–Year Book, 1992:311.

164. Holmberg L, Boman G, Bottiger IE, et al. Adverse reactions to nitrofurantoin: analysis of 921 reports. *Am J Med* 1980;69:733.

165. Sostman HD, Matthay RA, Putman CE, et al. Methotrexate-induced pneumonitis. *Medicine* 1976;55: 371.

166. Martin WJ II, Rosenow EC III. Amiodarone pulmonary toxicity. Part I. *Chest* 1988;93:1067.

167. Kennedy JI. Clinical aspects of amiodarone pulmonary toxicity. *Clin Chest Med* 1990;11:119.

168. Manicardi V, Bernini G, Bossini P, et al. Low-dose amiodarone-induced pneumonitis: evidence of an immunologic pathogenic mechanism. *Am J Med* 1989;86:134.

169. Kennedy JI, Myers JL, Plumb VJ, et al. Amiodarone pulmonary toxicity: clinical, radiologic, and pathologic correlations. *Arch Intern Med* 1987;147:50.

170. Evans RB, Ettensohn DB, Fawaz-Estrup F, et al. Gold lung: recent developments in pathogenesis, diagnosis, and therapy. *Semin Arthritis Rheumatol* 1987;16:196.

171. Cooper JAD Jr, White DA, Matthay RA. Drug-induced pulmonary disease. Part 1. Cytotoxic drugs. *Am Rev Respir Dis* 1986;133:321.

172. Holoye P, Luna M, Mackay B, et al. Bleomycin hypersensitivity pneumonitis. *Ann Intern Med* 1978;88:47.

173. Kavaru MS, Ahmad M, Amirthalingam KN. Hydrochlorothiazide-induced acute pulmonary edema. *Cleve Clin J Med* 1990;57:181.

174. Kline JN, Hirasuna JD. Pulmonary edema after free-base cocaine smoking—not due to an adulterant. *Chest* 1990;97:1009.

175. Brashear RE. Effects of heroin, morphine, methadone, and propoxyphene on the lung. *Semin Respir Med* 1980;2:59.

176. Heffner JE, Sahn SA. Salicylate-induced pulmonary edema: clinical features and prognosis. *Ann Intern Med* 1981;95:405.

177. Andersson BS, Luna MA, Yee C, et al. Fatal pulmonary failure complicating high-dose cytosine arabinoside therapy in acute leukemia. *Cancer* 1990;65:1079.

178. Ramesh S, Reisman RE. Noncardiogenic pulmonary edema due to radiocontrast media. *Ann Allergy Asthma Immunol* 1995;75:308–310.

179. Spry CJF. Eosinophilia and allergic reactions to drugs. *Clin Haematol* 1980;9:521.

180. Davis P. Significance of eosinophilia during gold therapy. *Arthritis Rheumatol* 1974;17:964.

181. Stafford BT, Crosby WH. Late onset of gold-induced thrombocytopenia. *JAMA* 1978;239:50.

182. Shulman NR. A mechanism of cell destruction in individuals sensitized to foreign antigens and its implications in autoimmunity. *Ann Intern Med* 1964;60:506.

183. Stricker RB, Shuman MA. Quinidine purpura: evidence that glycoprotein V is a target platelet antigen. *Blood* 1986;67:1377.

184. Chong BH. Heparin-induced thrombocytopenia. *Blood Rev* 1988;2:108.

185. Chong BH, Fawaz I, Cade J, et al. Heparin-induced thrombocytopenia: studies with a new low molecular weight heparinoid, Org 10172. *Blood* 1989;73:1592.

186. Salama A, Mueller-Eckhardt C. On the mechanisms of sensitization and attachment of antibodies to RBC in drug-induced immune hemolytic anemia. *Blood* 1987;69:1006.

187. Swanson MA, Chanmougan D, Swartz RS. Immunohemolytic anemia due to antipenicillin antibodies. *N Engl J Med* 1966;274:178.

188. Worlledge SM, Carstairs KC, Dacie JV. Autoimmune hemolytic anemia associated with alpha-methyldopa therapy. *Lancet* 1966;2:135.

189. Vincent PC. Drug-induced aplastic anemia and agranulocytosis incidence and mechanisms. *Drugs* 1986;31:52.

190. Kaufman DW, Kelly JP, Jurgelon JM, et al. Drugs in the aetiology of agranulocytosis and aplastic anemia. *Eur J Haematol* 1996;60:23–30.

191. Willson RA. The liver: its role in drug biotransformation and as a target of immunologic injury. *Immunol Allergy Clin North Am* 1991;11:555.

192. Lewis JH, Zimmerman HJ. Drug-induced liver disease. *Med Clin North Am* 1989;73:775.

193. Black M. Acetaminophen hepatotoxicity. *Ann Rev Med* 1984;34:577.

194. Zimmerman HJ, Lewis JH. Drug-induced cholestasis. *Med Toxicol* 1987;2:112.

195. Mitchell JR, Zimmerman HJ, Ishak KG, et al. Isoniazid liver injury: clinical spectrum, pathology and probable pathogenesis. *Ann Intern Med* 1976;84:181.

196. Kenna JG, Neuberger JM, Williams R. Evidence for expression in human liver of halothane induced neoantigens recognized by antibodies in sera from patients with halothane hepatitis. *Hepatology* 1988;8:1635.

197. Christ DD, Kenna JG, Satoh H, et al. Enflurane metabolism produces covalently bound liver adducts recognized by antibodies from patients with halothane hepatitis. *Anesthesiology* 1988;69:833.

198. Knobler H, Levij IS, Gavish D, et al. Quinidine-induced hepatitis: a common and reversible hypersensitivity reaction. *Arch Intern Med* 1986;146:526.

199. Zimmerman HJ. Drug-induced chronic hepatic disease. *Med Clin North Am* 1979;63:567.

200. Boulton-Jones M, Sissons JGP, Nash PF, et al. Self-induced glomerulonephritis. *Br Med J* 1974;3:387.

201. Treser G, Cherubin C, Longergan ET, et al. Renal lesions in narcotic addicts. *Am J Med* 1974;57:687.

202. Sternlieb I, Bennett B, Scheinberg H. D-penicillamine induced Goodpasture's syndrome in Wilson's disease. *Ann Intern Med* 1975;82:673.

203. Silverberg DS, Kidd EG, Shnilka TK, et al. Gold nephropathy: a clinical and pathological study. *Arthritis Rheumatol* 1970;13:812.

204. Case DB. Proteinuria during long-term captopril therapy. *JAMA* 1980;244:346.

205. Kleinknecht D, Vanhille P, Morel-Maroger L, et al. Acute interstitial nephritis due to drug hypersensitivity: an up-to-date review with a report of 19 cases. *Adv Nephrol* 1983;12:277.

206. Porile JL, Bakris GL, Garella S. Acute interstitial nephritis with glomerulopathy due to nonsteroidal anti-inflammatory agents: a review of its clinical spectrum and effects of steroid therapy. *J Clin Pharmacol* 1990;30:468.

207. Galpin JE, Shinaberger JH, Stanley TM, et al. Acute interstitial nephritis due to methicillin. *Am J Med* 1978;65:755.

208. Charleswarth, EN. Phenytoin induced pseudolymphomasyndrome: an immunologic study. *Arch Dermatol* 1977;113:477.

209. McCarthy LJ, Aguilar JC, Ransberg R. Fatal benign phenytoin lymphadenopathy. *Arch Intern Med* 1979;139:367.

210. Tomecki KH, Catalano CJ. Dapsone hypersensitivity. *Arch Dermatol* 1981;117:38.

211. Fenoglio JJ Jr, McAllister HA Jr, Mullick FG. Drug related myocarditis. I. Hypersensitivity myocarditis. *Hum Pathol* 1981;12:900.

212. Taliercio CP, Olney BA, Lie JT. Myocarditis related to drug hypersensitivity. *Mayo Clin Proc* 1985;60:463.

213. Kounis NG, Zavras GM, Soufras GD, et al. Hypersensitivity myocarditis. *Ann Allergy* 1989;62:71.

214. Ten RM, Klein JS, Frigas E. Allergy skin testing. *Mayo Clinic Proc* 1995;70:783.

215. Adkinson NF Jr. Diagnosis of immunologic drug reactions. *N Engl Rev Allergy Proc* 1984;5:104.

216. Calkin JM, Maibach HI. Delayed hypersensitivity drug reactions diagnosed by patch testing. *Contact Dermatitis* 1993;29:223.

217. Patterson R. Diagnosis and treatment of drug allergy. *J Allergy Clin Immunol* 1988;81:380.

218. Baldo BA, Harle DG. Drug allergenic determinants. *Monogr Allergy* 1990;28:11.

219. Weiss ME, Nyham D, Zhikang P, et al. Association of protamine IgE and IgG antibodies with life-threatening reactions to intravenous protamine. *N Engl J Med* 1989;320:886.

220. Dobozy A, Hunyadi J, Kenderessy ASZ, et al. Lymphocyte transformation test in the detection of drug hypersensitivity. *Clin Exp Dermatol* 1981;6:367.

221. Livini E, Halevy S, Stahl B, et al. The appearance of macrophage migration–inhibition factor in drug reactions. *J Allergy Clin Immunol* 1987;80:843.

222. Kalish RS, LaPorte A, Wood JA, et al. Sulfonamide-reactive lymphocytes detected at very low frequency in the peripheral blood of patients with drug-induced eruptions. *J Allergy Clin Immunol* 1994;94:465.

223. Schwartz LB. Tryptase, a mediator of human mast cells. *J Allergy Clin Immunol* 1990;86:594.

224. Appel GB. A decade of penicillin related acute intersititial nephritis: more questions than answers. *Clin Nephrol* 1980;13:151.

225. Rosenthal A. Followup study of fatal penicillin reactions. *JAMA* 1959;167:118.

226. Singer JZ, Wallace SL. The allopurinol hypersensitivity syndrome: unnecessary morbidity and mortality. *Arthritis Rheumatol* 1986;29:82.

227. Lawson DH, Jick H. Drug prescribing in hospitals: an international comparison. *Am J Public Health* 1976;66:644.

228. Pau AK, Morgan JE, Terlingo A. Drug allergy documentation by physicians, nurses, and medical students. *Am J Hosp Pharmacol* 1989;46:570.

229. Kuehm SL, Doyle MJ. Medication errors: 1977–1988. Experience in medical malpractice claims. *N J Med* 1990;87:27.

230. Blanca M, Fernandez J, Miranda A, et al. Cross-reactivity between penicillins and cephalosporins: clinical and immunologic studies. *J Allergy Clin Immunol* 1989;83:381–385.

231. Hanaford PC. Adverse drug reaction cards carried by patients. *Br Med J* 1986;292:1109.

232. Altman LC, Petersen PE. Successful prevention of an anaphylactoid reaction to iron dextran. *Ann Intern Med* 1988;109:346.

233. Chandler MJ, Ong RC, Grammer LC, et al. Detection, characterization, and desensitization of IgE to streptomycin. *J Allergy Clin Immunol* 1992;89:178.

234. Anné S, Middleton E Jr, Reisman RE. Vancomycin anaphylaxis and successful desensitization. *Ann Allergy* 1994;73:402.

235. Webster E, Panush RS. Allopurinol hypersensitivity in a patient with severe, chronic tophaceous gout. *Arthritis Rheumatol* 1985;28:707.

Part B: Allergic Reactions to Individual Drugs: Low Molecular Weight

1. Chandler MJ, Ong RC, Grammer LC, et al. Detection, characterization, and desensitization of IgE to streptomycin. *J Allergy Clin Immunol* 1992;89:178.

2. Anné S, Middleton E Jr, Reisman RE. Vancomycin anaphylaxis and successful desensitization. *Ann Allergy* 1994;73:402.

3. Greenberger PA. Desensitization and test-dosing for the drug-allergic patient. *Ann Allergy Asthma Immunol* 2000;85:250–251.

4. Kowalski ML. Management of aspirin-sensitive rhinosinusitis-asthma syndrome: what role for aspirin desensitization? *Allergy Proc* 1992;13:175–184.

5. Patterson R, DeSwarte RD, Greenberger PA, et al. Drug allergy and protocols for management of drug allergies. *Allergy Proc* 1994;15:239–264.

6. Bernstein IL, Gruchalla RS, Lee RE, et al. Disease management of drug hypersensitivity: a practice parameter. *Ann Allergy Asthma Immunol* 1999;83:665–700.

7. Webster E, Panush RS. Allopurinol hypersensitivity in a patient with severe, chronic tophaceous gout. *Arthritis Rheumatol* 1985;28:707.

8. Patterson R. Diagnosis and treatment of drug allergy. *J Allergy Clin Immunol* 1988;81:380.

9. DeSwarte RD, Patterson R. Drug allergy. In: Patterson R, Grammer LC, Greenberger PA, eds. *Allergic diseases: diagnosis and management.* 5th ed. Philadelphia: Lippincott-Raven 1997:317–412.

10. Adkinson NF Jr. Drug allergy. In: Middleton E Jr, Reed CE, Ellis EF, et al, eds. *Allergy: principles and practice.* 5th ed. St Louis: CV Mosby, 1998:1212–1224.

11. deShazo RD, Kemp SF. Allergic reactions to drugs and biologic agents. *JAMA* 1997;278:1895–1906.

12. Greenberger PA. Drug allergies. In: Rich RR, Fleisher TA, Schwartz BD, et al, eds. Clinical immunology: principles and practice. St. Louis: Mosby–Year Book, 1996:988.

13. Lee CE, Zembower TR, Fotis MA, et al. The incidence of antimicrobial allergies in hospitalized patients: implications regarding prescribing patterns and emerging bacterial resistance. *Arch Intern Med* 2000;160:2819–2899.

14. Sullivan TJ, Wedner HJ, Shatz GS, et al. Skin testing to detect penicillin allergy. *J Allergy Clin Immunol* 1981;68:171–180.

15. Solensky R, Earl HS, Gruchalla RS. Penicillin allergy: prevalence of vague history in skin test-positive patients. *Ann Allergy Asthma Immunol* 2000;85:195–199.

16. Shepherd GM. Allergy to B-Lactam antibiotics. *Immunol Allergy Clin North Am* 1991;11:611.

17. Idsoe O, Guthe T, Willcox RR, et al. Nature and extent of penicillin side-reactions with particular reference to fatalities from anaphylactic shock. *Bull WHO* 1968;38:159.

18. Neugut AI, Ghatak AT, Miller RL. Anaphylaxis in the

United States: an investigation into its epidemiology. *Arch Intern Med* 2001;161:15–21.

19. Weiss ME, Adkinson NF Jr. Immediate hypersensitivity reactions to penicillin and related antibiotics. *Clin Allergy* 1988;18:515.

20. Jerath Tatum A, Ditto AM, Patterson R. Severe serum sickness-like reaction to oral penicillin drugs: three case reports. *Ann Allergy Asthma Immunol* 2001;86:330–334.

21. Mackowiak PA, LeMaistre CF. Drug fever: a critical appraisal of conventional concepts. An analysis of 51 episodes in two Dallas hospitals and 97 episodes reported in the English literature. *Ann Intern Med* 1987;106:728–733.

22. Levenson DE, Arndt KA, Stern RS. Cutaneous manifestations of adverse drug reactions. *Immunol Allergy Clin North Am* 1991;11:493.

23. Wintroub BV, Stern R. Cutaneous drug reactions: pathogenesis and clinical classification. *J Am Acad Dermatol* 1985;13:167.

24. Platt R, Dreis MW, Kennedy DL, et al. Serum sickness-like reactions to amoxicillin, cefaclor, cephalexin, and trimethoprim-sulfamethoxazole. *J Infect Dis* 1988;158:474.

25. Joubert GI, Hadad K, Matsui D, et al. Selection of treatment of cefaclor-associated urticarial, serum sickness-like reactions and erythema multiforme by emergency pediatricians: lack of a uniform standard of care. *Can J Clin Pharmacol* 1999;6:197–201.

26. Grouhi M, Hummel D, Roifman CM. Anaphylactic reaction to oral cefaclor in a child. *Pediatrics* 1999;103:e50.

27. Pumphrey RSH, Davis S. Under-reporting of antibiotic anaphylaxis may put patients at risk. *Lancet* 1999;353:1157–1158.

28. Neu HD. The new beta-lactamase-stable cephalosporins. *Ann Intern Med* 1982;97:408.

29. Erffmeyer JE. Reactions to antibiotics. *Immunol Allergy Clin North Am* 1992;12:633.

30. Silviu-Dan F, McPhillips S, Warrington RJ. The frequency of skin test reactions to side-chain penicillin determinants. *J Allergy Clin Immunol* 1993;91:694.

31. Gonzalez J, Miranda A, Martin A, et al. Sensitivity to amoxycillin with good tolerance to penicillin. *J Allergy Clin Immunol* 1988;81:222(abst).

32. Harris AD, Sauberman L, Kabbash L, et al. Penicillin skin testing: a way to optimize antibiotic utilization. *Am J Med* 1999;107:166–168.

33. Arroliga ME, Wagner W, Bobek MB, et al. A pilot study of penicillin skin testing in patients with a history of penicillin allergy admitted to a medical ICU. *Chest* 2000;188:1106–1108.

34. Perencevich EN, Weller PF, Samore MH, et al. Benefits of negative penicillin skin test results persist during subsequent hospital admissions. *Clin Infect Dis* 2001;32:317–319.

35. Grieco MH. Cross-allergenicity of the penicillins and the cephalosporins. *Arch Intern Med* 1967;119:141.

36. Petz L. Immunologic cross-reactivity between penicillins and cephalosporins: a review. *J Infect Dis* 1978;137:574.

37. Blanca M, Fernandez J, Miranda A, et al. Cross-reactivity between penicillins and cephalosporins: clinical and immunological studies. *J Allergy Clin Immunol* 1989;83:381–385.

38. Anné S, Reisman RE. Risk of administering cephalosporin antibiotics to patients with histories of penicillin allergy. *Ann Allergy Asthma Immunol* 1995;74:167–170.

39. Moskovitz BL. Clinical adverse effects during ceftriaxone therapy. *Am J Med* 1984;8:84–88.

40. Saxon A, Beal GN, Rohr AS, et al. Immediate hypersensitivity reactions to B-lactam antibiotics. *Ann Intern Med* 1987;107:204.

41. Igea JM, Fraj J, Davila I, et al. Allergy to cefazolin: study of in vivo cross reactivity with other beta lactams. *Ann Allergy* 1992;68:515.

42. Saxon A, Adelman DC, Patel A, et al. Imipenem cross-reactivity with penicillin in humans. *J Allergy Clin Immunol* 1988;82:213.

43. Chen Z, Baur X, Kutscha-Lissberg F, et al. IgE-mediated anaphylactic reaction to imipenem. *Allergy* 2000;55:92–99.

44. Adkinson NF Jr. Immunogenicity and cross-allergenicity of aztreonam. *Am J Med* 1990;88:125.

45. Fernandez-Rivas M, Carral CP, Cuevas M, et al. Selective allergic reactions to clavulanic acid. *J Allergy Clin Immunol* 1995;95:748.

46. Hoffman DR, Hudson P, Carlyle SJ, et al. Three cases of fatal anaphylaxis to antibiotics in patients with prior histories of allergy to the drug. *Ann Allergy* 1989;62:91.

47. Sogn D, Evans R III, Shepherd G et al. Results of the NIAID collaborative clinical trial to test the predictive value of skin testing with major and minor penicillin derivatives in hospitalized adults. *Arch Intern Med* 1992;152:1025.

48. Greenberger PA. Patterns of anti-penicillin IgE antibodies in 634 penicillin allergic patients. *J Inv Med* 2001;49:303A.

49. Warrington RJ, Simons FER, Ho HW, et al. Diagnosis of penicillin allergy by skin testing: the Manitoba experience. *Can Med Assoc J* 1978;118:787.

50. Lin R. A perspective on penicillin allergy. *Arch Intern Med* 1992;152:930.

51. Adkinson NF Jr. Side-chain specific beta-lactam allergy. *Clin Exp Allergy* 1990;20:445.

52. Mendelson LM, Ressler C, Rosen JP, et al. Routine elective penicillin allergy skin testing in children and adolescents: study of sensitization. *J Allergy Clin Immunol* 1984;73:76.

53. Parker PJ, Parrinello JT, Condemi JJ, et al. Penicillin resensitization among hospitalized patients. *J Allergy Clin Immunol* 1991;88:213.

54. Bittner A, Greenberger PA. Incidence of penicillin resensitization in penicillin allergic patients. *J Allergy Clin Immunol* (in press).

55. Segreti J, Trenholme GM, Levin S. Antibiotic therapy in the allergic patient. *Med Clin North Am* 1995;79:935.

56. Bochner BS, Lichtenstein LM: Anaphylaxis. *N Engl J Med* 1991;324:1785.

57. Sullivan T, Yecies L, Shatz G, et al. Desensitization of patients allergic to penicillin using orally administered B-lactam antibiotics. *J Allergy Clin Immunol* 1982;69:275.

58. Borish L, Tamir R, Rosenwasser L. Intravenous desensitization to beta-lactam antibiotics. *J Allergy Clin Immunol* 1987;80:314.

59. Stark BJ, Earl HS, Gross GN, et al. Acute and chronic desensitization of penicillin-allergic patients using oral penicillin. *J Allergy Clin Immunol* 1987;79:523.

60. Brown LA, Goldberg ND, Shearer WT. Long-term ticarcillin desensitization by the continuous oral administration of penicillin. *J Allergy Clin Immunol* 1982;69:51.

61. Carrington DM, Earl HS, Sullivan TJ. Studies of human IgE to a sulfonamide determinant. *J Allergy Clin Immunol* 1987;79:442.

62. Gruchalla RS, Sullivan TJ. Detection of human IgE to sulfamethoxazole by skin testing with sulfamethoxazoyl-poly-L-tyrosine. *J Allergy Clin Immunol* 1991;88:784.

63. Shear NH, Spielberg SP, Grant DM, et al. Differences in metabolism of sulfonamides predisposing to idiosyncratic toxicity. *Ann Intern Med* 1986;105:179–184.

64. Rieder MJ, Vetrecht J, Shear NH, et al. Diagnosis of sulfonamide hypersensitivity reactions by *in vitro* "rechallenge" with hydroxylamine metabolites. *Ann Intern Med* 1989;110:286–289.

65. Carr A, Tindall B, Penny R, et al. *In vitro* cytotoxicity as a marker of hypersensitivity to sulphamethoxazole in patients with HIV. *Clin Exp Immunol* 1993;94:21.

66. Bayard PJ, Berger TG, Jacobson MA. Drug hypersensitivity reactions and human immunodeficiency virus disease. *J Acquir Immune Defic Syndr* 1992;5:1237.

67. Ryan CJ, McGeehan M, Graziano FM. Current controversies in the management of allergic disease in HIV-Positive patients. *Canadian J Allergy Clin Immunol* 1999;4:66–73.

68. Jick H. Adverse reactions to trimethoprim-sulfamethoxazole in hospitalized patients. *Rev Infect Dis* 1986;4:426.

69. Carr A, Cooper DA, Penny R. Allergic manifestations of human immunodeficiency virus infection. *J Clin Immunol* 1991;11:52.

70. Kovacs JA, Hiemenz JW, Macher AM, et al. *Pneumocystis carinii* pneumonia: a comparison between patients with the acquired immunodeficiency syndrome and patients with other immunodeficiencies. *Ann Intern Med* 1984;100:663–671.

71. Colebunders R, Izaley L, Bila K, et al. Cutaneous reactions to trimethoprim-sulfamethoxazole in African patients with acquired immunodeficiency syndrome. *Ann Intern Med* 1987;107:599.

72. Bijl AM, Van Der Klauw MM, Van Vliet AC, et al. Anaphylactic reactions associated with trimethoprim. *Clin Exp Allergy* 1998;28:510–512.

73. Cabañas R, Caballero M T, Veta A, et al. Anaphylaxis to trimethoprim. *J Allergy Clin Immunol* 1996;97:137–138.

74. Alonso MD, Marcos C, Dávilla I, et al. Hypersensitivity to trimethoprim. *Allergy* 1992;47:340–342.

75. Sattler FR, Cowan R, Nielson DM, et al. Trimethoprim-sulfamethoxazole with pentamidine for treatment of *Pneumocystis carinii* pneumonia in the acquired immunodeficiency syndrome. *Ann Intern Med* 1988;109:280.

76. Montgomery AB, Feigal DW Jr, Sattler F, et al. Pentamidine aerosol versus trimethoprim-sulfamethoxazole for Pneumocystis carinii in acquired immune deficiency syndrome. *Am J Respir Crit Care Med* 1995;151:1068–1074.

77. Greenberger PA, Patterson R. Management of drug allergy in patients with acquired immunodeficiency syndrome. *J Allergy Clin Immunol* 1987;79:484.

78. Absar N, Daneshvar H, Beall G. Desensitization to trimethoprim/sulfamethoxazole in HIV-infected patients. *J Allergy Clin Immunol* 1994;93:1001.

79. White MV, Haddad ZH, Brunner E, et al. Desensitization to trimethoprim-sulfamethoxazole in patients with acquired immunodeficiency syndrome and *Pneumocystis carinii* pneumonia. *Ann Allergy* 1989;62:177.

80. Yoshizawa S, Yasuoka A, Kikuchi Y, et al. A 5-day course of oral desensitization to trimethoprim/sulfamethoxazole (T/S) is successful in patients with human immunodeficiency virus type-1 infection who were previously intolerant to T/S but had no sulfamethoxazole-specific IgE. *Ann Allergy Asthma Immunol* 2000;85:241–244.

81. Baum CG, Sonnabend JA, O'Sullivan M. Prophylaxis of AIDS-related *Pneumocystis carinii* pneumonia with aerosolized pentamidine in a patient with hypersensitivity to systemic pentamidine. *J Allergy Clin Immunol* 1992;90:268.

82. Sher MR, Suchar C, Lockey RF. Anaphylactic shock induced by oral desensitization to trimethoprim/sulfamethoxazole (TMP/SMZ). *J Allergy Clin Immunol* 1986;77:133.

83. Wright DN, Nelson RP, Ledford DK, et al. Serum IgE and human immunodeficiency virus (HIV) infection. *J Allergy Clin Immunol* 1990;85:445.

84. Finegold I. Oral desensitization to trimethoprim-sulfamethoxazole in a patient with AIDS. *J Allergy Clin Immunol* 1985;75:137.

85. Hughes WT. Successful intermittent chemoprophylaxis for *Pneumocystis carinii* pneumonitis. *N Engl J Med* 1987;316:1627.

86. Martin MA, Cox PH, Beck K, et al. A comparison of the effectiveness of three regimens in the prevention of *Pneumocystis carinii* pneumonia in human immunodeficiency virus-infected patients. *Arch Intern Med* 1992;152:523.

87. Boxer MB, Dykewicz MS, Patterson R, et al. The management of patients with sulfonamide allergy. *N Engl Reg Allergy Proc* 1988;9:219.

88. Yango MC, Kim K, Evans R III. Oral desensitization to trimethoprim-sulfamethoxazole in pediatric patients. *Immunol Allergy Pract* 1992;14:56.

89. Caballer BH, Fernandez-Rivas M, Lazaro JF, et al. Management of sulfadiazine allergy in patients with acquired immunodeficiency syndrome. *J Allergy Clin Immunol* 1991;88:137.

90. Caballer BH, Fernandez-Rivas M, Lazaro JF, et al. Management of sulfadiazine allergy in patients with acquired immunodeficiency syndrome. *J Allergy Clin Immunol* 1991;88:137.

91. Belchí-Hernández J, Espinosa-Parra FJ. Management of adverse reactions to prophylactic trimethoprim-sulfamethoxazole in patients with human immunodeficiency virus infection. *Ann Allergy Asthma Immunol* 1996;76:355–358.

92. Kalanadhabhatta V, Muppidi D, Sahni H, et al. Successful oral desensitization to trimethoprim-sulfamethoxazole in acquired immune deficiency syndrome. *Ann Allergy Asthma Immunol* 1996;77:394–400.

93. Gluckstein D, Ruskin J. Rapid oral desensitization to trimethoprim-sulfamethoxazole (TMP-SMZ): use in prophylaxis for Pneumocystis carinii pneumonia in

patients with AIDS who were previously intolerant to TMP-SMZ. *Clin Infect Dis* 1995;20:849–853.

94. Duque S, de la Puente J, Rodríguez F. Zidovudine-related erythroderma and successful desensitization: a case report. *J Allergy Clin Immunol* 1996;98:234–235.

95. Douglas R, Spelman D, Czarny D, et al. Successful desensitization of two patients who previously developed Stevens-Johnson syndrome while receiving trimethoprim-sulfamethoxazole. *Clin Infect Dis* 1997;25:1480.

96. Meyers S, Sachar DB, Present DH, et al. Olsalazine sodium in the treatment of ulcerative colitis among patients intolerant of sulfasalazine: a prospective, randomized, placebo-controlled, double-blind, dose-ranging clinical trial. *Gastroenterology* 1987;93:1255.

97. Purdy BH, Philips DM, Summers RW. Desensitization for sulfasalazine rash. *Ann Intern Med* 1984;100:512.

98. Earl HS, Sullivan TJ. Acute desensitization of a patient with cystic fibrosis allergic to both B-lactam and aminoglycoside antibiotics. *J Allergy Clin Immunol* 1987;79:477.

99. Chandler MJ, Ong RC, Grammer LC, et al. Detection, characterization, and desensitization of IgE to streptomycin. *J Allergy Clin Immunol* 1992;89:178.

100. Polk RE, Healy DP, Schwartz LB, et al. Vancomycin and the red man syndrome: pharmacodynamics of histamine release. *J Infect Dis* 1988;157:502–507.

101. Lin RY. Desensitization in the management of vancomycin hypersensitivity. *Arch Intern Med* 1990;150:2197–2198.

102. Alexander II, Greenberger PA. Vancomycin-induced Stevens-Johnson syndrome. *Allergy Asthma Proc* 1996;17:75–78.

103. Forrence EA, Goldman MP. Vancomycin-associated exfoliative dermatitis. *DICP Ann Pharmacother* 1990;24:369–371.

104. Davis H, McGoodwin E, Reed TG. Anaphylactoid reactions reported after treatment with ciprofloxacin. *Ann Intern Med* 1989;111:1041.

105. Smythe MA, Cappelletty DM. Anaphylactoid reaction to levofloxacin. *Pharmacotherapy* 2000;20:1520–1523.

106. Palchick BA, Fink EA, McEntire JE, et al. Anaphylaxis due to chloramphenicol. *Am J Med Sci* 1984;288:43.

107. Gallardo M, Thomas I. Hypersensitivity reaction to erythromycin. *Cutis* 1999;64:375–376.

108. Jorro G, Morales C, Brasó JV, et al. Anaphylaxis to erythromycin. *Ann Allergy Asthma Immunol* 1996;77:456–458.

109. Yeu WW, Chau CH, Lee J, et al. Cholestatic hepatitis in a patient who received clarithromycin therapy for a *M. chelonae* lung infection. *Clin Infect Dis* 1994;18:1025.

110. Mazur N, Greenberger PA, Regalado J. Clindamycin hypersensitivity appears to be rare. *Ann Allergy Asthma Immunol* 1999;82:443–445.

111. Kurohara ML, Kwong FK, Lebherz TB, et al. Metronidazole hypersensitivity and oral desensitization. *J Allergy Clin Immunol* 1991;88:279

112. Kemp SF, Lockey RF. Amphotericin B: emergency challenge in a neutropenic, asthmatic patient with fungal sepsis. *J Allergy Clin Immunol* 1995;96:425.

113. Kauffman CA, Wiseman SW. Anaphylaxis upon switching lipid-containing amphotericin B formulations. *Clin Infect Dis* 1998;26:1237–1238.

114. Schneider P, Klein RM, Dietze L, et al. Anaphylactic reaction to liposomal amphotericin (Ambisome). *Br J Haematol* 1998;102:1107–1111.

115. Bittleman DB, Stapleton J, Casale TB. Report of successful desensitization to itraconazole. *J Allergy Clin Immunol* 1994;94:270.

116. Carr A, Penny R, Cooper DA. Allergy and desensitization to zidovudine in patients with acquired immunodeficiency syndrome (AIDS). *J Allergy Clin Immunol* 1993;91:683.

117. Kainer MA, Mijch A. Anaphylactoid reaction, angioedema and urticaria associated with lamivudine. *Lancet* 1996;348:1519.

118. Small PM, Schecter GF, Goodman PC, et al. Treatment of tuberculosis in patients with advanced human immunodeficiency virus infection. *N Engl J Med* 1991;234:289–294.

119. Wurtz RM, Abrams D, Becker S, et al. Anaphylactoid drug reactions due to ciprofloxacin and rifampicin in HIV-infected patients. *Lancet* 1989;1:955–956.

120. Moseley EK, Sullivan TJ. Allergic reactions to antimicrobial drugs in patients with a history of prior drug allergy. *J Allergy Clin Immunol* 1991;87:226.

121. Lumry WR, Curd JG, Zeiger RS, et al. Aspirin sensitive rhinosinusitis: the clinical syndrome and effects of aspirin administration. *J Allergy Clin Immunol* 1983;71:588.

122. Butterfield JH, Kao PC, Klee GG, et al. Aspirin idiosyncrasy in systemic mast cell disease: a new look at mediator release during aspirin desensitization. *Mayo Clin Proc* 1995;70:481.

123. Giraldo B, Blumenthal MN, Spink WW. Aspirin intolerance and asthma: a clinical and immunological study. *Ann Intern Med* 1969;71:479.

124. Spector SL, Wangaard CH, Farr RS. Aspirin and concomitant idiosyncrasies in adult asthmatic patients. *J Allergy Clin Immunol* 1979;64:500.

125. Weber RW, Hoffman M, Raine DA Jr, et al. Incidence of bronchoconstriction due to aspirin, azo dyes, non-azo-dyes and preservatives in a population of perennial asthmatics. *J Allergy Clin Immunol* 1979;64:32.

126. Pleskow WW, Stevenson DD, Mathison DA, et al. Aspirin-sensitive rhinosinusitis/asthma: spectrum of adverse reactions to aspirin. *J Allergy Clin Immunol* 1983;71:574.

127. Stevenson DD. Adverse reactions to nonsteroidal anti-inflammatory drugs. *Immunol Allergy Clin North Am* 1998;18:773–798.

128. Israel E, Fischer AR, Rosenberg MA, et al. The pivotal role of 5-lipoxygenase products in the reaction of aspirin-sensitive asthmatics to aspirin. *Am Rev Respir Dis* 1993;148:1447.

129. Christie PE, Tagari P, Ford Hutchinson AW, et al. Urinary LTE_4 concentrations increase after aspirin challenge in aspirin-sensitive asthmatic subjects. *Am Rev Respir Dis* 1991;143:1025–1029.

130. Dahlen B, Szczeklik A, Murray JJ. Celecoxib in patients with asthma and aspirin intolerance. *N Engl J Med* 2001;344:142.

131. Stevenson DD, Simon RA, Christensen SC, et al. Lack of cross-reactivity between selective COX-2 inhibitors and aspirin (ASA) in ASA, sensitive asthmatic subjects. *J Allergy Clin Immunol* 2000;105:S273.

132. Stevenson DD. Diagnosis, prevention, and treatment of adverse reactions to aspirin and nonsteroidal

anti-inflammatory drugs. *J Allergy Clin Immunol* 1984;74:617.

133. Mathison DA, Lumry WR, Stevenson DD, et al. Aspirin in chronic urticaria and/or angioedema: studies of sensitivity and desensitization. *J Allergy Clin Immunol* 1982;69:135.

134. Pleskow WW, Stevenson DD, Mathison DA, et al. Aspirin desensitization in aspirin-sensitive asthmatic patients: clinical manifestations and characterization of the refractory period. *J Allergy Clin Immunol* 1982;69:11.

135. Phillips GD, Foord R, Holgate ST. Inhaled lysine-aspirin as a bronchoprovocation procedure in aspirin-sensitive asthma: its repeatability, absence of late-phase reaction, and the role of histamine. *J Allergy Clin Immunol* 1989;84:232.

136. Stevenson DD. Aspirin and nonsteroidal anti-inflammatory drugs. *Immunol Allergy Clin North Am* 1995;15:529.

137. Settipane RA, Schrank PJ, Simon RA, et al. Prevalence of cross-reactivity with acetaminophen in aspirin-sensitive asthmatic subjects. *J Allergy Clin Immunol* 1995;96:480.

138. Fischer AR, Israel E. Identifying and treating aspirin-induced asthma. *J Respir Dis* 1995;16:304.

139. Stevenson DD, Hougham AJ, Schrank PJ, et al. Salsalate cross-sensitivity in aspirin-sensitive asthmatic patients. *J Allergy Clin Immunol* 1990;86:749.

140. Feigenbaum BA, Stevenson DD, Simon RA. Hydrocortisone sodium succinate does not cross-react with aspirin in aspirin-sensitive patients with asthma. *J Allergy Clin Immunol* 1995;96:545.

141. Stevenson DD, Simon RA, Lumry WR, et al. Adverse reactions to tartrazine. *J Allergy Clin Immunol* 1986;78:182.

142. Settipane GA. Aspirin and allergic diseases: a review. *Am J Med* 1983;74:102.

143. Stevenson DD, Mathison DA. Aspirin sensitivity in asthmatics: when may this drug be safe? *Postgrad Med* 1985;78:111.

144. Sweet JM, Stevenson DD, Mathison DA, et al. Long term effects of aspirin desensitization treatment for ASA sensitive patients with asthma. *J Allergy Clin Immunol* 1990;85:59.

145. Mathison DA, Lumry WR, Stevenson DD, et al. Aspirin in chronic urticaria and/or angioedema: studies of sensitivity and desensitization. *J Allergy Clin Immunol* 1982;69:135.

146. Settipane RA, Stevenson DD. Cross sensitivity with acetaminophen in aspirin-sensitive subjects with asthma. *J Allergy Clin Immunol* 1989;84:26–33.

147. Van Diem L, Grilliat JP. Anaphylactic shock induced by paracetamol. *Eur J Clin Pharmacol* 1990;38:389–390.

148. Vidal C, Pérez-Carral C, González-Quintela A. Paracetamol (acetaminophen) hypersensitivity. *Ann Allergy Asthma Immunol* 1997;79:320–321.

149. Doan T, Greenberger PA. Nearly fatal episodes of hypotension, flushing, and dyspnea in a 47-year-old woman. *Ann Allergy* 1993;70:439–444.

150. Schwarz N, Ham Pong A. Acetaminophen anaphylaxis with aspirin and sodium salicylate sensitivity: a case report. *Ann Allergy Asthma Immunol* 1996;77:473–474.

151. Katayama H, Yamaguchi K, Kozuka T, et al. Adverse reactions to ionic and nonionic contrast media: a report from the Japanese Committee on the safety of contrast media. *Radiology* 1990;175:621.

152. Wolf GL, Arenson RL, Cross AP. A prospective trial of ionic vs. nonionic contrast agents in routine clinical practice: comparison of adverse effects. *Am J Radiol* 1989;152:939.

153. Palmer FJ. The RACR survey of intravenous contrast media reactions: Final report. *Aust Radiol* 1988;32:426–428.

154. Steinberg EP, Moore RD, Powe NR, et al. Safety and cost effectiveness of high-osmolality as compared with low-osmolality contrast material in patients undergoing cardiac angiography. *N Engl J Med* 1992;326:425.

155. Committee on Drugs and Contrast Media, American College of Radiology. *Manual on contrast media.* 4th ed. Reston, VA: American College of Radiology 1998:1–46.

156. Caro JJ, Trindale E, McGregor M. The risk of death and of severe nonfatal reactions with high-versus low-osmolality contrast media: a meta-analysis. *AJR Am J Roentgenol* 1991;156:825.

157. Spring DB, Bettman MA, Barkan HE. Deaths related to iodinated contrast media reported spontaneously to the U.S. Food and Drug Administration 1978–1994: effect of the availability of low-osmolality contrast media. *Radiology* 1997;204:333–337.

158. Shellock FG, Hahn HP, Mink JH, et al. Adverse reaction to intravenous gadoteridol. *Radiology* 1993;189:151.

159. Greenberger PA, Patterson R. The prevention of immediate generalized reactions to radiocontrast media in high-risk patients. *J Allergy Clin Immunol* 1991;87:867.

160. Siegle RL, Halvosen R, Dillon J, et al. The use of iohexol in patients with previous reactions to ionic contrast material. *Invest Radiol* 1991;26:411–416.

161. Schrott KM, Behrends B, Clauss W, et al. Iohexol in excretory urography: results of the drug monitoring programs. *Fortschr Med* 1986;104:153–156.

162. Enright T, Chua-Lim A, Duda E, et al. The role of a documented allergic profile as a risk factor for radiographic contrast media reactions. *Ann Allergy* 1989;62:302.

163. Greenberger PA, Meyers SN, Kramer BL, et al. Effects of beta-adrenergic and calcium antagonists on the development of anaphylactoid reactions from radiographic contrast media during cardiac angiography. *J Allergy Clin Immunol* 1987;80:698.

164. Lang DM, Alpern MB, Visintainer PF, et al. Increased risk for anaphylactoid reaction from contrast media in patients on B-adrenergic blockers or with asthma. *Ann Intern Med* 1991;115:270.

165. Witten DM, Hirsch FD, Hartman GW. Acute reactions to urographic contrast medium: Incidence, clinical characteristics and relationship to history of hypersensitivity states. *AJR Am J Roentgenol* 1973;119:832–840.

166. Greenberger PA. Systemic reactions to radiocontrast media. *Immunol Allergy Clin North Am* (in press).

167. Greenberger PA, Patterson R, Tapio CM. Prophylaxis against repeated radiocontrast media reactions in 857 cases. *Arch Intern Med* 1985;145:2197.

168. Lasser EC, Berry CC, Mishkin MM, et al. Pretreatment with corticosteroids to prevent adverse reactions to nonionic contrast media. *AJR Am J Roentgenol* 1994;162:523.

169. Ramesh S, Reisman RE. Noncardiogenic pulmonary edema due to radiocontrast media. *Ann Allergy Asthma Immunol* 1995;75:308.

170. Tepel M, van der Geit M, Schwarzfeld C, et al.

Prevention of radiographic contrast-agent induced reductions in renal function by acetylcysteine. *N Engl J Med* 2000;343:180–184.

171. Chandler MJ, Grammer LC, Patterson R. Provocative challenge with local anesthetics in patients with a prior history of reaction. *J Allergy Clin Immunol* 1987;79:883–886.

172. deShazo RD, Nelson HS. An approach to the patient with a history of local anesthetic hypersensitivity: experience with 90 patients. *J Allergy Clin Immunol* 1979;63:387–394.

173. Incaudo G, Schatz M, Patterson R, et al. Administration of local anesthetics to patients with a history of a prior reaction. *J Allergy Clin Immunol* 1978;61:339–345.

174. Gall H, Kaufmann R, Kalveram CM. Adverse reactions to local anesthetics: analysis of 197 cases. *J Allergy Clin Immunol* 1996;97:933–937.

175. Schwartz HJ, Sher TH. Bisulfite sensitivity manifesting as allergy to local dental anesthesia. *J Allergy Clin Immunol* 1985;75:525–527.

176. Howard PA, Dunn MI. Is your patient's cough caused by an ACE inhibitor? *J Respir Dis* 1997;18:762–768.

177. Israili ZH, Hall WD. Cough and angioneurotic edema associated with angiotensin-converting enzyme inhibitor therapy: a review of the literature and pathophysiology. *Ann Intern Med* 1992;117:234–242.

178. Brown NJ, Snowden M, Griffin MR. Recurrent angiotensin-converting enzyme inhibitor-associated angioedema. *JAMA* 1997;278:232–233.

179. Brown NJ, Ray WA, Snowden M, et al. Black Americans have an increased rate of angiotensin converting enzyme inhibitor associated angioedema. *Clin Pharmacol Ther* 1996;60:8–13.

180. Abbosh J, Anderson JA, Levine AB, et al. Antiotensin converting enzyme inhibitor-induced angioedema more prevalent in transplant patients. *Ann Allergy Asthma Immunol* 1999;82:473–476.

181. Tielemans C, Madhoun P, Lenaers M, et al. Anaphylactoid reactions during hemodialysis on AN69 membranes in patients receiving ACE inhibitors. *Kidney Int* 1990;38:982–984.

182. Alvarez-Lara MA, Martin-Malo A, Espinosa M, et al. ACE inhibitors and anaphylactoid reactions to high-flux membrane dialysis [Letter]. *Lancet* 1991;337:370.

183. Tielemans C, Vanherweghem JL, Blumberg A, et al. ACE inhibitors and anaphylactoid reactions to high-flux membrane dialysis [Letter]. *Lancet* 1991;337: 370–371.

184. Acker CG, Greenberg A. Angioedema induced by the angiotensin II blocker losartan [Letter]. *N Engl J Med* 1995;333:1572.

185. van Rijnsoever EW, Kwee-Zuiderwijk WJM, Feenstra J. Angioneurotic edema attributed to the use of losartan. *Arch Intern Med* 1998;158:2063–2065.

186. Gutstein HB, Akil H. Opioid analgesics, In: Hardman JG, Limbird LE, Goodman Gilman A, eds. *Goodman & Gilman's the pharmacologic basis of therapeutics*, 10th ed. New York: McGraw Hill, 2001: 569–619.

187. Rosenow EC III, Myers JL, Swensen SJ, et al. Drug-induced pulmonary disease: an update. *Chest* 1992;102:239–250.

188. Zitnik RJ. Drug-induced lung disease: cancer chemotherapy agents. *J Resp Dis* 1995;16:855–865.

189. Shlebak AA, Clark PI, Green JA. Hypersensitivity and cross-reactivity to cisplatin and analogues. *Cancer Chemother Pharmacol* 1995;35: 349–351.

190. Goldberg A, Altaras MM, Mekori YA, et al. Anaphylaxis to cisplatin: diagnosis and value of pretreatment in prevention of recurrent allergic reactions. *Ann Allergy* 1994;73:271–272.

191. Vittorio CC, Muglia JJ. Anticonvulsant hypersensitivity syndrome. *Arch Intern Med* 1995;155:2285–2290.

192. Knowles SR, Shapiro LE, Shear NH. Anticonvulsant hypersensitivity syndrome: incidence, prevention and management. *Drug Safety* 1999;21: 489–501.

193. Roujeau J-C, Kelly JP, Naldi L, et al. Medication use and the risk of Stevens-Johnson syndrome or toxic epidermal necrolysis. *N Engl J Med* 1995;333:1600–1607.

194. Mahatma M, Haponik EF, Nelson S, et al. Phenytoin-induced acute respiratory failure with pulmonary eosinophilia. *Am J Med* 1989;87:93–94.

195. Gennis MA, Vemuri R, Burns EA, et al. Familial occurrence of hypersensitivity to phenytoin. *Am J Med* 1991;91:631–634.

196. Gonzalez FJ, Carvajal MJ, del Pozo V, et al. Erythema multiforme to phenobarbital: involvement of eosinophils and T cells expressing the skin homing receptor. *J Allergy Clin Immunol* 1997;100:135–137.

197. Chopra S, Levell NJ, Cowley G, et al. Systemic corticosteroids in the phenytoin hypersensitivity syndrome. *Br J Dermatol* 1996;134:1109–1112.

198. Tamayo E, Perez M, Gomez JI, et al. Allergy to anaesthetizing agents in Spain. *Br J Anaesth* 1999;83:336–337.

199. Matthey P, Wang P, Finegan BA, et al. Rocuronium anaphylaxis and multiple neuromuscular blocking drug sensitivities. *Can J Anesth* 2000;47:890–893.

200. Kant Pandey C, Mathur N, Singh N, et al. Fulminant pulmonary edema after intramuscular ketamine. *Can J Anesth* 2000;47:894–896.

Part C: Immunologic Reactions to High-Molecular-Weight Therapeutic Agents

1. Patterson R, Roberts M, Grammer LC. Insulin allergy: reevaluation after two decades. *Ann Allergy* 1990;64:459.

2. Lee TM, Grammer LC, Shaughnessy MA, et al. Evaluation and management of corticostropin allergy. *J Allergy Clin Immunol* 1987;79:964–968.

3. Grammer LC, Patterson R. Proteins: chymopapain and insulin. *J Allergy Clin Immunol* 1984;74:635.

4. Niblack G, Johnson K, Williams T, et al. Antibody formation following administration of antilymphocyte serum. *Transplant Proc* 1987;19:1896.

5. Grammer LC. Immunologic reaction to insulin and other proteins. *Immunol Allergy Clin North Am* 1998;18:809–816.

6. Rodgers JR, Rich RR. Antigens and antigen presentation. In: Fleisher TA, Schwartz BD, Shearer WT, et al, eds. *Clinical immunology*. St Louis, CV Mosby, 1996:114.

7. Fineberg SE, Galloway JA, Fineberg NS, et al. Immunogenicity of recombinant DNA human insulin. *Diabetologia* 1983;25:465.

8. Engler RJ, Weiss RB. Immediate hypersensitivity to human recombinant-macrophage colony-stimulating associated with a positive prick skin test reaction. *Ann Allergy Asthma Immunol* 1996;76:531.

9. Grammer LC, Roberts M. Cutaneous allergy to recombinant human type I IL-1 receptor (rhu IL-1RI). *J Allergy Clin Immunol* 1997;99:714–715.

10. Grammer LC, Metzger B, Patterson R. Cutaneous allergy to human (recombinant DNA) insulin. *JAMA* 1984;251:1459.

11. Grammer LC, Roberts M, Patterson R. IgE and I.G. antibody against human (recombinant DNA) insulin in patients with systemic insulin allergy. *J Lab Clin Med* 1985;105:108.

12. Grammer LC, Roberts M, Buchannan TA, et al. Specificity of IgE and I.G. against human (recombinant DNA) insulin in human (or DNA) insulin allergy and resistance. *J Lab Clin Med* 1987;109:141.

13. Alvarez-Thull L, Rosenwasser LJ, Brodie TD. Systemic allergy to endogenous insulin during therapy with recombinant DNA (rDNA) insulin. *Ann Allergy Asthma Immunol* 1996;76:253–256.

14. deShazo R, Boehm T, Kumar D, et al. Dermal hypersensitivity reaction to insulin: correlations of three patterns to their histopathology. *J Allergy Clin Immunol* 1982;69:229.

15. Grammer LC, Chen PY, Patterson R. Evaluation and management of insulin allergy. *J Allergy Clin Immunol* 1983;71:250.

16. Lluch-Bernal M, Fernandez M, Herraera-Pombo JL, et al. Insulin lispro, an alternative in insulin hypersensitivity. *Allergy* 1999;54:186–187.

17. Mattson JR, Patterson R, Roberts M. Insulin therapy in patients with systemic insulin allergy. *Arch Intern Med* 1975;135:818.

18. Sharath MD, Metzger WJ, Richerson HB, et al. Protamine-induced fatal anaphylaxis. *J Thorac Cardiovasc Surg* 1985;90:86.

19. Weiler JM, Gellhaus MA, Carter JG, et al. A prospective study of the risk of an immediate adverse reaction to protamine sulfate during cardiopulmonary bypass surgery. *J Allergy Clin Immunol* 1990;85:713.

20. Gottschlich GM, Graulee GP, Georgitis JW. Adverse reactions to protamine sulfate during cardiac surgery in diabetic and non-diabetic patients. *Ann Allergy* 1988;61:277.

21. Levy JH, Schwieger IM, Zaidan JR, et al. Evaluation of patients at risk for protamine reactions. *J Thorac Cardiovasc Surg* 1989;98:200.

22. Weiss ME, Adkinson NF Jr. Allergy to protamine. *Clin Rev Allergy* 1991;9:339.

23. McGrath KG, Patterson R. Anaphylactic reactivity to streptokinase. *JAMA* 1984;252:1314.

24. McGrath KG, Patterson R. Immunology of streptokinase in human subjects. *Clin Exp Immunol* 1985;62:421.

25. Dykewicz MS, McGrath KG, Davison R, et al. Identification of patients at risk for anaphylaxis due to streptokinase. *Arch Intern Med* 1986;146:305.

26. McGrath KG, Zeffren B, Alexander J, et al. Allergic reactions to streptokinase consistent with anaphylactic or antigen-antibody complex mediated damage. *J Allergy Clin Immunol* 1985;76:453.

27. Sherry S, Marder VJ. Streptokinase and recombinant tissue plasminogen activator (rt-PA) are equally effective in treating acute myocardial infarction. *Ann Intern Med* 1991;114:417.

28. Tsang TS, Califf RM, Stebbins AL, et al. Incidence and impact on outcome of streptokinase allergy in the GUSTO-I trial: global utilization of streptokinase and t-PA in occluded coronary arteries. *Am J Cardiol* 1997;79:1232–1235.

29. Manteiga R, Carlos Souto J, Altes A, et al. Short-course thrombolysis as the first line of therapy for cardiac valve thrombosis. *J Thorac Cardiovasc Surg* 1998;115:780–784.

30. Willis J, ed. Chymopapain approval. *FDA Bull* 1982;12(3):17.

31. Grammer LC, Patterson R. Chymopapain sensitivity testing. *Clin Chem News* 1985;11:6.

32. Poynton AR, O'Farrell DA, Mulcahy D, et al. Chymopapain chemonucleolysis: a review of 105 cases. *J R Coll Surg Edinb* 1998;43:407–409.

33. Slater JE. Allergic reactions to natural rubber. *Ann Allergy* 1992;68:203.

34. Nutter AE. Contact urticaria due to rubber. *Br J Dermatol* 1979;101:597.

35. Gelfand DW. Barium enemas, latex balloons, and anaphylactic reactions. *AJR Am J Roentgenol* 1991;156:1.

36. Yunginger JW, Jones RT, Fransway AF, et al. Extractable latex allergens and proteins in disposable medical gloves and other rubber products. *J Allergy Clin Immunol* 1994;93:836.

37. Kelly KJ, Kurup VP, Zacharisen M, et al. Skin and serological testing in the diagnosis of latex allergy. *J Allergy Clin Immunol* 1993;91:1140.

38. Turjanmaa K, Reunala T, Rasanen L. Comparison of diagnostic methods in latex surgical contact urticaria. *Contact Dermatitis* 1988;19:241.

39. Bubak ME, Reed CE, Fransway AF, et al. Allergic reactions to latex among health-care workers. *Mayo Clin Proc* 1992;67:1075.

40. Hunt LW, Fransway AF, Reed CE, et al. An epidemic of occupational allergy to latex involving health care workers. *J Occup Environ Med* 1995;37:1204–1209.

41. Allmers H, Brehler R, Chen Z, et al. Reduction of latex aeroallergens and latex-specific IgE antibodies in sensitized workers after removal of powdered natural rubber latex gloves in a hospital. *J Allergy Clin Immunol* 1998;102:841–846.

42. Winkelstein A, Kiss JE. Immunohematologic disorders. *JAMA* 1997;278:1982–1992.

43. Gupta RK, Siber GR. Use of in vitro Vero cell assay and ELISA in the United States potency test of vaccines containing adsorbed diphtheria and tetanus toxoids. *Dev Biol Stand* 1996;86:207–215.

44. Shapiro RL, Hatheway C, Swerdlow DL. Botulism in the United States: a clinical and epidemiologic review. *Ann Intern Med* 1998;129:221–228.

45. Dykewicz MS, Rosen ST, O'Connell MM, et al. Plasma histamine but not anaphylatoxin levels correlate with generalized urticaria from infusions of antilymphocyte monoclonal antibodies. *J Lab Clin Med* 1992;120:290.

46. Burks AW, Sampson HA, Buckley RH. Anaphylactic reactions after gamma globulin administration in patients with hypogammaglobulinemia: detection of IgE antibodies to IgA. *N Engl J Med* 1986;314:560.

47. Heard K, O'Malley GF, Dart RC. Antivenom therapy in the Americas. *Drugs* 1999;58:5–15.

48. Millar MM, Grammer LC. Case reports of evaluation and desensitization for anti-thymocyte globulin hypersensitivity. *Ann Allergy Asthma Immunol* 2000;85:311–316.

49. Dillman JB. Toxicity of monoclonal antibodies in treatment of cancer. *Semin Oncol Nurs* 1988;4:107–111.

50. Pai LH, Bookman MA, Ozols RF, et al. Clinical evaluation of IP *Pseudomonas* exotoxin immunoconjugate OVB3-PE in patients with ovarian cancer. *J Clin Oncol* 1991;9:2095–2103.

51. Hjelm Skog A, Ragnhammar P, Fagerberg J, et al. Clinical effects of monoclonal antibody 17-1A combined with granulocyte/macrophage-colony-stimulating factor and interleukin-2 for treatment of patients with advanced colorectal carcinoma. *Cancer Immunol Immunother* 1999;48:463–470.

52. Tsai D, Moore H, Hardy C, et al. Rituximab (anti-CD20 monoclonal antibody) therapy for progressive intermediate-grade non-Hodgkin's lymphoma after high-dose therapy and autologous peripheral stem cell transplantation. *Bone Marrow Transplant* 1999;24:521–526.

53. Winkler U, Jensen M, Manzke O, et al. Cytokine-release syndrome in patients with B-cell chronic lymphocytic leukemia and high lymphocyte counts after treatment with an anti-CD20 monoclonal antibody (rituximab, IDEC-C2B8). *Blood* 1999;94:2217–2224.

54. Guzzo JA, Nichols TC. Possible anaphylactic reaction to abciximab. *Cathet Cardiovasc Intervent* 1999;48:71–73.

55. Ricart E, Panaccione R, Loftus EV, et al. Successful management of Crohn's disease of the ileoanal pouch with infliximab. *Gastroenterology* 1999;117:429–432.

56. Moreland LW. Inhibitors of tumor necrosis factor: new treatment options for rheumatoid arthritis. *Cleve Clin J Med* 1999;66:367–374.

57. Sandborn WJ, Hanauer SB. Antitumor necrosis factor therapy for inflammatory bowel disease: a review of agents, pharmacology, clinical results, and safety. *Inflamm Bowel Dis* 1999;5:119–133.

58. Kahan BD, Rajagopalan PR, Hall M. Reduction of the occurrence of acute cellular rejection among renal allograft recipients treated with basiliximab, a chimeric anti- interleukin-2-receptor monoclonal antibody. United States Simulect Renal Study Group. *Transplantation* 1999;67:276–284.

59. Meissner HC, Groothuis JR, Rodriguez WJ, et al. Safety and pharmacokinetics of an intramuscular monoclonal antibody (SB 209763) against respiratory syncytial virus (RSV) in infants and young children at risk for severe RSV disease. *Antimicrob Agents Chemother* 1999;43:1183–1188.

60. Ball WJ Jr, Kasturi R, Dey P, et al. Isolation and characterization of human monoclonal antibodies to digoxin. *J Immunol* 1999;163:2291–2298.

61. Regan J, Campbell K, van Smith, et al. Characterization of antithymoglobulin, anti-Atgam and OKT3 IgG antibodies in human serum with an 11-min ELISA. *Transplant Immunol* 1997;5:49–56.

62. Jaiyesimi I, Giralt SS, Wood J. Subcutaneous granulocyte colony-stimulating factor and acute anaphylaxis. *N Engl J Med* 1991;325:587.

63. Stone HD Jr, DiPiro C, Davis PC, et al. Hypersensitivity reactions to *Escherichia coli*-derived polythylene glycolated-asparaginase associated with subsequent immediate skin test reactivity to *E. coli*-derived granulocyte colony-stimulating factor. *J Allergy Clin Immunol* 1998;101:429–431.

64. Scott GA. Reports of three cases of cutaneous reactions to granulocyte macrophage colony stimulating factor and a review of the literature. *Am J Dermatopathol* 1995;17:114.

65. Wadhwa M, Skog AL, Bird C, et al. Immunogenicity of granulocyte-macrophage colony-stimulating factor (GM-CSF) products in patients undergoing combination therapy with GM-CSF. *Clin Cancer Res* 1999;5:1353–1361.

66. Prabhakar SS, Muhlfelder T. Antibodies to recombinant erythropoietin causing pure red cell aplasia. *Clin Nephrol* 1997;47:331–335.

67. Urra JM, de la Torre M, Alcazar R, et al. Rapid method for detection of anti-recombinant human erythropoietin antibodies as a new form of erythropoietin resistance. *Clin Chem* 1997;43:848–849.

68. Antonelli G, Currenti M, Turriziani O, et al. Neutralizing antibodies to interferon-alpha: relative frequency in patients treated with different interferon preparations. *J Infect Dis* 1991;163:882–885.

69. Antonelli G, Giannelli G, Currenti M, et al. Antibodies to interferon (IFN) in hepatitis C patients relapsing while continuing recombinant IFN-α2 therapy. *Clin Exp Immunol* 1996;104:384–387.

70. Wussow PV, Jakschies D, Freund M, et al. Treatment of anti-recombinant interferon-alpha 2 antibody positive CML patients with natural interferon-alpha. *Br J Haematol* 1991;78:210–216.

71. Nolte KU, Gunther G, von Wussow P. Epitopes recognized by neutralizing therapy-induced human anti-interferon-alpha antibodies are localized within the N-terminal functional domain of recombinant interferon-alpha 2. *Eur J Immunol* 1996;26:2155–2159.

72. Bemiller LS, Roberts DH, Starko KM, et al. Safety and effectiveness of long-term interferon-γ therapy in patients with chronic granulomatous disease. *Blood Cells Molec Dis* 1995;21:239–247.

73. Ross C, Svenson M, Hansen MB, et al. High avidity IFN-neutralizing antibodies in pharmaceutically prepared human IgG. *J Clin Invest* 1995;95:1974–1978.

74. Prummer O, Fiehn C, Gallati H. Anti-interferon-γ antibodies in a patient undergoing interferon-γ treatment for systemic mastocytosis. *J Interferon Cytokine Res* 1996;16:519–522.

75. Phipps WR, Holden D, Sheehan RK. Use of recombinant human follicle-stimulating hormone for in vitro fertilization-embryo transfer after severe systemic immunoglobulin E-mediated reaction to urofollitropin. *Fertil Steril* 1996;66:148–150.

76. Whitman-Elia GF, Banks K, O'Dea LS. Recombinant follicle-stimulating hormone in a patient hypersensitive to urinary-derived gonadotropin. *Gynecol Endocrinol* 1998;12:209–212.

77. Helmer RE III, Alperin JB, Yunginger JW, et al. Anaphylactic reactions following infusion of factor VIII in a patient with classic hemophilia. *Am J Med* 1980;69:953–957.

78. Shopnick RI, Kazemi M, Brettler DB, et al. Anaphylaxis after treatment with recombinant factor VIII. *Transfusion* 1996;36:358–361.

79. White GC II, Courter S, Bray GL, et al. A multicenter study of recombinant factor VIII (Recombinate) in previously treated patients with hemophilia A. The

Recombinate Previously Treated Patient Study Group. *Thromb Haemost* 1997;77:660–667.

80. Pasi KJ. Previously untreated patients and recombinant factor VIII concentrate studies. *Blood Coagul Fibrinolysis* 1997:8[Suppl 1]:S29–32.

81. Prowse CV, MacGregor IR. Neoantigens and antibodies to factor VIII. *Blood Rev* 1998;12:99–105.

82. Scharrer I, Bray GL, Neutzling O. Incidence of inhibitors in haemophilia A patients: a review of recent studies of recombinant and plasma-derived factor VIII concentrates. *Haemophilia* 1999;5:145–154.

83. Yee TT, Williams MD, Hill FG, et al. Absence of inhibitors in previously untreated patients with severe haemophilia A after exposure to a single intermediate purity factor VIII product. *Thromb Haemost* 1997;78:1027–1029.

84. Rothschild C, Laurian Y, Satre EP, et al. French previously untreated patients with severe hemophilia A after exposure to recombinant factor VIII: incidence of inhibitor and evaluation of immune tolerance. *Thromb Haemost* 1998;80:779–783.

85. Bircher AJ, Czendlik CH, Messmer SL, et al. Acute urticaria caused by subcutaneous recombinant hirudin: evidence for an IgE-mediated hypersensitivity reaction. *J Allergy Clin Immunol* 1996;98:994–996.

86. Rudolf J, Grond M, Prince WS, et al. Evidence of anaphylaxis after alteplase infusion. *Stroke* 1999;30:1142–1143.

87. Eisenberg JD, Aitken ML, Dorkin HL, et al. Safety of repeated intermittent courses of aerosolized recombinant human deoxyribonuclease in patients with cystic fibrosis. *J Pediatr* 1997;131:118–124.

88. Milgrom H, Fick RB Jr, Su JQ, et al. Treatment of allergic asthma with monoclonal anti-IgE antibody. *N Engl J Med* 1999;341:1966–1973.

89. Edsall G, Elliot MW, Peebles TC, et al. Excessive use of tetanus toroid boosters. *JAMA* 1967;202:17–19.

90. Fulginiti VA, Eller JJ, Downie AW, et al. Altered reactivity to measles virus: atypical measles in children previously immunized with inactivated measles virus vaccine. *JAMA* 1967;202:1075–1080.

91. Peebles TC, Levine L, Eldred MC, et al. Tetanus-toxoid emergency boosters: a reappraisal. *N Engl J Med* 1969;280:575–581.

92. Nader PR, Horwitz MS, Rousseau J. Atypical exanthem following exposure to natural measles: 11 cases in children previously inoculated with killed vaccine. *J Pediatr* 1968;72:22–28.

93. Kapikian AZ, Mitchell RH, Chanock RM. An epidemiologic study of altered clinical reactivity to respiratory syncytial (RS) virus infection in children previously immunized with an inactivated RS virus vaccine. *Am J Epidemiol* 1969;89:405–421.

94. Kim HW, Canchola JG, Brandt CD, et al. Respiratory syncytial virus disease in infants despite prior administration of antigenic inactivated vaccine. *Am J Epidemiol* 1969;89:422–434.

95. Institute of Medicine. *Adverse events associated with childhood vaccines: evidence bearing on causality.* Washington, DC: National Academy of Sciences, 1994.

96. Jacobs RL, Lowe RS, Lanier BQ. Adverse reactions to tetanus toxoid. *JAMA* 1982;247:40.

97. Zaloga GP, Chernow B. Life-threatening anaphylactic reaction to tetanus toxoid. *Ann Allergy* 1982;49:107–108.

98. Carey AB, Meltzer EO. Diagnosis and "desensitization" in tetanus vaccine hypersensitivity. *Ann Allergy* 1992;69:336.

99. Mansfield LE, Ting S, Rawls DO, et al. Systemic reactions during cutaneous testing for tetanus toxoid hypersensitivity. *Ann Allergy* 1986;57:135–137.

100. Turktas I, Ergenekon E. Anaphylaxis following diphtheria-tetanus-pertussis vaccination: a reminder. *Eur J Pediatr* 1999;158:434.

101. Howson CP, Fineberg HV, Adverse events following pertussis and rubella vaccines. Summary of a report of the Institute of Medicine. *JAMA* 1992;267:392-6.

102. James JM, Burks AW, Roberson PK, et al. Safe administration of the measles vaccine to children allergic to eggs. *N Engl J Med* 1995;332:1262.

103. Watson JC, Hadler SC, Dykewicz CA, et al. Measles, mumps and rubella: vaccine use and strategies for elimination of measles, rubella, and congenital rubella syndrome and control of mumps. Recommendations of the Advisory Committee on Immunization Practices (ACIP). *MMWR Morb Mortal Wkly Rep* 1998;47: 1–57.

104. Sakaguchi M, Nakayama T, Inouye S. Food allergy to gelatin in children with systemic immediate-type reactions, including anaphylaxis, to vaccines. *J Allergy Clin Immunol* 1996;98:1058–1061.

105. Sakaguchi M, Yoshida T, Asahi T, et al. Development of IgE antibody to gelatin in children with systemic immediate-type reactions to vaccines. *J Allergy Clin Immunol* 1997;99:720–721.

106. Sakaguchi M, Hori H, Ebihara T, et al. Reactivity of the immunoglobulin E in bovine gelatin-sensitive children to gelatins from various animals. *Immunology* 1999;96:286–290.

107. Sakaguchi M, Yoshida M, Kuroda W, et al. Systemic immediate-type reactions to gelatin included in Japanese encephalitis vaccines. *Vaccine* 1997;15:121–122.

108. Trotter AC, Stone BD, Laszlo DJ, et al. Measles, mumps, rubella vaccine administration in egg-sensitive children: systemic reactions during vaccine desensitization. *Ann Allergy* 1994;72:25.

109. James JM, Zeiger RS, Lester MR, et al. Safe administration of influenza vaccine to patients with egg allergy. *J Pediatr* 1998;133:624–628.

110. Anonymous. Prevention and control of influenza: recommendations of the Advisory Committee on Immunization Practices (ACIP). *MMWR Morb Mortal Wkly Rep* 1999;48:1–28.

111. Campbell BG, Edwards RL. Safety of influenza vaccination in adults with asthma. *Med J Aust* 1984; 140:773.

112. Kelso JM, Mootrey GT, Tsai TF. Anaphylaxis from yellow fever vaccine. *J Allergy Clin Immunol* 1999;103:698–701.

113. Harvey RE, Posey WC, Jacobs RL. The predictive value of egg skin tests and yellow fever vaccine skin tests in egg-sensitive individuals. *J Allergy Clin Immunol* 1975;63:196.

114. *Yellow fever: disease and vaccine.* National Center for Infectious Diseases/Center for Disease Control and Prevention, June 10, 1999.

115. Kletz MR, Holland CL, Mendelson JS, et al. Administration of egg-derived vaccines in patients with history of egg sensitivity. *Ann Allergy* 1990;64:527.

116. Miller JR, Orgel A, Meltzer EO. The safety of egg-containing vaccines for egg-allergic patients. *J Allergy Clin Immunol* 1983;71:568.

117. Khan RI. Anaphylactoid reaction to typhoid-paratyphoid A and B vaccine. *Trop Geograph Med* 1971;23:115–116.

118. Kelleher PC, Kelley LR, Rickman LS. Anaphylactoid reaction after typhoid vaccination. *Am J Med* 1990;89:822–824.

119. Berg SW, Mitchell BS, Hanson RK, et al. Systemic reactions in U.S. Marine Corps personnel who received Japanese encephalitis vaccine. *Clin Infect Dis* 1997;24:265–266.

120. Yergeau A, Alain L, Pless R, et al. Adverse events temporally associated with meningococcal vaccines. *CMAJ* 1996;154:503–507.

121. Ventura A. Varicella vaccination guidelines for adolescents and adults. *Am Fam Physician* 1997;55:1220–1224.

122. Lear JT, English JS. Anaphylaxis after hepatitis B vaccination. *Lancet* 1995;345:1249.

123. Duclos P. Adverse events after hepatitis B vaccination. *CMAJ* 1992:147:1023–1026.

124. Availability of Hepatitis B vaccine that does not contain thimersol as a preservative. *MMWR Morb Mortal Wkly Rep* 1999;48:780–782.

18

Contact Dermatitis

Andrew J. Scheman

Department of Dermatology, Northwestern University Medical Center, Chicago, Illinois

A skin condition commonly encountered by physicians is allergic contact dermatitis. With new chemical sensitizers being introduced into our environment constantly, physicians will be evaluating more instances of this disease. Contact dermatitis is the most common occupational disease, and, as such, is of importance to both the individual and to society. The patient with allergic contact dermatitis may be very uncomfortable and have poor quality of life. Inability to pursue employment or recreation are common, especially if there is a delay in diagnosis and removal from exposure.

IMMUNOLOGIC BASIS

Allergic contact dermatitis is a type IVa_1, T-cell–mediated hypersensitivity. Type IVa_1 allergy is also referred to as delayed-type hypersensitivity, reflecting the fact that typical reactions occur 5 to 21 days after initial exposure and 12 to 96 hours after subsequent exposures. In contrast, immediate hypersensitivity is a type I immunoglobulin E (IgE) humoral antibody-mediated reaction.

Whereas the typical skin lesion in immediate hypersensitivity is urticarial, typical allergic contact dermatitis is eczematous (1). Thus, skin lesions can include vesicles, bullae, and poorly-demarcated erythematous scaly plaques acutely and, when chronic, lichenification. It is important to realize that contact allergy is often morphologically and histologically identical to other forms of eczema, including atopic dermatitis and irritant contact dermatitis, which is nonimmuno-

logic damage to the skin caused by a direct toxic effect. Therefore, patch testing is usually needed to distinguish contact allergy from other types of eczema.

Typically, immediate hypersensitivity is caused by parenteral exposure through ingestion or respiratory exposure through inhalation. An exception is immunologic contact urticaria, in which a type I reaction is induced by topical exposure. The typical contact allergy is induced by topical exposure. An exception occurs with systemic ingestion of a contact allergen that reproduces skin lesions caused by a previous external exposure to the same or a similar substance; this is termed systemic contact dermatitis. The list of substances capable of causing type I allergy is different from the list of substances capable of causing type IVa_1 allergy. There are a few substances, such as penicillin, quinine, sulfonamides, mercury, and arsenic that have caused simultaneous type IVa_1 contact hypersensitivity and type I anaphylactic reactions.

Although atopic individuals are prone to type I allergies, they have been generally considered not to be more likely to develop type IVa_1 allergy than nonatopic individuals. On the other hand, it has been clearly demonstrated that atopic persons are much more likely to have a lowered threshold for developing irritant contact dermatitis.

Sensitization

The inductive or afferent limb of contact sensitivity begins with the topical application to the skin of a chemically reactive substance called a hapten. The hapten may be organic or inorganic and is generally of low molecular weight (>500 daltons). Its ability to sensitize depends on penetrating the skin and forming covalent bonds with proteins. The degree of sensitization is directly proportional to the stability of the hapten–protein coupling. In the case of the commonly used skin sensitizer dinitrochlorobenzene, the union of the chemical hapten and the tissue protein occurs in the Malpighian layer of the epidermis, with the amino acid sites of lysine and cysteine being most reactive (2). It has been suggested that skin lipids might exert an adjuvant effect comparable with the myoside of mycobacterium tuberculosis.

There is strong evidence that Langerhans cells are of crucial importance in the induction of contact sensitivity (3). These dendritic cells in the epidermis cannot be identified on routine histologic sections of the skin by light microscopy, but they can be easily visualized using special stains. They possess Ia antigens and receptors for the Fc portion of IgG and complement, much like macrophages.

Elicitation

Langerhans cells are dendritic epidermal cells that possess HLA-DR antigen on their surface. The Langerhans cell ingests the hapten–protein complex, processes it, and then produces a resulting peptide that binds to the HLA-DR antigen on the surface of the cell. The peptide is then presented to a $CD4^+$ helper T cell type 1 (T_H1) with specific complementary surface receptors.

The binding of the T_H1 cell induces the Langerhans cell to release interleukin-1. Interleukin-1 in turn activates the bound T_H1 cell to release interleukin-2 which leads to T-cell proliferation. The proliferating T cells magnify the response by releasing interferon-γ, which leads to increased HLA-DR display on Langerhans cells and increased cytotoxicity of T cells, macrophages, and natural killer cells. The sensitized T_H1 cells also allow an anamnestic response to subsequent exposure to the same antigen. Type IVa_1 hypersensitivity can be transferred with sensitized T_H1 cells (4).

Contact allergy involves both T effector cells leading to hypersensitivity and T suppressor cells leading to tolerance. The net effect is the balance of these two opposing inputs. Cutaneous exposure tends to induce sensitization, whereas oral or intravenous exposure is more likely to induce tolerance. Once sensitivity is acquired, it usually persists for many years; however, it occasionally may be lost after only a few years. Hardening refers to either a specific or generalized loss of hypersensitivity due to constant low-grade exposure to an antigen. This type of deliberate desensitization has been successful only in rare instances.

Histopathology

The histologic picture in allergic contact dermatitis reveals that the dermis is infiltrated by mononuclear inflammatory cells, especially about blood vessels and sweat glands (2). The epidermis is hyperplastic with mononuclear cell invasion. Frequently, intraepidermal vesicles form, which may coalesce into large blisters. The vesicles are filled with serous fluid containing granulocytes and mononuclear cells. In Jones-Mote contact sensitivity, in addition to mononuclear phagocyte and lymphocyte accumulation, basophils are found. This is an important distinction from hypersensitivity reactions of the T_H1 type, in which basophils are completely absent.

CLINICAL FEATURES

History

Allergic contact dermatitis occurs most frequently in middle-aged and elderly persons, although it may appear at any age. In contrast to the classical atopic diseases, contact dermatitis is as common in the population at large as in the atopic population, and a history of personal or family atopy is not a risk factor.

The interval between exposure to the responsible agent and the occurrence of clinical manifestations in a sensitized subject is usually 12 to 96 hours, although it may be as early as 4 hours and as late as 1 week. The incubation or

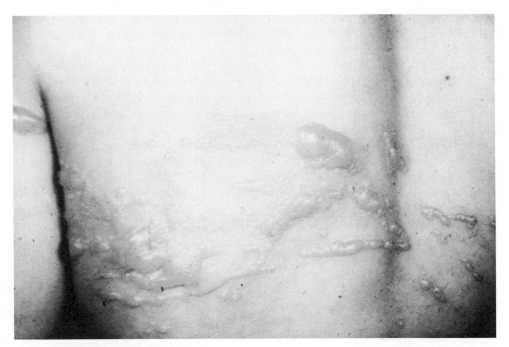

FIG. 18.1. The acute phase of contact dermatitis due to poison ivy. Note the linear distribution of vesicles (courtesy of Dr. Gary Vicik).

sensitization period between initial exposure and the development of skin sensitivity may be as short as 2 to 3 days in the case of a strong sensitizer such as poison ivy, or several years for a weak sensitizer such as chromate. The patient usually will note the development of erythema, followed by papules, and then vesicles. Pruritus follows the appearance of the dermatitis and is uniformly present in allergic contact dermatitis.

Physical Examination

The appearance of allergic contact dermatitis depends on the stage at which the patient presents. In the acute stage, erythema, papules, and vesicles predominate, with edema and occasionally bullae (Fig. 18.1). The boundaries of the dermatitis are generally poorly marginated. Edema may be profound in areas of loose tissue such as the eyelids and genitalia. Acute allergic contact dermatitis of the face may result in a marked degree of periorbital swelling that resembles angioedema. The presence of the associated dermatitis should allow the physician to make

the distinction easily. In the subacute phase, vesicles are less pronounced, and crusting, scaling, and early signs of lichenification may be present. In the chronic stage, few papulovesicular lesions are evident, and thickening, lichenification, and scaliness predominate.

Different areas of the skin vary in their ease of sensitization. Pressure, friction, and perspiration are factors that seem to enhance sensitization. The eyelids, neck, and genitalia are among the most readily sensitized areas, whereas the palms, soles, and scalp are more resistant. Tissue that is irritated, inflamed, or infected is more susceptible to allergic contact dermatitis. A clinical example is the common occurrence of contact dermatitis in an area of stasis dermatitis that has been topically treated.

Differential Diagnosis

The skin conditions most frequently confused with allergic contact dermatitis are seborrheic dermatitis, atopic dermatitis, psoriasis, and primary irritant dermatitis. In seborrheic dermatitis, there is a general tendency toward oiliness of the skin, and a predilection of the lesions for the scalp, the T-zone of the face, midchest, and inguinal folds.

Atopic dermatitis (see Chapter 15) often has its onset in infancy or early childhood. The skin is dry, although pruritus is a prominent feature, it appears before the lesions and not after them, as in the case of allergic contact dermatitis. The areas most frequently involved are the flexural surfaces. The margins of the dermatitis are indefinite, and the progression from erythema to papules to vesicles is not seen.

Psoriatic dermatitis is characterized by well demarcated erythematous plaques with white to silvery scales. Lesions are often distributed symmetrically over extensor surfaces such as the knee or elbow.

The dermatitis caused by a primary irritant is a simple chemical or physical insult to the skin. For example, what is commonly called "dishpan hands" is a dermatitis caused by household detergents. A prior sensitizing exposure to the primary irritant is not necessary, and the dermatitis develops in a large number of normal persons. The dermatitis begins shortly after exposure to the irritant, in contrast to the 12 to 96 hours after exposure in allergic contact dermatitis. Primary irritant dermatitis may be virtually indistinguishable in its physical appearance from allergic contact dermatitis. It should be emphasized that skin conditions may coexist. It is not unusual to see allergic contact dermatitis caused by topical medications applied for the treatment of atopic dermatitis and other dermatoses.

A variant of contact allergy is contact urticaria (5). This is an immediate wheal-and-flare response generated by a wide variety of contactants. There are three categories of contact urticaria, based on the mechanism of action. The first is nonimmunologic. It may affect nearly all individuals and occurs as a result of the direct release of inflammatory mediators. Urticariogenic agents causing this reaction include arthropod bodies, hairs, and nettles. The second category is allergic, and probably represents a type 1 hypersensitivity reaction with demonstration of antigen-specific IgE. Reported causes include foods (such as fish and eggs), medications

(such as penicillin G), silk, and animal saliva. The reaction may range from localized urticaria to urticaria and anaphylaxis. In the third category the mechanism is unknown but appears to combine features of both the allergic and nonallergic types. An example is ammonium persulfate, an oxidizing agent in hair bleach. Some patients with contact urticaria present with an immediate localized wheal and erythema response. Some appear with relapsing erythema or generalized urticaria. Some patients complain only of itching, burning, and tingling of the skin. The specific diagnosis is made with a patch test. One technique is to apply the substance in question on the forearm and observe for 30 minutes for the appearance of a macular erythematous reaction that evolves into a wheal. If the open test is negative, then a close patch test may be applied. In the allergic type of contact urticaria, a systemic reaction may occur to the patch test if the concentration is too high.

IDENTIFYING THE OFFENDING AGENT

History and Physical Examination

Once the diagnosis of allergic contact dermatitis is made, vigorous efforts should be directed toward determining the cause. A careful, thorough history is absolutely mandatory. The temporal relationship between exposure and clinical manifestations must be kept in mind as an exhaustive search is made for exposure to a sensitizing allergen in the patient's occupational, home, or recreational environment. The location of the dermatitis most often relates closely to direct contact with a particular allergen. At times this is rather straightforward, such as dermatitis of the feet, because of contact sensitivity to shoe materials or dermatitis from jewelry appearing on the wrist, the ear lobes, or the neck. The relationship of the dermatitis to the direct contact allergen may not be as obvious at other times, and being able to associate certain areas of involvement with particular types of exposure is extremely helpful. Contact dermatitis of the face, for example, is often due to cosmetics directly applied to the area. One must keep in mind other possibilities, however, such as hair dye, shampoo, and hair-styling preparations. Contact dermatitis of the eyelid, although often caused by eye shadow, mascara, and eye liner, also may be caused by nail polish. Involvement of the thighs may be caused by keys or coins in pants pockets. Therefore, it is vital that the physician be familiar with various distribution patterns of contact dermatitis that may occur in association with particular allergens.

Frequently, the distribution of the skin lesions may suggest a number of possible sensitizing agents, and patch testing is of special value. Certain allergens may be airborne, and exposure may occur by this route. Dermatitis among farmers caused by ragweed oil sensitivity occurs occasionally. Smoke from burning the poison ivy plant may contain the oleoresin as particulate matter, and thus expose the sensitive individual. Another route of acquiring poison ivy contact dermatitis without touching the plant is by indirect contact with clothing or animal fur containing the oleoresin. It should be remembered also that systemic administration of a drug or a related drug that has been previously used topically and to which the patient has been sensitized can elicit a localized or generalized eruption. An example is sensitivity to ethylenediamine. A patient may develop localized contact dermatitis to topically applied ethylenediamine hydrochloride used as a stabilizer in such compounds as Mycolog (Goldline, Hollywood, FL) cream; a localized or generalized eruption may occur when aminophylline is administered orally (6).

The oral mucosa also may be the site of a localized allergic contact reaction resulting in contact stomatitis or stomatitis venenata (7). The relatively low incidence of contact stomatitis compared with contact dermatitis is attributed to the brief duration of surface contact, the diluting and buffering action of saliva, and the rapid dispersal and absorption because of extensive vascularity. Agents capable of producing contact stomatitis include dentifrices, mouthwashes, dental materials such as acrylic and epoxy resins, and foods. The clinical response is most commonly inflammation of the lips, but cases of "burning mouth" syndrome have also been attributed to contact allergy.

Patch Testing

Principle

Patch testing or epicutaneous testing is the diagnostic technique of applying a specific substance to the skin with the intention of producing a small area of allergic contact dermatitis. It can be thought of as reproducing the disease in miniature. The patch test is generally kept in place for 48 to 96 hours (although reactions may appear after 24 hours in markedly sensitive patients), and then observed for the gross appearance of a localized dermatitis. The same principles of proper interpretation of a positive patch test apply as in the case of the immediate wheal and erythema skin test reaction (see Chapter 2). A positive patch test is not absolute proof that the test substance is the actual cause of dermatitis. It may reflect a previous episode of dermatitis, or it may be without any clinical relevance at all. The positive patch test must always correlate with the patient's history and physical examination.

Allergic Contact Dermatitis and Indications for Patch Testing

All unexplained cases of eczema that either do not respond to treatment or recur after treatment may be due to contact allergy and should be considered for patch testing (8). Currently, patch testing is the only accepted scientific proof of contact allergy. If patch testing is successful at identifying a causative allergen, avoidance will often be curative. Alternatively, if the causative agent is not identified, it is likely that the patient will need ongoing treatment and that treatment will be less than optimal.

A thorough history and physical examination should be performed with emphasis on the distribution and timing of the clinical lesions. Once this information is obtained, an exhaustive history should be taken to identify all potential allergens that had opportunity to come in contact with the skin of the patient. A tray of patch test materials is then assembled.

Most physicians doing patch testing use the True Test, a ready-made series of 23 common allergens that can be easily applied in a busy

TABLE 18.1. *Allergens on the true test standard tray listed by function*

Metals	Nickel sulfate, potassium dichromate Cobalt chloride
Medications	Benzocaine, neomycin sulfate
Cosmetic fragrances	Fragrance mix, balsam of Peru
Cosmetic preservatives	Paraben mix Quaternium 15, Kathon CG
Other cosmetic ingredients	Colophony (rosin), ethylenediamine, paraphenylenediamine, Lanolin (wool wax) alcohol, formaldehyde, thimerosol
Rubber ingredients	Mercaptobenzothiazole, mercapto mix, carba mix (carbamates), thiuram mix, black rubber paraphenylenediamine mix
Resins	Epoxy resin, paratertiarybutylphenol, formaldehyde resin

office setting (Table 18.1). Since a recent study reported that less than 26% of contact allergy problems will be fully solved using the True Test, patients often need referral to a physician specializing in patch testing. These specialists will generally have a wide array of allergens relevant to most occupations and exposures and are familiar with where these allergens are found and alternatives to avoid exposure. Testing is usually performed with an expanded standard tray and additional allergens individualized to the patient exposure.

The physician should become familiar with the potent sensitizers and with the various modes of exposure. It is important to keep in mind the possibility of cross-reactivity to other allergens because of chemical similarities. Sensitivity to paraphenylenediamine, for example, also may indicate sensitivity to para-amino-benzoic acid and other chemicals containing a benzene ring with an amino group in the "para" position.

The most common cause of allergic contact dermatitis in the United States is *Toxicodendron* (poison ivy, poison oak, poison sumac). Latex-induced contact dermatitis affects health-care workers, patients with spina bifida, and manufacturing employees who prepare latex-based products. Table 18.2 is a list of some of the most potent sensitizers and agents that contain them. It is by no means complete, and is not intended as a general survey. More detailed information on other sensitizers, environmental exposures, and preparation of testing material is contained in several standard texts (10–12).

Techniques

The two most common types of patch test chambers for patch testing, the aluminum Finn chamber and the plastic IQ chamber, come in strips that hold 10 allergens (9). Allergens are placed into the chambers as a drop of liquid on filter paper

TABLE 18.2. *Examples of antigens and exposure commonly causing contact dermatitis*

Contactant	Exposure
Carba mix	Rubber, lawn and garden fungicides
Copper	Coins, alloys, insecticides, fungicides
Epoxy resin	Adhesives
Formalin (formaldehyde)	Cosmetics, insecticides, wearing apparel (drip-dry, wrinkle resistant, water repellent)
Ethylenediamine hydrochloride	Mycolog cream (not ointment), aminophylline, hydroxyzine, antihistamines
Imidazolidinyl urea	Preservative in cosmetics
Mercaptobenzothiazole	Rubber compounds (accelerator), anticorrosion agent
Mercury	Topical ointments, disinfectants, insecticides
Nickel	Coins, jewelry, buckles, clasps, door handles
Paraben	Cosmetics, pharmaceuticals
Paraphenylenediamine	Hair dye, fur dye, black, blue, and brown clothing
Phenylbetanaphthylamine	Rubber compounds (antioxidant)
Potassium dichromate	Leather (chrome tanning), yellow paints
P-tert-butylphenol	Rubber, plastics, adhesives
Sodium hypochlorite	Bleach, cleansing agents
Thiouram	Rubber (accelerator), fungicides, wood preservatives

or as a 1-cm cylinder of allergen in petrolatum from a syringe.

With the patient standing erect, the patch test strips are applied starting at the bottom and pressing each allergen chamber firmly against the skin as it is applied. The skin surrounding the patch test strips is then typically outlined with either fluorescent ink or gentian violet marker. Reinforcing tape, and sometimes a medical adhesive such as Mastisol, is then used to further affix the patches in place. The patch test series is documented in the medical records clearly showing the position of each allergen. It is important that the patient be instructed to keep the patch test sites dry and avoid vigorous physical activity until after patch test reading is completed. The allergens are removed and read 48 hours after application and the patient returns for a second reading of the patch tests at 72 or 96 hours. Some physicians also do readings at 1 week after application to identify more delayed reactions.

It is essential that the skin of the back be free of eczema at the time of testing to avoid false-positive reactions due to what has been called the "angry back syndrome." It is also important that the testing site has not been exposed to topical steroids or ultraviolet light during the preceding week. Oral steroids should be avoided when possible; however, some strong patch test reactions can be obtained even when a patient is taking up to 30 mg prednisone daily.

Photoallergy and Photopatch Testing

When an eruption is observed in a sun-exposed distribution, photoallergic contact dermatitis should be considered. Photoallergy is identical to allergic contact dermatitis with the exception that the allergen in contact with the skin must be exposed to ultraviolet A (UVA) light for the reaction to occur. Photopatch testing is performed similar to routine patch testing, but a second identical set of allergens is also applied to the back. Approximately 24 hours after application, one set of allergens is uncovered and exposed to 15 joules of UVA light. The patches are then carefully reapplied. All patches are then removed at 48 hours and read at 72 hours. A photoallergy is confirmed if only the site exposed to

UVA light shows a reaction. If both the exposed and unexposed sites show equal reactions, a standard contact allergy is confirmed. A stronger reaction at the site exposed to UVA indicates contact allergy augmented by coexisting photoallergy.

Patch Testing Reading and Interpretation

The patch tests are read using a template that is aligned inside the marker lines on the back to show the exact position of each allergen. The sites are then graded as 1+ (erythema), 2+ (edema or vesiculation of <50% of the patch test site), 3+ (edema or vesiculation of >50% of the patch test site), ± or ? (questionable), or Ir (irritant). Strong irritant reactions sometimes result in a sharply demarcated, shiny, eroded patch test site. Weak irritant and allergic reactions are often morphologically indistinguishable.

One of the most important aspects of patch testing is to determine if patch test reactions are relevant to the patient's clinical condition. Some patch test reactions merely indicate an exposure that occurred many years prior. In addition, false-positive reactions are not uncommon. Pustular patch test reactions can occur with metal salts and do not indicate contact allergy. Some allergens, such as nickel, formaldehyde, and potassium dichromate, are tested at levels that can also cause an irritant reaction. Also, when a test site is strongly positive or if the patient experiences severe irritation from tape, nearby sites may show false-positive reactions due to the "angry back syndrome." When in doubt, a "use test" can be performed by applying a suspected substance twice daily for 1 week to the antecubital fossa to confirm an allergic reaction.

Reactions to Cosmetics and Skin Care Products

Although most skin care products available are quite safe, allergic reactions can occur occasionally to almost any cosmetic product. The most common causative agents are fragrance and preservative ingredients. A discussion of some common cosmetic allergens follows.

Fragrance

Fragrance is found in a wide variety of cosmetic products. It is responsible for a relatively large number of allergic reactions to cosmetics (13–15). This is partially because fragrance is not a single ingredient but is instead a general name that includes a variety of individual fragrance ingredients. Individual ingredients in fragrance are usually not listed on ingredient labels. It is important to read the actual ingredient list on products and avoid products that contain fragrance, perfume, or essential oils. Essential oils (i.e., cinnamon oil, clove oil, rosewood oil) are often used as fragrance ingredients. Labels that claim that the product is "unscented" or "fragrance free" can be misleading. Unscented products may contain masking fragrance designed to eliminate odors, and fragrance-free products can sometimes include essential oils that the manufacturer may not consider as fragrance. Also, consumers should beware of other less obvious fragrance ingredients that may be listed on the label, such as benzyl alcohol, benzaldehyde, and ethylene brassylate.

There are two materials in the standard patch test tray that screen for allergy to fragrance. The fragrance blend is a mixture of eight common fragrance ingredients and can corroborate the diagnosis in about 80% of individuals allergic to fragrance. Balsam of Peru is a tree extract from El Salvador containing many constituents used commonly in fragrances that will cause a reaction in approximately 50% of fragrance-allergic patients. Balsam of Peru is used in the artificial flavoring industry and individuals allergic to the substance may have reactions to sweet junk foods, condiments, mouthwashes, toothpaste, cough medicines, liqueurs, and spiced teas. It also can cross-react with citrus peels.

Formaldehyde-Releasing Preservatives

Formaldehyde is still the most effective cosmetic preservative against gram-negative bacteria. Substances that release formaldehyde are therefore still commonly used in skin care and cosmetic products (16). Currently used formaldehyde-releasing preservatives include quaternium 15, imidazolidinyl urea, diazolidinyl urea, DMDM hydantoin, and 2-bromo-2- nitropropane-1,3-diol (Bronopol). Individuals allergic to one of these ingredients may cross-react to any of the other formaldehyde-releasing preservatives. Therefore, it is often good advice to avoid all of these substances if patch testing results to one of them are clearly positive.

Parabens

Parabens are the most common preservatives in skin care products and cosmetics. A person who has an allergic reaction to parabens may still be able to use paraben-containing products if they are only applied to undamaged skin. That is, almost all paraben allergic reactions occur on inflamed or cracked skin; this has been termed the paraben paradox (17).

Parabens are also found in syrups, milk products, soft drinks, candies, jellies, and some systemic medications. However, no sensitization has been reported by ingestion of parabens. Foods containing various preservatives that are known to be topical contact allergens have been occasional causes of hand dermatitis in cooks and bakers.

Kathon CG

Kathon CG (methylisothiazolinone and methylchloroisothiazoline) is a relatively new preservative system that has now been used enough in products that it has become a common sensitizer (18).

Euxyl K400

Euxyl K400 (phenoxylethanol and methyldibromoglutaronitrile) is an even more recent preservative system that will probably become a more common cause of contact allergy once it is used more frequently (19). Methyldibromoglutaronitrile is the usual sensitizer.

Iodopropynylbutylcarbamate

Iodopropynylbutylcarbamate is the newest preservative to be used in skin care and cosmetic products (20). Case reports of contact allergy have been traced to this ingredient.

Sorbic Acid

Sorbic acid is another cosmetic preservative that occasionally causes allergic reactions (21). Persons allergic to sorbic acid also may react to potassium sorbate. Sorbic acid is often used to replace thimerosol in sensitive eye products. Sorbic acid can also cause nonimmunologic contact urticaria.

Thimerosol

Thimerosol is primarily in liquid products for use in the eyes, nose, and ears (22). In cosmetics, it is mostly used in mascaras. It is also found in vaccines, eye drops, contact lens products, nose sprays, nose drops, and ear drops.

Paraphenylenediamine

Paraphenylenediamine (PPD) is an ingredient in permanent, demipermanent, and semipermanent hair dyes (23). This ingredient can be avoided by use of temporary hair dyes, metallic hair dyes, henna, or occasional other dye products without PPD. Persons allergic to this ingredient also may react to similar "para compounds" such as paraaminobenzoic acid (PABA) and its derivatives (found in sunscreens), benzocaine (found in skin anesthetics such as sunburn medications), procaine, sulfonamides, paraaminosalicylic acid, carbutamide, and azo dyes (in synthetic clothing fabrics). Allergy to hair dye can be problematic for hair colorists because PPD penetrates readily through latex gloves.

Glyceryl Thioglycolate

Glyceryl thioglycolate is found in the acid permanent wave products used in salons (23). This is a common cause of contact allergy in hairdressers because latex gloves are not impermeable to it. The alkaline permanent waves predominate in retail stores and are also commonly used in salons. These products and many depilatories contain ammonium thioglycolate, which usually does not cross-react with glyceryl thioglycolate.

Lanolin

Lanolin is a moisturizing substance obtained from the sebaceous secretions of sheep (24). The alcohol fraction of lanolin is the sensitizing portion. Therefore, lanolin-allergic individuals only need to avoid lanolin and lanolin alcohol, synonymous with the European terms wool wax and wool wax alcohol, and not other lanolin derivatives.

Propylene Glycol

Propylene glycol is a versatile ingredient that is both a solvent and a humectant (25). It can be an irritant that stings when applied to inflamed or cracked skin. Less commonly, it can cause true allergic reactions.

Toluene Sulfonamide/Formaldehyde Resin

Toluene sulfonamide/formaldehyde resin is found in nail polish and is the most common cause of eyelid contact allergy (26). Nail polishes that use other resins in place of this ingredient can be used by persons who are allergic to this ingredient.

Cocamidopropyl Betaine

In recent years, there have been a number of reports of contact allergy to cocamidopropyl betaine (27). This ingredient is used in baby shampoos due to its gentleness and the fact that it does not sting when it gets onto the eyes. Recently, it has been used more widely in many types of shampoos and cleansers. The sensitizer appears to be an impurity formed in the manufacture of the ingredient.

Sunscreen Ingredients

Sunscreen ingredients that can cause allergic reactions include PABA and its derivatives, benzophenone, cinnamates, and Parsol 1789, also called avobenzone or butylmethoxydibenzoylmethane (28). These sunscreen ingredients are also found in many other cosmetic products, including foundations, pressed powders, antiaging products, lip and nail products, and toners.

One common cause of sunscreen allergy is PABA and its derivatives. The derivatives of PABA include glyceryl PABA and octyl dimethyl PABA, also called Padimate O. Most products on the market do not contain actual PABA. Unfortunately, there are products on the market that claim to be PABA free but which include PABA derivatives.

The benzophenones, which include oxybenzone and dioxybenzone, are now the most common cause of contact allergy to sunscreens. There are numerous cases of persons allergic to benzophenones who have assumed they were allergic to PABA and have switched to another PABA-free sunscreen only to discover they react poorly to the substitute because it also contains benzophenones. Benzophenones are also found in nail products, hair products, textiles, and plastics. Parsol 1789 is a newer UVA sunscreen that can cause both contact allergy and photoallergy. Cinnamates are occasional photosensitizers.

Colophony (Rosin)

Colophony or rosin is distilled oil of turpentine (29). It is used in some cosmetics, adhesives (commonly in shoe adhesives), tape, flypaper, epilating wax, rosin bags, furniture polish, price labels, varnish, glue, ink, recycled paper, and car or floor waxes. Colophony cross-reacts with abietic acid, abitol, and hydrobietic acid, which are also used in cosmetic products.

Medications that Are Sensitizers

A number of medications have been reported to cause allergic contact dermatitis. In the case of topical products, it is important to consider vehicle ingredients as possible contact allergens in addition to the active drug.

Topical Steroids

It is now appreciated that topical steroids are a fairly frequent cause of contact allergy (30–32). The two best screening ingredients for topical steroid allergy are believed to be tixocortol pivalate and budesonide. The European literature divides topical steroids into 4 structural groups: group A (tixocortol pivalate, hydrocortisone, prednisone); group B (budesonide and steroids ending in "-ide"); group C (betamethasone, dexamethasone, mometasone, desoximetasone, and steroids ending in "-one" that are not in group A); group D (steroids ending in "-ate" that are not in group A). Cross reactions between structural groups can occur; Groups B and D often cross-react.

Ethylenediamine-related Drugs

Ethylenediamine was most commonly found in Mycolog cream, but is not in the current Mycolog II. It is still found in a small number of topical products. Ethylenediamine cross-reacts with aminophylline (which contains 33% ethylenediamine by weight as a stabilizer), ethylenediamine and piperazine antihistamines such as hydroxyzine and cetirizine, ethylenediamine-related motion sickness medications and menstrual analgesics, and some antiparasitics. Ethylenediamine is also used as a stabilizer in the manufacture of dyes, rubber accelerators, fungicides, waxes, and resins. However, these sources of exposure are uncommon causes of contact dermatitis.

Neomycin and Bacitracin

These ingredients often cause contact allergy because they are used on injured skin with damaged barrier function (33). Neomycin may cross-react with gentamicin and other aminoglycosides. Bacitracin is now also known to be a frequent cause of contact allergy. Many patients are allergic to both neomycin and bacitracin. This probably does not represent a true cross-reaction but rather reflects the fact that these two ingredients are often in the same products.

Benzocaine

Benzocaine cross-reacts with other benzoate ester anesthetics, such as procaine, tetracaine, and cocaine (22). It also may cross-react with other para compounds such as paraaminosalicylic acid, PABA, paraphenylenediamine, procainamide, and sulfonamides. There is no cross-reaction with amide anesthetics, such as lidocaine, dibucaine, mepivacaine, and cyclomethycaine.

Mercurials

Mercurials are divided into organics or inorganics (34). Organics include Merthiolate (thimerosol) and Mercurochrome (merbromin). Inorganics include mercury (thermometers), yellow oxide of mercury, ammoniated mercury (found in Unguentum Bossi and Mazon cream for psoriasis) and phenylmercuric acetate (a spermicidal agent and an occasional preservative in eye solutions). Cross-reactions can occur between organic and inorganic mercury substances. Also, systemic administration of mercurials can induce a severe systemic allergic reaction in a person topically sensitized to mercury.

Metals

Metals can cause both allergic and irritant contact dermatitis. Reactions to metal are most common when sweat is present. Also, moisture under jewelry from repeated hand washing is a common cause of irritant dermatitis to metals. The most common cause of skin discoloration to metals is due to the abrasive action of powders in cosmetic products on metal jewelry. The resulting black powder creates what has been called black dermatographism.

Nickel

Nickel is the most common metal to cause allergic contact dermatitis (35). Sweat will act on nickel to create a green/black tarnish that can induce an allergic contact dermatitis. Sensitization often occurs via ear or body piercing. Metal jewelry that contains a significant amount of nickel turns red when a drop of 1% dimethylglyoxime from a nickel test kit is applied to the surface. All alloys of steel, except most stainless steel, can cause nickel contact allergy. The nickel in stainless steel is so firmly bound that sweat will often not liberate it and it will not react with dimethylglyoxime.

A significant amount of nickel is not only found in jewelry but also in bobby pins, safety pins, some non-U.S. coins, eyeglass frames, zippers, bra and garter snaps, doorknobs, scissors, pens, and shoelace eyelets. Nickel is also used in chrome, white gold, and 14 carat yellow gold.

Chromium

Chromium causes both allergic and irritant reactions; however, allergic reactions are more common (35). Allergy to chrome or chrome-plated objects is uncommon. When reactions to chrome products occur, the reaction is usually due to nickel in the product.

Most allergic reactions to chromium are to chromates in tanned leather or cement, and these reactions tend to be chronic dermatitis. Chromates are the most common cause of contact allergy to leather and are used in soft tanned leather of the type commonly found on shoe uppers. Potassium dichromate and other chromates are also found in cement, matches, bleach, phosphate-containing detergents, antirust compounds, varnish, orange or yellow paint, spackle, and green tattoos. Chromate reactions in cement workers are often severe, chronic, and may persist many years after exposure to cement has ended.

Cobalt

Objects containing nickel often also contain cobalt (35). It is found in the adhesive of flypaper, light brown hair colors, hard metals, polyester resins, paints, cements, pottery, ceramics, pigments, lubricating oils, and blue tattoos. Occupational exposure includes masons, construction workers, tile workers, dentists, printers, mechanics, and machinists.

Gold

Positive reactions to gold on patch testing are not uncommon (36). However, many individuals who test positive to gold will tolerate gold jewelry. Often, these individuals will only react to softer gold alloys or to gold objects subjected to perspiration and friction.

Tattoos

Several metals used in tattoos can cause allergic contact dermatitis: red tattoos contain mercury sulfide (red cinnabar); green tattoos contain chromium or chronic oxide; blue tattoos contain cobalt aluminate; yellow tattoos contain cadmium yellow (a possible cause of phototoxic reactions) (37).

Rubber-related Compounds

Latex products can cause type I allergy as well as type IVa_1 allergy (38). Type I latex allergy to gloves may present as a localized contact urticaria that can mimic an allergic contact dermatitis. Alternatively, latex protein can be inhaled on particles of powder from gloves and cause widespread urticaria and anaphylaxis. RAST can be used to screen for type I allergy to latex but does not have 100% sensitivity. Therefore, the skin-prick test is still the gold standard for type I latex allergy testing. Unfortunately, no U.S. Food and Drug Administration (FDA)-approved latex extract is available yet in the United States for skin-prick testing.

Alternatively, chemicals used to process rubber frequently cause type IVa_1 allergy to latex products and artificial rubber (nitrile rubber). Mercaptobenzothiazole and other mercapto compounds are rubber accelerators that frequently are allergic sensitizers.

Tetramethylthiuram and disulfiram are also rubber accelerators that can cause allergic contact dermatitis. Thiurams are also used in insecticides and fungicides and are often found on lawns and garden plants. Disulfiram is also the active ingredient in Antabuse. Carbamates are rubber accelerators that are common sensitizers and are closely related to thiurams. They are also found in similar products such as rubber and pesticides. Currently, carbamates are the most common accelerators used in latex and nitrile medical gloves.

Black rubber paraphenylenediamine is an antioxidant used in the manufacture of black rubber. This is fortunately a relatively uncommon sensitizer because avoidance of this ubiquitous substance is difficult. Thioureas and naphthyl compounds are rubber accelerators that are less common causes of allergy.

Clothing-related Dermatitis

Most clothing fibers are nonsensitizers or rare sensitizers (39). Dyes used in clothing and shoes can cause allergic reactions. The disperse dyes, such as azo and anthraquinone dyes, which are used on synthetic fabrics, are most problematic. Some persons reacting to azo dyes cross-react with paraphenylenediamine and PABA.

Fabrics containing cotton or rayon usually contain formaldehyde resins and a small amount of free formaldehyde. Allergy to free formaldehyde has become less common in recent years because manufacturers have reduced levels of free formaldehyde in fabrics. However, it is possible to have contact allergy to the formaldehyde resins used in these fabrics. These individuals may or may not react to formaldehyde.

Because allergy to clothing is not usually identified using a standard patch test, testing requires specialized nonstandard allergens. Other causes of clothing dermatitis include reactions to rubber used in elastic. Spandex (except some from Europe which contains mercaptobenzothiazole) and Lycra are good substitutes.

Plastic-related Dermatitis

Plastics that can sensitize include epoxies (before full hardening occurs), paratertiary butyphenol formaldehyde resin (commonly used in leather adhesives), and acrylate and methacrylate monomers (40,41). Household adhesives may contain both formaldehyde and epoxy.

Acrylic monomers, used in about 95% of dentures in the United States, are a common cause of contact allergy in dentists. The allergen can penetrate rubber gloves. Once the material polymerizes and hardens, it is no longer allergenic. Acrylic sculptured nails, nail products, and acrylic prostheses also can cause sensitization. Cyanoacrylate adhesives can occasionally cause contact allergy.

Plants

Allergic contact dermatitis to plants is most commonly due to the oleoresin fraction, especially the essential oil fraction. In contrast, type I reactions to plants are most commonly due to pollen and other plant proteins.

Rhus

Rhus dermatitis (poison ivy, oak, and sumac) is the most common form of allergic contact dermatitis seen in both children and adults in the United States (42,43). Rhus plants have now been reclassified as toxicodendron. Cross-reactions can occur with other anacardiacaeae such as Japanese lacquer tree, marking nut tree of India, cashew nutshells, mango, Ginkgo tree fruit pulp, and the Rengas (black varnish) tree.

Ragweed

Ragweed dermatitis generally affects older individuals and rarely occurs in children (44). Men are affected 20 times more often than women, primarily those who are dairy farmers. Affected persons are not usually atopic. The allergic contact reaction is a type IVa_1 hypersensitivity to the oil-soluble fraction. Type I reactions to the protein fraction lead to allergic rhinitis. Contact allergy occurs in Chicago from mid-August to late September. A rash involving exposed areas may develop from airborne ragweed exposure.

Compositae

Compositae are ubiquitous in many parts of the world (44). This large family of plants includes chrysanthemums, daisies, asters, arnica, artichokes, burdock, chamomile, chicory, cocklebur, feverfew, lettuce, marigold, marsh elder, pyrethrum, ragweed, sagebrush, sunflower, tansy, and yarrow. The sensitizers in these plants are sesquiterpene lactones. Although a sesquiterpene lactone mix is available for patch testing and will be positive in many cases of compositae allergy, it will miss some cases because sesquiterpene lactones may not be cross-reactive.

Alstromeria

Alstromeria (Peruvian lilly) is a common cause of allergy in florists and is due to tuliposide-A (α butyrolactone) (45). Cross-reactions may occur from handling tulip bulbs.

Photoreactions

Phototoxic reactions are due to nonimmunologic mechanisms, usually occur on first exposure, and tend to resemble sunburn (46). The action spectrum of the two most common causes, tar and psoralens, is primarily UVA. Other topical phototoxic agents include phenothiazines, sulfanilamide, anthraquinone dyes, eosin, and methylene blue.

Phytophotodermatitis

Phytophotodermatitis is a phototoxic reaction to UVA light due to furocoumarins in several families of plants, especially Umbelliferae (47). The Umbelliferae family includes carrots, celery, parsnips, fennel, dill, parsley, caraway, anise, coriander, and angelica. Also, Rutaceae plants (orange, lemon, grapefruit, lime, and bergamot lime) and some members of Compositae (yarrow) and Moraceae (figs) are also possible causes. Psoralens comes from an Egyptian Umbelliferae plant. Berloque dermatitis on the neck is caused by perfumes containing oil of bergamot (bergapten or 5-methoxy-psoralens). Bartenders handling Persian limes also can develop phytophotodermatitis.

Photoallergic Contact Reactions

Type IVa_1 hypersensitivity mediates photoallergic contact reactions (48). The most common cause in the past was halogenated salcylanides in soaps and cleansers; however, these are no longer used in the United States or Europe. Hexachlorophene, a halogenated phenol, also can cause photoallergy and can cross-react with these compounds.

Today sunscreen ingredients such as PABA, benzophenones, cinnamates, and avobenzone are the most common causes of photoallergy. Fragrances are another fairly common cause of photoallergy.

Phenothiazines are used in insecticides and can cause topical photoallergy and phototoxic reactions. This does not occur by the oral route, with the exception of chlorpromazine, which can cause phototoxic reactions.

Most topical sulfonamides are not photosensitizers, but sulfanilamide can cause both photoallergic and phototoxic reactions. Oral sulfonamides, tetracyclines, fluoroquinolones, hypoglycemics, and thiazides can cause both photoallergic and phototoxic reactions.

Precautions

Several precautions must be observed in patch testing. The application of the test material itself may sensitize the patient. Potent materials that may sensitize on the first application include plant oleoresins, paraphenylenediamine, and methylsalicylate. Patch testing and especially repeated patch testing should not be performed unnecessarily. In testing, one has to avoid provoking nonspecific inflammation. The testing material must be dilute enough to avoid a primary irritant effect. This is especially important when testing with a contactant not included in the standard patch test materials. To be significant, a substance must elicit a reaction at a concentration that will not cause reactivity in a suitable number of normal controls. Patch testing should never be performed in the presence of an acute or widespread contact dermatitis. False-positive reactions may be obtained because of increased reactivity of the skin. In addition, a positive patch test reaction with the offending agent may cause a flare-up of the dermatitis. The patient should be carefully instructed at the time of patch test application to remove any patch that is causing severe irritation. If the patch is left on for the full

48 hours, such an area actually may slough. As mentioned earlier, an anaphylactoid reaction can occur when testing for contact urticaria.

COMPLICATIONS

The most common complication of allergic contact dermatitis is secondary infection caused by the intense pruritus and subsequent scratching. An interesting but poorly understood complication is the occasional occurrence of the nephrotic syndrome and glomerulonephritis in severe generalized contact dermatitis caused by poison ivy or poison oak (49).

MANAGEMENT

General management strategies are outlined in Table 18.3 (50).

SYMPTOMATIC TREATMENT

The inflammation and pruritus of allergic contact dermatitis necessitate symptomatic therapy. For limited, localized allergic contact dermatitis, cool tap water compresses and a topical corticosteroid are the preferred modalities. It is safest to use hydrocortisone on the face.

When the dermatitis is particularly acute or widespread, systemic corticosteroids should be used. In instances when further exposure can be avoided, such as poison ivy dermatitis, there should be no hesitation in administering systemic corticosteroids. This is a classic example of a self-limited disease that will respond to a course of oral corticosteroid therapy. The popular use of a 4- to 5-day decreasing steroid regimen often results in a flare-up of the dermatitis several days

TABLE 18.3. *Management of the allergic contact dermatitis*

Limited, localized reaction	Cool tap water compress Topical corticosteroid cream
Extensive, acute reaction	Oral prednisone: 40–60 mg per day initially (adult); allow taper over 2 weeks
Prophylaxis	Antigen avoidance Protective clothing Barrier cream

after discontinuing the steroids. It is probably best to continue the treatment for 10 to 14 days. There seems to be no need for prolonged antihistamine therapy in such instances. The response to systemic corticosteroids is generally dramatic, with improvement apparent in only a few hours. Three rules that might be applied to systemic corticosteroid therapy in acute contact dermatitis are (a) use an inexpensive preparation such as prednisone; (b) use enough (1 mg/kg); and (c) avoid prolonged administration (rarely more than 2 weeks of therapy is required).

For secondary infection resulting from scratching because of the pruritus of allergic contact dermatitis, antibiotics may be needed. Because of the risk involved in sensitization from topical antibiotics, the oral or injectable forms are preferred.

PROPHYLAXIS

The physician has a responsibility to his or her patients not only to treat disease but also to prevent it. For that reason, avoid topical applications of medications that have a high index of sensitization. Included in this group are benzocaine, antihistamines, neomycin, penicillin, sulfonamides, and ammoniated mercury.

When the offending agent causing allergic contact dermatitis is discovered, careful instruction must be given to the patient so as to avoid it in the future. The physician should discuss all of the possible sources of exposure, and when dealing with occupational dermatitis, should have knowledge about suitable jobs for patients. In the case of chemical sensitivity, this list of sources may be quite extensive. When dealing with a plant sensitizer, the patient should be instructed in the proper identification of the offending plant.

If sensitization has occurred, the amount of information about the allergen is correlated with the condition of the skin. It has been reported that if the patient is aware of the allergen and informed about the variety of substances that contain it, the skin condition is much more satisfactory that if the patient knows little about the allergen (51).

There may be instances in which exposure cannot be avoided, either because of the patient's occupation or because of the ubiquitous nature of the allergen. The use of protective clothing is beneficial, as are newly available barrier creams. Early diagnosis and evidence of further allergen exposure are critical if chronic, debilitating dermatitis is to be avoided (52).

REFERENCES

1. Rietschel RL, Fowler JF. The pathogenesis of allergic contact hypersensitivity. In: Rietschel RL, Fowler JF, eds. *Fisher's contact dermatitis,* 4th ed. Baltimore: Williams & Wilkins, 1995:1–10.
2. Ray MC, Tharp MD, Sullivan TJ, et al. Contact hypersensitivity reactions to dinitrofluorobenzene mediated by monoclonal IgE anti-DNP antibodies. *J Immunol* 1983;131:1096.
3. Silberberg-Sinakin I, Gigli I, Baer RL, et al. Langerhans cells: role in contact hypersensitivity and relationship to lymphoid dendritic cells and to macrophages. *Immunol Rev* 1980;53:203.
4. Belsito DV. The pathophysiology of allergic contact dermatitis. *Clin Rev Allergy* 1989;7:347.
5. Von Kroch G, Maibach HI. The contact urticaria syndrome: an update review. *J Am Acad Dermatol* 1981;6:328.
6. Fisher AA. New advances in contact dermatitis. *Int J Dermatol* 1977:16:552.
7. Archard HO. Common stomatologic disorders. In: Fitzpatrick TB, Arndt KA, Clark WH, et al., eds. *Dermatology in general medicine.* New York: McGraw-Hill,1971.
8. Scheman AJ. Patch testing and photopatch testing. In: Chan L, ed. *American Academy of Dermatology core curriculum.* Schaumberg, IL: American Academy of Dermatology (in press).
9. Rietschel RL, Fowler JF. The role of patch testing. In: Rietschel RL, Fowler JF, eds. *Fisher's contact dermatitis,* 4th ed. Baltimore: Williams & Wilkins, 1995:11–32.
10. Belsito DV. The diagnostic evaluation treatment, and prevention of allergic contact dermatitis in the new millennium. *J Allergy Clin Immunol* 2000;3: 409–420.
11. Krasteva M, Kehren J, Sayag M, et al. Contact dermatitis: clinical aspects and diagnosis. *Eur J Dermatol* 1999;9:144–159.
12. Beltrani VS, Beltrani VP. Contact dermatitis. Ann Allergy Asthma Immunol 1997:2:160–173
13. Scheinman PL. Allergic contact dermatitis to fragrance: a review. *Am J Contact Dermatitis* 1996;7:65–76.
14. Johansen JD, Menne T. The fragrance mix and its constituents: a 14 year material. *Contact Dermatitis* 1995;32:18–23.
15. Larsen W, Nakayama H, Lindberg M, et al. Fragrance contact dermatitis: a worldwide multicenter investigation (Part I). *Am J Contact Dermatitis* 1996;7:77–83.
16. Fransway AF. The problem of preservation in the 1990s. I. Statement of the problem, solution(s) of the industry, and the current use of formaldehyde and formaldehyde-releasing biocides. *Am J Contact Dermatitis* 1991;2: 6–22.
17. Jackson EM. Paraben paradoxes. *Am J Contact Dermatitis* 1993;4:69–70.

18. Mowad CM. Methylchloro-isothiazolinone revisited. *Am J Contact Dermatitis,* 2000;11:115–118.

19. De Groot AC, Van Ginkel CJW, Weijland JW. Methyl-dibromoglutaronitrile (Euxyl K 400): an important "new" allergen in cosmetics. *J Am Acad Dermatol* 1996;35:743–747.

20. Bryld LE, Agner T, Rastogi SC, et al. Iodopropynylbutyl-carbamate: a new contact allergen. *Contact Dermatitis* 1997;36:156–158.

21. Fisher AA. Sorbic acid: a cause of immediate nonaller-genic facial erythema: an update. *Cutis* 1998;61:17.

22. Scheman AJ. Contact allergy alternatives 1996. *Cutis* 1996;57:235–240.

23. Scheman AJ. New trends in hair products: an update for dermatologists. *Cosmetic Derm* 1998;11:17–21.

24. Matthieu L, Dockx P. Discrepancy in patch test results with wool wax alcohols and Amerchol L-101. *Contact Dermatitis* 1997;36:150–151.

25. Jackson EM. Propylene glycol: irritant, sensitizer or nei-ther? *Cosmetic Derm* 1995;8:43–45.

26. Rosenzweig R, Scher RK. Nail cosmetics: adverse reac-tions. *Am J Contact Dermatitis* 1993;4:71–77.

27. Fowler JF, Fowler LM, Hunter JE. Allergy to cocami-dopropyl betaine may be due to amidoamine: a patch test and product use test study. *Contact Dermatitis* 1997;37:276–281.

28. Schauder S, Ippen H. Contact and photocontact sensitiv-ity to sunscreens: review of a 15-year experience and of the literature. *Contact Dermatitis* 1997;37:221–232.

29. Downs AMR, Sansom J. Colophony allergy: a review. *Contact Dermatitis* 1999;41:305–310.

30. Isaksson M, Andersen KE, Brandão FM, et al. Patch testing with corticosteroid mixes in Europe: a multicen-tre study of the EECDRG. *Contact Dermatitis* 2000;42: 27–35.

31. Lepoittevin JP, Drieghe J, Dooms-Goossens A. Studies in patients with corticosteroid contact allergy: understand-ing cross-reactivity among different steroids. *Arch Der-matol* 1995;131:31–37.

32. Lutz ME, el-Azhary A, Gibson LE, et al. Contact hyper-sensitivity to tixocortol pivalate. *J Am Acad Dermatol* 1998;38:691–695.

33. Gette MT, Marks JG, Maloney ME. Frequency of postop-erative allergic contact dermatitis to topical antibiotics. *Arch Dermatol* 1992;128:365–367.

34. Wekkeli M, Hippman G, Rosenkranz AR, et al. Mer-cury as a contact allergen. *Contact Dermatitis* 1990; 22:295.

35. Kiec-Swierczynska M. Allergy to chromate, cobalt and nickel in Lodz 1977–1988. *Contact Dermatitis* 1990;8:95–104.

36. Bruze M, Edman B, Björkner B, Müller H. Clinical rele-vance of contact allergy to gold sodium thiosulfate. *J Am Acad Dermatol* 1994;31:579–583.

37. Levy J, Sewell M, Goldstein N. II. A short history of tattooing. *J Derm Surg Oncol* 1979;5:851.

38. Cohen DE, Scheman AJ, Stewart L, et al. American Academy of Dermatology's position paper on latex allergy. *J Am Acad Dermatol* 1998;39:98–106.

39. Scheman AJ, Carroll PA, Brown KH, et al. Formaldehyde-related textile allergy: an update. *Contact Dermatitis* 1998;38:332–336.

40. Holness DL, Nethercott JR. Results of patch testing with a specialized collection of plastic and glue allergens. *Am J Contact Dermatitis* 1997;8:121–124.

41. Kanerva L, Jolanki R, Estlander T. Ten years of patch testing with the (meth)acrylate series. *Contact Dermatitis* 1997;37:255–258.

42. Fisher AA. Poison ivy/oak dermatitis. Part I: prevention—soap and water, topical barriers, hyposen-sitization. *Cutis* 1996;57:384–386.

43. Fisher AA. Poison ivy/oak/sumac. Part II: specific fea-tures. *Cutis* 1996;58:22–24.

44. Warshaw EM, Zug KA. Sesquiterpene lactone allergy. *Am J Contact Dermatitis* 1996;7:1–23.

45. Marks JG. Allergic contact dermatitis to *Alstromeria.* *Arch Dermatol* 1988;124:914–916.

46. MacFarlane DF, DaLeo VA. Phototoxic and photoaller-gic dermatitis. In: Guin JD, ed. *Practical contact der-matitis.* New York: McGraw-Hill, 1995:83–92.

47. Pathak MA. Phytophotodermatitis. *Clin Dermatol* 1986;4:102–121.

48. DaLeo VA, Suarez SM, Maso MJ. Photoallergic contact dermatitis: results of photopatch testing in New York, 1985 to 1990. *Arch Dermatol* 1992;128: 1513–1518.

49. Rytand DA. Fatal anuria, the nephrotic syndrome and glomerular nephritis as sequels of the dermatitis of poi-son oak. *Am J Med* 1968;5:548.

50. Slavin RG. Allergic contact dermatitis. In: Fireman P, Slavin RG, eds. *Atlas of allergies.* Philadelphia: JB Lippincott, 1991.

51. Breit R, Turk RBM. The medical and social fate of the dichromate allergic patient. *Br J Dermatol* 1976;94:349.

52. Rietschel RL. Occupational contact dermatitis. *Lancet* 1997;349:1093–1095.

19

Nasal Polyposis, Sinusitis, and Nonallergic Rhinitis

David I. Bernstein

Division of Immunology, University of Cincinnati; Department of Medicine, University of Cincinnati College of Medicine, Cincinnati, Ohio

NASAL POLYPS

Nasal polyps have been recognized and treated since ancient times (1). The "aspirin triad" or occurrence of nasal polyps in association with asthma and aspirin sensitivity was first identified in 1911 (2). Nasal polyps represent a consequence of chronic mucosal inflammation; this condition also has been referred to as hypertrophic rhinitis. In most cases, nasal polyps arise from the middle meatus and clefts of the ethmoid region (3). Histologic sections of nasal polyp tissue exhibit infiltration with eosinophils, plasma cells, lymphocytes, and mast cells (4). Polypoid tissue is rich in ground substance containing acid mucopolysaccharide (5,6).

The overall incidence or prevalence of nasal polyposis is unknown. Nasal polyps are diagnosed more frequently in men and during the third and fourth decades of life. Most clinical data indicate that there is no greater prevalence of nasal polyps among atopic compared with normal populations (2,7,8). A population-based study was conducted in Finland to determine the prevalence of asthma, aspirin intolerance, nasal polyposis, and chronic obstructive pulmonary disease in the adult population. The overall prevalence of nasal polyposis was 4.3%. Overall prevalence of aspirin intolerance and aspirin-induced asthma was 5.7% and 1.2%, respectively (9). In an adult allergy clinic population, 211 (4.2%) had nasal polyps; 71% had

asthma. Nasal polyps occur in 7% of patients with asthma (10). Approximately 14% of polyp patients reported aspirin intolerance. The prevalence could be underestimated in that 8% of nasal polyp patients without histories of salicylate sensitivity exhibit aspirin intolerance when challenged with aspirin (10,11). Nasal polyps are much less common in children than in adults. If nasal polyps are recognized in a child, the clinician must exclude cystic fibrosis, a disease in which the occurrence of nasal polyps ranges between 6.7% and 26% (12,13). A recent study of 211 adults with cystic fibrosis, who underwent intranasal endoscopy, reported a 37% prevalence of nasal polyps (14).

Clinical Presentation

Perennial nasal congestion, rhinorrhea, and anosmia (or hyposmia) are common presenting symptoms. Nasal and osteomeatal obstruction may result in purulent nasal discharge and sinusitis. Enlargement of nasal polyps may lead to broadening of the nasal bridge (15), and rarely, nasal polyps can encroach into the orbit, causing compression of ocular structures and resulting in unilateral proptosis, which falsely suggests the presence of an orbital malignancy (16).

A thorough examination with a nasal speculum is necessary for identification of nasal polyps. More complete visualization of nasal polyps can be accomplished by flexible rhinoscopy. Nasal polyps appear as bulbous translucent to opaque growths, and are best visualized extending from the middle and inferior nasal turbinates, causing partial or complete obstruction of the nasal canals. Frontal, ethmoidal, and maxillary-tenderness with purulent nasal discharge from the middle meatus indicate concurrent acute or chronic paranasal sinusitis. Sinus radiographic studies are rarely necessary for identification of nasal polyps. Common radiographic changes observed in patients with chronic nasal polyposis include the following: widening of the ethmoid labyrinths; mucoceles or pyoceles within the paranasal sinuses; and generalized loss of translucence in the maxillary, ethmoid, and frontal sinuses (15).

Causes

The pathogenesis of nasal polyposis has not been defined. Allergic mechanisms have been investigated, but no consistent association has been established between atopy and nasal polyposis. Mast cells and their mediators could play a role in that mast cells as well as eosinophils are abundantly present in nasal polyp tissue. Bunstead and colleagues (17) detected measurable amounts of histamine, a mast cell and basophil mediator, in nasal polyp fluid. Allergen-induced release of histamine and proinflammatory mediators (e.g., leukotrienes) has been demonstrated after passive sensitization of nasal polyp tissue with allergic serum (18). Interestingly, a recent study reported that 40% of patients with nasal polyps exhibited prick test reactivity to *Candida albicans*. However, the significance of *Candida* hypersensitivity in the pathogenesis of nasal polyps is uncertain (19). Polypoid tissue has been reported to produce growth factors and cytokines that stimulate in vitro proliferation of basophils, mast cells, and eosinophils, which could amplify and sustain tissue inflammation (20–22). Increased numbers of CD8[+] T cells are found in nasal polyps (23), and immunoglobulin G (IgG), IgM, IgA, and IgE levels are elevated in polyp fluid (24).

A variety of other factors may contribute to the pathogenesis of nasal polyps. In culture, nasal polyp tissue readily supports the growth of influenza A virus, although this does not establish a causative role for viral infection (25). Autonomic imbalance, endocrine abnormalities, and abnormal vasomotor responses may contribute to the formation of nasal polyps. Although nasal polyposis seems to be an acquired condition, a higher than expected prevalence of nasal polyps, asthma, and aspirin intolerance have been reported in certain families (26). For many years, it was hypothesized that aspirin sensitivity associated with asthma and nasal polyps were linked by an abnormality in arachidonic acid metabolism, resulting in enhanced leukotriene synthesis using the lipoxygenase pathway. This hypothesis has been supported by demonstration of increased levels of leukotrienes in nasal secretions of nasal polyp patients after oral aspirin challenge (14). Nasal polyp–derived epithelial cells cultured from aspirin-sensitive patients generate the eicosanoid 15-HETE after *in vitro* stimulation with aspirin; no such effect was demonstrated in aspirin-insensitive patients (27). In summary, it is postulated but not proven that allergic, infectious, environmental irritant, genetic, or metabolic factors may alone or in combination result in formation of nasal polyps.

Treatment

The surgical treatment of nasal polyposis often is unsatisfactory. Simple nasal polypectomy results in temporary relief of nasal obstructive symptoms but is often followed by recurrence. Medical treatment with topical intranasal glucocorticoids has been reported to be more effective than surgical polypectomy (28). Aggressive treatment of nasal polyps with nasal corticosteroids can reduce the requirement for nasal sinus surgery. Intranasal steroids significantly reduce the size of polyps, nasal congestion, and rhinorrhea, and increase nasal airflow. Among the various mechanisms of action, topical corticosteroids have been reported to reduce secretion of proinflammatory cytokines such as granulocyte-macrophage colony-stimulating factor (GM-CSF) from nasal polyp epithelial cells (16) and reduce tissue eosinophils (29). Optimal delivery is achieved by positioning of the head in the downward and forward position. There is evidence that higher doses of a potent nasal corticosteroid are more effective; fluticasone propionate administered as 400 μg twice daily was more effective than 400 μg once daily in improving nasal inspiratory flow and reducing polyp size (30). Unfortunately, intranasal steroids have marginal effects in improving olfactory function. The latter result is best achieved with brief courses of systemic corticosteroids. Intranasal steroids exert little effect on associated sinus disease, as evidenced by lack of improvement in sinus radiographs over a 12-month interval (31). Leukotriene antagonists are effective antiasthmatic agents and are particularly effective in aspirin-sensitive patients. However, there have been no published controlled clinical trials of antileukotriene agents in the treatment of nasal polyps (32). Long-term treatment with daily intranasal glucocorticoids is safe and has not been reported to result in atrophic changes in nasal mucosa (33). If polyps fail to respond to intranasal glucocorticoids, a brief 5- to 7-day course of oral prednisone (30–35 mg/day) may be effective. The long-term use of oral glucocorticoids should be avoided. Once nasal polyps have been reduced in size with prednisone, maintenance dosages of intranasal glucocorticoids should be resumed to prevent recurrence. Coexistent sinus infection may render individuals refractory to intranasal glucocorticoids and therefore should be treated with an appropriate course of antibiotics.

If all attempts at medical management have failed, surgical intervention should be recommended, particularly in the presence of chronic sinusitis that has been refractory to antibiotics. Simple polypectomy may be indicated for complete nasal obstruction, which causes extreme discomfort. If nasal polyps are associated with persistent ethmoid sinusitis with obstruction of the osteomeatal complex, a more extensive surgical procedure is required. Sphenoethmoidectomy with complete marsupialization of the ethmoid sinus and resection of the middle turbinate is a definitive procedure that has been reported to effectively prevent recurrence of nasal polyps in approximately 85% of treated patients (34). Outcomes of endoscopic sinus surgery are less favorable among aspirin triad patients compared with patients with chronic sinusitis who are aspirin insensitive. In a retrospective study reported by Amar et al., patients with aspirin

triad have more extensive sinus disease based on radiologic findings and 39% required revision nasal surgeries compared with 9% in a group of sinusitis patients without the aspirin triad (35).

Asthmatic patients undergoing nasal polypectomy or sinus surgery had previously been regarded to be at risk for postoperative bronchospasm, but this outcome rarely occurs. Nonspecific airway responsiveness determined by methacholine challenge does not increase significantly in patients with asthma after nasal polypectomy (36). After recovery from polypectomy or sphenoethmoidectomy, maintenance intranasal glucocorticoids should be instituted to prevent recurrence of nasal polyps (37). In patients with the aspirin triad (i.e., asthma, rhinosinusitis, and aspirin sensitivity), long-term aspirin desensitization has been reported to be effective in reducing the number of episodes of acute sinusitis, corticosteroid use, and requirements for polypectomies and sinus surgery (76). This procedure should be performed exclusively by a subspecialist and considered only in aspirin-sensitive patients refractory to conventional therapies.

The effect of sinus surgery on asthma has been debated. Lamblin reported results of a 4-year longitudinal study in two groups of patients with nasal polyposis. Nasal polyps were responsive to nasal steroids in the first group, whereas the other group required nasal surgical intervention (ethmoidectomy). Interestingly, the steroid unresponsive group exhibited a significant decline in forced expiratory volume in 1 second (FEV_1) and the FEV_1/FVC (forced vital capacity) ratio over 4 years compared with the steroid-responsive group, despite the observation that there was no substantial difference in clinical asthma severity between groups. This suggests that ethmoidectomy does not result in long-term benefit for asthma in steroid-unresponsive patients with nasal polyposis (38).

SINUSITIS

Sinusitis affects approximately 14% of the population, with estimated annual costs exceeding $2 billion (39). Sinusitis is an inflammatory disorder of the mucosal lining of the paranasal sinuses that may be initiated by either infectious or noninfectious factors. Regardless of initiating events, the four physiologic derangements that contribute to the evolution of infectious sinusitis are as follows: (a) decreased patency of the sinus ostia; (b) a decrease in the partial pressure of oxygen within the sinus cavities caused by impairment of ventilatory exchange; (c) diminished mucociliary transport; and (d) compromise of mucosal blood flow. Edematous obstruction of the sinus ostia is a consistent finding in both acute and chronic sinusitis; this condition causes a low-oxygen environment within the sinus cavity, which results in decreased mucociliary transport (40) and favors the growth of common bacterial pathogens, including *Streptococcus pneumoniae, Haemophilus influenzae*, and anaerobic bacteria.

Viral upper respiratory infections often precede acute bacterial sinus infections. Clinically, it is difficult to distinguish viral from bacterial sinusitis. Sinusitis may follow environmental exposure to fumes or chemical vapors. Bacterial sinusitis has long been considered a complication of seasonal or perennial allergic rhinitis, although no good data support this assumption. Cigarette smokers and individuals with vasomotor rhinitis are more susceptible to recurrent or chronic sinusitis.

The microbial pathogens implicated in acute maxillary sinusitis have been studied extensively. Identification of bacterial pathogens has been achieved by culturing antral aspirates obtained by needle puncture of the maxillary sinus. Gwaltney et al. reported pretreatment sinus puncture culture results in 339 patients with acute sinusitis. Bacterial species represented included *Streptococcus pneumoniae* in 92 (41%); *Haemophilus influenzae* in 79 (35%); anaerobes in 17 (7%); streptococcal species in 16 (7%); *Moraxella catarrhalis* in 8 (4%); *Staphylococcus aureus* in 7 (33%); and other miscellaneous organisms in 8 (4%) (41). Cultures of nasopharyngeal specimens are useless because they do not reflect bacterial isolates in the sinuses. Viruses are cultured from 8% of aspirates, whereas 15% to 40% of antral aspirates are sterile. Common isolates include rhinovirus, influenza type A, and parainfluenza viruses (42).

In children with acute maxillary sinusitis, *S. pneumoniae, H. influenzae*, and *M. catarrhalis* have been identified as the predominant pathogens (43). Viruses were isolated from 4% of pediatric patients, and 20% of cultured aspirates were sterile. Anaerobic bacteria have been cultured from 88% of antral aspirates of adult patients with chronic sinusitis but are seldom identified in children (44,45).

Mucormycotic sinusitis is caused by fungus of the genus *Mucor*, a zygomycete (46). This organism is saprophytic, is abundant in the natural environment, and may be isolated easily from the throat and stools of normal individuals. *Mucor* can become an invasive pathogen in diabetic, leukemic, or otherwise immunosuppressed patients. Similarly, invasive aspergillosis may involve the paranasal sinuses in the immunocompromised host (47). Allergic fungal sinusitis is an increasingly recognized syndrome occurring in nonimmunocompromised atopic patients with hypertrophic rhinitis and nasal polyps, which may result from local hypersensitivity responses to a variety of mold spores colonizing the sinus cavities. Abundant mucin found within the sinuses demonstrates numerous eosinophils and Charcot-Leyden crystals; fungal stains reveal the presence of noninvasive hyphae (48,77). Rarely, tuberculosis or syphilis has been reported to cause infectious sinusitis. Atypical mycobacteria can cause sinusitis in patients with acquired immunodeficiency syndrome (49).

Clinical Presentation

Episodes of acute sinusitis are most commonly preceded by symptoms suggestive of viral upper respiratory tract infections or other environmental stimuli, which can cause mucosal inflammation, hypertrophy, and obstruction of the sinus ostia. Common presenting symptoms include frontal or maxillary head pain, fever, and mucopurulent or bloody nasal discharge. Other clinical features include general malaise, cough, hyposmia, mastication pain, and changes in the resonance of speech. Pain cited as coming from the upper molars may be an early symptom of acute maxillary sinusitis. Children with acute maxillary sinusitis present most often with cough, nasal discharge, and fetid breath, whereas fever is less common (43).

Symptoms associated with chronic sinusitis are less fulminant; facial pain, headache, and postnasal discharge are common symptoms. The clinician should be aware that chronic maxillary sinusitis may result from primary dental infections (i.e., apical granuloma of the molar teeth, periodontitis) (42). Pain associated with temporomandibular dysfunction may be incorrectly diagnosed as chronic sinusitis. Individuals with sinusitis may experience severe facial pain associated with rapid changes in position (e.g., lying supine or bending forward) or with rapid changes in atmospheric pressure that occur during air travel.

Episodes of acute or chronic sinusitis may be manifestations of other underlying problems. Local obstruction by a deviated nasal septum, nasal polyps, or occult benign or malignant neoplasm may explain recurrent sinus infections. Patients presenting with frequent sinus infections that respond poorly to antibiotics should be examined for primary or acquired immunodeficiency states. Common variable hypogammaglobulinemia and selective IgA deficiency combined with IgG2 and IgG4 subclass deficiencies are humoral immunodeficiencies that should be considered (50). Disorders of ciliary dysmotility usually occur in male patients. Kartagener syndrome is characterized by recurrent sinusitis, nasal polyps, situs inversus, infertility, and bronchiectasis (51). Incomplete forms of ciliary dysmotility may occur without associated pulmonary or cardiac involvement. Nasal mucosal biopsy and electron microscopic examination can identify abnormalities in ciliary structure. Wegener granulomatosis is a necrotizing vasculitis that presents with epistaxis, refractory sinusitis, serous otitis, nodular pulmonary infiltrates, and focal necrotizing glomerulonephritis (52). Notice that chronic sinusitis or otitis media can precede pulmonary and renal manifestations for years before the disease becomes fulminant. Thus, early diagnosis and treatment of this condition before development of renal disease can be life saving.

Diagnosis

Palpable tenderness, erythema, and warmth may be appreciated over inflamed frontal, ethmoid, or maxillary sinuses. Clinical history and physical examination can reliably identify purulent sinusitis in more than 80% of cases (53,54). Sinus imaging should be reserved for difficult diagnostic problems or for patients with sinusitis unresponsive to an initial course of antibiotics. Rhinoscopy can be useful in identifying purulent discharge in the middle meatus compatible with acute maxillary sinusitis. Radiologic changes of sinus mucosal thickening of 8 mm or greater is a sensitive diagnostic marker of bacterial sinusitis. Minimal radiologic changes are common in many cases of sterile sinusitis as well as in asymptomatic individuals. Computed tomography (CT) of the sinuses is a valuable method for defining pathologic changes in the paranasal sinuses (55,56). CT is particularly useful for defining abnormalities in the anterior ethmoid and middle meatal areas (osteomeatal unit), which cannot be visualized well on sinus roentgenograms. The CT coronal views (Fig. 19.1) are much less costly than a complete sinus CT and are adequate for determining the patency of the osteomeatal complex, which includes the ethmoid and maxillary ostia and infundibulum. Such information is essential for assessing the need for surgical intervention in the treatment of chronic sinusitis.

Complications

In the age of antibiotics, severe life-threatening complications of acute sinusitis are relatively uncommon. However, the clinician must be able to recognize clinical manifestations of potentially fatal complications of sinusitis so that prompt medical and surgical treatments can be initiated in a timely fashion.

Symptoms commonly associated with acute frontal sinusitis include frontal pain, local erythema and swelling, fever, and purulent nasal discharge. Serious complications of frontal sinusitis may be attributed to the proximity of the frontal sinus to the roof of the orbit and anterior cranial fossa. Osteomyelitis can result from acute

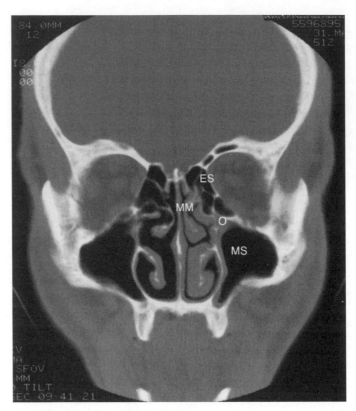

FIG. 19.1. Computed tomographic image of the paranasal sinuses. A coronal section exhibits significant sinus disease on the left with a relatively normal appearance on the right. The left middle meatus (*MM*) and maxillary ostium (*O*) are obstructed by inflamed tissue, causing significant obstruction of the left ethmoid (*ES*) and maxillary (*MS*) sinuses.

frontal sinusitis and may present as a localized subperiosteal abscess (Pott puffy tumor). Sinus radiographs exhibit sclerotic changes in the bone contiguous to the frontal sinus. Intracranial complications of frontal sinusitis include extradural, subdural, and brain abscesses as well as meningitis and cavernous sinus thrombosis (57). Acute ethmoiditis is encountered most commonly in children. Extension of inflammation into the orbit can result in unilateral orbital and periorbital swelling with cellulitis. This presentation can be distinguished from cavernous sinus thrombosis by the lack of focal cranial neurologic deficits, absence of retroorbital pain, and no meningeal signs. Affected patients usually respond to antibiotics, and surgical drainage is rarely necessary.

Cavernous sinus thrombosis is a complication of acute or chronic sinusitis, which demands immediate diagnosis and treatment (57). The cavernous sinuses communicate with the venous channels draining the middle one third of the face. Cavernous sinus thrombosis often arises from a primary infection in the face or paranasal sinuses. Vital structures that course through the cavernous sinus include the internal carotid artery and the third, fourth, fifth, and sixth cranial nerves. Symptoms of venous outflow obstruction caused by cavernous sinus thrombosis include retinal engorgement, retrobulbar pain, and visual loss. Impingement of cranial nerves in the cavernous sinus can result in extraocular muscle paralysis and trigeminal sensory loss. If not treated promptly with high doses of parenteral antibiotics, septicemia and central nervous system involvement lead to a fatal outcome.

Acute sphenoid sinusitis is difficult to diagnose (54,57). Affected patients report occipital and retroorbital pain, or the pain distribution may be nonspecific. Because of the posterior location of the sphenoid sinus, diagnosis of sphenoiditis may be delayed until serious complications are recognized. Extension of infections to contiguous structures may result in ocular palsies, orbital cellulitis, subdural abscess, meningitis, or hypopituitarism. Sinus radiographs often are unsatisfactory for evaluating sphenoiditis; sinus CT is a more effective diagnostic tool.

It long has been recognized that chronic or recurrent sinusitis may exacerbate asthma. Successful prevention and treatment of chronic sinusitis can be effective in controlling patients with difficult or refractory asthma. Slavin (58) described a group of steroid-dependent asthmatics with sinusitis in whom sinus surgery (i.e., the Caldwell-Luc procedure or sphenoidectomy) was performed. Asthma symptoms, steroid requirements, and nonspecific airway reactivity were reduced after surgery.

Treatment

Medical treatment of acute sinusitis should be initiated promptly. The primary goal of treatment should be facilitation of drainage of affected sinuses and elimination of causative organisms. Gwaltney studied 31 patients who presented with upper respiratory infection with significant CT abnormalities consistent with sinusitis (59). Despite no antibiotic treatment, CT abnormalities had resolved in most patients 2 weeks later. These data suggest that antibiotics are being used unnecessarily in many patients who could also have viral infections. Judicious use of antibiotics is essential, especially in light of increasing problems with antibiotic resistance. Oral decongestants alone or combined with antihistamines may diminish nasal mucosal edema and enhance sinus drainage. A 12-hour sustained-release oral preparation containing pseudoephedrine or phenylpropanolamine combined with antibiotics is recommended. Topical nasal vasoconstrictors (e.g., oxymetazoline) used judiciously over the initial 2 to 3 days of treatment of acute sinusitis can facilitate drainage. Frequent nasal lavage with saline can be effective for improvement of sinus

drainage. Intranasal glucocorticoids may be a useful adjunctive treatment for decreasing mucosal inflammation and edema.

Antibiotics should be considered in those who fail the aforementioned drainage measures. The emergence of penicillin-resistant strains must be recognized. For treating acute sinusitis, amoxicillin (250–500 mg three times daily) is still the antibiotic of choice. In chronic sinusitis, amoxicillin should be administered for a duration of 21 to 28 days; briefer courses are associated with a greater probability of recurrence. In the penicillin-allergic patient, the alternative antibiotic of choice is trimethoprim-sulfamethoxazole (45). In 1997, β-lactamase production was found in 34% of *H. influenza,* 92% of *M. catarrhalis,* and 25% of *S. pneumoniae* strains. Infection with penicillinase-producing organisms should be suspected in those patients who fail 14- to 21-day courses of amoxicillin (44,60). In this situation, amoxicillin—clavulanic acid or an appropriate cephalosporin (e.g., cefuroxime), both of which are active against penicillinase-producing bacteria, should be substituted. Newer modified macrolide antibiotics (e.g., clarithromycin, azithromycin), which have a broad spectrum of activity against pathogens implicated in sinusitis, can be used either in the penicillin- and sulfonamide-allergic patient or for treating patients who are unresponsive to amoxicillin (61). Despite an increase in antibiotic resistance, a recent review of clinical trials comparing amoxicillin to newer penicillins and nonpenicillin drugs failed to show significant differences in cure rates (62). Thus, antibiotic resistance data based on MIC studies are not always predictive of unfavorable responses to amoxicillin. In addition to equivalent efficacy, amoxicillin is favored due to lower overall costs (63).

Intensive medical therapy may be unsuccessful in treating acute sinusitis. When fever, facial pain, and sinus imaging changes persist, surgical drainage of infected sinuses may be indicated. Direct puncture and aspiration of affected sinuses should be performed by an otolaryngologist under local anesthesia. Parenteral antibiotics should be instituted if local extension of infection (i.e., cellulitis or osteomyelitis) occurs, or if the infection is suspected to have spread to vital ocular or central nervous system structures. For patients with maxillary sinusitis who do not respond to conservative drainage measures and aggressive antibiotic therapy, resection of diseased tissue within the sinuses is recommended (58). Similar principles apply to the treatment of frontal, ethmoid, or sphenoid sinusitis. Adequate open drainage of frontal sinuses can be achieved by trephination through the roof of the orbit. If acute ethmoiditis is refractory to antibiotics, intranasal or external ethmoidectomy may be required. Sphenoid sinusitis, which often occurs with ethmoid sinusitis, may require a surgical aspiration and drainage procedure.

Patients with asthma who undergo sinus surgery should receive a thorough evaluation. Asthma must be under optimal control before the operation. In steroid-dependent patients, a brief course of oral steroids should be administered before surgery.

Intracranial complications of sinusitis (e.g., subdural emphysema or brain abscess) must be treated with prompt open surgical drainage and parenteral antibiotics. Diffuse extension of osteomyelitis requires high-dose antibiotic treatment. Surgical debridement of localized osteomyelitis is recommended if a bony sequestrum of infection exists.

The treatment approach to chronic sinusitis and recurrent sinusitis should begin with identifying contributing factors such as underlying conditions (i.e., chronic allergic rhinitis, deviated nasal septum, polyps, condra bullosa, rhinitis medicamentosa) and environmental factors (e.g., active or passive exposure to tobacco smoke, exposure to toxic irritants at work). In many cases, recurrent infections can be prevented by daily maintenance therapy with an oral 12-hour sustained-release decongestant (i.e., pseudoephedrine or phenylpropanolamine). Oral phenylpropanolamine increases ostial and nasal patency, facilitating mucus drainage and thereby preventing infection (64). Chronic use of topical glucocorticoids in combination with topical decongestants reduces nasal airway resistance and ameliorates radiographic changes in patients with chronic sinusitis (65). Based on these reports, concurrent administration of nasal topical glucocorticoids and a 12-hour slow-release oral sympathomimetic (pseudoephedrine

or phenylpropanolamine) is a rational strategy for prevention of recurrent sinusitis.

When all attempts at pharmacologic management have failed, surgery may be required for chronic or recurrent sinusitis. Functional endoscopic sinus surgery has supplanted older surgical procedures such as maxillary Caldwell-Luc antrostomy. The basic principle of endoscopic techniques is to resect the inflamed tissues that obstruct the osteomeatal complex and the anterior ethmoids, and thus directly interfere with normal physiologic drainage. Inflammation or scarring of the latter structures obstructs drainage, resulting in spread of infection to the maxillary and frontal sinus cavities. As mentioned, sinus CT is essential in defining the specific disease in this area. Surgical resection of ethmoidal and osteomeatal structures is performed through the nose under guidance of a rigid endoscope. Diseased mucosa is resected, and narrow or stenotic areas, including the maxillary ostia, are widened (66,67). This type of surgery is far more effective than the Caldwell-Luc procedure, which failed to restore normal physiologic drainage through the ostia. Because nasal endoscopic surgery is less invasive, postoperative morbidity has been reduced markedly in comparison with formerly used surgical techniques. A 4-year follow-up of 100 patients reported general improvement in over 90% of patients. Recurrence of symptoms occurred as late as 3 years after surgery and primarily in patients who initially presented with nasal polyps, aspirin sensitivity, and reactive airways disease (37).

NONALLERGIC RHINITIS

Symptoms of nonallergic rhinitis often are indistinguishable from those associated with perennial allergic rhinitis. Therefore, the evaluation and treatment of nonallergic rhinitis can be challenging. *Nonallergic rhinitis* is defined as inflammation of the nasal mucosa that is not caused by sensitization to inhalant aeroallergens. Lack of allergic causation must be proven by the absence of skin test reactivity to a panel of common aeroallergens.

Table 19.1 presents a classification for the nonallergic nasal disorders, which has been

TABLE 19.1. *Classification scheme of nonallergic rhinitis*

Inflammatory
  Infectious rhinitis
    Viral
    Bacterial
  Atrophic rhinitis
  Nonallergic rhinitis with eosinophilia (NARES)
  Rhinitis associated with nasal polyposis
  Nasal mastocytosis
Noninflammatory
  Rhinitis medicamentosa caused by:
    Topical drugs
    Systemic drugs
  Vasomotor rhinitis
  Hormonal induced vasomotor instability
    Endocrine diseases (e.g., hypothyroidism)
    Pregnancy
  Rhinopathy associated with structural defects
    Deviated septum
    Head trauma resulting in cerebrospinal fluid
      rhinorrhea
    Tumors
    Foreign bodies

Adapted from Middleton E. Chronic rhinitis in adults. *J Allergy Clin Immunol* 1988;81:971; with permission.

subdivided into inflammatory and noninflammatory disorders (68).

Nonallergic vasomotor rhinitis or idiopathic nonallergic rhinitis is the most common of these disorders. This is an idiopathic condition characterized by perennial nasal congestion, rhinorrhea, and postnasal discharge. Ocular itching is noticeably absent. Typically, symptoms are increased early in the morning and aggravated by tobacco smoke, irritants, chemicals, perfumes, and various noxious odors. Symptoms are triggered by rapid changes in temperature. *Mixed perennial rhinitis* is diagnosed in allergic patients with prominent vasomotor symptoms. The pathophysiology of this condition is not well understood. However, a recent study reported that as compared with normal individuals, affected patients exhibited enhanced nasal responses to histamine; no increase in inflammatory cells; and nasal mucosal swelling after cold stimulation. Although cold stimulation of the feet normally causes mucosal contraction due to sympathomimetic stimulation, the opposite was observed in vasomotor rhinitis patients. This study suggests that vasomotor rhinitis patients have nasal sympathetic hyposensitivity resulting in unopposed parasympathetic stimulation (69).

Infectious rhinitis is suspected when purulent nasal discharge is present. Sinusoidal tenderness may indicate coexistent acute or chronic sinusitis. Atrophic rhinitis is a disorder of unknown origin, which often is seen in the elderly and is characterized by formation of thick, malodorous, dry crusts that obstruct the nasal cavity (70). The nonallergic rhinitis with eosinophilia syndrome (NARES) is an inflammatory nasal disorder in which eosinophils are detectable in nasal secretions. The cause of this condition is unknown. Patients have negative skin test reactions to common inhalant aeroallergens (71). The turbinates are pale with a purplish hue, edematous, or similar in appearance to what is observed in allergic rhinitis. NARES could represent a precursor to nasal polyposis. Nasal mastocytosis is a rare disorder that can be confirmed by the finding of increased mast cells in the nasal mucosa.

Nasal symptoms can result from the chronic use or abuse of topical and systemic medications, a syndrome referred to as *rhinitis medicamentosa*. A list of causative oral medications is provided in Table 19.2 (68). In addition to older antihypertensive agents, angiotensin-converting enzyme inhibitors have been reported to cause rhinorrhea and vasomotor symptoms in association with chronic cough, which resolve after withdrawal of the drug (72). Excessive use of topical vasoconstrictor agents such as phenylephrine or oxymetazoline can result in epistaxis, "rebound" nasal congestion, and rarely cause nasal septal perforation. Intranasal cocaine use can result in the same signs and symptoms.

Prominent nasal congestion is recognized in patients with hypothyroidism and myxedema. Approximately one third of pregnant women

TABLE 19.2. *Rhinitis medicamentosa: causative agents*

Antihypertensives	Psychotropic drugs
Reserpine	Thioridazine
Hydralazine	Chlordiazepoxide-
Guanethidine	amitryptiline
Methyldopa	**Ovarian hormonal agents**
Prazosin	Oral contraceptives
β blockers	Illicit agent
Angiotensin-	Cocaine
converting	
enzyme (ACE)	
inhibitors	

report nasal congestion and rhinorrhea during gestation (73). This could be related to progester one or estrogen-induced nasal vasodilation and enhancement of mucus secretion. Other causes of nasal obstruction must be considered in the differential diagnosis. A grossly deviated nasal septum, nasal tumors, or a foreign body can be the source of unilateral nasal obstruction refractory to medical treatment. Cerebral spinal fluid (CSF) rhinorrhea is characterized by clear nasal discharge. It occurs in 5% of all basilar skull fractures but can be present in patients with no history of trauma. The use of glucose oxidase paper tests may result in an erroneous diagnosis. Detection of beta 2 transferrin in the CSF is useful in confirming the diagnosis.

Evaluation begins with a careful history and examination with a nasal speculum. Nasal septal deviation is usually obvious. Pale, boggy nasal turbinates characteristic of allergic rhinitis may be seen in a patient with NARES or nasal polyps. The nasal mucosa appear beefy red or hemorrhagic in patients with rhinitis medicamentosa. Cytologic examination of a nasal mucus smear may reveal an abundance of neutrophils, which is suggestive of infectious rhinitis (74). Nasal eosinophils are consistent with allergic rhinitis, NARES, or nasal polyposis. The absence of inflammatory cells on nasal smear should direct the physician to consider noninflammatory rhinopathies.

Treatment

The therapeutic approach to nonallergic nasal disorders is determined by findings derived from the diagnostic evaluation. Differentiation between inflammatory and noninflammatory nasal conditions is useful in selecting appropriate therapy.

Treatment of Noninflammatory Rhinopathy

Patients with rhinitis medicamentosa should discontinue offending medications. Intranasal glucocorticoids may be of considerable benefit in these patients in decreasing mucosal edema. For vasomotor instability associated with endocrinologic changes during pregnancy, medications should be withheld if possible. If necessary, nasal topical steroids (e.g., beclomethasone diproprionate) may be safe and effective for controlling chronic symptoms encountered during pregnancy. Nasal congestion associated with hypothyroidism and myxedema responds to thyroid hormone replacement. Nasal obstruction caused by a deviated septum requires septoplasty. Fifty percent of patients with CSF rhinorrhea recover spontaneously. When persistent, intravenous antibiotics should be started to prevent meningitis, and surgery often is required to repair a dural tear.

The treatment of vasomotor rhinopathy is problematic. Selection of therapy for vasomotor rhinitis is empiric, and there are variable responses to different regimens. Oral decongestants often are effective when given as 12-hour slow-release preparations (e.g., pseudoephedrine.) Antihistamines alone or in combination with decongestants often are effective therapy for patients with concurrent allergic and vasomotor rhinitis. Pseudoephedrine is contraindicated in patients receiving monoamine oxidase inhibitors and should be administered cautiously in patients with hypertension, thyroid disease, coronary artery disease, or glaucoma. When the disease is refractory to oral decongestants, topical intranasal steroids should be added. Ipratropium, 80 μg four times daily, an anticholinergic agent, is proven to be effective in treating perennial nonallergic rhinitis (75). The effect of anticholinergic agents has been attributed to inhibition of cholinergic nasal hyperresponsiveness, which is a feature of vasomotor rhinitis. In most patients, vasomotor symptoms can be controlled successfully with oral sympathomimetic agents combined with intranasal steroids or ipratropium. Although the mechanism of action is uncertain, two sprays (274 μg) of the intranasal antihistamine azelastine twice daily is often effective in controlling symptoms of vasomotor rhinitis. Environmental triggers such as cigarette smoke and other irritants should be avoided.

Treatment of the Inflammatory Rhinitis

The syndrome of nonallergic rhinitis with eosinophilia responds best to intranasal glucocorticoids. Once initial control of daily symptoms has been achieved, doses can be reduced to the minimal levels required to prevent recurrence of symptoms. Infectious rhinitis and concurrent sinus infections should be treated with appropriate antibiotics. Viral-induced nasal symptoms can be treated symptomatically with antihistamine-decongestant preparations.

REFERENCES

1. Vancil ME. A historical survey of treatments for nasal polyposis. *Laryngoscope* 1969;79:435–445.
2. Moloney JR, Colins J. Nasal polyps and bronchial asthma. *Br J Dis Chest* 1977;71:1–6.
3. Stammberger H. Surgical treatment of nasal polyps: past, present, and future. *Allergy* 1999; 54(suppl 53): 7–11.
4. Cauna N, Manzetti GW, Hinderer KH, et al. Fine structure of nasal polyps. *Ann Otolaryngol* 1972;81: 41–58.
5. Weisskopf A, Burn HF. Histochemical studies of the pathogenesis of nasal polyps. *Ann Otol Rhinol Laryngol* 1959;68:509.
6. Taylor M. Histochemical studies on nasal polypi. *J Laryngol Otol* 1973;77:326.
7. Blumstein GI, Tuft L. Allergy treatment in recurrent nasal polyposis. *Am J Med Sci* 1957;234:269.
8. Settipane GA. Nasal polyps and immunoglobulin E (IgE). *Allergy Asthma Proc* 1996;17:269–273.
9. Hedman J, Kaprio J, Poussa T, et al. Prevalence of asthma, aspirin intolerance, nasal polyposis and chronic obstructive pulmonary disease in a population-based study. *Int J Epidemiol* 1999;28:717–722.
10. Settipane GA, Chafee FH. Nasal polyps in asthma and rhinitis. A review of 6,037 patients. *J Allergy Clin Immunol* 1977;59:17–21
11. Ferreri NR, Howland WC, Stevenson DD, et al. Release of leukotrienes, prostaglandins, and histamine into nasal secretions of aspirin-sensitive asthmatics during reaction to aspirin. *Am Rev Respir Dis* 1988;137:847–854.
12. English GM. Nasal polyps and sinusitis. In: Middleton E, Reed CE, Ellis EF, eds. *Allergy principles and practices.* St. Louis, MO: CV Mosby, 1983:1215.
13. Cuyler JP, Monaghan AJ. Cystic fibrosis and sinusitis. *J Otolaryngol* 1989;18:173–175.
14. Hadfield PJ, Rowe-Jones JM, Mackay IS. The prevalence of nasal polyps in adults with cystic fibrosis. *Clin Otolaryngol* 2000;25:19–22.
15. Lund VJ, Lloyd GAS. Radiological changes associated with benign nasal polyps. *J Laryngol Otol* 1983;97: 503–510.
16. Rawlings EF, Olson RJ, Kaufman HE. Polypoid sinusitis mimicking orbital malignancy. *Am J Ophthalmol* 1979;87:694–697.
17. Bunstead RM, El-Ackad T, Smith JM, et al. Histamine, norepinephrine and serotonin content of nasal polyps. *Laryngoscope* 1979;89:832–843.
18. Kaliner M, Wasserman SI, Austen KF. Immunologic release of chemical mediators from human nasal polyps. *N Engl J Med* 1973;289:277–281.
19. Asero R, Bottazzi G. Hypersensitivity to molds in patients with nasal polyposis: a clinical study. *J Allergy Clin Immunol* 2000;105:186–188.
20. Rudack C, Stoll W, Bachert C. Cytokines in nasal polyposis, acute and chronic sinusitis. *Am J Rhinol* 1998;12: 383.
21. Ohnishi M, Ruhno J, Bienenstock J, et al. Hematopoietic growth factor production by cultured cells of human nasal polyp epithelial scraping: kinetics, cell source and relationship to clinical status. *J Allergy Clin Immunol* 1989;83:1091–1100.
22. Sakaguchi K, Okuda M, Ushijima K, et al. Study of nasal surface basophilic cells in patients with nasal polyp. *Acta Otolaryngol (Stockh)* 1986;430(suppl):28–33.
23. Stoop AE, Hameleers DMH, v. Run PE, et al. Lymphocyte and nonlymphoid cells in the nasal mucosa of patients with nasal polyps and of healthy subjects. *J Allergy Clin Immunol* 1989;84:734–741.
24. Chandra RK, Abol BM. Immunopathology of nasal polypi. *J Laryngol Otol* 1974;88:1019–1024.
25. Ginzburg VP, Rosina EE, Sharova OK, et al. The replication of influenza A viruses in organ cultures of human nasal polyps. *Arch Virol* 1982;74:293–298.
26. Falliers CJ. Familial coincidence of asthma, aspirin intolerance and nasal polyposis. *Ann Allergy* 1974;32: 65–69.
27. Kowalski ML, Pawliczak R, Wozniak J, et al. Differential metabolism of arachidonic acid in nasal polyp epithelial cells cultured from aspirin-sensitive and aspirin-tolerant patients. *Am J Respir Crit Care Med* 2000;161:391–398.
28. Lildholdt T, Fogstrup J, Gammelguard N, et al. Surgical versus medical treatment of nasal polyps. *Acta Otolaryngol* 1988;105:140–143.
29. Mulloi J, Roca-Ferrer J, Xaubet A, et al. Inhibition of GM-CSF secretion by topical corticosteroids and nedocromil sodium. A comparison study using nasal polyp epithelial cells. *Respir Med* 2000; 94:428–431.
30. Penttila M, Poulsen P, Hollingworth K, et al. Dose-related efficacy and tolerability of fluticasone propionate nasal drops 400 microg once daily and twice daily in the treatment of bilateral nasal polyposis: a placebo-controlled randomized study in adult patients. *Clin Exp Allergy* 2000; 30:94–102.
31. Hardy JG, Lee SW, Wilson CG. Intranasal drug delivery by sprays and drops. *J Pharmacol* 1985; 37:294–297.
32. Mygind N. Advances in the medical treatment of nasal polyps. *Allergy* 1999;54:12–16.
33. Mygind N, Sorensen H, Pedersen CB. The nasal mucosa during long-term treatment with beclomethasone dipropionate aerosol. *Acta Otolaryngol* 1978;85:437–443.
34. Friedman WH, Katsantonis GP, Rosenblum BN, et al. Sphenoethmoidectomy: the case for ethmoid marsupialization. *Laryngoscope* 1986;96:473–479.
35. Amar YG, Frenkiel S, Sobol SE. Outcome analysis of endoscopic sinus surgery for chronic sinusitis in patients having Samter's triad. *J Otolaryngol* 2000;29:7–12.
36. Miles-Lawrence R, Kaplan M, Chang K. Methacholine sensitivity in nasal polyposis and the effects of polypectomy. *J Allergy Clin Immunol* 1982;69:102–109.
37. Schaitkin B, May M, Shapiro A, et al. Endoscopic sinus surgery: 4 year follow-up on the first 100 patients. *Laryngoscope* 1993;103:1117–1120.
38. Lamblin C, Brichet A, Perez T, et al. Long-term follow-up of pulmonary function in patients with nasal polyposis. *Am J Respir Crit Care Med* 2000;161:406.

39. Poole MD. A focus on acute sinusitis in adults: changes in disease management. *Am J Med* 1999;106(suppl): 38–47.

40. Drettner B. Pathophysiology of paranasal sinuses with clinical implications. *Clin Otolaryngol* 1980;5:227.

41. Evans FD, Syndor JB, Moore WEC, et al. Sinusitis of the maxillary antrum. *N Engl J Med* 1975;293:735.

42. Gwaltney JM Jr, Scheld WM, Sande MA, et al. The microbial etiology and antimicrobial therapy of adults with acute community-acquired sinusitis: a fifteen-year experience at the University of Virginia and review of other selected studies. *J Allergy Clin Immunol* 1992;90 (Part 2):457–461.

43. Wald ER, Milmoe GJ, Bowen A, et al. Acute maxillary sinusitis in children. *N Engl J Med* 1981;304:749–754.

44. Brook I. Bacteriology of chronic maxillary sinusitis in adults. *Ann Otol Rhinol Laryngol* 1989;98:46.

45. Wald ER, Byers C, Guerra N, et al. Subacute sinusitis in children. *J Pediatr* 1989;115:28–32.

46. Lewis DR, Thompson DH, Fetter TW. Mucormycotic sphenoid sinusitis. *Ear Nose Throat J* 1981;60: 398–403.

47. Stevens MH. Aspergillosis of the frontal sinus. *Arch Otolaryngol* 1978;104:153.

48. Katzenstein AL, Sale SR, Greenberger PA. Allergic *Aspergillus* sinusitis: a newly recognized form of sinusitis. *J Allergy Clin Immunol* 1983;79:89–93.

49. Naguib MT, Byers JM, Slater L. Paranasal sinus infection due to atypical mycobacteria in two patients with AIDS. *Clin Infect Dis* 1994;19:789.

50. Oxelius V, Laural A, Lindquist B, et al. IgG subclass in selective IgA deficiency. *N Engl J Med* 1981;304: 1476–1477.

51. Eliasson R, Mossberg B, Camner P, et al. The immotile cilia syndrome. *N Engl J Med* 1977;291:1–6.

52. Abraham-Inpijn L. Wegener's granulomatosis, serous otitis media and sinusitis. *J Laryngol Otol* 1980;94:785.

53. Berg O, Berostedt H, Carenfelt C, et al. Discrimination of purulent from nonpurulent maxillary sinusitis. *Ann Otolaryngol* 1981;90:272.

54. Abramovich S, Smelt GJ. Acute sphenoiditis: alone and in concert. *J Laryngol Otol* 1982;96:751–757.

55. Bhattacharyya N. Test-retest reliability of computed tomography in the assessment of chronic rhinosinusitis. *Laryngoscope* 1999;109(Part 1):1055–1058.

56. Forbes W, Fawcitt RA, Isherwood I, et al. Computed tomography in the diagnosis of diseases of the paranasal sinuses. *Clin Radiol* 1978;29:501–511.

57. Yarington CT. Sinusitis as an emergency. *Otolaryngol Clin North Am* 1979;12:447–454.

58. Slavin RG. Relationship of nasal disease and sinusitis to bronchial asthma. *Ann Allergy* 1982;49:76–79.

59. Gwaltney JM Jr, Phillips CD, Miller RD, et al. Computed tomographic study of the common cold. *N Engl J Med* 1994;330:25–30.

60. Goldenhersh MJ, Rachelefsky G, Dudley J, et al. The microbiology of chronic sinus disease in children with respiratory allergy. *J Allergy Clin Immunol* 1990;85:1030–1039.

61. Casiano R. Azithromycin and amoxicillin in the treatment of acute maxillary sinusitis. *Am J Med* 1991;91(suppl 3A):27.

62. Williams JW Jr, Aguilar C, Makela M, et al. Antibiotics for acute maxillary sinusitis. Cochrane Database Systems Review, 2000; CD000243.

63. Laurier C, Lachaine J, Ducharme M. Economic evaluation of antibacterials in the treatment of acute sinusitis. *Pharmacoeconomics* 1999;97:113.

64. Melen I, Friberg B, Andreasson L, et al. Effects of phenylpropanolamine on ostial and nasal patency in patients treated for chronic maxillary sinusitis. *Acta Otolaryngol (Stockh)* 1986;101:494–500.

65. Sykes DA, Wilson R, Chan KL, et al. Relative importance of antibiotic and improved clearance in topical treatment of chronic mucopurulent rhinosinusitis. *Lancet* 1986;2:359–360.

66. Kennedy DW. Functional endoscopic sinus surgery. *Arch Otolaryngol* 1985;111:643–649.

67. Stammberger H. Endoscopic surgery for mycotic and chronic recurring sinusitis. *Ann Otol Rhinol Laryngol* 1985;94:1–11.

68. Middleton E Jr. Chronic rhinitis in adults. *J Allergy Clin Immunol* 1988;81:971–975.

69. Numata T, Konno A, Hasegawa S, et al. Pathophysiological features of the nasal mucosa in patients with idiopathic rhinitis compared to allergic rhinitis. *Int Arch Allergy Immunol* 1999;119:304–313.

70. Goodman WS, de Souza FM. Otolaryngology. In: English GM, ed. *Atrophic rhinitis.* Philadelphia: JB Lippincott, 1990.

71. Mullarkey MF. Eosinophilic nonallergic rhinitis. *J Allergy Clin Immunol* 1988;82:941–949.

72. Berkin KE. Respiratory effects of angiotensin converting enzyme inhibitors. *Eur Respir J* 1989;2:198–201.

73. Schatz M, Hoffman CP, Zeiger RS, et al. Course and management of asthma. In: Middleton E, Reed C, et al, eds. *Allergy: principles and practice.* St. Louis, MO: CV Mosby, 1988:1093.

74. Meltzer EO. Evaluating rhinitis: clinical, rhinomanometric and cytologic assessments. *J Allergy Clin Immunol* 1988;82:900–908.

75. Kirkegaard J, Mygind N, Melgaard F, et al. Ordinary and high dose ipratropium in perennial allergic rhinitis. *J Allergy Clin Immunol* 1987;79:585–590.

76. Sweet JM, Stevenson DD, Simon RA, et al. Long term effects of aspirin desensitization. Treatment for aspirin sensitive rhinosinusitis asthma. *J Allergy Clin Immunol* 1990;85:59–65.

77. Schubert MS, Goetz DW. Evaluation and treatment of allergic fungal sinusitis. I. Demographics and diagnosis. J Allergy Clin Immunol 1998;102:387–394.

20

Anaphylaxis

Kris G. McGrath

Division of Allergy-Immunology, Department of Medicine, Northwestern University Medical School, Saint Joseph Hospital, Chicago, Illinois

DEFINITION AND HISTORY

Anaphylaxis is the clinical manifestation of immediate hypersensitivity. This adverse event occurs rapidly, often dramatically, and is unanticipated. Anaphylaxis is the most severe form of allergy and must always be considered a medical emergency. Death may occur suddenly through airway obstruction or irreversible vascular collapse.

The first such fatality was discovered by archaeologists unearthing an Egyptian funerary tablet dated 2641 B.C. Pharaoh Menes died following an allergic reaction to a wasp sting (1). Portier and Richet in 1901 observed that injecting a previously tolerated sea anemone antigen into a dog produced a fatal reaction as opposed to the anticipated prophylaxis. They called this phenomenon anaphylaxis, the antonym of prophylaxis (Greek *ana*, backward, and *phylaxis*, protection). They observed two factors likely essential for anaphylaxis: increased sensitivity to a toxin after previous injection of the same toxin and an incubation period of at least 2 to 3 weeks necessary for this state of increased sensitivity to develop. Richet was recognized as the founder of the new science of allergy and was awarded the Nobel Prize in 1913 and honored on a French stamp issued in 1987 (1–3). Other publications noteworthy for similar observations occurred within a 9-year period before Portier and Richet's pivotal work. In 1893, von Behring injected immunized pigs with diphtheria toxin and believed they became "hypersensitive" (German, *uberenpfindlichkeit*). Hericourt in 1898 reported similar findings in dogs injected with eel serum. The first published observations of anaphylaxis in experimental animals following injections of egg albumin was by Francois Magendie in 1839 (4–6).

True anaphylaxis is caused by immunoglobulin E (IgE)-mediated release of mediators from mast cells and basophils. Anaphylactoid (anaphylaxis-like) or pseudoallergic reactions are similar to anaphylaxis. However, they are not mediated by antigen–antibody interaction, but result from substances acting directly on mast cells and basophils, causing mediator release or acting on tissues such as anaphylotoxins of the complement cascade.

Idiopathic (nonallergic) anaphylaxis occurs spontaneously and is not caused by an unknown allergen. Munchausen's anaphylaxis is a purposeful self-induction of true anaphylaxis. All forms of anaphylaxis present the same and require the same rigorous diagnostic and therapeutic intervention.

The development of modern drugs, as well as therapeutic and diagnostic agents, and the use of herbal and natural remedies have resulted in increased incidence of anaphylaxis. These agents used by physicians, pharmacists, and the general public require acute awareness of the problem and knowledge of preventative and therapeutic measures.

The following factors are associated with an increased incidence of anaphylaxis (7–11):

- The nature of the antigen affects the risk for anaphylaxis (certain antigens more often are the cause of anaphylaxis, e.g., penicillin among drugs, and nuts and shellfish among foods).
- Parenteral administration of a drug is more likely to result in anaphylaxis than its oral ingestion.
- An atopic history is associated with an increased incidence of anaphylaxis to latex, ingested antigens, exercise, and radiographic contrast media (RCM). Idiopathic anaphylaxis patients have a higher prevalence of atopy. Atopic persons are not at increased risk for anaphylaxis from insulin penicillin and Hymenoptera stings.
- Repeated interrupted courses of treatment with a specific substance and long durations between doses increase the risk for anaphylaxis.
- Immunotherapy extract injection to a symptomatic patient (especially under treated asthma) during increased natural exposure to extract components may increase the risk for anaphylaxis.

EPIDEMIOLOGY

The incidence of anaphylaxis in the general population has been underestimated because it is commonly unrecognized and undiagnosed by physicians and patients. Mild episodes, although potentially fatal, often are not evaluated by a physician, especially an allergist (12–14).

Previous attempts to determine the incidence of anaphylaxis investigated narrow subtypes (15–22). Yocum et al., however, examined the overall incidence of anaphylaxis from all causes in a defined community, reflective of the general population. The incidence of anaphylaxis was 21 cases per 100,000. The case-fatality rate was 0.65% (12). Many other studies suggest a lower incidence of anaphylaxis. In Munich, Germany, the incidence of anaphylaxis was reported as 9.8 per 100,000 (23). Sorensen reported an incidence of anaphylaxis as 3.2 cases per 100,000 (24). The number of cases of idiopathic anaphylaxis in the United States was estimated by

Patterson to be between 20,592 and 47,024 (25). Hospital studies estimate anaphylaxis to occur in one of every 3,000 patients and is responsible for more than 500 deaths per year (26–28). Weiler estimated that of 300 individuals expected to have anaphylaxis each year in a community of 1 million, 3 are expected to die (14). The National Office of Vital Statistics estimated an average death rate of 0.28 per 1 million persons per year from Hymenoptera stings alone (29). The Boston Collaborative Drug Surveillance Program reported 0.87 anaphylactic fatalities per 10,000 patients (30).

Occupation, race, season of the year, and geographic location are not predisposing factors for anaphylaxis. However, they may provide the nature of the inciting agent. There are exceptions to the belief that gender is not a significant factor. For instance, anaphylaxis occurs more frequently in women exposed to intravenous muscle relaxants (31), latex (32), and aspirin (33). Insect sting anaphylaxis can occur more frequently in men (34). Most studies conclude that an atopic person is at no greater risk than the nonatopic person for developing IgE-mediated anaphylaxis from penicillin (10), insect stings (11), insulin (35), and muscle relaxants (36). Atopy is a risk factor for anaphylaxis from ingested antigens (8), latex (32,37,38), exercise anaphylaxis (39), idiopathic anaphylaxis (22), and RCM reactions (40). The frequency of anaphylaxis is increased during pollen season for individuals (atopics) receiving immunotherapy (41). In the population-based study of Yocum et al., 53% of Olmstead County residents with an anaphylactic episode from all causes were atopic (12). He concluded that atopy is probably more prevalent among individuals having anaphylaxis than the general population. Generally, a cause is suspected in two thirds of anaphylaxis cases, with the remaining one third being idiopathic (12,15,42). Food appears to be the most common cause of anaphylaxis and is likely the single most common cause presenting to the emergency departments (15,42). Approximately 100 individuals per year die from food-induced anaphylaxis in the United States (43). Foods have surpassed antibiotics (especially penicillin) as the most common cause of anaphylaxis.

Penicillin has been reported to cause fatal anaphylaxis at a rate of 0.002% (27,44). The most common cause of anaphylactoid reactions are from RCM. Life-threatening reactions after administration of RCM occur in approximately 0.1% of procedures. Fatal reactions occur in about 1:10,000 to 1:50,000 intravenous procedures. As many as 500 deaths per year occur after RCM administration (45–47). Fatal reactions occur less frequently with lower osmolar RCM agents (48). The next most common cause of anaphylaxis is Hymenoptera stings, with an incidence of 23 deaths per 150 million stings (27,49–52). Fatalities from allergen immunotherapy and skin testing are rare, with 6 fatalities from allergen skin testing and 24 fatalities from immunotherapy reported from 1959 to 1984 (53). In another study, 17 fatalities associated with immunotherapy occurred from 1985 to 1989 (54).

Not all persons who have had anaphylaxis have it again on reexposure to the same substance. Those who do may react less severely than at the initial event. Factors suggested to explain this include the interval between exposures, the route of exposure, and the amount of the substance received (27). The percentage of persons at risk for recurrent anaphylactic reactions has been estimated to be 10% to 20% for penicillins (55), 20% to 40% for RCM (56), and 40% to 60% for insect stings (27,57). A growing concern are persons with idiopathic anaphylaxis with distinct subtypes (see Chapter 21).

CLINICAL MANIFESTATIONS OF ANAPHYLAXIS

The manifestations of anaphylaxis vary with animal species. The guinea pig typically has acute respiratory obstruction; the rat, circulatory collapse with increased peristalsis; the rabbit, acute pulmonary hypertension; and the dog, circulatory collapse.

Humans vary greatly in the onset and course of anaphylaxis (22,42,58–61). The skin, conjunctivae, upper and lower airways, cardiovascular system, and gastrointestinal tract may be affected solely or in combination. Neurologic involvement also may occur. Involvement of the respira-

tory and cardiovascular systems is of the most concern. In one series of anaphylactic deaths, 70% died of respiratory complications and 24% of cardiovascular failure (62). Symptoms generally begin in seconds to minutes after exposure to the inciting agent. However, symptoms may be delayed for up to an hour. Anaphylaxis from an ingested antigen can occur immediately, but usually occurs within the first 2 hours and can be delayed for several hours (8). Initial signs and symptoms may include cutaneous erythema and pruritus, especially of the hands, feet, and groin. There can be a sense of oppression, impending doom, cramping abdominal pain, and a feeling of faintness or "light headedness." The skin findings of urticaria and angioedema are the most frequent manifestations and usually last less than 24 hours. Respiratory symptoms, the next most common manifestation, may progress to include mild airway obstruction from laryngeal edema and, more severely, to asphyxia. Early laryngeal edema may manifest as hoarseness, dysphonia, or "lump in the throat." Edema of the larynx, epiglottis, or surrounding tissues can result in stridor and suffocation. With lower airway obstruction and bronchospasm, the individual may complain of chest tightness or wheezing. Gastrointestinal manifestations include nausea, vomiting, abdominal pain, and intense diarrhea, which may be bloody. Of grave concern is the concurrent appearance of both airway obstruction and cardiovascular symptoms. Clinical findings may include hypotension and vascular collapse (shock) followed by complications of asphyxia or cardiac arrhythmia. Myocardial infarction may be a complication of anaphylaxis (63,64). Other frequent manifestations include nasal, ocular, and palatal pruritus; sneezing; diaphoresis; disorientation; and fecal or urinary urgency or incontinence. The initial manifestation of anaphylaxis even may be loss of consciousness. Dizziness, syncope, seizures, confusion, and loss of consciousness may occur as a result of cerebral hypoperfusion or as a direct toxic effect of mediator release (27). Death may follow in minutes (65). Late deaths may occur days to weeks after anaphylaxis, but are often manifestations of organ damage experienced early in the course of anaphylaxis (49). In general, the later the onset of anaphylaxis, the less severe the reaction (66). In some patients, an early anaphylactic reaction may resolve only to be followed by another (biphasic, multiphasic) episode of anaphylaxis (67–71).

PATHOLOGIC FINDINGS

The anatomic and microscopic findings must be examined relative to the underlying illness from which the patient was being treated, the drugs administered, and the effect of secondary changes related to hypoxia, hypovolemia, and postanaphylaxis therapy (26). Anaphylactic death is usually caused by respiratory obstruction with or without cardiovascular collapse (72–77). The prominent pathologic features of fatal anaphylaxis in humans are acute pulmonary hyperinflation, laryngeal edema, upper airway submucosal transudate, pulmonary edema and intraalveolar hemorrhage, visceral congestion, urticaria, and angioedema. In some patients no specific pathologic findings are found, especially if death is from cardiovascular collapse.

Microscopic examination reveals noninflammatory fluid in the lamina propria of the areas just described, increased airway secretions, and eosinophilic infiltrates in bronchial walls (65,77), the laminae propria of the gastrointestinal tract, and sinusoids of the spleen.

Sudden vascular collapse usually is attributed to vessel dilation or cardiac arrhythmia, but myocardial infarction may be sufficient to explain the clinical findings (78). Myocardial damage may occur in up to 80% of fatal cases (76).

The diagnosis of anaphylaxis is clinical, but the following laboratory findings help in unusual cases or in ongoing management. A complete blood count may show an elevated hematocrit secondary to hemoconcentration. Blood chemistries may reveal elevated creatinine phosphokinase, troponin, aspartate aminotransferase, or lactate dehydrogenase if myocardial damage has occurred. Acute elevation of serum histamine, urine histamine, and serum tryptase can occur, and complement abnormalities have been observed (79). Plasma histamine has a short half-life and is not reliable for postmortem diagnosis of anaphylaxis. Mast cell–derived tryptase with a half-life of several hours, however, has

been reported to be elevated for up to 24 hours after death from anaphylaxis and not from other causes of death. Serum tryptase may not be detected within the first 15 to 30 minutes of onset of anaphylaxis; therefore, persons with sudden fatal anaphylaxis may not have elevated tryptase in their postmortem sera (80). The radioallergosorbent test (RAST) may be used on postmortem serum to measure specific IgE to antigens such as Hymenoptera or suspected foods. Together the postmortem serum tryptase and the determination of specific IgE may elucidate the cause of an unexplained death. Serum should be obtained antemortem and within 15 hours of postmortem for tryptase and specific IgE assays, with sera frozen and stored at $-20°C$ (80,81). A chest radiograph may show hyperinflation, atelectasis, or pulmonary edema. The most common electrographic changes other than sinus tachycardia or infarction include T-wave flattening and inversion, bundle branch blocks, supraventricular arrhythmia, and intraventricular conduction defects (65,82).

PATHOPHYSIOLOGY OF ANAPHYLAXIS

Anaphylactic reactions are initiated when a host interacts with a foreign material. The exposure can be topical, inhaled, ingested, or parenteral. Classic anaphylaxis occurs when an allergen combines with specific IgE antibody bound to the surface membranes of mast cells and circulating basophils. Cross-linking of the high-affinity IgE receptor FcεRI occurs through antigen–antibody interaction. This leads to the initiation of a signal transduction cascade mediated by lyn and syk kinases, analogous to that induced by T-cell and B-cell receptors. This mast cell and basophil activation leads to rapid degranulation release of histamine, followed by synthesis and release of leukotrienes, prostaglandins, cytokines, and other mediators of the allergic response (83–86). These chemical mediators are discussed in detail in Chapter 4.

Anaphylactoid (pseudoallergic) reactions are not IgE antibody/antigen mediated, but are induced by substances acting directly on mast cells and basophils causing mediator release. This non–IgE-mediated mast cell and basophil activation occurs with drugs such as opioids, vancomycin, and etoposide, RCM, extracts of some foods, dextran, and complement components (C3a, C5a).

Histamine is a preformed and stored vasoactive mediator in mast cell and basophil cytoplasmic granules. Upon its release, histamine acts on histamine (H_1 and H_2) receptors on target organs to increase vascular permeability, cause vasodilation, enhance mucus secretion, and cause bronchial constriction and gastrointestinal smooth muscle constriction. Other mast cell preformed mediators include neutral proteases (tryptase, chymase, carboxypeptidase), acid hydrolase (arylsulphatase), oxidative enzymes (superoxide, peroxidase), chemotactic factors (eosinophils, neutrophils), and proteoglycans (heparin). Mediators that are generated and released from mast cell membranes by arachidonic acid metabolism include prostaglandin D_2, leukotrienes B_4, C_4, and E_4, and platelet-activating factor. These membrane-derived mediators also cause bronchoconstriction, mucus secretion, and changes in vascular permeability. Platelet-activating factor can alter pulmonary mechanics and lower blood pressure in animals (87), as well as activate clotting, and produce disseminated intravascular coagulation (88). In humans it causes bronchoconstriction if inhaled and causes a wheal and flare reaction when injected into human skin. Its release also has been reported in cold urticaria, but whether platelet-activating factor participates in anaphylaxis remains speculative (89).

Other proinflammatory pathways are activated by mast cell and basophil mediators. Basophil kallikrein, mast cell kininogenase, and tryptase can all activate the kinin system (90–93). Chymase release may enhance the compensatory response to hypotension by converting angiotensin I to angiotensin II (8).

Nitric oxide synthesis occurs during anaphylaxis (94). This is induced by mast cells and vascular endothelium. Its synthesis is triggered by hypoxia, substance P, bradykinin, leukotriene C_4, and histamine. Hypotension occurs by nitric oxide increasing vascular permeability and causing smooth muscle relaxation (94–97).

Chemotactic mediators attract eosinophils and neutrophils prolonging the inflammatory response. In summary, anaphylactic and anaphylactoid events occur as a result of multimediator release and recruitment with a potential for a catastrophic outcome.

DIAGNOSIS AND DIFFERENTIAL DIAGNOSIS

Because of the profound and dramatic presentation, the diagnosis of anaphylaxis is usually readily apparent. When sudden collapse occurs in the absence of urticaria or angioedema, other diagnoses must be considered, although shock may be the only symptom of Hymenoptera anaphylaxis. These include cardiac arrhythmia, myocardial infarction, other types of shock (hemorrhagic, cardiogenic, endotoxic), severe cold urticaria, aspiration of food or foreign body, insulin reaction, pulmonary embolism, seizure disorder, vasovagal reaction, hyperventilation, globus hystericus, and factitious allergic emergencies. The most common is vasovagal collapse after an injection or a painful stimulation. In vasovagal collapse, pallor and diaphoresis are common features associated with presyncopal nausea. There is no pruritus or cyanosis. Respiratory difficulty does not occur, the pulse is slow, and the blood pressure can be supported without sympathomimetic agents. Symptoms are almost immediately reversed by recumbency and leg elevation. Hereditary angioedema must be considered when laryngeal edema is accompanied by abdominal pain. This disorder usually has a slower onset, and lacks urticaria and hypotension, and there is often a family history of similar reactions. There is also a relative resistance to epinephrine, but epinephrine may have life-saving value in hereditary angioedema.

Idiopathic urticaria occurring with the acute onset of bronchospasm in an asthmatic patient may make it impossible to differentiate from anaphylaxis. Similarly, a patient experiencing a sudden respiratory arrest from asthma may be thought to be experiencing anaphylaxis because of severe dyspnea and facial fullness and erythema.

"Restaurant syndromes" may mimic anaphylaxis such as from monosodium glutamate, histamine fish poisoning, and saurine, a histamine-like chemical also from spoiled fish (98–101).

Many patients suffer from flush reactions that mimic anaphylaxis and may blame monosodium glutamate incorrectly. These include carcinoid flush, postmenopausal flush, chlorpropamide flush, flush due to medullary carcinoma of the thyroid, flush related to autonomic epilepsy, and idiopathic flush (98). Excessive endogenous production of histamine may mimic anaphylaxis such as systemic mastocytosis, urticaria pigmentosa, certain leukemias, and ruptured hydrated cysts (98). Other disorders in the differential diagnosis include panic attacks, vocal cord dysfunction syndrome, Munchausen stridor, undifferentiated somatoform anaphylaxis, and other factitious allergic diseases (98,102, 103).

Laboratory tests can help in the differential diagnosis; for example, blood serotonin and the urinary 5-hydroxy-indoleacetic acid level will be elevated in carcinoid syndrome. Measurement of plasma histamine levels may not be helpful because of its rapid release and short half-life. However, a 24-hour urine collection or spot sample for histamine or histamine metabolites can be helpful, because urinary histamine levels usually are elevated for longer periods. Measurement of serum tryptase levels are useful, if elevated, peaking 1 to 1.5 hours after the onset of anaphylaxis with elevated levels persisting for 5 to 24 hours (80,104). During controlled studies of immunotherapy for insect hypersensitivity, investigators noted in patients experiencing shock dramatic increases in plasma histamine concentrations and a decrease in concentrations levels of factor V, factor VIII, fibrinogen, and high-molecular-weight kininogen. In one patient a decrease in C3 and C4 occurred (105,106). A subsequent study demonstrated an increase in C3a, a clearing product of C3 supporting activation of the complement cascade (107).

Munchausen stridor patients can be distracted from their vocal cord adduction by maneuvers such as coughing. There also will be no cutaneous signs. In vocal cord dysfunction patients, the involuntary vocal cord adduction can be confirmed by video laryngoscopy during episodes and absence of cutaneous signs (98,102,103).

A history of recent antigen or substance exposure and clinical suspicion are the most important diagnostic tools. IgE antibody can be demonstrated *in vivo* by skin-prick testing. Skin-prick testing can be useful in predicting anaphylactic sensitivity to many antigens. Caution must be exercised, beginning with very dilute antigens. Anaphylaxis has followed skin-prick testing with penicillin, insect sting extract, and foods. Passive transfer to human skin carries the risk for transmitting viral illnesses (i.e., hepatitis, human immunodeficiency virus) and should not be done. The RAST can quantitate nanogram quantities of specific antibody but is not as sensitive as skin testing. Other *in vitro* techniques include the release of histamine from leukocytes of sensitive individuals on antigen challenge, and the ability of a patient's serum to passively sensitize normal tissues such as leukocytes for the subsequent antigen-induced release of mediators (26). Complement consumption has not yet been used routinely to define anaphylactic mechanisms. The only currently reliable test for agents that alter arachidonic acid metabolism such as aspirin and other nonsteroidal antiinflammatory agents and other suspected non–IgE-mediated agents is carefully graded oral challenge with close clinical observation and measurement of pulmonary function, nasal patency, and vital signs, following informed patient consent.

Substances that can directly release histamine from mast cells and basophils may be identified *in vitro* using washed human leukocytes or by *in vivo* skin testing. These agents must release histamine in the absence of IgG or IgE antibody (26).

FACTORS INCREASING THE SEVERITY OF ANAPHYLAXIS OR INTERFERING WITH TREATMENT

There are many factors that increase the severity of anaphylaxis or interfere with treatment (Table 20.1). Concomitant therapy with β-adrenergic–blocking drugs or the presence of asthma exacerbate the responses of the airways in anaphylaxis and inhibit resuscitative efforts (27,108–111). Furthermore, epinephrine use in patients on β-adrenergic–blocking drugs may induce unopposed α-adrenergic effects, resulting in severe hypertension. Rapid intravenous infusion of an allergen in a patient with a preexisting cardiac disorder may increase the risk for severe anaphylaxis (27). β-adrenergic–blocking drugs

TABLE 20.1. *Factors that intensify anaphylaxis or interfere with treatment*

Presence of asthma
Underlying cardiac disease
Concomitant therapy with:
    β-adrenergic blockers
    Monoamine oxidase inhibitors
    Angiotensin-converting enzyme inhibitors
Delay in epinephrine administration

should be used with caution, and preferably avoided in patients receiving immunotherapy and for idiopathic anaphylaxis. The difficulty in reversing anaphylaxis may occur in part from underlying cardiac disease for which β-adrenergic blockers have been given.

Angiotensin-converting enzyme (ACE) inhibitors prevent the mobilization of angiotensin II, an endogenous compensatory mechanism, and can cause life-threatening tongue or pharyngeal edema themselves (112,113). Monoamine oxidase inhibitors can increase the hazards of epinephrine by interfering with its degradation (112).

Systemic reactions occur more frequently in undertreated asthma patients receiving immunotherapy. It has been recommended that measurements of forced expiratory volume in 1 second (FEV_1) be performed before immunotherapy, with injections withheld if the FEV_1 is below 70% of the predicted volume (53,114,115). However, this recommendation is not standard practice.

CAUSES OF ANAPHYLAXIS

Many substances have been reported to cause anaphylaxis in humans. These antigens are subdivided into proteins, polysaccharides, and haptens. A hapten is a low-molecular-weight organic compound that becomes antigenic when it or one of its metabolites forms a stable bond with a host protein. With penicillin, both the parent hapten and nonenzymatic degradation products may form bonds with host proteins to form an antigen.

The route of antigen exposure causing human anaphylaxis may be oral, parenteral, topical, or inhalational. An example of an agent that can cause anaphylaxis by any of four ways of entry is penicillin.

Table 20.2 lists common causes of anaphylaxis and anaphylactoid reactions in humans. This list is not all-inclusive. The following discussion is a review of some important and interesting causes of anaphylaxis.

Penicillin

Surpassed by food, penicillin is no longer the most frequent cause of anaphylaxis in humans (116,117). Estimates of nonfatal allergic reactions vary, ranging from 0.7% to 10%, and fatal reactions have been estimated at a frequency of 0.002%, or 1 fatality per 7.5 million injections (7), and 1 per 50,000 to 100,000 penicillin courses (8,18).

The most likely mode of administration to induce anaphylaxis is parenteral. Oral, inhalation, and diagnostic skin testing can cause anaphylaxis. Cross-reactivity exists between the various penicillins. If an individual is allergic to penicillin G, he or she must be considered allergic to other natural and synthetic penicillins. Cross-reactivity, challenged by some (118), also exists with cephalosporin and carbapenam antibiotics.

Penicillin haptens of importance are benzylpenicillin and semisynthetic penicillins. The benzylpenicilloyl group of benzylpenicillin quantitatively is the major haptenic determinant (119,120). There is much cross-reactivity with α-aminobenzyl (ampicillin) penicilloyl hapten, but only minimal cross-reactivity with dimethoxyphenyl (methicillin) or oxacilleyl (oxacillin) penicilloyl haptens (121). Penicillin therapy also induces the formation of antibodies for minor determinants derived from benzylpenicillin (122). Cephalosporins induce the formation of a major determinant, the cephaloyl group, and minor determinants cross-reacting with those of benzylpenicillin (121,123,124). Clinical cross-reactivity between penicillin and a first- through third-generation cephalosporin ranges from about 16% (first-generation) to less than 5% (third-generation). Aztreonam, a β-lactam with a monobactam structure can be used safely in patients with penicillin allergy.

Heterologous Antiserum

Before frequent penicillin and antitoxin use, horse serum was the most common cause of

TABLE 20.2. *Some causes of anaphylactic and anaphylactoid reactions in humans*

Substance	Immunologic Mediator (IgE Antibody)	Substance	Immunologic Mediator (IgE Antibody)
Antibiotics		**Allergy extracts**	
Penicillins	Yes	Ragweed	Yes
Cephalosporins	Yes	Grass	Yes
Tetracyclines	Yes	Molds	Yes
Sulfonamides	Yes	Epidermals	Yes
Nitrofurantoin	Possible	Hymenoptera	Yes
Streptomycin	Possible	**Hormones**	
Vancomycin	No	Insulin	Yes
Chloramphenicol	No	Corticotropin	Yes
Ciprofloxacin	No	Parathormone	Yes
Amphotericin B	No	Adrenocorticotrophic hormone (ACTH)	Yes
Miscellaneous drugs/ therapeutic agents		Synthetic ACTH	Yes
Acetylsalicylic acid	No	Thymostimulin	Yes
Nonsteroidal antiinflammatory agents	Possible	**Enzymes**	
Progesterone	Uncertain	Trypsin	Yes
Suxamethonium	Yes	Chymotrypsin	Yes
Succinylcholine	Uncertain	Penicillinase	Yes
Thiopental	Uncertain	Asparaginase	Yes
d-Tubocurarine	Uncertain	Chymopapain	Yes
Mechlorethamine	Uncertain	Streptokinase	Yes
Opiates	No	**Diagnostic agents**	
Vaccines	Yes	Sodium dehydrocholate	No
Antitoxins (horse)	Yes	Sulfobromophthalein	No
Protamine sulfate	Varies	Radiographic contrast media	No
OKT3 monoclonal antibody	Yes	Benzylpenicilloyl-polylysine	Yes
Foods		Pre-Pen	Yes
Nuts (peanut most common)	Yes	**Blood products**	
Shellfish	Yes	Whole blood	Possible
Fish	Yes	Gamma globulin	Possible
Milk (raw)	Yes	Cryoprecipitate	Possible
Buckwheat	Yes	IgA	Possible
Egg white	Yes	Plasma	Possible
Chamomile tea (ragweed crossreacts)	Yes	**Dialysis exposure**	
Pinto bean	Yes	Ethylene oxide gas	Yes
Rice	Yes	AN69 membrane	No (Bradykinin)
Potato	Yes	**Venoms and saliva**	
Orange	Yes	Hymenoptera	Yes
Tangerine	Yes	Deerfly	Yes
Sunflower seed	Yes	Snake venom	Yes
Banana	Yes	Fire ant	Yes
Mustard	Yes	Triatoma	Yes
Pistachio, cashew	Yes	**Polysaccharides/volume expanders**	
Tree nuts	Yes	Dextran	Uncertain
Food additive		Acacia	Uncertain
Carmine	Yes	**Seminal plasma**	Yes
		Latex	Yes

anaphylaxis (125,126). The use of horse serum is less common since the advent of human tetanus antitoxin and rabies vaccine. Heterologous preparations were used at one time for numerous infections other than tetanus caused by pneumococci, meningococci, staphylococci, and the tubercle bacillus. Heterologous sera are used in the treatment of snake bite, botulism, gangrene, diphtheria, spider bite, and organ transplant rejection. The incidence of horse antilymphocyte globulin anaphylaxis is near 2% (127). Skin testing should precede use of such preparations to identify the presence of IgE antibodies (128).

Insect Stings

Systemic allergic reactions to insect stings occur in an estimated 3.3% of the population, and approximately 40 deaths occur annually in the United States due to insect stings (52,129). The most common species are members of the order Hymenoptera, which includes hornets, wasps, honey bees, and yellow jackets. Fire ant stings also cause human anaphylaxis, particularly in the southern United States, at an estimated annual rate of 0.6% to 16%, with greater than 80 fatalities (130–135).

The victim may not accurately identify the specific insect necessitating confirmation of hypersensitivity by skin testing with purified venoms or whole-body fire ant extracts. *In vitro* tests, such as enzyme-linked immunosorbent assay and RAST, can be used to confirm a clinical history of hymenoptera or fire ant hypersensitivity. Severe reactions to insect stings with confirmed positive skin tests warrant the physician to advise the patient to undergo highly effective venom (Hymenoptera) or whole-body vaccine (fire ant) immunotherapy in addition to carrying epinephrine and practicing avoidance (129,136,137). See Chapter 12 for complete discussion of insect allergy.

Food

Foods are likely the most common cause of anaphylaxis, and the sequence of events generally makes the diagnosis (15,42,116,138–141). However, occasionally the physician and the patient may not suspect the offending antigen. Any food may cause anaphylaxis. The most frequent causes of food anaphylaxis include peanuts, tree nuts, fish, shellfish, some fruits (kiwi), and seeds (116). With some foods, microgram quantities are enough to induce anaphylaxis. If the cause of food-induced anaphylaxis is not apparent from the patient's history, skin testing or RAST determination with food extracts may demonstrate

IgE antibody and help determine the cause (142). Skin testing with foods may cause anaphylaxis, necessitating the use of diluted solutions, the skin-prick technique, physician presence, and emergency materials and equipment. Factors that predispose a person's severity of food-induced anaphylaxis include a personal history of atopy, older age, previous particular food allergy, poorly controlled asthma, and delay in epinephrine administration (143–147). Food antigenicity can be altered by cooking and processing, which may prevent a reaction such as occurs with heat-labile antigens. Food handling such as reported with kiwi fruit can cause anaphylaxis (148). Cross-reactivity between foods exists, such as with sunflower seeds and chamomile tea, which are in the ragweed family (149,150). Food ingestion followed by exercise has been reported to cause two subsets of anaphylaxis. Nonspecific food-dependent anaphylaxis occurs when a meal is ingested before exercise (153–155). Specific food-induced anaphylaxis (food-dependent exercise-induced anaphylaxis) occurs when exercise follows ingestion of a particular food. Such foods have included celery (158), shellfish (116,155–158), wheat (159–163), grapes (164), nuts (164), peaches (164), eggs (165–167), oranges (163), apples (151), hazelnuts (169), cheese (170), and cabbage (171). These foods may be tolerated without exercise.

Food Additives

Papain in meat tenderizers has caused serious allergic reactions. Results of skin-prick testing with papain and meat tenderizer have been positive. The reaction may be confirmed by oral challenge and prevented with oral cromolyn sodium premedication (172). Avoidance is the treatment of choice.

Anaphylactic-type reactions have been reported to occur from metabisulfites. No IgE-mediated mechanism has been demonstrated (173–175), and the relationship with anaphylaxis is questionable. Sulfites have been used for centuries to preserve food and are cheaper and more effective than ascorbic acid. Sulfiting agents include sulfur dioxide, sodium or potassium sulfite, bisulfite, and metabisulfite. In addition to food preservation, these agents are used as sanitizers for containers, as antioxidants to prevent food discoloration, and as fresheners. They are found in foods such as beer, wine, shellfish, salad, fresh fruits and vegetables, potatoes, and avocados. The highest levels occur in restaurant foods, with federal regulations restricting their use in fresh served foods.

Anaphylaxis has occurred following ingestion of the food colorant carmine, confirmed by positive skin-prick test results and positive RAST results to carmine. One individual had serum IgE antibodies to a carmine–acid albumin conjugate (176,177).

Latex Anaphylaxis

The incidence of anaphylaxis to latex has yet to be determined or estimated. Increased reports parallel the increased use of latex gloves following increased precaution to reduce the spread of acquired immunodeficiency syndrome. Between 1988 and 1992 the U.S. Food and Drug Administration received more than 1,000 reports of latex anaphylaxis, 15 of which were fatal (178,179). Children with spinabifida or severe urogenital defects, health-care workers, and rubber industry workers appear to be at greater risk than the general population (179). Risk factors for health-care workers include a personal history of atopy, frequent use of disposable latex gloves, and hand dermatitis (8,180). These reactions are mediated by IgE antibody to residual rubber tree proteins in latex gloves, condoms, and medical devices (179,181). Exposure can be topical, inhalation, mucosal during condom use, surgery, and dental procedures, and intravenous. It has been suggested that any person at high risk should be tested (182). Skin tests are more sensitive than serologic tests, but no approved skin test reagent is available in the United States. Extracts have been made from raw latex and from finished rubber products. Systemic reactions to latex skin testing have been reported; thus, care must be exercised when skin testing with uncharacterized extracts (182). *In vitro* testing is available by some commercial and university laboratories. High-risk individuals should be tested. If they test positive for latex-specific IgE or have a history

of latex anaphylaxis, they should be identified as having a latex allergy. Latex must be avoided by these individuals, and when in the hospital, a latex-free environment should be provided. Injectable epinephrine should be carried in case of accidental exposure.

Drugs Used in General Anesthesia

The reported incidence of anaphylaxis in general anesthesia varies and is approximately one in 5,000 to one in 15,000 operations (one study estimated 1 in 980 to 1 in 22,000), with death varying in reports from 0.05% to 4% to 6% (183–191). Induction agents and neuromuscular relaxants have caused reactions. These reactions have been anaphylactic (IgE mediated) and anaphylactoid. The implicated induction agents include propanidid, alfathesin, thiopentone, methohexitone, propofol, and midazolam. Muscle relaxants are predominantly implicated, including D-tubocurarine, alcuronium, suxamethonium, gallamine, succinylcholine, pancuronium, vecuronium, and atracurium. Alcuronium is primarily used in Australia, and suxamethonium is used in France (182). The main antigenic determinants of suxamethonium are two molecules of quaternary ammonium (NH_4), which are also found in other muscle relaxants (190). An IgE-mediated process is likely based on skin tests, passive transfer, and histamine release studies (190–193). Anaphylaxis typically occurs following previous sensitization to the drug or related agent. Researchers have cautioned that hydrophobic IgE can be responsible for nonspecific cross-reactions, necessitating IgE inhibition studies (191). The induction agent propofol can interact with a muscle relaxant and potentiate mediator release by unknown mechanisms in some cases (191).

Other mechanisms of anesthetic drug-induced mediator release include osmotic release of histamine, basophil determination complement activation, the kinin-kallikrein system, and a direct membrane effect of the drug (186,190,191,195, 196). Cross-reactivity among these drugs exists, and variable results occur when intradermal and radioimmunoassay tests are conducted (185,188, 194).

The presence of skin manifestations may help indicate an allergic reaction during general anesthesia to avoid confusion with other causes of bronchospasm, hypotension, and cardiac arrhythmias. Some immediate type reactions have occurred because of bolus injection of muscle relaxants rather than infusions over 1 minute, which are not associated with reactions.

Blood Components, Related Biologics, and Chemotherapy

Blood transfusions have induced anaphylactic reactions. A nonatopic recipient may be passively sensitized by transfusion of donor blood containing elevated titers of IgE (197). Conversely, in rare cases, transfusion of an allergen or drug into an atopic recipient has caused plasma anaphylaxis.

Antihuman IgA antibodies are present in about 40% of individuals with selective IgA deficiency. Some of the patients have allergic reactions varying from mild urticaria to fatal anaphylaxis, usually after numerous transfusions (198). These antibodies are usually IgG mediated but may be IgE mediated. These reactions can be prevented by using sufficiently washed red blood cells or by using blood from IgA-deficient donors (199–202).

Serum protein aggregates (nonimmune complex) such as human albumin, human γ globulin, and horse antihuman lymphocyte globulin can cause anaphylactoid reactions. These complexes apparently activate complement, resulting in release of bioactive mediators (202,203).

Cryoprecipitate and factor VIII concentrate have been reported as causes of anaphylaxis. An IgE-mediated mechanism was demonstrated in one patient by leukocyte histamine release, positive skin test results to factor VIII, factor IX, and cryoprecipitate, and positive RAST results to factor VIII. An attempt at pretreatment with corticosteroids and diphenhydramine and an attempt to desensitize did not prevent future reactions (203,204).

Plasma expanders composed of modified fluid gelatins, plasma proteins, dextran, and hydroxyethyl starch have caused anaphylaxis. Skin testing and leukocyte histamine release may aid in predicting those at risk, but an immunologic mechanism is not clear (204–209).

Protamine sulfate derived from salmon testes caused an anaphylactic reaction in a patient allergic to fish, with such a risk suggested to be higher in infertile men or in those who have had vasectomies (210). However, fish hypersensitivity does not necessarily imply an increased risk for protamine reactions, which may not always be IgE mediated. IgE antibodies to salmon obtained from patients who had experienced salmon anaphylaxis were not inhibited by protamine, suggesting lack of cross-reactivity (211). There has been an increased use of protamine for medicinal purposes. These include the reversal of heparin anticoagulation during vascular surgery, cardiac catheterization, and the retardation of insulin absorption. Included are isophane, protamine zinc, and human insulins. Diabetic patients receiving daily subcutaneous injections of insulin containing protamine appear to have a 40- to 50-fold increased risk for life-threatening reactions when given protamine intravenously (212,213). The mechanism appears to be caused by antibody-mediated mechanisms. In diabetic patients who had received protamine insulin injections, the presence of antiprotamine IgE antibody is a significant risk factor for acute protamine reactions, as was antiprotamine IgG. Patients having reactions to protamine without previous protamine insulin injections had no antiprotamine IgE antibodies. But in this group, antiprotamine IgG was a risk factor for protamine reactions (214).

Streptokinase is an enzymatic protein produced by group C β-hemolytic streptococci. Streptokinase has been used as a thrombolytic agent. Allergic reactions range in frequency from 1.7% to 18%. This includes anaphylaxis supported by *in vitro* and *in vivo* evidence. Intradermal skin testing with 100 IU of streptokinase is recommended before infusion. This dose causes an immediate reaction without a large delayed reaction in sensitive subjects. In those patients with positive immediate cutaneous reactivity, an alternative thrombolytic agent such as urokinase or alteplase (recombinant rt-PA) should be substituted, even though they cost significantly more than streptokinase (215–217). An anaphylactoid reaction to recombinant rt-PA has been reported (218,219). Chemotherapy agents have caused hypersensitivity reactions, including anaphylaxis. An IgE mechanism has been implicated in some reactions, including L-asparaginase, cisplatin, cytarabine, cyclophosphamide, and possibly methotrexate. Etoposide, its congener teniposide, and paclitaxel hypersensitivity reactions are non–IgE mediated, necessitating a pretreatment regimen if use is essential (220–224).

Miscellaneous IgE-mediated and Non–IgE-mediated Anaphylaxis

The injection of chymopapain into herniated vertebral discs is called chemonucleolysis. This procedure has been associated with anaphylaxis in 1.2% of women and 0.4% of men with a death rate of 0.01% (225). Chymopapain is administered rarely. Chymopapain is obtained from papain, a crude fraction from the papaya, *Carcia papaya* (226). It is used industrially as a meat-tenderizing agent and to clarify beer and sterilize soft contact lenses. These exposures likely sensitize individuals who then receive and react to chymopapain injections. IgE-mediated allergy to papain has been reported in both occupational and nonoccupational settings (172). Cutaneous skin testing by investigators has a 1% incidence of positive reactivity approaching the historical incidence of anaphylaxis (227,228). There were no instances of defined anaphylaxis due to chymopapain in skin test–negative patients. Bernstein et al. (229) compared the incidence of positive skin test results with chymopapain and positive RAST results with chymopapain and found that RAST was less sensitive. This concurs with the concept that cutaneous testing is more sensitive than *in vitro* assays. Furthermore, cutaneous testing provides immediate results. Therapeutic injection of chymopapain in only skin test–negative patients can reduce the incidence of anaphylaxis below the historical rate of 1%.

Anaphylaxis has occurred after using ciprofloxacin (230), cytarabine (231), tetanus toxoid (232), yellow fever vaccine (233), trichophytin skin testing (234), ranitidine (235), psyllium (236), cromolyn sodium (237), and proton pump inhibitors (238). Severe allergic reactions have been associated with ethylene oxide gas (239) used to sterilize supplies for chronic hemodialysis patients. IgE and IgG antibodies have been demonstrated against human serum albumin linked to ethylene oxide. Grammer and Patterson (240) demonstrated IgE antibodies against ethylene oxide–altered proteins as a likely explanation for some hemodialysis anaphylaxis. The ethylene oxide–human serum albumin (ETO-HSA) antigen was characterized by immunoelectrophoresis, gel filtration chromatography, and immunologic inhibition assays. During dialysis, anaphylactoid reactions (possibly mediated by bradykinin) have occurred due to AN69 membranes, especially in patients receiving ACE inhibitor drugs (241,242). Anaphylactoid reactions may occur with all types of dialyzer membranes (243).

Anaphylaxis following sexual intercourse has been reported in women (244–245). One women's serum contained a heat-labile antibody that conferred anaphylactic sensitivity to human and monkey skin. The IgE antibody was directed against a glycoprotein in her husband's seminal fluid. In another woman, a defined antigen could not be determined, but her serum contained IgE antibodies to partially purified seminal fraction IV. Elevated levels of serum-specific IgE antibodies to human seminal plasma (HuSePl) have also been demonstrated. In one such patient, immunotherapy with HuSePl fractions prevented postcoital anaphylaxis (246). Artificial insemination with sperm devoid of seminal plasma induced pregnancy in a woman with human seminal plasma atopy (247).

Allergic reactions to insulin are less common using human insulin produced by recombinant DNA methods, but reactions still occur (248). This is probably due to tertiary structure differences between endogenous insulin and insulin obtained by recombinant DNA. Skin testing will exclude insulin allergy when doubt exists and enable selection of the least allergenic insulin preparation.

Desensitization protocols are available if no alternatives exist and insulin must be given to the allergic patient (249). The incidence of allergic reactions to insulins appears to be decreasing. In nearly all cases of systemic allergy, the patient experiences a local wheal and erythema at the site of insulin injection and there has been a hiatus in therapy.

Life-threatening reactions following the administration of RCM occur in approximately 0.1% of procedures. Fatal reactions with RCM administration occur in about 1:10,000 to 1:50,000 intravenous procedures (45–47). As many as 500 deaths per year may occur following RCM administration (250,251). The immediate-type, generalized reactions after RCM simulate anaphylaxis clinically but are not IgE mediated.

No method is available to identify individuals at risk for an initial reaction, but it is known that a person who had a previous reaction is at higher risk for a repeat reaction. Thus, individuals with previous adverse allergic reactions to RCM should be pretreated to reduce risk (251). This should be done only if RCM administration is absolutely essential. A complete review of RCM allergy is provided in Chapter 17. The introduction of lower osmolality RCM has reduced but not eliminated the problem of RCM reactions.

Idiopathic anaphylaxis is discussed in Chapter 21.

EXERCISE-INDUCED ANAPHYLAXIS

Exercise-induced anaphylaxis (EIA) occurs with vigorous exercise and may produce shock or loss of consciousness. Symptoms include urticaria, angioedema, nausea, vomiting, abdominal cramps, diarrhea, laryngeal edema, bronchospasm, and respiratory distress (168,252, 253). The reaction typically begins during or after exercise is completed and may occur only when exercise is performed shortly after a meal. Specific foods have been linked to EIA, including celery, shrimp, apples, squid, abalone, wheat, hazelnuts (154,155,169), grapes (154), eggs (164,167), oranges (163), cabbage (171), and chicken, but most cases are not associated with prior food ingestion (143,154–156,255,259). These foods have been tolerated without exercise, and exercising without eating these foods does not cause anaphylaxis. Nonspecific food-dependent EIA also can occur (153–155). EIA does not occur with each period of exercise, and

the same amount of exercise on each occasion may not lead to anaphylaxis. About two thirds of patients with EIA have a family history of atopy, and about half have a personal history of atopy (253). Familial EIA also has been reported (256). One death has been reported from EIA (257). Elevated concentrations of plasma histamine, serum lactate, and CPK have been demonstrated during episodes (258). The exact mechanism is unknown, and it has been speculated that release of endogenous opioid peptides with vigorous exercise may release bioactive mediators in susceptible individuals (128). There is evidence for mast cell activation from skin biopsy specimens. Reproducibility in the laboratory using plastic occlusive suits does not always occur, in contrast to raising core body temperature in patients with cholinergic urticaria (252). Treatment is best provided by limiting exercise, especially on warm humid days or stopping at the first sign of prodromal symptoms. Pretreatment with H_1 antihistamines may not always be effective. The "buddy system" of exercise and self-discipline are required along with the availability of injectable epinephrine (259).

TREATMENT AND PREVENTION

The treatment of anaphylaxis should follow established principles for emergency resuscitation. Anaphylaxis has a highly variable presentation, and treatment must be individualized for a patient's particular symptoms and their severity. Treatment recommendations are based on clinical experience, understanding pathologic mechanisms, and the known action of various drugs (260). Rapid therapy is of utmost importance. The approach outlined in Table 20.3 is required to counteract the effects of mediator release, support vital functions, and prevent further release of mediators.

At the first sign of anaphylaxis the patient should be treated with epinephrine. Next, the clinician should determine whether the patient is dyspneic or hypotensive. Airway patency must be assessed, and if the patient has suffered cardiopulmonary arrest, basic cardiopulmonary resuscitation must be instituted immediately. If shock is present or impending, the legs should

TABLE 20.3. *Management of anaphylaxis*

1. Immediate: Epinephrine 1:1,000 0.3 mL i.m. (deltoid)
2. Record blood pressure and pulse
3. Depending on severity, degree of response and the individual patient:
   a. Benadryl 50 mg i.v. slowly
   b. Nasal oxygen
4. Repeat epinephrine every 15 min
5. Be prepared for intubation; hypotension
6. For severe bronchospasm:
   a. i.v. aminophylline
   b. Solu-cortef 200 mg i.v. push
7. For systolic blood pressure <90 mm Hg:
   a. 2 i.v. lines wide open
   b. Dopamine 400 mg (2 amps) in 500 mL D5W Infuse until systolic blood pressure is 90 mm Hg, then titrate (alternatives: norepinephrine, metaraminol)
8. For patients taking β-adrenergic blocking drugs:
   a. Glucagon 1–5 mg i.v. bolus, then titrate at 5–15 μg/min
   b. Atropine if bradycardia; 0.3–0.5 mg i.m. or i.v. every 10 min, maximum of 2 mg

be elevated and intravenous fluids administered. Epinephrine is the most important single agent in the treatment of anaphylaxis, and its delay in or failure to be administered is more problematic than its administration. Epinephrine in an aqueous solution at a 1:1,000 dilution (0.30–0.50 mL; 0.01 mL/kg in children, up to 0.30 mL) is administered intramuscularly in the upper extremity or thigh. If anaphylaxis resulted from an injection or sting, as long as the sting is not on the head, neck, hands, or feet, a second injection of epinephrine may be given at the injection or sting site to reduce antigen absorption (260).

Intravenous epinephrine should be used only in a terminal patient (1 mL of 1:1,000 solution of epinephrine diluted in 10 mL of saline solution, doses are 0.1 to 0.2 mL every 5–20 minutes). If the reaction is from an injection or sting (not if sting or injection was in the head, neck, hands, or feet), a tourniquet should be placed proximal to the site of the injection. The tourniquet should be released for 1 to 2 minutes every 10 minutes. Oxygen should be given in patients with cyanosis, dyspnea, or wheezing with oximetric monitoring. Caution must be exercised if the patient has preexisting chronic obstructive pulmonary disease.

Diphenhydramine can be administered intravenously (slowly over 20 seconds), intramuscularly, or orally (1–2 mg/kg) up to 50 mg in a single dose. Continue to administer diphenhydramine orally every 6 hours for 48 hours to reduce the risk for recurrence. Other rapidly absorbed antihistamines can be substituted.

If the patient does not respond to the above measures and remains hypotensive or in persistent respiratory distress, hospitalization in an intensive care unit is essential. In these circumstances, intravenous fluids should be given through the largest gauge line available at a rate necessary to maintain a systolic blood pressure above 100 mm Hg in adults and 50 mm Hg in children. If intravenous fluids are not effective, vasopressors such as dopamine (norepinephrine) or metaraminol may be necessary. If bronchospasm persists, aminophylline can be cautiously administered intravenously, with serum theophylline monitoring. Intubation and tracheostomy are necessary if airway obstruction is so severe that the patient cannot maintain adequate ventilation.

Corticosteroids are not helpful in the acute management of anaphylaxis. They should be used in moderate or severe reactions to prevent protracted or recurrent anaphylaxis. Aqueous hydrocortisone should be given (5 mg/kg, up to 200 mg; higher doses are also acceptable), immediately followed by 2 to 5 mg/kg every 4 to 6 hours. An equivalent dose of other corticosteroid preparations can be used intravenously, intramuscularly, or orally. Glucagon may be the drug of choice for adult patients taking β-adrenergic blockade medications because of its positive inotropic and chronotropic effects on the heart that are independent of catechol receptors. The dose is an intravenous bolus of 1 to 5 mg followed by a 5 to 15 μg/min titration. Atropine may be useful in these patients if they are bradycardic; the dose is 0.3 to 0.5 mg (subcutaneously, intramuscularly, intravenously) repeated every 10 minutes to a maximum of 2 mg (112).

After the patient's condition has been stabilized, supportive therapy should be maintained with fluids, drugs, and ventilation as long as it is needed to support vital signs and functions.

TABLE 20.4. *Rules to reduce the risk of anaphylaxis*

1. Know the patient's allergy and medical history with medical record documentation.
2. Know the patient's concurrent therapy.
3. Administer drugs orally rather than parenterally if possible.
4. Observe immunotherapy patients in the physician's office 30 min after the injection.
5. Hold immunotherapy in the presence of undertreated asthma.
6. The patient should carry, at all times, a statement of allergy in the form of a bracelet, necklace, or wallet card.
7. Patients with a history of an anaphylactoid reaction, such as radiographic contrast media (see Chapter 17), should be pretreated if use of the agent is essential.
8. Patients with exercise and idiopathic anaphylaxis or those at risk of accidental exposure to known anaphylactic agents should carry an emergency treatment kit.

A careful history of previous adverse reactions to suspected antigens is mandatory. As in all allergic diseases, avoidance of a known antigen is the single most effective prophylactic measure. Avoidance of a known food should be advised, but accidental exposure may still occur from food mixtures or utensils. General measures including avoidance, repellents, and protective clothing can help avoid some stinging insect reactions. Drug avoidance is paramount based on a detailed history. Alternative drugs must be used. If the drug is absolutely essential, skin testing, test dosing, desensitization, or premedication may be attempted with great caution, depending on the drug's allergic mechanisms of action. Substances requiring pretreatment regimens include RCM, protamine sulfate, and etoposide. Skin testing before drug use may be required, such as with chymopapain, streptokinase, and local (some systemic) anesthetics. Oral food and substance challenge was discussed earlier in this chapter and in Chapter 17. Washed red blood cells, predeposited blood, and IgA-deficient blood are choices for IgA-deficient patients who have anti-IgA antibodies. Skin testing and RAST were discussed earlier in this chapter. General rules to reduce the risk for anaphylaxis are listed in Table 20.4.

EMERGENCY DRUGS AVAILABLE TO PATIENTS

Certain patients are at risk for unpredictable anaphylaxis. This includes stinging insect exposure, food allergy, latex allergy, and idiopathic anaphylaxis. These patients should carry injectable epinephrine with them at all times, an oral antihistamine, and a tourniquet (for stinging insects). Examples of commercial kits are Ana-kit (Bayer Corp.), a prefilled syringe that can deliver two doses of 0.3 mL 1:1,000 aqueous epinephrine, and an Epi-Pen regular or junior (Dey Medical Technologies), a prefilled automatic injection device with 0.3 mL or 0.15 mL of 1:1,000 aqueous epinephrine. A medic alert card or jewelry may be useful. Patient education and instruction is required. After using these devices the patient should go to the nearest medical facility and seek further definitive therapy.

REFERENCES

1. Wasserman SI. The allergist in the new millennium. *J Allergy Clin Immunol* 2000;105:3–8.
2. Portier P, Richet C. De l'action anaphylactique de certaines venins. *Compt Rend Soc Biol* 1902;54:170–172.
3. Shafrir E. Pioneers in allergy and anaphylaxis. *Isr J Med Sci* 1999;32:344.
4. Saavedra-Delgado AM. Francois Magendie on anaphylaxis (1839). *Allergy Proc* 1991;12:355–356.
5. Hericourt J, Richet C. Effects lointains des injections de serum d'anguille. *Soc Biol* 1898;50:137.
6. Magendie F. *Lectures on the blood; and on changes it undergoes during diseases.* Philadelphia: Haswell, Barington & Haswell 1893:244–249.
7. Weiszer I. Allergic emergencies. In: Patterson R, ed. *Allergic diseases: diagnosis and management.* Philadelphia: JB Lippincott, 1985:418.
8. Liberman P. Anaphylaxis. In: Middleton E Jr, Reed CE, Ellis EF, eds. *Allergy: principles and practice.* St. Louis, MO: CV Mosby, 1998:1079–1092.
9. Wiggins CA, Dykewicz MS, Patterson R. Idiopathic anaphylaxis: classification, evaluation, and treatment of 123 patients. *J Allergy Clin Immunol* 1988;82:849–855.
10. Horowitz L. Atopy as factor in penicillin reactions. *N Engl J Med* 1975;292:1243–1244.
11. Settipane GA, Klein DE, Boyd GK. Relationship of atopy and anaphylactic sensitization: a bee sting allergy model. *Clin Allergy* 1978;8:259–265.
12. Yocum MW, Butterfield JH, Klein JS, et al. Epidemiology of anaphylaxis in Olmstead County: a population-based study. *J Allergy Clin Immunol* 1999;104:452–456.
13. Klein JS, Yocum MW. Underreporting of anaphylaxis in

a community emergency room. *J Allergy Clin Immunol* 1995;95:637–638.

14. Weiler JM. Anaphylaxis in the general population: a frequent and occasionally fatal disorder that is under-recognized. *J Allergy Clin Immunol* 1999;104:271–273.

15. Yocum MW, Khan DA. Assessment of patients who have experienced anaphylaxis: a 3 year survey. *Mayo Proc* 1994;69:16–23.

16. Bacal E, Patterson R, Zeiss CR. Evaluation of severe (anaphylactic) reactions. *Clin Allergy* 1978;8:295–304.

17. Sorenson HT, Nielson B, Nielson JO. Anaphylactic shock occurring outside hospitals. *Allergy* 1989;44:288–290.

18. Idsoe O, Guthe T, Willcox RR, et al. Nature and extent of penicillin side-reactions, with particular reference to fatalities from anaphylactic shock. *Bull WHO* 1968;38:159–188.

19. van der Klauw MM, Stricker BH, et al. A population based case-cohort study of drug-induced anaphylaxis. *Br J Clin Pharmacol* 1993;35:400–408.

20. Amornman L, Berard L, Kumar N, et al. Anaphylaxis admissions to a university hospital. *J Allergy Clin Immunol* 1992;89:349.

21. Settipane GA, Newstead GJ, Boyd GK. Frequency of hymenoptera allergy in an atopic and normal population. *J Allergy Clin Immunol* 1972;50:146–150.

22. Orfan NA, Stoffoff RS, Harris KE, et al. Idiopathic anaphylaxis: total experience with 225 patients. *Allergy Proc* 1992;13:35–43.

23. Biesser H. Sandner C, Rakoski J. Anaphylactic emergencies in Munich in 1992 [Abstract]. *J Allergy Clin Immunol* 1995;95:363.

24. Sorenson HT, Nielsen B, Ostergaard NJ. Anaphylactic shock occurring outside the hospital. *Allergy* 1989;44:288–290.

25. Patterson R. Hogan MB, Yarnold PR, et al. Idiopathic anaphylaxis: an attempt to estimate the incidence in the United States. *Arch Intern Med* 1995;155:869–871.

26. Marquardt DL, Wasserman SI. Anaphylaxis. In: Middleton E Jr, Reed CE, Ellis EF, et al., eds. *Allergy: principles and practice.* St. Louis, MO: CV Mosby, 1993:1525–1526.

27. Bochner BS, Lichtenstein LM. Anaphylaxis. *N Engl J Med* 1991;324:1785–1790.

28. Boston Collaborative Drug Surveillance Program. Drug-induced anaphylaxis. *JAMA* 1973;224:613–615.

29. Parrish HM. Analysis of 460 fatalities from venomous animals in the United States. *Am J Med Sci* 1963;245:129–141.

30. Porter J, Jick H. Boston collaborative drug surveillance programs: drug induced anaphylaxis, convulsions, deafness and extrapyramidal symptoms. *Lancet* 1977;1:587.

31. Vervloet D, Arnaud A, Vellieux P, et al. Anaphylactic reactions to muscle relaxants under general anesthesia. *J Allergy Clin Immunol* 1979;63:348–353.

32. Hamann CP. Natural rubber latex protein sensitivity. *Rev Am J Contact Dermatitis* 1993;4:4–11.

33. Harnett JC, Spector SL, Farr RS. Aspirin idiosyncrasy: asthma and urticaria. In: Middleton E Jr, Reed CE, Ellis EF, eds. *Allergy: principles and practice.* St. Louis, MO: CV Mosby, 1978:1004.

34. Reisman RE. Insect allergy. In: Middleton E Jr, Reed CE, Ellis EF, eds. *Allergy: principles and practice.* St. Louis: CV Mosby, 1978:100.

35. Lieberman P, Patterson R, Metz R, et al. Allergic reactions to insulin. *JAMA* 1971;215:1106.

36. Vervloet D, Dorri F, Lemiere C, et al. Prevalence of muscle relaxant sensitization in a health care center [Abstract]. *J Allergy Clin Immunol* 1995;95:289.

37. Slater J. Latex allergies. *Ann Allergy* 1993;70:1–2.

38. Fernandez de Corres L, Moneo I, Munoz D, et al. Sensitization from chestnuts and bananas in patients with urticaria and anaphylaxis from contact with latex. *Ann Allergy* 1993;7:35–39.

39. Horan RF, Sheffer AL. Exercise-induced anaphylaxis. *Immunol Allergy Clin North Am* 1992;12:559–570.

40. Katayama H, Yamaguchi K, Kozuka T, et al. Adverse reactions to ionic and nonionic contrast media: a report from the Japanese Committee on the Safety of Contrast Media. *Radiology* 1990;175:621–628.

41. van Meter T, Adkinson NF. Immunotherapy for allergic disease. In: Middleton E Jr, Reed CE, Ellis E, et al., eds. *Allergy: principles and practice,* 3rd ed. St. Louis, MO: CV Mosby, 1988:1338.

42. Kemp SF, Lockey RF, Wolf BL, et al. Anaphylaxis: a review of 266 cases. *Arch Intern Med* 1995;155:1749–1754.

43. Sampson HA, Mandelson LM, Rosen JP. Fatal and near-fatal anaphylactic reactions to food in children and adolescents. *N Engl J Med* 1992;327:380–384.

44. Idsoe O, Gruthe T, Wilcox RR, et al. Nature and extent of penicillin side-reactions with particular references to fatality from anaphylactic shock. *Bull WHO* 1968;38:159.

45. Shehadi WH. Adverse reactions to intravascularly administered contrast media. *AJR* 1975;124:145.

46. Ansell G. Adverse reactions to contrast agents. Scope of problem. *Invest Radiol* 1970;6:374–391.

47. Witten DM. Reactions to urographic contrast media. *JAMA* 1975;231:974–977.

48. Katayama H, Yamaguchi K, Kozuka T, et al. Adverse reactions to ionic and nonionic contrast media: a report from the Japanese Committee on the safety of contrast media. *Radiology* 1990;175:621–628.

49. Parrish HM. Analysis of 460 fatalities from venomous animals in the United States. *Am J Med Sci* 1965;245:129–134.

50. Patterson R, Valentine M. Anaphylaxis and related allergic emergencies, including reactions due to insect stings. *JAMA* 1982;248:2632–2636.

51. Golden DBK, Lichtenstein LM. Insect sting allergy. In: Kaplan AP, ed. *Allergy.* New York: Churchill Livingstone 1985:507.

52. Golden DBK. Epidemiology of allergy to insect venoms and stings. *Allergy Proc* 1989;10:103–107.

53. Lockey RF, Benedict IM, Turkeltauk PC, et al. Fatalities from immunotherapy (IT) and skin testing (ST). *J Allergy Clin Immunol* 1987;79:660–677.

54. Reid MJ, Lockey RF, Turkeltaub PC, et al. Survey of fatalities from skin testing and immunotherapy 1985–1989. *J Allergy Clin Immunol* 1993;92:6–15.

55. Weiss ME, Adkinson NF. Immediate hypersensitivity reactions to penicillin and related antibiotics. *Clin Allergy* 1988;18:515–540.

56. Greenberger PA, Patterson R, Kelly J, et al. Administration of radiographic contrast media in high-risk patients. *Invest Radiol* 1980;15(suppl 6):40.

57. Hunt KJ, Valentine MD, Sobotka AK, et al. A controlled

trial of immunotherapy in insect hypersensitivity. *N Engl J Med* 1978;299:157–161.

58. Wade JP, Liang MH, Sheffer AL. Exercise-induced anaphylaxis: epidemiological observations. *Prog Clin Biol Res* 1989;297:175–182.

59. Ditto A, Harris K, Krasnick J, et al. Idiopathic anaphylaxis: a series of 335 cases. *Ann Allergy Asthma Immunol* 1996;77:285–291.

60. Wiggins CA. Characteristics and etiology of 30 patients with anaphylaxis. *Immunol Allergy Pract* 1991;13:313–316.

61. Perez C, Tejdor M, de la Hoz B, et al. Anaphylaxis: a descriptive study of 182 patients [Abstract]. *J Allergy Clin Immunol* 1995;95:368.

62. Barnard JH. Studies of 400 hymenoptera sting deaths in the United States. *J Allergy Clin Immunol* 1973;52:525–530.

63. Levine HD. Acute myocardial infarction following wasp sting: report of two cases and critical survey of the literature. *American Heart J* 1976;91:365–374.

64. Miline MD. Unusual case of coronary thrombosis. *BMJ* 1949;1:1123.

65. James LP, Austen KF. Fatal systemic anaphylaxis in man. *N Engl J Med* 1967;270:597–601.

66. Siegel SC, Heimlich EM. Anaphylaxis. *Pediatr Clin North Am* 1962;9:29–34.

67. Stark BJ, Sullivan TJ. Biphasic and protracted anaphylaxis. *J Allergy Clin Immunol* 1986;78:76–83.

68. Brady WJ, Luber S, Joyce TP. Multiphasic anaphylaxis: report of a cause of a case with prehospital and emergency department considerations. *J Emerg Med* 1997;15:477–481.

69. Brady WJ, Luber S, Carter CT, et al. Multiphasic anaphylaxis: an uncommon event in the emergency department. *Acad Emerg Med* 1997;4:193–197.

70. Douglas DM, Sukenick E, Andrade WP, et al. Biphasic systemic anaphylaxis: an inpatient and outpatient study. *J Allergy Clin Immunol* 1994;93:977–985.

71. Stark BJ, Sullivan TJ. Biphasic and protracted anaphylaxis. *J Allergy Clin Immunol* 1986;78:76–83.

72. Delange C, Irey NS. Anaphylactic deaths: a clinical pathologic study of 43 cases. *J Forensic Sci* 1972;17:525–530.

73. Hunt EL. Death from allergic shock. *N Engl J Med* 1993;228:502–504.

74. Lamson RW. So-called fatal anaphylaxis in man with a special reference to diagnosis and treatment of clinical allergies. *JAMA* 1929;93:1775–1779.

75. Sheppe WM. Fatal anaphylaxis in man. *J Lab Clin Med* 1980;16:372–375.

76. Delage C, Mullick FG, Irey NS. Myocardial lesions in anaphylaxis. *Arch Patholog Lab Med* 1973;95:185–189.

77. Delage C, Ivey WS. Anaphylactic deaths: a clinicopathic study of 43 cases. *J Forensic Sci* 1972;17:525–540.

78. Criep LH, Wochler TR. The heart in human anaphylaxis. *Ann Allergy* 1971;29:399.

79. Smith PL, Kagey-Sobotka A, Bleecker ER, et al. Physiologic manifestations of human anaphylaxis. *J Clin Invest* 1980;66:1072–1080.

80. Yunginger JW, Nelson DR, Squillace DL, et al. Laboratory investigation of deaths due to anaphylaxis. *J Forensic Sci* 1991;36:857–865.

81. Becker A, Mactavrish G, Frith E, et al. Postmortem tryptase and immunoglobulin E [Abstract]. *J Allergy Clin Immunol* 1995;95:369.

82. Booth BH, Patterson R. Electrocardiographic changes during human anaphylaxis. *JAMA* 1970;211:627–631.

83. Garmen SC, Wurzburg BA, Tarcheuskaya SS. Structure of the Fc fragment of human IgE bound to its high-affinity receptor Fce R/x. *Nature* 2000;406:259–266.

84. Daeron M. Fc receptor biology. *Annu Rev Immunol* 1997;15:203–234.

85. Turner H, Kinet JP. Signaling through the high-affinity IgE receptor FceRI. *Nature* 1999;402(suppl B):24–30.

86. Ravetch JV, Clynes RA. Divergent roles for Fc receptors and complement in vivo. *Annu Rev Immunol* 1998;16:421–432.

87. McManus LM, Hanahan DJ, Demopoulos CA, et al. Pathobiology of intravenous infusion of acetyl glyceryl ether phosphorylcholine (AGEPC), a synthetic platelet activating factor (PAF), in the rabbit. *J Immunol* 1980;124:2919–2924.

88. Choi IH, Ha T, Lee D, et al. Occurrence of disseminated intravascular coagulation in active systemic anaphylaxis: role of platelet activating factor. *Clin Exp Immunol* 1995;100:390–394.

89. Grandel KE, Farr RS, Wanderer AA, et al. The association of platelet activating factor with primary acquired cold urticaria. *N Engl J Med* 1985;313:405–409.

90. Proud D, Macglashan DW, Newball HH, et al. Immunoglobulin E–mediated release of a kininogenase from purified human lung mast cells. *Am Rev Respir Dis* 1985;132:405–408.

91. Goetzl EJ, Wasserman SI, Ansten KF. Eosinophil polymorphonuclear leukocyte function in immediate hypersensitivity. *Arch Pathol Lab Med* 1975;99:1–4.

92. Newball HH, Berninger RW, Talamo RC, et al. Anaphylactic release of a basophil kallikrein-like activity. I. Purification and characterization. *J Clin Invest* 1979;64:457–465.

93. Holgate ST, Robinson C, Church M. Mediators of immediate hypersensitivity. In: Middleton E Jr, Reed CE, Ellis E, et al., eds. *Allergy: principles and practice,* 3rd ed. St. Louis, MO: CV Mosby, 1993:267–301.

94. Yokokawa K, Mankus R, Saklayen M, et al. Increased nitric oxide production in patients with hypotension during hemodialysis. *Ann Intern Med* 1995;123:35–37.

95. Mayhan W. Nitric oxide accounts for histamine induced increases in macromolecular extravasation. *Am J Physiol* 1994;266:H2369–H2373.

96. Anggard E. Nitric oxide: mediator, murderer and medicine. *Lancet* 1994;343:1199–1206.

97. Mitsuhata H, Saiton J, Hasome N, et al. Nitric oxide synthesis inhibitor is detrimental to cardiac function and promotes bronchospasm in rabbits. *Shock* 1995;4:143–148.

98. Lieberman P. Distinguishing anaphylaxis from other serious disorders. *J Respir Dis* 1995;16:411–420.

99. Settipane GA. The restaurant syndromes. *Arch Intern Med* 1986;146:2129–2130.

100. Morrow SD, Margolies GR, Rowland BS, et al. Evidence that histamine is the causative toxin of scombroidfish poisoning. *N Engl J Med* 1991;324:716–720.

101. Hughes JM, Potter ME. Scombroid-fish poisoning from pathogenesis to prevention. *N Engl J Med* 1991;324:766–768.

102. Patterson R, Schatz M. Factitious allergic emergencies: anaphylaxis and laryngeal "edema." *J Allergy Clin Immunol* 1975;56:152–159.

103. McGrath KG, Greenberger PA, Zeiss CR. Factitious allergic disease: multiple factitious illness and familial Munchausen's stridor. *Immunol Allergy Pract* 1984;6:41–47.

104. LaRoche D, Vergnand M, Sillard B, et al. Biochemical markers of anaphylactoid reactions to drugs: comparison of plasma histamine and tryptase. *Anesthesiology* 1991;75:945–949.

105. Smith PL, Kagey-Sobotka A, Bleecker ER, et al. Physiologic manifestations of human anaphylaxis. *J Clin Invest* 1980;66:1072–1080.

106. Kaplan AP, Hunt KJ, Sobotka AK, et al. Human anaphylaxis: a study of mediator systems [Abstract]. *Clin Res* 1977;25:361.

107. van der Linden PW, Hack CE, Kerckhaert J, et al. Preliminary report: compliment activation in wasp-sting anaphylaxis. *Lancet* 1990;336:904–906.

108. Newman RB, Schultz LK. Epinephrine-resistant anaphylaxis in a patient taking propranolol hydrochloride. *Ann Allergy* 1981;47:35–37.

109. Harmany PJ, Hopper GDK. Severe anaphylaxis and drug-induced beta blockade [Letter]. *N Engl J Med* 1983;308:1536.

110. Jacobs RL, Rake GW Jr, Fournier DC, et al. Potentiated anaphylaxis in patients with drug induced beta-adrenergic blockade. *J Allergy Clin Immunol* 1981;68:125–127.

111. Toogood JH. Risk of anaphylaxis in patients receiving beta-blocker drugs. *J Allergy Clin Immunol* 1988;81:1–5.

112. Lieberman P. Anaphylaxis: guidelines for prevention and management. *J Respir Dis* 1995;16:456–462.

113. Kemp SF, Lieberman P. Inhibitors of angiotensin II: potential hazards for patients at risk for anaphylaxis? *Ann Allergy Immunol* 1997;78:527–529.

114. Bousquet J. Hejjaeni A, Dhivert H, et al. Immunotherapy with a standardized *Dermatophagoides pteronyssinus* extract IV. Systemic reactions according to the immunotherapy schedule. *J Allergy Clin Immunol* 1990;85:473–479.

115. Shortened version of a World Health Organization/International Union of Immunological Societies Working Group Report. Current status of allergen immunotherapy. *Lancet* 1989;1:259.

116. Sampson HA. Fatal food-induced anaphylaxis. *Allergy* 1998;53(suppl 46):125–130.

117. Erffmeyer JE. Reactions to antibiotics. *Immunol Allergy Clin North Am* 1992;12:633–648.

118. Suresh A, Reisman RE. Risk of administering cephalosporin antibiotics to patients with histories of penicillin allergy. *Ann Allergy Asthma Immunol* 1995;74:167–170.

119. Austen KF. The anaphylactic syndrome. In: Sampter M, Talmage DW, Frank MM, et al., eds. *Immunologic diseases.* Boston: Little, Brown, 1988:1119.

120. Parker CW. Allergic drug responses: mechanisms and unsolved problems. *CRC Crit Rev Toxicol* 1972;1:261–267.

121. Levine BB. Antigenicity and crossreactivity of penicillins and cephalosporins. *J Infect Dis* 1973;128:364–366.

122. Levine BB, Redmond AP. Minor haptenic determinant-specific reagins of penicillin hypersensitivity in man. *Int Arch Allergy Appl Immunol* 1969;35:445–455.

123. Hamilton-Miller JMT, Newton GGP, Abraham EP. Products of aminolysis and enzymatic hydrolysis of the cephalosporins. *Biochem J* 1970;116:371–384.

124. Girard JP. Common antigenic determinants of penicillin G, ampicillin and the cephalosporins demonstrated in men. *Int Arch Allergy Appl Immunol* 1968;33:428–438.

125. Lamson RW. Fatal anaphylaxis and sudden death associated with injection of foreign substances. *JAMA* 1924;82:1091.

126. Vaughn WT, Pipes DM. On the probable frequency of allergic shock. *Am J Dig Dis* 1936;3:558–563.

127. Ring J, Seifert J, Lob G, et al. Allergic reactions to horse globulin therapy and their prevention by induction of immunologic tolerance. *Allergol Immunopathol* 1974;2:93–121.

128. Bonner JR. Anaphylaxis. Part I. Etiology and pathogenesis. *Alabama J Med Sci* 1988;25:283–287.

129. Hunt KJ, Valentine MD, Sobotka AK, et al. A controlled trial of immunotherapy in insect hypersensitivity. *N Engl J Med* 1978;299:157–161.

130. Adams CT, Lofgren CS. Red imported fire ants (*Hymenoptera formicidae*): frequency of sting attacks on residents of Sumter County, Georgia. *Georgia J Med Entomol* 1981;18:378–382.

131. Stafford CT. Hypersensitivity to fire ant venom. *Ann Allergy Asthma Immunol* 1996;77:87–95.

132. Caldwell ST, Schuman SH, Simpson WM Jr. Fire ants: a continuing community threat in South Carolina. *J S C Med Assoc* 1999;95:231–235.

133. Rhoades RB, Stafford CT, James FK Jr. Survey of fatal anaphylactic reactions to imported fire ant stings: report of the Fire Ant Subcommittee of the American Academy of Allergy and Immunology. *J Allergy Clin Immunol* 1989;84:159–162.

134. Prahlow JA, Barnard JJ. Fatal anaphylaxis due to fire ant stings. *Am J Forensic Med Pathol* 1998;19:137–142.

135. Kemp SF, deShazo RD, Moffit JE, et al. Expanding habitat of the imported fire ant (*Solenopsis invecta*): a public health concern. *J Allergy Clin Immunol* 2000;105:683–691.

136. Freeman TM, Hylander R, Ortiz A, et al. Imported fire ant immunotherapy: effectiveness of whole body extracts. *J Allergy Clin Immunol* 1992;9:210–215.

137. Duplantier JE, Freeman TM, Bahna SL, et al. Successful rush immunotherapy for anaphylaxis to imported fire ants. *J Allergy Clin Immunol* 1998;101:855–856.

138. Golbert TM, Patterson R, Pruzansky JJ. Systemic allergic reactions to ingested antigens. *J Allergy* 1969;44:96–107.

139. Pumphrey RSH, Stanworth SJ. The clinical spectrum of anaphylaxis in north-west England. *Clin Exp Allergy* 1996;26:1364–1370.

140. Stewart AG, Ewan P. The incidence, etiology and management of anaphylaxis presenting to an accident and emergency department. *Q J Med* 1996;89:859–864.

141. Novembre E, Cianferoni A, Bernardini R, et al. Anaphylaxis in children: clinical and allergologic features. *Pediatrics* 1998;101:e8/1–e8/8.

142. Stricker WE, Anorve-Lopez E, Reed CE. Food skin testing in patients with idiopathic anaphylaxis. *J Allergy Clin Immunol* 1986;77:516–519.

143. Yunginger JW, Sweeney KG, Sturner WQ, et al. Fatal

food-induced anaphylaxis. *JAMA* 1988;260:1450–1452.

144. Sampson HA, Mendelson LM, Rosen JP. Fatal and near-fatal anaphylactic reactions to food in children and adolescents. *N Engl J Med* 1992;327:380–384.

145. Atkins FM, Steinberg SS, Metcalfe DD. Evaluation of immediate adverse reactions to foods in adult patient. I. Correlation of demographic, laboratory, and prick skin test data with response to controlled oral food challenges. *J Allergy Clin Immunol*, 1985;75:348–355.

146. DeMartino M, Novembre E, Gozza G, et al. Sensitivity to tomato and peanut allergens in children monosensitized to grass pollen. *Allergy* 1988;43:206–213.

147. Settipane GA, Klein DE, Boyd GK. Relationship of atopy and anaphylactic sensitization: a bee sting allergy model. *Clin Allergy* 1978;8:259–264.

148. Fine AJ. Hypersensitivity reactions to kiwi fruit (Chinese gooseberry, *Actinidiachinesis*). *J Allergy Clin Immunol* 1981;68:235–237.

149. Noyes JH, Boyd GK, Settipane GA. Anaphylaxis to sunflower seed. *J Allergy Clin Immunol* 1979;63:242–244.

150. Benner MH, Lee HJ. Anaphylactic reaction to chamomile tea. *J Allergy Clin Immunol* 1973;52:307–308.

151. Añibarro B, Dominguez C, Diaz JM, et al. Apple-dependent exercise-induced anaphylaxis. *Allergy* 1994;49:481–482.

152. Tanaka S. An epidemiological survey on food dependent exercise-induced anaphylaxis in kindergartners, school children and junior high school students. *Asian Pacific J Public Health* 1994;7:26–30.

153. Caffarelli C, Vittono T, Perrone F, et al. Food related exercise induced anaphylaxis. *Arch Dis Child* 1996;75:141–144.

154. Kidd JM, Cohen SH, Sosman AJ, et al. Food-dependent exercise-induced anaphylaxis. *J Allergy Clin Immunol* 1983;71;403–411.

155. Novey HS, Fairshter RD, Solness K, et al. Postprandial exercise-induced anaphylaxis. *J Allergy Clin Immunol* 1983;71:498–504.

156. Maulitz RM, Pratt DS, Schoiket AL. Exercise-induced anaphylactic reactions to shellfish. *J Allergy Clin Immunol* 1979;63:433–434.

157. Dahl M, Syko M, Sugiyama H, et al. Food-dependent exercise-induced anaphylaxis: a study on 11 Japanese cases. *J Allergy Clin Immunol* 1991;87:34–40.

158. McNeil D, Strauss R. Exercise-induced anaphylaxis related to food intake. *Ann Allergy* 1988;61:440–442.

159. Aoki T, Kushimoto H. Masked type I wheat allergy. *Arch Dermatol* 1985;121;355–357.

160. Armentia A, Martin-Santos JM, Blanco M, et al. Exercise- induced anaphylactic reaction to grain flours. *Ann Allergy* 1990;64:149–151.

161. Juji F, Suko M. Effectiveness of disodium cromoglycate in food-dependent, exercise-induced anaphylaxis: a case report. *Ann Allergy* 1994;72:452–454.

162. Okazaki M, Kitani H, Mifune T, et al. Food-dependent exercise-induced anaphylaxis. *Intern Med* 1992;31:1052–1055.

163. Akutsu I, Motojima S, Ikeda Y, et al. Three cases of food-dependent exercise induced anaphylaxis. *Arerugi* 1988;38:277–284.

164. Buchbinder EM, Bloch KJ, Moss J, et al. Food-dependent exercise-induced anaphylaxis. *JAMA* 1983;250:2973–2974.

165. Fukutomi O, Kondo N, Agata H, et al. Abnormal response of the autonomic nervous system in food-dependent exercise-induced anaphylaxis. *Ann Allergy* 1992;68:438–445.

166. Longley S, Panush RS. Familial exercise-induced anaphylaxis. *Ann Allergy* 1987;58:257–259.

167. Asero R, Mistrello G, Roncarolo D, et al. Exercise-induced egg anaphylaxis. *Allergy* 1997;52:687–689.

168. Debavelaere C, De Blic J, Bodermer C, et al. Syndrome d'anaphylaxie induite par l'exercise. *Arch Fr Pediatr* 1989;46:281–283.

169. Martin Munoz F, Lopez Cazana JM, Villas F, et al. Exercise-induced anaphylactic reaction to hazelnut. *Allergy* 1994;49:314–316.

170. Tilles S, Schocket A, Milgrom H. Exercise-induced anaphylaxis related to specific foods. *J Pediatr* 1995;127:587–589.

171. Wade JP, Liang MH, Sheffer AL. Exercise-induced anaphylaxis: epidemiologic observations. In: Tauber AL, Wintroub BU, Stolper-Simon AS, eds. *Progress in clinical and biological research: biochemistry of acute allergic reactions.* New York: Alan R. Liss, 1989:175–182.

172. Mansfield LE, Bowers CH. Systemic reaction to papain in a nonoccupational setting. *J Allergy Clin Immunol* 1983;71:371–374.

173. Prenner BM, Stevens JJ. Anaphylaxis after ingestion of sodium bisulfite. *Ann Allergy* 1976;37:180–182.

174. Schwartz HJ. Sensitivity to ingested metabisulfite: variations in clinical presentation. *J Allergy Clin Immunol* 1983;71:487–489.

175. Tarlo SM, Sussman GL. Asthma and anaphylactoid reactions to food additives. *Can Fam Physician* 1993;39:1119–1123.

176. Wuthrich B, Kagi MK, Stucker W. Anaphylactic reactions to ingested carmine. *Allergy* 1997;52:1133–1137.

177. DiCello MC, Myc A, Baker JR Jr, et al. Anaphylaxis after ingestion of carmine colored foods: two case reports and a review of the literature. *Allergy Asthma Proc* 1999;20:377–382.

178. Nicklas RA, Bernstein IL, Li JT, et al. The diagnosis and management of anaphylaxis. *J Allergy Clin Immunol* 1998;101(suppl):5465–5497.

179. Sussman GL, Beezhold DH. Allergy to latex rubber. *Ann Intern Med* 1995;122:43–46.

180. Hamann CP. Natural rubber latex protein sensitivity. *Rev Am J Contact Dermatitis* 1993;4:4–21.

181. Oei HD, Tjiook SB, Chang KC. Anaphylaxis due to latex allergy. *Allergy Proc* 1992;13:121–122.

182. Polen GE Jr, Slater JE. Latex allergy. *J Allergy Clin Immunol* 2000;105:1054–1062.

183. Fisher MM, Baldo BA. Anaphylactoid reactions during general anesthesia. *Clin Anesth* 1984;2:677–683.

184. Vervloet D, Nizankowska E, Arnaud A, et al. Adverse reactions to suxamethonium and other muscle relaxants under general anesthesia. *J Allergy Clin Immunol* 1983;71:551–559.

185. Monevet-Vautrin DA, Guéant JL, Kamel L, et al. Anaphylaxis to muscle relaxants: cross sensitivity studied by radioimmunoassays compared to intradermal tests in 34 cases. *J Allergy Clin Immunol* 1988;82:745–752.

186. Moscicki RA, Sockin SM, Corsello BF, et al. Anaphylaxis during induction of general anesthesia: subsequent

evaluation and management. *J Allergy Clin Immunol* 1990;86:325–332.

187. Laxenaire MC, Monevet-Vautrin DA, Vervloet D. The French experience of anaphylactoid reactions. In: Sage DJ, ed. *International anesthesiology clinics: anaphylactoid reactions in anesthesia.* Boston: Little, Brown, 1985:145–149.

188. Fisher M, Baldo BA. Anaphylaxis during anesthesia: current aspects of diagnosis and prevention. *Eur J Anaesth* 1994;11:263–284.

189. Anonymous. Cardiac arrest and anaphylaxis with anesthetic agents. *JAMA* 1985;254:2741–2742.

190. Martinez FU, Joral A, Garmendia FJ, et al. Anaphylactic reactions to syxgmethonium (succinylcholine). *Invest Allergol Clin Immunol* 1999;9:126–128.

191. Gueant JL, Aimone-Gastin I, Namone F, et al. Diagnosis and pathogenesis of the anaphylactic and anaphylactoid reactions to anesthetics. *Clin Exp Allergy* 1998;28:65–70.

192. Fisher MM. Intradermal testing in the diagnosis of acute anaphylaxis during anaesthesia. Results of five years experience. *Anaesth Intens Care* 1979;7:58–61.

193. Gueugniaud PY, Peverelli E, Vaudelin T, et al. Bradycardies relatives au cas des chocs anaphylactoides. *Presse Med* 1989;18:726.

194. Harle DG, Baldo BA, Fisher MM. Cross-reactivity of metocurine, atracurium vecuronium, and fazadinium with IgE antibodies from patients unexposed to these drugs but allergic to other myoneural blocking drugs. *Br J Anesth* 1985;57:1073–1076.

195. McKinnon RP, Wildsmith JAW. Histaminoral reactions to anaesthesia. *Br J Anesth* 1995;74:217–218.

196. Monneret G, Benoit Y, Gutowski MC, et al. Detection of basophil activation by flow cytometry in patients with allergy to muscle-relaxant drugs. *Anesthesia* 2000;92:275–277.

197. Routledge RC, DeKretser DMH, Wadsworth LD. Severe anaphylaxis due to passive sensitization by donor blood. *BMJ* 1976;1:434.

198. Wells JV, Buckley RH, Schanfield MS, et al. Anaphylactic reactions to plasma infusions in patients with hypogammaglobulinemia and anti-IgA antibodies. *Clin Immunol Immunopathol* 1977;8:265–271.

199. Vyas GN, Perkins HA, Yang YM, et al. Healthy blood donors with selective absence of immunoglobulin A: prevention of anaphylactic transfusion reactions caused by antibodies to IgA. *J Lab Clin Med* 1975;85:838–842.

200. Martinez-Sanz R, Marsal L, De La Llana R, et al. Anaphylactic reaction associated with anti-IgA antibodies. Description of one case successfully treated by means of extracorporeal circulation. *J Cardiovasc Surg* 1990;31:247–248.

201. Kumar ND, Sharma S, Sethi S, et al. Anaphylactoid transfusion reaction with anti-IgA antibodies in an IgA deficient patient: a case report. *Ind J Pathol Microbiol* 1993;36:282–284.

202. Ellis EF, Henny CS. Adverse reactions following administration of human gamma-globulin. *J Allergy* 1969;43:45–54.

203. Burman D, Hodson AK, Wood CBS, et al. Acute anaphylaxis, pulmonary edema and intravascular hemolysis due to cryoprecipitate. *Arch Dis Child* 1973;48:483–485.

204. Helmer RE, Alperin JR, Yunginger JW, et al. Anaphylactic reactions following infusion of factor VIII

in a patient with classic hemophilia. *Am J Med* 1980;69:953–957.

205. Vervloet D, Senft M, Dugne P, et al. Anaphylaxis reactions to modified fluid gelatins. *J Allergy Clin Immunol* 1983;71:535–540.

206. Ring J. Anaphylactoid reactions to intravenous solutions used for volume substitution. *Clin Rev Allergy* 1991;9:397–414.

207. Renck H, Ljungström KG, Rosberg B, et al. Prevention of dextran-induced anaphylactic reactions by hapten inhibition. *Acta Chir Scand* 1983;149:349–353.

208. McHugh GJ. Anaphylactoid reaction to penta starch. *Can J Anaesth* 1998;45:270–272.

209. Kannan S, Milligan KR. Moderately severe anaphylactoid reaction to penta starch (200/0.5) in a patient with acute severe asthma. *Intens Care Med* 1999;25:220–222.

210. Knape JTA, Schuller JC, Dehaas P, et al. An anaphylactic reaction to protamine in a patient allergic to fish. *Anesthesiology* 1981;55:324–325.

211. Greenberger PA, Patterson R, Tobin ML, et al. Lack of cross reactivity between IgE to salmon and protamine sulfate. *Am J Med Sci* 1989;296:104–108.

212. Stewart WS, McSweeney SM, Kellet MA, et al. Increased risk of severe protamine reactions in NPH insulin-dependent diabetics undergoing cardiac catheterization. *Circulation* 1984;70:788–792.

213. Goftschlich GM, Cravlee GP, Georgitis JW. Adverse reactions to protamine sulfate during cardiac surgery in diabetic and non-diabetic patients. *Ann Allergy* 1988;61:277–281.

214. Weiss ME, Nyhan D, Zhikang P, et al. Association of protamine IgE and IgG antibodies with life-threatening reactions to intravenous protamine. *N Engl J Med* 1989;320:886–892.

215. McGrath KG, Patterson R. Anaphylactic reactivity to streptokinase. *JAMA* 1984;252:1314–1317.

216. McGrath KG, Zeffren B, Alexander J, et al. Allergic reactions to streptokinase consistent with anaphylactic or antigen-antibody complex mediated damage. *J Allergy Clin Immunol* 1985;76:453–457.

217. Dykewicz MS, McGrath KG, Davison R, et al. Identification of patients at risk for anaphylaxis from streptokinase. *Arch Intern Med* 1986;146:305–307.

218. Massei D, Gill JB, Cairns JA. Anaphylactoid reaction during an infusion of recombinant tissue-type plasminogen activator for acute myocardial infarction. *Can J Cardiol* 1991;7:298–302.

219. Hill MD, Barber PA, Takahashi J, et al. Anaphylactoid reactions and angioedema during alteplase treatment of acute ischemic stroke. *Can Med Assoc J* 2000;162:1281–1284.

220. Weis BB. Hypersensitivity reactions. *Semin Oncol* 1992;19;454–477.

221. de Souza P, Frielander M, Wilde C, et al. Hypersensitivity reactions to etoposide. *Am J Clin Oncol* 1994;17:387–389.

222. Hoptelmams RMW, Schornagel JH, Wten Bokkel Huinink W, et al. Hypersensitivity reactions to etoposide. *Ann Pharmacother* 1996;30:367–371.

223. Kasperek C, Black CD. Two cases of suspected immunologic-based hypersensitivity reactions to etoposide therapy. *Ann Pharmacother* 1992;26:1227–1229.

224. Ogle KM, Kennedy BJ. Hypersensitivity reactions to etoposide. *Am J Clin Oncol* 1988;11:663–665.

225. Willis J, ed. Chymopapain approval. *FDA Drug Bull* 1982;12:17.
226. Novey HS, Marchioli LE, Sokol WN, et al. Papain-induced asthma: physiological and immunologic features. *J Allergy Clin Immunol* 1979;63:98–103.
227. Grammer LC, Schafer M, Bernstein D, et al. Prevention of chymopapain anaphylaxis by screening chemonucleolysis candidates with cutaneous chymopapain testing. *Clin Orthop Rel Res* 1988;234:12–15.
228. McCulloch JA, Canham WD, Dolovish J. Skin tests for chymopapain allergy. *Ann Allergy* 1985;55:609–611.
229. Bernstein DI, Gallagher JS, Ulmer A, et al. Prospective evaluation of chymopapain sensitivity in patients undergoing chemonucleolysis. *J Allergy Clin Immunol* 1985;76:458–465.
230. Davis H, McGoodwin E, Reed TG. Anaphylactoid reactions after treatment with ciprofloxacin. *Ann Intern Med* 1989;111:1041–1043.
231. Rassiga AL, Schwartz HJ, Forman WB, et al. Cytarabine-induced anaphylaxis. *Arch Intern Med* 1980;140:425–426.
232. Zaloga GP, Chernow B. Life-threatening anaphylactic reactions to tetanus toxoid. *Ann Allergy* 1982;49:107–108.
233. Kelso JM, Mootrey GT, Tsai TF. Anaphylaxis from yellow fever vaccine. *J Allergy Clin Immunol* 1999;103:698–701.
234. Klotz SD, Sweeny MJ, Dienst S, et al. Systemic anaphylaxis immediately after delayed hypersensitivity skin tests. *Ann Allergy* 1982;49:142–145.
235. Lazaro M, Comparied JA, De la Hoz B, et al. Anaphylactic reaction to ranitidine. *Allergy* 1993;48:385–387.
236. Sussman GL, Dorian W. Psyllium anaphylaxis. *Allergy Proc* 1990;11:241–242.
237. Brown LA, Kaplan RA, Benjamin PA, et al. Immunoglobulin E–mediated anaphylaxis with inhaled cromolyn sodium. *J Allergy Clin Immunol* 1981;68:416–420.
238. Natsch S, Matthews HV, Voogt AK, et al. Anaphylactic reactions to proton-pump inhibitors. *Ann Pharmacother* 2000;34:474–476.
239. Dolovich J, Bell B. Allergy to products of ethylene oxide gas. Demonstration of IgE and IgG antibodies and hapten specificity. *J Allergy Clin Immunol* 1978;762:30–32.
240. Grammer LC, Patterson R. IgE against ethylene oxide-altered human serum albumin (ETO- HSA) as an etiologic agent in allergic reactions of hemodialysis patients. *Artif Organs* 1987;11:97–99.
241. Schafer RM, Fink E, Schaefer L, et al. Role of bradykinin in anaphylactoid reactions during hemodialysis with AN 69 dialyzers. *Am J Nephrol* 1993;13:473–477.

242. Verresen L, Fink E, Lemke H, et al. Bradykinin is a mediator of anaphylactoid reactions during hemodialysis with AN 69 membranes. *Kidney* 1994;45:1497–1503.
243. Salem MM, Brennan JF. Anaphylactoid reactions in dialysis patients: pathogenesis and management. *Semin Dialysis* 1995;8:212–219.
244. Frankland AW, Parish WE. Anaphylactic sensitivity to human seminal fluid. *Clin Allergy* 1974;4:249–253.
245. Kooistra JB, Yunginger JW, Santrach PJ, et al. In vitro studies of human seminal plasma allergy. *J Allergy Clin Immunol* 1980;66:148–154.
246. Mittman RJ, Bernstein DI, Adler TR, et al. Selective desensitization to seminal plasma protein fractions after immunotherapy for postcoital anaphylaxis. *J Allergy Clin Immunol* 1990;86:954–960.
247. Iwahashi K, Miyasaki T, Kuji N, et al. Successful pregnancy in a woman with human seminal plasma allergy. A case report. *J Reprod Med* 1999;44:391–393.
248. Grammer LC, Metzger BE, Patterson R, et al. Cutaneous allergy to human (rDNA) insulin. *JAMA* 1984;251:1459–1460.
249. Grammer LC. Insulin allergy. *Clin Rev Allergy* 1986;4:189–200.
250. Lasser EC, Lang J, Sovak M, et al. Steroids: theoretical and experimental basis for utilization in prevention of contrast media reactions. *Radiology* 1977;125:1–9.
251. Greenberger PA. Prophylaxis against repeat radiographic media reactions in 857 cases: adverse experience with cimetidine and safety of beta adrenergic antagonists. *Arch Intern Med* 1985;145:2197–2200.
252. Sheffer AL, Soter NA, McFadden ER Jr., et al. Exercise-induced anaphylaxis: a distinct form of physical allergy. *J Allergy Clin Immunol* 1983;71:311–316.
253. Briner WW, Scheffer AL. Exercise-induced anaphylaxis. *Med Sci Sports Exerc* 1992;24:849–850.
254. Horan RF, Sheffer AL. Food-dependent exercise-induced anaphylaxis. *Immunol Allergy Clin North Am* 1991;11:757–763.
255. Maulitz RM, Pratt DS, Schocket AL. Exercise induced anaphylactic reactions to shellfish. *J Allergy Clin Immunol* 1979;63:433–434.
256. Longley S, Panush RS. Familial exercise-induced anaphylaxis. *Ann Allergy* 1987;58:257–259.
257. Ausdenmoore RW. Fatality in a teenager secondary to exercise-induced anaphylaxis. *Pediatr Asthma Allergy Immunol* 1991;5:21–23.
258. Tse KS, Yeung M, Ferrlera P. A study of exercise induced urticaria and angioedema [Abstract]. *J Allergy Clin Immunol* 1980;65:227.
259. Volcheck GW, Li JTC. Exercise-induced urticaria and anaphylaxis. *Mayo Clin Proc* 1997;72:140–147.
260. Bonner JR. Anaphylaxis. Part I. Etiology and pathogenesis. *Alabama J Med Sci* 1988;25:283–287.

21

Idiopathic Anaphylaxis

Roy Patterson and Kathleen E. Harris

Division of Allergy-Immunology, Department of Medicine, Northwestern University Medical School, Chicago, Illinois

Of the many unusual features of idiopathic anaphylaxis (IA), the following are some of the most striking. The disease was described about two decades ago (1), and in the next 15 years IA was classified (2), treatment regimens were established, and remission was induced in most cases. Fatalities have been described (3), and the number of cases of IA in the United States is estimated at 20,000 to 30,000 (4). Patients with frequent episodes have multiple emergency service visits and hospitalizations and usually are very frightened. IA is not limited to the United States (5) and is likely to be worldwide in distribution. When IA is identified and the treatment regimens are instituted, the prognosis for control and remission is far better than for prednisone-dependent asthma in adults, which generally persists for years with control but no remission. The questions about IA thus become obvious. What were the explanations for recurrent IA before the disease was described? For such a costly, frightening, potentially fatal disease, why has there been so little interest on the part of the federal government and the major national allergy societies? Fortunately, the diagnostic methodology and treatment regimens are now sufficiently successful that the alert physician who is aware of IA as the explanation for single or recurrent episodes of anaphylaxis with no apparent external cause can competently and successfully manage IA in pediatric or adult populations.

DESCRIPTIONS AND DEFINITIONS

Idiopathic anaphylaxis is an immediate-type, life-threatening event with no external allergen triggering the onset through an IgE antibody-mediated reaction. Thus, foods, drugs, and venoms are not related to the onset of episodes of IA, but must be excluded during initial evaluation. The two major types of IA are IA-angioedema (IA-A), in which airway obstruction occurs, or IA-generalized (IA-G), in which the various other systemic manifestations of anaphylaxis occur. The classification of IA relative to clinical manifestations and frequency is shown in Table 21.1.

TREATMENT REGIMENS

These regimens evolved from our experience in treating or preventing anaphylactic-type reactions such as those due to radiographic contrast media (6). As increasing numbers of patients were referred for management or opinions about management of IA, an algorithm was developed for guidance in management. This is depicted in Fig. 21.1.

Outcome of Treatment Regimens for Idiopathic Anaphylaxis

After initiation of the regimen for IA-G–frequent, consisting of prednisone, hydroxyzine,

TABLE 21.1. *Classification of idiopathic anaphylaxis*

Disease	Symptoms
Idiopathic anaphylaxis-generalized-infrequent (IA-G-I)	Urticaria or angioedema with bronchospasm, hypotension, syncope, or gastrointestinal symptoms with or without upper airway compromise with infrequent episodes (fewer than 6 episodes occurring per year)
Idiopathic anaphylaxis-generalized-frequent (IA-G-F)	Clinical manifestations as for IA-G-I but occurring more than 6 times per year
Idiopathic anaphylaxis-angioedema-infrequent (IA-A-I)	Urticaria or angioedema with upper airway compromise such as laryngeal edema, severe pharyngeal edema, or massive tongue edema without other systemic manifestations with infrequent episodes (fewer than 6 episodes occurring per year)
Idiopathic anaphylaxis-angioedema-frequent (IA-A-F)	Clinical manifestations as for IA-A-I but occurring more than 6 times per year
Idiopathic anaphylaxis-questionable (IA-Q)	This diagnosis is applied for a patient who is referred for management with a presumptive diagnosis of IA for which repeated attempts at documentation of objective findings are unsuccessful, response to appropriate doses of prednisone do not occur and the diagnosis of IA becomes uncertain
Idiopathic anaphylaxis-variant (IA-V)	This diagnosis is applied when symptoms and physical findings of IA vary from classic findings of IA; IA-V may subsequently be classified as IA-Q or IA-excluded or IA-A or IA-G
Undifferentiated somatoform IA	Symptoms mimic IA but no objective findings are seen and there is no response to the regimen for IA

and albuterol (Fig. 1), the episodes of IA should cease while the patient is receiving daily prednisone. This may require 1 to 6 weeks of daily prednisone. If longer daily prednisone is required, the diagnosis of IA becomes questionable and alternate diagnoses must be considered, including those in the differential diagnosis of IA (Table 21.2). If the patient's condition is not controlled by prednisone (adult dose of 60 mg daily) for 6 weeks, the diagnosis is likely not IA and undifferentiated somatoform IA (7) must be considered seriously.

After IA is controlled with daily prednisone, an alternate-day regimen of prednisone at a

TABLE 21.2. *Differential diagnosis of idiopathic anaphylaxis*

Hereditary angioedema
Systemic mastocytosis
Hidden allergen (e.g., latex)
Munchausen's anaphylaxis (purposeful self-exposure to antigen)
Undifferentiated somatoform idiopathic anaphylaxis

higher dose is initiated, and if the IA remains controlled, the dose of prednisone is reduced cautiously. If, after a reduction of alternate-day prednisone, an episode of IA occurs, daily prednisone must be resumed followed by alternate-day prednisone at a higher dose and slower reduction. The long-term result of this regimen will be an induction of remission, and in most patients the use of prednisone can then be terminated (Fig. 21.2). If a dose of alternate-day prednisone is reached below which episodes of IA recur, this is corticosteroid-dependent IA (CSD-IA). Patients with CSD-IA may respond to montelukast (Singulaire, Merck, Westpoint, PA), oral cromolyn (Gastrocom, Medera, Rochester, NY), or ketotifin (Zaditen, Novartis, Hanover, NJ) (in countries in which this drug is available), which can allow reduction and eventual discontinuation of prednisone use, and possibly induce a remission. Alternatively, these medications may not alter the prednisone requirement, in which case they should be tapered and

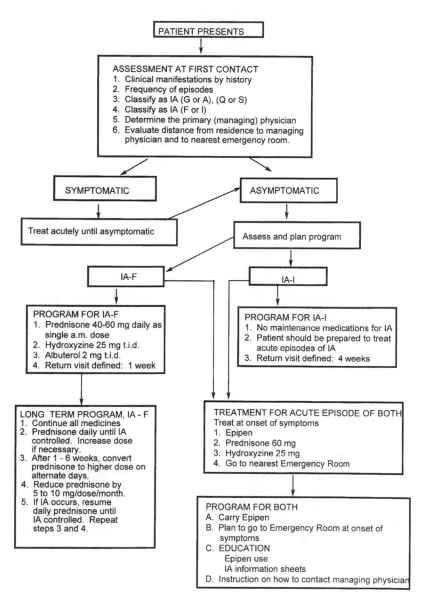

FIG. 21.1. The algorithm for initial assessment and management of idiopathic anaphylaxis (*IA*) of frequent (*F*) or infrequent (*I*) types at the first visit of the patient. *G,* generalized; *A,* angioedema; *Q,* questionable; *S,* somatoform; *a.m.,* morning; *t.i.d.,* three times per day.

discontinued, and the diagnosis would remain CSD-IA.

IDIOPATHIC ANAPHYLAXIS–SINGLE EPISODE OR IDIOPATHIC ANAPHYLAXIS–INFREQUENT

The patient with a single episode of IA should carry emergency therapy in the event of recur-rence (Fig. 21.1). When a single episode has been recent and sufficiently severe to suggest the like-lihood of a fatality, the treatment course for IA–frequent (IA-F) (Fig. 21.1) can be considered. Patients with IA–infrequent (IA-I) are managed with the availability of emergency therapy. How-ever, these patients also may be considered for a course of prednisone, as indicated for IA-F, to at-tempt to induce a remission of the IA syndrome.

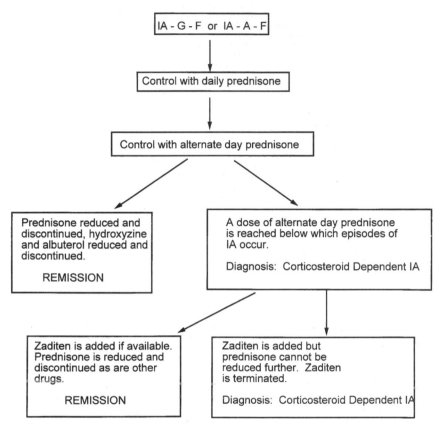

FIG. 21.2. The outcome and continued management of patients with idiopathic anaphylaxis (*IA*) at subsequent visits. For long-term management, patients should be seen initially at least every 4 weeks for reduction of prednisone dose. Clinical judgment is necessary to avoid excess prednisone or too rapid a reduction of prednisone dose. *G*, generalized; *A*, angioedema; *F*, frequent; *I*, infrequent.

PATIENT EDUCATION

A major goal in management of IA has to be the education of the patient, family, and sometimes the referring physician. It is important that they understand several aspects of the disease. First, there is not an external agent; therefore, attention must be given to pharmacologic induction of a remission. Second, patients should understand the risks and benefits of prednisone so that they will be able to make informed choices about their management. Finally, it is important to explain to patients that we are performing research to determine why mast cells and basophils are releasing mediators and cytokines. Among the hypotheses are that there are autoimmune (anti–immunoglobulin E) factors or the inappropriate release of chemokines such as histamine-releasing factors, which are modified by prednisone therapy (8).

UNDIFFERENTIATED SOMATOFORM IDIOPATHIC ANAPHYLAXIS

This is the term applied when patients describe symptoms consistent with IA but they have no organic disease. It would seem that

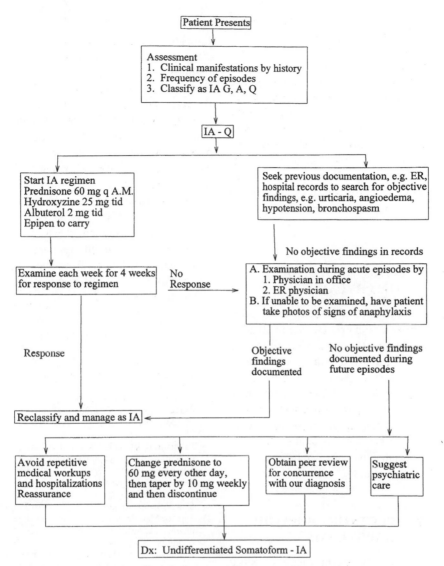

FIG. 21.3. An algorithm for diagnosis of undifferentiated somatoform idiopathic anaphylaxis. *A.M.,* morning; *G,* generalized; *A,* angioedema; *Q,* questionable; *ER,* emergency room; *Dx,* diagnosis. (Reprinted from Choy AC, Patterson R, Patterson DR, et al. Undifferentiated somatoform idiopathic anaphylaxis: nonorganic symptoms mimicking idiopathic anaphylaxis. *J Allergy Clin Immunol* 1995;96:893; with permission.)

the differentiation of organic from hysterical IA would be relatively simple, but this has not been the case. In reports of nine cases (7,9), the following general characteristics have been observed. The referring physician generally has not recognized the nonorganic nature of the problem. The medical costs of hospitalizations, emergency service visits, and laboratory tests can be extremely high, and these patients may be treated excessively with unnecessary corticosteroids. An algorithm for the diagnosis of undifferentiated somatoform IA is shown in Fig. 21.3. When the managing physician arrives at this conclusion, further management may become difficult. Approaching the basis of the problem as psychological in origin with referral to a psychiatrist is the logical approach. Among the psychological diagnoses the patient may have are globus hystericus, panic disorder, or conversion reactions. This may be accepted by the patient. Alternatively, the patient may reject the concept of a psychological disorder as the explanation, often with hostility. Some of these cases can be managed by the allergist and generalist with safe, low doses of antihistamines and supportive ambulatory visits at increasing intervals. Other patients may continue appearing at hospital emergency services and be admitted. They continue playing their role of a patient in anaphylaxis with unimaginable skill.

PEDIATRIC IDIOPATHIC ANAPHYLAXIS

In our service, the ratio of pediatric IA to adult IA cases is about 1 pediatric IA case to 20 adult cases. For this reason, the diagnosis of IA in children may be more delayed than would the diagnosis in adults. Fortunately, in our series, the response to the regimen for IA (with adjustment of doses for the pediatric population) appears equally successful and the prognosis equally favorable as in the majority of adults (10). In a series of 22 pediatric patients, we have reported successful outcomes (11).

OTHER ASPECTS OF IDIOPATHIC ANAPHYLAXIS

We have reported long-term follow-up studies and a cost analysis for IA patients. Using our management programs, we estimated that $11 million per year can be saved in the United States (12). We have reviewed the problems with managing patients from distant cities. The primary issues of concern were severity, guidance for treatment, and advice to local physicians (13). Two contrasting patients with anaphylaxis, one with IA and one with undifferentiated somatoform IA, were compared (14). Finally, a comprehensive review of all types of anaphylaxis was reported comparing and contrasting various types of anaphylaxis (15).

SUMMARY

Idiopathic anaphylaxis was identified over 20 years ago. It was classified, and treatment regimens were adopted, tested, and proven effective. The prognosis for the individual patient is good, and reassurance of a newly diagnosed patient is justified when the regimen described here is used. This is of particular value when patients and their families are extremely frightened (16). The number of patients with IA evaluated at the Northwestern Allergy-Immunology Service approximates 400, with the last publication describing 335 of those patients (17). One fatality has been documented (18). Unfortunately, the prognosis for undifferentiated somatoform IA is not as good, but a diagnosis is important to attempt to prevent unnecessary medication and hospitalizations.

REFERENCES

1. Bacal E, Patterson R, Zeiss CR. Evaluation of severe (anaphylactic) reactions. *Clin Allergy* 1978;8:295–304.
2. Wiggins CA, Dykewicz MS, Patterson R. Idiopathic anaphylaxis: classification, evaluation, and treatment of 123 patients. *J Allergy Clin Immunol* 1988;82:849–855.
3. Patterson R, Booth BH, Clayton DE, et al. Fatal and near fatal idiopathic anaphylaxis. *Allergy Proc* 1995;16:103–108.
4. Patterson R, Hogan MB, Yarnold P, et al. Idiopathic anaphylaxis: an attempt to estimate the incidence in the United States. *Arch Intern Med* 1995;155:869–871.
5. Tejedor MA, Perez C, de la Hoz B, et al. Idiopathic anaphylaxis. Clinical differences [Abstract]. *J Allergy Clin Immunol* 1992;89:349.
6. Greenberger PA, Patterson R. The prevention of immediate generalized reactions to radiocontrast media in high-risk patients. *J Allergy Clin Immunol* 1991;87:867–872.
7. Choy AC, Patterson R, Patterson DR, et al. Undifferentiated somatoform idiopathic anaphylaxis: non-organic symptoms mimicking idiopathic anaphylaxis. *J Allergy Clin Immunol* 1995;96:893–900.
8. Patterson R, Harris KE. Idiopathic anaphylaxis: management and theories of pathogenesis. *Clin Immunother* 1995;4:265–269.
9. Patterson R, Greenberger PA, Orfan NA, et al. Idiopathic anaphylaxis: diagnostic variants and the problem of nonorganic disease. *Allergy Proc* 1992;13:133–137.
10. Patterson R, Ditto A, Dykewicz MS, et al. Pediatric idiopathic anaphylaxis: additional cases and extended observations. *Pediatr Asthma Allergy Immunol* 1995;9:43–47.

11. Ditto AM, Krasnick J, Greenberger PA, et al. Pediatric idiopathic anaphylaxis: experience with 22 patients. *J Allergy Clin Immunol* 1997;100:320–326.

12. Krasnick J, Patterson R, Harris KE. Idiopathic anaphylaxis: long-term follow-up, cost, and outlook. *Allergy* 1996;51:724–731.

13. Patterson R, Harris KE. Distant referrals for idiopathic anaphylaxis. *Medscape Pulmonary Medicine* 1997;1: http://www.medscape.com/Medscape/Respiratory care/journal/1997/v01.n09/mrc3047.patterson/mrc3047.patterson.html

14. Sikora RA, Ricaurte K, Ditto AM, Patterson R. Two contrasting cases of anaphylaxis seen simultaneously. *Ann Allergy Asthma Immunol* 2000;84:15–18.

15. Millar MM, Patterson R. Anaphylaxis. In: Altman LC, Becker JW, Williams PV, eds. *Allergy in primary care.* Philadelphia:WB Saunders, 2000:265–279.

16. Patterson R, ed. *Idiopathic anaphylaxis.* Providence, RI: Oceanside Publications, 1997.

17. Ditto AM, Patterson R, Harris KE, et al. Idiopathic anaphylaxis: a series of 335 cases. *Ann Allergy Asthma Immunol* 1996;77:285–291.

18. Krasnick J, Patterson R, Meyers GL. A fatality from idiopathic anaphylaxis. Ann Allergy Asthma Immunol 1996;76:376–378.

22

Asthma

Paul A. Greenberger

*Division of Allergy-Immunology, Department of Medicine, Northwestern University
Medical School, Chicago, Illinois*

OVERVIEW

Asthma is a disease characterized by hyper-responsiveness of bronchi to various stimuli as well as changes in airway resistance, lung volumes, and inspiratory and expiratory flow rates, with symptoms of cough, wheezing, dyspnea, or shortness of breath. In 1991, a National Institutes of Health Expert Panel suggested that asthma was a disease characterized by (a) airway obstruction that is reversible—partially or completely, (b) airway inflammation, and (c) airway hyperresponsiveness (1). In 1997, another panel described asthma as follows:

> A chronic inflammatory disorder of the airways in which many cells and cellular elements play a role, in particular, mast cells, eosinophils, T lymphocytes, macrophages, neutrophils, and epithelial cells. In susceptible individuals, this inflammation causes recurrent episodes of wheezing, breathlessness, chest tightness, and coughing, particularly at night or in the early morning (2).

Asthma has been defined by other designations, including allergic bronchitis, asthmatic bronchitis, allergic asthma, atopic asthma, non-allergic asthma, cough equivalent asthma (3), and cardiac asthma (4–6). A central feature of asthma from a physiologic viewpoint is bronchial hyperresponsiveness to stimuli such as histamine or methacholine, as compared with patients without asthma. In population screening, such nonspecific hyperresponsiveness has been reported as sensitive but not specific (6). Surprisingly, in a study of children 7 to 10 years of age, 48% of those with a diagnosis of asthma did not have bronchial hyperresponsiveness (7). Asthma is characterized by wide variations of resistance to airflow on expiration (and inspiration) with remarkable transient increases in certain lung volumes, such as residual volume, functional residual capacity, and total lung capacity.

Asthma is considered a reversible obstructive airways disease as compared with chronic obstructive pulmonary disease (COPD). Many patients with asthma experience symptom-free periods of days, weeks, months, or years in between episodes, whereas chronic symptoms and fixed dyspnea characterize COPD. When daily symptoms of cough, wheezing, and dyspnea have been present for months in a patient with asthma, bronchodilator nonresponsiveness may be present. However, appropriate antiinflammatory therapy reduces symptoms and improves the quality of life significantly along with improvement in pulmonary function status.

Immunoglobulin E (IgE)-mediated bronchospasm can be demonstrated in many patients with asthma, but not all cases of asthma are "allergic"; it is thought that about 75% of patients have allergic asthma. Some evidence does exist for IgE antibodies to respiratory syncytial virus (RSV) (8) and parainfluenza virus (9); however, as our understanding of nonallergic asthma increases, perhaps our description of viral infection triggered asthma will change. Nevertheless, serologic tests and nasopharyngeal or sputum cultures were positive for viruses in 23 of 29

(80%) adult patients who reported a recent respiratory tract infection and were hospitalized for asthma (10). Influenza A and rhinovirus (9) were found most often. Overall, 37% of adults admitted for asthma had reported a recent respiratory tract infection (10). In children, viral infections (RSV in infants younger than 2 years of age and rhinovirus in children 2 to 16 years of age) were associated with acute wheezing episodes resulting in emergency department treatment or hospitalization (11). The sudden onset of wheezing dyspnea that occurs after ingestion of aspirin or other nonsteroidal antiinflammatory drugs (NSAIDs) (12,13) is not an IgE-mediated reaction but represents alterations of arachidonic acid metabolism, such as blockage of the cyclooxygenase pathway with shunting of arachidonic acid into the lipoxygenase pathway. Potent lipoxygenase pathway products, such as leukotriene D4 (LTD4), cause acute bronchospasm in aspirin- and NSAID-sensitive patients (14,15). Most patients with asthma may have symptoms precipitated by nonspecific, non–IgE-mediated triggers, such as cold air, air pollutants, exercise, crying or laughing, and changes in barometric pressure. Fortunately, pharmacologic therapy can minimize the effects of these nonspecific triggers.

GENETIC AND ENVIRONMENTAL FACTORS

Genetic and environmental factors are important in terms of development of asthma (16). The approximate risk for an allergic-type disease in a child is 20%, but if one parent is allergic, this risk increases to 50% (17–19). If both parents are allergic, there is a 66% chance of the child developing an allergic condition (17–19). In a prospective study of children evaluated during the first 6 years of life, the risk for a boy developing asthma was 14.3%, compared with 6.3% for girls (20). These data support the notion of polygenic inheritance with greater prevalence in boys. In twin studies, the concordance for asthma in monozygotic twins reared together was similar to that for twins reared apart (21). In addition, in a study of 5,864 twins who were evaluated from infancy to age 25 years, the cumulative incidence

of asthma was 6% in males and 5.4% in females. If one twin developed asthma, the relative risk of the co-twin developing asthma was 17.9 for identical twins, compared with 2.3 for fraternal twins (22). More than 80% of cases of asthma began by 15 years of age, when nearly all of the study subjects lived in the same home environment (22). These data support a strong genetic effect on development of asthma. Methacholine responsiveness, total serum IgE concentration, and immediate skin test reactivity have been found to be more concordant in monozygotic twins than in dizygotic twins (23), which supports a genetic influence over an environmental influence. Both factors should be considered as contributory, and production of specific antiallergen IgE appears to be affected by environmental and local allergic exposures in the genetically susceptible subject. The onset of early childhood asthma has and has not been associated with parental smoking (20,24). However, once asthma begins, evidence exists for increased childhood respiratory symptoms from passive smoking (25–27) or actively by the adolescent who smokes (26).

Environmental factors have been associated with development of IgE antibodies. Frick and co-workers (28) demonstrated development of antiallergen IgE in association with increasing antiviral antibodies in a prospective study of high-risk infants whose parents both had allergic diseases. Croup in early childhood has been associated with subsequent development of asthma (29), as have RSV and parainfluenza virus infections (27). Seemingly in contrast, a history of pneumonia in the first 7 years of life was associated with reduced forced expiratory volume in 1 second (FEV_1) and forced vital capacity (FVC) by 35 years of age, but this effect (102 mL and 173 mL, respectively, compared with controls) was independent of any history of wheezing (30).

Indoor allergen exposures from house dust mites (31), cats (32), and cockroaches (33) have been associated with the development of asthma, emphasizing that both viral infections (27) and allergens are involved in emergence of childhood asthma. New-onset asthma in older men (aged 61 years or older) was associated with detectable serum IgE antibodies to cat allergen but not dust mites, ragweed, or mouse urinary antigen (34). In this study, IgE antibodies to dog dander and cockroach excreta were not measured.

Environmental factors other than infections, allergens, and occupational exposures favor development of asthma by altering the predominant cytokines generated by $CD4^+$ lymphocytes. A process that favors asthma includes generation of the helper T-cell subset T_H2, which is central to IgE production, as opposed to T_H1, which would diminish an "atopic" pattern and contribute to a classic delayed-type hypersensitivity response (type IVa_1). In a study of 867 children in Japan who had received bacille Calmette Guérin (BCG) immunization after birth and at 6 and 12 years of age, the presence of and induration of tuberculosis skin tests were studied in relation to the emergence of atopy (asthma, rhinitis, and atopic dermatitis) (35). By age 12 years, 58% of the children had developed positive (≥ 10 mm in duration) responses to tuberculin testing, and 36% of children had reported atopic symptoms (35). Asthma symptoms and atopy were associated negatively with positive tuberculin responses, and presence of tuberculin reactivity was associated with remission from asthma by years 6 or 12 (35). The data raise the possibility that the T_H1 response produced by BCG immunization resulted in increases in the T_H1 cytokines, interferon-γ (IFN-γ), and interleukin-12 (IL-12) and decreases in incidence of asthma, possibly even inducing remissions of atopy. In addition, there were reduced quantities of the T_H2 cytokines IL-4, IL-13, and IL-10, compared with the BCG nonresponders, who had more atopy and asthma. Alternatively, these data might be interpreted that children likely to become atopic have a reduced ability to develop T_H1 memory lymphocytes after BCG immunization (36) or, by analogy, reduced response to measles vaccination (37). The latter stems from data revealing less atopy when there was a previous episode of measles (37). These studies and the association between RSV infections (which cause a T_H2 profile) and childhood asthma suggest that the critical link may be the predominance of the T_H1 cytokines, which would be protective. The notion that asthma is "an epidemic in the absence of infection" has been suggested (38) and might be supported by the finding that house dust containing endotoxin (which activates macrophages) was associated with wheezing in infants (39).

COMPLEXITY OF ASTHMA

The cause of asthma remains unknown, although asthma is considered a very complex inflammatory disease (40,41). Some important pathologic findings include a patchy loss of bronchial epithelium, usually associated with eosinophil infiltration (42,43), contraction and hypertrophy of bronchial smooth muscles, bronchial mucosa edema and increased blood flow (44), bronchial gland hyperplasia and hypersecretion of thick bronchial mucus, and basement membrane thickening (41,45). Collagen synthesis may result from stimulation or injury to airway epithelial cells (46). The key cell is the myofibroblast, which is a hybrid cell of fibroblast and smooth muscle cell origins. These cells produce type III and I collagen (46). Epithelial cells obtained during bronchoalveolar lavage (BAL) from patients with asthma have been found to be much less viable than in subjects without asthma (47). However, the epithelial cells from patients with asthma produced much more (a) fibronectin, a glycoprotein involved with cell attachment, cell growth, and chemotaxis; and (b) 15- hydroxyeicosatetraenoic acid (15-HETE) a metabolite of arachidonic acid (47). The increased metabolic activity of epithelial cells appears to contribute to airway damage and remodeling. There is subepithelial "fibrosis" that is composed of collagen types I, II, and V, which contributes to the basement membrane thickening of asthma.

When bronchial biopsy samples were obtained from 14 patients who had asthma for 1 year or less, increases in numbers of mast cells, eosinophils, lymphocytes, and macrophages were found in the epithelium (48). Deeper in the lamina propria, eosinophils, lymphocytes, macrophages, and plasma cells were present, suggesting that patients with mild asthma who had not received antiinflammatory therapy had marked cellular infiltration in the bronchial mucosa (48).

Human bronchial epithelium from patients with asthma express Fas ligand (Fas L) and Fas on eosinophils and T lymphocytes (49). Activation of Fas by Fas L induces apoptosis. Biopsy samples from patients who had not received inhaled corticosteroids had reduced numbers of apoptotic eosinophils and reduced expression Fas L and *Bcl-2,* which help regulate apoptosis. Conversely, inhaled corticosteroid–treated patients had fewer eosinophils and increased numbers of apoptotic eosinophils (49). In a study of BAL of 12 newly diagnosed and untreated patients with asthma, reduced expression of Fas in messenger RNA (mRNA) and the Fas receptor (CD95) on CD3$^+$ T lymphocytes was found (50). These findings are consistent with a persisting inflammatory cell infiltrate that characterizes asthma.

Some physiologic characteristics of asthma include bronchial hyperresponsiveness to stimuli such as histamine (51), methacholine (52), or LTD4 (53) and at least a 12% improvement in FEV$_1$ after inhalation of a β_2-adrenergic agonist, unless the patient is experiencing status asthmaticus or has had severe, ineffectively treated airway obstruction. There are large changes in lung compliance, depending on severity of the disease.

On a cellular level, during acute episodes of asthma, activated or hypodense eosinophils are present in increased numbers (43,54), and eosinophil products such as major basic protein (MBP) can be identified in sputum (55) and in areas where bronchial epithelium has been denuded (56). Eosinophil cationic protein has been identified in areas of denuded bronchial epithelium. This cationic protein has been reported to be even more cytotoxic than MBP (57). Mast cells in the bronchial lumen and submucosa are activated, and their many cell products are released, whether preformed or synthesized *de novo.* Macrophages, lymphocytes, and epithelial cells participate as well, as mentioned earlier.

Evidence supports the concept of neuroimmunologic abnormalities in asthma, such as the lack of the bronchodilating nonadrenergic noncholinergic vasoactive intestinal peptide in lung sections from patients with asthma (58). Substance P concentrations in induced sputum have been reported to be markedly elevated, compared with that in controls (59). The free radical nitric oxide is known to be detectable in expired air in patients with asthma, and its concentration increases further after allergen challenge (60). A free radical generated from arachidonic acid, 8-isoprostane, is increased in asthma and reflects ongoing oxidative stress (61). There are progressively greater amounts in expired air as asthma severity increases from mild to severe (61). These findings demonstrate the complexity of asthma, which decades ago was considered a psychological condition. Asthma is not a psychological disorder. Nevertheless, the burden of asthma as a chronic disease, especially when the patient has experienced repeated hospitalizations or emergency department visits, may result in psychological disturbances that coexist with asthma (62–65).

INCIDENCE AND SIGNIFICANCE

Asthma affects more than 18 million people in the United States (66). Acute asthma is the most common childhood medical emergency (67), with a distinct subset of patients (16%) accounting for 36% of emergency department visits (68). Often, adults and children requiring acute treatment of asthma have not received or are not using optimal antiinflammatory therapy. The prevalence of asthma and asthma mortality rates are greater in urban than in rural areas, in boys than in girls, and in blacks than in whites or Hispanic children (66). The prevalence of asthma in children up to 17 years of age has been increasing by about 5% annually from 1980 to 1995 (66). The prevalence of childhood asthma has been estimated to be 5% or 6% (22,66) to as high as 22% (26). Such information was generated from questionnaire surveys in the United States and United Kingdom. Asthma prevalence has increased in many countries; Australia and New Zealand also have a high prevalence of asthma (69). Methodology is important; for example, in a study of children 8 to 11 years of age in Australia, the prevalence of current asthma in 1991 was 9.9%, but 30.8% of children had asthma diagnosed by a physician, and 40.7% had wheezing reported by a parent (69). Current bronchial hyperresponsiveness was found in 16% of such children (69). The prevalence of asthma in Oregon was lower and more in line with total U.S. data, with a childhood (school-aged) prevalence of 6% and an adult prevalence of 7% (70). Self-reported asthma prevalence, however, in adults was 11% (70).

The onset of asthma occurs in the first two decades of life, especially the first few years of age (71), or in patients older than 40 years of age. However, intermittent respiratory symptoms may exist for years before the actual diagnosis of asthma is made in patients older than 40 years of age (71). The diagnosis of asthma may be more likely made in women and nonsmokers, whereas men may be labeled as having chronic bronchitis, when in fact they do not have chronic sputum production for 3 months each year for 2 consecutive years. Asthma may have its onset in the geriatric population (72) and usually begins during or after an upper respiratory tract infection. The prevalence of asthma was found to be 6.5% in patients at least 70 years of age living in South Wales (73).

Asthma morbidity can be enormous from a personal and family perspective as well as from the societal aspect. It has been estimated that in the United States there were more than 100 million days with restricted activity by patients with asthma (69). The number of hospitalizations in the United States for asthma increased almost fourfold from 1965 to 1983, with absolute numbers growing from 127,000 to 459,000 per year (74). This number had stabilized at about 470,000 as of 1996 (69). The number of days of school missed from asthma is excessive, as is work absenteeism. In adults, about 15% to 33% of patients receiving emergency department treatment are hospitalized for status asthmaticus (75). In a study of 3,223 patients aged 28 years and older receiving emergency department treatment, 60% of Hispanic patients with asthma were hospitalized, compared with 30% of white and 35% African American patients (75).

Asthma was thought to be related to occupation in 2% of the 6 million people with asthma in the United States in 1960. As of 2000, it was estimated that 5% to 15% of newly diagnosed asthma in working adults is caused by an occupational exposure (76,77). In a survey of 2,646 workers in Spain aged 20 to 44 years, it was estimated that the prevalence of asthma was 5% to 6.7% (78). The public health and economic issues are complex in that some 250 different chemicals have been recognized as causes of asthma (76,77).

The asthma death rate remains about 5,000 annually in the United States (79). The number and percentage of fatalities from asthma has increased in the United States from 0.8 deaths per 100,000 general population in 1977 to 2.0 in 1989 and still 2.0 in 1997 (79). The death rate has increased in other countries, including the United Kingdom (80), New Zealand (81), Denmark (82), France (83), Germany (83), and to a lesser extent, Canada (84,85). The extraordinarily high death rate in New Zealand (7 per 100,000 population) that occurred in the 1980s has been reduced to 4 per 100,000, similar to that in Australia (84). The asthma death rates in the United States and Canada are about 2 per 100,000 population even though the health care systems differ (79,86). The exact number of people who die from asthma is not known, but increases in death rates in patients aged 5 to 34 years had been noted in the 1980s (87). This age range was used to minimize the number of confounding diagnoses, such as COPD or chronic bronchitis. Four locations—New York City, Chicago, Phoenix, and Fresno, California—experienced very high mortality rates, in part associated with lower socioeconomic conditions (87). Surprisingly, 21.1% of all asthma deaths occurred in New York City and Chicago, despite having 6.8% of all 5- to 34-year-olds in the United States (87). The fatality rate among nonwhites remains higher than among whites, with death rates of 3.5 per 100,00 population in blacks, compared with 1.0 per 100,000 in whites as of 1997 (79). A disturbing finding that blacks received or filled fewer prescriptions for inhaled corticosteroids and oral steroids was reported in the Detroit area (88) in a managed care setting in which physician prescribing and advice (referral to an asthma specialist) appeared to be different depending on the ethnicity of the patient. All the patients in this study were enrolled in the same large health maintenance organization; thus, lack of insurance or access to medications were not issues seemingly.

The costs of asthma include direct costs of medications, hospitalizations, and physician charges in addition to indirect costs for time lost from work and loss of worker productivity. The totals in 1987 and 1990 in the United States were estimated at $5.8 to $6.2 billion (87,89). Some 20% of the patients used 80% of the resources ($2,584, compared with $140 per patient) (89). Some patients have been labeled as the "$100,000 asthmatic patients" because of repeated hospitalization and emergency department visits (90). Emotional costs of asthma are great for the sufferer and the family if asthma is managed ineffectively or if the patient refuses to adhere to appropriate medical advice. The death of a family member from asthma is shocking; the person may be young, and the fatal attack may not have been anticipated by others or even the patient. It must be kept in mind that with current understanding and treatment of asthma, all fatalities should be avoidable and asthma need not be a fatal disease. More than half of deaths from asthma occur outside of a hospital (74). This finding has led some physicians to conclude that emergency medical services should be improved. One cannot dispute such an argument, but it is advisable for the physician managing the patient with asthma to have an emergency plan available for the patient or family so that asthma is not managed from a crisis orientation but rather on a preventive basis. Further, an education program or patient instructions can identify what patients should do when their medications are not effective, such as with a flare of asthma.

The number of prescriptions for asthma or COPD medications was estimated in 1985 to be 3% to 4%, or 51 million, of 1.5 billion prescriptions written in the United States for all medications (91). From 1972 to 1985, the number of asthma and COPD prescriptions increased from 17 to 51 million (91). Substantial increases in cromolyn by metered-dose inhaler had occurred as well as increases in inhaled corticosteroids. The sales of inhaled corticosteroids increased 12-fold from 1976 to 1991, whereas sales of β-adrenergic agonist inhalers increased threefold (91). Using data from a 1987 study in the United States, 55.8% of children (aged 1 to 17 years) with asthma reported not using asthma medications,

whereas chronic users, defined as those obtaining three or more prescriptions for asthma, characterized 10.7% of children with asthma (92). At that time, there was little combined use of inhaled corticosteroids and β-adrenergic agonists. Overall health care expenditures in children with asthma were 2.8 times higher than in children without asthma (92). In a study of more than 25,000 patients with asthma in four health maintenance organizations, there was an inverse relationship between pharmaceutical costs and acute care charges, as one might expect (93). In summary, the incidence of asthma continues to increase. The hospitalization rates and fatality rates have increased, as have medication prescriptions.

ANATOMY AND PHYSIOLOGY

The central function of the lungs is gas exchange with delivery into the blood stream of oxygen and removal of carbon dioxide. The lung is an immunologic organ and has endocrine and drug-metabolizing properties that affect respiration. The lung consists of an alveolar network with capillaries passing near and through alveolar walls and progressively larger intrapulmonary airways, including membranous bronchioles (1 mm or smaller noncartilaginous airways) and larger cartilaginous bronchi and upper airways. Inspired air must reach the gas exchange network of alveoli. The first 16 airway divisions of the lung are considered the conducting zone, whereas subsequent divisions from 17 to 23 are considered transitional and respiratory zones. The conducting zone consists of trachea, bronchi, bronchioles, and terminal bronchioles and produces what is measured as airway resistance. The terminal bronchioles as a rule have diameters as small as 0.5 mm. Respiratory bronchioles, alveolar ducts, and sacs compose the transitional and respiratory zones (94) and are the sites of gas exchange.

The structures of bronchi and trachea are similar, with cartilaginous rings surrounding the bronchi completely until the bronchi enter the lungs, at which point there are cartilage plates that surround the bronchi. When bronchioles are about 1 mm in diameter, the cartilage plates are not present. Smooth muscle surrounds bronchi

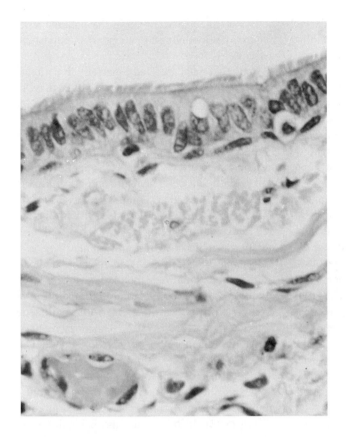

FIG. 22.1. Microphotograph of the wall of a normal bronchus. Note the uniform ciliated epithelium and their bands of smooth muscle. (H& E stain, magnification × 250.)

and is present until the end of the respiratory bronchioles.

The lining mucous membrane of the trachea and bronchi is composed of pseudostratified ciliated columnar epithelium (Fig. 22.1). Goblet cells are mucin-secreting epithelial cells and are present in airways until their disappearance at the level of terminal bronchioles. In the terminal bronchioles, the epithelium becomes that of cuboidal cells with some cilia, clara (secretory) cells, and goblet cells until the level of respiratory bronchioles, where the epithelium becomes alveolar in type. The cilia move in a watery lining layer proximally to help remove luminal material (debris, cells, mucus) by the ciliary "mucus escalator." Above the watery lining layer is a mucus layer. Other cells have been identified, including histamine-containing bronchial lumen cells (95), alveolar macrophages, polymorphonuclear leukocyte lymphocytes, eosinophils, and airway smooth muscle cells, which contribute to lung pathology in different ways. The bronchial wall is characterized by mucosa, lamina propria, smooth muscle, submucosa, submucosal glands, and then cartilaginous plates. Submucosal glands produce either mucous or serous material depending on their functional type. Mast cells can be identified in the bronchial lumen or between the basement membrane and epithelium. Mast cells have been recovered from BAL samples but are low in number in these samples (96). Mast cell heterogeneity has been recognized based on contents and functional properties (97). Briefly, mucosal mast cells are not recognized in a formalin-fixed specimen, but connective tissue mast cells are. Mucosal mast cells are present in the lung and contain tryptase, whereas connective tissue mast cells contain tryptase and chymotryptase. Mast cells may participate in airway remodeling because they activate fibroblasts (98), and mast cell–derived tryptase is a mitogen for epithelial cells and stimulates synthesis of collagen (98). In addition to mast cell generation of histamine, prostaglandin D_2 (PGD_2), LTD4, and tryptase, they secrete IL-4, which upregulates vascular cell adhesion molecule (VCAM) on vessel endothelial surfaces. Eosinophil entry into tissues is facilitated by VCAM. IL-4 also favors isotype switching within the nucleus to cause production of IgE antibodies. The mast cell has multiple effects, from mediator release and cytokine production to fibrogenic activity, and can express CD40 ligand (97,98). Because CD40 is present on epithelial cells, perhaps mast cells result in epithelial cell activation or dysfunction.

Neutrophils have been recovered in induced sputum using 3.5% saline in an ultrasonic nebulizer (99) from patients with asthma. The numbers were increased in patients with severe asthma (53%) compared with moderate (49%) and mild (35%) asthma. Sputum from nonatopic, nonasthmatic subjects had 28% neutrophils (99). The concentrations of IL-8, which is chemoattractant for neutrophils and is an angiogenic cytokine, and of myeloperoxidase were increased in sputum from patients with moderate and severe asthma (99). Neutrophils have been identified in some (100) but not all (101) patients with sudden (<3 hours) death from asthma.

Macrophages serve as accessory cells–presenting antigens and are present in patients with asthma but are found in greater numbers in patients with chronic bronchitis (98). Macrophages have been detected during both early and late bronchial responses to allergens. These cells are metabolically active in that they can generate prostaglandins and leukotrienes, cytokines, free radicals, and mucus secretagogues (98). Alveolar macrophages from asthma patients have been found to release increased quantities of transforming growth factor-β, which could contribute to remodeling and fibrosis.

Increased numbers of eosinophils in bronchial biopsy specimens (98) and sputum (99) can be expected in patients with asthma. It has been estimated that for every 1 eosinophil in peripheral blood, there are 1,000 in the tissue. Patients with mild asthma have eosinophils detected in bronchial biopsy samples, and eosinophils can be found in postmortem histologic sections (100,101). Eosinophils produce MBP, eosinophil cationic protein, free radicals, leukotrienes, and T_H2 cytokines. Eosinophils are proinflammatory

cells that likely participate in the pathogenesis of airway remodeling in patients with persistent asthma.

Epithelial cells are shed especially in patients with severe asthma but also in patients with mild asthma. There are many recognized functions of epithelial cells (98), but because they produce neutral endopeptidase, which degrades substance P, the loss of functioning epithelium could lead to potentiated effects of this neuropeptide. Similarly, epithelial cells generate smooth muscle–relaxing factors that could be decreased in amount as epithelium is denuded (98). Epithelial cell fluid obtained during BAL was analyzed for a gelatinase, which is in the family of matrix metalloproteinases (102). Mechanically ventilated patients with asthma were found to have very high quantities of a 92-kDa gelatinase, compared with patients with mild asthma and with ventilated, nonasthmatic subjects (102). This enzyme may damage collagen and elastin and the subepithelial basal lamina region (102). Increased permeability could result because of epithelial cell shedding and alterations of types IV and V collagens that are present in this basement membrane region (102). In this study, mechanically ventilated patients with status asthmaticus had increased numbers of eosinophils and neutrophils, compared with nonventilated patients with mild asthma (102). There was no difference in numbers of epithelial cells in BAL between patients with mild asthma and the mechanically ventilated patients with asthma, but both groups had twice the percentage as the nonasthmatic subjects, emphasizing that epithelial cell denudation occurs in mild as well as severe asthma.

Innervation

The nervous system and various muscle groups participate in respiration. Table 22.1 lists muscles; their innervation; other respiratory responses, such as smooth muscle cell and bronchial glands; and nonadrenergic, noncholinergic responses. Efferent parasympathetic (vagal) nerves innervate smooth muscle cells and bronchial glands. The vagus nerve also provides for afferent innervation of three types of sensory responses. The irritant (cough) reflex is rapidly adapting

TABLE 22.1. *Examples of innervation, muscles, and respiratory responses*

Efferents	
Muscles, cells, or responses	Innervation
Sternocleidomastoid	C2, C3
Trapezius	C3, C4, spinal accessory nerve XI
Diaphragm	C3–C5
Scaleni	C4–C8
Intercostals	T1–T11
Smooth muscle cells	Vagus X
Bronchial glands	Vagus X, rare thoracic sympathetic
Epithelial sensory nerves (source of substance P, neurokinins, and vasoactive intestinal polypeptide, etc.)	Nonadrenergic, noncholinergic
Afferents	
Special function or site	Innervation
Irritant—cough (rapidly adapting) in trachea and main bronchi	Vagus X
Pulmonary stretch (slowly adapting) in trachea and main bronchi	Vagus X
C fibers in small airways or alveolar wall interstitium	Vagus X
Carotid body	Glossopharyngeal IX
CNS chemoreceptors	Medulla

and originates in the trachea and main bronchi. Pulmonary stretch or slowly adapting afferents are also located in the trachea and main bronchi, whereas C fibers are located in small airways and alveolar walls. Afferent stimulation occurs through the carotid body (sensing oxygen tension) and nervous system chemoreceptors in the medulla (sensing hypercapnia).

Efferent respiratory responses include cervical and thoracic nervous system innervation of respiratory muscles, such as those listed in Table 22.1. Fortunately, not all respiratory muscles are essential for respiration should a spinal cord injury occur. In addition to efferent parasympathetic innervation of smooth muscle cells and bronchial glands, another source of efferent stimulation is through the nonadrenergic, noncholinergic epithelial sensory nerves. Stimulation of these nerves by epithelial cell destruction that occurs in asthma can trigger release of bronchospastic

agonists, such as substance P and neurokinins (A and B), through an antidromic axon reflex. The bronchodilating nonadrenergic, noncholinergic neurotransmitter vasoactive intestinal polypeptide may oppose effects of other bronchoconstricting agonists, such as substance P. An epithelium-relaxing factor has been identified that may not be present when bronchial epithelium has been shed (103). The absence of vasoactive intestinal polypeptide or an epithelium-relaxing factor could cause bronchoconstriction.

Smooth muscle cells participate in the Hering-Breuer inflation reflex, in which inspiration leading to inflation of the lung causes bronchodilation. This reflex has been described in animals and humans. The clinical significance in human respiratory disease may be minimal. For example, when a patient with asthma experiences bronchoconstriction when inhaling methacholine or histamine, there is increased airway resistance during a deep inspiration (104). In contrast, patients without asthma and those with rhinitis demonstrate bronchodilation and reduced airway resistance at total lung capacity. During a bronchial challenge procedure in a patient with rhinitis, if the patient performs a FVC maneuver by inhaling to total lung capacity after inhaling the bronchoconstricting agonist in question, the resultant bronchodilation may mask any current airway obstruction. To obviate this possibility, the initial forced expiratory maneuver should be a partial flow volume effort, not a maximal one, which requires maximal inspiration. Otherwise, the dose of agonist necessary to achieve finally a 20% decline in FEV_1 will be higher than necessary.

PATHOPHYSIOLOGIC CHANGES IN ASTHMA

From a pathophysiologic perspective, the changes that occur in asthma are multiple, diverse, and complex. Further, some of the abnormalities, such as bronchial hyperresponsiveness and mucus obstruction of bronchi, can be present when patients do not have symptoms. Major pathophysiologic abnormalities in asthma are (a) widespread smooth muscle contraction, (b) mucus hypersecretion, (c) mucosal and submucosal edema, (d) bronchial hyperresponsiveness, and (e) inflammation of airways. Obstruction to airflow during expiration and inspiration results in greater limitation during expiration. Hypertrophy and even hyperplasia of smooth muscle have been recognized in asthma. Smooth muscle contraction occurs in large and or small bronchi. Challenge of patients with asthma by inhalation of histamine demonstrated two abnormal responses compared with patients without asthma (105). First, the patients with asthma have increased sensitivity to histamine (or methacholine) because a smaller-than-normal dose of agonist is usually necessary to produce a 20% decline in FEV_1. Second, the maximal response to the agonist in asthma is increased over that which occurs in nonasthmatic, nonrhinitis subjects. In fact, the maximal bronchoconstrictive response (reduction of FEV_1) that occurs in the nonasthmatic, nonrhinitis subject, if one occurs at all, reaches a plateau beyond which increases in agonist produce no further bronchoconstriction. In contrast, were it possible (and safe) to give a patient with asthma increasing amounts of an agonist such as histamine, or methacholine, increasing bronchoconstriction would occur. In an analysis of 146 patients with mild asthma who had undergone bronchial provocation challenge with histamine, two patterns were identified (106). The first was the decline of FEV_1 and FEV_1/FVC without a change in FVC at the dose of histamine causing a 20% decline in FEV_1 (PC_{20}). The second pattern detected at the time of the PC_{20} response had reductions in FVC and FEV_1 but not FEV_1/FVC. It was concluded that the latter subjects experienced excessive bronchoconstriction (106). The authors identified a clinical connection in that there was a moderate correlation between the percentage decline in FVC at the PC_{20} and patients necessitating prescriptions for oral corticosteroids (but not β-adrenergic agonists) (106). In the patients who develop a declining FVC and FEV_1 after bronchoprovocation challenge, there is a concurrent increase in residual volume, which is detrimental if it continues.

Hypersecretion of bronchial mucus may be limited or extensive in patients with asthma. Autopsy studies of patients who died from asthma after having symptoms for days or weeks classically reveal extensive mucus plugging of airways. Large and small airways are filled with viscid mucus that is so thick that the plugs must be cut for examination (107). Reid (107) has described this pattern as consistent with endobronchial mucus suffocation. Other patients have mild amounts of mucus, suggesting that perhaps the fatal asthma episode occurred suddenly (over hours) and that severe bronchial obstruction from smooth muscle contraction contributed to the patient's death. A virtual absence of mucus plugging, called *empty airways* or *sudden asphyxic asthma*, has been reported (107,108). Desquamation of bronchial epithelium can be identified on histologic examination (109) or when a patient coughs up clumps of desquamated epithelial cells (creola bodies). Bronchial mucus contains eosinophils, which may be observed in expectorated sputum. Charcot-Leyden crystals (lysophospholipase) are derived from eosinophils and appear as dipyramidal hexagons or needles in sputum. Viscid mucus plugs, when expectorated, can form a cast of the bronchi and are called *Curschmann spirals*.

Clinically, mucus hypersecretion is reduced or eliminated after treatment of acute asthma or inadequately controlled chronic asthma with systemic and then inhaled corticosteroids. Mucus from patients with asthma has tightly bound glycoprotein and lipid, compared with mucus from patients with chronic bronchitis (110). Macrophages have been shown to produce a mucus secretagogue as well as generate mediators and cytokines (98,111).

The bronchial mucosa is edematous, as is the submucosa, and both are infiltrated with mast cells, activated eosinophils, and $CD4^+$ T_H2 lymphocytes (98,112,113). Venous dilation and plasma leakage occur along with the cellular infiltration. In addition to its presence on mast cells, basophils, and eosinophils, IgE has been identified in bronchial glands, epithelium, and basement membrane. Because plasma cell staining for IgE was not increased in number, it has been thought that IgE is not produced locally. However, because the lung is recognized as an immunologic organ, further work may that show IgE is produced in the lung.

TABLE 22.2. *Conditions of patients that may demonstrate bronchial hyperresponsiveness*

1. After a viral upper respiratory infection for 6 weeks in nonasthma patients
2. In absence of changes in FEV_1 in patients with asthma
3. In chronic bronchitis
4. In left ventricular failure
5. In allergic rhinitis in absence of asthma
6. In apparently normal subjects
7. In subjects exposed to irritants
8. In smokers
9. In some normal infants
10. In first-degree relatives of asthma patients
11. In sarcoidosis
12. In patients with quadriplegia or high paraplegia (lesions T1 to T6)

FEV_1, forced expiratory volume in 1 second.

The mechanism of bronchial hyperresponsiveness in asthma is unknown but is perhaps the central abnormality physiologically. Bronchial hyperresponsiveness occurs in patients with asthma to agonists, such as histamine, methacholine, leukotriene D_4, allergens, platelet-activating factor (PAF), and PGD_2 (short-lived response), and adenosine monophosphate (AMP). Bronchial hyperresponsiveness is sensitive for asthma if one considers a maximum dose of methacholine of 8 mg/mL, which is necessary to cause a decline in FEV_1 of 20%. Patients with active symptomatic asthma often experience such a decline in FEV_1 when the dose of methacholine is 2 mg/mL or less. However, bronchial hyperresponsiveness is not specific for asthma because it occurs in other patients without asthma (Table 22.2).

Bronchial hyperresponsiveness is measured physiologically by reductions in expiratory flow rates (FEV_1) or decreases in specific conductance. Nevertheless, hyperresponsiveness consists of bronchoconstriction, hypersecretion, and hyperemia (mucosa edema). It has been easier to measure airway caliber by changes in FEV_1 than to measure changes in bronchial gland secretion, cellular infiltration, or blood vessels (dilation and increased permeability) that also contribute to hyperresponsiveness and cause airways obstruction. Indeed, there has yet to be an "inflammamometer" for asthma. The bronchial responsiveness detected after challenge with his-

tamine or methacholine measures bronchial sensitivity or ease of bronchoconstriction (106). As stated, an additional finding in some patients with asthma is excessive bronchoconstriction, which can be attributable to associated increases in residual volume and possibly more rapid clinical deterioration (106).

Often, on opening the thorax of a patient who has died from status asthmaticus, the lungs are hyperinflated and do not collapse (Fig. 22.2). Mucus plugging and obstruction of bronchi and bronchioles are present. In some cases, complicating factors, such as atelectasis or acute pneumonia, are identified. Upon histologic examination, there is a patchy loss of bronchial epithelium with desquamation and denudation of mucosal epithelium. Eosinophils are present in areas of absent epithelium, and immunologic staining has revealed evidence of eosinophil MBP at sites of bronchial epithelium desquamation. Activated (EG2-positive) eosinophils are present in the mucosa, submucosa, and connective tissue. Other histologic findings include hyperplasia of bronchial mucus glands, bronchial mucosal edema, smooth muscle hypertrophy, and basement membrane thickening (Fig. 22.3). The latter occurs from collagen deposition (types I, III, and V) immunoglobulin deposition and cellular infiltrates as evidence of inflammation. The mucus plugs may contain eosinophils. Occasionally, bronchial epithelium is denuded, but histologic studies do not identify eosinophils. In some cases, neutrophils have been present (100). Other mechanisms of lung damage are present but not understood completely. Similarly, although many autopsy examinations reveal the classic pattern of mucus plugging (Fig. 22.4) of large and smaller bronchi and bronchioles leading to mucus suffocation or asphyxia as the terminal asthmatic event, some autopsies reveal empty bronchi (101,107,108). Eosinophils have been identified in such cases in airways or in basement membranes, but a gross mechanical explanation, analogous to mucus suffocation, is not present. A third morphologic pattern of patients dying from asthma is that of mild to moderate mucus plugging (107).

Some patients dying from asthma have evidence of myocardial contraction band necrosis,

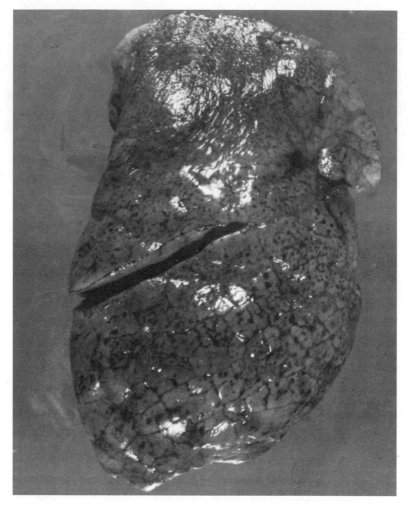

FIG. 22.2. Distended lung of patient who died in status asthmaticus.

which is different from myocardial necrosis associated with infarction. Contraction bands are present in necrotic myocardial smooth muscle cell bands in asthma and curiously the cells are thought to die in tetanic contraction whereas in cases of fatal myocardial infarction, cells die in relaxation.

In patients who experience acute severe asthma but do not die from it, it can be expected that when the patient presents with an FEV_1 of 50% of predicted value, there may be a 10-fold increase in inspiratory muscle work. Pleural pressure becomes more negative, so that as inspiration occurs, the patient is able to apply sufficient radial traction on the airways to maintain their potency. Air can get in more easily than

it can be expired, which results in progressively breathing at higher and higher lung volumes. The residual volume increases several-fold, and functional residual capacity expands as well. Expiratory flow rates decrease in large and small airways. The lung hyperinflation is not distributed evenly, and some areas of the lung have a high or low ventilation-perfusion ratio ($\dot{V}/\dot{Q}$). Overall, the hypoxemia that results from status asthmatics occurs from reduced $\dot{V}/\dot{Q}$, not from shunting of blood. The lung hyperinflation also results in "dynamic autopeep" as the patient attempts to maintain airway caliber by applying some endogenous positive airway pressure.

There is no evidence of chest wall (inspiratory muscle) weakness in patients with asthma.

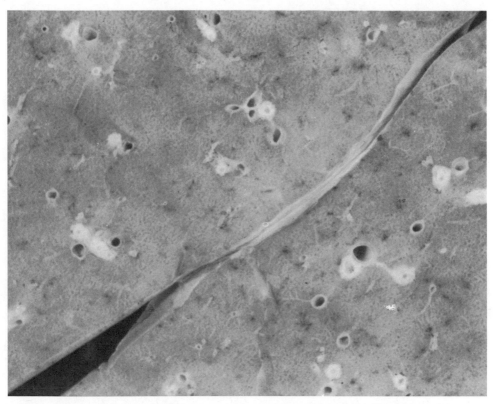

FIG. 22.3. Close-up view of pulmonary parenchyma in a case of status asthmaticus. Bronchi are dilated and thickened.

Nevertheless, some patients who have received prolonged courses of daily or twice-daily prednisone or who have been mechanically ventilated with muscle relaxants and corticosteroids can be those who have respiratory muscle fatigue.

After successful treatment of an attack of status asthmaticus, the increases in lung volume may remain present for 6 weeks. The changes are primarily in residual volume and functional residual capacity. Small airways may remain obstructed for weeks or months; in some patients, they do not become normal again. At the same time, it can be expected that the patient has no sensation of dyspnea within 1 week of treatment of status asthmaticus despite increases in residual volume and reduced small airways caliber. This divergence between symptom recognition in asthma and physiologic measurements has been demonstrated in ambulatory patients who did not have status asthmaticus (114). When patients with an FEV_1 percentage of 60% were

studied, 31% overestimated and 17% underestimated the extent of airway obstruction (114). Some patients reported fewer symptoms despite no improvement in FEV_1 or peak expiratory flow rate (PEFR). The reduction in trapped gas in the lung can result in symptom reduction even without improvement in expiratory flow rates.

In summary, asthma pathophysiology includes poor or impaired symptom perception in some patients. There may be poor sensitivity or discrimination (recognizing improvement or worsening status) (115).

CONTROL OF AIRWAY TONE

The patency of bronchi and bronchioles is a function of many factors not fully understood (116). Bronchomotor patency is affected by mediators secreted by mast cells, the autonomic nervous system, the nonadrenergic noncholinergic nervous system, circulating humoral substances, the

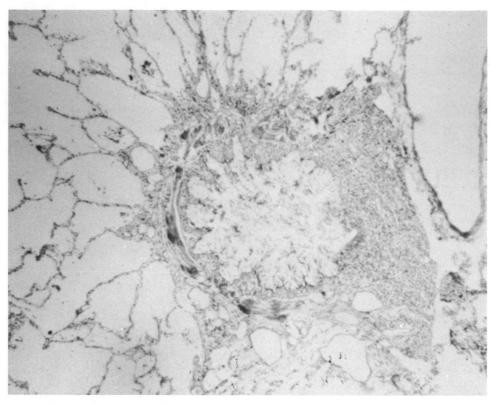

FIG. 22.4. Microphotograph of a dilated bronchus filled with a mucous plug. There is hypertrophy of the muscle layer, and the alveolar spaces are dilated.

respiratory epithelium, smooth muscle cells, and effects of cellular infiltration and glandular secretions (Tables 22.3 and 22.4). Even this list is oversimplified because asthma must be considered a very complex condition in terms of airway caliber and tone.

Mediator release caused by mast cell activation results in acute and late bronchial smooth muscle contraction, cellular infiltration, and mucus production. Autonomic nervous stimulation contributes through vagal stimulation. The neurotransmitter for postganglionic parasympathetic nerves is acetylcholine, which causes smooth muscle contraction. Norepinephrine is the neurotransmitter for postganglionic sympathetic nerves. However, there appears to be little if any significant smooth muscle relaxation through stimulation of postganglionic sympathetic nerves. Exogenously administered epinephrine can produce smooth muscle relaxation. Circulating endogenous epinephrine apparently does not serve to produce relaxation of smooth muscles. Sensory nerves in the respiratory epithelium are stimulated and lead to release of a host of neuropeptides that may be potent bronchoconstrictors or bronchodilators. Respiratory epithelium itself may contain bronchirelaxing factors that may become unavailable when epithelium is denuded. Tables 22.2 and 22.3 list some chemical mediators derived from mast cells and neuropeptides that may contribute to pathogenesis of asthma.

Although much attention has been directed at understanding the contribution of IgE and mast cell activation in asthma, triggering or actual regulation of some of the inflammation of asthma may occur because of other cells in lungs of patients. Low-affinity IgE receptors are known to exist on macrophages, eosinophils, monocytes, lymphocytes, and platelets. These cells, as well

TABLE 22.3. *Selected mast cell mediators and cytokines and their proposed actions in asthma*

Mediator	Preformed	Newly synthesized	Actions
Histamine	+		Smooth muscle contraction (H_1 and via vagus); increased vascular permeability; vasodilator; mucus production (H_2).
Tryptase	+		Degrades vasoactive intestinal polypeptide; cleaves kininogen to form bradykinin, cleaves C3
Eosinophil chemotactic factor	+		Eosinophil chemoattractant
Neutrophil chemotactic factor	+		Neutrophil chemoattractant
Peroxidase	+		Inactivates leukotrienes
Bradykinin		+	Smooth muscle contraction
Leukotriene D_4 (generated from leukotriene C_4)		+	Smooth muscle contraction; increases vascular permeability, mucus secretion
Prostaglandin D_2, $F_{2\alpha}$		+	Smooth muscle contraction; increases vascular permeability, mucus secretion
Platelet-activating factor		+	Smooth muscle contraction; increases vascular permeability, neutrophil and eosinophil chemoattractant; aggregates platelets; sensitizes airways to the agonists
Leukotriene B_4 Cytokine		+	Neutrophil and eosinophil chemoattractant
Interleukin-3 (IL-3)		+	Eosinophil growth factor and chemoattractant, stem cell growth, mast cell growth
IL-5		+	Eosinophil growth factor and chemoattractant
Granulocyte-macrophage colony-stimulating factor		+	Eosinophil growth factor and chemoattractant
IL-1		+	Cytokine production; B-cell differentiation and proliferation
IL-2		+	Proliferation of T cells
IL-4		+	Growth of B cells; class switching from immunoglobulin M (IgM) to IgE production; increases VCAM on endothelium. Favors T_H2 phenotype of CD_4^+ T cells
Tumor necrosis factor-α		+	Activation of macrophages with increased major histocompatibility complex (MHC) molecules (increased antigen presentation)
Interferon-γ		+	Increased MHC molecules on macrophages

TABLE 22.4. *Selected neuropeptides and their proposed actions in asthma*

Neuropeptide	Actions
Vasoactive intestinal polypeptide	Smooth muscle relaxation Pulmonary vasodilator Stimulates adenylate cyclase Suppresses mucus secretion May be deficient in asthma
Substance P	Smooth muscle contraction Vasodilator Mucus secretion Increases capillary permeability
Neurokinin A	Smooth muscle contraction
Peptide histamine methionine	Inhibits vagus-induced bronchoconstriction; stimulates adenylate cyclase
Calcitonin gene–related peptide	Smooth muscle contraction

as mast cells in the bronchial mucosa or lumen, can be activated in the absence of classic IgE-mediated asthma.

Bronchial biopsy specimens from patients with asthma demonstrate mucosal mast cells in various stages of activation in patients with and without symptoms (117,118). Mast cell hyper-releasibility may occur in asthma, in that bronchoalveolar mast cells recovered during lavage contain and release greater quantities of histamine when stimulated by allergen or anti-IgE *in vitro* (119,120).

Eosinophils are thought to contribute to proinflammatory effects by secretion of damaging cell products, such as MBP, that can result in bronchial epithelial denudation, exposing sensory nerves and leading to smooth muscle contraction. Eosinophils are proinflammatory in that they cause eosinophil and neutrophil chemotaxis, which produces positive feedback in terms of leukotriene and PAF production from attracted and newly activated eosinophils. The latter can be demonstrated by their reduced density upon centrifugation that occurs during acute episodes of asthma.

Experimental data suggest a possible role of histamine-releasing factor (HRF) in asthma (121). HRF has been generated from mononuclear cells, neutrophils, pulmonary macrophages, and platelets. *In vitro*, for example, peripheral blood mononuclear cells from patients with asthma are stimulated with allergen, and the supernatant is obtained. Subsequent incubation of supernatant with basophils results in histamine release. If basophils are representative of bronchial mast cells, HRF may affect airway tone by facilitating mast cell mediator release. On a cellular level, the control of airway tone is influenced by even more fundamental factors, including IL-1, IL-2, IL-3, IL-4, IL-6, IL-10, IL-12, and IL-16 and IFN-γ, among others, that influence lymphocyte development and proliferation. IL-3 and IL-5 are eosinophil growth factors. IL-8, detected in bronchial epithelium, binds to secretory IgA and serves to chemoattract eosinophils that generate PAF and LTC4. IL-8 is also a potent chemotactic substance for neutrophils.

During an acute attack of asthma, there is an increase in inspiratory efforts, which apply greater radial traction to airways. Patients with asthma have great ability to generate increases in inspiratory pressures. Unfortunately, patients who have experienced nearly fatal attacks of asthma have blunted perception of dyspnea and impaired ventilatory responses to hypoxia (115,122).

Severe asthma patients have been divided into eosinophil-positive (and macrophage-positive) and eosinophil-negative categories based on results on bronchial biopsy findings (123). Both subgroups of patients were prednisone dependent (average, 28 mg daily) and had asthma for about 20 years (123). The residual volume measurements were about 200% of predicted and FEV$_1$ percentage was 56% in eosinophil-positive and 42% in eosinophil-negative patients (123). The ratio of the FVC to slow vital capacity was 88%, indicating more airway collapsibility in eosinophil-positive patients, compared with 97% in eosinophil-negative patients. Perhaps the former patients who had somewhat higher FEV$_1$ percentages had more loss of elastic recoil in their lungs, so that their airways collapsed more easily (123). On biopsy assessments, sub–basement membrane thickening was higher in these eosinophil-predominant patients than in eosinophil-negative patients. These findings were associated with eosinophil-predominant patients with severe asthma having an increased number of CD3$^+$ lymphocytes and activated eosinophils (EG2$^+$) in biopsy samples and an increased quantity of β-tryptase in BAL (123). It is likely that the cellular inflammation and cell products participate in control or perturbation of airway tone, and continued investigations should help clarify this difficult issue.

CLINICAL OVERVIEW

Clinical Manifestations

Asthma results in coughing, wheezing, dyspnea, sputum production, and shortness of breath. Symptoms vary from patient to patient and within the individual patient depending on the activity of asthma. Some patients experience mild, nonproductive coughing after exercising or exposure to cold air or odors as examples of transient mild bronchospasm. The combination of coughing and wheezing with dyspnea is common in patients who have a sudden moderate to severe episode (such as might occur within 3 hours after aspirin ingestion in an aspirin-intolerant patient). Symptoms of asthma may be sporadic and are often present on a nocturnal basis. Some patients with asthma present with a persistent nonproductive cough as a main symptom of asthma (124). Typically, the cough has occurred on a daily basis and may awaken the patient at night. Repetitive spasms of cough from asthma are refractory to treatment with expectorants, antibiotics, and antitussives. The patient likely will respond to antiasthma therapy, such as inhaled β-adrenergic agonists; if that is unsuccessful, inhaled corticosteroids or the combination may work. At times, oral corticosteroids are necessary to stop the coughing and are very useful as a diagnostic therapeutic trial (124). Pulmonary physiologic studies usually reveal large airway obstruction, as illustrated by reductions in FEV_1 with preservation of forced expiratory flow, midexpiratory phase ($FEF_{25\%-75\%}$) or small airways function (125). The latter may be reduced in patients with this variant form of asthma. Conversely, some patients present with isolated dyspnea as a manifestation of asthma. Some of these patients have small airways obstruction with preservation of function of larger airways. The recognition of variant forms of asthma emphasizes that not all patients with asthma have detectable wheezing on auscultation. The medical history is invaluable, as is a diagnostic-therapeutic trial with antiasthma medications. Pulmonary physiologic abnormalities, such as reduced FEV_1 that responds to therapy, or bronchial hyperresponsiveness to methacholine can provide additional supportive data.

During an acute, moderately severe episode of asthma or in longer-term ineffectively controlled asthma, patients typically produce clear, yellow, or green sputum that can be viscid. The sputum contains eosinophils, which supports the diagnosis of asthma. Because either polymorphonuclear leukocytes or eosinophils can cause the sputum to be discolored, it is inappropriate to consider such sputum as evidence of a secondary bacterial infection. Patients with nonallergic asthma also produce eosinophil-laden sputum. An occasional patient with asthma presents with cough syncope, a respiratory arrest that is perceived as anaphylaxis, chest pain, pneumomediastinum, or pneumothorax, or with symptoms of chronic bronchitis or bronchiectasis.

The physical examination may consist of no coughing or wheezing if the patient has stable chronic asthma or if there has not been a recent episode of sporadic asthma. Certainly, patients with variant asthma may not have wheezing or other supportive evidence of asthma. Usually, wheezing is present in other patients and can be associated with reduced expiratory flow rates. A smaller number of patients always have wheezing on even tidal breathing, not just with a forced expiratory maneuver. Such patients may not have symptoms and may or may not have expiratory airflow obstruction when FVC and FEV_1 are measured. The physical examination must be interpreted in view of the patient's clinical symptoms and supplemental tests, such as the chest radiograph or pulmonary function tests. There may be a surprising lack of correlation in some ambulatory patients between symptoms and objective evidence of asthma (physical findings and spirometric values) (114,115).

An additional physical finding in patients with asthma is repetitive coughing on inspiration. Although not specific for asthma, it is frequently present in unstable patients. In normal patients, maximal inspiration to total lung capacity results in reduced airway resistance, whereas in patients with asthma, increased resistance occurs with a maximal inspiration. Coughing spasms can be precipitated in patients who otherwise may not be heard to wheeze. This finding is transient and, after effective therapy, will not occur. The patient with a very severe episode of asthma may be found to have pulsus paradoxus and use of accessory muscles of respiration. Such findings correlate with an FEV_1 of less than 1.0 L and air trapping as manifested by hyperinflation of the functional residual capacity and residual volume (126). The most critically ill patients have markedly reduced tidal volumes, and their maximal ventilatory efforts are not much higher than their efforts during tidal breathing. A silent chest with absence of or greatly reduced breath sounds indicates likely alveolar hypoventilation (normal or elevated arterial PCO_2) and hypoxemia. Such patients may require intubation or, in most cases, admission to the intensive care unit. Great difficulty in speaking more than a half sentence before needing another inspiration is likely present in such patients.

Asthma may be occurring in patients who have concurrent gastroesophageal reflux disease (GERD), sinusitis, and rhinitis, all of which can cause a cough or worsen ongoing asthma (127).

Radiographic and Laboratory Studies

In about 90% of patients, the presentation chest radiograph is considered within normal limits (128–130). The most frequently found abnormality is hyperinflation. The diaphragm is flattened, and there may be an increase in the anteroposterior diameter and retrosternal air space. The chest radiograph is indicated because it is necessary to exclude other conditions that mimic asthma and to search for complications of asthma.

Congestive heart failure, COPD, pneumonia, and neoplasms are just some other explanations for acute wheezing dyspnea that may mimic or co-exist with asthma. Asthma complications include atelectasis as a result of mucus obstruction of bronchi, mucoid impaction of bronchi (often indicative of allergic bronchopulmonary aspergillosis), pneumomediastinum, and pneumothorax. Atelectasis often involves the middle lobe, which may collapse. The presence of pneumomediastinum or pneumothorax may have associated subcutaneous emphysema with crepitus on palpation of the neck, supraclavicular areas, or face (Figs. 22.5 and 22.6). Sharp pain in the neck or shoulders should be a clue to the presence of a pneumomediastinum in status asthmaticus.

Depending on the patients examined, abnormal findings on sinus films may be frequent (131). Screening computed tomography (CT) examinations of the sinuses are not indicated routinely but may identify unrecognized findings, such as air-fluid levels, indicative of infection; mucoperiosteal thickening, which is consistent with current or previous infection; and opacification of a sinus or presence of nasal polyps (see Chapters 19 and 29.)

Clinical research studies of acutely ill patients with asthma have been carried out with $\dot{V}/\dot{Q}$ scans. These procedures are not indicated in most cases and, in the markedly hypoxemic patient, may be harmful because the technetium-labeled albumin macrospheres injected for the perfusion scan can lower arterial Po_2. Ventilation is extremely uneven (132). Perfusion scans reveal abnormalities such that there may or may not be matched $\dot{V}/\dot{Q}$ inequalities. In some patients, the $\dot{V}/\dot{Q}$ in the superior portions of the lungs has declined from its relatively high value (132). The explanation for such a finding is increased perfusion of upper lobes presumably from reduced

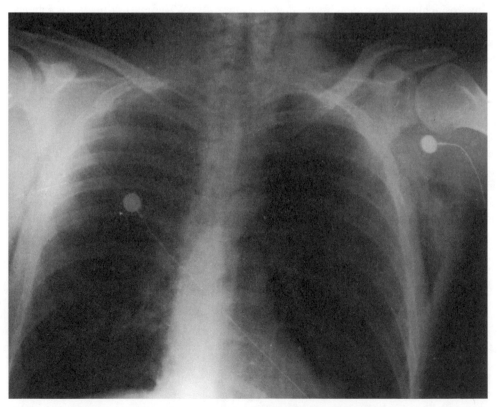

FIG. 22.5. Anteroposterior view of the chest of a 41-year-old woman demonstrated hyperinflation of both lungs, with pneumomediastinum and subcutaneous emphysema.

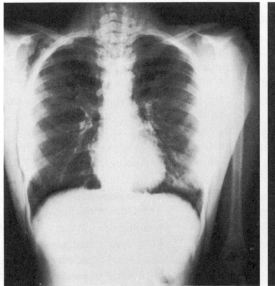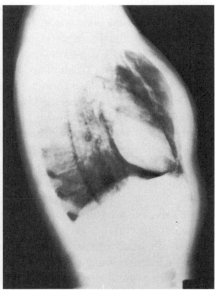

FIG. 22.6. Posteroanterior (**A**) and lateral (**B**) chest films of a 13-year-old asthmatic patient demonstrate hyperinflated lungs with bilateral perihilar infiltrates, pneumomediastinum, and subcutaneous emphysema in soft tissue of the chest and neck.

resistance relative to lower lobes that receive most of the pulmonary blood flow. Little evidence for shunting exists (132). When a pulmonary embolus is suspected, the $\dot{V}/\dot{Q}$ scan may be nondiagnostic in the patient with an exacerbation of asthma. In some patients with asthma and pulmonary emboli, areas of ventilation but not perfusion are identified, so that the diagnosis may be made. Spiral CT examinations of the lung may demonstrate evidence of pulmonary emboli, but acute asthma is not typically complicated by pulmonary emboli.

In the assessment of the emergency department patient with acute severe wheezing dyspnea, the measurement of arterial PO_2, PCO_2, and pH can be invaluable. Although hypoxemia is a frequent and expected finding and is identified by measuring the pulse oximetry, the PCO_2 provides information on the effectiveness of alveolar ventilation. This latter status will not be assessed if just oxygen saturation is determined. The PCO_2 should be decreased initially during the hyperventilation stage of acute asthma. A normal or elevated PCO_2 is evidence of alveolar hypoventilation and may be associated with subsequent need for intubation to try to prevent a fatal outcome.

Pulmonary function measurements can help to establish patient status. However, such measurements must be correlated with the physical examination. In the emergency room or ambulatory setting, many physicians determine spirometric values for expiratory flow rates with either PEFR or FEV_1. These tests are effort dependent, and patients with acute symptoms may be unable to perform the maneuver satisfactorily. This finding could be from severe obstruction or patient inability or unwillingness to perform the maneuver appropriately. When properly performed, spirometric measurements can be of significant clinical utility in assessing patient status. For example, as a rule, patients presenting with spirometric determinations of 20% to 25% of predicted value should receive immediate and intensive therapy and nearly always be hospitalized. Frequent measurements of PEFR or FEV_1 in ambulatory patients can establish a range of baseline values for day and night. Declines of more than 20% from usual low recordings can alert the patient to the need for more intensive pharmacologic therapy. Nevertheless, such measurements can be insensitive in some patients. Pulmonary physiologic values such as PEFR and FEV_1 have demonstrated value in clinical research studies, such as in documenting a 12% increase in expiratory flow rates after bronchodilator. Such a response (including a 200-mL increase in FEV_1) meets criteria for a bronchodilator response (2). Similarly, in testing for bronchial hyperresponsiveness, a 20% decline in FEV_1 is a goal during incremental administration of methacholine or histamine.

Some patients may benefit from measuring PEFR daily at home (2). Unfortunately, some patients do not continue to measure this PEFR or may fabricate results (133). Other patients manipulate spirometric measurements to make a convincing case for occupational asthma. Thus, the physician must correlate pulmonary physiologic values with the clinical assessment. A complete set of pulmonary function tests should be obtained in other situations, such as in assessing the degree of reversible versus nonreversible obstruction in patients with heavy smoking histories. The diffusing capacity for carbon monoxide (DLCO) is reduced in the COPD patient but normal or elevated in the patient with asthma. Such tests should be obtained after 2 to 4 weeks of intensive therapy to determine what degree of reversibility exists. In acutely ill patients with asthma, the DLCO may be reduced. Thus, its usefulness in differentiating COPD from asthma will be obscured if the wrong time is chosen to obtain this test. Flow-volume loops will demonstrate intrathoracic obstruction in patients with asthma (134) or extrathoracic obstruction in those with vocal cord dysfunction (VCD) (135) (Fig. 22.7).

The complete blood count should be obtained in the emergency setting. First, the hemoglobin and hematocrit provide status regarding anemia, which if associated with hypoxemia can compromise oxygen delivery to tissues. Conversely, an elevated hematocrit is consistent with hemoconcentration such as occurs from dehydration or polycythemia. The latter does not occur in asthma in the absence of other conditions. The white blood count may be elevated from epinephrine (white blood cell demargination from vessel walls), systemic corticosteroids (demargination and release from bone marrow), or infection. In the absence of prior systemic corticosteroids, the acutely ill patient with allergic or nonallergic asthma often has peripheral blood eosinophilia. For best accuracy, an absolute eosinophil count is required. However, in the management of most patients with asthma, both those with acute symptoms and long-term sufferers, eosinophil counts are not of value. The presence of eosinophilia in patients receiving long-term systemic corticosteroids should suggest noncompliance or possibly rare conditions, such as Churg-Strauss syndrome, allergic bronchopulmonary aspergillosis, or chronic eosinophilic pneumonia (136). Usually, the eosinophilia in asthma does not exceed 10% to 20% of the differential. Higher values should suggest an alternative diagnosis.

Sputum examination reveals eosinophils, eosinophils plus polymorphonuclear leukocytes (asthma and purulent bronchitis or bacterial pneumonia), or absence of eosinophils. In mild asthma, no sputum is produced. In severely ill patients with asthma, the sputum is thick, tenacious, and yellow or green. MBP from eosinophils has been identified in such sputum (55). Dipyramidal hexagons from eosinophil cytoplasm may be identified and are called Charcot-Leyden crystals. These crystals contain lysophospholipase. Curschmann spirals are expectorated yellow or clear mucus threads that are remnants or casts of small bronchi. Expectorated ciliated and nonciliated bronchial epithelial cells can also be identified that emphasize the patchy loss of bronchial epithelium in asthma. On a related basis, high-molecular-weight neutrophil chemotactic activity has been identified in sera from patients with status asthmaticus (137). This activity declined with effective therapy.

Serum electrolyte abnormalities may be present and should be anticipated in the patient presenting to the emergency department. Recent use of oral corticosteroids can lower the potassium concentration (as can β_2-adrenergic agonists) and cause a metabolic alkalosis. Oral corticosteroids may raise the blood glucose in some patients, as can systemic administration of β-adrenergic agonists. Elevations of atrial natriuretic peptide (antidiuretic hormone) can occur in acute asthma or COPD (138,139). Clinically, few patients have large declines of serum sodium. Because intravenous fluids will be administered, it is necessary to determine the current status

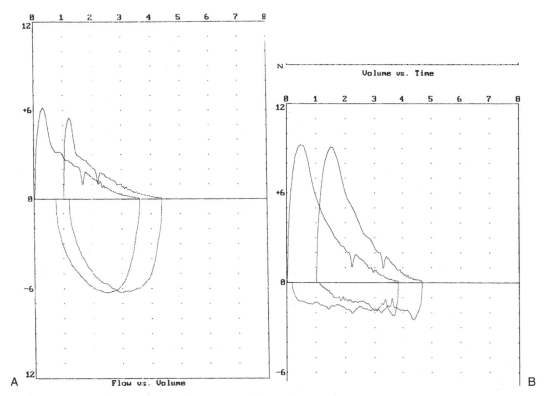

FIG. 22.7. A: A 46-year-old man with asthma since childhood. He had been taking prednisone, 60 mg daily for 6 weeks; salmeterol, 2 puffs twice a day; and budesonide, 800 μg twice a day. He had mild expiratory wheezes on examination. The pattern is that of intrathoracic obstruction from asthma. The forced vital capacity (FVC) was 3.6 L (72%), and the forced expiratory volume in 1 second (FEV$_1$) was 2.3 (62%). The FEV$_1$ percentage was 64%. The forced expiratory flow, midexpiratory phase (FEF$_{25\%-75\%}$) was 1.36 L/sec (36%). The inspiratory loop is not altered. **B:** A 47-year-old man with adult-onset asthma and intermittent sinusitis, nonallergic rhinitis, and gastroesophageal reflux disease. Medications included prednisone, 35 mg on alternate days; budesonide, 800 μg twice a day; salmeterol, 2 puffs twice a day; omeprazole, 40 mg daily; fexofenadine, 60 mg twice daily; and triamcinolone nasal spray. He had mild end-expiratory wheezes and a hoarse voice. No stridor was present. The FVC was 3.9 L (78%), the FEV$_1$ was 2.9 L (77%), and the FEV$_1$ percentage was 74%. The FEF$_{25\%-75\%}$ was 2 L/sec (56%). The inspiratory loop is truncated, consistent with vocal cord dysfunction.

of electrolytes and serum chemistry values. After prolonged high-dose corticosteroids, hypomagnesemia or hypophosphatemia may occur.

Rarely, a patient younger than 30 years of age may be thought to have asthma when the underlying condition is α_1-antitrypsin deficiency. More commonly, patients with wheezing dyspnea have asthma and cystic fibrosis. The sweat chloride should be elevated markedly in such patients. A properly performed sweat chloride test is essential, as is proper performance of other laboratory tests.

In the outpatient management of asthma, determination of the presence or absence of antiallergen IgE is of value. For decades, skin testing for immediate cutaneous reactivity has been the most sensitive and specific method. Some physicians prefer *in vitro* tests. One cannot emphasize enough the need for high quality control for both skin testing and *in vitro* testing. Both tests are subject to misinterpretation. The experienced physician should use either method of demonstration of antiallergen IgE as adjunctive to, rather than a substitute for, the narrative history of asthma. More patients have immediate cutaneous reactivity or detectable *in vitro* IgE than have asthma that correlates with exposure to the specific allergen.

Complications

Complications from asthma include death, adverse effects of hypoxemia or respiratory failure on other organ systems, growth retardation in children, pneumothorax or pneumomediastinum, rib fractures from severe coughing, cough syncope, and adverse effects of medications or therapeutic modalities used to treat asthma. Some patients develop psychological abnormalities because of the burden of a chronic illness such as asthma. Ineffectively treated asthma in children can result in chest wall abnormalities, such as "pigeon chest," because of sustained hyperinflation of the chest. Further, the annual rate of decline of FEV_1 is increased; for example, it may be 38 mL/year in patients with asthma, compared with 22 mL/year in patients without asthma (140).

In general, long-term asthma does not result in irreversible obstructive lung disease. However, an occasional patient with long-term asthma develops apparently irreversible disease in the absence of cigarette smoking, α_1-antitrypsin disease, or other obvious cause (141). Usually, these patients have childhood-onset asthma and are dependent on oral corticosteroids. Intensive therapy with oral and inhaled corticosteroids does not result in an FEV_1 that is 80% of the predicted value (mean, 57%) (141). In contrast to the few patients with irreversible asthma, patients with asthma do not become "respiratory cripples," as might occur from COPD. Nevertheless, pulmonary physiologic studies do not reveal return of parameters to the expected normal ranges. Asthma patients are not deficient in antiproteases that can be measured, and they do not have bullous abnormalities on chest radiographs. CT demonstrates gas trapping, especially on expiration, as well as bronchial wall thickening caused by increased smooth muscle mass and elastic and collagenous tissue (142).

Pneumomediastinum or pneumothorax can occur in patients presenting in status asthmaticus. Neck, shoulder, or chest pain is common, and crepitations can be detected in the neck or supraclavicular fossae. Rupture of distal alveoli results in dissection of air proximally through bronchovascular bundles. The air can then travel superiorly in the mediastinum to the supraclavicular or cervical areas. At times, the air dissects to the face or into the subcutaneous areas over the thorax. Treating the patient's asthma with systemic corticosteroids is indicated to reduce the likelihood of hyperinflation and continued air leak. Unless the pneumothorax is very large, conservative treatment is effective. Otherwise, thoracostomy with tube placement is necessary.

Fatalities from asthma are unnecessary because asthma is not an inexorably fatal disease. Fatalities do occur, however, and many factors have been suggested as explanations (2,101,127,143–149). Some deaths from asthma are unavoidable despite appropriate medical care. A high percentage of deaths from asthma should be considered preventable. Survivors of major asthma events, such as respiratory failure or arrest, patients with pneumodiastinum or pneumothorax on two occasions, and those with repeated status asthmaticus despite oral corticosteroids have potentially fatal asthma and are at higher risk for fatality than other patients with asthma (63,150).

Uncontrolled asthma can lead to mucus plugging of airways and frank collapse of a lobe or whole lung segment. The middle lobe can collapse, especially in children. Repeated mucoid impactions should raise the possibility of allergic bronchopulmonary aspergillosis (ABPA) or cystic fibrosis.

Cough syncope or cough associated cyanosis occurs in patients whose respiratory status has deteriorated and in whom status asthmaticus or need for emergency therapy has occurred. During severe airway obstruction from asthma, during inspiration, intrathoracic pressure is negative because the patient must generate very high negative pressures to apply radial traction on bronchi in an attempt to maintain their patency. During expiration, the patient must overcome severe airway resistance and premature airways collapse. Increases in intrathoracic pressure during expiration with severe coughing, as compared with intraabdominal pressure, causes a decline in venous return to the right atrium. There may also be increased blood flow to the lung during a short inspiration, but that is accompanied by pooling in the pulmonary vasculature from the markedly elevated negative inspiratory pressure. There will be reduced blood flow to the left ventricle with temporary decreases in cardiac output and cerebral blood flow.

Pulsus paradoxus is present when there is greater than a 10-mm Hg decline in systolic blood pressure during inspiration. It is associated with severe airway obstruction and hyperinflation (151). The most frequent electrocardiographic findings during acute asthma are sinus tachycardia followed by right axis deviation, clockwise rotation, prominent R in lead V_1 and S in lead V_5, and tall peaked P waves consistent with cor pulmonale (151).

Linear growth retardation can occur from ineffectively controlled asthma. Administration of oral corticosteroids is indicated to prevent repeated hospitalizations and frequent episodes of wheezing dyspnea. The child often responds with a growth spurt. Alternate-day prednisone and recommended doses of inhaled corticosteroids do not result in growth retardation, especially when the dose is 30 mg on alternate days or less. Even high alternate-day doses in children can be tolerated reasonably well as long as status asthmaticus is prevented. Similarly, depot corticosteroids given every 2 to 3 weeks in high doses may result in growth retardation. Despite efficacy in asthma, such corticosteroid administration causes hypothalamic-pituitary-adrenal (HPA) suppression (152). The use of depot corticosteroids should be considered only in the most recalcitrant children in terms of asthma management. Ineffective parental functioning or poor compliance usually accompanies such cases in which reliable administration of prednisone and inhaled corticosteroids is impossible. The term *malignant, potentially fatal asthma* has been suggested for such patients (153).

Psychological Factors

Asthma has evolved from a disorder considered to be psychological to one recognized as extremely complex (127) and of unknown etiology. Psychological stress can cause modest reductions in expiratory flow rates such as occur during watching a terrifying movie (154). Laughing and crying or frank emotional upheaval, such as an argument with a family member, can result in wheezing. Some patients require additional antiinflammatory medication. Usually, if the patient has stable baseline respiratory status, severe asthma necessitating emergency hospital care does not result. Nevertheless, some fatal episodes of asthma have been reported as associated with a high level of emotional stress. In an absence of how to quantitate stress and determine whether there is a dose-response effect in asthma, such information must be considered speculative. Specific personality patterns have not been identified in patients with asthma.

The patient with asthma may develop strategies to function with the burden of asthma as a chronic, disruptive, and potentially fatal disease. A variety of behavior patterns have been recognized, including (a) disease denial, with complacency or outright denial of symptoms, refusal to alert the managing physician about a major change in respiratory symptoms, or personally decreasing medications; (b) using asthma for obvious secondary gain, such as to not attend school or work, or to gain compensation; (c) developing compulsive or manipulative patterns of behavior that restrict the lifestyle of the patient and family members excessively; and (d) resorting to quackery. Some patients display hateful behavior toward physicians and their office staff personnel (155,156). Psychiatric care can be of value in some cases, but often patients refuse appropriate psychiatric referrals. The use of PEFR monitoring devices can be misleading because patients can generate expected but truly inaccurate measurements. Obviously, in contrast to theories implying that wheezing dyspnea in patients with asthma was primarily psychological, the physician must now decide how much of a patient's symptoms and signs are from asthma and how much might be psychological as a result of asthma. Indeed, a psychologist, psychiatrist, or social worker may help identify what the patient might lose should asthma symptoms be controlled better.

Major management problems occur when asthma patients also have schizophrenia, delusional behavior, neurosis, depression, or manic-depressive disorders (157). Suicidal attempts are recognized from theophylline overdosage and unjustified cessation of prednisone. Repeated episodes of life-threatening status asthmaticus are difficult to avoid in the setting of untreated major psychiatric conditions.

The presence of factitious asthma indicates significant psychiatric disturbance (158). Initially, there must be trust established between the patient and physician. Abrupt referral of the patient to a psychiatrist can result in an unanticipated suicidal gesture or attempt. Psychiatric care can be valuable if the patient is willing to participate in therapy.

TABLE 22.5. *Classification of asthma*

Allergic asthma
Nonallergic asthma
Mixed asthma
Potentially fatal asthma
Malignant potentially fatal asthma
Aspirin-intolerant asthma
Occupational asthma
Exercise-induced asthma
Variant asthma
Factitious asthma
Vocal cord dysfunction and asthma
Coexistent asthma and chronic obstructive
    pulmonary disease
Irreversible asthma

sented. It can be helpful to determine that patients have "moderate persistent allergic asthma" and use the classifications from Table 22.5 and 22.6 together when applicable.

CLASSIFICATION

Some types of asthma are listed in Table 22.5. It is helpful to categorize the type of asthma because treatment programs vary depending on the type of asthma present. Some patients have more than one type of asthma. The National Institutes of Health Expert Panel Report 2 has suggested assessing signs and symptoms of asthma in association with spirometry or peak flow measurements (2). Asthma severity is classified as intermittent (implying mild asthma) or persistent (mild, moderate, or severe). In Table 22.6, a simplified version of this classification system is pre-

Allergic Asthma

Allergic asthma is caused by inhalation of allergen that interacts with IgE present in high-affinity receptors on bronchial mucosal mast cells. Allergic asthma often occurs from ages 4 to 40 years but has been recognized in the geriatric population (159) and in adult patients attending a pulmonary clinic for care (160). Some physicians believe that many patients with asthma must have some type of allergic asthma because of elevated total serum IgE concentrations (161), antiallergen IgE (162) and the frequent finding of peripheral blood or sputum eosinophilia. The use of

TABLE 22.6. *An asthma classification system*

Designation	Symptoms	Nocturnal symptoms	Pulmonary function
Intermittent (mild)	≤ 2 times a week; asymptomatic with normal PEFR between exacerbations	≤ 2 times a month	PEFR or FEV_1 ≥ 80%
Persistent (mild)	≥ 2 times a week but <1 time a day; may have exertional asthma	≥ 2 times a month	PEFR or FEV_1 ≥ 80%
Persistent (moderate)	Daily symptoms; exacerbations ≥ 2 days a week or lasting days	≥ 1 time a month	PEFR or FEV_1 ≥ 60% but <80%
Persistent (severe)	Continual symptoms; Reduced physical activity; frequent exacerbations	Frequent	PEFR or FEV_1 ≤ 60%

PEFR, peak expiratory flow rate; FEV_1, forced expiratory volume in 1 second.
From National Heart, Lung, and Blood Institute. *Expert Panel Report 2: guidelines for the diagnosis and management of asthma.* NIH publication No. 97-4051. Bethesda, MD: National Institutes of Health, 1997, with permission.

the term *allergic asthma* implies that a temporal relationship exists between respiratory symptoms and allergen exposure and that antiallergen IgE antibodies can be demonstrated or suspected. Perhaps 75% of patients with persistent asthma have an allergic basis.

Respiratory symptoms may develop within minutes or in an hour after allergen exposure or may not be obvious when there is uninterrupted allergen exposure. Common allergens associated with IgE-mediated asthma include pollens, such as from trees, grasses, and weeds; fungal spores; dust mites; animal dander; and in some settings, animal urine or cockroach excreta. IgE-mediated occupational asthma is considered under the category of occupational asthma. Allergen particle size must be less than 10 μm to penetrate into deeper parts of the lung because larger particles, such as ragweed pollen (19 μm), impact in the oropharynx. However, submicronic ragweed particles have been described that could reach smaller airways (163). Particles smaller than 1 μm, however, may not be retained in the airways. Fungal spores, such as *Aspergillus* species, are 2 to 3 μm in size, and the major cat allergen (*Fel d 1*) has allergenic activity from 0.4 μm to 10 μm in size (164). Another study demonstrated that 75% of *Fel d 1* was present in particles of at least 5 μm and that 25% of *Fel d 1* was present in particles of less than 2.5 μm (165). Cat dander allergen can be present in indoor air, on clothes, and in schoolrooms where no cats are present (166).

The potential severity of allergic asthma should not be minimized because experimentally, after an antigen-induced early bronchial response, bronchial hyperresponsiveness to an agonist such as methacholine or histamine can be demonstrated. This hyperresponsiveness precedes a late (3- to 11-hour) response (167). In addition, fungus-related (mold-related) asthma may result in a need for intensive antiasthma pharmacotherapy, including inhaled corticosteroids and even alternate-day prednisone in some patients. Exposure to *A. alternata*, a major fungal aeroallergen, was considered an important risk factor for respiratory arrests in 11 patients with asthma (168). In children undergoing long-term evaluation for development of atopic conditions who have one parent with asthma or

allergic rhinitis, asthma by age 11 years was associated with exposure to high concentrations of *Dermatophagoides pteronyssinus*, a major mite allergen (169). Similar results seem likely when children of atopic parents are exposed to animals in the house. Cockroaches are another indoor allergen associated with childhood asthma (33).

The diagnosis of allergic asthma should be suspected when symptoms and signs of asthma correlate closely with local patterns of pollinosis and fungal spore recoveries. For example, in the upper midwestern United States after a hard freeze in late November, which reduces (but does not eliminate entirely) fungal spore recoveries from outdoor air, patients suffering from mold-related asthma note a reduction in symptoms and medication requirements. When perennial symptoms of asthma are present, potential causes of asthma include animal dander, dust mites, cockroach excreta, and depending on the local conditions, fungal spores and pollens. Cockroach allergen (*Bla g 1*) is an important cause of asthma in infected buildings, usually in low socioeconomic areas. High indoor concentrations of mouse urine protein (*Mus d 1*) have been identified with volumetric sampling, and monoclonal antibodies directed at specific proteins suggested additional indoor allergens. The physician should correlate symptoms with allergen exposures, support the diagnosis by demonstration of antiallergen IgE antibodies, and institute measures when applicable to decrease allergen exposure. Some recommendations for environmental control have been made (170,171), but these may not be practical to implement for many patients and their families. Detection of cat allergen (*Fel d 1*) in homes or schools never known to have cat exposure is consistent with transport of *Fel d 1* into such premises and sensitivity of immunoassays for cat allergen. The removal of an animal from a home and covering a mattress and pillow properly are interventions known to decrease the concentration of allergen below which many patients do not have clinical asthma symptoms.

Although food ingestion can result in anaphylaxis, persistent asthma is not explained by food ingestion with IgE-mediated reactions. Food production exposure, such as occurs in bakers (172), egg handlers, flavoring producers, and workers exposed to vegetable gums, dried fruits, teas (173), or enzymes (174), is known to produce occupational asthma mediated by IgE antibodies.

Nonallergic Asthma

In nonallergic asthma, IgE-mediated airway reactions to common allergens are not present. Nonallergic asthma occurs at any age range, as does allergic asthma, but the former is generally more likely to occur in subjects with asthma younger than 4 years of age or older than 60 years of age. Episodes of nonallergic asthma are triggered by ongoing inflammation or by upper respiratory tract infections, purulent rhinitis, or sinusitis. Most patients have no evidence of IgE antibodies to common allergens. In some patients, skin tests are positive, but despite the presence of IgE antibodies, there is no temporal relationship between exposure and symptoms. Often, but not exclusively, the onset of asthma occurs in the setting of a viral upper respiratory tract infection. Virus infections have been associated with mediator release and bronchial epithelial shedding, which could lead to ongoing inflammation and asthma symptoms. Commonly recovered viruses that cause asthma are picornaviruses (rhinoviruses), coronaviruses, RSV, parainfluenza viruses, influenza viruses, and adenovirus (175). Chronic sinusitis can be identified in some patients with asthma, as can nasal polyps with or without aspirin sensitivity.

Some experimental data exist on the presence of antiviral IgE antibodies and asthma (176). As our knowledge of mast cell activation grows, antiviral IgE antibodies or viral infection of lymphocytes causing cytokine production with triggering of asthma may be considered nonallergic. Indeed, the T_H2 theory of asthma was supported in part by a study finding that protection against developing asthma in children aged 6 to 13 years was associated with day care attendance during the first 6 months of life or with having two or more older siblings at home (177). The "protected" children by age 13 years had a 5% incidence of asthma, compared with 10% in children who had not attended day care or who had 1 or no sibling (177). Of note is that at 2 years of age, the ultimately protected children had a 24% prevalence of wheezing, compared with 17% in nonprotected children. Overall, the frequent exposure to other children in early childhood, which is presumably associated with more viral infections, could result in a T_H1 predominance as opposed to a T_H2 or allergy profile of $CD4^+$ lymphocytes.

Allergen immunotherapy is not indicated and will not be beneficial in patients with nonallergic asthma despite any presence of antiallergen IgE antibodies.

Mixed Asthma

The term *mixed asthma* characterizes combined allergic and nonallergic triggers of asthma. These patients experience both classic IgE-mediated asthma and nonallergic asthma that may or may not be explained by recent viral upper respiratory tract infections, purulent rhinitis, or sinusitis. An example is a patient with grass- and ragweed-induced asthma, which in the particular geographic area is a recognized cause of asthma for 5 months of the year, but asthma is perennial.

Potentially Fatal Asthma

The term *potentially fatal asthma* refers to the patient who is at high risk for an asthma fatality (63,150). These patients have one of the following criteria: (a) respiratory acidosis or failure from asthma, (b) endotracheal intubation from asthma, (c) two or more episodes of status asthmaticus despite use of oral corticosteroids and other antiasthma medications, or (d) two or more episodes of pneumomediastinum or pneumothorax from asthma. Other factors have been associated with a potentially fatal outcome from asthma, and these criteria may not identify all high-risk patients (2). The physician managing the high-risk patient should be anticipating a potential fatality and trying to prevent this outcome (127). The impossible-to-manage (because of noncompliance) patient is said to have malignant, potentially fatal asthma (153).

Aspirin-induced Asthma

Selected patients with asthma, often nonallergic, have unusual bronchial responses to aspirin and or nonselective NSAIDs (178,179). The onset of acute bronchoconstrictive symptoms after ingestion of such agents can be within minutes (such as after chewing Aspergum) to within 3 hours. Some physicians accept a respiratory response that occurs within 8 to 12 hours after aspirin or NSAID ingestion; however, a shorter time interval seems more appropriate, such as up to 3 to 4 hours. In persistent asthma, variations in expiratory flow rates occur frequently, so that confirming that aspirin produces a reaction at 8 hours requires carefully controlled studies. The most severe reactions occur within minutes to 2 hours after ingestion. With indomethacin, 1 mg or 5 mg oral challenges resulted in acute responses (180). Cross-reaction exists, such that certain nonselective NSAIDs (indomethacin, flufenamic acid, and mefenamic acid) have a higher likelihood of inducing bronchospastic responses in aspirin-sensitive subjects than other NSAIDs. Because fatalities have occurred in aspirin-sensitive subjects with asthma, challenges should be carried out only with appropriate explanation to the patient, with obvious need for the challenge (such as presence of rheumatoid arthritis), and by experienced physicians. Interestingly, some aspirin-sensitive patients can be desensitized to aspirin after experiencing early bronchospastic responses (180). Subsequent regular administration of aspirin does not cause acute bronchospastic responses (180).

The *aspirin triad* refers to aspirin-sensitive patients with asthma who also have chronic nasal polyps (181). The onset of asthma often precedes the recognition of aspirin sensitivity by years. Tartrazine (FD& C Yellow No.5) was reported to result in immediate bronchospastic reactions in 5% of patients with the aspirin triad (181). Contrary results in double-blind studies have been reported in that none of the patients responded to tartrazine (182). The risk for inadvertent exposure to tartrazine by the aspirin-sensitive patient appears to be smaller than initially reported and ranges from nonexistent (182) to 2.3% (183).

The drugs that produce such immediate respiratory responses share the ability to inhibit the enzyme cyclooxygenase-1, which is known to metabolize arachidonic acid into PGF_2 and thromboxanes. Structurally, these drugs are different but they have a common pharmacologic effect. Data suggest that the blockade of cyclooxygenase diverts arachidonic acid away from production of the bronchodilating PGE_2 and into the lipoxygenase pathway with resultant production of LTC4 and LTD4 (184,185). The latter is a potent bronchoconstrictive agonist. Aspirin-sensitive patients have higher resting $PGF_{2\alpha}$ concentrations and higher urinary LTE4 concentrations (185) than aspirin-tolerant patients with asthma. After aspirin ingestion, intolerant patients have profound increases in urinary LTE4 compared with aspirin-tolerant subjects (185). When bronchial biopsy specimens were obtained from aspirin-intolerant and aspirin-tolerant patients with asthma, there were many more cells (primarily EG2 and eosinophils, but also mast cells and macrophages) that expressed LTC4 synthase in the aspirin-intolerant patients (186). This critical finding supports the urinary LTE4 results, which are the marker for the bronchoconstrictor LTD4 that requires LTC4 synthase for generation. It has been suggested that after aspirin or NSAID ingestion, besides LTD4 production, there is a decline in the bronchodilator PGE_2. However, there is no evidence that resting (baseline) BAL fluid concentrations of PGE_2 are reduced (186). Bronchial biopsies have not identified differential staining for cycloxygenase-1, cyclooxygenase-2, 5-lipoxygenase, LTA4 hydrolase, or 5-lipoxygenase–activating protein in aspirin-intolerant versus aspirin-tolerant patients (186). The overexpression of LTC4 synthase primarily by eosinophils results in profound increases in LTD4 after aspirin or a nonselective cyclooxygenase inhibitor is ingested.

Emerging evidence suggests that selective cyclooxygenase-2 inhibitors will be tolerated safely in aspirin-intolerant patients (187). None of 27 patients with aspirin-intolerant asthma developed acute bronchospasm during an incremental challenge protocol with celecoxib (10 mg, 30 mg, 100 mg every 2 hours on day 1 and 200 mg twice on day 2) (187). Similarly negative results have been found in 15 additional patients, 12 receiving celecoxib and 3 refecoxib (188).

Occupational Asthma

Occupational asthma has been estimated to occur in 5% to 15% of all patients with asthma (76–78). Specific industry prevalence may be even higher (e.g., 16%) in snow crab processors in Canada (189). Occupational asthma may or may not be IgE mediated. When it is IgE mediated, accumulating longitudinal data support a time of sensitization followed by development of bronchial hyperresponsiveness and then bronchoconstriction (76,189). After removal from the workplace exposure, the reverse sequence has been recorded. Malo and colleagues documented that spirometry and bronchial hyperresponsiveness in patients no longer working with snow crabs reached a plateau of improvement by 2 years after cessation of work exposure (189). The assessment of patients with possible occupational asthma is discussed in detail in Chapter 25. Some workers have early, late, dual, or irritant bronchial responses, such as occur to trimellitic anhydride, which is used in the plastics industry as a curing agent in the manufacture of epoxy resins.

The differential diagnosis of occupational asthma is complex and includes consideration of irritants, smoke, toxic gases, metal exposures, insecticides, organic chemicals and dusts, infectious agents, and occupational chemicals. In addition, one must differentiate true occupational asthma from exposed workers who have coincidental adult-onset asthma not affected by workplace exposure. Some workers have chemical exposure and a compensation syndrome, but no objective asthma despite symptoms and usually a poor response to medications. One must exclude work-related neuroses with fixation on an employer as well as a syndrome of reactive airways dysfunction, which occurs after an accidental exposure to a chemical irritant or toxic gas (190,191). Atopic status and smoking do not predict workers who will become ill to lower-molecular-weight chemicals. Atopic status and smoking are predictors of IgE-mediated occupational asthma to high-molecular-weight chemicals (76). For example, Western red cedar workers display bronchial hyperresponsiveness during times of exposure, with reductions in hyperresponsiveness during exposure-free periods. It is still undetermined whether anti–plicatic acid IgE is necessary for development of Western red cedar asthma because immediate skin tests are negative and bronchial responses are present. An

in vitro assay to detect IgE to plicatic acid–human serum albumin demonstrated elevated antibodies to this conjugate in workers (192).

The complexity of diagnosing occupational asthma cannot be underestimated in some workers. Respiratory symptoms may intensify when a worker returns from a vacation but may not be dramatic when deterioration occurs during successive days at work. In patients with preexisting asthma, fumes at work may cause an aggravation of asthma without having been the cause of asthma initially.

Avoidance measures and temporary pharmacologic therapy can suffice to help confirm a diagnosis in some cases. Resumption of exposure should produce objective bronchial obstruction and clinical changes. The physician must be aware that workers may return serial peak expiratory flow rate measurements that coincide with expected abnormal values during work or shortly thereafter. Such values should be assessed critically because they are effort dependent and may be manipulated. Demonstration of IgE or IgG antibodies to the incriminated workplace allergen or to an occupational chemical bound to a carrier protein has been of value in supporting the diagnosis of occupational asthma and even in prospective use to identify workers who are at risk for occupational asthma (193). Such assays are not commonly available but are of discriminatory value when properly performed.

If a bronchial provocation challenge is deemed necessary, it is preferable to have the employee perform a job-related task that exposes him or her to the usual concentration of occupational chemicals. Subsequent blinding may be necessary as well, and successive challenges may be needed. The PC_{20} to histamine can decrease after an uneventful challenge, but the next day, when the employee is exposed to the incriminated agent again, a 30% decline in FEV_1 can occur, which confirms the diagnosis (194).

Exercise-induced Asthma

Exercise-induced asthma occurs in response to either an isolated disorder in patients with mild asthma or an inability to complete an exercise program in symptomatic patients with chronic asthma. Control of the latter often permits successful participation in a reasonable degree of exercise. In patients with mild asthma whose only symptoms might be triggered by exercise, the pattern of bronchoconstriction is as follows: during initial exercise, the FEV_1 is slightly increased (about 5%), unchanged, or slightly reduced, but no symptoms occur. This is followed by declines of FEV_1 and onset of symptoms 5 to 15 minutes after cessation of exercise. The decline of FEV_1 is at least 15% (195). Airway hyperresponsiveness does not occur, but there is an increase in expired nitric oxide (196). A subsequent decline in $FEV_{1.0}$ has been documented in 1 study at 5 hours, consistent with a dual respiratory response. However, such declines also occurred on days in which no exercise challenge was conducted (197). The greater than 32% declines in FEV_1 5 hours after exercise in association with clinical symptoms were part of variations in pulmonary physiology of asthma and might be from loss of airway caliber from withdrawal of medications (197).

Exercise-induced asthma resulting in a decline in FEV_1 of at least 15% is associated with inspiration of cold or dry air. In general, greater declines in spirometry and the presence of respiratory symptoms are seen directly proportional to the level of hyperventilation and inversely proportional to inspired air temperature and extent of water saturation. The exact mechanism of bronchoconstriction remains controversial, but it is thought that postexertional airway rewarming causes increased bronchial mucosal blood flow as a possible mechanistic explanation (198). Clinically, it has been recognized that running outdoors while inhaling dry, cold air is a far greater stimulus to bronchospasm than running indoors while breathing warmer humidified air or than swimming. It is thought that the hyperventilation of exercise causes a loss of heat from the airway, which is followed by cooling of the bronchial mucosa. The "resupply" of warmth to the mucosa causes hyperemia and edema of the airway wall (198).

Exercise-induced bronchospasm can occur in any form of asthma on a persistent basis but also can be prevented completely or to a great extent by pharmacologic treatment. In prevention of isolated episodes of exercise-induced bronchospasm, medications such as inhaled β-adrenergic agonists inspired 10 to 15 minutes before exercise often prevent significant exercise-induced bronchospasm. Cromolyn by inhalation is effective, as to a lesser extent are oral β-adrenergic agonists and theophylline. Leukotriene antagonists have a positive but more modest protective effect but suggest that LTD4 participates in exercise-induced bronchospasm (199). For patients with chronic asthma, overall improvement in respiratory status by avoidance measures and regular pharmacotherapy can minimize exercise symptoms. Pretreatment with β-adrenergic agonists in addition to regular antiasthma therapy can allow asthma patients to participate in exercise activities successfully.

Variant Asthma

Although most patients with asthma report symptoms of coughing, chest tightness, and dyspnea, and the physician can auscultate wheezing or rhonchi on examination, *variant asthma* refers to asthma with the primary symptoms of paroxysmal and repetitive coughing or dyspnea in the absence of wheezing. The coughing often occurs after an upper respiratory infection, exercise, or exposure to odors, fresh paint, or allergens. Sputum is usually not produced, and the cough occurs on a nocturnal basis. Antitussives, expectorants, antibiotics, and use of intranasal corticosteroids do not suppress the coughing. The chest examination is free of wheezing or rhonchi. McFadden (125) documented increases in large airways resistance, moderate to severe reductions in FEV_1 (mean, 53%), and bronchodilator responses. The mean residual volume was 152%, consistent with air trapping. In addition, patients with exertional dyspnea as the prime manifestation of asthma had an FEV_1 value still within normal limits but a residual volume of 236% (125) and not greatly increased airways resistance. Both types of patients had reduced small airways flow rates. Some patients can be heard to wheeze after exercise or after performing an FVC maneuver.

Pharmacologic therapy can be successful to suppress the coughing episodes or sensation of dyspnea, but often, when inhaled, β-adrenergic agonists have not been effective; the best way to suppress symptoms is with an inhaled corticosteroid. If using an inhaler produces coughing, a 5- to 7-day course of oral corticosteroids often stops the coughing (124). At times, even longer courses of oral corticosteroids and antiasthma therapy are necessary.

Factitious Asthma

Factitious asthma presents diagnostic and management problems that often require multidisciplinary approaches to treatment (158,200). The diagnosis may not be suspected initially because patient history, antecedent triggering symptoms, examination, and even abnormal pulmonary physiologic parameters may appear consistent with asthma. Nevertheless, there may be no response to appropriate treatment or in fact worsening of asthma despite what would be considered effective care. Some patients are able to adduct their vocal cords during inspiration and on expiration emit a rhonchorous sound, simulating asthma. Other patients have repetitive coughing paroxysms or "seal barking" coughing fits. A number of patients with factitious asthma are physicians and paramedical or nursing personnel or have an unusual degree of medical knowledge. Psychiatric disease can be severe, yet patients seem appropriate in a given interview. Factitious asthma episodes do not occur during sleep, and the experienced physician can distract the patient with factitious asthma and temporarily cause an absence of wheezing or coughing. Invasive procedures may be associated with conversion reactions or even respiratory "arrests" from breath holding.

Vocal Cord Dysfunction and Asthma

VCD (also called *laryngeal dyskinesia*) may coexist with asthma (134) (Fig. 22.7B). In a series of 95 patients with VCD, 53 patients had asthma. The level of medication prescriptions can be very high in patients with VCD with or without asthma (134). Of great concern is the prolonged use of oral corticosteroids for dyspnea that in fact is from VCD and not from asthma. Patients with VCD and asthma may or may or may not have insight into the VCD. Some patients

can be taught to avoid vocal cord adduction during inspiration. The diagnosis can be suspected when there is a truncated inspiratory loop on a flow-volume loop and when direct visualization of the larynx identifies vocal cord adduction on inspiration, on CT examination of the neck (201), or by bedside examination. In the latter case, the patient may have a diagnosis of asthma and be hospitalized, but although symptoms are present, the patient has limited wheezing to a quiet chest (but blood gases or pulse oximetry are not abnormal for the degree of symptoms) and unwillingness to phonate the vowel "e" for more than 3 seconds. Also, when prompted, there is no large inspiratory effort made. In the series of 95 patients, many were health care providers and females who were obese (134). GERD was present in 15 of 40 (37.5%) patients who had both VCD and asthma, compared with 11 of 33 (33%) with VCD without asthma (134). Thirty-eight percent of the 95 patients had a history of abuse, such as physical, sexual, or emotional (134). VCD should be suspected in difficult-to-control patients with asthma, in patients whose symptoms or medical requirements do not concur with the modest spirometric abnormalities or arterial blood gas findings, and in those who have prolonged hoarseness with dyspnea, wheezing, or coughing, with or without asthma.

Coexistent Asthma and Chronic Obstructive Pulmonary Disease

Usually, in the setting of long-term cigarette smoking (at least 40 pack-years), asthma may coexist with COPD. Obviously, the patients with asthma or COPD should not smoke. Multiple medications may be administered in patients with asthma and COPD to minimize signs and symptoms. However, some dyspnea likely will be fixed and not transient because of underlying COPD. The component of asthma can be significant, perhaps 25% to 50% initially. However, with continued smoking, the reversible component, even using oral and inhaled corticosteroids, β-adrenergic agonists, theophylline, anticholinergic agents, and leukotriene antagonists, diminishes or becomes nonexistent. At that point, the fewest medications possible should be used.

When there is no benefit from oral corticosteroids, it is advisable to taper and discontinue them.

Initially, such as after hospitalization for asthma, the patient with combined asthma and COPD may benefit from a 2- to 4-week course of oral corticosteroids. The effort to identify the maximal degree of reversibility should be made even when asthma is a modest component of COPD. The lack of bronchodilator responsiveness or peripheral blood eosinophilia does not preclude a response to a 2-week course of prednisone.

Long-term care of patients with coexistent asthma and COPD can be successful in improving quality of life and reducing or eliminating disabling wheezing. However, eventually, patients may succumb to end-stage COPD or coexisting cardiac failure.

NONANTIGENIC PRECIPITATING STIMULI

Hyperresponsiveness of bronchi in patients with asthma is manifested clinically by responses to various nonantigenic triggers. Examples include odors such as cigarette smoke, fresh paint, cooking, perfumes (202), cologne, insecticides, and household cleaning agents (203). In addition, sulfur dioxide, ozone, nitrogen dioxide, and carbon monoxide and combustion products, both indoors and outdoors, can trigger asthma signs and symptoms. Emergency department visits for asthma in adults in New York City were found to peak 2 days after increases in ozone in ambient air (204). The effect was most in patients who had smoked more than 14 pack-years of cigarettes (204). There was no ozone effect for adult nonsmokers or light smokers (<13 pack-years) with asthma. In this study, most patients had severe asthma, and there was no effect of relative humidity on emergency department visits. These data support an effect of ozone on patients with severe asthma who were cigarette smokers. Adverse effects of ozone were not found on light or nonsmokers. Bronchoconstriction likely occurs on an irritant basis. Effective management of patients with asthma may permit patients to tolerate most inadvertent exposures with little troubling effects. Diesel exhaust particles have been shown to stimulate increases in allergen-specific IgE antibodies and increase IL-4 and IL-13 production. Further, these particles were able to induce isotype switching from IgM to IgE antibodies in B cells (205). The public health effects of diesel exhaust particles may be very great on emergence of allergen responses.

GERD has been a recognized trigger of asthma episodes (206,207). Frank GERD with aspiration into the bronchi has been associated with chronic cough, episodic wheezing, rhonchi, and even cyanosis if aspiration is severe. Reflux of gastric acid into the lower esophagus can precipitate symptoms of asthma or cough without frank aspiration, perhaps by an esophagobronchial vagal reflex (206). Patients with asthma and GERD who underwent esophageal acid infusion have demonstrated increases in airways resistance and decreases in PEFR (206), but patients with asthma without GERD can also have these changes (206). An acute episode of asthma can cause increased negative intrathoracic pressures, which can increase reflux. Medical therapy, such as avoiding meals for 3 hours before sleeping, weight reduction, cessation of cigarette smoking, discontinuation of drugs that decrease gastroesophageal sphincter pressure (theophylline), diet manipulation, and raising the head of the bed 6 inches, may be of value. Pharmacotherapy with protein-pump inhibitors for 3 months is advisable (206). Surgical intervention is indicated rarely but has been successful in varying degrees with either laparoscopic fundoplication or open procedures in patients with large hiatal hernias or strictures or previous surgery (206).

Left-sided congestive heart failure has been associated with exacerbations of asthma. Bronchial hyperresponsiveness has been recognized in nonasthmatic patients who developed left ventricular failure. When patients with asthma develop congestive heart failure, at times, sudden episodes of wheezing dyspnea can occur in the absence of neck vein distention or peripheral edema, which would support a diagnosis of left ventricular failure. Differentiating pulmonary edema from acute asthma may be difficult in brittle cardiac patients who have severe asthma or asthma, COPD, and left ventricular failure.

Sinusitis is discussed in Chapters 19, 29 and 40 and may be associated with deterioration of respiratory status and status asthmaticus in some patients.

DIFFERENTIAL DIAGNOSIS OF WHEEZING

There are many causes of wheezing, dyspnea, and coughing individually and collectively. A partial listing follows:

I. Commonly encountered diseases or conditions
   A. Asthma
   B. Upper respiratory tract infection
      1. Bronchiolitis
      2. Croup
      3. Viruses (e.g., RSV, rhinovirus, influenza, parainfluenza)
      4. Acute and chronic bronchitis
      5. Acute pneumonia
      6. Bronchiectasis
      7. Sinusitis
      8. Purulent rhinitis
   C. Congestive heart failure
      1. Left ventricular failure
      2. Mitral stenosis
      3. Congenital heart disease
   D. COPD
   E. Hyperventilation syndrome
   F. Pulmonary infarction or embolism
   G. Cystic fibrosis
   H. Laryngotracheomalacia
   I. Bronchopulmonary dysplasia
   J. Vascular rings
   K. GERD
II. Less common conditions
   A. Tuberculosis
   B. Hypersensitivity pneumonitis
   C. Inhalation of irritant gases, odors, or dusts
   D. Physical obstruction of the upper airways
      1. Neoplasms (benign or malignant)
      2. Foreign bodies
      3. Acute laryngeal or pharyngeal angioedema
      4. Bronchial stenosis
         a. Postintubation
         b. Granulomatous
         c. Postburn
   E. Interstitial lung disease
   F. *Pneumocystis carinii* pneumonia
   G. Sarcoidosis
III. Uncommon conditions
   A. Restrictive lung disease
   B. Churg-Strauss vasculitis
   C. Mediastinal enlargement
   D. Diptheria
   E. Carcinoid tumor of main-stem bronchi
   F. Thymoma
   G. Tracheoesophageal fistula
   H. Allergic bronchopulmonary aspergillosis
   I. α_1-Antitrypsin deficiency
   J. Factitious coughing, wheezing, or stridor
   K. VCD

TREATMENT

The treatment of an episode of asthma varies according to its clinical severity. Similarly, long-term treatment regimens depend on the type of asthma and its severity. The basic objective of treatment, as in other chronic illnesses, is to achieve significant control of symptoms to prevent physical as well as psychological impairment. In addition to clinical improvement, the practical goals of treatment are best measured by avoidance of fatalities, hospitalizations, and school or work absenteeism and the ability of the patient to lead a normal, functional life with little or no impairment of exercise activities and sleep habits. The Expert Panel Report 2 of the National Heart, Lung, and Blood Institute suggested specific management protocols for patients categorized with mild, moderate, and severe asthma (2). The goals should be to maximize control of symptoms of asthma, permit as normal a lifestyle as possible, avoid nocturnal asthma, and achieve as best respiratory status as possible. Preservation of lung function to avoid excessive loss of FEV_1 per year should be another goal as a practical approach to overcoming inflammation in asthma.

Principles

The treatment of asthma consists of therapeutic measures to control inflammatory changes and to reverse bronchial mucosal edema, bronchospasm, hypersecretion of mucus, and $\dot{V}/\dot{Q}$ imbalance. Depending on the severity of the attack, various degrees of hypocarbia or hypercarbia with their resultant acid-base changes may also require specific therapy. Finally, other emergency measures may be necessary to prevent or treat acute respiratory failure.

Preventive measures are very important in the proper management of asthma. In exercise-induced asthma, appropriate premedication can prevent symptoms. In allergic asthma, removing the offending allergen or allergens is of primary importance because it can reduce symptoms, decrease the need for medication, and eventually decrease bronchial hyperresponsiveness. If this is impossible, immunotherapy should be considered (171,208,209). Protective measures must also be included to lessen the deleterious effects of certain aggravating factors, such as dust mites and fungi. In addition, drugs that precipitate asthma should be avoided.

The best approach to asthma treatment consists of determining the clinical classification (Table 22.5), the functional classification (Tables 22.6 and 22.7), necessary avoidance measures, drug therapy, allergen immunotherapy when indicated, and other conditions that may affect the patient (Table 22.8).

TABLE 22.7. *Acute asthma tips*

In the emergency department

1. Establish severity of asthma
   Cannot speak in a sentence
   Accessory muscle use?
   Cyanotic?
   Heart rate 120 beats/min or greater
   Cannot perform spirometry or peak flow
      is less than 200 L/mm
   β_2-adrenergic agonist overuse
   Marked nocturnal symptoms
2. Send the patient who clears after emergency therapy home with a short course of oral corticosteroids. Arrange follow-up care.

In the office

1. Does the patient need hospitalization or emergency therapy?
2. A combination of regular β_2-adrenergic agonist and inhaled corticosteroid may suffice. Otherwise add a short course of an oral corticosteroid.
3. Check inhaler technique.
4. Schedule follow-up care.
5. Consider referral to an allergist-immunologist.

TABLE 22.8. *Chronic asthma tips*

1. Appreciate limitations of inhaled β_2-adrenergic agonists, theophylline, and cromolyn.
2. Check and improve inhaler technique even in patients using spacer devices.
3. Reassess the patient after initial therapy and change management if satisfactory improvement has not occurred.
4. Emphasize antiinflammatory therapy as opposed to scheduled β_2-adrenergic agonists (and possibly theophylline).
5. Address allergic factors at home, school, and workplace. Consider referral to an allergist-immunologist.
6. Exclude allergic bronchopulmonary aspergillosis.
7. Many patients are managed successfully with inhaled corticosteroids and β_2-adrenergic agonists.
8. Avoid excessively demanding medication regimens.
9. Arrange for emergencies or deteriorations in respiratory status by involving the patient or family, if possible.
10. Use oral corticosteroids early to decrease asthma symptoms in a patient who has deteriorated after an upper respiratory tract infection rather than as a "last resort."
11. Identify patients with potentially fatal asthma.

Drug Therapy

β-Adrenergic Receptor Antagonists

The effects of an adrenergic agonist depend on its specific (α or β) receptor-stimulating capacity as well as on the type and density of receptor present in the organ or tissue stimulated (Table 22.9). The bronchi contain predominantly β_2-adrenergic receptors, which promote bronchodilation. β Receptors themselves may differ from organ to organ. Those in the heart are primarily β_1-adrenergic receptors, which increase cardiac contractibility and heart rate. Thus, adrenergic drugs possessing β_2-stimulating activity are most effective in the treatment of asthma (see Chapter 35).

Biochemical mechanisms of action (Fig. 22.8) of the β-stimulating adrenergic drugs have not been completely clarified, but they are known to increase the rate of formation of $3'5'$-cyclic adenosine monophosphate (cAMP) from adenosine triphosphate (ATP) in the presence of adenylyl cyclase (formerly called *adenylate* or *adenyl cyclase*). The increased cAMP in turn triggers other intermediate reactions, which ultimately result in both bronchodilation and inhibition of

TABLE 22.9. *Some effects of adrenergic stimulation*

α Stimulation	β_1 Stimulation	β_2 Stimulation	β_3 Stimulation
Vasoconstriction	Cardiac stimulation	Bronchial relaxation	Lipolysis (brown adipose tissue); heat generation
Intestinal relaxation	Chronotropic	Uterine relaxation	
Contraction of uterus	Inotropic	Vascular smooth muscle relaxation	
Contraction of ureter	Lipolysis	Stimulates skeletal muscle (tremor)	
Contraction of dilator papillae		Stimulates liver and muscle glycogenolysis	
Inhibition of insulin secretion		Stimulates skeletal muscle Na^+K^+- ATPase (hypokalemia)	

the mediator release in immediate hypersensitivity reactions. These effects reverse or inhibit some of the pathophysiologic events known to occur in asthma.

β_2-Adrenergic agonists have great value in management of asthma but limitations as well. For example, as with inhaled corticosteroids and theophylline, the dose-response curve for β_2-adrenergic agonists becomes flattened as the dose of medication is increased. In addition, aside from increasing function of cilia in epithelial cells, there seem to be almost no antiinflammatory effects from β_2-adrenergic agonists. In a study of 11 patients with allergic asthma who had dual responses upon bronchoprovocation challenges, 1 week's use of albuterol by metered-dose inhaler, 200 μg 4 times daily, was associated with a larger late asthmatic response (210). With placebo inhaler, there was a decline in FEV_1 during the early response of 17.9%, and with albuterol 21.1%, a nonsignificant trend was noted (210). However, the late asthmatic response was affected in that the placebo response was a decline in FEV_1 of 13.2%, compared with 23.1% after 1 week of albuterol (210). The conclusion was that regular, scheduled use of albuterol could cause continued airway inflammation. In this study, nonspecific bronchial responsiveness changed modestly from 1.9 mg/mL with placebo to 2.4 mg/mL with albuterol treatment (210). How much clinical effect these data have on asthma control and management has been controversial. For patients with persistent asthma, however, it has been advisable to use antiinflammatory therapy and a β-adrenergic agonist together,

trying not to use additional scheduled short-acting β_2-adrenergic agonists. Similarly, if patients receive the 12-hour β_2-adrenergic agonists salmeterol or formoterol, concurrent antiinflammatory therapy, such as inhaled corticosteroids, is advised (2). The combination of an inhaled corticosteroid and 12-hour β_2-adrenergic agonist, even scheduled, provides effective asthma control. As patients improve, less β_2-adrenergic agonist can be used, whether short acting or long acting.

A medication may be a bronchodilator, and it may or may not have bronchoprotective properties. As regards salmeterol, 24 patients with mild asthma received either salmeterol 50 μg twice daily or placebo for 8 weeks (211). Methacholine challenges were performed initially and at the end of the study. Salmeterol caused a steady, almost 10% increase in FEV_1 throughout the 8 weeks (211). There was no evidence for tachyphylaxis. Nevertheless, there was a 10-fold shift (from 1.5 to 16 mg/mL) in the PC_{20} to methacholine 1 hour after the initial salmeterol dose, meaning less responsive airways. By 4 weeks, the PC_{20} was 3 mg/mL and remained at that concentration at 8 weeks (211). Thus, although a bronchodilator effect continued, bronchoprotection was temporary and associated with tolerance (211). Somewhat similar findings have been reported with terbutaline, 500 μg given four times daily (212).

In a 16-week study of 255 patients with mild asthma, "as-needed" and "scheduled" albuterol produced similar degrees of bronchodilation and symptom control (213). Patients with moderate

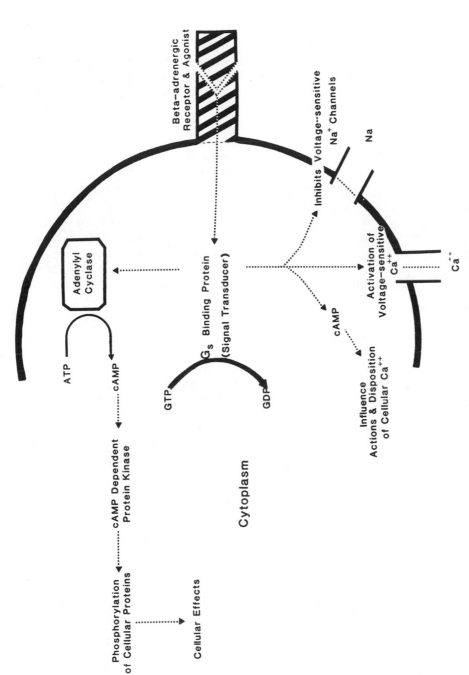

FIG. 22.8. A simplified schematic of β-adrenergic receptor stimulation. β-Adrenergic agonist stimulation of its receptor causes a conformational change in the guanine nucleotide-binding regulatory protein G_S. There is increased guanosine triphosphatase (GTPase) activity and then a transduced signal, resulting in activation of adenyl cyclase. The sequence raises the concentration of cyclic adenosine monophosphate (camp). The regulatory protein G_S couples β-adrenergic receptors to adenyl cyclase and calcium channels. G_S interacts with the sodium channel, resulting in its inhibition.

or severe persistent asthma may require scheduled salmeterol or formoterol and intermittent albuterol or other short-acting β_2-adrenergic agonist. Responses of FEV_1 to albuterol were preserved for 6 hours despite regular use of salmeterol (214). Such patients should receive antiinflammatory therapy, but even in its absence, in this study, tachyphylaxis to albuterol did not occur (214).

Excessive use of β_2-adrenergic agonists has been associated with fatalities from asthma (63,80,81,84,91,148,149) (see Chapter 35). Physicians (and pharmacists) need to be aware of overuse of metered-dose inhalers, dry-powder inhalers, or nebulizers by patients. Unlimited or unsupervised prescription refills cannot be recommended because patient self-management when asthma is worsening may result in a fatality. As an asthma attack worsens and continued β_2-adrenergic agonist therapy is used in the absence of inhaled or oral corticosteroids, there may be development of arterial hypoxemia, carbon dioxide retention, and acidosis not recognized by the patient.

Various alterations of the molecular structure of the catecholamine nucleus have resulted in a variety of antiasthma drugs (Fig. 22.9).

Epinephrine

Epinephrine, administered intramuscularly, because of its potent bronchodilating effect and rapid onset of action, is an alternative therapy but is not recommended for ambulatory use by inhalation in acute asthma. It directly stimulates both α- and β-adrenergic receptors. The recommended adult dose is 0.30 mL of a 1:1000 solution administered intramuscularly. In infants and children, the dose is 0.01 mL/kg, with a maximum of 0.25 mL. The dose may be repeated in 15 to 30 minutes if necessary. Nebulized racemic epinephrine is also effective but is used less commonly today unless a patient has upper airway obstruction (epiglottitis or stridor).

Some side effects of epinephrine include agitation, tremulousness, tachycardia, and palpitation. Hypertension in the presence of acute asthma often resolves with epinephrine administration.

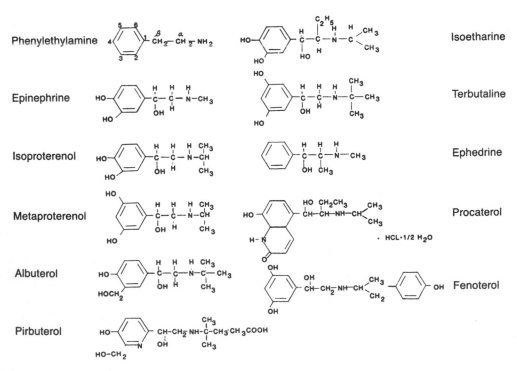

FIG. 22.9. The chemical structures of sympathomimetic drugs compared with those of phenylethylamine.

This occurs because of a decrease in bronchospasm and as a result of a decrease in peripheral vascular resistance by stimulation of β_2 receptors in smooth muscle of blood vessels in skeletal muscle. Epinephrine must be administered with caution in patients with cardiovascular disease and hypertension but should not be considered contraindicated when bronchospasm is significant if albuterol is not being used. Epinephrine is rapidly metabolized and in the emergency setting can be administered once and repeated once or twice to determine whether wheezing can be cleared. The maximum bronchodilator effect of epinephrine given intramuscularly is not less than that of inhaled β-adrenergic agonists and occasionally in the severely obstructed patient exceeds what can be gained by aerosol therapy. Although epinephrine is an old drug, it is expedient, effective, and rapidly metabolized. In patients experiencing an episode of anaphylaxis, epinephrine remains the drug of choice.

Ephedrine

Ephedrine, although less potent than isoproterenol, albuterol, and epinephrine, was used for decades because it was effective by oral administration and possessed a longer duration of action (3 to 6 hours). Its onset of action is about 1 hour, with a peak effect of 2 to 3 hours. Ephedrine stimulates α- and β-adrenergic receptors directly and indirectly. Ephedrine is an integral component of some nonprescription combination oral preparations available for treatment of asthma. The adult dose is 25 mg four times daily. Adverse effects of ephedrine include central nervous system stimulation. Ephedrine is an outdated drug for antiasthma therapy. The 25-mg ephedrine capsule has been shown to have about the same efficacy as 2.5 mg of terbutaline. Unfortunately, 50 mg of ephedrine is used by motor vehicle drivers as a central nervous system stimulant, not a bronchodilator.

Albuterol

Albuterol is the leading short-acting β_2-adrenergic agonist. Comparable bronchodilation occurs with use of metered-dose inhalers and nebulizers, although larger doses of albuterol are necessary during nebulization because of the nebulizer's inefficiency (215). In acute asthma, adults may receive three 2.5-mg doses every 30 minutes by nebulization. This protocol was compared with two 5-mg aerosolized treatments given 40 minutes apart (216). Both protocols were effective. The initial PEFR was 35% to 39% in the two groups. Both treatment groups were able to improve the PEFR to about 60%, although the 5-mg doses produced a somewhat faster bronchodilator response. The outcomes from treatment were separated by whether patients were released from the emergency department or whether hospitalization occurred. Discharged patients whose presentation PEFR was 43% improved their PEFR to 72.5%, whereas hospitalized patients whose initial PEFR was 29% improved to about 40% (216) (Table 22.10). These data differentiate the patients with an adequate response to emergency department treatment from those who have status asthmaticus, defined by an inadequate response to two or three albuterol treatments.

Continuously nebulized albuterol solution for treatment of acute episodes of asthma has consisted of preparing 7.7 mL of 0.5% albuterol in 100 mL of saline. A pump infuses the solution initially from 14 to 26 mL/h while the nebulizer supplies 100% oxygen. However, initial studies have not demonstrated superior results compared with repeated nebulized albuterol administration (217).

Fenoterol

Fenoterol is structurally similar to metaproterenol and is a β_2-selective adrenergic agonist. Fenoterol is not approved for use in the United States. It is available as a metered-dose inhaler, and the dosage is 2 inhalations every 6 hours. A 0.5% solution is available for nebulization. Because an excess number of fatalities have been reported in patients who used more than 1 canister per month (149), caution is advised (81).

Salmeterol

Salmeterol is a potent β_2-adrenergic agonist with a long half-life, so that administration is 1 to

TABLE 22.10. *Effect of two dosage regimens of albuterol in patients treated for acute asthma in the emergency department*

	Presentation PEFR (%)	Posttreatment PEFR (%)	
		After albuterol 7.5 mg[a]	After albuterol 10 mg[b]
Patients	40		73
Discharged	43	72	
Patients	33		41
Hospitalized	26	35	

PEFR, peak expiratory flow rate.
[a] Nebulized albuterol, 2.5 mg, given at 20-min intervals.
[b] Nebulized albuterol, 5.0 mg, given initially and at 40 min.
Data abstracted from McFadden ER, Strauss L, Hejal R, et al. Comparison of two dosage regimens of albuterol in acute asthma. *Am J Med* 1998;105:12–17, with permission.

2 inhalations every 12 hours. It is 50 times more potent experimentally than albuterol but provides similar peak bronchodilation as albuterol. Each metered-dose inhaler provides the equivalent of 25 µg salmeterol per actuation. Units contain either 60 or 120 actuations. A shorter-acting β_2-adrenergic agonist may be added 4 to 6 hours after use of salmeterol. However, antiinflammatory (bronchoprotective) therapy should be administered concurrently. A combination salmeterol and fluticasone diskus is available as Advair, containing 50 µg of salmeterol and 100, 250, or 500 µg of fluticasone.

Formoterol

Formoterol is similar to salmeterol in that the bronchodilator effect is for 12 hours. The drug is administered by inhalation and has its onset of action within 5 minutes. Its maximum bronchodilator effects are similar to those of salmeterol or albuterol administered every 6 hours. For patients with moderate or persistent asthma, formoterol should be used with antiinflammatory therapy, such as inhaled corticosteroids.

Levalbuterol

Levalbuterol is available as a nebulized inhalation solution of either 0.63 or 1.25 mg. It can be administered three times a day. Levalbuterol is about 4 times as potent as albuterol nebulized solution; 0.63 mg of levalbuterol provided comparable bronchodilation to 2.5 mg of albuterol (218). Its place in therapy remains to be established. It is indicated for children 12 years of age and older and for adults.

The variety of β_2-adrenergic agonists and their formulations are listed in Table 22.11.

Adverse Effects of β_2-Adrenergic Therapy

Aerosols containing adrenergic drugs have been used in the treatment of asthma for 45 years. The immediate relief of this form of therapy has made it widely acceptable to both patients and physicians. Unfortunately, some patients develop an almost addictive relationship with their inhalers, which results in excessive use and risk. The most common side effects are related to β_1 stimulation, resulting in cardiac symptoms as listed previously with epinephrine. Potential adverse effects from β_2-adrenergic agonists include overuse, systemic absorption across bronchial mucosa, delay in receiving antiinflammatory therapy, and fatality.

Although subjective and objective improvement of airway obstruction is produced by inhaled β agonists, the associated hypoxemia of asthma is not improved and may be increased. This probably results from enhancing the already existing $\dot{V}/\dot{Q}$ imbalance by either increasing aeration of those alveoli already overventilating in relation to their perfusion or by reestablishing ventilation to nonperfused alveoli. Absorption of β-adrenergic agonists from bronchial mucosa may result in systemic effects, such as increased

TABLE 22.11. *β-Adrenergic agonists*

Name	Single entity formulation
Albuterol	Proventil, Ventolin inhalation aerosol
	Proventil HFA inhalation aerosol
	Proventil, Ventolin inhalation solution 0.5%
	Ventolin rotocaps 200 μg
	Ventolin syrup 2 mg/5 mL
	Proventil tablets 2 mg, 4 mg
	Proventil repetabs 4 mg
	Volmax extended-release tablets 4 mg, 8 mg
Salmeterol	Serevent inhalation aerosol
	Serevent Diskus
Levalbuterol	Xopenex inhalation aerosol 0.63 mg, 1.25 mg
Pirbuterol	Maxair inhaler
	Maxair Autohaler
Metaproterenol	Alupent inhalation aerosol
	Alupent syrup, tablets 10 mg/5 mL, 10 mg, 20 mg
Terbutaline	Brethine Ampuls 1 mg/mL
	Brethine tablets 2.5 mg, 5 mg
Formoterol	Foradil aerolizer inhalation powder
Fenoterol	Berotec inhalation solution 0.5%
	Berotec inhalation aerosol
	Combinations
Albuterol	Combivent inhalation aerosol
Ipratropium bromide	
Salmeterol	Advair Diskus 100/50, 250/50, 500/50
Fluticasone	Fluticasone 100 μg, salmeterol 50 μg
	Fluticasone 250 μg, salmeterol 50 μg
	Fluticasone 500 μg, salmeterol 50 μg

cardiac output (219). $\dot{V}/\dot{Q}$ mismatching would occur by perfusion of underventilated alveoli. The resultant hypoxemia is usually clinically insignificant, unless the initial PO_2 is on the steep portion of the oxygen–hemoglobin dissociation curve (i.e., less than 60 mm Hg). In moderately severe acute asthma, oxygen should be administered to correct the hypoxemia.

Of concern is the paradoxical response of increased bronchial obstruction seen in occasional patients using β_2-adrenergic agonists by inhalation. With an exacerbation of asthmatic symptoms, these patients may overuse inhalation therapy because of a decreasing response to proceeding inhalations. A cycle begins of increasing obstruction with increasing use of the aerosol. This pattern precedes status asthmaticus or asthma fatality. Patients identified as using β-adrenergic agonist inhalation or nebulizers excessively should have this therapy terminated or monitored more aggressively. The physician should begin a short course of prednisone to control underlying bronchoconstriction and airway inflammation. Overuse of β-adrenergic agonists

can be defined as more than manufacturer's recommendations or perhaps daily scheduled use even at manufacturer's recommendations. For short- to moderate-duration bronchodilators such as albuterol, pirbuterol, or terbutaline, I believe that the recommended scheduled use is neither dangerous nor unsafe in terms of control of asthma. However, as stated previously, as-needed but not overused β_2-adrenergic therapy should be a goal. Unanticipated fatality in patients with asthma who rely on β_2-adrenergic agonists remains a source of concern and a public health issue.

Practical Considerations in Using β_2-Adrenergic Receptor Agonists

Proper technique is essential. Patients may fail to expire fully to functional residual capacity (FRC) before actuating their metered-dose inhaler or dry-powder inhaler. Other patients may inhale too rapidly to total lung capacity (TLC), take a submaximal inspiration, flex the neck during inspiration, forget to shake the canister before actuation, or not hold breath for 8 to 10 seconds after a full inspiration. Some patients activate the inhaler twice during 1 inhalation. All of these variables may decrease drug delivery to the lung periphery and explain poor therapeutic responses. Rarely, the inhaler cap can be inhaled inadvertently, or coins, paper clips, or capsules stored inside the metered-dose inhaler cap may be inhaled. When effective synchronization of inhalation with actuation of the air inhaler cannot be corrected, improvement in patient care may be achieved by discontinuing the inhaler and using dry-power inhalers or spacer devices.

A number of devices have been developed in an effort to improve the dynamics of aerosol administration by a pressurized inhaler. (See Chapter 37) Some of these include the tube spacer (10 × 3.2 cm), aerochamber, and collapsible reservoir aerosol system (when inflated, it is 11.5 cm long and 9 cm in diameter), among others. These devices attempt to minimize aerosol deposition in the oropharynx and increase delivery to the airways. Further, by necessitating a slower inspiration, more drug may be distributed to obstructed peripheral airways than with a rapid inspiration, which favors central airway deposition at the expense of the peripheral airways.

Motor-driven nebulizers do not result in greater bronchodilation than that achieved with pressurized metered-dose aerosol canisters (220). Drug delivery by motor-driven nebulizers has been considered more efficacious because the patient inhales a relatively large concentration of drug from the nebulizer. For example, the dose of albuterol added to the nebulizer is 5 mg, which is 56 times the dose generated by the pressured canister (90 μg). However, it has been demonstrated that perhaps 15% to 20% of the drug is actually nebulized during inspiration, and only 10% of the nebulized dose would reach the bronchi (220). Thus, the dose delivered to the lung from the nebulizer may be similar to that given by a pressurized aerosol canister. The delivery system can also cause nosocomial infections. On the other hand, it has been suggested that motor-driven nebulizers formalize the process of drug administration and do not require the patient to learn correct inhalation technique as for the metered-dose inhalers (220).

In summary, the physician should become familiar with a few bronchodilators and emphasize proper inhalation technique. In some patients, spacer devices or breath-activated units improve drug delivery. Physicians should recheck the patient's inhaler technique periodically because errors are made frequently that impede drug delivery and because some patients use delivery devices improperly. The goal should be to have the patient use β_2-adrenergic agonists intermittently rather than on a scheduled basis.

It must be recognized that, useful as the β_2-adrenergic agonists are, even combined with inhaled corticosteroids, leukotriene antagonists, cromolyn, theophylline, and nedocromil, they are not capable of controlling some cases of severe, persistent asthma. This limitation must be kept in mind, and oral corticosteroids should be used when appropriate.

Corticosteroids

Overview

Corticosteroids are the most effective drugs in the treatment of asthma (see Chapter 34). Parenteral corticosteroids are indicated for the treatment of status asthmaticus, but objective evidence of improvement in flow rates and FEV_1 requires about 12 hours of therapy (221). In some patients, beneficial effects occur by 6 hours (222,223). Short-term outpatient administration decreases the incidence of return visits to emergency medical facilities (224,225). High-dose budesonide (1,600 μg daily) resulted in almost a 50% reduction in relapses (12.8% versus 24.5%) over a 21-day follow-up period in a study in which all patients received prednisone, 50 mg daily for the first 7 days after treatment in the emergency department (226). Chronic administration prevents work and school absenteeism, disabling wheezing, and episodes of status asthmaticus or respiratory failure in patients with severe asthma. A double-blind study in acutely ill children supported their efficacy as well (227). Because of their potentially serious side effects, their systemic use is advised only when other measures have not provided sufficient control of acute or chronic symptoms. Their indiscriminate employment in mild asthma is not indicated.

Failure to use them when indicated, however, may result in unwarranted morbidity and mortality. In life-threatening asthma, corticosteroids are essential, but because of their delayed onset of action, they cannot replace other necessary emergency measures, including β-adrenergic agonists, patent airway, and oxygen. Patients who are still wheezing after initial emergency treatment with β_2-adrenergic agonists are in status asthmaticus and should receive systemic corticosteroids. Patients who must be hospitalized for exacerbations of asthma should receive systemic corticosteroids immediately without attempting to determine whether continued β-adrenergic agonists (or theophylline) will work without systemic corticosteroids.

Oral corticosteroids are of value in prevention of repeated emergency room visits or office visits in acutely ill patients who respond to β-adrenergic agonists and do not require hospitalization. A prednisone dosage regimen of 30 to 50 mg each morning for 5 to 7 days is often effective in adults, and in children 1 to 2 mg/kg prednisone is necessary, often the latter dosage for the first few days.

The exact mode of action of corticosteroids is complex (see Chapter 34 and references 112 and 228), but they have many antiinflammatory effects (Table 22.12). As valuable as inhaled corticosteroids are, they cannot "do everything." For example, after allergen bronchoprovocation challenges, there are increases in bone marrow CD34[+] (mast cell) progenitor cells and eosinophil and basophil colony-forming units (229). These findings suggest that asthma is truly a systemic disorder, but budesonide, 400 μg inhaled daily for 8 days could not prevent this activation of the bone marrow. In this study, budesonide did inhibit the early and late bronchial responses to allergen challenge and the number of eosinophils in sputum, but not the bone marrow responses. Not to minimize their important effects in the treatment of asthma, in a study of 16,941 subjects enrolled in a health maintenance organization, inhaled corticosteroids and cromolyn in children were associated with about a 50% reduction in risk for hospitalization, compared with patients who did not receive inhaled corticosteroids (230). There was no dose-

TABLE 22.12. *Antiinflammatory effects of corticosteroids in asthma*

- Reduction of symptoms (cough, wheezing, dyspnea) from asthma
- Decreases mucus production and sputum eosinophilia
- Increases the ratio of ciliated columnar cells to goblet cells in the bronchial epithelium
- Improves oxygenation and time to discharge after status asthmaticus
- Reduces recidivism to emergency departments after acute therapy
- Can prevent deterioration leading to status asthmaticus
- Reduces need for β_2-adrenergic agonists in persistent asthma
- Improvement in morning expiratory flow rates and intraday variation
- Partial inhibition of the late bronchoconstrictive responses to aerosol allergen provocation after one dose of inhaled corticosteroid
- Partial inhibition of the early and late bronchoconstrictive responses to aerosol allergen provocation after 1 week of inhaled corticosteroids and early response after 1 week of prednisone
- Modest lessening of nonspecific bronchial hypersensitivity
- Reduction in recovery of eosinophils and mast cells in bronchoalveolar lavage
- Reduction of eosinophils, mast cells in the respiratory epithelium and lamina propria
- Reduction of numbers of activated (CD25[+] and HLA-DR[+]) lymphocytes in bronchoalveolar lavage and mucosa
- Reduction of *ex vivo* bronchoalveolar (macrophage) cell synthesis of leukotriene B$_4$ and thromboxane B$_2$
- Reduction in bronchoalveolar lavage cells expressing mRNA for interleukin-4 (IL-4) and IL-5 with an increase in interferon-γ–positive cells
- Increased numbers of intraepithelial nerves
- Regeneration of bronchial epithelium

response relationship noted for inhaled corticosteroids regarding avoidance of hospitalizations from asthma (230).

In addition to their therapeutic importance, corticosteroids may be useful as a diagnostic tool. Often, it is helpful to document the extent of reversibility of a patient's signs and symptoms to establish whether the basic underlying process is asthma or irreversible obstructive airways disease. Therapeutic doses of corticosteroids for 7 to 14 days should significantly reverse the airway obstruction of asthma in almost all patients but would result in little or no reversal in most patients with chronic bronchitis or emphysema. The initial therapeutic dose of prednisone in children is 1 to 2 mg/kg/day and in adults is 40 to 80 mg per day.

To minimize side effects, it is important to use these drugs for the shortest time necessary to achieve the clinical goal. A 3- to 5-day course of prednisone in therapeutic doses may be sufficient to reverse an occasional acute episode of asthma that has not responded adequately to the common modes of therapy, such as inhaled corticosteroids and β_2-adrenergic agonists. If oral corticosteroids are required for longer periods, abrupt discontinuation may be followed by the return of acute symptoms. Until significant clearing of signs and symptoms of asthma occur, prednisone or the equivalent should be administered at a steady dosage rate over the first 1 to 2 weeks. In a small group of patients who have abruptly discontinued corticosteroids after prolonged use, a withdrawal syndrome may occur, consisting of malaise, emotional lability, myalgia, and low-grade fever.

In patients requiring maintenance oral therapy, the lowest possible dose (preferably, alternate-day dosing) compatible with adequate control of symptoms should be used, and there should be use of inhaled corticosteroids as well. There is a relatively flat dose-response curve for inhaled corticosteroids, especially when increases in FEV_1 are used as an end point (231). Perhaps it is not surprising that adding a long-acting β_2-adrenergic agonist to a moderate dose of inhaled steroid achieved greater increases in FEV_1 and PEFR than did doubling the inhaled corticosteroid dose (232–234). Some patients have better control of asthma on moderate- to high-dose inhaled corticosteroids and can have prednisone tapered or discontinued. These patients should have little need for β_2-adrenergic agonists over time as the airway inflammation recedes.

Measures to prevent or correct abnormalities in bone mineral metabolism induced by oral corticosteroids or high-dose inhaled corticosteroids require cooperative patients and physician expertise. Estrogen replacement therapy has proven value in prevention of bone loss in postmenopausal women and should be administered. Regular gynecologic examinations are necessary. Prevention of osteopenia is of paramount importance and should begin early because bone mass increases until about 45 years of age (or earlier) and then declines over years. Exercise, lack of sedentary lifestyle, avoidance of cigarette smoking, excessive alcohol consumption, and overuse of thyroxine in euthyroid or possibly hypothyroid patients are some additional factors to address in terms of bone formation. In addition, adequate calcium intake of 1,000 mg or more and of vitamin D, 400 to 1,000 IU daily, are advisable (235). Oral corticosteroids, if necessary on a long-term basis, should be administered as alternate-day therapy with short-acting agents such as prednisone or methylprednisolone. Split daily doses should be avoided in stable ambulatory patients. Maximal dosage inhaled corticosteroids should be used, but not to a degree that would affect bone density. Patients with established osteoporotic fractures may require biphosphonates, fluorides, estrogens, and calcium supplementation.

A potentially serious side effect from corticosteroids is suppression of the HPA axis. This results in an impaired ability to tolerate stress, and for this reason, patients must receive increased doses of corticosteroids during stressful situations such as surgery, infectious illness, and even exacerbations of asthma. The extent of suppression, however, is variable from patient to patient. The time required for a return to normal HPA activity after discontinuation of corticosteroids also varies and is unpredictable. In a rare patient, inability of the HPA axis to respond to stress may continue for up to 1 year after the cessation of therapy; in other patients, normal HPA reactivity may persist despite their taking corticosteroids for as long as 10 years. Fortunately, surgery with modern anesthesia techniques rarely results in maximal adrenal output of about 300 mg cortisol; output is more likely 100 mg (236).

Maximal doses of inhaled corticosteroids on a daily basis should be used when indicated. To minimize the occurrence of adverse side effects from oral corticosteroids, the use of alternate-day prednisone therapy is recommended. The total daily dose of a short-acting corticosteroid preparation (prednisone, prednisolone) should be taken in the morning every 48 hours, as long as underlying airways obstruction is controlled adequately. Daily prednisone is indicated in the acutely ill patient. Often, a short course (5 to 7 days) of daily prednisone is required to control asthma. Alternate-day prednisone therapy should be considered for patients who still require corticosteroids after 3 weeks of daily medication of severe asthma. Most patients obtain adequate control of symptoms by this form of therapy, with little, if any, deterioration in pulmonary function on the alternate-day schedule (237).

Although major side effects are not usually observed in patients receiving less than 20 mg of prednisone daily (administered as a single morning dose), the physician should convert to an alternate-day regimen. One common mistake is to attempt to accomplish the conversion too rapidly. If a patient has been receiving split doses of prednisone on a daily basis, the first goal should be to establish control of the severe asthma with a single morning dose of prednisone. Once the patient is stable, tripling the daily dose on alternate days may be adequate for control of the disease. Close patient supervision is essential during this critical changeover period. Some patients will not tolerate alternate-day steroid therapy even with very large doses of prednisone and should be managed on daily steroids using a single morning prednisone dose. The half-life of prednisolone is about 200 minutes in patients requiring daily prednisone or alternate-day prednisone, and other pharmacokinetic parameters are similar (238).

Parenteral Corticosteroids

Intravenous corticosteroids are employed generally for status asthmaticus. Hydrocortisone (Hydrocortone Phosphate), methylprednisolone, and dexamethasone (Decadron Phosphate) are available. (It is possible to manage status asthmaticus with oral corticosteroids if access is difficult or if there are shortages of parenteral agents.)

For malignant, potentially fatal asthma, intramuscular Depo-Medrol can be a short-term consideration. It is available in 20-, 40-, and 80-mg/mL preparations. For adults who can be considered unreliable, a dose of 40 to 120 mg can be given to try to prevent a hospitalization or potential fatality from asthma. Regular administration should be avoided unless there is no other alternative.

Inhaled Corticosteroids

Bronchial mucosa atrophy has not been described in patients who have used topical corticosteroids in recommended doses, even for decades. Because of the absence of serious side effects and with the impressive array of antiinflammatory effects (Table 22.12), primary monotherapy of asthma with inhaled corticosteroids continues to be recommended (see Chapter 34). In newly diagnosed patients with mild asthma, budesonide, 600 μg twice daily, was considered superior to inhaled terbutaline, 375 μg twice daily (239). Patients were treated for 2 years with this moderately high dose of budesonide and then received budesonide, 400 μg/day or placebo (240). Not surprisingly, patients who received budesonide had better asthma control (FEV$_1$, peak flow, and bronchial responsiveness) than patients who received the placebo. Further, patients who initially had received terbutaline improved after therapy with 1,200 μg/day of budesonide (240). (The physician should individualize the therapeutic options for patients with persistent asthma and verify that IgE-mediated triggering allergens are avoided.)

Theophylline

Theophylline is not essential in the management of asthma for the ambulatory patient or for the hospitalized patient (see Chapter 36). The most important pharmacologic action of theophylline (1,3-dimethylxanthine) is bronchodilation. Other properties of the drug include central respiratory stimulation, inotropic and chronotropic cardiac effects, diuresis, relaxation of vascular smooth muscles, improvement in ciliary action, and reduction of diaphragmatic muscle fatigue.

Theophylline has been shown *in vitro* to increase cAMP concentrations by inhibiting phosphodiesterase, the enzyme that converts 3'5'-cAMP to 5'-AMP. However, the inhibition of phosphodiesterase by theophylline was accomplished with concentrations that would be toxic *in vivo*; thus, theophylline's mechanism of action is unclear but is unlikely attributable to phosphodiesterase inhibition. A possible explanation for bronchodilation from theophylline is adenosine antagonism (241) (see Chapter 36).

Optimal bronchodilation from theophylline is a function of the serum concentration. Maximal bronchodilation is usually achieved with concentrations between 8 and 15 μg/mL. Some patients achieve adequate clinical improvement with serum theophylline levels at 5 μg/mL or even lower. The explanation for this phenomenon is that the bronchodilator effect of theophylline, as measured by percentage increase in FEV_1, is related to and fairly dependent on the logarithm of the serum level concentration (242). A dose-related improvement in pulmonary function was reported in six patients. The mean improvement in FEV_1 was 19.7% with theophylline concentration 5 μg/mL, 30.9% at 10 μg/mL, and 42.2% at 20 μg/mL. Two methods of graphic presentation of these data are shown in Figure 22.10. At these concentrations, improvement in pulmonary function occurs in linear fashion with the log of the theophylline concentration. However, using an arithmetic scale on the abscissa, improvement in pulmonary function occurs in a hyperbolic manner. Thus, although continued improvement occurs with increasing serum concentrations, the incremental increase with each larger dose decreases. About half of the improvement in FEV_1 that is achievable with a theophylline concentration of 20 μg/mL is reached with concentration of 5 μg/mL and 75% of the improvement is reached with a concentration of 10 μg/mL.

Theophylline is of value in mild to moderate asthma and may be well tolerated if peak concentrations are 8 to 15 μg/mL. It can be of help in patients with asthma and COPD. Compared with inhaled β-adrenergic agonists administered with inhaled corticosteroids, theophylline may add no apparent additional benefit (243,244). In treatment of acute asthma, however, metaanalysis of 13 studies did not reveal a benefit of aminophylline over adrenergic agonists (245). The indications for theophylline or aminophylline remain problem patients with asthma and COPD, steroid-phobic patients, and perhaps patients who cannot afford inhaled corticosteroids.

Cromolyn

Cromolyn sodium (Intal) was shown to be effective in preventing bronchospasm from inhaled

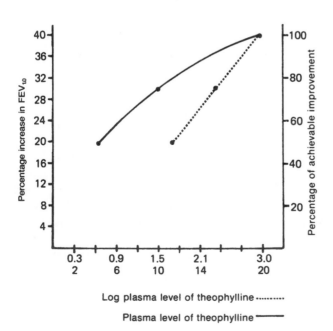

Log plasma level of theophylline ··········

Plasma level of theophylline ——

FIG. 22.10. Percentage of increase in forced expiratory volume in 1 second (FEV_1) plotted against increasing concentration of theophylline. The log of the corresponding theophylline concentration is plotted on an arithmetic scale.

allergens and exercise for 35 years (see Chapter 36). It has been used in the United States since 1973 and has a very high therapeutic index. It is available as a metered-dose inhaler containing 112 or 200 actuations or by nebulized aerosol inhalation. Ampules contain 20 mg of cromolyn in 2 mL of diluent. Intal can be added to a nebulizer containing a β-adrenergic agonist such as albuterol for inhalation. An HFA formulation of the metered-dose inhaler was found comparable to the older inhaler, and patients had a 28% to 33% reduction in asthma symptoms after cromolyn administration, compared with placebo (246).

Nedocromil

Nedocromil (Tilade) is an NSAID that experimentally inhibited both early and late bronchial responses to allergen (see Chapter 36). Nedocromil inhibits afferent nerve transmission from respiratory nerves, so that substance P may be limited in its effect as a bronchoconstrictor or trigger of cough. It can also decrease nonspecific bronchial hyperresponsiveness (247). Nedocromil is administered by metered-dose inhaler, with each actuation delivering 1.75 mg. The canister contains 112 inhalations, and the initial dosage for children aged 12 years and older and adults is 2 inhalations four times daily. The dosage may be reduced as improvement (cessation of coughing) occurs. Some adverse effects include unpleasant (bitter) taste and slight temporary yellowing of teeth from the inhaler contents. Use of a spacer device is helpful.

Nedocromil is efficacious in patients with mild to moderate asthma and in patients who require inhaled corticosteroids (248). If it does not help reduce the dose of inhaled corticosteroids or reduce symptoms after 1 to 2 months of use, it should be discontinued.

Leukotriene Antagonists

Montelukast (Singulair) and zafirlukast (Accolate) are leukotriene receptor antagonists, and zileuton (Zyflo) is an inhibitor of the 5-lipoxygenase enzyme that catalyzes synthesis of leukotrienes. All these medications can block de-clines in FEV_1 from exercise, allergen challenge, and aspirin administration (199,249,250) (see Chapter 36). Administration of montelukast or zafirlukast to adults with persistent mild to moderate asthma results in reduced symptoms and increased FEV_1 up to 13%, compared with a placebo response of 4.2% (251). Comparable results were reported in children 6 to 14 years of age (252). These findings support the concept that leukotrienes contribute to airway tone. In adult patients "incompletely controlled" with inhaled beclomethasone dipropionate, $200 \mu g$ twice daily, montelukast 10 mg or placebo was added. The combination drugs produced 6% increases in FEV_1, compared with no change with continued beclomethasone dipropionate (253). Days with asthma symptoms decreased by 25%, and asthma attacks decreased by 50% (253). These findings demonstrate that control of asthma extends beyond bronchodilator responses. The leukotriene receptor antagonists can help some patients lower their dosage of inhaled corticosteroids.

Zileuton can also cause bronchodilation (14.6% versus 0% for placebo using FEV_1 after 60 minutes) (254). Because zileuton must be administered frequently, it is much less convenient than zafirlukast or montelukast, and liver function must be measured.

Next-generation leukotriene receptor antagonists or 5-lipoxygenase inhibitors presumably will be even more effective than the currently available products.

Anticholinergic Agents

Anticholinergic agents diminish cyclic guanosine monophosphate concentrations and inhibit vagal efferent pathways. Bronchodilation then could occur in a multiplicative fashion when ipratropium bromide is administered with albuterol (Combivent inhalation aerosol). Monotherapy with anticholinergic bronchodilators will not replace β_2-adrenergic agonists in acute asthma, in that the onset of action is slower and effect smaller than with β_2 adrenergic agonists. Combination therapy in acute asthma possibly is superior to albuterol alone, but whether this approach is clinically important is not clear. Combivent is useful for patients with asthma and COPD, perhaps because of the relative influence of cholinergic tone in COPD.

Nonspecific Measures

Protection from Meteorologic Factors

Increasing air pollution is a known worldwide health hazard. It is considered to be a major causative factor in certain conditions such as bronchitis, emphysema, and lung cancer. Urban surveys have demonstrated the deleterious effect of pollution on patients with chronic cardiopulmonary disease. The alarming morbidity and mortality rates resulting from thermal inversions in cities in the United States and elsewhere have dramatized the seriousness of stagnating pollution. The patient with asthma, because of inherent bronchial hyperreactivity, may be more vulnerable to air pollution. However, asthma death rates have increased over time when air quality has improved (144).

Industrial smog results from incomplete combustion of fossil fuels, and it consists of sulfuric acid, sulfur dioxide, nitrogen dioxide, carbon monoxide, and particulate material. Photochemical smog occurs from the action of ultraviolet radiation on nitrogen oxides or hydrocarbons from automobile exhaust. Ozone is the major constituent of photochemical smog. Clinical and immunologic effects of excessive diesel fumes are under investigation.

Other meteorologic factors, such as sudden changes in temperature, increases in relative humidity, and increasing or decreasing barometric pressure, may also aggravate asthmatic symptoms in some patients. It is impossible to protect patients from these changes entirely. Why weather changes should aggravate asthma remains completely understood. The breathing of cold, dry air is a potent stimulus that precipitates symptoms in many patients. The use of scarves or facemasks may be beneficial in these patients.

Home Environment

Certain controls of the internal environment of the home (especially the bedroom) are benefi-cial. Extremes of humidity can adversely affect the patient with asthma; the optimal humidity should range from 40% to 50%. Low humidity dries the mucous membranes and can be an irritative factor, although it helps to desiccate house dust mites.

Most patients benefit from air conditioning, but in a few patients, the cold air may increase symptoms. The reduction in spore counts in air-conditioned homes in part results from simply having the windows closed to reduce the influx of outdoor spores (255).

Mechanical devices that purify circulating air may be helpful but are not essential. Conventional air filters such as those in a typical furnace vary in their effectiveness but in general remove only particles larger than 5 μm (e.g., pollens). Many inhalant particles, such as dust mites, fumes, smoke, some fungal spores, some rat urinary proteins, some cat allergen, bacteria, and viruses, are smaller than 5 μm. Efficient air-cleaning devices include the electrostatic precipitator, which attracts particles of any size by high-voltage plates; nonelectronic precipitators, useful for forced air heating systems; other, more efficient furnace filters; and air cleaners that use a high-efficiency particulate accumulator filtering system. The latter have helped reduce clinical symptoms, which is the primary requirement of any filtering system (256). In general, an animal in the home environment produces too great a quantity of dander to be removed or reduced by air cleaners. Sensitive immunoassays have documented presence of mouse urinary protein (*Mus d 1*) in indoor environment air samples. Similar findings occur with cockroach fecal particles or saliva (*Bla g 1*) (33). Control measures can be difficult in such conditions but should be encouraged. It is not possible to reduce indoor concentrations of house dust mite (*Der p 1*) to a mite-free level. Clinical benefit to dust mite–sensitive patients, however, occurs if some avoidance measures are instituted. It is advisable that the mattress, box spring, and pillow be covered with special zippered encasings. Window blinds should be cleaned regularly or not installed, and attention to other dust collection sites should be given. Rugs should be vacuumed each week, and dust mite–trapping vacuum sweeper bags should be used. In that *Der p 1* is heat labile (but *Der p 2* is not), some benefit has been reported of steam-cleaning carpets and upholstery along with applying dry heat (>100°C) to mattresses and blinds (257). Concentrations of both *Der p 1* and *Der p 2* were reduced for 1 year with that intensive treatment (257).

The presence of moist basements and crawl spaces may provoke acute or chronic symptoms in certain patients allergic to fungal spores. Dehumidification and more effective drainage are advised. Patients with mold-induced asthma should not sleep or work in moldy basements.

Smoking

Cigarette smoking must be discouraged in all patients and their family members. Its deleterious effects probably result from bronchial irritation and impairment of antibacterial defense mechanisms. Cigarette smoke has been shown to impair mucociliary transport and to inhibit alveolar macrophage phagocytosis. Patients with asthma who continue to smoke often require progressive increments in medication. Keeping a patient with asthma controlled with medication while the patient continues to smoke is not good practice of medicine. When emphysema occurs, episodes of asthma may be tolerated poorly and may result in frequent hospitalizations or in respiratory failure.

Passive smoking by nonasthmatic subjects has been associated with statistically significant reductions in expiratory flow rates. This finding raises the possibility that some patients with asthma may experience increased symptoms in smoke-filled office rooms or homes.

Exercise

The subjective and psychological value of physical conditioning can be a helpful adjunct in treatment. A unique feature of asthma is the occurrence of exercised-induced bronchospasm. Many children or adults may be discouraged by their inability to participate in sports or to withstand other normal exertional activities. These feelings of inferiority or anger promote additional physical and psychological incapacitation. An exercise program, once asthma has been stabilized with appropriate therapy, will result in a noticeable increase in physical capacities and hopefully self-image and self-confidence. Inhaled β_2-adrenergic agonists, inhaled cromolyn, or inhaled nedocomil taken 15 to 30 minutes before exercise will decrease postexercise bronchospasm. Some patients require two medications to suppress symptoms. It is advisable to inquire about the patient's current exercise tolerance and participation in sports because this is a good guide to overall therapy. Some patients find that use of an inhaled corticosteroid or leukotriene antagonist on a regular basis allows full exercise or sports activities without need for other medications.

Drugs to Use Cautiously or to Avoid

Antidepressants of the monoamine oxidase inhibitor class are not recommended because these substances may induce a hypertensive crisis when taken with sympathomimetic drugs that are commonly used in the medical treatment of asthma. The tricyclic antidepressants are much less likely to produce this complication and can be used with asthma medications.

Narcotics, such as morphine and meperidine, and other sedating medications are contraindicated during exacerbations of asthma. Moreover, morphine can activate mast cells to release histamine. Asthma should not be considered primarily as an expression of an underlying psychological disturbance, and its diagnosis alone is not an indication for the use of antidepressant or anxiolytic medications.

Excessive use of hypnotics for sleep must also be discouraged. Nocturnal reductions in PO_2 occur regularly in normal subjects and in patients with asthma. Status asthmaticus is a contraindication for the use of soporific drugs. In this situation, even small doses of these drugs may cause respiratory depression.

Drugs possessing anticholinesterase properties may potentiate wheezing. This results from their parasympathomimetic-enhancing effect due to the inhibition of acetylcholine catabolism. These drugs represent the primary drug treatment of myasthenia gravis; if asthma coexists, a therapeutic problem arises. When anticholinesterases are necessary, maximal doses of β_2-adrenergic agonists and inhaled corticosteroids may be necessary. The addition of oral corticosteroids may be indicated for more adequate control of asthma, but it must be remembered that, in some patients, myasthenic symptoms may initially worsen with addition of oral corticosteroids (258).

β-Adrenergic blocking drugs have gained wide clinical use in the treatment of cardiac arrhythmias, angina, hypertension, asymmetric septal hypertrophy, myocardial infarction, thyrotoxicosis, and migraine. These drugs exert blocking properties on both cardiac and pulmonary β receptors. As a result of the effect on the latter, β blockers may enhance or trigger wheezing in overt and latent asthmatic patients. The adrenergic receptors of the lung are predominantly β_2 in type, and they subserve bronchodilation. When these receptors are blocked, bronchoconstriction may result. Should selective or nonselective β_2-adrenergic antagonists be required in a patient with asthma, cautious increase in dose with close supervision is recommended. Acute bronchospasm has been associated with conjunctival instillation of timolol for glaucoma (259).

Bronchoconstriction has been described even for betaxolol, a β_1-adrenergic antagonist, which is less likely to cause declines in FEV_1 than timolol (260). Occasionally, parasympathomimetic agents, such as pilocarpine, administered in the conjunctival sac can cause bronchospasm (260). It is advisable to make certain that the patient with persistent asthma is first stabilized, such as with inhaled β_2-adrenergic agonists and inhaled corticosteroids, so that any possible effects from necessary ophthalmic drugs are minimized.

Angiotensin-converting enzyme inhibitors have been associated with cough and asthma (or pharyngeal or laryngeal angioedema), even after the first dose (261,262). Discontinuation of the angiotensin-converting enzyme inhibitor is associated with rapid resolution of symptoms. This class of drugs and angiotensin II antagonists are not contraindicated in patients with asthma in the absence of prior adverse reactions such as cough or acute angioedema.

Specific Measures

Allergic Asthma

Specific allergy management must be included in the treatment regimen of allergic asthma. When one allergen is the primary cause (e.g., animal dander) and can be removed from the environment, symptomatic relief is achieved, often within 1 to 2 months. Most allergic patients, however, are sensitive to more than one allergen, and many allergens cannot be removed completely. In adults, inhalant allergens are the most frequent causative agents. Foods are almost never the cause of asthma, except occasionally in children and infants, but they often are incriminated erroneously.

Patients may attribute their respiratory symptoms to aspartame or monosodium glutamate when such associations are not justified. Exposure to sulfur dioxide from sodium or potassium metabisulfite used as an antioxidant in foods can cause acute respiratory symptoms in patients with asthma. However, patients with stable asthma who are managed by antiinflammatory medications will not be affected significantly by metabisulfite.

Certain basic environmental controls in the house are advisable. Dacron (or hypoallergenic) pillows are preferred and should be enclosed in zippered encasings. Box springs and mattresses should be enclosed similarly. In some situations, additional cleaning or removal of rugs (especially old ones) is beneficial.

Other aspects may be considered with regard to the environmental control in the home. Basement apartments, because of increased moisture, are most likely to have higher levels of airborne fungi and mite antigens. For the highly dust-allergic patient, appropriate furnace filters and precipitators should be used and maintained properly. In patients with perennial symptoms, it is generally advisable that pets (e.g., cats, dogs, and birds) be removed from the house if there are symptoms from contact or if there is a positive skin test. Nevertheless, most patients do not remove the pet as advised. The physician and patient must then rely on pharmacologic therapies.

When environmental control is either impossible or insufficient to control symptoms, allergen immunotherapy should be included as a form of immunomodulation. Efficacy in asthma has been documented for pollens, dust mite, and *Cladosporium* species (171,208). Other than very modest effects, immunotherapy with cat dander extracts has not been impressive in reducing symptoms when the cat remains in the home environment.

Johnstone and Dutton (263), in a 14-year prospective study of allergen immunotherapy for asthmatic children, have shown that 72% of the treated group were free of symptoms at 16 years of age, as compared with only 22% of the placebo group. Similar data have been generated again in that rhinitis patients who received allergen immunotherapy had less emergence of asthma than rhinitis patients who did not receive allergen immunotherapy (264).

Nonallergic Asthma

Treatment of nonallergic asthma primarily involves the judicious use of pharmacologic therapy.

Convincing evidence is available that virus-induced upper respiratory infections initiate exacerbations of asthma. Important agents for children 1 to 5 years of age include RSV, parainfluenza virus, and rhinovirus; for older children and adults, influenza virus, parainfluenza virus, and rhinovirus are important. Adenovirus infection rarely acts to initiate asthma attacks.

Annual influenza vaccination should be administered according to the Centers for Disease Control and Prevention recommendations for children and adults. Prompt treatment of secondary bacterial infections, such as purulent bronchitis, rhinitis, or sinusitis, is desirable. Pneumococcal vaccine can be administered to patients with persistent asthma, although pneumococcal pneumonia is an infrequent occurrence.

Aspirin-sensitive Asthma

Treatment of aspirin-sensitive asthma is similar to that of nonallergic asthma, except for those patients in whom there is clinical and skin test evidence of contributing inhalant allergy. It is important to avoid aspirin and NSAIDs, which may also produce adverse reactions. Patients must be informed that numerous proprietary mixtures contain aspirin, and they must be certain to take no proprietary medication that contains acetylsalicylic acid. Acetaminophen may be used as a safe substitute for aspirin, and other salicylates, such as sodium salicylate, choline magnesium trisalicylate, or salsalate, can be taken safely. The ingestion of aspirin or NSAIDs by these patients commonly causes acute bronchoconstriction. Other patients respond with urticaria, angioedema, or a severe reaction resembling anaphylaxis. Some physicians include both groups of patients as aspirin reactors, but others consider that the group in whom aspirin causes asthma differs from the group in whom urticaria, angioedema, or the anaphylactic type of reaction occurs. Emerging data suggest that the mechanisms include the blockade of cyclooxygenase-1, reduced production of the bronchodilating PGE_2, and production of LTD4. Reduced risk appears to be the case with the cyclooxygenase-2 inhibitors (187,188).

The exact mechanism by which these patients become intolerant to aspirin and the other substances is not known, but there is overexpression of LTC4 synthase (186). The relationship that this intolerance bears to rhinitis, nasal polyposis, and asthma is unclear. A property common to all these substances is their antiinflammatory effect. Aspirin and nonspecific NSAIDs inhibit cyclooxygenase-1, which metabolizes arachidonic acid into prostaglandins and thromboxanes. Compared with patients with asthma, patients with aspirin-sensitive asthma have increased baseline urinary concentrations of LTE4, a marker of 5-lipoxygenase products. After aspirin ingestion, there is even greater increase in urinary LTE4 concentrations, consistent with synthesis of the potent agonist LTD4 (184,185).

In aspirin-sensitive asthma, potentially dangerous drugs must be avoided. In some situations, provocative dose testing with either aspirin or NSAIDs may be carried out to confirm the diagnosis. The physician should be in attendance at all times because of the explosiveness and severity of these reactions. Pulmonary function parameters and vital signs should be measured. Aspirin should be administered in serial doubling doses, beginning with 3 or 30 mg (12,265). If 650 mg of aspirin has been given and there is not a 20% decrease in FEV_1, it is unlikely that aspirin is significant in the patient's condition. When test dosing with tartrazine, FD& C Yellow No. 5, begin 1 mg, 5 mg, 15 mg, and 29 mg every hour (266). Tartrazine sensitivity is not found in the absence of aspirin sensitivity. The aspirin (or NSAID) challenge as described previously may be dangerous and should not be done without a clear indication. The physician should be experienced in this type of challenge, and the patient should be fully informed about potential risks and benefits.

Serial test dosing with aspirin in patients with aspirin-sensitive asthma has been reported as a possible specific therapeutic modality. Patients received increasing doses of aspirin as follows every 2 hours: 3 or 30 mg, 60 mg, 100 mg, 150 mg, 325 mg, and 650 mg. When a decrease in FEV_1 of 25% was achieved, the provoking dose was repeated every 3 to 24 hours until no bronchospastic response occurred. Patients then were treated for 3 months with aspirin and, as a group, experienced fewer nasal symptoms, but unfortunately only half of patients had a reduction in asthma symptoms (267). The use of prednisone and other antiasthmatic medications was not different after aspirin desensitization. Thus, although it is possible to administer aspirin cautiously to patients with proven bronchospastic responses to aspirin, the subsequent administration of aspirin for a 3-month period did not alter the severity of asthma, with only a few exceptions. The administration of aspirin or NSAIDs to aspirin-sensitive patients should be reserved for selected patients when it is necessary to confirm the diagnosis of aspirin hypersensitivity or to administer aspirin or related drugs for another disease (such as rheumatoid arthritis) for which suitable alternatives are not satisfactory.

Potentially Fatal Asthma

The diagnosis of potentially fatal asthma (defined earlier) is helpful because it identifies high-risk patients who are more likely to die from asthma (63). Despite aggressive intervention, such as early and intensive pharmacotherapy,

allergen avoidance, and psychological evaluation, the death rate was found to be 7.1%, which is much greater than the asthma death rate overall of 0.0017% (63). Potentially fatal asthma patients do not have an inexorably fatal condition, in that stabilization and clinical improvement can occur if patients are managed effectively and are compliant with office appointments and other factors. Some patient factors that complicate care of potentially fatal asthma and result in noncompliance include psychological or psychiatric conditions (schizophrenia, bipolar disorder, personality disorders), chaotic dysfunctional family, denial, anger, lack of insight, ignorance, and child abuse by proxy. In the latter situation, some parents refuse to permit essential medications such as prednisone to be administered to their children despite previous episodes of respiratory arrest or repeated status asthmaticus. Some physician factors that can contribute to ineffectively managed patients and potential fatalities include (a) lack of appreciation for limitations in effectiveness of β-adrenergic agonists, theophylline, and the combination in increasingly severe asthma; (b) fear of prednisone; (c) failure to increase the dosage of prednisone or to administer prednisone when asthma exacerbations occur, such as during an upper respiratory tract infection; (d) lack of availability; (e) excessively demanding regimens; and (f) limited understanding of importance of a quiet chest on auscultation in severely dyspneic patients.

In survivors of episodes of *nearly fatal asthma*, defined as acute respiratory arrest, presentation with PCO_2 of at least 50 mm Hg, or impaired level of consciousness, blunted perceptions of dyspnea were identified when patients were hospitalized, but these normalized (268). Similarly, the ventilatory response to inhalation of carbon dioxide was not different from that of other patients with less severe asthma or nonasthmatic subjects (268). However, abnormal respiratory responses to decreases in inspired oxygen were identified (115). This group of patients with potentially fatal asthma does not demonstrate persistent physiologic abnormalities that identify them as having intrinsically precarious asthma.

Potentially fatal asthma can be treated with inhaled corticosteroids, inhaled β_2-adrenergic agonists, and usually alternate-day or rarely daily prednisone in compliant patients. It is advisable to institute the nonspecific general areas of care discussed previously. In contrast, in patients with malignant, potentially fatal asthma, depot corticosteroids (Depo-Medrol) can be administered after appropriate documentation is made in the medical record and the patient is informed. As for other types of asthma, prevention of fatalities and status asthmaticus involves understanding asthma, knowing the patient, instituting stepwise but effective therapy, establishing a physician–patient relationship, and emphasizing early therapy for increasingly severe asthma.

Personal peak flow monitoring will not help the unreliable, noncompliant patient. A personal peak flow monitor possibly will improve asthma if it can formalize antiasthma therapy in the otherwise noncompliant patient.

CLINICAL MANAGEMENT

Treatment of the Acute Asthmatic Attack

In mild attacks, the use of inhaled or oral bronchodilators every 4 to 6 hours may suffice. Inhaled β_2-adrenergic agonists can be administered by metered β_2-adrenergic dose inhaler with or without a spacer device, depending on patient technique, or by nebulizer. Patients must be advised about their proper use and warned against overuse. However, aqueous epinephrine, 1:1,000 given intramuscularly, is an acceptable alternative. The dose should be repeated in 15 to 20 minutes if necessary. More than three doses are not recommended. After the acute attack has subsided, regular and continuous use of bronchodilators should follow for at least 3 to 5 days. Most patients benefit from concurrent inhaled corticosteroids with or without a short course of oral corticosteroid (e.g., prednisone, 1 to 2 mg/kg for children and 40 to 60 mg for adults). When signs and symptoms of asthma are refractory to two treatments with inhaled β_2-adrenergic agonists or epinephrine, status asthmaticus exists, a medical emergency requiring corticosteroids. Its treatment is presented later and Chapter 28) (Tables 22.13 and 22.14).

Because tachyphylaxis to β_2-adrenergic agonists has been demonstrated *in vivo* and *in vitro* in some studies, concern has been expressed that prior administration of β-adrenergic agonists may abrogate clinical response from

---

TABLE 22.13. *Initial treatment of status asthmaticus*

1. Corticosteroid therapy (give immediately in the office or emergency department). Methylprednisolone (Solu-Medrol), 0.5–1.0 mg/kg intravenously every 6 hours; or hydrocortisone (Solu-Cortef), 4 mg/kg intravenously every 6 hours; or prednisone, 1 mg/kg orally every 6 hours.
2. β-Adrenergic agonists
   Choice of approaches available:
   a. Aerosolized therapy; albuterol, levabuterol, metaproterenol, terbutaline, or other agent. Repeat in 30 minutes, then at reduced frequency. May use continuous nebulization of albuterol.
   b. Epinephrine, 0.01 mL/kg of 1:1000 solution, intramuscularly not to exceed 0.3–0.4 mL in adults. May repeat twice at 20-minute intervals, then at reduced frequency.
   c. If a patient does not respond to a, try b.
3. Hospitalize
4. Laboratory studies
   White blood cell count with differential
   Chest radiograph
   Pulse oximetry or arterial blood gas
   Serum electrolytes and chemistries
   Sputum Gram stain, culture, and sensitivities (some cases)
   Bedside spirometer may be useful, but not essential
   Electrocardiogram
5. Oxygen therapy; 2–3 L/min nasal cannula (best guided by arterial blood gas determination)
6. Correct dehydration
7. Aminophylline therapy (controversial.) Check theophylline concentration if chronic therapy. Administration is discouraged because efficacy has been questioned during emergency use.
8. Antibiotic therapy. When indicated for purulent rhinitis, bronchitis, or sinusitis.
9. Impending or acute respiratory failure. Repeat β-adrenergic agonists; endotracheal intubation with assisted or controlled ventilation.

TABLE 22.14. *Spirometry and blood gases in asthma as related to the stage or severity*

	FEV$_1$	Vital capacity	Po$_2$(normal, 90–100 mm Hg)	Pco$_2$(normal, 35–40 mm Hg)	pH (normal, 7.35–7.43 mm Hg)
Stage I (respiratory alkalosis)	↓	Normal	Normal	↓	>7.43
Stage II (respiratory alkalosis)	↓↓	↓	↓	↓↓	>7.43
Stage III	↓↓↓	↓↓	↓↓	35–40	7.35–7.43
Stage IV (respiratory acidosis)	↓↓↓↓	↓↓↓	↓↓↓	↑↑↑	<7.35

FEV$_1$, forced expiratory volume in 1 second; ↑, increased; ↓, reduced.

current emergency treatment of asthma. Failure of a patient to improve suggests increasingly severe asthma (bronchospasm, hyperinflation, mucus plugging of airways), not tachyphylaxis to β-adrenergic agonists. Conversely, in patients using salmeterol regularly but for whom emergency department care for asthma was required, nebulized albuterol at 2.5 or 5.0 mg produced similar improvement in PEFR, compared with patients who had not been using salmeterol (269). The responses to albuterol were not impaired. Typically, the PEFR improved from about 200 L/min (40% predicted) to 300 L/min (60% predicted) (269). The patients who were hospitalized (32%) did not respond to albuterol, which is the definition of status asthmaticus.

There may be a modest benefit of using ipratropium bromide with nebulized albuterol (270–272), but other studies have found no advantage (273,274). Although ipratropium bromide is safe, its bronchodilating effect is small. In a study of children, when asthma was stratified into severe asthma and moderate asthma, fewer hospitalizations occurred in the former patients (52.6% versus 37.5%) when ipratropium bromide, 500 μg, was included with albuterol and prednisone or prednisolone, 2 mg/kg (271).

Treatment of Persistent Asthma

The management of persistent asthma entails a continuous broad control that should be tailored to each patient. Features of general management, as discussed previously, must be included in the treatment regimen. Significant allergic factors are treated by environmental control combined with appropriately administered allergen immunotherapy. In each patient, secondary contributing factors must be evaluated and controlled as best as possible. Some of these factors include

cessation of smoking, compliance with medications, and treatment of concurrent medical conditions, such as sinusitis, GERD, COPD, congestive heart failure, and medication intolerance.

Patients with persistent asthma require some form of antiinflammatory therapy (preferably inhaled corticosteroids, but cromolyn, nedocromil, and leukotriene receptor antagonists or inhibitors are acceptable in some situations). In those patients with mild intermittent symptoms, inhaled or oral β_2-adrenergic agonists taken only when or before symptoms occur may suffice. A patient who has asthma only with infection should be instructed to begin β_2-adrenergic agonists and inhaled corticosteroids at the first sign of coryza. Some children who wheeze only with upper respiratory infections may need to use bronchodilators or inhaled corticosteroids (or both) regularly because of the chronicity of pulmonary function abnormalities in asthma and frequent viral upper respiratory syndromes in children. This point needs to be explained clearly to the parents to obtain maximal benefit of the antiasthma medications. Patients with persistent symptoms clearly require chronic daily medication (2) used properly (with or without a spacer device). Some plan for regular or intensified therapy is indicated, as for times when symptoms are not controlled by ongoing medications.

If the patient has corticosteroid-dependent asthma with nocturnal symptoms, effective control of these symptoms may be achieved either by increasing the morning prednisone dose or by increasing the use of inhaled corticosteroids.

A patient being treated with chronic bronchodilator therapy using either β_2-adrenergic agonists, theophylline, ipratropium bromide, or a combination of these agents may have an exacerbation of asthma. For these patients, additional

β_2-adrenergic agonists may result in side effects. Additional theophylline may result in toxicity. Short-term oral corticosteroid therapy may be the most appropriate therapy. If longer use of corticosteroids or more frequent courses are required, inhaled corticosteroids and alternate-day prednisone should be considered after the patient has improved (Table 22.14).

Cromolyn, nedocromil, leukotriene receptor antagonists, or a combination of these should be tried in some patients. When cromolyn is used properly in persistent asthma, certain patients show definite improvement. Cromolyn can also be used prophylactically for intermittent but unavoidable animal exposure. If added to inhaled corticosteroid therapy on a scheduled basis, the additional benefit of cromolyn may or may not be seen. However, a 1- to 2-month trial of cromolyn, nedocromil, or leukotriene antagonist should be attempted. If unsuccessful, inhaled corticosteroid and alternate-day prednisone should be administered.

Because of their frequent recurrence, it is generally advisable that surgical removal of nasal polyps be considered only after local corticosteroid aerosol treatment, coupled with good medical and allergy management, have not been effective in decreasing obstruction and infection. Sinus surgery should also be considered when more conservative treatment (medical and allergic) has resulted in little or no success in preventing recurrent sinusitis. Referral for surgery typically occurs when patients have four sinus infections per year, asthma episodes clearly triggered by acute sinusitis, or sinusitis resistant to medical therapy and in patients in whom allergic fungal sinusitis is suspected (see Chapter 24).

Anxiety or depression may aggravate asthma. When these conditions are present, antidepressants may be necessary. Psychological or psychiatric evaluation should be obtained. Occasionally, it has been assumed by the lay public as well as by some members of the medical profession that asthma is primarily an expression of an underlying psychological disturbance. This attitude has inappropriately prevented proper medical and allergy management in some patients. In most patients, psychiatric factors are of little to no significance in the cause of the disease.

Psychological factors may be a contributory aggravating factor in asthma, but this point should not be construed as evidence that asthma is predominantly psychological. Asthma is a chronic disease that also may be associated with significant impairment of physical and social activity. These factors in themselves may lead to the development of psychological dysfunction. Often, when symptoms of asthma are brought under control, concomitant improvement of psychological dynamics occurs. When schizophrenia and corticosteroid-dependent asthma coexist, the physician may become frustrated because of the patient's prednisone phobia, medication or appointment noncompliance, and abuse of emergency medical facilities (64,157). Depot methylprednisolone (Depo-Medro) may be beneficial or lifesaving in patients if they keep their medical appointments.

The decision to use a peak flow meter should be kept in perspective. If the patient is under effective control of asthma such that exercise tolerance is satisfactory, nocturnal wheezing is absent or infrequent, emergency room visits are not happening, and symptoms of asthma are uncommon or mild, little benefit from a peak flow meter will occur. If the peak flow meter can help emphasize patient compliance with antiasthma measures and medication, its addition to a regimen will be valuable. Some patients submit peak flow diaries consistent with their expectations or perceptions of asthma. Other patients do not contact their physicians or intensify therapy for peak flow rates of 30% of predicted, nullifying any value to the patient or physician. There may be discrepancies between measurements of PEFR and FEV_1, resulting in overestimation or underestimation of the FEV_1 (275).

Treatment of Intractable or Refractory Asthma

Intractable asthma refers to persistent, incapacitating symptoms that have become unresponsive to the usual therapy, including moderate to large doses of oral corticosteroids and high-dose inhaled corticosteroids. These cases fortunately are few, and most involve patients with the nonallergic or mixed type of asthma. Their constant medical and nonmedical requirements are heavy social and financial burdens on their families. Further, these patients may have cushingoid features from daily prednisone use. Most patients with intractable asthma, however, are not deficient in antiproteases. Their asthma may represent an intense inflammatory process with marked bronchial mucosal edema, mucus plugging of airway, and decreased lung compliance and more easily collapsible airways instead of a primary bronchospastic state. In cases of intractable asthma, a home visit by the physician may be beneficial for the patient as well as for the physician. For example, the finding that an animal resides in the home of a patient with atopic intractable asthma may explain the apparent failure of corticosteroids to control severe asthma. Also, when speaking to the patient by telephone, a physician's overhearing of a barking dog may provide the explanation for the difficulty controlling the asthma.

Some cases of intractable asthma include those patients with severe, corticosteroid-dependent asthma in whom adequate doses of corticosteroids have not been used, either by physician or patient avoidance. After initiation of appropriate doses of prednisone and clearing of asthma, many cases can be controlled with alternate-day prednisone and inhaled corticosteroids or with corticosteroids alone. Others require moderate to even high doses of daily prednisone for functional control. Fortunately, this latter group is small. Occasionally, it includes patients with severe lung damage from allergic bronchopulmonary aspergillosis or with irreversible asthma (141). Other patients may have asthma and COPD, with most or their disease being COPD. Improvement of asthma can be achieved pharmacologically, but the irreversible obstructive component cannot be altered significantly.

In an attempt to reduce the prednisone dosage in patients with intractable asthma (severe corticosteroid-dependent asthma), some physicians have recommended using methylprednisolone (Medrol) and the macrolide antibiotic troleandomycin in an effort to decrease the prednisone requirement. Although prednisone dosage can be reduced, the decreased clearance of methylprednisolone by the effect of troleandomycin on the liver still may result in cushingoid obesity or corticosteroid side effects, at times exceeding prednisone alone. Therefore, methylprednisolone and troleandomycin are reduced as the patient improves. This approach has little to offer. The antifungal drug itraconazole also decreases metabolism of methylprednisolone.

High doses of intramuscular triamcinolone have been recommended and are effective therapy but were associated with expected adverse effects, such as cushingoid facies, acne, hirsutism, and myalgias (276). In adults, methotrexate (15 mg/week) was found to be steroid sparing in a group of patients whose daily prednisone dosage was reduced by 36.5% (277). A double-blind placebo-controlled trial over a shorter period, 13 weeks, did not disclose a benefit of methotrexate, in that both methotrexate and placebo-treated patients had prednisone reductions of about 40% (278). Such a finding is consistent with the observation that entry into a study itself can have a beneficial effect. The use of methotrexate (and drugs like azathioprine) remains experimental. Cyclosporine has also been disappointing and appears to provide only prednisone-sparing effects that are not sustainable after cyclosporine is discontinued (279).

In a study of the natural history of severe asthma in patients who required at least 1 year of prednisone in addition to other pharmacotherapy (β-adrenergic agonists, theophylline, and high-dose inhaled corticosteroids), avoidance measures, and possibly immunotherapy, prednisone-free intervals occurred that even lasted for several years (280). It was uncommon to have greater prednisone requirements, although usually, in these severe cases of asthma, prednisone dosages were stable over time, or reductions occurred. Adequate "wash-in" periods are needed in studies of such patients; otherwise, credit may be given to a new therapy inappropriately.

The administration of gold therapy for asthma has been described but is associated with recognized toxicity (281).

Studies with dapsone, hydroxychloroquine, and intravenous gammaglobulin (282–284) are not convincing in the management of difficult cases of asthma. Nebulized lidocaine (40 to 160 mg, 4 times daily) has been investigated in adults (285) and children (286). Its role remains to be established. In steroid-dependent patients, a confounding factor is unrecognized respiratory or skeletal muscle weakness. Although this may result from use of intravenous corticosteroids and muscle relaxants (287–289), it can have residual effects (289). Every attempt must be made to reduce the prednisone dose and eventually to use alternate-day prednisone if possible.

The term *glucocorticoid-resistant* has been applied to patients with asthma who did not improve after 2 weeks of prednisone or prednisolone administration (40 mg daily for week 1, 20 mg daily for week 2) (290,291). Experimentally, glucocorticoid receptor downregulation on T lymphocytes has been identified, suggesting that such patients may have impaired inhibition of activated T lymphocytes in asthma. For example, dexamethasone *in vitro* did not inhibit T-lymphocyte proliferation to the mitogen phytohemagglutinin in glucocorticoid-resistant subjects (291).

STATUS ASTHMATICUS

Status asthmaticus is defined as severe asthma unresponsive to emergency therapy with β_2-adrenergic agonists. It is a medical emergency for which immediate recognition and treatment are necessary to avoid a fatal outcome. For practical purposes, status asthmaticus is present in the absence of meaningful response to two aerosol treatments with β_2-adrenergic agonists or with intramuscular epinephrine (two or three injections).

A number of factors have been shown to be important in inducing status asthmaticus and contributing to the mortality of asthma. About half of patients have an associated respiratory tract infection. Some have overused sympathomimetics before developing refractoriness. In the aspirin-sensitive asthmatic patient, ingestion of aspirin or related cyclooxygenase-1 inhibitors may precipitate status asthmaticus. Exposure to animal dander (especially cat dander) in the highly atopic patient may contribute to development of status asthmaticus, particularly when this is associated with a respiratory infection. Withdrawal or too sudden reduction of corticosteroids may be associated with the development of status asthmaticus. In many situations, both the patient and physician are unaware of the severity of progression of symptoms, and often earlier and more aggressive medical management would have prevented status asthmaticus. The inappropriate use of soporific medications in the treatment of status asthmaticus has contributed to the development of respiratory failure. Overdose of theophylline has been cited as a cause of death or cardiac arrest in some patients.

Status asthmaticus requires immediate treatment with high-dose corticosteroids (292) either parenterally or orally. Patients with status asthmaticus must be hospitalized where close observation and ancillary treatment by experienced personnel are available. If respiratory failure occurs, optimal treatment often involves the combined efforts of the allergist-immunologist, pulmonary disease critical care physician, and anesthesiologist.

Initial laboratory studies should include a complete blood count, Gram stain with culture and sensitivity of the sputum, chest radiograph, serum electrolytes, and chemistries, pulse oximetry, and perhaps arterial blood gas studies (Table 22.14). A bedside spirometer may be helpful in determining and following ventilatory parameters. However, there may be considerable improvement during treatment of status asthmaticus without improvement in FEV_1 or vital capacity. This apparent lack of spirometric improvement occurs even though the hyperinflation of lung volumes is diminishing in association with a reduction in the elastic work of breathing. Of these laboratory aids, blood gas determinations are probably the most valuable. They are important not only in guiding therapy but also in providing a true assessment of severity.

These determinations allow the classification of asthma into four stages of severity (Table 22.14). Stage I signifies the presence of airway obstruction only. Because of the associated hyperventilation, the PCO_2 is low, and the pH is therefore slightly alkalotic (respiratory alkalosis). The PO_2 in stage I is normal. Spirometric study shows only a decrease in FEV_1, with a normal vital capacity. As symptoms progress, obstruction of the airway increases, compliance decreases, and air trapping and hyperinflation develop. As a result of the latter changes, the FRC increases, and the vital capacity is decreased. In stage II, $\dot{V}/\dot{Q}$ imbalance with hypoxemia occurs. These changes, however, are not enough to impair net alveolar ventilation; thus, although PO_2 is lowered, PCO_2 remains low, and an alkalotic pH persists. With progressive severity, net alveolar ventilation decreases, and a transitional period exists (stage III), in which the PCO_2 increases and the pH decreases, so that now both values appear to be normal. When the blood gas study shows hypoxemia in the presence of a normal PCO_2 and pH, close supervision and frequent determinations of pH and PCO_2 are essential to evaluate the adequacy of treatment and the possible progression to respiratory failure characterized by hypoxemia and elevated PCO_2 (stage IV). Clinical observation alone is inadequate in determining the seriousness of status asthmaticus (292).

Treatment

Although many patients with status asthmaticus manifest signs of fright, restlessness, and anxiety, the use of anxiolytic drugs is contraindicated. Appropriate therapy for status asthmaticus eventually controls the anxiety as the asthma improves. Even small doses of soporific medications may suppress respiratory drive to an extent sufficient to induce respiratory failure.

Some patients in status asthmaticus are dehydrated. The hyperventilation and increased work of breathing cause water loss through the lungs and skin. Also, because of their respiratory distress, many patients have not maintained an adequate fluid intake.

Intravenous solutions of 5% dextrose, alternating with 5% dextrose in normal saline, constitute basic caloric, sodium, and chloride requirements. In patients with a compromised cardiovascular system, sodium and water overload must be avoided. Because a high dose of corticosteroids is used in these patients, adequate potassium supplementation must be included in the intravenous therapy. In some adults, 80 mEq of potassium chloride per 24 hours (not to exceed 20 mEq/hour) is indicated. Frequent serum electrolyte determinations provide the best guide for continued electrolyte therapy.

It is no longer considered that aminophylline should be administered. If it is used, which would be an unusual situation, aminophylline should be given intravenously using constant infusion and being cognizant of serum theophylline concentrations and drug interactions.

Because nearly all patients are hypoxemic, oxygen therapy is required. Ideally, blood gas determinations should guide proper therapy. Therapeutically, a PO_2 of 60 mm Hg or slightly higher is sufficient. This often can be accomplished with low flow rates of 2 to 3 L/min by nasal cannula. Ventimasks calibrated to deliver 24%, 28%, and 35% oxygen may also be used. The necessity for higher concentration of oxygen to maintain a PO_2 of 60 mm Hg usually signifies the presence of thick tracheobronchial secretions and of $\dot{V}/\dot{Q}$ mismatch. Also, β_2-adrenergic agonists initially may cause a mild decrease in PO_2 by increasing pulmonary blood flow to poorly ventilated alveoli, increasing $\dot{V}/\dot{Q}$ mismatch. Oxygen helps protect against this effect. It is cautioned that, in patients with asthma complicated by COPD, chronic hypercapnia may be present, and hypoxemia remains the only respiratory stimulus. Oxygen therapy during an acute respiratory insult in these patients may enhance progression to respiratory failure. Close clinical observation and frequent blood gas monitoring are important in preventing this complication. In infants and young children, fine mist tents in an oxygen-enriched atmosphere should be avoided because they obscure the patient from view, may frighten the patient, and may not deliver adequate oxygen.

With evidence of infection (i.e., purulent sputum containing polymorphonuclear leukocytes, fever, sinusitis, or radiographic evidence of pneumonia), antibiotics should be administered. In some instances, infection may be present in the absence of these suggestive findings but, conversely, after patients have purulent sputum containing eosinophils. Thus, antibiotics should not be prescribed routinely (292). Results of sputum culture should dictate change in antibiotic therapy. If sinusitis is present, other antibiotics, such as amoxicillin-clavulanate, azithromycin, clarithromycin, or trimethoprim-sulfamethoxazole, can be administered.

Large doses of corticosteroids are essential immediately in status asthmaticus. The exact dose of corticosteroids necessary for treatment of status asthmaticus is unknown, but the doses must be high. Methylprednisolone (Solu-Medrol), 0.5 to 1 mg/kg, should be given intravenously and repeated every 6 hours. Hydrocortisone (Solu-Cortef), 4 mg/kg, may be given intravenously and repeated every 6 hours as an alternative. With improvement, oral doses of prednisone can be substituted at 60 to 80 mg/day in an adult and 2 mg/kg/day in children. There is no benefit to 1,000-mg doses of methylprednisolone. It is possible to manage status asthmaticus without giving intravenous corticosteroids. For example, when prednisone, 2 mg/kg twice daily, was compared in children with methylprednisolone, 1 mg/kg four times daily given intravenously, equal efficacy was found for hospital length of stay and respiratory parameters (293). For adults, prednisone, 60 mg immediately and every 6 hours, can be administered. Chemistries, including glucose and potassium, should be determined. Magnesium rarely can be decreased in ambulatory patients and may contribute to respiratory muscle dysfunction but should be considered in some situations, especially after mechanical ventilation.

For acute dyspnea, nebulized or aerosolized β_2-adrenergic agonists may be administered every 4 hours or continuously (a fad that does not produce superior results); however, little or no effect may be seen in the first 24 hours. For most patients in status asthmaticus, postural drainage and chest percussion are not necessary as part of the treatment. Treatment of status asthmaticus is summarized in Table 22.13 and Chapter 28. There remains no defined role for magnesium (unless the patient has hypomagnesemia) or heliox (292).

RESPIRATORY FAILURE

Most patients with status asthmaticus respond favorably to the management described previously. In those who continue to deteriorate, other aggressive measures must be included to prevent respiratory failure, which may be defined as a PCO_2 of greater than 50 mm Hg or a PO_2 of less than 50 mm Hg. The important features of treatment at this stage include measures to maintain adequate alveolar ventilation and to protect from the severe acid-base disturbances that may arise. It is suggested that, at this point, the coordinated efforts of the critical care specialist, chest physician, anesthesiologist, and allergist are important in providing proper and effective treatment.

Signs of impending respiratory failure result from the combined effects of hypercapnia, hypoxia, and acidosis. Clinically, because of fatigue, inability to talk, and exhaustion, thoracic excursion is decreased, and auscultation of the chest may show decreased respiratory sounds because there is a decrease in air flow (294). Because of accompanying stupor, the patient may appear to be struggling less to breathe. These two features may give a false impression of improvement. Signs and symptoms of hypoxia include restlessness, confusion or delirium, and central cyanosis, which is present when arterial saturation is less than 70% and arterial PO_2 is less than 40 mm Hg. Hypercapnia is associated with headache or dizziness, confusion, unconsciousness, asterixis, miosis, papilledema, hypertension, and diaphoresis. Other danger signs in the patient with status asthmaticus include the presence of pulsus paradoxus, marked inspiratory retractions, inability to speak in full sentences, and cardiac arrhythmias that may lead to cardiac arrest.

Acute chest pain is consistent with myocardial ischemia or infarction, pulmonary infarction (emboli usually cause dyspnea without chest wall pain), or rib fractures. When subcutaneous emphysema is present, chest pain suggests pneumomediastinum or pneumothorax. Acidosis and hypoxemia contribute to pulmonary vasoconstriction, with resultant pulmonary hypertension and right ventricular strain. The acidosis is primarily respiratory in origin, but with severe hypoxemia, aerobic metabolism is impaired, and there is an accumulation of pyruvic and lactic acid (end products of anaerobic metabolism). These result in a superimposed metabolic acidosis.

The presence of these signs and symptoms associated with development of acidosis and hypercapnia usually demands the institution of mechanical ventilation. Electrocardiographic

monitoring is advised to facilitate the early detection and treatment of arrhythmias that may
occur during or immediately after intubation.
The monitoring should continue throughout the
entire time of mechanical ventilation. For intubation, midazolam (1 mg given intravenously
slowly), ketamine (1 to 2 mg/kg/min given intravenously at 0.5 mg/kg/min), or propofol (60
to 80 mg given intravenously up to 2 mg/kg)
is recommended (292). Preoxygenation with humidified 100% oxygen is administered with the
use of mask and bag. A neuromuscular blocking
drug (atracurium, vecuronium, or pancuronium)
may be administered to facilitate intubation and
mechanical ventilation (292).

In status asthmaticus, high pulmonary pressures are present, and it can be difficult to deliver the tidal volume. There should be adequate
time for expiration in mechanically ventilated
patients. Initial tidal volume settings can be 8 to
10 mL/kg (292). Controlled ventilation with permissive hyperapnea is achieved using high frac-
tional concentration of oxygen, peak pressures
under 40 cm H_2O, and low respiratory frequency.

Overtreatment with sodium bicarbonate must
be avoided. With efficient mechanical ventilation, sudden removal of carbon dioxide may result in acute alkalosis because the elevated levels
of bicarbonate remain uncompensated. Hyperex-
citability and convulsions may then occur. This
complication is best treated by temporarily decreasing ventilation. Other factors such as depletion of potassium (from corticosteroids or diuretics) and chloride may occur in status asthmaticus
and may also contribute to alkalosis. Adequate
replacement of these ions must be included in
therapy.

The only possible contraindication to the use
of mechanical ventilation is the presence of
pneumothorax or pneumomediastinum. In view
of the potential lethality of acute respiratory
failure, these conditions are considered relative contraindications. Mechanical ventilation
may be undertaken, provided all other measures
have been unsuccessful. Pneumothorax must be
treated with a chest tube under water seal before
ventilation is attempted.

Patients who survive an episode of status
asthmaticus and undergo mechanical ventilation
should be considered to have potentially fatal

asthma (40). Attempts should be made to identify reasons for the episode of status asthmaticus.
Some examples include allergic asthma from animal exposure, such as cats, dogs, gerbils, or hamsters; molds (fungi); upper respiratory infections;
acute sinusitis; noncompliance with outpatient
advice; undertreatment on an ambulatory basis
(failure to receive a short course of prednisone
when the deterioration began); use of aspirin
or cyclooxygenase-1 inhibitor within 3 hours of
onset of severe asthma symptoms; or substance
abuse, such as cocaine use (101,127,295). Some
patients have surprise attacks (108), but these
patients should undergo allergy-immunology
evaluation and receive more intensive pharmacotherapy. Acute respiratory failure may occur
seemingly without apparent explanation and can
be fatal. Furthermore, not all patients with acute
respiratory failure report moderate to severe persistent symptoms of asthma. However, some of
these patients are poor perceivers of dyspnea and
decreases in FEV_1 and are not recognized as having more than mild symptoms.

COMPLICATIONS OF
MECHANICAL VENTILATION

Mechanical ventilation, although lifesaving in
acute respiratory failure, may be associated
with specific complications (292). Sudden occurrence of tachypnea, hypotension, tachycardia,
and cyanosis usually indicates a serious complication, such as kinking of the endotracheal tube
with obstruction of a major bronchus, disconnec-
tion from the ventilator, pneumothorax or pneumomediastinum, or obstruction of the endotracheal tube by secretions.

Oxygen toxicity from the chronic use of a
high concentration of oxygen (50% to 100% for
48 hours or longer) is another complication that
can occur with the use of mechanical ventilation. Frequent checks of the inspired oxygen concentration can prevent this from happening. The
pulmonary changes found with oxygen toxicity
are capillary congestion, interstitial edema, alveolar edema, fibrin deposition, hemorrhage, and
atelectasis. These changes may impair oxygen
transport and contribute to hypoxemia. Later and
irreversible changes of oxygen toxicity include
capillary proliferation and fibrosis.

Abnormal fluid retention and weight gain also may occur with prolonged mechanical ventilation. The chest radiograph may assume the appearance of pulmonary edema. As expected, a decrease in vital capacity and compliance, with a tendency toward hypoxemia, results. The cause of the water retention is not known, but subclinical heart failure and antidiuretic hormone release have been suggested mechanisms. Water restriction and diuretic therapy constitute treatment of this complication.

Tracheal stenosis is a complication of cuffed endotracheal or tracheostomy tubes. This occurs as a result of the mucosal injury arising from cuff-induced pressure necrosis. Other factors, such as local infection and hypotension, may be contributory. The occurrence of stridor or loud wheezing, heard best at the mouth, suggests the possibility of this complication in a patient recently intubated. Modifications in tube design may lower the incidence of this complication. Fortunately, mechanical ventilation, even for severe episodes of status asthmaticus, is not required for more than 7 days, and thus this complication is less likely to occur.

A potentially fatal complication of mechanical ventilation is *Pseudomonas aeruginosa* pneumonia or other nosocomial infection. The ventilators are often the source of infection, but the concomitant use of antibiotics and corticosteroids, along with an impaired bronchopulmonary defense mechanism, are important predisposing factors. The radiologic picture of this type of pneumonia is variable and may consist of bilateral or unilateral consolidation, nodular lesions, or abscess formation. The diagnosis is established by repeated cultures from tracheal and bronchial secretions, and specific antibiotic therapy is best determined by sensitivity studies.

Prolonged use of neuromuscular-blocking drugs combined with corticosteroids can cause severe myopathy that requires rehabilitation measures.

PREPARATION OF THE ASTHMATIC PATIENT FOR SURGERY

For elective surgery, the patient with asthma ideally should be evaluated 1 to 2 weeks in advance as an ambulatory patient so that adequate treatment can be instituted to ensure optimal bronchopulmonary status. If the patient is a corticosteroid-dependent asthmatic patient currently on a maintenance dose of prednisone, increase the dose of prednisone instead of relying on increased use of bronchodilators or inhaled corticosteroids to ensure complete control of asthma. See the patient on an ambulatory basis the day before surgery if necessary. If the patient is dependent on inhaled corticosteroids, a short course (4 to 5 days) of prednisone (25 to 40 mg/day) before surgery is recommended to maximize pulmonary function. Pulmonary function testing should be obtained, at least FVC and FEV_1. The main need for corticosteroids, however, is prevention of intraoperative or postoperative asthma rather than adrenal crisis.

Hydrocortisone, 100 mg intravenously, should be started before surgery and continued every 8 hours until the patient can tolerate oral or inhaled medications (296). Often, just one dose of hydrocortisone is necessary. If no postoperative asthma occurs, the hydrocortisone dose can be discontinued. The doses of prednisone and hydrocortisone needed to control asthma do not increase postoperative complications, such as wound infection or dehiscence (296).

In patients with asthma, optimal respiratory status should be achieved before surgery occurs. Manipulation of the upper airway (e.g., suction, pharyngeal airways) may cause bronchoconstriction during light stages of sedation or anesthesia.

After surgery, the patient should be examined carefully. Aerosol bronchodilators, deep-breathing exercises, adequate hydration, and gentle coughing should be instituted to avoid accumulation of secretions and atelectasis. Use of epidural or spinal anesthesia is not necessarily safer than general anesthesia (297).

COMPLICATIONS OF ASTHMA

Although they are rare, pneumothorax, pneumomediastinum, and subcutaneous emphysema can occur during an attack of severe asthma. These complications are thought to result from the rupture of overdistended peripheral alveoli. The escaping air then follows and dissects through bronchovascular sheaths of the lung parenchyma. Usually, the amount of air is minimal, and no specific intervention is required. When severe tension symptoms occur, insertion of a chest tube under a water seal for pneumothorax may be needed. Tracheostomy may be required for severe tension complications of pneumomediastinum. A common feature of these conditions is chest pain; this is not expected with uncomplicated asthma, and when present should suggest the possibility of the extravasation of air. On auscultation of the heart, a crunching sound synchronous with the heartbeat may be present with pneumomediastinum (Hamman sign).

Minimal areas of atelectasis may occur in asthma. Atelectasis of the middle lobe is a common complication of asthma in children. It is often reversible with bronchodilators and prednisone, given immediately to avoid the risk of bronchoscopy, or at least to prepare for this examination. It probably results from mucus plugging and edema of the middle lobe bronchus. When the atelectasis does not respond to the above treatment within a few days, bronchoscopy is indicated for both therapeutic and diagnostic reasons. Occasionally, children may develop atelectasis of other lobes or of an entire lung. Allergic bronchopulmonary aspergillosis (see Chapter 24) and cystic fibrosis must be excluded in these patients, as in any patient with asthma.

Rib fracture and costochondritis may occur as a result of coughing during attacks of asthma. In a few patients, severe coughing from asthma may result in cough syncope.

Chronic bronchitis and emphysema are not complications of asthma. These conditions occur with irreversible destruction of lung tissue, whereas asthma is at least a partially to completely reversible inflammatory condition. In some patients, asthma and emphysema or chronic bronchitis may coexist. The identification of bronchiectasis in a patient with asthma should raise the possibility of allergic bronchopulmonary aspergillosis, undiagnosed cystic fibrosis, or hypogammaglobulinemia. Hypoxemia from uncontrolled asthma has been associated with adverse effects on other organs, such as myocardial ischemia or infarction.

Another complication of asthma is excessive loss of FEV_1 compared with patients without asthma (141). Although this effect typically produces no clinical ramifications, in the exceptional patient, "irreversible asthma" occurs (141). These patients do not have COPD, allergic bronchopulmonary aspergillosis, cystic fibrosis, occupational asthma, or other lung disease, and α_1-antitrypsin concentrations are not reduced. High-resolution CT scanning of the lungs does not demonstrate fibrosis or other explanations. Most of these patients do not have steroid-resistant asthma because they have more than 15% bronchodilator response to 2 weeks of daily prednisone. However, their ultimate FEV_1 after prednisone and other pharmacotherapy is markedly impaired, with a mean FEV_1 percentage of 57 (141). Treatment of asthma in the future should help overcome excessive loss of FEV_1 and preserve lung function in patients with severe and mild persistent asthma.

MORTALITY

Death from asthma commonly occurs either as a result of status asthmaticus progressing to respiratory failure or suddenly and unexpectedly from severe bronchoconstriction and hypoxia, perhaps with a terminal cardiac arrhythmia. The increase in mortality rate from asthma that occurred in the 1980s in the United States appeared to stabilize by 1996 but has not declined (298). The use of repeated doses of β_2-adrenergic aerosols has been suspected to be a contributing factor in some of these deaths but is unlikely to be a satisfactory explanation. Fatality rates are lower in the United States and Canada than in many countries, including as New Zealand and Australia. Efforts in these two latter countries have helped to reduce deaths from asthma.

A 1980s surge in deaths in New Zealand and the availability of albuterol inhalers without prescription in that country has been considered possibly analogous to the earlier epidemics of the 1960s. Undue reliance on inhaled β_2-adrenergic agonists by patients and physicians may contribute to fatalities in patients with severe exacerbations of asthma because essential corticosteroid therapy is not being administered. In addition, excessive deaths associated with the potent β_2-adrenergic agonist fenoterol have been reported. This has led to the recommendation that, in persistent asthma, inhaled corticosteroids should be used in conjunction with β_2-adrenergic agonists.

Some factors that have been implicated in contributing to asthma deaths include the use of sedation in the hospital or illicit drugs and substance abuse outside of the hospital, the failure to use adequate doses of oral corticosteroids, theophylline toxicity, excessive use of β_2-adrenergic agonists, noncompliance with physician instructions, failure to initiate oral corticosteroids for exacerbations of asthma, and ineffective (lack of aggressive) outpatient management of asthma (127). The latter phenomenon may be exemplified by the use of inhaled corticosteroids, which will not substitute for oral corticosteroids acutely. High-risk patients include those who have had severe wheezing (often since the first year of life), frequent episodes of prolonged asthma necessitating hospitalization or chronic oral corticosteroid use, chest deformities such as pigeon breast, wheezing in between exacerbations of asthma, or gross pulmonary function abnormalities when asymptomatic (poor perceivers) and patients previously requiring mechanical ventilation during respiratory failure, such as those with potentially fatal asthma (150). Patients with underlying restrictive lung disease, because of reduction in functional residual capacity, tolerate status asthmaticus poorly as well because baseline lung function favors more easy collapsibility of bronchi. Some fatalities occur in the setting of no medical care or are associated with substance abuse even without a history of a previous nearly fatal attack (101).

FUTURE CONSIDERATIONS

Asthma management will be improved by continued improvements in therapy, implementation of these advances, health care system improvement, and stability of the family. Specific curative therapy can be realized only when basic pathologic mechanisms are understood. Then, therapeutic modalities can be devised rationally to reverse the underlying pathogenetic processes.

Many patients with persistent asthma can be managed successfully with an inhaled corticosteroid and intermittent but not excessive use of β_2-adrenergic agonists. Additional antiinflammatory therapies include cromolyn, nedocromil, and LTD4 antagonists. None of the medications can substitute for prednisone in patients with oral corticosteroid—dependent asthma. Future therapies can be assessed for their ability to (a) decrease symptoms, (b) allow for withdrawal for prednisone or inhaled corticosteroids, (c) preserve lung function, and (d) permit improved quality of life without unacceptable adverse effects. Physicians managing patients with asthma should consider allergic triggers in all patients with persistent asthma because about 75% of patients have IgE antibodies by skin testing. Allergen vaccine therapy, especially with trees, grasses, ragweed, and dust mites, remains effective as an immunomodulatory therapy. Some patients respond to injection of molds (fungi).

Humanized monoclonal antibody therapy, such as anti-IgE, may be of value in the management of persistent asthma (299). The antibody is primarily human IgG4 and thus does not activate complement. Immediate and late bronchial responses to inhaled allergen challenge can be reduced by intravenous anti-IgE infusions (299). However, by aerosol delivery, there was no effect (300). In a study using a soluble IL-4 receptor to inactivate IL-4, apparent benefit was reported (301). The requirement for β_2-adrenergic agonists and asthma symptom scores were reduced. Theoretically, such a "decoy" therapy, which binds free IL-4, would be of value in asthma therapy. The true measure of an agonist in asthma is the effect when antagonists interact with the agonist and disease severity is reduced.

Fundamental principles of asthma management include (a) trying to minimize mast cell activation, smooth muscle contraction, inflammatory airway changes, and pulmonary physiologic abnormalities; (b) preventing death, disability, and school or work absenteeism; and (c) using medications effectively and as safely as possible. It is expected that our treatment modalities will continue to improve and that more specific therapies, whether pharmacologic, vaccine based, or immunologically targeted, will be of help to patients and their physicians.

REFERENCES

1. National Institutes of Health, National Heart, Lung, and Blood Institute, Expert Panel Report, National Asthma Education Program, Executive Summary. *Guidelines for the diagnosis and management of asthma.* Bethesda, MD: Public Health Service, U.S. Department of Health and Human Services, NIH Publication No. 91-3042A, 1991.

2. National Heart, Lung, and Blood Institute, Expert Panel Report 2. *Guidelines for the diagnosis and management of asthma.* Bethesda, MD: U.S. Department of Health and Human Services, 1997, NIH publication No. 97-4051.

3. Carrao WM, Braman SS, Irwin RS. Chronic cough as the sole presenting manifestation of bronchial asthma. *N Engl J Med* 1979;30:633.

4. Quesenberry PJ. Cardiac asthma: a fresh look at an old wheeze. *N Engl J Med* 1989;320:1346.

5. Cabanes LR, Weber SN, Matran R, et al. Bronchial hyperresponsiveness to methacholine in patients with impaired left ventricular function. *N Engl J Med* 1989;320:1317.

6. Samet JM. Epidemiologic approaches for the identification of asthma. *Chest* 1987;91:74S.

7. Pattermore PK, Asher MI, Harrison AC, et al. The interrelationship among bronchial hyperresponsiveness, the diagnosis of asthma, and asthma symptoms. *Am Rev Respir Dis* 1990;142:549–554.

8. Welliver RC, Sun M, Rinaldo D, et al. Predictive value of respiratory syncytial virus-specific IgE responses for recurrent wheezing following bronchiolitis. *J Pediatr* 1986;109:776.

9. Welliver RC, Duffy L. The relationship of RSV-specific immunoglobulin E antibody responses in infancy, recurrent wheezing, and pulmonary function at age 7–8 years. *Pediatr Pulmonol* 1993;15:19.

10. Teichtahl H, Buckmaster N, Pernikovs E. The incidence of respiratory tract infection in adults requiring hospitalization for asthma. *Chest* 1997;112:591–596.

11. Rakes GP, Arruda E, Ingram JM, et al. Rhinovirus and respiratory syncytial virus in wheezing children requiring emergency care. *Am J Respir Crit Care Med* 1999;159:785–790.

12. Stevenson DD. Adverse reactions to nonsteroidal antiinflammatory drugs. *Immunol Allergy Clin North Am* 1998;18:773–798.

13. Babu KS, Salvi SS. Aspirin and asthma. *Chest* 2000;118:1470–1476.

14. Israel E, Fischer AR, Rosenberg MA, et al. The pivotal role of 5-lipoxygenase products in the reaction of aspirin-sensitive asthmatic subjects to aspirin. *Am Rev Respir Dis* 1993;148:1447.

15. Shuaib Nasser SM, Patel M, Bell GS, et al. The effect of aspirin desensitization on urinary leukotriene E$_4$ concentrations in aspirin-sensitive asthma. *Am J Respir Crit Care Med* 1995;151:1326.

16. Ownby DR. Environmental factors versus genetic determinants of childhood inhalant allergies. *J Allergy Clin Immunol* 1990;86:279.

17. Luoma R, Koirvkko A, Viander M. Development of asthma, allergic rhinitis, and atopic dermatitis by the age of five years. *Allergy* 1983;38:339.

18. Ratner B, Silberman DE. Allergy: its distribution and hereditary concept. *Ann Allergy* 1952;9:1.

19. Wittig HJ, McLaughlin ET, Leifer KL, et al. Risk factors for the development of allergic disease: analysis of 2190 patient records. *Ann Allergy* 1978;41:84.

20. Horwood LJ, Fergusson DM, Hons BA, et al. Social and familial factors in the development of early childhood asthma. *Pediatrics* 1985;75:859.

21. Blumenthal MN, Yunis E, Mendell N, et al. Preventive allergy: genetics of IgE-mediated diseases. *J Allergy Clin Immunol* 1986;78:962.

22. Harris JR, Magnus P, Samuelson SO, et al. No evidence for effects of family environment on asthma: a retrospective study of Norwegian twins. *Am J Respir Crit Care Med* 1997;156:43–49.

23. Hopp RJ, Bewtra AK, Watt GD, et al. Genetic analysis of allergic disease in twins. *J Allergy Clin Immunol* 1984;73:265.

24. Tager IB. Smoking and childhood asthma: where do we stand? *Am J Respir Crit Care Med* 1998;158:349–351.

25. Murray AB, Morrison BJ. Passive smoking by asthmatics: its greater effect on boys than on girls and on older than on young children. *Pediatrics* 1989;84:451.

26. Withers NJ, Low L, Holgate ST, et al. The natural history of respiratory symptoms in a cohort of adolescents. *Am J Respir Crit Care Med* 1998;158:352–357.

27. Martinez FD, Wright AL, Taussig LM, et al. Asthma and wheezing in the first six years of life. *N Engl J Med* 1995;332:133–138.

28. Frick OL, German DF, Mills J. Development of allergy in children. I. Association with virus infections. *J Allergy Clin Immunol* 1979;63:228.

29. Weiss ST, Tager IB, Munoz A, et al. The relationship of respiratory illness in childhood to the occurrence of increased levels of bronchial responsiveness and atopy. *Am Rev Respir Dis* 1985;141:573.

30. Johnston IDA, Strachan DP, Anderson HR. Effect of pneumonia and whooping cough in childhood on adult lung function. *N Engl J Med* 1998;338:581–587.

31. Price JA, Pollock I, Little SA, et al. Measurement of airborne mite antigen in homes of asthmatic children. *Lancet* 1990;336:895.

32. von Mutius E. The environmental predictors of allergic disease. *J Allergy Clin Immunol* 2000;105:9–19.

33. Rosenstreich DL, Eggleston P, Kattan M, et al. The role of cockroach allergy and exposure to cockroach allergen in causing morbidity among inner-city children with asthma. *N Engl J Med*, 1997;336:1356–1363.

34. Litonjua AA, Sparrow D, Weiss ST, et al. Sensitization to cat allergen is associated with asthma in older men and predicts new-onset airway hyperresponsiveness. *Am J Respir Crit Care Med* 1997;156:23–27.

35. Shirakawa T, Enomoto T, Shimazu S, et al. The inverse association between tuberculin responses and atopic disorder. *Science* 1997;275:77–79.

36. Douglas JA, O'Hehir RE. What determines asthma phenotype? Respiratory infections and asthma. *Am J Respir Crit Care Med* 2000;161:S211–214.

37. Shaheen SO, Aaby P, Hall AJ, et al. Measles and atopy in Guinea-Bissau. *Lancet* 1996;347:1792–1796.

38. Cookson WOCM, Moffat MF. Asthma: an epidemic in the absence of infection? *Science* 1997;275:41–42.

39. Park J-H, Gold DR, Spiegelman DL, et al. House dust endotoxin and wheeze in the first year of life. *Am J Respir Crit Care Med* 2001;163:322–328.

40. Greenberger PA, Patterson R. Potentially fatal asthma

and asthma deaths: knowledge is greater but implementation appears problematic. *Ann Allergy Asthma Immunol* 2000;84:563–564.

41. Busse WW, Lemanske RF. Asthma. *N Engl J Med* 2001;344:350–362.

42. Gleich GJ, Motojima S, Frigas E, et al. The eosinophilic leukocyte and the pathology of fatal bronchial asthma: evidence for pathologic heterogeneity. *J Allergy Clin Immunol* 1987;80:412.

43. Bousquet J, Chanej P, Lacoste JY, et al. Eosinophilic inflammation in asthma. *N Engl J Med* 1990;323:1033.

44. Kuman SD, Emery MJ, Atkins ND, et al. Airway mucosal blood flow in bronchial asthma. *Am J Respir Crit Care Med* 1998;158:153–156.

45. Kleinerman J, Adelson L. A study of asthma death in a coroner's population. *J Allergy Clin Immunol* 1987;80:406.

46. Morishima Y, Nomura A, Uchida Y, et al. Triggering the induction of myofibroblast and fibrogenesis by airway epithelial shedding. *Am J Respir Cell Mol Biol* 2001;24:1–11.

47. Campbell AM, Chanez P, Bignola AM, et al. Functional characteristics of bronchial epithelium obtained by brushing from asthmatic and normal subjects. *Am Rev Respir Dis* 1993;147:529–534.

48. Laitinin LA, Laitinin A, Haahtela A. Airway mucosal inflammation even in patients with newly diagnosed asthma. *Am Rev Respir Dis* 1993;147:697–704.

49. Druilhe A, Wallaert B, Tsicopoulos A, et al. Apoptosis, proliferation, and expression of Bcl-2, Fas, and Fas ligand in bronchial biopsies from asthmatics. *Am J Respir Cell Mol Biol* 1998;19:747–757.

50. Spinozzi F, Fizzotti M, Agea E, et al. Defective expression of Fas messenger RNA and Fas receptor on pulmonary T cells from patients with asthma. *Ann Intern Med* 1998;128:363–369.

51. Salome CM, Peat JK, Britton WJ, et al. Bronchial hyperresponsiveness in two populations of Australian schoolchildren. I. Relation to respiratory symptoms and diagnosed asthma. *Clin Allergy* 1987;17:271.

52. Cookson WOCM, Musk AW, Ryan G. Associations between asthma history, atopy and non-specific bronchial responsiveness in young adults. *Clin Allergy* 1986;16:425.

53. Smith LJ, Greenberger PA, Patterson R, et al. The effect of inhaled leukotriene D4 in humans. *Am Rev Respir Dis* 1985;131:368.

54. Frick WE, Sedgwick JB, Busse WW. The appearance of hypodense eosinophils in antigen-dependent late phase asthma. *Am Rev Respir Dis* 1989;139:1401.

55. Frigas E, Loegering DA, Solley GO, et al. Elevated levels of eosinophil granule major basic protein in the sputum of patients with bronchial asthma. *Mayo Clin Proc* 1981;56:345.

56. Filley WV, Holley KE, Kephart GM, et al. Identification by immunofluorescence of eosinophil granule major basic protein in lung tissues of patients with bronchial asthma. *Lancet* 1982;2:11.

57. Fredens K, Dahl P, Venge P. Eosinophils and cellular injury: the Gordon Phenomenon as a model. *Allergy Proc* 1985;6:346.

58. Ollerenshaw S, Jarvis D, Woolcock A, et al. Absence of immunoreactive vasoactive intestinal polypeptide in tissue from the lungs of patients with asthma. *N Engl J Med* 1989;320:1244.

59. Tomaki M, Ichinose N, Miura M, et al. Elevated substance P content in induced sputum from patients with asthma and patients with chronic bronchitis. *Am J Respir Crit Care Med* 1995;151:613.

60. Sanders SP. Nitric oxide in asthma: pathogenic, therapeutic or diagnostic? *Am J Respir Cell Mol Biol* 1999;21:147–149.

61. Montuschi P, Corradi M, Ciabattoni G, et al. Increased 8-isoprostane, a marker of oxidative stress, in exhaled condensate of asthma patients. *Am J Respir Crit Care Med* 1999;160:216–220.

62. Miller BD. Depression and asthma: a potentially lethal mixture. *J Allergy Clin Immunol* 1987;80:481.

63. Walker CL, Greenberger PA, Patterson R. Potentially fatal asthma. *Ann Allergy* 1990;64:487.

64. Sonin L, Patterson R. Corticosteroid dependent asthma and schizophrenia. *Arch Intern Med* 1984;144:554.

65. Yellowlees PM, Ruffin RE. Psychological defenses and coping styles in patients following a life-threatening attack of asthma. *Chest* 1989;95:1298.

66. Measuring childhood asthma prevalence before and after the 1997 redesign of the national health interview survey-United States. *MMWR Morb Mortal Wkly Rep* 2000;49:908–911.

67. Kerem E, Eibshirani R, Canny G, et al. Predicting the need for hospitalization in children with acute asthma. *Chest* 1990;98:1355.

68. Friday Jr GA, Khine H, Lin MS, et al. Profile of children requiring emergency treatment for asthma. *Ann Allergy Asthma Immunol* 1997;78:221–224.

69. Global Initiative for Asthma. *Global strategy for asthma management and prevention NHLBI/WHO workshop report.* NIH Publication No. 95-3659, January 1995.

70. Ertle AR, London MR. Insights into asthma prevalence in Oregon. *J Asthma* 1998;35(3):281–289.

71. Burrows B. The natural history of asthma. *J Allergy Clin Immunol* 1987;80:373.

72. Apter A, Grammer LC, Naughton B, et al. Asthma in the elderly: a brief report. *N Engl Reg Allergy Proc* 1988;9:153.

73. Burr MC, Charles D, Roy K, et al. Asthma in the elderly: an epidemiological survey. *Br Med J* 1979;1:1041.

74. Evans R III. Recent observations reflecting increase in mortality from asthma. *J Allergy Clin Immunol* 1987;80:337.

75. Stanford R, McLaughlin T, Okamoto LJ. The cost of asthma in the emergency department and hospital. *Am J Respir Crit Care Med* 1999;160:211–215.

76. Chan-Yeung M, Malo J-L. Occupational asthma. *N Engl J Med* 1995;333:107.

77. Beckett WS. Occupational respiratory diseases. *N Engl J Med* 2000;342:406–413.

78. Kogevinas M, Antó JM, Soriano JB, et al. The risk of asthma attributable to occupational exposures: a population-based study in Spain. *Am J Respir Crit Care Med* 1996;154:137–143.

79. Sly RM. Decreases in asthma mortality in the United States. *Ann Allergy Asthma Immunol* 2000;85:121–127.

80. Burney PGJ. Asthma mortality: England and Wales. *J Allergy Clin Immunol* 1987;80:379.

81. Sears MR. Changing patterns in asthma morbidity and mortality. *J Invest Allergol Clin Immunol* 1995;5:66.

82. Juel K, Pedersen PA. Increasing asthma mortality in Denmark 1969–88 not a result of a changed coding practice. *Ann Allergy* 1992;68:180.

83. Bousquet J, Hatton F, Godard P, et al. Asthma mortality in France. *J Allergy Clin Immunol* 1987;80:389.

84. Sly RM. Changing asthma mortality. *Ann Allergy* 1994;73:259.

85. Fitzgerald JM, Macklem PT. Proceedings of a workshop on near fatal asthma. *Can Respir J* 1995;2:113–126.

86. Current trends: asthma–United States, 1982–1992. *MMWR Morb Mortal Wkly Rep* 1995;43:952.

87. Weiss KB, Wagener DK. Changing patterns of asthma mortality: identifying target populations at high risk. *JAMA* 1990;264:1683–1687.

88. Zoratti EM, Havstad S, Rodriguez J, et al. Health service use by African Americans and Caucasians with asthma in a managed care setting. *Am J Respir Crit Care Med* 1998;158:371–377.

89. Smith DH, Malone DC, Lawson KA, et al. A national estimate of the economic costs of asthma. *Am J Respir Crit Care Med* 1997;156:787–793.

90. Greenberger PA. Preventing the emergence of the $100,000 asthmatic. *Medscape Respir Care* 1998;2(1).

91. Sly MR. Changing asthma mortality and sales of inhaled bronchodilators and anti-asthmatic drugs. *Ann Allergy* 1994;73:439.

92. Lozano P, Sullivan SD, Smith DH, et al. The economic burden of asthma in US children: estimates from the National Medical Expenditure Survey. *J Allergy Clin Immunol* 1999;104:957–963.

93. Stempel DA, Hedblom EC, Durcanin-Robbins JF, et al. Use of a pharmacy and medical claims database to document cost centers for 1993 annual asthma expenditures. *Arch Fam Med* 1996;5:36–40.

94. Bates DV. Airway structure and function. In: *Respiratory function in disease.* Philadelphia: WB Saunders, 1989:1.

95. Patterson R, McKenna JM, Susko IM, et al. Living histamine containing cells from the bronchial lumens of humans: description and comparison of histamine content with cells of rhesus monkeys. *J Clin Invest* 1977;59:217.

96. Fick RB, Richerson HB, Zavala DC, et al. Bronchoalveolar lavage in allergic asthmatics. *Am Rev Respir Dis* 1987;135:1204.

97. Friedman MM, Kaliner MA. Human mast cells and asthma. *Am Rev Respir Dis* 1987;135:1157.

98. Bousquet J, Jeffery PK, Busse WW, et al. Asthma: from bronchoconstriction to airways inflammation and remodeling. *Am J Respir Crit Care Med* 2000;161:1720–1745.

99. Jatakanon A, Uasuf C, Maziak W, et al. Neutrophilic inflammation in severe persistent asthma. *Am J Respir Crit Care Med* 1999;160:1532–1539.

100. Sur S, Crotty TB, Kephart GM, et al. Sudden-onset fatal asthma: a distinct clinical entity with few eosinophils and relatively more neutrophils in the airway submucosa? *Am Rev Respir Dis* 1993;148:713–719.

101. Jerath Tatum A, Greenberger PA, Mileusnic D, et al. Clinical, pathologic, and toxicologic findings in asthma deaths in Cook County, Illinois. *Allergy Asthma Proc* 2001;22:285–291.

102. Lemjabbar H, Gosset P, Lamblin C, et al. Contribution of 9 kDa gelatinase/type IV collagenase in bronchial inflammation during status asthmaticus. *Am J Respir Crit Care Med* 1999;159:1298–1307.

103. Barnes PJ, Cuss FM, Palmer JB. The effect of airway epithelium on smooth muscle contractability in bovine trachea. *Br J Pharmacol* 1985;86:685.

104. Burns GP, Gibson GJ. Airway hyperresponsiveness in asthma: not just a problem of smooth muscle relaxation with inspiration. *Am J Respir Crit Care Med* 1998;158:203–206.

105. Woolcock AJ, Salmone CM, Yan K. The shape of the dose response curve to histamine in asthmatic and normal subjects. *Am Rev Respir Dis* 1984;130:71.

106. Gibbons WJ, Sharma A, Lougheed D, et al. Detection of excessive bronchoconstriction in asthma. *Am J Respir Crit Care Med* 1996;153:582–589.

107. Reid LM. The presence or absence or bronchial mucus in fatal asthma. *J Allergy Clin Immunol* 1987;80:415.

108. Robin ED, Lewiston N. Unexpected, unexplained sudden death in young asthmatic subjects. *Chest* 1989;96:790.

109. Hamid QA, Minshall EM. Molecular pathology of allergic disease I. Lower airway disease. *J Allergy Clin Immunol* 2000;105:20–36.

110. Bhaskar KR, Reid L. Application of density gradient methods for the study of mucus glycoprotein and other macromolecular components of the sol and gel phases of asthmatic sputa. *J Biol Chem* 1981;256:7583.

111. Maron Z, Shelhamer JG, Kaliner M. Human pulmonary macrophage-derived mucus secretagogue. *J Exp Med* 1984;189:844–860.

112. Proceedings of the ATS workshop on refractory asthma: Current understanding, recommendations, and unanswered questions. *Am J Respir Crit Care Med* 2000;162:2341–2351.

113. Laitinen LA, Laitinen A, Haahtela T. A comparative study of the effects of an inhaled corticosteroid, budesonide, and a B_2-agonist, terbutaline, on airway inflammation in newly diagnosed asthma: a randomized, double-blind, parallel-group controlled trial. *J Allergy Clin Immunol* 1992;90:32.

114. Teeter JG, Bleecker ER. Relationship between airway obstruction and respiratory symptoms in adult asthmatics. *Chest* 1998;113:272–277.

115. Banzett RB, Dempsey JA, O'Donnell DE, et al. Symptom perception and respiratory sensation in asthma. *Am J Respir Crit Care Med* 2000;162:1178–1182.

116. Leff AR. Endogenous regulation of bronchomotor tone. *Am Rev Respir Dis* 1988;137:1198.

117. Beasley R, Rocke ER, Roberts JA, et al. Cellular events in the bronchi in mild asthma and after bronchial provocation. *Am Rev Respir Dis* 1989;139:806.

118. Cutz E, Levison H, Cooper DM. Ultrastructure of airways in children with asthma. *Histopathology* 1978;2:407.

119. Flint KC, Leung KBP, Hudspith BN, et al. Bronchoalveolar mast cells in extrinsic asthma: a mechanism for the inhalation of antigen specific bronchoconstriction. *Br Med J* 1985;291:923.

120. Pearce FL, Flint KC, Leung KBT, et al. Some studies on human pulmonary mast cells obtained by bronchoalveolar lavage and by enzymatic dissociation of whole lung tissue. *Int Arch Allergy Applied Immunol* 1987;82:507.

121. Lian T-N, Hsieh K-H. Altered production of histamine-releasing factor (HRF) activity and responsiveness to HRF after immunotherapy in children with asthma. *J Allergy Clin Immunol* 1990;86:894.

122. Kikuchi Y, Okabe S, Tamura G, et al. Chemosensitivity and perception of dyspnea in patients with a history of near-fatal asthma. *N Engl J Med*, 1994;330:1329–1334.

123. Wenzel SE, Schwartz LB, Langmack EL, et al. Evidence that severe asthma can be divided pathologically into two inflammatory subtypes with distinct physiologic and clinical characteristics. *Am J Respir Crit Care Med* 1999;160:1001–1008.

124. Cheriyan S, Greenberger PA, Patterson R. Outcome of cough variant asthma treated with inhaled steroids. *Ann Allergy* 1994;73:478.

125. McFadden ER Jr. Exertional dyspnea and cough as preludes to acute attacks of bronchial asthma. *N Engl J Med* 1975;292:555.

126. Rebuck S, Pengelly LD. Development of pulsus paradoxus in the presence of airways obstruction. *N Engl J Med* 1973;288:66.

127. Greenberger PA. Preventing hospitalizations for asthma by improving ambulatory management. *Am J Med* 1996;100:381–382.

128. Petheram IS, Kerr IH, Collins JB. Value of chest radiographs in severe acute asthma. *Clin Radiol* 1981; 32:281.

129. Findley LJ, Sahn SA. The value of chest roentgenograms in acute asthma in adults. *Chest* 1981;80:535.

130. Sherman S, Skoney JA, Ravikrishnan KP. Routine chest radiographs in exacerbations of chronic obstructive pulmonary disease: Diagnostic value. *Arch Intern Med* 1989;149:2493.

131. Slavin RG. Sinusitis in adults and its relation to allergic rhinitis, asthma and nasal polyps. *J Allergy Clin Immunol* 1988;82:950.

132. Rodriquez-Roisin R, Ballester E, Roca J, et al. Mechanisms of hypoxemia in patients with status asthmaticus. *Am Rev Respir Dis* 1989;139:732.

133. Cote J, Cartier A, Malo J-L, et al. Compliance with peak expiratory flow monitoring in home management of asthma. *Chest* 1998;113:968–972.

134. Newman KB, Mason UG III, Schmaling KB. Clinical features of vocal cord dysfunction. *Am J Respir Crit Care Med* 1995:152:1382–1386.

135. Bacharier LB, Strunk RC. Vocal cord dysfunction: a practical approach to diagnosis. *J Respir Dis* 2001;22:93–103.

136. Allen JN, Davis WB. Eosinophilic lung diseases. *Am J Respir Crit Care Med* 1994;150:1423.

137. Buchanan DR, Crowell O, Kay AB. Neutrophil chemotactic activity in acute severe asthma. *Am Rev Respir Dis* 1987;136:1397.

138. Backer JW, Yerger S, Segar WE. Elevated plasma antidiuretic hormone levels in status asthmaticus. *Mayo Clin Proc* 1976;51:31.

139. Adnot S, Chabrier PE, Andrivet P, et al. Atrial natriuretic peptide concentrations and pulmonary hemodynamics in patients with pulmonary artery hypertension. *Am Rev Respir Dis* 1987;136:951.

140. Lange P, Perner J, Vestbo J, et al. A 15-year follow-up study of ventilatory function in adults with asthma. *N Engl J Med* 1998;339:1194–1200.

141. Backman KS, Greenberger PA, Patterson RP. Airways obstruction in patients with long-term asthma consistent with 'irreversible asthma.' *Chest* 1997;112:1234–1240.

142. King GC, Müller NL, Paré PD. Evaluation of airways in obstructive pulmonary disease using high-resolution computed tomography. *Am J Respir Crit Care Med* 1999;159:992–1004.

143. Strunk RC. Death due to asthma: new insights into sudden unexpected deaths, but the focus remains on prevention. *Am Rev Respir Dis* 1992;148:550.

144. Lang DM. Trends in US asthma mortality: good news and bad news. *Ann Allergy Asthma Immunol* 1997;78:333–337.

145. Birkhead G, Attaway NJ, Strunk RC, et al. Investigation of a cluster of deaths of adolescents from asthma: evidence implicating inadequate treatment and poor patient adherence with medications. *J Allergy Clin Immunol* 1989;84:484.

146. Robertson CF, Rubinfeld AR, Bowes G. Deaths from asthma in Victoria: a 12-month survey. *Med J Aust* 1990;152:511.

147. Esdaile JM, Feinstein AR, Horwitz RI. A reappraisal of the United Kingdom epidemic of fatal asthma: can general mortality data implicate a therapeutic agent? *Arch Intern Med* 1987;147:543.

148. Suissa S, Ernst P, Boivin J-F, et al. A cohort analysis of excess mortality in asthma and the use of inhaled B-agonists. *Am J Respir Crit Care Med* 1994;149:604.

149. Spitzer WO, Suissa S, Ernst P, et al. The use of B-agonists and the risk of death and near death from asthma. *N Engl J Med* 1992;326:501.

150. Greenberger PA. Potentially fatal asthma. *Chest* 1992;l101:401S.

151. Rebuck AS, Read J. Assessment and management of severe asthma. *Am J Med* 1971;51:788.

152. Axelrod L. Glucocorticoids. In: Kelly WN, Harris ED, Ruddy S, et al, eds. *Textbook of rheumatology.* 4th ed. Philadelphia: WB Saunders, 1993:779.

153. Lowenthal M, Patterson R, Greenberger PA, et al. Malignant potentially fatal asthma: achievement of remission and the application of an asthma severity index. *Allergy Proc* 1993;14:333.

154. Huckauf H, Mach AN. Behavioral factors in the etiology of asthma. *Chest* 1987;91:141S.

155. Groves JE. Taking care of the hateful patient. *N Engl J Med* 1976;293:883.

156. Fitzsimons T, Patterson D, Patterson R. The allergic patient who is non-compliant and abusive: dealing with the adverse experience. *Ann Allergy* 1991;66:311.

157. Chandler MJ, Grammer LC, Patterson R. Noncompliance and prevarication in life-threatening adolescent asthma. *N Engl Reg Allergy Proc* 1986;7:367.

158. McGrath KG, Greenberger PA, Patterson R, et al. Factitious allergic disease: multiple factitious illness and familial Munchausen's stridor. *Immunol Allergy Pract* 1984;7:263.

159. Apter A, Grammer LC, Naughton B, et al. Asthma in the elderly: a brief report. *N Engl Reg Allergy Proc* 1988;9:153.

160. Kalliel JN, Goldstein BM, Braman SS, et al. High frequency of atopic asthma in a pulmonary clinic population. *Chest* 1989;96:1336.

161. Sporik R, Ingram JM, Price W, et al. Association of asthma with serum IgE and skin test reactivity to allergens among children living at high altitude: tickling the dragon's breath. *Am J Respir Crit Care Med* 1995:151:1388–1392.

162. Christie GL, Helms PJ, Godden DJ, et al. Asthma, wheezy bronchitis, and atopy across two generations. *Am J Respir Crit Care Med* 1999;159:125–129.

163. Habenicht HA, Burge HA, Muilenberg MC, et al. Allergen carriage by atmospheric aerosols. II. Ragweed-pollen determinants in submicronic atmospheric aerosols. *J Allergy Clin Immunol* 1984;74:64.

164. Findley SR, Stotsky E, Lieterman K, et al. Allergens detected in association with airborne particles capable of penetrating into the peripheral lung. *Am Rev Respir Dis* 1983;128:1008.

165. Luczynska CM, Yin L, Chapman MD, et al. Airborne concentrations and particle size distribution of allergen derived from domestic cats (Felis domesticus). *Am Rev Respir Dis* 1990;141:361.

166. Patchett K, Lewis S, Crane J, et al. Cat allergen (Fel d 1) levels on school children's clothing and in primary school classrooms in Wellington, New Zealand. *J Allergy Clin Immunol* 1997;100:755–759.

167. Cockcroft DW. The bronchial late response in the pathogenesis of asthma and its modulation by therapy. *Ann Allergy* 1985;55:857.

168. O'Hollaren MT, Yunginger JW, Offord KP, et al. Exposure to an aeroallergen as a possible precipitating factor in respiratory arrest in young patients with asthma. *N Engl J Med*, 1991;321:359–363.

169. Sporik R, Holgate ST, Platts-Mills TAE, et al. Exposure to house-dust mite allergen (Der p I) and the development of asthma in childhood: a prospective study. *N Engl J Med* 1990;323:502–507.

170. American Thoracic Society. Environmental control and lung disease. *Am Rev Respir Dis* 1990;142:915.

171. Practice parameters for the diagnosis and treatment of asthma. *J Allergy Clin Immunol* 1995;96:S707–870.

172. Houba R, Heederik D, Doekes G. Wheat sensitization and work-related symptoms in the baking industry are preventable. *Am J Respir Crit Care Med* 1998;158:1499–1503.

173. Zuskin E, Kanceljak B, Schacter EN, et al. Respiratory function and immunologic status in workers processing dried fruits and teas. *Ann Allergy Asthma Immunol* 1996;77:417–422.

174. Houba R, Heederik JJ, Doekes G, et al. Exposure: sensitization relationship for α-amylase allergens in the baking industry. *Am J Respir Crit Care Med* 1996;154:130–136.

175. Atmar RL, Guy E, Guntupalli KK, et al. Respiratory tract viral infections in inner-city asthmatic adults. *Arch Intern Med* 1998;158:2453–2459.

176. Welliver RC, Wong DT, Sun M, et al. The development of respiratory syncytial virus-specific IgE and the release of histamine in nasopharyngeal secretions after infection. *N Engl J Med* 1981;305:841.

177. Ball TM, Castro-Rodriguez JA, Griffith KA, et al. Sibling, day-care attendance, and the risk of asthma and wheezing during childhood. *N Engl J Med*, 2000; 343:538–543.

178. Szczeklik A. Mechanisms of aspirin-induced asthma. *Allergy* 1997;52:613–619.

179. Szczeklik A, Sanak M. Molecular mechanisms in aspirin-induced asthma. *ACI Int* 2000;12:171–176.

180. Stevenson DD, Pleskow WW, Simon RA, et al. Aspirin-sensitive rhinosinusitis asthma: a double-blind crossover study of treatment with aspirin. *J Allergy Clin Immunol* 1984;73:500.

181. Samter M, Beers RF. Intolerance to aspirin: clinical studies and consideration to its pathogenesis. *Ann Intern Med* 1968;69:975.

182. Mathison DA, Stevenson DD, Simon RA. Precipitating factors in asthma: aspirin, sulfites, and other drugs and chemicals. *Chest* 1985;87:50S.

183. Szczeklik A, Gryglewski RJ, Czerniawska-Mysik G, et al. Aspirin sensitive asthma and arachidonic acid transportation. *N Engl Reg Allergy Proc* 1986;7:21.

184. Israel E, Fischer AR, Rosenberg MA, et al. The pivotal role of 5-lipoxygenase products in the reaction of aspirin-sensitive asthmatic subjects to aspirin. *Am Rev Respir Dis* 1993;148:1447.

185. Shuaib Nasser SM, Patel M, Bell GS, et al. The effect of aspirin desensitization on urinary leukotriene E$_4$ concentrations in aspirin-sensitive asthma. *Am J Respir Crit Care Med* 1995;151:1326.

186. Cowburn AS, Sladek K, Soja J, et al. Overexpresssion of leukotriene C$_4$ synthase in bronchial biopsies from patients with aspirin-intolerant asthma. *J Clin Invest* 1998;101:834–846.

187. Dahlén B, Szczeklik A, Murray JJ. Celecoxib in patients with asthma and aspirin intolerance. *N Engl J Med* 2001;344:142.

188. Stevenson DD, Simon RA, Christensen SC, et al. Lack of cross-reactivity between selective COX-2 inhibitors and aspirin (ASA), in ASA sensitive asthmatic subjects. *J Allergy Clin Immunol* 2000;105;S273.

189. Malo J-L, Cartier A, Ghezzo H, et al. Patterns of improvement in spirometry, bronchial hyperresponsiveness and specific IgE antibody levels after cessation of exposure in occupational asthma caused by snow-crab processing. *Am Rev Respir Dis* 1988;138:807.

190. Brooks SM, Weiss MA, Bernstein IL. Reactive airway dysfunction syndrome (RADS): persistent asthma syndrome after high level irritant exposure. *Chest* 1985;88:376.

191. Promisloff PA, Lenchner GS, Cichelli AV. Reactive airway dysfunction syndrome in three police officers following a roadside chemical spill. *Chest* 1990;98: 928.

192. Vedal S, Enarson DA, Chan H, et al. A longitudinal study of the occurrence of bronchial hyperresponsiveness in Western red cedar workers. *Am Rev Respir Dis* 1988;137:651.

193. Zeiss CR, Mitchell JH, Van Peenin PFD, et al. A twelve-year clinical and immunologic evaluation of workers involved in the manufacture of trimellitic anhydride (TMA). *Allergy Proc* 1990;11:71.

194. Malo J-L, Cartier A, Desjardins A, et al. Occupational asthma caused by oak wood dust. *Chest* 1995;108:856–858.

195. McFadden ER, Gilbert IA. Exercise-induced asthma. *N Engl J Med* 1994;330:1362–1367.

196. Kotaru C, Coreno A, Skowronski M, et al. Exhaled nitric oxide and thermally induced asthma. *Am J Respir Crit Care Med* 2001;163:383–388.

197. Rubenstein I, Levinson H, Slutsky AS, et al. Immediate and delayed bronchoconstriction after exercise in patients with asthma. *N Engl J Med* 1987;317:482.

198. McFadden ER, Nelson JA, Skowronski ME, et al. Thermally induced asthma and airway drying. *Am J Respir Crit Care Med* 1999;160:221–226.

199. Leff JA, Busse WW, Pearlman D, et al. Montelukast, a leukotriene-receptor antagonist, for the treatment of mild asthma and exercise-induced bronchoconstriction. *N Engl J Med* 1998;339:147–152.

200. Patterson R, Schatz M. Factitious allergic emergencies:

anaphylaxis and laryngeal "edema." *J Allergy Clin Immunol* 1975;56:152.

201. Beckman DB, Greenberger DA. Diagnostic dilemma. Vocal cord dysfunction. *Am J Med* 2001;101:731, 741.

202. Kumar P, Caradonna-Graham VM, Gupta S, et al. Inhalation challenge effects of perfume scent strips in patients with asthma. *Ann Allergy Asthma Immunol* 1995;75:429–433.

203. Shim C, Williams MH. Effects of odors in asthma. *Am J Med* 1986;80:18.

204. Cassino C, Ito K, Bader I, et al. Cigarette smoking and ozone-associated emergency department use for asthma by adults in New York City. *Am J Respir Crit Care Med* 1999;159:1773–1779.

205. Fujieda S, Diaz-Sanchez D, Saxon A. Combined nasal challenge with diesel exhaust particles and allergen induces *in vivo* IgE isotope switching. *Am J Respir Cell Mol Biol* 1998;19:507–512.

206. Harding SM, Richter JE. The role of gastroesophageal reflux in chronic cough and asthma. *Chest* 1997;111:1389–1402.

207. Richter JE. Asthma and gastroesophageal reflux disease: the truth is difficult to define. *Chest* 1999:116:1150–1152.

208. Brown JE, Greenberger PA. Immunotherapy and asthma. *Immunol Allergy Clin North Am* 1993;13:939.

209. Abramson MJ, Puy RM, Weiner JM. Is allergen immunotherapy effective in asthma? A meta-analysis of randomized controlled trials. *Am J Respir Crit Care Med* 1995;151:969.

210. Cockcroft DW, O'Byrne PM, Swystun VA, et al. Regular use of inhaled albuterol and the allergen-induced late asthmatic response. *J Allergy Clin Immunol* 1995;96:44–49.

211. Cheung D, Timmers MC, Zwinderman AH, et al. Long-term effects of a long-acting β_2-adrenoceptor agonist, salmeterol, on airway hyperresponsiveness in patients with mild asthma. *N Engl J Med*, 1992;327:1198–1203.

212. O'Connor BJ, Aikman SL, Barnes PJ. Tolerance to the nonbronchodilator effects of inhaled β_2-agonists in asthma. *N Engl J Med* 1992;327:1204–1208.

213. Drazen JM, Israel E, Boushey HA, et al. Comparison of regularly scheduled with as-needed use of albuterol in mild asthma. *N Engl J Med* 1996;335:841–847.

214. Nelson HS, Berkowitz RB, Tinkelman DA, et al. Lack of subsensitivity to albuterol after treatment with salmeterol in patients with asthma. *Am J Respir Crit Care Med* 1999;159:1556–1561.

215. Turner MO, Patel A, Ginsburg S, et al. Bronchodilator delivery in acute airflow obstruction: a meta-analysis. *Arch Intern Med* 1997;157:1736–1744.

216. McFadden ER, Strauss L, Hejal R, et al. Comparison of two dosage regimens of albuterol in acute asthma. *Am J Med* 1998;105:12–17.

217. Baker EK, Willsie SK, Marinac JS, et al. Continuously nebulized albuterol in severe exacerbations of asthma in adults: a case-controlled study. *J Asthma* 1997;34:521–530.

218. Handley DA, Tinkelman D, Noonan M, et al. Dose-response evaluation of levabuterol versus racemic albuterol in patients with asthma. *J Asthma* 2000;37:319–327.

219. Chapman KR, Smith DK, Rebuck AS. Hemodynamic effects of an inhaled beta-2 agonist. *Clin Pharmacol Ther* 1984;35:762.

220. Shim CS, Williams MH. Effects of bronchodilator therapy administered by canister versus jet nebulizer. *J Allergy Clin Immunol* 1984;73:387.

221. Fanta CH, Rossing TH, McFadden ER. Glucocorticoids in acute asthma: critical controlled trial. *Am J Med* 1983;74:845.

222. Svedmyr N. Action of corticosteroids on beta-adrenergic receptors. *Am Rev Respir Dis* 1990;141:S31.

223. Rodrigo G, Rodrigo C. Corticosteroids in the emergency department therapy of acute adult asthma: an evidence-based evaluation. *Chest* 1999;116:285–295.

224. Fiel SB, Swartz MA, Glanz K, et al. Efficacy of short-term corticosteroid therapy in outpatient treatment of acute bronchial asthma. *Am J Med* 1983;75:259.

225. Chapman KR, Verbeek PR, White JG, et al. Effect of a short course of prednisone in the prevention of early relapse after the emergency room treatment of acute asthma. *N Engl J Med* 1991;324:788.

226. Rowe BH, Bota GW, Fabris L, et al. Inhaled budesonide in addition to oral corticosteroids to prevent asthma relapse following discharge from the emergency department: a random controlled trial. *JAMA* 1999;281:2119–2126.

227. Shapiro GG, Furukawa CT, Pierson WE, et al. Double-blind evaluation of methylprednisolone versus placebo for acute asthma episodes. *Pediatrics* 1983;71:510.

228. Jaffuel D, Demoly P, Gougat C, et al. Transcriptional potencies of inhaled glucocorticoids. *Am J Respir Crit Care Med* 2000;162:57–63.

229. Wood LJ, Sehmi R, Gauvreau GM, et al. An inhaled corticosteroid, budesonide, reduces baseline but not allergen-induced increases in bone marrow inflammatory cell progenitors in asthmatic subjects. *Am J Respir Crit Care Med* 1999;159:1457–1463.

230. Donahue JG, Weiss ST, Livingston JM, et al. Inhaled steroids and the risk of hospitalization for asthma. *JAMA* 1997;277:887–891.

231. Kamada AK, Szefler SJ, Martin RJ, et al. Issues in the use of inhaled glucocorticoids. *Am J Respir Crit Care Med* 1996;153:1739–1748.

232. Pauwels RA, Löfdahl C-G, Postma DS, et al. Effect of inhaled formoterol and budesonide on exacerbations of asthma. *N Engl J Med*, 1997;337:1405–1411.

233. Verberne AAPH, Frost C, Duiverman EJ, et al. Addition of salmeterol versus doubling the dose of beclomethasone in children with asthma. *Am J Respir Crit Care Med* 1998;158:213–229.

234. Shrewsbury S, Pyke S, Britton M. Meta-analysis of increased dose of inhaled steroid or addition of salmeterol in symptomatic asthma (MIASMA). *Br Med J* 2000;320:1368–1373.

235. NIH Consesus Development Panel on Osteoporosis Prevention, Diagnosis and Therapy. Osteoporosis prevention, diagnosis, and therapy. *JAMA* 2001;285:785–795.

236. Chernow B, Alexander R, Smallridge RC, et al. Hormonal responses to graded surgical stress. *Arch Intern Med* 1987;147:1273.

237. Falliers CJ, Chai H, Molk L, et al. Pulmonary and adrenal effects of alternate-day corticosteroid therapy. *J Allergy Clin Immunol* 1972;49:156.

238. Greenberger PA, Chow MJ, Adkinson AJ Jr, et al. Comparison of prednisolone kinetics in patients receiving

daily or alternate-day prednisone for asthma. *Clin Pharmacol Ther* 1986;39:163.

239. Haahtela T, Jarvinen M, Kava T, et al. Comparison of a B₂-agonist, terbutaline, with an inhaled corticosteroid, budesonide, in newly detected asthma. *N Engl J Med* 1991;325:388–392.

240. Haahtela T, Jarvinen M, Kava T, et al. Effects of reducing or discontinuing inhaled budesonide in patients with mild asthma. *N Engl J Med* 1994;331:770.

241. Rall TW. Drugs used in the treatment of asthma. In: Gilman AG, Rall TW, Nies AS, et al, eds. *The pharmacologic basis of therapeutics.* 8th ed. New York: Pergamon, 1990:618.

242. Mitenko PA, Ogilvie RI. Rational intravenous doses of theophylline. *N Engl J Med* 1973;289:600.

243. Newhouse MT. Is theophylline obsolete? *Chest* 1990;98:1.

244. Lam A, Newhouse MT. Management of asthma and chronic airflow limitation. Are methylxanthines obsolete? *Chest* 1990;98:44.

245. Littenberg B. Aminophyllin treatment in severe acute asthma: a meta-analysis. *JAMA* 1988;259:1678.

246. Furukawa C, Atkinson D, Forster TJ, et al. Controlled trial of two formulations of cromolyn sodium in the treatment of asthmatic patients 12 years of age. *Chest* 1999;116:65–72.

247. DeJong JW, Teengs JP, Postma DS, et al. Nedocromil sodium versus albuterol in the management of allergic asthma. *Am J Respir Crit Care Med* 1994;149:91.

248. O'Hickey SP, Rees PJ. High-dose nedocromil sodium as an addition to inhaled corticosteroids in the treatment of asthma. *Respir Med* 1984;88:499.

249. Wenzel SE. New approaches to anti-inflammatory therapy for asthma. *Am J Med* 1998;104:287–300.

250. Edelman JM, Turpin JA, Bronsky EA, et al. Oral montelukast compared with inhaled salmeterol to prevent exercise-induced bronchoconstriction. *Ann Intern Med* 200;132:97–104.

251. Reiss TF, Chervinsky P, Dockhorn RJ, et al. Montelukast, a once-daily leukotriene receptor antagonist, in the treatment of chronic asthma: a multicenter, randomized, double-blind trial. *Arch Intern Med* 1998;158:1213–1220.

252. Knorr B, Matz J, Bernstein JA, et al. Montelukast for chronic asthma in 6- to 14-year-old children: a randomized double-blind trial. *JAMA* 1998;279:1181–1186.

253. Laviolette M, Malmstrom K, Lu S, et al. Montelukast added to inhaled beclomethasone in treatment of asthma. *Am J Respir Crit Care Med* 1999;160:1862–1868.

254. Israel E, Rubin P, Kemp JP, et al. The effect of inhibition of 5-lipoxygenase by zileuton in mild-to moderate asthma. *Ann Intern Med* 1993;119:1059–1066.

255. Hirsch DJ, Hirsch SR, Kalbfleisch JH. Effect of central air conditioning and meteorologic factors on indoor spore counts. *J Allergy Clin Immunol* 1978;62:22.

256. Reisman RE, Mauriello PM, Davis DB, et al. A double-blind study of the effectiveness of a high efficiency particulate air (HEPA) filter in the treatment of patients with perennial allergic rhinitis and asthma. *J Allergy Clin Immunol* 1990:85;1050.

257. Htut T, Higenbottam TW, Gill GW, et al. Eradication of house dust mite from homes of atopic asthmatic subjects: a double-blind trial. *J Allergy Clin Immunol* 2001;107:55–60.

258. Dunn TL, Gerber MJ, Shen AS, et al. The effect of topical ophthalmic instillation of timolol and betaxolol on lung function in asthmatic subjects. *Am Rev Respir Dis* 1986;133:264.

259. Prakish VBS, Rosenow EC III. Pulmonary complications from ophthalmic preparations. *Mayo Clin Proc* 1990;65:521.

260. Lipworth BJ, McMurray JJ, Clark RA, et al. Development of persistent late onset asthma following treatment with captopril. *Eur Respir J* 1989;2:586.

261. Levey BA. Angiotensin-converting enzyme inhibitors and cough. *Chest* 1990;98:1052.

262. May CD. Objective clinical laboratory studies of immediate hypersensitivity reactions to foods in asthmatic children. *J Allergy Clin Immunol* 1976;58:500.

263. Johnstone DE, Dutton A. The value of hyposensitization therapy for bronchial asthma in children: a 14 year study. *Pediatrics* 1968;42:793.

264. Jacobsen L, Nüchel Petersen B, Wihl JA, et al. Immunotherapy with partially purified and standardized tree pollen extracts. IV. Results from long-term (6-year) follow-up. *Allergy* 1997;52:914–920.

265. Stevenson DD. Oral challenge to detect aspirin and sulfite sensitivity in asthma. *N Engl Reg Allergy Proc* 1988;9:135.

266. Patterson R, DeSwarte RD, Greenberger PA, et al. Drug allergy and protocols for management of drug allergies. *Allergy Proc* 1994;15:243.

267. Stevenson DD, Pleskow WW, Simon RA, et al. Aspirin-sensitive rhinosinusitis asthma: a double-blind crossover study of treatment with aspirin. *J Allergy Clin Immunol* 1984;73:500.

268. Ruffin RE, Latimer KM, Schembri DA. Longitudinal study of near fatal asthma. *Chest* 1991;99:77.

269. Koresec M, Novak RD, Myers E, et al. Salmeterol does not compromise the bronchodilator response to albuterol during acute episodes of asthma. *Am J Med* 1999;107:209–213.

270. Rodrigo GJ, Rodrigo C. First-line therapy for adult patients with acute asthma receiving a multiple-dose protocol of ipratropium bromide plus albuterol in the emergency department. *Am J Respir Crit Care Med* 2000;161:1862–1868.

271. Qureshi F, Pestian J, Davis P, et al. Effect of nebulized ipratropium on the hospitalization rates of children with asthma. *N Engl J Med* 1998;339:1030–1035.

272. Lanes SF, Garrett JE, Wentworth CE III, et al. The effect of adding ipratropium bromide to salbutamol in the treatment of acute asthma: a pooled analysis of three trials. *Chest* 1998;144:365–372.

273. Fitzgerald JM, Grunfeld A, Pare PD, et al. The clinical efficacy of combination nebulized anticholinergic and adrenergic bronchodilators vs nebulized adrenergic bronchodilator alone in acute asthma. *Chest* 1997;111:311–315.

274. Karpel JP, Schackter EN, Fanta C, et al. A comparison of ipratropium and albuterol vs albuterol alone for the treatment of acute asthma. *Chest* 1996;110:611–616.

275. Gautrin P, D'Aquino LC, Gagnon G, et al. Comparison between peak expiratory flow rates (PEFR) and FEV₁ in the monitoring of asthmatic subjects at an outpatient clinic. *Chest* 1994;106:1419.

276. Ogirala RG, Aldrich TK, Prezant DJ, et al. High-dose intramuscular triamcinolone in severe, chronic, life-threatening asthma. *N Engl J Med* 1991;324:585.

277. Mullarkey MF, Blumenstein BA, Andrade WP, et al. Methotrexate in the treatment of corticosteroid-dependent asthma: a double blind crossover study. *N Engl J Med* 1988;318:603.

278. Ezrurum SC, Leff JA, Cochran JE, et al. Lack of benefit of methotrexate in severe, steroid-dependent asthma. *Ann Intern Med* 1991;114:353.

279. Lock SH, Kay AB, Barnes NC. Double-blind, placebo-controlled study of cyclosporin A as a corticosteroid-sparing agent in corticosteroid-dependent asthma. *Am J Respir Crit Care Med* 1996;153:509–514.

280. Dykewicz MS, Greenberger PA, Patterson R, et al. Natural history of asthma in patients requiring long-term systemic corticosteroids. *Arch Intern Med* 1986;146:2369.

281. Klaustermeyer WB, Noritake DT, Kwong FK. Cryotherapy in the treatment of corticosteroid-dependent asthma. *J Allergy Clin Immunol* 1987;79:720.

282. Kishiyama JL, Valacer D, Cunningham-Rundles C, et al. A multicenter, randomized, double-blind, placebo-controlled trial of high-dose intravenous immunoglobulin for oral corticosteroid-dependent asthma. *Clin Immunol* 1999;91:126–133.

283. Salmun LM, Barlan I, Wolf HM, et al. Effect of intravenous immunoglobulin on steroid consumption in patients with severe asthma: a double-blind, placebo-controlled, randomized trial. *J Allergy Clin Immunol* 1999;103:810–815.

284. Landwehr LP, Jeppson JD, Katlan MG, et al. Benefits of high-dose IV immunoglobulin in patients with severe steroid-dependent asthma. *Chest* 1998;114:1349–1356.

285. Hunt LW, Swedlund HA, Gleich GJ. Effect of nebulized lidocaine on severe glucocorticoid-dependent asthma. *Mayo Clin Proc* 1996;71:361–368.

286. Decco ML, Neeno TA, Hunt LW, et al. Nebulized lidocaine in the treatment of severe asthma in children: a pilot study. *Ann Allergy Asthma Immunol* 1999;82:29–32.

287. Leatherman JW, Fluegel WL, David WS, et al. Muscle weakness in mechanically ventilated patients with severe asthma. *Am J Respir Crit Care Med* 1996;153:1686–1690.

288. Behbehani NA, Al-Mane F, D'yachkova Y, et al. Myopathy following mechanical ventilation for acute severe asthma: the role of muscle relaxants and corticosteroids. *Chest* 1999;115:1627–1631.

289. Manthous CA, Chatlia W. Prolonged weakness after the withdrawal of atracurium. *Am J Respir Crit Care Med* 1994;150:1441–1443.

290. Corrigan CJ, Brown PH, Barnes NC, et al. Glucocorticoid resistance in chronic asthma: Glucocorticoid pharmacokinetics, glucocorticoid receptor characteristics, and inhibition of peripheral blood T cell proliferation by glucocorticoids in vitro. *Am Rev Respir Dis* 1991;144:1016.

291. Corrigan CJ, Brown PH, Barnes NC, et al. Glucocorticoid resistance in chronic asthma: peripheral blood T lymphocyte activation and comparison of the T lymphocyte inhibitory effects of glucocorticoids and cyclosporin A. *Am Rev Respir Dis* 1991;144:1026.

292. Corbridge TC, Hall JB. The assessment and management of adults with status asthmaticus. *Am J Respir Crit Care Med* 1995;151:1296.

293. Becker JM, Arora A, Scarfone RJ, et al. Oral versus intravenous corticosteroids in children hospitalized with asthma. *J Allergy Clin Immunol* 1999;103:586–590.

294. Mountain RD, Sahn SA. Clinical features and outcome in patients with acute asthma presenting with hypercapnia. *Am Rev Respir Dis* 1988;138:535.

295. Levenson T, Greenberger PA, Donoghue ER, et al. Asthma deaths confounded by substance abuse: an assessment of fatal asthma. *Chest* 1996;110:604–610.

296. Steichen Kabalin C, Yarnold PR, Grammer LC. Low complication rate of corticosteroid-treated asthmatics undergoing surgical procedures. *Arch Intern Med* 1995;155:1379.

297. Smetana GW. Preoperative pulmonary evaluation. *N Engl J Med* 1999;340;937–944.

298. Moorman JE, Mannino DM. Increasing U.S. asthma mortality rates: who is really dying? *J Asthma* 2001;38:65–71.

299. Milgrom H, Fick RB Jr, Su JQ, et al. Treatment of allergic asthma with monoclonal anti-IgE antibody. *N Engl J Med* 1999;341:1966–1973.

300. Fahy JV, Cockcroft DW, Boulet L-P, et al. Effect of aerosolized anti-IgE (E25) on airway responses to inhaled allergen in asthmatic subjects. *Am J Respir Crit Care Med* 1999;160:1023–1027.

301. Borish LC, Helson HS, Lanz MJ, et al. Interlukin-4 receptor in moderate atopic asthma: a phase I/II randomized, placebo-controlled trial. *Am J Respir Crit Care Med* 1999;160:1816–1823.

23

Hypersensitivity Pneumonitis

Michael C. Zacharisen and Jordan N. Fink

Allergy/Immunology Section, Departments of Pediatrics and Medicine
Medical College of Wisconsin and Children's Hospital of
Wisconsin, Milwaukee, Wisconsin

Hypersensitivity pneumonitis, also known as extrinsic allergic alveolitis, is a complex immunologically mediated lung disease with associated constitutional symptoms. It is characterized by non–immunoglobulin E (IgE)-mediated inflammation of the pulmonary interstitium, terminal airways, and alveoli. A wide variety of inhaled organic dusts or ingested medications has been implicated in this disorder. This syndrome occurs in both atopic and nonatopic individuals and may present in several clinical forms depending on the duration, frequency, and intensity of antigen exposure, the antigenicity of the offending agent, and the patient's age and immunologic responsiveness. The majority of cases occur in the occupational and agricultural setting. However, various hobbies and medications are also associated with hypersensitivity pneumonitis. Despite the many antigens recognized to cause hypersensitivity pneumonitis, the clinical, immunologic, and pathophysiologic findings are generally similar.

ALLERGENS OF HYPERSENSITIVITY PNEUMONITIS

Hypersensitivity pneumonitis was first recognized by Ramazzini in 1713 in grain workers (1). As awareness of this pulmonary disease has increased, there has been identification of new antigens implicated in the disease. Although the immunopathophysiology is becoming clarified, there continue to be cases of hypersensitivity pneumonitis in which the specific antigen has not been defined. The primary exposures for the development of hypersensitivity pneumonitis are occupational, agricultural, and those related to hobbies. To reach the terminal airways and alveoli, the allergenic particles must be smaller than 3 to 5 μm. The causative antigens include airborne microbial antigens, animal or plant products, and low-molecular-weight chemicals (Table 23.1). Many of these same antigens, such as diisocyanates, mammalian and insect proteins, and wood dusts, also can induce IgE-mediated asthma.

Thermophilic actinomycetes were recognized as the causative agent in farmer's lung in 1932 in England (2). These bacteria thrive at temperatures of 70°C and can be found in high concentrations in compost piles or in silos where animal fodder is stored and becomes a culture medium for the organism. Identification and clarification of the responsible antigens have been described by a number of investigators (3,4). Increased awareness of the environmental factors favoring disease and changes in farming techniques have reduced the incidence of this disorder (5).

Both commercial and residential exposures to mold-contaminated substances have been implicated in many cases of hypersensitivity pneumonitis. The descriptive names of many of these diseases reflect the source of exposure. For example, ventilation pneumonitis, caused by contaminated heating or cooling units, is probably the most common building-related form of

TABLE 23.1. *Some antigens of hypersensitivity pneumonitis*

Antigens	Source of antigen	Disease name
Bacteria		
Thermophilic actinomycetes	Moldy hay, compost, silage, grain, moldy sugarcane	Farmer's lung, mushroom picker's lung, bagassosis
Bacillus, Klebsiella	Air conditioner, humidifier, moldy wood floors	Ventilation pneumonitis Floor finisher's lung
Pseudomonas, Acinetobacter	Contaminated metal-working fluids	Machine operator's lung
Bacillus subtilis	Enzyme dust	Enzyme worker's lung
Mycobacterium	Hot tub, metal working fluid	Hot tub lung
Fungi		
Aspergillus	Moldy malt used in brewing, moldy Esparto grass dust (stucco)	Malt worker's lung, stipatosis
Alternaria, Pullaria	Moldy redwood	Wood workers lung, sequoiosis
Penicillium	Moldy cheese, moldy cork dust	Cheese worker's/washer's lung, suberosis, residential composter's lung
Penicillium, Monocillium	Moldy peat moss	Peat moss processor's lung
Cryptostroma corticale	Moldy maple bark	Maple bark disease
Trichosporum species	Moldy homes in Japan	Summer pneumonitis, mushroom picker's lung
Candida	Moldy reed	Saxophonist's lung
Pezizia domiciliana	Moldy home	El Niño lung
Other		Hot tub lung/sauna taker's lung
Amebae		
Naegleria, Acanthamoeba	Contaminated humidifier	Ventilation pneumonitis
Animal protein		
Avian proteins (pigeon, duck, goose, turkey, chicken, dove, parakeet, parrot, lovebird, owl)	Droppings, feather bloom	Bird/pigeon breeder's lung/disease, bird fanciers disease, budrigerar's disease
Rodent urine protein	Rat or gerbil urine	Laboratory worker's lung, gerbil keepers' lung
Pearl oyster/mollusk shell protein	Shell dust	Oyster shell lung/sericulturist lung
Animal fur dust (e.g., cat)	Animal pelts, fur	Furrier's lung
Insect	*Sitophilus granarius*	Wheat wheevil disease
Drugs		
Amiodarone, chlorambucil, clozapine, cyclosporin, gold, β blocker, sulfonamide, nitrofurantoin, minocycline, procarbazine, methotrexate, HMG-CoA reductase inhibitor	Oral drug ingestion	Drug-induced hypersensitivity pneumonitis
Heroin	Nasal	
Chemicals		
Isocyanates (TDI, HDI, MDI)	Paint/chemical catalyst, varnish, lacquer, polyurethane foam plasticizer	Bathtub refinisher's disease, paint refinisher's disease, plastic workers' lung
Phthalic anhydride	Heated epoxy resin	Epoxy resin lung
Others	Tobacco leaves	Tobacco grower's lung
	Insecticide	Pyrethrum lung
	Coffee and tea dust	Coffee worker's lung, tea grower's lung
	Pinewood sawdust	Wood worker's lung

HMG-CoA, 3-Hydroxy-3-methyl-glutaryl–coenzyme A; TDI, toluene diisocyanate; HDI, hexamethylene diisocyanate; MDI, methylene diphenyl diisocyanate.

hypersensitivity pneumonitis (11,12). This syndrome may occur from aerosols containing antigens found in small home ultrasonic humidifiers to large industrial units (13). More recently, respiratory illness related to inhalation of metal working fluids has been reported; this has far-reaching consequences for industry (14,15).

Pigeon breeders and bird fanciers have long been recognized to develop hypersensitivity pneumonitis to inhaled antigens in dried avian droppings and feather bloom (6,7). A variety of exotic, wild, and domestic birds have been identified as causing bird breeder's disease (8–10).

As new cases of hypersensitivity pneumonitis are recognized, measures to identify the antigen and decrease antigen exposure can be implemented. This recognition as well as changes in exposure environments have made some hypersensitivity diseases such as smallpox handler's lung and pituitary snuff taker's lung (porcine and bovine allergens) of historical interest only (16).

Medications are an important cause of pulmonary disease that resembles hypersensitivity pneumonitis (17–20). Among the implicated medications are nitrofurantoin, amiodarone, minocycline, and sulphasalazine. Recently, intranasal heroin has been reported to cause the syndrome (21).

Specific syndromes of hypersensitivity pneumonitis occur in different parts of the world. For example, esparto grass is used in the production of rope, matting, paper pulp, and plaster in the Mediterranean countries. Individuals such as stucco makers have developed hypersensitivity pneumonitis to *Aspergillus fumigatus*–contaminated esparto fiber dust in their workplace environments (22). Workers in Eastern Canada who are employed in peat moss processing plants are frequently exposed to loose dry material which may contain many microorganisms, of which molds have been implicated in causing hypersensitivity pneumonitis (23). Summer-type hypersensitivity pneumonitis due to Trichosporon is an important example of a disease not found in the United States, but is the most prevalent form of hypersensitivity pneumonitis in Japan (24).

EPIDEMIOLOGY

The exact incidence of hypersensitivity pneumonitis is unknown, but it has been identified in 2% to 8% of farmers (25) and in 6% to 21% of pigeon breeders (26). Of 36 cases of chronic hypersensitivity pneumonitis identified by a hospital survey in Japan, reported etiologies were summer-type hypersensitivity pneumonitis (10 cases), other home-related causes (5 cases), bird fancier's disease (7 cases), isocyanate (5 cases), farmer's lung (4 cases), and five miscellaneous cases (27). The "healthy worker effect" and high employee turnover may be partly responsible for the underreporting or underrecognition of work-related cases of hypersensitivity pneumonitis.

DIAGNOSTIC CRITERIA AND CLINICAL FEATURES

The criteria for the diagnosis of hypersensitivity pneumonitis consists of recognizing the clinical features with supporting exposure history, laboratory, pulmonary function, and radiographic characteristics (28). There is no single confirmatory test for hypersensitivity pneumonitis, not even lung biopsy. This makes the diagnosis challenging. The only essential criteria are exposure, sensitization, and clinical response to organic dust or low-molecular-weight compounds. The clinical presentation follows repeat exposure and can vary from sudden and explosive systemic and respiratory symptoms to an insidious, progressive course of dyspnea, fatigue, and weight loss. Based on these clinical presentations, hypersensitivity pneumonitis has been divided into acute, subacute, and chronic forms (29).

The patient with the acute form presents with nonproductive cough, dyspnea, sweating, myalgia, and malaise occurring 6 to 12 hours after intense exposure to the inciting allergen. Acute viral or bacterial infections may mimic this presentation, leading to treatment with antibiotics. With avoidance of the allergen, the symptoms spontaneously resolve over 18 hours, with complete resolution within days. On repeat exposure, the symptoms recur. The chronic form is characterized by the insidious onset of dyspnea that especially occurs with exertion. Other symptoms include productive cough, fatigue, and anorexia with weight loss. Fever is not typical unless there is a high-dose allergen exposure superimposed on the chronic symptoms. This form is usually related to continuous low-level antigen exposure. The subacute form is characterized by symptoms intermediate to the acute and chronic form with progressive lower respiratory symptoms. The acute and subacute forms may overlap clinically, just as the subacute and chronic forms may.

PHYSICAL EXAMINATION

The physical examination may be normal in the asymptomatic patient between widely spaced episodes of acute hypersensitivity pneumonitis. Fine, dry rales may be present, depending on the degree of lung disease present and the timing following the most recent exposure. Wheezing is not a prominent symptom. An acute flare-up of hypersensitivity pneumonitis is associated with an ill-appearing patient in respiratory distress with temperature elevation up to 40°C 6 to 12 hours after antigen exposure. Rash, lymphadenopathy, or rhinitis should prompt investigation for causes other than hypersensitivity pneumonitis. With extensive fibrosis that occurs in the chronic form of the disease, dry rales, and decreased breath sounds predominate. Some patients with end-stage disease may have digital clubbing (30). Deaths due to hypersensitivity pneumonitis have been reported.

PULMONARY FUNCTION TESTS

The classic pulmonary function abnormality in the acute form is restriction with decreased forced vital capacity (FVC) and forced expiratory volume in 1 second (FEV_1) occurring 6 to 12 hours after exposure to the offending antigen. A biphasic obstructive response similar to that seen in asthma has been observed in patients who develop both asthma and hypersensitivity pneumonitis to the same antigen. Peripheral airways obstruction as determined by decreased FEV_1 and/or forced midrange flow measurements ($FEF_{25-75\%}$) has been reported frequently. Decreased gas transfer across the alveolar wall as measured by the diffusion capacity of carbon monoxide (DLCO) is often detected. This is in contrast to asthma, a disease in which an elevated DLCO commonly occurs. Although hypoxemia at rest may be observed with severe lung damage, hypoxemia with exercise is common and can be documented by pre- and postexercise arterial blood gas measurements. Bronchial hyperresponsiveness as determined by methacholine challenge is present in a majority of patients with hypersensitivity pneumonitis and is likely due to the inflammatory response of the airways. In subacute and chronic hypersensitivity pneumonitis, there is usually a combination of obstruction and restriction.

RADIOGRAPHIC FEATURES

Chest Radiographs

Radiographic abnormalities may be transient or permanent depending on the form or stage of disease. Transient radiographic changes occur primarily in the acute form with patchy, peripheral, bilateral interstitial infiltrates with a fine, reticulonodular pattern (31) as seen in Fig. 23.1. There may be bilateral ground-glass opacities in the middle to lower lung fields that are indistinguishable from other interstitial lung disorders. Central lymphadenopathy also may be present. These changes usually resolve spontaneously with avoidance or with corticosteroid therapy. Between acute attacks, the chest radiograph is usually normal. In the chronic form, fibrotic changes with honeycombing and areas of emphysema may be seen. In the subacute form, nodular, patchy infiltrates as well as fibrosis may be observed. Findings not characteristic of hypersensitivity pneumonitis include calcification, cavitation, atelectasis, solitary pulmonary nodules, pneumothorax, and pleural effusions.

Computed Tomograpy Scans

High-resolution chest computed tomography (CT) scans may be helpful when vague parenchymal changes are present on plain chest radiographs. Findings include ground-glass opacification and diffuse consolidation suggestive of alveolar disease. A normal chest CT scan does not rule out acute hypersensitivity pneumonitis

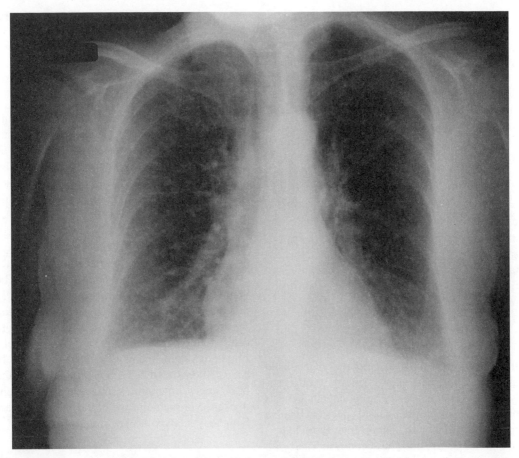

FIG. 23.1. Chest radiograph of a patient with hypersensitivity pneumonitis demonstrating bilateral lower lobe patchy infiltrates and a reticulonodular pattern.

because the sensitivity of this technique may be only 55% (32). In subacute disease, 1- to 3-mm ill-defined centrilobular nodules with superimposed areas of ground-glass opacity may be seen (33). The CT findings of the chronic form are honeycombing, pulmonary fibrosis, and traction bronchiectasis. CT features to suggest hypersensitivity pneumonitis are predominantly middle lung involvement, extensive ground-glass opacities, and small nodules often in the central and peripheral compartments. The role of magnetic resonance imaging has been limited due to respiratory and cardiac motion artifact. Similarly, gallium lung scan and the clearance rate from the alveolar epithelium using a technetium-label are being investigated in the early detection of inflammation or damage to the alveolar-capillary unit, respectively, in infiltrative lung diseases, but studies specifically in hypersensitivity pneumonitis are lacking (34).

LABORATORY

Routine laboratory studies are typically normal in the asymptomatic patient. In the acute form, leukocytosis with a white blood cell count to 25,000 mm^3 and a left shift, an elevated erythrocyte sedimentation rate, and decreased DLCO are common. Eosinophilia is uncommon. Total serum IgE levels are normal unless the patient has coexisting atopic disease (35). Quantitative immunoglobulin measurements are normal, or at times serum IgG may be elevated.

The characteristic immunologic feature of hypersensitivity pneumonitis is the presence of high titers of precipitating IgG and other classes of antibodies directed against the offending antigen in the sera of affected patients (36). Serum precipitating antibodies, as detected by the Ouchterlony double-gel immunodiffusion technique, indicate antigen exposure, but not necessarily disease. In pigeon breeders, as many as 50% of similarly exposed but asymptomatic individuals may have detectable precipitins (37). Enzyme-linked immunosorbent assay and complement fixation techniques for antibody measurements may be too sensitive. If these tests are negative despite a suggestive history, additional testing with antigens specifically prepared from the suspect environment may be necessary. Depending on the exposure, an airborne mist, fluid, dust, or soil sample may be obtained and cultured for contaminating microorganisms. This cultured material can then be used as an antigen in gel diffusion reactions.

SKIN TESTING

In contrast to asthma and other IgE-mediated diseases, immediate skin reactivity to allergens is not useful because the immunopathogenesis of hypersensitivity pneumonitis does not involve IgE. Skin testing with antigens that cause hypersensitivity pneumonitis has been associated with late-onset skin reactions that histologically resemble Arthus-type reactions with mild vasculitis. On gross inspection, necrosis also has been described. When differentiating IgE-mediated occupational asthma from hypersensitivity pneumonitis, skin testing can aid in the diagnosis. Both asthma and hypersensitivity pneumonitis may occur in the same individual; in that case, both immediate and delayed reactions to cutaneous testing may occur.

BRONCHOALVEOLAR LAVAGE

Pulmonary consultation for bronchoscopy and bronchoalveolar lavage may be indicated when other studies are normal or other diagnoses are entertained, such as tuberculosis, pulmonary sarcoidosis, alveolar proteinosis, or idiopathic pulmonary fibrosis. Bronchoalveolar lavage fluid (BALF) is helpful in the diagnosis of hypersensitivity pneumonitis when it demonstrates a lymphocytosis with preponderance of CD8$^+$ T lymphocytes over CD4$^+$ T cells (38). Cultures of BALF can help exclude infectious disorders.

PATHOLOGIC FEATURES

If a biopsy is deemed necessary, open lung biopsy is recommended to obtain an adequate tissue sample. Transbronchial biopsy could be attempted, but studies suggest that the sample may not be adequate. Lung biopsy findings depend on the form of the disease and extent of lung damage that has occurred. Specimens classically reveal interstitial and alveolar noncaseating granulomas, activated "foamy" macrophages, marked predominance of lymphocytes, plasma cells, and neutrophils (39). The granulomas differ from pulmonary sarcoidosis in that they appear smaller, dispersed in interstitial fibrosis, loosely arranged, poorly formed, and are distributed away from bronchioles and vessels. Immunoglobulin or complement have only rarely been demonstrated in pulmonary biopsies. In the later stages, interstitial fibrosis with collagen-thickened bronchiolar walls and less prominent lymphocytic alveolitis is common.

SPECIFIC INHALATION CHALLENGE

Although purposeful inhalation challenge is not required for diagnosis, it can be helpful in situations in which the history is convincing but other data are lacking and the diagnosis is unclear. An allergen challenge can be performed in two ways. First, the patient can return to the workplace or the suspect environment where the antigen is present. In conjunction with pulmonary function and laboratory studies, this approach can implicate the suspect environment, but it will not necessarily identify the allergen. In evaluating these individuals, vital signs, including temperature, spirometry, diffusing capacity, and white blood cell counts with differentials, should be monitored before exposure and at intervals up to 12 hours later.

An inhalation challenge also can be performed in the hospital pulmonary function laboratory. In this situation, vital signs, including temperature,

TABLE 23.2. *Clinical presentation of hypersensitivity pneumonitis*

Features	Acute	Subacute	Chronic
Fever, chills	+	−	−
Dyspnea	+	+	+
Cough	Nonproductive	Productive	Productive
Malaise, myalgia	+	+	+
Weight loss	−	+	+
Rales	Bibasilar	Diffuse	Diffuse
Chest film	Nodular infiltrates	Nodular infiltrates	Fibrosis
PFTs	Restrictive	Mixed	Mixed
DLCO	Decreased	Decreased	Decreased

Adapted from Grammer LC. Occupational allergic alveolitis. *Ann Allergy Asthma Immunol* 1999;83:602–606; with permission.

spirometry, and complete blood count should be monitored before, during, and after exposure. Unfortunately, there generally is no specified concentration of allergen or commercially available allergen preparations for this use. The concentration of antigen used can be determined by using air sampling data, which reflects usual exposure. This inhalation test requires careful observation by trained personnel because severe systemic febrile and respiratory reactions requiring intervention may occur.

DIFFERENTIAL DIAGNOSIS

Hypersensitivity pneumonitis should be considered in any patient with acute or chronic respiratory distress or interstitial pneumonia (Table 23.2). Like other occupational respiratory diseases, a detailed knowledge of the work environment is required. Documentation of cross-shift lung function changes can be detected in some individuals. Furthermore, a detailed history that includes hobbies and the home environment is critical.

The acute form is commonly confused with atypical, community-acquired pneumonia. A group of conditions referred to as organic dust toxic syndrome (ODTS) is also often confused with hypersensitivity pneumonitis (40). Table 23.3 outlines key differences between asthma, ODTS, and hypersensitivity pneumonitis. ODTS occurs in the agricultural setting, presents in individuals exposed to grain, silage, or swine materials, and primarily affects younger age groups and those without prior sensitization to offending agents. In contrast to hypersensitivity pneumonitis, ODTS is thought to be due to inhalation of endotoxin and other phlogistic agents. Diseases such as humidifier fever also can occur in outbreaks and may be related to inhalation of endotoxin from gram-negative bacteria that contaminate ventilation and humidification systems (41).

The differential diagnosis of the subacute form of hypersensitivity pneumonitis includes chronic bronchitis, recurrent episodes of influenza, and idiopathic pulmonary fibrosis. The chronic form of hypersensitivity pneumonitis must be differentiated from many chronic interstitial lung diseases, including idiopathic pulmonary fibrosis, chronic eosinophilic pneumonia, collagen vascular disorders, emphysema, lymphogenous spread of carcinoma, sarcoid, desquamative interstitial pneumonia, and Hamman-Rich syndrome. Extrapulmonary findings of liver or spleen enlargement, generalized or local lymphadenopathy, severe sinusitis, or myositis are not consistent with hypersensitivity pneumonitis.

PATHOGENESIS

Although the mechanisms of inflammation are complex and still not fully clarified, the Gell and Coombs type III and IV reactions are not the best paradigm for explaining the immunologic mechanisms that result in hypersensitivity pneumonitis. Several animal models and many animal studies have been conducted to elucidate the complexity of the inflammation of hypersensitivity pneumonitis (42–45). Unfortunately, the

TABLE 23.3. *Evaluating chronic interstitial lung disorders in the differential diagnosis of chronic hypersensitivity pneumonitis*

Disease	Etiology	Diagnostic Testing			Lung Biopsy	Other
		Blood	BAL			
Pulmonary sarcoidosis	Unknown	↑ ACE level, ↑ IgG, ↑ Calcium	CD4+ alveolitis		Diffuse uniform granulomas	Hilar adenopathy, skin test anergy, gallium scan
Chronic bronchitis	Tobacco smoke	Normal	PMNs increased		Centrilobular emphysema	Reversible obstruction
Byssinosis	Cotton, flax, or hemp dust	Normal	Inflammation		NA	
Histiocytosis X/eosinophilic granuloma	Unknown	Normal			Cytoplasmic Birbeck granules	Pneumothorax
Coal worker's pneumoconiosis	Coal dust	Normal			Focal emphysema, "dust macules"	
Pulmonary alveolar proteinosis	Unknown	Normal	Saline lavage can improve function		PAS staining alveolar material, no interstitial changes	PAS material in sputum
Chronic eosinophilic pneumonia	Unknown	Eosinophilia	Eosinophils		Eosinophils	
Alpha-1-antitrypsin deficiency	Genetic deficiency	Pi typing-ZZ phenotype	NA		Alveolar wall destruction	Panacinar emphysema
Sick building syndrome	Irritants	Normal	Normal		Normal	
Idiopathic pulmonary fibrosis	Unknown	Normal	Lymphocytes		Fibrosis	
Drug reactions	Drug	Eosinophils	Eosinophils, lymphs, PMNs		Variable	
Chronic granulomatous infections	Tuberculosis	Normal	Positive AFB culture		Caseating granulomas	Positive PPD
Inorganic respiratory dust syndromes	Berylliosis, silicosis	BeLPT	CD4+ alveolitis, BeLPT		Granulomas, nodular silica deposits	
Chronic aspergillosis	*Aspergillus* species	Precipitating antibody, eosinophilia, elevated total and specific IgE	Few degenerating eosinophils and fungal hyphae		Exudative bronchiolitis, marked eosinophils, central saccular bronchiectasis	Positive SPT, positive sputum culture, asthma

BAL, bronchoalveolar lavage; PPD, purified protein derivative; PAS, periodic acid-Schiff stain; BeLPT, beryllium lymphocyte proliferation test; ACE, angiotensin-converting enzyme; SPT, skin puncture test; NA, not available; PMNs, polymorphonuclear cells; AFB,___.

findings do not appear to directly parallel the cellular infiltrate seen in human disease. Also, there is difficulty evaluating exposed but asymptomatic animals, as can be done in human studies. Animal models suggest that hypersensitivity pneumonitis is facilitated by the overproduction of interferon-γ (IFN-γ, a helper T cell type 1 (T$_H$1) response (46). This is supported by observations that interleukin-10 (IL-10), a T$_H$1 suppressor molecule, ameliorates the severity of the disease.

Human studies are more difficult to perform, relying on patients who have already experienced symptoms and therefore not truly evaluating the course of inflammation from the onset. The relative contributions of cellular versus humoral immunity in the pathogenesis are not entirely defined. A case report of a patient with hypogammaglobulinemia and hypersensitivity pneumonitis supports the central role of cellular immunity in mediating the disease (47).

The study data are frequently based on bronchoalveolar lavage findings compared with biopsy or peripheral blood. The data suggest that the most important elements in the inflammatory process are the activation of alveolar macrophages CD8$^+$ cells and of T$_H$1 lymphocytes. The hypothesized mechanism for hypersensitivity pneumonitis is depicted in Fig. 23.2. When antigens 2 to 10 μm in size are inhaled, they

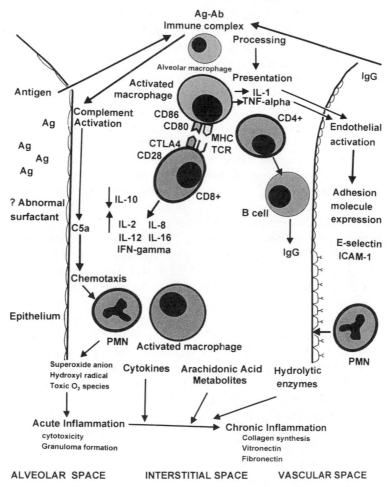

FIG. 23.2. Immunopathogenesis of hypersensitivity pneumonitis. (Modified from Kaltreider HB. Hypersensitivity pneumonitis. *West J Med* 1993;159:575–576; with permission.)

are engulfed and processed by activated alveolar macrophages that can be detected by an increase in surface IL-2R (CD25). The activated macrophages release proinflammatory cytokines such as IL-1 and tumor necrosis factor α (TNF-α) (48). This in turn activates endothelial cells to increase adhesion molecules by upregulating intracellular adhesion molecule type 1 (ICAM-1) and e-selectin (49).

Antigens also may combine with antibodies, forming immune complexes that directly activate complement releasing C3a and C5a, which promote chemotaxis of neutrophils. The neutrophils release superoxide anions, hydroxyl radicals, and toxic oxygen radicals, which contribute to the inflammation.

Alveolar macrophages have cognate interaction with regulatory CD8$^+$ T lymphocytes through the T-cell receptor (TCR) in the presence of B7 costimulatory molecules CD80 and CD86 on macrophages, which act as an accessory signal (50). In healthy subjects, alveolar macrophages have a normal suppressive activity. In contrast, the activated alveolar macrophages in hypersensitivity pneumonitis increase the antigen-presenting capacity through the increased expression of CD80 and CD86, thus enhancing the lymphocytic alveolitis. Cigarette smoking may provide a protective effect from hypersensitivity pneumonitis by decreasing the expression of B7 costimulatory molecules, whereas viral infections could enhance hypersensitivity pneumonitis by increasing B7 expression. BALF CD8$^+$ T lymphocytes release multiple T_H1 cell type cytokines, including IL-2, IL-8, IL-12, IL-16, and IFN-γ. These cytokines are associated with an intense inflammatory process. In direct contrast to asthma, there is an imbalance of IL-10 and IL-12. Stimulated by TNF-α, IL-10 normally functions to inhibit ICAM-1 and B7 molecule expression to prevent the alveolar macrophage from interacting with the T cell, thus preventing activation. In hypersensitivity pneumonitis there is a decreased production of IL-10, leading to activated macrophages and ongoing inflammation.

BALF T cells from patients with hypersensitivity pneumonitis have high levels of functioning IL-12R compared with peripheral blood T cells. When stimulated with recombinant IL-12, lung T cells significantly increased IFN-γ production (51).

Increased expression of the integrin $\alpha^E\beta_7$ on the surface of T cells function as mucosal homing receptors for the selective retention of T lymphocytes in lung mucosa (52). The chemokines IL-8 and monocyte chemoattractant protein-1/monocyte chemotactic and activating factor (MCP-1/MCAF) are significantly increased in BALF, suggesting a role in the accumulation of cells such as neutrophils, lymphocytes, and monocyte/macrophages into the alveoli of patients with hypersensitivity pneumonitis (53). Arachidonic acid metabolites are released from many cell types. Along with hydrolytic enzymes, these further contribute to inflammation.

Surfactant is responsible for the regulatory activities of lung lymphocytes and alveolar macrophages. Alveolar macrophages from patients with hypersensitivity pneumonitis enhance PHA-induced peripheral blood mononuclear cell (PBMC) proliferation, whereas normal alveolar macrophages suppress this proliferation. Surfactant from normal individuals decreases mitogen-induced proliferation of PBMC greater than surfactant from patients with hypersensitivity pneumonitis in the presence of alveolar macrophages (54). Thus, the alveolitis in hypersensitivity pneumonitis also may be due in part to alteration in the surfactant immunosuppressive effect.

Viruses including influenza A have been demonstrated by polymerase chain reaction in the lower airways of patients with acute hypersensitivity pneumonitis. In experimental murine models infected with respiratory syncytial virus, both the early and late inflammatory responses are augmented in hypersensitivity pneumonitis. Further studies are required to clarify the nature of this relationship between viral infection and the modulation of pulmonary immune response (55,56).

MANAGEMENT

Avoidance

The most important element of management, as in any allergic lung disease, is avoidance of the offending antigen. This can occur in two ways: removal of the individual from the antigen or removal of the antigen exposure from the individual's environment. Workplace reassignment is a reasonable means of managing affected employees. Although this straightforward approach is simple to recommend, adherence by patients can be more difficult. For example, farmers afflicted with farmer's lung may be unable to change careers. Machinists with metal-working fluid–induced lung disease may be unable to work in other capacities. Pigeon breeders frequently continue intermittent pigeon exposure. Although elimination of the antigen seems essential for a long-term solution to the problem, continued antigen exposure may not lead to clinical deterioration for some persons (57). Depending on the source of the antigen and the conditions surrounding its generation, various industrial hygiene measures have been proposed. For instance, reducing the humidity in silos has resulted in a decline in the prevalence and incidence of farmer's lung. Other measures include alterations in plant management, increased automation, improved exhaust ventilation, and personal protective face masks. Frequently, assays for the presence of the material in the environment are lacking, or the minimum concentration to provoke symptoms or initiate sensitization is not known.

Pharmacologic Treatment

Few data exist on the various pharmacologic treatments for hypersensitivity pneumonitis. Corticosteroid therapy should be instituted in the acute and subacute forms because this has been reported to reduce symptoms and detectable inflammation and improve pulmonary function. Oral corticosteroids are recommended for acute disease starting at prednisone doses of 40 to 80 mg daily until clinical and laboratory improvements are observed, then decreased stepwise to 5 to 10 mg every other day for six weeks. Indefinite corticosteroid therapy is not necessary. Unfortunately, the long-term outcome of patients treated with a course of prednisone for acute farmer's lung has not always been complete recovery (58). Ongoing follow-up visits should include pulmonary function studies, not peak flow measurements, because they are not sensitive enough. Inhaled corticosteroid therapy is not as effective as oral drug. If obstructive pulmonary function changes are present, then treatment with bronchodilators can be attempted.

PREVENTION AND SCREENING

The presence of occupational lung disease in a worker usually represents a sentinel event. As in other occupational lung diseases, a systematic evaluation and investigation of the work environment and exposed cohort is recommended, although not mandated by law or always conducted (59). The investigation for additional cases may include a screening questionnaire survey with positive responses undergoing chest radiographs, serum precipitins, and lung function testing. Questionnaire surveys can be used to screen for further cases of disease, and to compare rates of symptoms between different locations in the same plant. If possible, the numbers of workers on medical leave should be reviewed. Survey questions should include demographics, risk factors, and protective factors in the home and workplace, including tobacco use and the presence of a humidifier/dehumidifier. Industrial hygiene surveys should include reviewing building maintenance records, visual inspection for standing water, mold growth, stained ceiling tile or carpet, roof drainage patterns, measurement of temperature and humidity, and measurement and culture of airborne, soil, or water microorganisms.

PROGNOSIS

There have been limited studies on the factors determining prognosis of hypersensitivity pneumonitis. Factors identified as having predictive value in the likelihood of recovery from pigeon breeder's disease and farmer's lung include age at diagnosis, duration of antigen exposure after onset of symptoms, and total years of exposure before diagnosis. The effect of other factors including the nature of the allergen, especially its inflammatory potential, host susceptibility, severity of lung function at diagnosis, and form of the disease are not well clarified. Although most cases of acute disease improve, those patients with ongoing exposure continue to experience symptoms, and have abnormal lung function and abnormal chest radiographs. Deaths from farmer's lung and pigeon breeders disease have been reported (60).

CONCLUSION

The diagnosis of hypersensitivity pneumonitis requires a high index of suspicion, because the primary focus of treatment is avoidance of the offending allergen even if the specific allergen is not identified. Efforts are needed to prevent recurrent and progressive disease in individuals already sensitized and prevent potential epidemics in occupational settings. Because the diagnosis is difficult and occupational evaluation complex, a team approach including the collaborative efforts of allergists, pulmonologists, occupational physicians, industrial hygienists, and microbiologists is important.

REFERENCES

1. Ramazzini B. *De morbus artificum diatriba* (originally published 1713). Chicago: University of Chicago Press, 1940.
2. Campbell JM. Acute symptoms following work with hay. *BMJ* 1932;2:1143–1144.
3. Dickie HA, Rankin J. Farmer's lung: an acute granulomatous interstitial pneumonitis occurring in agricultural workers. *JAMA* 1958;167:1069–1076.
4. Emanuel DA, Wenzel FJ, Bowerman CI, et al. Farmer's lung: clinical, pathologic and immunologic study of twenty-four patients. *Am J Med* 1964;37:392–401.
5. Ranalli G, Grazia L, Roggeri A. The influence of hay-packing techniques on the presence of saccharopolyspora rectivirgula. *J Appl Microbiol* 1999;87:359–365.
6. Reed CE, Sosman AJ, Barbee RA. Pigeon breeder's lung. *JAMA* 1965;193:261–265.
7. Tebo T, Moore V, Fink JN. Antigens in pigeon breeder's disease. *Clin Allergy* 1977;7:103–108.
8. Cunningham A, Fink JN, Schlueter D. Hypersensitivity pneumonitis due to doves. *Pediatrics* 1976;58:436–442.
9. Saltoun CA, Harris KE, Mathisen TL, et al. Hypersensitivity pneumonitis resulting from community exposure to Canada goose droppings: when an external environmental antigen becomes an indoor environmental antigen. *Ann Allergy Asthma Immunol* 2000:84:84–86.
10. Boyer RS, Klock LE, Schmidt CD, et al. Hypersensitivity lung disease in the turkey-raising industry. *Am Rev Respir Dis* 1974;109:630–635.
11. Fink JN, Banaszak EF, Thiede WH, et al. Interstitial pneumonitis due to hypersensitivity to an organism contaminating a heating system. *Ann Intern Med* 1971;74:80–83.
12. Banaszak EF, Thiede WH, Fink JN. Hypersensitivity pneumonitis due to contamination of an air conditioner. *N Engl J Med* 1970;283:271–276.
13. Volpe BT, Sulavik SB, Tran P, et al. Hypersensitivity pneumonitis associated with a portable home humidifier. *Conn Med* 1991;55:571–573.
14. Bernstein D, Lummus Z, Santilli G, et al. Machine operator's lung, hypersensitivity pneumonitis disorder associated with exposure to metalworking fluid aerosols. *Chest* 1995;108:636–641.
15. Fox J, Anderson H, Moen T, et al. Metal working fluid-associated hypersensitivity pneumonitis: an outbreak investigation and case-control study. *Am J Industrial Med* 1999;35:58–67.
16. Mahon WE, Scott DJ, Ansell G, et al. Hypersensitivity to pituitary snuff with miliary shadowing in the lungs. *Thorax* 1967;22:13–20.
17. Akoun GM, Cadranel JL, Blanchette G, et al. Bronchoalveolar lavage cell data in amiodarone-associated pneumonitis. *Chest* 1991;99:1177–1182.
18. Leino R, Liipo K, Ekfors T. Sulphasalazine-induced reversible hypersensitivity pneumonitis and fatal fibrosing alveolitis: report of two cases. *J Intern Med* 1991;229:553–556.
19. Guillon JM, Joly P, Autran B, et al. Minocycline-induced cell mediated hypersensitivity pneumonitis. *Ann Intern Med* 1992;117:476–481.
20. Ridley MG, Wolfe CS, Mathews JA. Life threatening acute pneumonitis during low dose methotrexate treatment for rheumatoid arthritis: a case report and review of the literature. *Ann Rheum Dis* 1988; 47:784–788.
21. Suresh K, D'Ambrosio C, Einarsson O, et al. Hypersensitivity pneumonitis induced by intranasal heroin use. *Am J Med* 1999;107:392–395.
22. Quirce S, Hinojosa M, Blanco R, et al. *Aspergillus fumigatus* is the causative agent of hypersensitivity pneumonitis caused by esparto dust. *J Allergy Clin Immunol* 1998;102:147–148.
23. Cormier Y, Israil-Assayag E, Bedard G, et al. Hypersensitivity pneumonitis in peat moss processing plant workers. *Am J Respir Crit Care Med* 1998;158:412–417.
24. Kawai T, Tamura M, Murao M. Summer type hypersensitivity pneumonitis: a unique disease in Japan. *Chest* 1984; 85:311–317.
25. Madsen D, Kloch LE, Wenzel FJ, et al. The prevalence of farmer's lung in an agricultural population. *Am Rev Respir Dis* 1976;113:171–174.
26. Lopez M, Salvaggio JE. Epidemiology of hypersensitivity pneumonitis/allergic alveolitis. *Monogr Allergy* 1987;21:70–86.
27. Yoshizawa Y, Ohtani Y, Hayakawa H, et al. Chronic hypersensitivity pneumonitis in Japan: a nationwide epidemiologic survey. *J Allergy Clin Immunol* 1999; 103:315–320.
28. Richerson H, Berstein IL, Fink JN, et al. Guidelines for the clinical evaluation of hypersensitivity pneumonitis. *J Allergy Clin Immunol* 1989;84:839–844.
29. Fink JN, Sosman AJ, Barboriak JJ, et al. Pigeon breeder's disease: a clinical study of a hypersensitivity pneumonitis. *Ann Intern Med* 1968;68:1205–1219.
30. Sansores R, Salas J, Chapela R et al. Clubbing in hypersensitivity pneumonitis. *Arch Intern Med* 1990;150: 1849–1851.

31. Unger JD, Fink JN, Unger GF. Pigeon breeder's disease: roentgenographic lung findings in a hypersensitivity pneumonitis. *Radiology* 1968;90:683–687.

32. Lynch DA, Rose CS, Way D, King TE. Hypersensitivity pneumonitis: sensitivity of ARCT in a population based study. *Am J Radiol* 1992;159:469–472.

33. Buschman DL, Gamsu G, Waldron JA, et al. Chronic hypersensitivity pneumonitis: use of CT in diagnosis. *Am J Radiol* 1992;159:957–960.

34. Uh S, Lee SM, Kim HT, et al. The clearance rate of alveolar epithelium using 99mTc- DTPA in patients with diffuse infiltrative lung diseases. *Chest* 1994; 106:161–165.

35. Patterson R, Fink JN, Pruzansky JJ, et al. Serum immunoglobulin levels in pulmonary allergic aspergillosis and certain other lung diseases, with special reference to immunoglobulin E. *Am J Med* 1973;54:16–22.

36. Moore VL, Fink JN, Barboriak JJ, et al. Immunologic events in pigeon breeder's disease. *J Allergy Clin Immunol* 1974;53:319–328.

37. Fink JN, Schlueter DP, Sosman AJ et al. Clinical survey of pigeon breeder's. *Chest* 1972; 62:277–281.

38. Leatherman JW, Michael AF, Schwartz BA, et al. Lung T-cells in hypersensitivity pneumonitis. *Ann Intern Med* 1984;100:390–392.

39. Kawanami O, Basset F, Barrios R, et al. Hypersensitivity pneumonitis in man. Light and electron microscope studies of 18 lung biopsies. *Am J Pathol* 1983;110:275–289.

40. Parker JE, Petsonk LE, Weber SL. Hypersensitivity pneumonitis and organic dust toxic syndrome. *Immunol Allergy Clin North Am* 1992;12:279–290.

41. Rylander R, Haglind P. Airborne endotoxins and humidifier disease. *Clin Allergy* 1984;14:109–112.

42. Fink JN, Hensley GT, Barboriak JJ. An animal model of hypersensitivity pneumonitis. *J Allergy* 1970;46:156–161.

43. Moore VL, Hensley GT, Fink JN. An animal model of hypersensitivity pneumonitis in the rabbit. *J Clin Invest* 1975;56:937–944.

44. Takizawa H, Ohta K, Horiuchi T, et al. Hypersensitivity pneumonitis in athymic nude mice. *Am Rev Respir Dis* 1992;146:479–484.

45. Bice D, Salvaggio J, Hoffman E. Passive transfer of experimental hypersensitivity pneumonitis with lymphoid cells in the rabbit. *J Allergy Clin Immunol* 1976;58:250–262.

46. Denis M, Ghadirian E. Murine hypersensitivity pneumonitis: bidirectional role of interferon-gamma. *Clin Exp Allergy* 1992;22:783–792.

47. Schkade PA, Routes JM. Hypersensitivity pneumonitis in a patient with hypogamma-globulinemia. *J Allergy Clin Immunol* 1996;98:710–712.

48. Denis M. Interleukin-1 (IL-1) is an important cytokine in granulomatous alveolitis. *Cell Immunol* 1994;157:70–80.

49. Pforte A, Schiessler A, Gais P, et al. Expression of the adhesion molecule ICAM-1 on alveolar macrophages and in serum in extrinsic allergic alveolitis. *Respiration* 1993;60:221–226.

50. Israil-Assayag E, Dakhama A, Lavigne S, et al. Expression of costimulatory molecules on alveolar macrophages in hypersensitivity pneumonitis. *Am J Respir Crit Care Med* 1999;159:1830–1834.

51. Yamasaki H, Ando M, Brazer W, et al. Polarized type 1 cytokine profile in bronchoalveolar lavage T cells of patients with hypersensitivity pneumonitis. *J Immunol* 1999;163:3516–3523.

52. Lohmeyer J, Friedrich J, Grimminger F, et al. Expression of mucosa-related integrin $\alpha^E \beta_7$ on alveolar T cells in interstitial lung diseases. *Clin Exp Immunol* 1999;116:340–346.

53. Sugiyama Y, Kasahara T, Mukaida N, et al. Chemokines in bronchoalveolar lavage fluid in summer-type hypersensitivity pneumonitis. *Eur Respir J* 1995;8:1084–1090.

54. Israel-Assayag E, Cormier Y. Surfactant modifies the lymphoproliferative activity of macrophages in hypersensitivity pneumonitis. *Am J Physiol* 1997;273:L1258–L1264.

55. Dakhama A, Hegele RG, Laflamme G, et al. Common respiratory viruses in lower airways of patients with acute hypersensitivity pneumonitis. *Am J Respir Crit Care Med* 1999;159:1316–1322.

56. Gudmundsson G, Monick M, Hunninghake G. Viral infection modulates expression of hypersensitivity pneumonitis. *J Immunol* 1999;162:7397–7401.

57. Cuthbert OD, Gordon MF. Ten year follow-up of farmers with farmer's lung. *Br J Industrial Med* 1983;40:173–176.

58. Kokkarinen JI, Tukiainen HO, Terho EO. Effect of corticosteroid treatment on the recovery of pulmonary function in farmer's lung. *Am Rev Respir Dis* 1992;145:3–5.

59. Weltermann BM, Hodgson M, Storey E, et al. Hypersensitivity pneumonitis: a sentinel event investigation in a wet building. *Am J Industrial Med* 1998;34:499–505.

60. Greenberger PA, Pien LC, Patterson R, et al. End-stage lung and ultimately fatal disease in a bird fancier. *Am J Med* 1989;86:119–122.

24

Allergic Bronchopulmonary Aspergillosis

Paul A. Greenberger

Division of Allergy-Immunology, Department of Medicine, Northwestern University Medical School, Northwestern Memorial Hospital, Chicago, Illinois

INTRODUCTION

Allergic bronchopulmonary aspergillosis (ABPA) is characterized by immunologic reactions to antigens of *Aspergillus fumigatus* that are present in the bronchial tree and result in pulmonary infiltrates and proximal bronchiectasis. Allergic bronchopulmonary aspergillosis was first described in England in 1952 in patients with asthma who had recurrent episodes of fever, roentgenographic infiltrates, peripheral blood and sputum eosinophilia, and sputum production containing *A. fumigatus* hyphae (1). The first adult with ABPA in the United States was described in 1968 (2), and the first childhood case was reported in 1970 (3). Since then, the increasing recognition of ABPA in children (4–8), adults (9,10), corticosteroid-dependent asthmatic patients (11), patients with cystic fibrosis (CF) (11–22), and patients with allergic fungal sinusitis (23,24) is probably the result of the increasing awareness by physicians of this complication of asthma or CF. Diagnosis has been helped by serologic aids such as total serum immunoglobulin E (IgE) (25), serum IgE, IgG antibodies to *A. fumigatus* (26,27), precipitating antibodies (28), and familiarity with chest radiography and high-resolution computed tomography (CT) findings. Some atypical patients seemingly have no documented history of asthma and present with chest roentgenographic infiltrates and peripheral blood eosinophilia (29).

Allergic bronchopulmonary aspergillosis was identified in 6.0% of 531 patients in Chicago with asthma and immediate cutaneous reactivity to an *Aspergillus* mix (30), whereas 28% of such patients in Cleveland had ABPA (31). These surprisingly high prevalence figures were generated from the ambulatory setting of the allergist-immunologist clinic and suggest that the overall prevalence of ABPA in patients with persistent asthma is 1% to 2% (31). Allergic bronchopulmonary aspergillosis has been identified on an international basis, and because of its destructive potential should be confirmed or excluded in all patients with persistent asthma.

Aspergillus species are ubiquitous, thermotolerant, and can be recovered on a perennial basis (32,33). Spores measure 2 to 3.5 μm and can be cultured on Sabouraud's agar slants incubated at 37° to 40°C. *Aspergillus* hyphae may be identified in tissue by hematoxylin and eosin staining, but identification and morphology are better appreciated with silver methenamine or periodic acid-Schiff stains. Hyphae are 7 to 10 μm in diameter, septate, and classically branch at 45 degree angles. *Aspergillus* spores, which often are green, are inhaled from outdoor and indoor air and can reach terminal airways. They then could grow as hyphae. Alveolar macrophages ingest and kill the spores (conidia) by a nonoxidative process (33). Polymorphonuclear leukocytes do not ingest hyphae but bind to them and kill the hyphae by damaging their cell walls with an oxidative burst (33). Protection against invasive aspergillosis occurs due to multiple factors, but most crucial is the presence of functioning polymorphonuclear cells because prolonged neutropenia (<500 cells/mm^3), possibly thrombocytopenia (as platelets bind to hyphae and become activated), and injured pulmonary epithelium (from chemotherapy) contribute to invasive disease.

Aspergillus species, particularly *A. flavus* and *A. fumigatus*, produce some toxic metabolites, of which aflatoxin is the most widely known. Another toxic metabolite, gliotoxin, inhibits macrophage phagocytosis and lymphocyte activation (33). *A. fumigatus* produces proteolytic enzymes and ribosome toxins (RNAses) (34) that possibly may contribute to lung damage when *A. fumigatus* hyphae are present in bronchial mucus. Epithelial cells could be damaged by proteases from *A. fumigatus* that also would decrease ciliary function (33). *A. flavus* and *A. fumigatus* have been incriminated in avian aspergillosis, a major economic concern in the poultry industry. For example, aspergillosis is common in turkey poults and can cause 5% to 10% mortality rates in production flocks (35). *Aspergillus* infections as a cause of abortions and mammary gland infections in sheep are recognized, as are infections in horses (pneumonia), cattle (pneumonia), camels (ulcerative tracheobronchitis), and dolphins (pneumonias including a condition resembling ABPA with cough, weight loss, and pulmonary infiltrates).

Aspergillus terreus is used in the pharmaceutical industry for synthesis of the cholesterol-lowering drug levostatin. For use in the baking industry, *Aspergillus* species produce amylase, cellulase, and hemicellulase. Because these enzymes are powdered, some bakery workers may develop IgE-mediated rhinitis and asthma (36).

The genus *Aspergillus* may produce different types of disease, depending on the immunologic status of the patient. In nonatopic patients, *Aspergillus* hyphae may grow in damaged lung and cause a fungus ball (aspergilloma). Morphologically, an aspergilloma contains thousands of tangled *Aspergillus* hyphae in pulmonary cavities, and can complicate sarcoidosis, tuberculosis, old histoplasmosis, carcinoma, CF, or ABPA (37). Hypersensitivity pneumonitis may result from inhalation of large numbers of *A. fumigatus* or *A. clavatus* spores by malt workers. These spores also may produce farmer's lung disease. *Aspergillus* species may invade tissue in the immunologically compromised (neutropenic and thrombocytopenic) host, causing sepsis and death. A rare patient who seemingly is immunocompetent may develop acute respiratory failure from bilateral "community acquired" pneumonia due to *A. fumigatus* infection. *Aspergillus* species have been associated with emphysema, colonization of cysts, pulmonary suppurative reactions, and necrotizing pneumonia in other patients (38). In the atopic patient, fungal spore–induced asthma may occur from IgE-mediated processes in response to inhalation of *Aspergillus* spores. About 25% of patients with persistent asthma have immediate cutaneous reactivity to *A. fumigatus* or a mix of *Aspergillus* species. Why some of these patients with asthma develop ABPA remains unclear. In patients without asthma, *Aspergillus* hyphae have been identified in mucoid impactions of sinuses, a condition that morphologically resembles mucoid impaction of bronchi in ABPA (39–46). Such allergic *Aspergillus* sinusitis may occur in patients with ABPA (23,24,47).

There are over 180 *Aspergillus* species and an additional 18 variants. When *A. fumigatus* is grown in culture, changing media components and conditions alter the characteristics of the resultant strains of *A. fumigatus*. The International Union of Immunological Societies has accepted 18 allergens of *A. fumigatus,* which are listed as *Asp f* 1, 2, 3, and so forth.

DIAGNOSTIC CRITERIA AND CLINICAL FEATURES

The criteria used for diagnosis of classic ABPA consist of five essential criteria and other criteria that may or may not be present, depending on the classification and stage of disease. The minimal essential criteria are (a) asthma, even cough variant asthma or exercise-induced asthma; (b) central (proximal) bronchiectasis; (c) elevated total serum IgE ($\geq 1,000$ ng/mL); (d) immediate cutaneous reactivity to *Aspergillus*; and (e) elevated serum IgE and/or IgG antibodies to *A. fumigatus*. Central (proximal) bronchiectasis in the absence of distal bronchiectasis, as occurs in CF or chronic obstructive pulmonary

TABLE 24.1. *Diagnostic criteria for allergic bronchopulmonary aspergillosis (ABPA)*

Asthma
Chest roentgenographic infiltrates
Immediate cutaneous reactivity to *Aspergillus*
Elevated total serum IgE concentration (>1,000 ng/mL or 417 IU/mL)
Elevated serum IgE-Af and/or IgG-Af antibodies
Serum precipitating antibodies to Af
Proximal bronchiectasis
Peripheral blood eosinophilia (≥1,000/mm^3)

Minimal Essential Criteria for ABPA-CB[a]

Asthma
Immediate cutaneous reactivity to *Aspergillus*
Elevated total IgE concentration
Elevated serum IgE-Af and or IgG-Af antibodies
Proximal bronchiectasis

[a]Suitable for diagnosis of ABPA in cystic fibrosis.
Af, *Aspergillus fumigatus.*

disease, is virtually pathognomonic for ABPA. Such patients are labeled ABPA-CB, for central bronchiectasis. Other features of ABPA are often present. For example, the expected diagnostic criteria (Table 24.1) of ABPA-CB include (a) asthma; (b) immediate cutaneous reactivity to *A. fumigatus*; (c) precipitating antibodies to *A. fumigatus*; (d) elevated total serum IgE; (e) peripheral blood eosinophilia (≥1,000/mm^3); (f) a history of either transient or fixed roentgenographic infiltrates; (g) proximal bronchiectasis; and (h) elevated serum IgE–*A. fumigatus* and IgG–*A. fumigatus* (48). These diagnostic criteria may not apply to ABPA-S (seropositive), where bronchiectasis cannot be detected by high-resolution chest tomography. Patients who have all the criteria for ABPA but in whom central bronchiectasis is not present have ABPA-S (10,49). The minimal essential criteria for ABPA-S include (a) asthma; (b) immediate cutaneous reactivity to *Aspergillus*; (c) elevated total serum IgE; and (d) elevated serum IgE and IgG antibodies to *A. fumigatus* compared with sera from patients with asthma without ABPA (10).

Other features of ABPA may include positive sputum cultures for *A. fumigatus* and a history of expectoration of golden brown plugs containing *A. fumigatus* hyphae. Patients with asthma without ABPA may have positive cutaneous tests for *A. fumigatus*, peripheral blood eosinophilia, and a history of roentgenographic infiltrates (due to atelectasis from inadequately controlled asthma). *Aspergillus* precipitins are not diagnostic of ABPA, and sputum cultures may be negative for *A. fumigatus* or even unobtainable if the patient has little bronchiectasis. In ABPA-S, bronchiectasis cannot be detected by high-resolution CT. Serologic measurements have proven useful in making the diagnosis of ABPA. A marked elevation in total serum IgE and IgE and IgG antibodies to *A. fumigatus* is of value in making the diagnosis (27). Furthermore, the decline in total serum IgE by at least 35% by 6 weeks after institution of prednisone has been shown to occur in ABPA (50).

Allergic bronchopulmonary aspergillosis should be suspected in all patients with asthma who have immediate cutaneous reactivity to *A. fumigatus* (30). The absence of a documented chest roentgenographic infiltrate or mucoid infiltrates demonstrable by CT does not exclude ABPA-CB. Familial ABPA has been described occasionally, which emphasizes the need for screening family members for evidence of ABPA if they have asthma. Clearly, ABPA should be suspected in patients with a history of roentgenographic infiltrates, pneumonia, or abnormal chest films and in patients with allergic fungal sinusitis. Increasing severity of asthma without other causes may indicate evolving ABPA, but some patients present solely with asymptomatic pulmonary infiltrates. Consolidation on the chest roentgenogram caused by ABPA often is not associated with the rigors, chills, as high a fever, and overall malaise as with a bacterial pneumonia causing the same degree of roentgenographic consolidation. The time of onset of ABPA may precede recognition by many years (51), or there may be early diagnosis of ABPA before significant lung destruction and roentgenographic infiltrates have occurred (10). Allergic bronchopulmonary aspergillosis must be considered in the patient over 40 years of age with chronic bronchitis, bronchiectasis, or interstitial fibrosis. Further lung damage may be prevented by prednisone treatment of ABPA exacerbations. The dose of prednisone necessary for controlling persistent asthma may be inadequate to prevent the emergence of ABPA, although the total serum

IgE concentration may be elevated only moderately because of suppression by prednisone.

Patients with ABPA manifest multiple allergic conditions. For example, just 1 of the first 50 patients diagnosed and managed at Northwestern University Medical School had isolated cutaneous reactivity to *A. fumigatus* (50). Other atopic disorders (rhinitis, urticaria, atopic dermatitis) may be present in patients with ABPA (50). The severity of asthma ranges from intermittent asthma to mildly persistent, to severe corticosteroid-dependent persistent asthma. Four patients denied developing wheezing or dyspnea on exposure to raked leaves, moldy hay, or damp basements, but they noted nonimmunologic triggering factors such as cold air, infection, or weather changes. The findings in these patients emphasize that ABPA may be present in patients who appear to have no obvious IgE-mediated asthma.

The number of diagnostic criteria vary depending on the classification (ABPA-CB or ABPA-S) and stage of ABPA. Furthermore, prednisone therapy causes clearing of the chest roentgenographic infiltrates, decline of the total serum IgE concentration, disappearance of precipitating antibodies, peripheral blood or sputum eosinophilia, and absence of sputum production.

PHYSICAL EXAMINATION

The physical examination in ABPA may be completely unremarkable in the asymptomatic patient, or the patient may have crackles, bronchial breathing, or wheezing, depending on the degree and quality of lung disease present. An acute flare-up of ABPA may be associated with temperature elevation to 103°F (although this is most uncommon), with malaise, wheezing, and sputum production. Viral or bacterial infections in patients with asthma may simulate exacerbations of ABPA. In some cases of ABPA, extensive pulmonary consolidation on roentgenography may be accompanied by few or no clinical symptoms, in contrast to the usual manifestations of a patient with a bacterial pneumonia and the same degree of consolidation. When extensive fibrosis has occurred from ABPA, posttussive crackles will be present. Allergic bronchopulmonary aspergillosis has been associated with collapse of a lung from a mucoid impaction, and in one patient it was associated with a spontaneous pneumothorax (51). The physical examination yields evidence for these diagnoses. When ABPA infiltrates affect the periphery of the lung, pleuritis may occur and it may be associated with restriction of chest wall movement on inspiration and a pleural friction rub. Some patients with end-stage ABPA (fibrotic stage V) have digital clubbing and cyanosis (52,53). The latter findings should suggest concomitant CF as well.

RADIOLOGY

Chest roentgenographic changes may be transient or permanent (Figs. 24.1 to 24.6) (54–59). Transient roentgenographic changes, which may clear with or without oral corticosteroid therapy, appear to be the result of parenchymal infiltrates, mucoid impactions, or secretions in damaged bronchi. These nonpermanent findings include (a) perihilar infiltrates simulating adenopathy; (b) air-fluid levels from dilated central bronchi filled with fluid and debris; (c) massive consolidation that may be unilateral or bilateral; (d) roentgenographic infiltrates; (e) "toothpaste" shadows that result from mucoid impactions in damaged bronchi; (f) "gloved-finger" shadows from distally occluded bronchi filled with secretions; and (g) "tramline" shadows, which are two parallel hairline shadows extending out from the hilum. The width of the transradiant zone between the lines is that of a normal bronchus at that level (54). Tramline shadows, which represent edema of the bronchial wall, may be seen in asthma without ABPA, in CF, and in left ventricular failure with elevated pulmonary venous pressure. Permanent roentgenographic findings related to proximal bronchiectasis have been shown to occur in sites of previous infiltrates, which are often, but not exclusively, in the upper lobes. This is in contrast to postinfectious bronchiectasis, which is associated with distal abnormalities and normal proximal bronchi. When permanent lung damage occurs to large bronchi, parallel line shadows and ring shadows are seen. These do not change with oral corticosteroids. Parallel line shadows are dilated

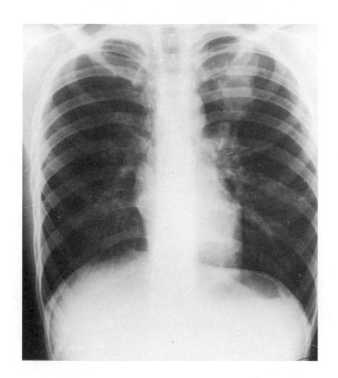

FIG. 24.1. An 11-year-old boy with far-advanced allergic bronchopulmonary aspergillosis. Presensation chest radiograph shows massive homogeneous consolidation in left upper lobe. (Reprinted from Mintzer RA, Rogers LF, Kruglick GD, et al. The spectrum of radiologic findings in allergic bronchopulmonary aspergillosis. *Radiology* 1978;127:301; with permission.)

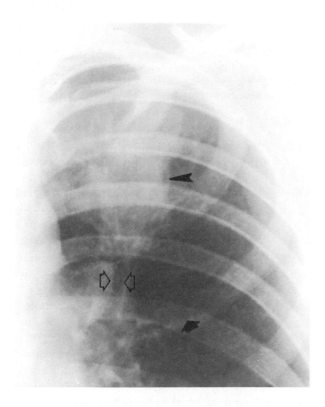

FIG. 24.2. Magnified view of the left upper lobe shows massive homogenous consolidation (*narrow arrowhead*), parallel lines (*open broad arrowheads*), and ring shadows (*closed broad arrowheads*). (Reprinted from Mintzer RA, Rogers LF, Kruglick GD, et al. The spectrum of radiologic findings in allergic bronchopulmonary aspergillosis. *Radiology* 1978;127:301; with permission.)

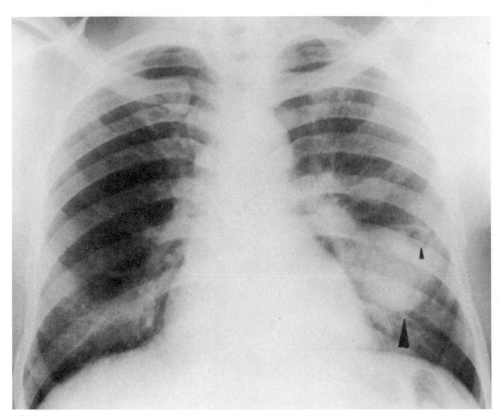

FIG. 24.3. A 31-year-old man with far-advanced allergic bronchopulmonary aspergillosis. Presentation chest radiograph. Note massive homogeneous consolidation (*large arrowhead*) and air-fluid level (*small arrowhead*). (Reprinted from Mintzer RA, Rogers LF, Kruglick GD, et al. The spectrum of radiologic findings in allergic bronchopulmonary aspergillosis. *Radiology* 1978;127:301; with permission.)

tramline shadows that result from bronchiectasis; the transradiant zone between the lines is wider than that of a normal bronchus. These shadows are believed to be permanent, representing bronchial dilation. The ring shadows, 1 to 2 cm in diameter, are dilated bronchi *en face*. Pulmonary fibrosis may occur and might be irreversible. Late findings in ABPA include cavitation, contracted upper lobes, and localized emphysema. When bullous changes are present, a spontaneous pneumothorax may occur (52).

With high clinical suspicion of ABPA (bronchial asthma, high total serum IgE concentration, immediate cutaneous reactivity to *A. fumigatus*, precipitating antibody against *A. fumigatus*) and a negative chest roentgenogram, central bronchiectasis may be demonstrated by high-resolution chest tomography (56–59). This examination should be performed as an initial radiologic test beyond the chest roentgenogram (Figs. 24.7 through 24.9). If findings are normal, studies should be repeated in 1 to 2 years for highly suspicious cases.

High-resolution CT using 1.5-mm section cuts has proved valuable in detecting bronchiectasis in ABPA (56). The thin-section cuts were obtained every 1 to 2 cm from the apex to the diaphragm. Bronchial dilatation was present in 41% of lung lobes in eight ABPA patients compared with 15% of lobes in patients with asthma without ABPA. Bronchiectasis may be cylindrical, cystic, or varicose (56–58). From the axial perspective, central bronchiectasis was present when it occurred in the inner two thirds of the lung.

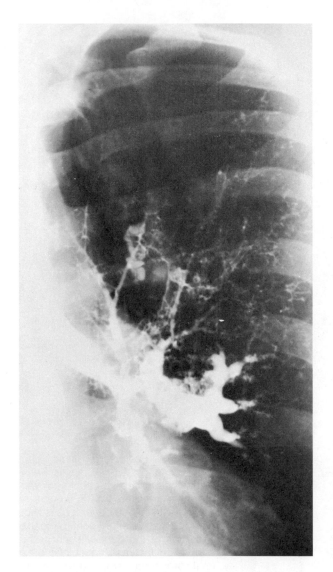

FIG. 24.4. Bronchogram showing classic proximal bronchiectasis with normal peripheral airways in a 25-year-old woman with allergic bronchopulmonary aspergillosis. (Reprinted from Mintzer RA, Rogers LF, Kruglick GD, et al. The spectrum of radiologic findings in allergic bronchopulmonary aspergillosis. *Radiology* 1978;127:301; with permission.)

When high-resolution CT using 1 to 3 mm of collimation (thin sections) was performed in 44 patients with ABPA and compared with 38 patients with asthma without ABPA, bronchiectasis was identified in both patient groups (58). Bronchiectasis was present in 42 (95%) ABPA patients compared with 11 (29%) patients with asthma. The CT scans revealed bronchiectasis in 70% of lobes examined in ABPA versus 9% of lobes from patients with asthma (58). Some 86% of ABPA patients had three or more bronchiectatic lobes, whereas 91% of the patients with asthma had bronchiectasis in one or two lobes. In the ABPA patients, bronchiectasis was varicose in 41% of patients, cystic in 34% of patients, and cylindrical in 23% of patients. Consolidation was identified in 59% of ABPA patients, primarily being located peripherally, whereas consolidation was present in 9% of patients with asthma (58).

STAGING

Five stages of ABPA have been identified (9). These stages are acute, remission, exacerbation, corticosteroid-dependent asthma, and fibrotic.

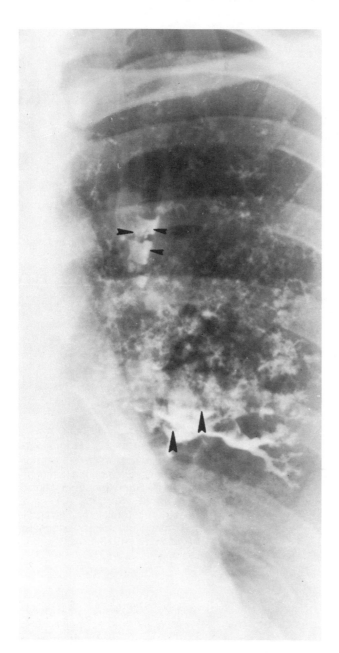

FIG. 24.5. Posttussive films after bronchography. Air-fluid levels (*large arrowheads*) are present in several partially filled ectatic bronchi. A bronchus in the left upper lobe is filled after the tussive effort, confirming that a portion of the density seen in this area is in fact a filled ectatic proximal bronchus (*small arrowheads*). (Reprinted from Mintzer RA, Rogers LF, Kruglick GD, et al. The spectrum of radiologic findings in allergic bronchopulmonary aspergillosis. *Radiology* 1978;127:301; with permission.)

The acute stage (stage I) is present when all the major criteria of ABPA can be documented. These criteria are asthma, immediate cutaneous reactivity to *A. fumigatus*, precipitating antibody to *A. fumigatus*, elevated serum IgE, peripheral blood eosinophilia, history of or presence of roentgenographic infiltrates, and proximal bronchiectasis, unless the patient has ABPA-S. If measured, sera from stage I patients have elevated serum IgE and IgG antibodies to *A. fumigatus* compared with sera from patients with asthma and immediate cutaneous reactivity to *Aspergillus* but not sufficient criteria for ABPA. After therapy with prednisone, the chest

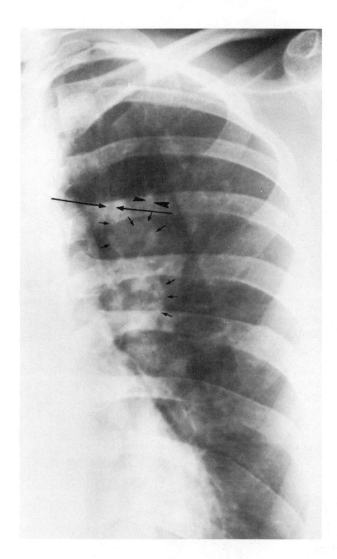

FIG. 24.6. Magnified view of the left upper lung of the patient shown in Figs. 24.4 and 24.5 demonstrates parallel lines (*long arrows*) and toothpaste shadows (*arrowheads*). Perihilar infiltrates (pseudohilar adenopathy) and a gloved-finger shadow also are seen (*small arrows*). (Reprinted from Mintzer RA, Rogers LF, Kruglick GD, et al. The spectrum of radiologic findings in allergic bronchopulmonary aspergillosis. *Radiology* 1978;127:301; with permission.)

roentgenogram clears and the total serum IgE declines substantially. Remission (stage II) is defined as clearing of the roentgenographic lesions and decline in total serum IgE for at least 6 months. Exacerbation (stage III) of ABPA is present when, after the remission that follows prednisone therapy, the patient develops a new roentgenographic infiltrate, total IgE rises over baseline, and the other criteria of stage I appear. Corticosteroid-dependent asthma (stage IV) includes patients whose prednisone cannot be terminated without occurrence of severe asthma or new roentgenographic infiltrates. Despite

prednisone administration, most patients have elevated total serum IgE concentration, precipitating antibody, and elevated serum IgE and IgG antibodies to *A. fumigatus*. Roentgenographic infiltrates may or may not occur. Stage V ABPA is present when extensive cystic or fibrotic changes are demonstrated on the chest roentgenogram. Patients in the fibrotic stage have some degree of irreversible obstructive flow rates on pulmonary function testing. A reversible obstructive component requires prednisone therapy, but high-dose prednisone does not reverse the roentgenographic lesions

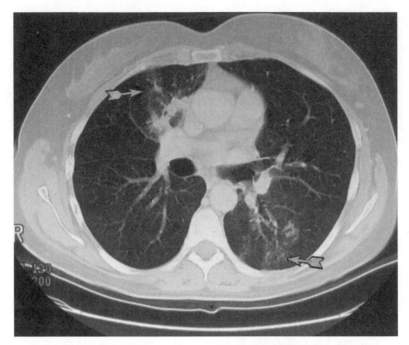

FIG. 24.7. Computed tomography scan of a 42-year-old woman demonstrating right upper lobe and left lower lobe infiltrates, the latter not seen on the posteroanterior and lateral radiographs. Dilated bronchioles are present in areas of infiltrates (*arrows*).

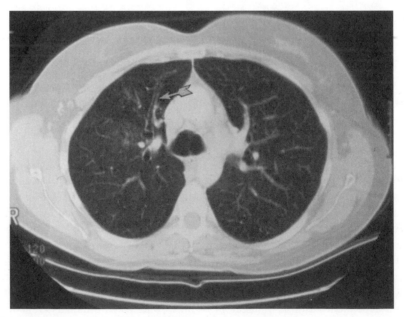

FIG. 24.8. Dilated bronchi from an axial longitudinal orientation (*arrow*) consistent with bronchiectasis (same patient as in Fig. 24.7).

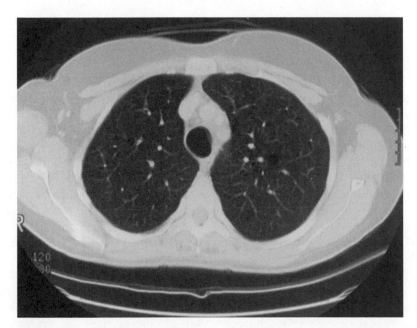

FIG. 24.9. Cystic (dilated) bronchi and bronchioles (same patient as in Fig. 24.7).

or irreversible obstructive disease. At the time of the initial diagnosis, the stage of ABPA may not be defined, but it becomes clear after several months of observation and treatment.

Patients with ABPA-S can be in stages I through IV, but not stage V. Patients with ABPA and CF often are in stage III (recurrent exacerbation) but may be in any stage.

LABORATORY FINDINGS

All patients exhibit immediate cutaneous reactivity (wheal and flare) to *A. fumigatus* antigen. Because of the lack of standardized *A. fumigatus* antigens for clinical testing, differences in skin reactivity have been reported by different researchers (Table 24.2) (48,60–63). Approximately 25% of patients with asthma without ABPA demonstrate immediate skin reactivity to *A. fumigatus*, and about 10% show precipitating antibodies against *A. fumigatus* (63,64). Conversely a nonreactive skin test (prick and intradermal) to reactive extracts of *A. fumigatus* essentially excludes the diagnosis of ABPA.

Some ABPA patients display a diphasic skin response to the intradermal injection of *Aspergillus* antigen. This consists of a typical

TABLE 24.2. *Incidence of immunologic reactions to* Aspergillus fumigatus

Patients studied	Immediate skin reactivity (%)	Precipitins (%)
Normal population	1–4	0–3
Hospitalized patients		2.5–6
Asthma without aspergillosis	12–38	9–25
Asthma without aspergillosis[a]		
London	23	10.5
Cleveland	28	7.5
Allergic bronchopulmonary aspergillosis	100	100[b]
Aspergilloma	25	100
Cystic fibrosis	39	31

[a] Similar antigenic material used for both groups.
[b] May be negative at times.
   Data from Hoehne JH, Reed CE, Dickie HA. Allergic bronchopulmonary aspergillosis is not rare. *Chest* 1973;63:177; Longbottom JL, Pepys J. Pulmonary aspergillosis; diagnostic and immunologic significance of antigens and C-substance in *Aspergillus fumigatus. J Pathol Bacteriol* 1964;88:141; Reed C. Variability of antigenicity of *Aspergillus fumigatus. J Allergy Clin Immunol* 1978;61:227; Rosenberg M, Patterson R, Mintzer R, et al. Clinical and immunologic criteria for the diagnosis of allergic bronchopulmonary aspergillosis. *Ann Intern Med* 1977;86:405; and Schwartz HJ, Citron KM, Chester EH et al. A comparison of the prevalence of sensitization to *Aspergillus* antigens among asthmatics in Cleveland and London. J Allergy Clin Immunol 1978;62:9; with permission.

immediate wheal and flare seen within 20 minutes, which subsides, to be followed in 4 to 8 hours by erythema and induration that resolves in 24 hours. IgG, IgM, IgA, and C3 have been reported on biopsies of these late reactions, suggesting an Arthus (type III) immune response (65). IgE antibodies also likely participate in the late reactions. Few ABPA patients treated at Northwestern University Medical School have biphasic skin reactivity despite the presence of anti–*A. fumigatus* IgE antibodies and precipitating antibodies. Conversely, these patients are not tested by intradermal injection, because skin-prick test results are positive in virtually all patients. As shown in Table 24.2, precipitating antibody to *A. fumigatus* is not uncommon in patients without ABPA and likely represents previous exposure to *A. fumigatus* antigens. In ABPA, however, these antibodies appear to be important in the pathogenesis of the disease, although exactly how they contribute is unclear.

Aspergillus fumigatus extracts are a mixture containing over 200 proteins and glycoproteins (33,66). There is marked heterogeneity of immunoglobulin and lymphocyte binding or stimulation with these potential allergens (33,66). For example, after rocket immunoelectrophoresis of *A. fumigatus* mycelia and addition of *A. fumigatus* antisera raised in rabbits, 35 different bands can be detected by that methodology. More sophisticated methodology (immunoblotting) has resulted in identification of 100 proteins (glycoproteins) that bind to immunoglobulins (33,66,67).

The use of crossed immunoelectrophoresis of an *Aspergillus* culture filtrate with sera from patients with ABPA demonstrated 35 arcs, of which 8 to 10 had reactivity with IgE antibodies (68). Concanavalin A nonbinding components of *A. fumigatus* culture filtrates or mycelium have been found to react with sera from ABPA patients, and other components have molecular weights of up to 200,000 daltons (69,70). There are more than 40 known components of *A. fumigatus* extracts that bind to IgE antibodies.

One example is an *A. fumigatus* polypeptide called *Asp f* 1, which has a molecular weight of 18,000 daltons and is generated from a culture filtrate that was found to react with IgE and IgG antibodies and was toxic to lymphocytes (34,70). *Asp f* 1 is a member of the mitogillin family, which demonstrates ribonuclease (ribotoxic) activity. Sera from ABPA patients react with several ribotoxins, and far greater quantities of IgE and IgG antibodies to ribotoxins from *Aspergillus* are present in patients with ABPA as compared with nonatopic patients with asthma (34). As stated, *A. fumigatus* allergens have been identified and labeled up to *Asp f* 18. Some peptides (12–16 amino acids from *Asp f* 1) induce Th1, and others produce Th2 cytokine responses in spleen cells from immunized mice. Peptides that are three to seven amino acids long have been obtained from the IgE binding region of *Asp f* 2 and evaluated for IgE binding with sera from ABPA patients. Overall, just a few amino acids of *Asp f* 2 provide the conformation to react with IgE, whereas these short IgE-specific peptides did not react with IgG antibodies (67,71,72). These assays are research based and emphasize the complexities to be addressed in the future (33). Reactive epitopes of *A. fumigatus* are under investigation for use in skin testing and *in vitro* assays (67). It is hoped that more precise skin testing and *in vitro* test results using recombinant allergens will lead to more accurate diagnoses. However, such an approach, at least with ragweed proteins, was unsuccessful in that a particular "immunologic fingerprint" did not occur as proposed. The genotypes were different for the "hay fever" phenotype.

In the double-gel diffusion technique, most patients' sera have at least one to three precipitin bands to *A. fumigatus*. Some sera must be concentrated five times to demonstrate precipitating antibody. A precipitin band with no immunologic significance may be seen, caused by the presence of C-reactive protein in human sera that cross-reacts with a polysaccharide antigen in *Aspergillus*. This false-positive band can be avoided by adding citric acid to the agar gel.

Because of the high incidence of cutaneous reactivity and precipitating antibodies to *A. fumigatus* in patients with CF and transient roentgenographic infiltrates attributed to *Aspergillus*, there is concern that *Aspergillus* could contribute to the ongoing lung damage of

CF. Use of high-dose tobramycin by nebulization might favor the growth of *A. fumigatus* in the bronchial mucus of CF patients. The question also has been raised whether ABPA might be a variant form of the latter. Genetic testing has identified the ΔF508 mutation in one allele of some ABPA patients or other variant patterns (73). Eleven patients with ABPA who had normal sweat electrolytes ($\leq$40 mM) had extensive genetic analysis of the coding region for the cystic fibrosis transmembrane regulator (CFTR). Five patients had one CF mutation (ΔF508 in four and R117H in one), whereas another patient had two CF mutations (ΔF508/R347H). In comparison were 53 patients with chronic bronchitis who did not have any with the ΔF508 mutation, demonstrating clear-cut differences and suggesting that ABPA in some patients includes CF heterozygosity. In a study of 16 patients with ABPA, 6 (37.5%) patients were homozygous for ΔF508 and 6 were heterozygous with other mutations in 4 patients (22). In our patient population, all but one patient tested had normal sweat chloride concentrations in the absence of CF. Nevertheless, there is increasing evidence that ABPA can complicate CF, and it must be considered in that population because 1% to 10% of patients with CF have ABPA (12–21).

Serum IgE concentrations in patients with ABPA are elevated, but the degree of elevation varies markedly. In most patients, the total serum IgE concentration is greater than 1,000 ng/mL (1 IU/mL = 2.4 ng/mL). It has been demonstrated that *A. fumigatus* growing in the respiratory tract without tissue invasion, as in ABPA, can provide a potent stimulus for production of total "nonspecific" serum IgE (74). The serum IgE antibody to *A. fumigatus* can be determined by radioimmunoassay or enzyme-linked immunoassay. When serum IgE or serum IgG antibodies, or both, against *A. fumigatus* are elevated compared with sera from skin-prick–positive asthmatic patients without evidence for ABPA, ABPA is highly probable or definitely present (75). With prednisone therapy and clinical improvement, the total IgE and IgE–*A. fumigatus* decrease, although at different rates. Seemingly, this decrease is associated with a decrease in the number of *A. fumigatus* organisms in the bronchi. It is

possible, but unlikely, that the reduction in IgE concentration is due directly to prednisone without an effect on *A. fumigatus* in the lung, because in other conditions, such as atopic dermatitis and asthma, corticosteroids did not lower total serum IgE concentrations significantly (76,77).

Because of the wide variation of total serum IgE concentrations in atopic patients with asthma, some difficulty exists in differentiating the patient with ABPA from the patient with asthma and cutaneous reactivity to *A. fumigatus*, with or without precipitating antibody to *A. fumigatus* and a history of an abnormal chest roentgenogram. Detection of elevated serum IgE and IgG antibodies to *A. fumigatus* has proved useful to identify patients with ABPA (6,7,16,31). Sera from patients with ABPA have at least twice the level of antibody to *A. fumigatus* than do sera from patients with asthma with skin-prick–positive reactions to *A. fumigatus*. During other stages of ABPA, the indices have diagnostic value if results are elevated, but are not consistently positive in all patients (78). In patients with suspected ABPA, serodiagnosis should be attempted before prednisone therapy is started. Hyperimmunoglobulinemia E should raise the possibility of ABPA in any patient with asthma, although other causes besides asthma include parasitism, atopic dermatitis, hyper-IgE syndrome, immune deficiency, Churg-Strauss syndrome, allergic bronchopulmonary mycosis, and, remotely, IgE myeloma.

Lymphocyte transformation is present in some cases but is not a diagnostic feature of ABPA (48). Delayed hypersensitivity (type IV) reactions occurring 48 hours after administration of intradermal *Aspergillus* antigens typically are not seen (79).

T- and B-cell analysis of selected patients with ABPA has not shown abnormal numbers of B cells, CD4 (helper), or CD8 (suppressor) cells. However, some patients have evidence for B-cell activation (CD19$^+$ CD23$^+$) or T-cell activation (CD25$^+$). T-cell clones from peripheral blood from three ABPA patients, two of whom had been in remission, were generated and analyzed (80). The clones were specific for *Asp f* 1 and were reported to be HLA class II molecules restricted to HLA-DR2 or HLA-DR5 alleles.

Furthermore, the T-cell clones produced high quantities of interleukin 4 (IL-4) and little interferon-γ, consistent with helper T cell type 2 (T_H2 subtype of CD4$^+$ cells). Additional experiments explored major histocompatibility complex (MHC) class II restriction in 15 additional ABPA patients to determine whether specific HLA class II molecules were likely associated with *A. fumigatus* presentation (81). Sixteen of 18 (88.8%) patients overall were either HLA-DR2 or HLA-DR5 compared with 42.1% frequency in normal individuals (81). Using polymerase chain reaction techniques to investigate HLA-DR subtypes, it was determined that three HLA-DR2 alleles (identified as subtypes DRB1 1501, 1503, and 1601) and three HLA-DR5 alleles (identified as subtypes DRB1 1101, 1104, and 1202) were recognized by T cells in their activation (81). In other words, T-cell activation after binding to *Asp f* 1 was restricted to certain subtypes of class II molecules HLA-DR2 or HLA-DR5, raising the possibility that selective HLA-DR alleles might provide the genetic disadvantage that permits T-cell activation and possibly ABPA to evolve.

Circulating immune complexes have been described during an acute flare-up of ABPA with activation of the classic pathway (82). Although Clq precipitins were present in patient sera, it was not proven that *Aspergillus* antigen was present in these complexes. ABPA is not considered to be characterized by circulating immune complexes as in serum sickness. But it has been demonstrated that *A. fumigatus* can convert C3 proactivator to C3 activator, a component of the alternate pathway (83). It is known that secretory IgA can activate the alternate pathway, and that *Aspergillus* in the bronchial tract can stimulate IgA production (84).

In vitro basophil histamine release resulted from exposure to an *Aspergillus* mix, anti-IgE, and other fungi in patients with ABPA and fungi-sensitive asthma (with immediate cutaneous reactivity to *A. fumigatus*) (85). There was much greater histamine release to *Aspergillus* and anti-IgE from basophils of patients with ABPA than there was from fungi-sensitive asthmatic patients. Furthermore, patients with stage IV and stage V ABPA demonstrated greater histamine release to *Aspergillus* than did patients in stages I, II, or III. There was greater histamine release to other fungi from cells taken from ABPA patients than there was from patients with asthma. These data document a cellular difference in ABPA patients when compared with fungi-sensitive asthmatic patients. There was no difference between ABPA patients and patients with asthma in terms of cutaneous end-point titration using a commercially available *Aspergillus* mix.

A positive sputum culture for *A. fumigatus* is a helpful, but not pathognomonic, feature of ABPA. Repeated positive cultures may be significant. Whereas some patients produce golden brown plugs or "pearls" of mucus containing *Aspergillus* mycelia, others produce no sputum at all, even in the presence of roentgenographic infiltrates. Sputum eosinophilia usually is found in patients with significant sputum production, but is not essential for diagnosis and clearly is not specific.

Peripheral blood eosinophilia is common in untreated patients, but need not be extremely high, and often is about 10% to 25% of the differential in patients who have not received oral corticosteroids.

Bronchial inhalational challenges with *Aspergillus* are not required to confirm the diagnosis, and are not without risk. Nevertheless, a dual reaction usually occurs after bronchoprovocation. An immediate reduction in flow that resolves, to be followed in some cases by a recurrence of obstruction after 4 to 10 hours, has been described (65). Pretreatment with β agonists prevents the immediate reaction; pretreatment with corticosteroids prevents the late reaction; and cromolyn sodium has been reported to prevent both. Inhalational challenge with *A. fumigatus* in a patient with asthma sensitive to *Aspergillus* produces the immediate response only. Aspergilloma patients may respond only with a late pattern.

LUNG BIOPSY

Because of the increasing recognition of ABPA, and the availability of serologic tests, the need for lung biopsy in confirming the diagnosis appears unnecessary unless other diseases must be

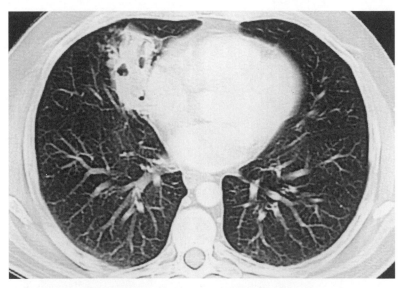

FIG. 24.10. Computed tomography scan demonstrating a cavitary mass in the right lower lobe in a 56-year-old man. The total serum IgE was 4,440 ng/mL. His only symptom was a mild nonproductive cough.

excluded. Bronchiectasis in the affected lobes in segmental and subsegmental bronchi, with sparing of distal branches, characterizes the pattern of proximal or central bronchiectasis (86–88). Bronchi are tortuous and very dilated. Histologically, bronchi contain tenacious mucus, fibrin, Curschmann spirals, Charcot-Leyden crystals, and inflammatory cells (mononuclear cells and eosinophils). Fungal hyphae can be identified in the bronchial lumen, and *Aspergillus* can be isolated in culture. Except for a few unusual case reports, no evidence exists for invasion of the bronchial wall, despite numerous hyphae in the lumen. Bronchial wall damage is associated with the presence of mononuclear cells and eosinophils, and in some cases with granulomata. Organisms of *Aspergillus* may be surrounded by necrosis, or acute or chronic inflammation. In other areas, there is replacement of submucosa with fibrous tissue. It is not known why bronchial wall destruction is focal with uninvolved adjacent areas.

A variety of morphologic lesions have been described in patients meeting criteria of ABPA (86–88). These include *Aspergillus* hyphae in granulomatous bronchiolitis, exudative bronchiolitis, *Aspergillus* hyphae in microabscess,

eosinophilic pneumonia, lipid pneumonia, lymphocytic interstitial pneumonia, desquamative interstitial pneumonia, pulmonary vasculitis, and pulmonary fibrosis. Some patients with ABPA may show pathology consistent with bronchocentric granulomatosis. Mucoid impaction related to ABPA may cause proximal bronchial obstruction with distal areas of bronchiolitis obliterans. Examples of microscopic sections from ABPA patients are shown in Figures 24.10 through 24.13.

PATHOGENESIS

On a historical basis in some asthma patients who had a normal bronchogram before they developed ABPA, bronchiectasis has been found to occur at the sites of roentgenographic infiltrates. This phenomenon has been confirmed by repeated CT examinations as well. Currently, it is thought that inhaled *Aspergillus* spores grow in the patient's tenacious mucus and release antigenic glycoproteins and perhaps other reactants that activate bronchial mast cells, lymphocytes, macrophages, and eosinophils, and generate antibodies, followed by tissue damage that is associated with subsequent bronchiectasis or

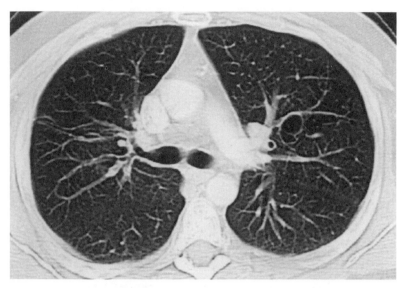

FIG. 24.11. The same patient as in Fig. 24.10. The computed tomography scan at the level of the carina demonstrates cystic bronchiectasis (*arrows*).

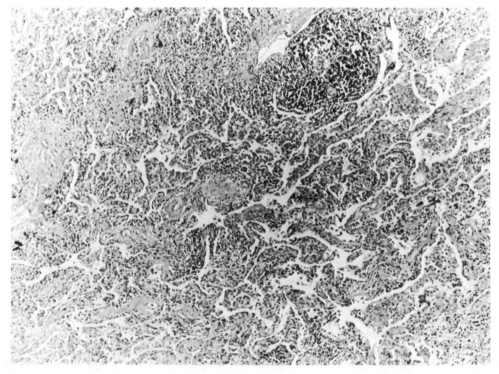

FIG. 24.12. Typical microscopic appearance representing eosinophilic pneumonia. The collapsed alveolus contains a predominance of large mononuclear cells, few lymphocytes, plasma cells, and clumps of eosinophils; similar cells infiltrate the alveolar walls. Superior segment of the upper lobe was resected for a cavitary and infiltrative lesion. (Reprinted from Imbeau SA, Nichols D, Flaherty D, et al. Allergic bronchopulmonary aspergillosis. *J Allergy Clin Immunol* 1978;62:243; with permission. Photographs from the specimen collection of Enrique Valdivia; magnification ×120, hematoxylin and eosin stain.)

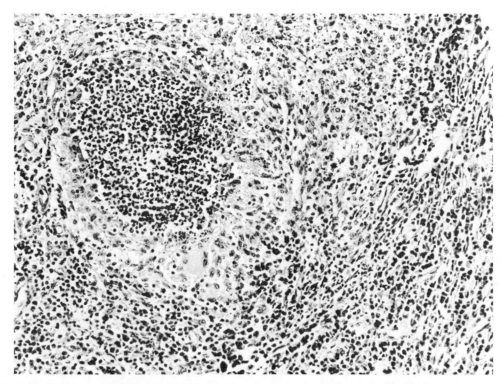

FIG. 24.13. Right lower lobectomy. The lung has prominent cellular infiltration and an area of early bronchocentric granulomatosis, with leukocytes and a crown of epithelioid cells. *Aspergillus* was demonstrated in the center of the lesions with special stains. (Reprinted from Imbeau SA, Nichols D, Flaherty D, et al. Allergic bronchopulmonary aspergillosis. *J Allergy Clin Immunol* 1978:62:243; with permission. Photographs from the specimen collection of Enrique Valdivia; magnification ×240, hematoxylin and eosin stain.)

roentgenographic infiltrates. *Aspergillus* spores are thermophilic; therefore, growth is feasible in bronchi. It is unclear whether *Aspergillus* spores are trapped in the viscid mucus, or whether they have a special ability to colonize the bronchial tree and result in development of tenacious mucus. The latter is such that during bronchoscopy, the mucoid material may remain impacted after 30 minutes of attempted removal. In contrast, in patients with CF without ABPA, such difficulty is not encountered. Proteolytic enzymes and possibly ribotoxins produced by *A. fumigatus* growing in the bronchial tree may contribute to lung damage on a nonimmunologic or immunologic basis. Immunologic injury could occur because the release of antigenic material is associated with production of IgE, IgA, and IgG antibodies and activation of the pulmonary immune response with a panoply of harmful effects.

Although peripheral blood lymphocytes from stable ABPA patients have not been reported to form excess IgE *in vitro* compared with nonatopic patients, at the time of an ABPA flare-up, these cells produced significantly increased amounts of IgE (89). This suggests that during an ABPA flare-up, IgE-forming cells are released into the systemic circulation, presumably from the lung. The biphasic skin reaction requires IgE and possibly IgG, and it has been suggested that a similar reaction occurs in the lung. Nevertheless, the lack of immunofluorescence in vascular deposits is evidence against an immune complex vasculitis as a cause of bronchial wall damage.

The passive transfer of serum containing IgG and IgE antibodies from a patient with ABPA to a monkey, followed by bronchial challenge with *Aspergillus*, has been associated with pulmonary lesions in the monkey (2). When monkeys were immunized with *A. fumigatus* and generated IgG antibodies, normal human serum was infused into both immunized and nonimmunized monkeys, and allergic human serum from a patient with ABPA (currently without any precipitating antibody) was infused into other monkeys, immunized and nonimmunized (90). All animals were challenged with aerosolized *A. fumigatus*, and lung biopsy samples were obtained on the fifth day. Only the monkey with precipitating antibody (IgG) to *Aspergillus* who received human allergic serum (IgE) showed biopsy changes consistent with ABPA (90). Mononuclear and eosinophilic infiltrates were present, with thickening of alveolar septa, but without evidence of vasculitis. These findings confirm that IgE and IgG directed against *Aspergillus* are necessary for the development of pulmonary lesions.

Similarly, a murine model of ABPA was developed that resulted in blood and pulmonary eosinophilia (91) using *A. fumigatus* particulates simulating spores that were inoculated by the intranasal route. However, if *A. fumigatus* in alum was injected into the peritoneal cavity, anti–*A. fumigatus*-IgG1 and total IgE concentrations increased, but pulmonary and peripheral blood eosinophilia did not occur. In contrast, intranasal inoculation of *A. fumigatus* resulted in perivascular eosinophilia, as well as pulmonary lymphocytes, plasma cells, histocytes, and eosinophils consistent with ABPA. A true model of ABPA where animals develop spontaneously occurring pulmonary infiltrates has yet to be described.

It is likely that lymphocytes produce IL-4 (or IL-13) and IL-5 to support IgE synthesis and eosinophilia, respectively. Elevated soluble IL-2 receptors suggest CD4$^+$ lymphocyte activation (92), and CD4$^+$-T$_H$2 type clones have been produced from ABPA patients (80). It appears as if presentation of *Asp f* 1 is restricted to certain class II MHC molecules, HLA-DR2 and -DR5 (81). The demonstration of hyperreleasability of mediators from basophils of patients with stage IV and V ABPA (85) is consistent with the hypothesis that a subgroup of patients may be most susceptible to immunologic injury if peripheral blood basophils are representative bronchial

mast cells. The fact that basophils from patients with any stage of ABPA have increased *in vitro* histamine release as compared with basophils from *A. fumigatus* skin-prick–positive patients with asthma suggests that mast cell mediator release to various antigens (fungi) may contribute to lung damage in ABPA if these findings can be applied to bronchial mast cells.

Analysis of bronchoalveolar lavage from stages II and IV ABPA patients who had no current chest roentgenographic infiltrates revealed evidence for local antibody production of IgA–*A. fumigatus* and IgE–*A. fumigatus* compared with peripheral blood (93). Bronchial lavage IgA–*A. fumigatus* was 96 times that of peripheral blood, and IgE–*A. fumigatus* in lavage was 48 times that found in peripheral blood. Although total serum IgE was elevated, there was no increase in bronchial lavage total IgE corrected for albumin. These results suggest that the bronchoalveolar space is not the source of the markedly elevated total IgE in ABPA. Perhaps pulmonary interstitium or nonpulmonary sources (tonsils or bone marrow) serve as sites of total IgE production in ABPA.

In a serial analysis of serum IgA–*A. fumigatus* in 10 patients, there were sharp elevations over baseline before (five cases) or during (five cases) roentgenographic exacerbations of ABPA for IgA1–*A. fumigatus* (84). Serum IgA2–*A. fumigatus* was elevated before the exacerbation in two cases and during the exacerbation in five cases. Heterogeneous polyclonal antibody responses to seven different molecular weight bands of *A. fumigatus* were present on immunoblot analysis of sera (94). Band intensity increased during ABPA exacerbations, and patient's sera often had broader reactivity with *A. fumigatus* bands from 24- to 90-kDa molecular weights during disease flare-ups. Some patients had immunoblot patterns consistent with increases in IgE, IgG, or IgA antibodies binding to different *A. fumigatus* antigens but no consistent binding to a particular *A. fumigatus* band.

The many immunologic and other abnormalities identified in ABPA likely participate directly or indirectly in lung destruction both in bronchi and distally (67). The basis of the effectiveness of prednisone in treatment of ABPA requires greater clarification as well.

DIFFERENTIAL DIAGNOSIS

The differential diagnosis of ABPA includes disease states associated primarily with transient or permanent roentgenographic lesions, asthma, and peripheral blood or sputum eosinophilia. The asthma patient with a roentgenographic infiltrate may have atelectasis from inadequately controlled asthma. Bacterial, viral, or fungal pneumonias must be excluded in addition to tuberculosis and the many other causes of roentgenographic infiltrates. Eosinophilia may occur with parasitism, tuberculosis, Churg-Strauss vasculitis, pulmonary infiltrates from drug allergies, neoplasm, eosinophilic pneumonia, and, rarely, avian-hypersensitivity pneumonitis. Mucoid impaction of bronchi may occur without ABPA. All patients with a history of mucoid impaction syndrome or with collapse of a lobe or lung, however, should have ABPA excluded. Similarly, although the morphologic diagnosis of bronchocentric granulomatosis is considered by some to represent an entity distinct from ABPA, ABPA must be excluded in such patients. Although the sweat test for CF is within normal limits in ABPA patients, unless concomitant CF is present, the patient with CF and asthma or changing roentgenographic infiltrates should have ABPA excluded or confirmed. The genetics of ABPA are beginning to be studied to determine similarities with CF. Some patients with asthma who develop pulmonary infiltrates with eosinophilia are likely to have ABPA.

In the patient without a history of roentgenographic infiltrates, ABPA should be suspected on the basis of (a) a positive, immediate cutaneous reaction to *Aspergillus*, (>1,000 ng/mL or 417 IU/mL); (b) elevated total serum IgE; (c) increasing severity of asthma; (d) abnormalities on chest roentgenogram or CT; (e) repeatedly positive sputum cultures for *Aspergillus* species; or (f) bronchiectasis.

A rare patient with asthma, roentgenographic infiltrates, and bronchiectasis or a history of surgical resection for such may present with peripheral eosinophilia, elevated total serum IgE, but other negative serologic results for ABPA. Some other species of *Aspergillus* may be responsible, such as *A. oryzae*, *A. ochraceus*, or *A. niger*. Perhaps a different allergic bronchopulmonary mycosis may be present. For example, illnesses consistent with allergic bronchopulmonary candidiasis, curvulariosis, dreschleriosis, stemphyliosis, fusariosis, and pseudallescheriasis have been described (95–97). Positive sputum cultures, precipitating antibodies, or *in vitro* assays for a fungus other than *Aspergillus* or for different *Aspergillus* species could suggest a causative source of the allergic bronchopulmonary fungosis.

The presence of bronchiectasis from ABPA has been associated with colonization of bronchi by atypical mycobacteria (98). It appears that the identification of atypical mycobacteria in the sputum should at least raise the possibility of ABPA in patients with asthma who do not have acquired immunodeficiency syndrome. Similarly, bronchiectatic airways may become colonized by *Pseudomonas aeruginosa* in ABPA patients who do not have CF.

NATURAL HISTORY

Although most patients arc diagnosed before the age of 40 years, and an increasing number are diagnosed before the age of 20 years, one must not overlook the diagnosis of ABPA in older patients previously characterized as having chronic asthma or chronic bronchiectasis. Some patients as old as 80 have had the diagnosis of ABPA made. Late sequelae of ABPA include irreversible pulmonary function abnormalities, symptoms of chronic bronchitis, and pulmonary fibrosis (51). Death results from respiratory failure and cor pulmonale. Allergic bronchopulmonary aspergillosis has been associated with respiratory failure in the second or third decade of life. Most patients who have ABPA do not progress to the end-stage disease, especially if there is early diagnosis and appropriate treatment. Patients who present in the acute stage (stage I) of ABPA may enter remission (stage II), recurrent exacerbation (stage III), or may develop corticosteroid-dependent asthma (stage IV). One patient who had a single roentgenographic infiltrate when her ABPA was diagnosed entered a remission stage that lasted for 8 years until an exacerbation occurred (99). Thus, a remission does not imply permanent cessation of disease activity. This patient may be the exception, but serves to emphasize the need for longer term observation of patients with ABPA. Patients who have corticosteroid-dependent asthma (stage IV) at the time of diagnosis may evolve into having pulmonary fibrosis (stage V). Because prednisone does not reverse bronchiectasis or the pulmonary fibrotic changes in the lung, every effort should be made by physicians managing patients with asthma to suspect and confirm cases of ABPA before significant structural damage to the lung has developed.

In managing patients with ABPA, there is a lack of correlation between clinical symptoms and chest roentgenographic lesions. Irreversible lung damage including bronchiectasis may occur without the patient seeking medical attention. In Great Britain, ABPA exacerbations were reported to occur between October and February during elevations of fungal spore counts (28). In Chicago, 38 of 49 (77.5%) ABPA exacerbations (new roentgenographic infiltrate with elevation of total serum IgE) occurred from June through November in association with increased outdoor fungal spore counts (100).

Acute and chronic pulmonary function changes have been studied in a series of ABPA cases, during which time all patients received corticosteroids and bronchodilators (101). There appeared to be no significant correlation between duration of ABPA (mean follow-up period, 44 months), duration of asthma, and diffusing capacity of the lungs for carbon monoxide (DLCO), total lung capacity (TLC), vital capacity (VC), forced expiratory volume in 1 second (FEV_1), and $FEV_1\%$. In six patients with acute exacerbations of ABPA, a significant reduction in TLC, VC, FEV_1, and DLCO occurred, which returned to baseline during steroid treatment. Thus, early recognition and prompt effective treatment of flare-ups appears to reduce the likelihood of irreversible lung damage. Other patients may have reductions in FEV_1 and $FEV_1\%$ consistent with an obstructive process during an ABPA exacerbation.

The prognosis for stage V patients is less favorable than for patients classified into stages I through IV (53). Although prednisone has proven useful in patients with end-stage lung disease, 6 of 17 stage V patients, observed for a mean 4.9 years, died. When the FEV_1 was 0.8 L or less after aggressive initial corticosteroid administration, the outcome was poor (53). In contrast, when stage IV patients are managed effectively, deterioration of respiratory function parameters or status asthmaticus has not occurred.

Safirstein et al. (102), in a 5-year follow-up of ABPA cases, reported that a daily prednisone dose of 7.5 mg was required to maintain clinical improvement and roentgenographic clearing in 80% of patients, compared with 40% of those treated with either cromolyn or bronchodilators alone (102). In a study of patients from Northwestern University who had periodic blood sampling, both immunologic and clinical improvement occurred with prednisone therapy. Individuals with ABPA have high presentation (stages I and III) total serum IgE concentrations, and those patients previously never requiring oral steroids for control of asthma have the highest concentrations. Treatment with prednisone causes roentgenographic and clinical improvement, as well as decreases in total serum IgE. Total serum IgE and IgE–*A. fumigatus* may increase before and during a flare-up, but the serum IgE–*A. fumigatus* does not fluctuate to the extent that total serum IgE concentration does.

Prognostic factors remain to be established that may identify patients at risk for developing stage IV or V ABPA. The roentgenographic lesion at the time of diagnosis does not appear to provide prognostic data about long-term outcome unless the patient is stage V.

The effect of untreated ABPA exacerbations has produced stage V ABPA. In addition, at least some patients with CF who develop ABPA have a worse prognosis. Lastly, the effect of allergic fungal sinusitis (Table 24.3) on the natural history of ABPA is unknown.

TREATMENT

Prednisone is the drug of choice but need not be administered indefinitely (Table 24.4). Multiple

TABLE 24.3. *Criteria for diagnosis of allergic fungal sinusitis*

Chronic sinusitis—at least 6 months duration with nasal polyposis

Allergic mucin (histologic examination with eosinophils and fungal hyphae and "putty" material by rhinoscopy)

Computed tomography of sinuses shows opacification and magnetic resonance imaging shows fungal findings[a]

Absence of invasive fungal disease, diabetes mellitus, HIV

[a]T_1-weighted imaging reveals isointense or hypointense findings of mucin in sinuses; T_2-weighted imaging demonstrate a "signal void" where there is inspissated mucin.

agents have been tried, including intrabronchial instillation of amphotericin B, nystatin, itraconazole, cromolyn, beclomethasone dipropionate, and triamcinolone by inhalation. Itraconazole may have an adjunctive role, but prednisone therapy typically eliminates or diminishes sputum plug production. Although the exact pathogenesis of ABPA is unknown, oral corticosteroids have been demonstrated to reduce the clinical symptoms, incidence of positive sputum cultures, and roentgenographic infiltrates. Oral corticosteroids may be effective by decreasing sputum volume, by making the bronchi a less

suitable culture media for *Aspergillus* species, and by inhibiting many of the *Aspergillus*–pulmonary immune system interactions. The total serum IgE declines by at least 35% within 2 months of initiating prednisone therapy (25). Failure to observe this reduction suggests noncompliance of patients or an exacerbation of ABPA.

Our current treatment regimen is to clear the roentgenographic infiltrates with daily prednisone, usually at 0.5 mg/kg. Most infiltrates clear within 2 weeks, at which time the same dose, given on a single alternate-day regimen, is begun and maintained for 2 months until the total serum IgE, which should be followed up every 4 to 8 weeks for the first year, has reached a baseline concentration. The baseline total serum IgE concentration can remain elevated despite clinical and radiographic improvement. Slow reductions in prednisone, at no faster than 10 mg/month, can be initiated once a stable baseline of total IgE has been achieved. Acute exacerbations of ABPA often are preceded by a 100% increase in total serum IgE and must be treated promptly with increases in prednisone and reinstitution of daily steroids. Certainly, the physician must exclude other causes for roentgenographic infiltrates. Pulmonary

TABLE 24.4. *Treatment of allergic bronchopulmonary aspersillosis (ABPA)*

1. Prednisone is drug of choice; 0.5 mg/kg daily for 2 wk, then on alternate days for 6–8 wk, then attempt tapering by 5 mg on alternate days every 2 wk
2. Repeat chest roentgenogram and or high-resolution computed tomography of lung at 2–4 wk to document clearing of infiltrates
3. Serum IgE concentration at baseline and at 4 and 8 wk, then every 8 wk for first year to establish range of total IgE concentrations (a 100% increase can identify a silent exacerbation)
4. Baseline spirometry or full pulmonary function tests depending on the clinical setting
5. Environmental control for fungi and other allergens at home or work
6. Determine if prednisone-dependent asthma (stage IV ABPA) is present; if not, manage asthma with antiinflammatory medications and other medications as indicated
7. Future ABPA exacerbations may be identified by
    a. Asymptomatic sharp increases in the total serum IgE concentration
    b. Increasing asthma symptoms or signs
    c. Deteriorations in FVC and/or FEV_1
    d. Cough, chest pain, new production of sputum plugs, dyspnea not explained by other causes
    e. Chest roentgenographic or high-resolution computed tomography findings (patient may be asymptomatic)
8. Document in chart that prednisone side effects were discussed and address bone density issues (e.g., adequate calcium, exercise, hormone replacement and antiosteopenia medication if indicated)
9. Persistent sputum expectoration should be cultured to identify *Aspergillus fumigatus, Staphylococcus aureus, Pseudomonas aeruginosa,* atypical mycobacteria, etc.
10. If new ABPA exacerbations occur, repeat step 1

FVC, forced vital capacity; FEV_1, forced expiratory volume in 1 second.

functions should be measured yearly or as necessary for stages IV and V and as required for asthma.

If prednisone can be discontinued, the patient is in remission (stage II), and perhaps just an inhaled corticosteroid will be needed for management of asthma. Alternatively, if the patient has asthma that cannot be managed without prednisone despite avoidance measures and maximal antiinflammatory medications, alternate-day prednisone will be necessary. The dose of prednisone required to control asthma and to prevent ABPA radiologic exacerbations is usually less than 0.5 mg/kg on alternate days. For corticosteroid-dependent patients (stages IV or V) with ABPA, an explanation of prednisone risks and benefits is indicated, as is the discussion that untreated ABPA infiltrates result in bronchiectasis (54,57) and irreversible fibrosis. Specific additional recommendations regarding estrogen supplementation for women, adequate calcium ingestion, bronchial hygiene, and physical fitness and bone density measurements should be considered.

In ABPA patients receiving prednisone, itraconazole, 200 mg twice daily or placebo, was administered for 16 weeks (103). A response was defined as (a) at least a 50% reduction in oral corticosteroid dose, and (b) a decrease of 25% or more of the total serum IgE concentration and at least one of three additional parameters: a 25% improvement in exercise tolerance or similar 25% improvement in pulmonary function tests or resolution of chest roentgenographic infiltrates if initially present with no subsequent new infiltrates, or if no initial chest roentgenographic infiltrates were present, no emergence of new infiltrates. Oral corticosteroids were tapered during the study, although it was not certain that all patients had an attempt at steroid tapering. With that consideration, itraconazole administration was associated with a response as defined. Unfortunately, less than 25% of patients had chest roentgenographic infiltrates at the beginning of the study. More responders (60%) occurred in patients without bronchiectasis (ABPA-S) versus ABPA-CB (31%), compared with 8% in placebo-treated patients (103). Eleven isolates from sputum cultures were analyzed for antifungal susceptibility, and five were susceptible to intraconazole (103). None of the patients whose isolates of *A. fumigatus* were resistant or tolerant *in vitro* to itraconazole had responses to treatment. The conclusions from this study were that patients with ABPA "generally benefit from concurrent itraconazole" (103). The difficulties and complexities in such studies are apparent, and ideally the drug would be of value in patients with ABPA-CB, who are the patients more frequently seen in the office.

Itraconazole's absorption is reduced if there is gastric hypochlorhydria, so it should be ingested 1 hour before or 2 hours after meals. It slows hepatic metabolism of drugs that use the CYP 3A4 pathway, including methylprednisolone, statins, coumadin, oral hypoglycemics, tacrolimus, cyclosporines, and benzodiazepines, as examples. Itraconazole itself is potentiated by clarithromycin and some protease inhibitors used for human immunodeficiency virus infection.

Antifungal agents have been administered for 30 years to ABPA patients and are not a substitute for oral corticosteroids. They are adjunctive at best (104,105). The primary pharmacologic therapy remains prednisone, which, if the patient is in stage IV or V, often can be administered on an alternate-day basis. Perhaps itraconazole has antiinflammatory effects or a delaying effect on corticosteroid elimination. If so, then its effects might resemble those of the macrolide troleandomycin, delaying the metabolism of methylprednisolone. I have seen failures of itraconazole and excessive reliance on it without clearing of chest roentgenographic infiltrates. Nevertheless, as adjunctive therapy in patients who have susceptible strains of *A. fumigatus*, itraconazole could be considered in ABPA. Some studies have reported reductions in daily prednisone use and clearance of *A. fumigatus* from sputum.

In CF patients with ABPA, itraconazole was reported to result in a 47% reduction in oral steroid dose and a 55% reduction in ABPA exacerbations (22). The study group was composed of 16 (9%) patients from a pool of 122 CF patients. Itraconazole was administered to 12 of the 16 patients, who also received inhaled corticosteroids and prednisone and treatment for CF. Elevated serum aspartate aminotransferase (AST) or alanine aminotransferase (ALT) results of greater than three times the upper limit of normal were contraindications to the use of itraconazole. Although there were reductions in acute ABPA exacerbations and oral steroid doses, there were no differences in total cumulative prednisone doses (22). Moss et al. suggested trying intraconazole in "properly selected" patients with CF, especially because ABPA seems to cause a faster deterioration of FEV_1 per year in CF patients compared with CF without ABPA (22). Whether this antifungal therapy will be effective on a longer term basis remains uncertain. Indeed, just as it is possible that the increasing frequency of ABPA occurring in CF may be a consequence of high-dose nebulized tobramycin allowing for emergence of *A. fumigatus* in bronchial mucus, perhaps resistance to antifungals will occur and create additional issues that complicate the clinical care of patients with CF who have ABPA.

Immunotherapy with *Aspergillus* species probably should not be administered in patients with ABPA, but examples of adverse effects aside from injection reactions have not been reported. It is not expected that immunotherapy with *Aspergillus* extracts would result in immune complex formation. Immunotherapy can be administered with pollens and mites and possibly fungi, but not those in the *Aspergillus* genus.

Inhaled corticosteroids should be used in an effort to control asthma but one should not depend on them to prevent exacerbations of ABPA. Similarly, the leukotriene D_4 antagonists have antieosinophil actions *in vitro* and theoretically might be of value for use in ABPA patients. They can be administered for a trial of 1 to 3 months.

The exact role of environmental exposure of *Aspergillus* spores in the pathogenesis of ABPA remains unknown. *Aspergillus* spores are found regularly in crawl spaces, "unfinished" compost piles, manure, and fertile soil. Some patients have developed acute wheezing dyspnea and recognized ABPA exacerbations after inhalation of heavy spore burdens such as moldy wood chips or after exposure to closed up cottage homes. Attempts should be made to repair leaky basement walls and floors to minimize moldy basements. Because spores of *Aspergillus* species, including *A. fumigatus*, are detected regularly both indoors and outside, a common sense approach seems advisable.

REFERENCES

1. Hinson KFW, Moon AJ, Plummer NS. Bronchopulmonary aspergillosis: a review and report of eight new cases. *Thorax* 1952;73:317–333.
2. Patterson R, Golbert T. Hypersensitivity disease of the lung. *Univ Michigan Med Center J* 1968;34:8–11.
3. Slavin RG, Laird TS, Cherry JD. Allergic bronchopulmonary aspergillosis in a child. *J Pediatr* 1970;76:416–421.
4. Chetty A, Bhargava S, Jain RK. Allergic bronchopulmonary aspergillosis in Indian children with bronchial asthma. *Ann Allergy* 1985;54:46–49.
5. Turner ES, Greenberger PA, Sider L. Complexities of establishing an early diagnosis of allergic bronchopulmonary aspergillosis in children. *Allergy Proc* 1989;10:63–69.
6. Kiefer TA, Kesarwala HH, Greenberger PA, et al. Allergic bronchopulmonary aspergillosis in a young child: diagnostic confirmation by serum IgE and IgG indices. *Ann Allergy* 1986;56:233–236.
7. Greenberger PA, Liotta JL, Roberts M. The effects of age on isotypic antibody responses to *Aspergillus fumigatus*: implications regarding *in vitro* measurements. *J Lab Clin Med* 1989;114:278–284.
8. Imbeau SA, Cohen M, Reed CE. Allergic bronchopulmonary aspergillosis in infants. *Am J Dis Child* 1977;131:1127–1130.
9. Patterson R, Greenberger PA, Radin RC, et al. Allergic bronchopulmonary aspergillosis: staging as an aid to management. *Ann Intern Med* 1982;96:286–291.
10. Greenberger PA, Miller TP, Roberts M, et al. Allergic bronchopulmonary aspergillosis in patients with an without evidence of bronchiectasis. *Ann Allergy* 1993;70:333–338.
11. Basich JE, Graves TS, Baz MN, et al. Allergic bronchopulmonary aspergillosis in steroid dependent asthmatics. *J Allergy Clin Immunol* 1981;68:98–102.
12. Laufer P, Fink JN, Bruns W, et al. Allergic bronchopulmonary aspergillosis in cystic fibrosis. *J Allergy Clin Immunol* 1984;73:44–48.
13. Maguire S, Moriarty P, Tempany E, et al. Unusual clustering of allergic bronchopulmonary aspergillosis in children with cystic fibrosis. *Pediatrics* 1988;82:835–839.
14. Nelson LA, Callerame ML, Schwartz RH. Aspergillosis and atopy in cystic fibrosis. *Am Rev Respir Dis* 1979;120:863–873.
15. Zeaske R, Bruns WT, Fink JN, et al. Immune responses to *Aspergillus* in cystic fibrosis. *J Allergy Clin Immunol* 1988;82:73–77.
16. Knutsen AP, Hutchinson PS, Mueller KR, et al. Serum immunoglobulins E and G anti–*Aspergillus fumigatus* antibody in patients with cystic fibrosis who have allergic bronchopulmonary aspergillosis. *J Lab Clin Med* 1990;116:724–727.
17. Hutcheson PS, Knutsen AP, Rejent AJ, et al. A 12-year old longitudinal study of *Aspergillus* sensitivity in patients with cystic fibrosis. *Chest* 1996;110:363–366.

18. Geller DE, Kaplowitz H, Light MJ, et al. Allergic bronchopulmonary aspergillosis: reported prevalence, regional distribution, and patient characteristics. *Chest* 1999;116:639–646.

19. Becker JW, Burke W, McDonald G, et al. Prevalence of allergic bronchopulmonary aspergillosis and atopy in adult patients with cystic fibrosis. *Chest* 1996;109:1536–1540.

20. Fitzsimons EJ, Aris R, Patterson R. Recurrence of allergic bronchopulmonary aspergillosis in the post-transplant lungs of a cystic fibrosis patient. *Chest* 1997;112:281–282.

21. Skov M, Koch C, Reinert CM, et al. Diagnosis of allergic bronchopulmonary aspergillosis (ABPA) in cystic fibrosis. *Allergy* 2000;55:50–58.

22. Nepomuceno IB, Esrig S, Moss BB. Allergic bronchopulmonary aspergillosis in cystic fibrosis: role of atopy and response to itraconazole. *Chest* 1999;115:364–370.

23. Bhagat R, Shah A, Jaggi OP, et al. Concomitant allergic bronchopulmonary aspergillosis and allergic *Aspergillus* sinusitis with an operated aspergilloma. *J Allergy Clin Immunol* 1993;91:1094–1096.

24. Shah A, Bhagat R, Panchal N, et al. Allergic bronchopulmonary aspergillosis with middle lobe syndrome and allergic *Aspergillus* sinusitis. *Eur Respir J* 1993;6:917–918.

25. Rosenberg M, Patterson R, Roberts M, et al. The assessment of immunologic and clinical changes occurring during corticosteroid therapy for allergic bronchopulmonary aspergillosis. *Am J Med* 1978;64:599–606.

26. Wang JLF, Patterson R, Rosenberg M, et al. Serum IgE and IgG antibody activity against *Aspergillus fumigatus* as a diagnostic aid in allergic bronchopulmonary aspergillosis. *Am Rev Respir Dis* 1978;117:917–927.

27. Greenberger PA, Patterson R. Application of enzyme linked immunosorbent assay (ELISA) in diagnosis of allergic bronchopulmonary aspergillosis. *J Lab Clin Med* 1982;99:288–293.

28. Pepys J. Hypersensitivity disease of the lungs due to fungi and organic dusts. In: *Karger monographs in allergy*. Vol. 4. Basel: Karger, 1969:63–68.

29. Glancy JJ, Elder JL, McAleer R. Allergic bronchopulmonary fungal disease without clinical asthma. *Thorax* 1981;36:345–349.

30. Greenberger PA, Patterson R. Allergic bronchopulmonary aspergillosis and the evaluation of the patient with asthma. *J Allergy Clin Immunol* 1988;81:646–650.

31. Schwartz HJ, Greenberger PA. The prevalence of allergic bronchopulmonary aspergillosis in patients with asthma, determined by serologic and radiologic criteria in patients at risk. *J Lab Clin Med* 1991;117:138–142.

32. Solomon WR, Burge HP, Boise JR. Airborne *Aspergillus fumigatus* levels outside and within a large clinical center. *J Allergy Clin Immunol* 1978;62:56–60.

33. Latge J-P. *Aspergillus fumigatus* and aspergillosis. *Clin Microbiol Rev* 1999;12:310–350.

34. Kurup VP, Kumar A, Kenealy WR, et al. *Aspergillus* ribotoxins react with IgE and IgG antibodies of patients with allergic bronchopulmonary aspergillosis. *J Lab Clin Med* 1994;123:749–756.

35. Morris MP, Fletcher OJ. Disease prevalence in Georgia turkey flocks in 1986. *Avian Dis* 1988;32:404–406.

36. Quirce S, Cuevas M, Diez-Gomez ML, et al. Respiratory allergy to *Aspergillus*-derived enzymes in bakers' asthma. *J Allergy Clin Immunol* 1992;90:970–978.

37. Rosenberg IL, Greenberger PA. Allergic bronchopulmonary aspergillosis and aspergilloma: long-term followup without enlargement of a large multiloculated cavity. *Chest* 1984;85:123–125.

38. Binder RE, Faling LJ, Pugatch RE, et al. Chronic necrotizing pulmonary aspergillosis: a discreet clinical entity. *Medicine* 1982;151:109–124.

39. Katzenstein AL, Sale SR, Greenberger PA. Allergic *Aspergillus* sinusitis: a newly recognized form of sinusitis. *J Allergy Clin Immunol* 1983;72:89–93.

40. Goldstein MF, Atkins PC, Cogan FC, et al. Allergic *Aspergillus* sinusitis. *J Allergy Clin Immunol* 1985;76:515–524.

41. DeShazo RD, Chapin K, Swain RE. Fungal sinusitis. *N Engl J Med* 1997;337:254–259.

42. Kohn FA, Javer AR. Allergic fungal sinusitis: a four-year follow-up. *Am J Rhinol* 2000;14:149–156.

43. Chrzanowski RR, Rupp NT, Kuhn FA, et al. Allergenic fungi in allergic fungal sinusitis. *Ann Allergy Asthma Immunol* 1997;79:431–435.

44. Houser SM, Corey JP. Allergic fungal sinusitis: pathophysiology, epidemiology, and diagnosis. *Otolaryngol Clin North Am* 2000;33:390–408.

45. Marple BF. Surgical fungal sinusitis: surgical management. *Otolaryngol Clin North Am* 2000;33:409–418.

46. Marple BF, Mabry RL. Comprehensive management of allergic fungal sinusitis. *Am J Rhinol* 1998;12:263–268.

47. Sher TH, Schwartz HJ. Allergic *Aspergillus* sinusitis with concurrent allergic bronchopulmonary *Aspergillus*: report of a case. *J Allergy Clin Immunol* 1988;81:844–846.

48. Rosenberg M, Patterson R, Mintzer R, et al. Clinical and immunologic criteria for the diagnosis of allergic bronchopulmonary aspergillosis. *Ann Intern Med* 1977;86:405–414.

49. Patterson R, Greenberger PA, Halwig JM, et al. Allergic bronchopulmonary aspergillosis: natural history and classification of early disease by serologic and roentgenographic studies. *Arch Intern Med* 1986;146:916–918.

50. Ricketti AJ, Greenberger PA, Patterson R. Immediate type reactions in patients with allergic bronchopulmonary aspergillosis. *J Allergy Clin Immunol* 1983;71:541–545.

51. Ricketti AJ, Greenberger PA, Glassroth J. Spontaneous pneumothorax in allergic bronchopulmonary aspergillosis. *Arch Intern Med* 1984;144:181–182.

52. Greenberger PA, Patterson R, Ghory AC, et al. Late sequelae of allergic bronchopulmonary aspergillosis. *J Allergy Clin Immunol* 1980;66:327–335.

53. Lee TM, Greenberger PA, Patterson R, et al. Stage V (fibrotic) allergic bronchopulmonary aspergillosis: a review of 17 cases followed from diagnosis. *Arch Intern Med* 1987;147:319–323.

54. Mintzer RA, Rogers LF, Kruglick GD, et al. The spectrum of radiologic findings in allergic bronchopulmonary aspergillosis. *Radiology* 1978;127:301–307.

55. Mendelson EB, Fisher MR, Mintzer RA, et al. Roentgenographic and clinical staging of allergic bronchopulmonary aspergillosis. *Chest* 1985;87:334–339.

56. Neeld DA, Goodman LR, Gurney JW, et al. Computerized tomography in the evaluation of

allergic bronchopulmonary aspergillosis. *Am Rev Respir Dis* 1990;142:1200–1205.

57. Goyal R, White CS, Templeton PA, et al. High attenuation mucous plugs in allergic bronchopulmonary aspergillosis: CT appearance. *J Comput Assist Tomogr* 1992;16:649–650.

58. Ward S, Heyneman L, Lee MJ, et al. Accuracy of CT in the diagnosis of allergic bronchopulmonary aspergillosis in asthmatic patients. *AJR* 1999;173:937–942.

59. Mitchell TAM, Hamilos DL, Lynch DA, et al. Distribution and severity of bronchiectasis in allergic bronchopulmonary aspergillosis (ABPA). *J Asthma* 2000;37:65–72.

60. Hoehne JH, Reed CE, Dickie HA. Allergic bronchopulmonary aspergillosis is not rare. *Chest* 1973;63:177–181.

61. Kurup VP, Fink JN. Immunologic tests for evaluation of hypersensitivity pneumonitis and allergic bronchopulmonary aspergillosis. In: Rose NR, Conway de Macario E, Folds JD, et al., eds. *Manual of clinical laboratory immunology,* 5th ed. Washington, DC: ASM Press, 1997:908–915.

62. Reed C. Variability of antigenicity of *Aspergillus fumigatus. J Allergy Clin Immunol* 1978;61:227–229.

63. Schwartz HJ, Citron KM, Chester EH, et al. A comparison of the prevalence of sensitization to *Aspergillus* antigens among asthmatics in Cleveland and London. *J Allergy Clin Immunol* 1978;62:9–14.

64. Novey HS. Epidemiology of allergic bronchopulmonary aspergillosis. *Immunol Allergy Clin North Am* 1998;18:641–653.

65. McCarthy DS, Pepys J. Allergic bronchopulmonary aspergillosis: clinical immunology: II. Skin, nasal, and bronchial tests. *Clin Allergy* 1971;1:415–432.

66. Sarma PU, Banerjee B, Bir N, et al. Immunodiagnosis of allergic bronchopulmonary aspergillosis. *Immunol Allergy Clin North Am* 1998;18:525–547.

67. Kurup VP, Banerjee B, Greenberger PA, et al. Allergic bronchopulmonary aspergillosis: challenges in diagnosis. *Medscape Respir Care* 1999;3(6).

68. Kurup VP, Ramasamy M, Greenberger PA, et al. Isolation and characterization of a relevant *Aspergillus fumigatus* antigen with IgG and IgE binding activity. *Int Arch Allergy Appl Immunol* 1988;86:176–182.

69. Longbottom JL, Austwick PKC. Antigens and allergens of *Aspergillus fumigatus*: I. Characterization by quantitative immunoelectrophoretic techniques. *J Allergy Clin Immunol* 1986;78:9–17.

70. Arruda LK, Mann BJ, Chapman MD. Selective expression of a major allergen and cytotoxin, *Asp fI,* in *Aspergillus fumigatus*: implications for the immunopathogenesis of *Aspergillus*-related diseases. *J Immunol* 1992;149:3354–3359.

71. Banerjee B, Kurup VP, Phadnis S, et al. Molecular cloning and expression of a recombinant *Aspergillus fumigatus* protein Asp fII with significant immunoglobulin E reactivity in allergic bronchopulmonary aspergillosis. *J Lab Clin Med* 1996;127:253–262.

72. Banerjee B, Greenberger PA, Fink JN, et al. Immunologic characterization of Asp f2, a major allergen from *Aspergillus fumigatus* associated with allergic bronchopulmonary aspergillosis. *Infect Immun* 1998;66:5175–5182.

73. Weiner Miller P, Hamosh A, Macek Jr M, et al.

Cystic fibrosis transmembrane conductance regulator (CFTR) gene mutations in allergic bronchopulmonary aspergillosis. *Am J Hum Genet* 1996;59:45–51.

74. Patterson R, Rosenberg M, Roberts M. Evidence that *Aspergillus fumigatus* growing in the airway of man can be a potent stimulus of specific and nonspecific IgE formation. *Am J Med* 1977;63:257–262.

75. Patterson R, Greenberger PA, Harris KE. Allergic bronchopulmonary aspergillosis. *Chest* 2000;118:7–8.

76. Gunnar S, Johansson O, Juhlin L. Immunoglobulin E in "healed" atopic dermatitis and after treatment with corticosteroids and azathioprine. *Br J Dermatol* 1970;82:10–13.

77. Settipane GA, Pudupakkam RK, McGowan JH. Corticosteroid effect on immunoglobulins. *J Allergy Clin Immunol* 1978;62:162–166.

78. Patterson R, Greenberger PA, Ricketti AJ, et al. A radioimmunoassay index for allergic bronchopulmonary aspergillosis. *Ann Intern Med* 1983;99:18–21.

79. Slavin RG, Hutcheson PS, Knutsen AP. Participation of cell-mediated immunity in allergic bronchopulmonary aspergillosis. *Int Arch Allergy Appl Immunol* 1987;83:337–340.

80. Chauhan B, Knutsen AD, Hutcheson PS, et al. T cell subsets, epitope mapping, and HLA restriction in patients with allergic bronchopulmonary aspergillosis. *J Clin Invest* 1996;97:2324–2331.

81. Chauhan B, Santiago L, Kirschmann DA, et al. The association of HLA-DR alleles and T cell activation with allergic bronchopulmonary aspergillosis. *J Immunol* 1997;159:4072–4076.

82. Geha RS. Circulating immune complexes and activation of the complement sequence in acute allergic bronchopulmonary aspergillosis. *J Allergy Clin Immunol* 1977;60:357–359.

83. Marx JJ, Flaherty DK. Activation of the complement sequence by extracts of bacteria and fungi associated with hypersensitivity pneumonitis. *J Allergy Clin Immunol* 1976;57:328–334.

84. Apter AJ, Greenberger PA, Liotta JL, et al. Fluctuations of serum IgA and its subclasses in allergic bronchopulmonary aspergillosis. *J Allergy Clin Immunol* 1989;84:367–372.

85. Ricketti AJ, Greenberger PA, Pruzansky JJ, et al. Hyperreactivity of mediator releasing cells from patients with allergic bronchopulmonary aspergillosis as evidenced by basophil histamine release. *J Allergy Clin Immunol* 1983;72:386–392.

86. Chan-Yeung M, Chase WH, Trapp W, et al. Allergic bronchopulmonary aspergillosis. *Chest* 1971;59:33–39.

87. Imbeau SA, Nichols D, Flaherty D, et al. Allergic bronchopulmonary aspergillosis. *J Allergy Clin Immunol* 1978;62:243–255.

88. Bosken CH, Myers JL, Greenberger PA, et al. Pathologic features of allergic bronchopulmonary aspergillosis. *Am J Surg Pathol* 1988;12:216–222.

89. Ghory AC, Patterson R, Roberts M, et al. In vitro IgE formation by peripheral blood lymphocytes from normal individuals and patients with allergic bronchopulmonary aspergillosis. *Clin Exp Immunol* 1980;40:581–585.

90. Slavin RG, Fischer VW, Levin EA, et al. A primate model of allergic bronchopulmonary aspergillosis. *Int Arch Allergy Appl Immunol* 1978;56:325–333.

91. Kurup VP, Mauze S, Choi H, et al. A murine model of allergic bronchopulmonary aspergillosis with elevated eosinophils and IgE. *J Immunol* 1992;148:3783–3788.

92. Brown JE, Greenberger PA, Yarnold PR. Soluble serum interleukin 2 receptors in patients with asthma and allergic bronchopulmonary aspergillosis. *Ann Allergy Asthma Immunol* 1995;74:484–488.

93. Greenberger PA, Smith LJ, Hsu CCS, et al. Analysis of bronchoalveolar lavage in allergic bronchopulmonary aspergillosis: divergent responses in antigen-specific antibodies and total IgE. *J Allergy Clin Immunol* 1988;82:164–170.

94. Bernstein JA, Zeiss CR, Greenberger PA, et al. Immunoblot analysis of sera from patients with allergic bronchopulmonary aspergillosis: correlation with disease activity. *J Allergy Clin Immunol* 1990;86:532–539.

95. Greenberger PA. Allergic bronchopulmonary aspergillosis and funguses. *Clin Chest Med* 1988;9:599–608.

96. Miller MA, Greenberger PA, Palmer J, et al. Allergic bronchopulmonary pseudallescheriasis in a child with cystic fibrosis. *Am J Asthma Allergy Pediatr* 1993;6:177–179.

97. Miller MA, Greenberger PA, Amerian R, et al. Allergic bronchopulmonary mycosis caused by *Pseudoallescheria boydii*. *Am J Respir Crit Care Med* 1993;148:810–812.

98. Greenberger PA, Katzenstein A-LA. Lipoid pneumonia with atypical mycobacterial colonization in allergic bronchopulmonary aspergillosis: a complication of bronchography and a therapeutic dilemma. *Arch Intern Med* 1983;143:2003–2005.

99. Halwig JM, Greenberger PA, Levin M, et al. Recurrence of allergic bronchopulmonary aspergillosis after seven years of remission. *J Allergy Clin Immunol* 1984;74:738–740.

100. Radin R, Greenberger PA, Patterson R, et al. Mold counts and exacerbations of allergic bronchopulmonary aspergillosis. *Clin Allergy* 1983;13:271–275.

101. Nichols D, Dopico GA, Braun S, et al. Acute and chronic pulmonary function changes in allergic bronchopulmonary aspergillosis. *Am J Med* 1979;67:631–637.

102. Safirstein BH, D'Souza MF, Simon G, et al. Five-year follow-up of allergic bronchopulmonary aspergillosis. *Am Rev Respir Dis* 1973;108:450–459.

103. Stevens DA, Schwartz HJ, Lee JY, et al. A randomized trial of itraconazole in allergic bronchopulmonary aspergillosis. *N Engl J Med* 2000;342:756–762.

104. Denning DW, Van Wye JE, Lewiston NJ, et al. Adjunctive therapy of allergic bronchopulmonary aspergillosis with itraconazole. *Chest* 1991;100:813–819.

105. Leon EE, Craig TJ. Antifungals in the treatment of allergic bronchopulmonary aspergillosis. *Ann Allergy Asthma Immunol* 1999;82:511–517.

25

Occupational Immunologic Lung Disease

Leslie C. Grammer

Division of Allergy-Immunology, Department of Medicine, Northwestern University Medical School and Northwestern Memorial Hospital Chicago, Illinois

It has been known for many years that a wide variety of occupational respiratory disorders are caused by immunologic mechanisms (1). Moreover, increasing industrialization has led to the production of numerous materials capable of inducing immunologically mediated lung disease in the working population. This is of concern to physicians who diagnose and treat these diseases and to labor, management, and various governmental agencies.

There are two major subdivisions of diseases that constitute occupational immunologic lung disease (OILD): immunologically mediated asthma and hypersensitivity pneumonitis (2). In addition, there is an asthma syndrome that can occur after one high-irritant exposure; this is called *reactive airways dysfunction syndrome* (RADS). This chapter organizes the various exposures into the most relevant disease category. However, various overlaps and uncertainties exist in OILD. First, some exposures can cause more than one disease. For instance, some antigens, such as trimellitic anhydride (TMA) and various fungal antigens, can cause more than one immunologic pulmonary disease, including asthma or hypersensitivity pneumonitis (3). Second, many reactive chemicals, such as toluene diisocyanate (TDI), can cause disease by inducing either RADS or immunologic asthma (4). Finally, pulmonary responses to some antigens have not been definitely established as immunologically or nonimmunologically mediated. An example would be Western red cedar.

EPIDEMIOLOGY

Incidence and prevalence figures for OILD are difficult to obtain for several reasons. First, there is often a high turnover rate in jobs associated with OILD, thus selecting workers who have not become sensitized. For instance, there is a high turnover rate among platinum workers. In a study of an electronics industry, a substantial proportion of workers who left reported respiratory disease as the reason (5). Second, occupationally related diseases generally are underreported (6). For instance, although the incidence of work-related illness is thought to be upward of 20 per 100, only 2% of these illnesses were recorded in employers' logs, as required by the Occupational Safety and Health Administration (OSHA) (7). Finally, the incidence of disease varies with the antigen exposure involved. For example, the incidence of occupational lung disease among animal handlers is estimated at 8% (8), whereas that of workers exposed to proteolytic enzymes can be as high as 45% (9).

It has been estimated that 2% of all cases of asthma in industrialized nations are occupationally related. In a U.S. Social Security Disability survey, about 15% of asthma cases were classified as occupational in origin (10). In another study of adult asthma in general medical practice, it was reported that more than 1 in 10 patients has a work history strongly suggestive of a potential relationship between work exposure and asthma (11).

A health maintenance organization (HMO) study of individuals aged 15 to 55 years reported that the incidence of asthma attributable to occupational exposures is significantly higher than previously reported and that accounts for a sizable proportion of adult-onset asthma (12). The European Community Respiratory Health Survey Study Group reported the highest risk for asthma was in farmers (odds ratio, 2.62), painters (2.34), plastic workers (2.20), cleaners (1.97), and spray painters (1.96) (13). In an American study of work-related asthma in California, Massachusetts, Michigan, and New Jersey, the most common industries were transportation manufacturing equipment (19.3%), health services (14.2%) and educational services (8.7%) (14).

MEDICOLEGAL ASPECTS

Most sensitizing agents that have been reported to cause occupational asthma are proteins of plants, animal, or microbial derivation and are therefore not specifically regulated by OSHA. Some of the low-molecular-weight sensitizers, such as isocyanates, anhydrides, and platinum, are regulated by OSHA; published standards for airborne exposure can be found in the Code of Federal Regulations (CFR 29.1910.1000) (15). OSHA, a division of the U.S. Department of Labor, is responsible for determining and enforcing these legal standards. The National Institute of Occupational Health and Safety (NIOSH), a division of the U.S. Department of Health and Human Services, is responsible for reviewing available research data on exposure to hazardous agents and providing recommendations to OSHA relative to airborne exposure limits. However, NIOSH has no regulatory or enforcement authority in this regard. More than 200 different substances have been reported to act as respiratory sensitizers and causes of occupational asthma (1). In only a few European countries are such occupational respiratory illnesses recognized by law with rights of compensation. In France, such etiologic agents as isocyanates, biologic enzymes, and tropical wood dusts are recognized (16). In the United Kingdom, such

agents as platinum salts, isocyanates, colophony, and epoxy resins are recognized. It has been reported that in countries where legislation involving compensation exists, implementation may still be difficult because of the lack of explicit criteria for the diagnosis of a given occupational disease (17).

About three decades ago in the United States, there was passage of hazard communication, also called "worker right-to-know," legislation at the federal, state, and local level (18). Substances that are capable of inducing respiratory sensitization are generally considered hazardous, and thus workers exposed to such substances are covered in most legislation. The common elements that exist in most hazard communication legislation are (a) that the employer apprise a governmental agency relative to its use of hazardous substances; (b) that the employer inform the employee of the availability of information on hazardous substances to which the employee is exposed; (c) that there be availability to the employee of alphabetized lists of material safety data sheets for hazardous substances in the workplace; (d) that there be labeling of containers of hazardous substances; and (e) that training be provided to employees relative to health hazards, methods of detection, and protective measures to be used in handling hazardous substances. This sort of hazard communication legislation may make workers more aware of the potential that exists to develop respiratory sensitization and OILD syndromes due to certain exposures. Whether this awareness will have an effect on the incidence of OILD remains to be seen.

Legal and ethical aspects of management of individuals with occupational asthma are major problems (17,19). Guidelines for assessing impairment and disability from occupational asthma continue to evolve (20,21). The ATS has proposed criteria based on a possible 4 points for each of the following: forced expiratory volume in 1 second (FEV_1), methacholine challenge, and medication. After totaling the points, degree of impairment can be determined (21). Depending on the occupation, disability can then be assessed.

ASTHMA

Pathophysiology

The pathophysiology of asthma is reviewed in Chapter 22. The major pathophysiologic abnormalities of asthma, occupational or otherwise, are bronchoconstriction, excess mucus production, and bronchial wall inflammatory infiltration, including activated T cells, mast cells, and eosinophils (22). Neutrophilic occupational asthma has also been described (23). There is evidence that these abnormalities may be at least in part explained by neurogenic mechanisms and release of inflammatory mediators and cytokines such as interleukins and interferons. Type I hypersensitivity involving cross-linking immunoglobulin E (IgE) on the surface of mast cells and basophils, resulting in release of mediators such as histamine and leukotrienes and of cytokines such as interleukin-3 (IL-3), IL-4, and IL-5, is believed to be the triggering mechanism in most types of immediate-onset asthma. There is increasing evidence that cellular mechanisms are very important in asthma (22). An updated paradigm of the Gell and Coombs classification is improving our understanding of some of those cellular mechanisms (24). There are now four types of type IV, or cellular, mechanisms. Type IV_{a2} involves T_H2 cells and is probably responsible for late asthmatic responses.

There are also nonsensitizing causes of occupational asthma (25). RADS was originally described two decades ago by Brooks and Lockey. The criteria for RADS are listed in Table 25.1. Several aspects of RADS are very characteristic (26). First, it results from a very high level of exposure to a toxic substance. Second, the asthma-like condition starts with that exposure. Third, the patient has symptoms that persist for at least 3 months. Finally, because of airway hyperreactivity, the patient develops bronchospasm from a variety of stimuli, including exercise, cold air, fumes, and household chemicals.

Reaction Patterns

A number of patterns of asthma may occur after a single inhalation challenge, as shown in Table 25.2 (22). The immediate reaction is mediated by IgE, occurs within minutes of challenge, presents as large airway obstruction, and is preventable with cromolyn and reversible by bronchodilators. The late response occurs several hours after inhalation challenge, presents as small airway obstruction in which wheezing may be mild and cough and dyspnea may predominate, lasts for several hours, is usually preventable with steroids (27) or cromolyn, and is only partly reversed by most bronchodilators. It may well result from a type IV_{a2} reaction.

The dual response is a combination of the immediate and late asthmatic responses. It is partially prevented by steroids or bronchodilators. After a single challenge study with certain antigens like Western red cedar, the patient may have repetitive asthmatic responses occurring over several days. This repetitive asthmatic response can be reversed with bronchodilators.

Other atypical patterns—square wave, progressive, and progressive and prolonged immediate—have been described after diisocyanate challenges; the mechanisms resulting in these patterns have not been elucidated (28). There is increasing evidence implicating immunologic mechanisms, in particular cellular mechanisms, in the pathophysiology of asthmatic responses to isocyanates (29–31).

Etiologic Agents

Most of the 200 agents that have been described to cause occupational asthma are high-molecular-weight (≥ 3 kDa) heterologous proteins of plant, animal, or microorganism origin.

TABLE 25.1. *Criteria for reactive airways dysfunction syndrome*

1. No history of bronchospastic respiratory disease
2. Onset of symptoms follows a high-level exposure to a respiratory irritant
3. Onset of symptoms is abrupt, within minutes to hours
4. Symptoms must persist for at least 3 months
5. Methacholine challenge is positive
6. The symptoms are asthma-like, such as cough and wheeze
7. Other respiratory disorders have been excluded

TABLE 25.2. *Types of respiratory response to inhalation challenge*

Asthma	Immediate	Late	Repetitive
Onset	10–20 min	4–6 hr	Periodic after initial attack
Duration	1–2 hr	2–6 hr	Days
Abnormality	FEV_1	FEV_1	FEV_1
Immune mechanism	IgE	IgE (IgG)	?
Symptoms	Wheezing	Wheezing, dyspnea	Recurrent wheezing
Therapy	Bronchodilators	Bronchodilators, corticosteroids	Bronchodilators

FEV_1, forced expiratory volume in 1 second; IgE, immunoglobulin E; IgG, immunoglobulin G.

Low-molecular-weight chemicals can act as irritants and aggravate preexisting asthma. They may also act as allergens if they are capable of haptenizing autologous proteins in the respiratory tract. Numerous reviews of occupational asthma have information on etiologic agents (1,6,16,32). A representative list of agents and industries associated with OILD can be found in Table 25.3.

Etiologic Agents of Animal Origin

Proteolytic enzymes are known to cause asthmatic symptoms on the basis of type I immediate hypersensitivity. Examples are pancreatic enzymes, hog trypsin (33) used in the manufacture of plastic polymer resins, *Bacillus subtilis* enzymes (34) incorporated into laundry detergents, and subtilisin. Positive skin test results, *in vitro* IgE antibody, and inhalation challenges have been demonstrated with *B. subtilis* enzymes, which are no longer used in the United States (35). Papain, which is a proteolytic enzyme of vegetable origin used in brewing beer and manufacturing meat tenderizer, has been noted to cause similar symptoms by IgE-mediated mechanisms (36).

Animal dander can cause asthma in a variety of workers, including veterinarians, laboratory workers, grooms, shepherds, breeders, pet shop owners, farmers, and jockeys (37). This can even be a problem for people whose work takes them to homes of clients who have pets, such as real estate salespeople, interior designers, and domestic workers.

Immediate asthmatic reactions and late interstitial response have been reported after inhalation challenge with avian proteins in people who raise birds for profit (38). Positive skin test results and *in vitro* IgE have been demonstrated.

A variety of insect scales have been associated with asthma. Occupational exposure to insect scales occurs in numerous circumstances (1). Bait handlers can become sensitized to mealworms used as fishing bait (39). Positive skin test results, *in vitro* IgE antibody, and inhalation challenges have been demonstrated to mealworms. Positive skin test results have been shown in various workers who have asthma upon insect exposure: to screw worm flies in insect control personnel (40), to moths in fish bait workers (41), and to weevils in grain dust workers (42).

Asthma has been noted in workers who crush oyster shells to remove the meat (43). On the basis of skin tests to various allergens, the authors determined that the allergen was actually the primitive organisms that attached to the oyster shell surface. Similarly, asthma may occur from sea squirt body fluids in workers who gather pearls and oysters and in snow crab workers (44).

Etiologic Agents of Vegetable Origin

In terms of plant protein antigens, exposure to latex antigens, particularly those dispersed by powder in gloves, has become an important cause of occupational asthma in the health care setting (45). People working in a number of other occupations, including seamstresses, may develop latex hypersensitivity (46). In the baking industry, flour proteins are well recognized to cause occupational asthma (47). A new occupational allergen, xylanase, has been reported to be the antigen in some cases of baker's asthma (48). Numerous other plant foodstuff proteins have

TABLE 25.3. *Examples of occupational allergens*

Agent	Industries and occupations
Animal proteins	
Proteolytic enzymes	Plastic polymer resin manufacturing; detergent industry; pharmaceutical industry; meat tenderizer manufacturing; beer clearing
Animal dander, saliva, urine	Lab researchers; veterinarians; grooms; breeders; pet shop owners; farmers
Avian protein	Poultry breeders; bird fanciers
Insect scales	Beekeepers; insect control workers; bait handlers; mushroom workers; entomologists
Vegetables proteins	
Latex	Health care workers
Flour or contaminants (insects, molds)	Bakers
Green coffee beans, tea, garlic, other spices, soybeans	Workers in processing plants
Grain dust	Farmers; workers in processing plants
Castor beans	Fertilizer workers
Guar gum	Carpet manufacturing
Wood dusts: boxwood, mahogany, oak, redwood, Western red cedar	Carpenters; sawyers, wood pulp workers; foresters; cabinet makers
Penicillium caseii	Cheese workers
Orris root, rice flour	Hairdressers
Thermophilic molds	Mushroom workers
Chemicals	
Antibiotics	Hospital and pharmaceutical personnel
Other drugs; piperazine hydrochloride, α-methyldopa, amprolium hydrochloride	Hospital and pharmaceutical personnel
Platinum	Workers in processing plants
Nickel	Nickel-plating workers
Anhydrides (TMA, PA, TCPA)	Workers in manufacture of curing agents, plasticizers, anticorrosive coatings
Azo dyes	Dye manufacturers
Ethylenediamine	Shellac and lacquer industry workers
Isocyanates	Production of paints, surface coatings, insulation polyurethane foam
Soldering fluxes, colophony	Welders
Chloramine-T	Sterilization
Acrylates	Surgical personnel

TMA, trimellitic anhydride; PA, phthalic anhydride; TCPA, tetrachlorophthalic anhydride.

been described to cause occupational asthma with inhalational exposure. These include tea (49), garlic, coffee beans (50), spices (51), and soybeans (52). Other plant protein sources reported to cause occupational asthma include vegetable gums (50), castor bean (53), guar gum (54), grain dust (55), wood dust (56), and dried flowers (57). Wood dust from Western red cedar is a well-recognized cause of occupational asthma, but the antigen appears to be the low-molecular-weight chemical, plicatic acid, not a high-molecular-weight plant protein (58).

A variety of microbes have been reported to be sensitizing agents in occupational asthma. Among these are molds (59) and bacteria such as thermophilic actinomycetes (60). Sensitization to *Aspergillus oryzae*–derived lactase has been reported in pharmaceutical workers (61).

Chemicals

Asthma has been described in pharmaceutical workers and hospital personnel exposed to pharmacologic products. Numerous antibiotics, including ampicillin, penicillin, spiramycin, and sulfas (60), are known to cause asthma, positive skin test results, or specific IgE. Other pharmaceuticals, including amprolium hydrochloride,

TABLE 25.4. *Trimellitic anhydride–induced respiratory diseases and immunologic correlates*

Disease	Mechanism	Immunologic tests
Asthma or rhinitis	Immunoglobulin E (IgE)	Immediate skin test IgG against TM-protein conjugate
Late respiratory systemic syndrome	IgG and IgA	IgG, IgA, or total antibody against TM-protein conjugate
Pulmonary disease, anemia syndrome	Complement-fixing antibodies	Complement-fixing antibodies against TM cells

TM, trimellityl.

α-methyldopa, and piperazine hydrochloride, cause asthma on an immunologic basis (6).

Workers in platinum-processing plants may have rhinitis, conjunctivitis, and asthma (62). Positive bronchial challenges and specific IgE have been demonstrated in affected workers. Another metal, nickel sulfate, has also been reported to cause IgE-mediated asthma (63).

The manufacture of epoxy resins requires a curing agent, usually an acid anhydride or a polyamine compound. Workers may thus be exposed to acid anhydrides in the manufacture of curing agents, plasticizers, and anticorrosive coating material. Studies have reported that three different patterns of immunologic respiratory response may occur (3) (Table 25.4).

Initially, it was presumed that the antibody in affected workers would be directed only against the trimellityl (TM) haptenic determinant. However, studies of antibody specificity have demonstrated that there is antibody directed against both hapten and TM-protein determinants that are considered new antigen determinants (NADs). Other acid anhydrides that have been described to cause similar problems include phthalic anhydride (PA), hexahydrophthalic anhydride (HHPA), and pyromellitic anhydride (PDMA) (3).

Isocyanates are required catalysts in the production of polyurethane foam, vehicle spray paint, and protective surface coatings. It is estimated that about 5% to 10% of isocyanate workers develop asthma from exposure to subtoxic levels after a variable period of latency (64). The isocyanates that have been described to cause occupational asthma include TDI, hexamethylene diisocyanate (HDI), diphenylmethyl diisocyanate (MDI), and isopherone diisocyanate (IPDI) (64). The histology of bronchial biopsy specimens from workers with isocyanate asthma appears very similar to that from patients with immunologic asthma and thus is suggestive of an immunologic mechanism (65). Compared with those isocyanate workers with negative bronchial challenges, workers with positive challenges have a higher incidence and level of antibody against isocyanate–protein conjugates (66). However, in most studies, isocyanate workers with positive challenges did not have detectable specific IgE in their serum. In a more recent study, an association between isocyanate asthma and specific IgE was again reported (67). Hypersensitivity pneumonitis (68) and hemorrhagic pneumonitis (69) due to isocyanates have been reported to be caused by immunologic mechanisms. Human leukocyte antigen (HLA) class II alleles have been studied in isocyanate asthma; a positive association was reported in one study and negative in another (70,71). Formaldehyde, a respiratory irritant at ambient concentrations of 1 ppm or more, is often cited as a cause of occupational asthma; however, documented instances of formaldehyde-induced IgE-mediated asthma are almost nonexistent (72). A bifunctional aldehyde, glutaraldehyde, has been reported to cause occupational asthma (73). Ethylenediamine, a chemical used in shellac and photographic developing industries, has been reported to cause occupational asthma (74). Chloramine T (75), reactive azo dyes (76), piperazine acrylates (77), and dimethyl ethanolamine are other chemicals that have also been reported to be causes of occupational asthma (78).

HYPERSENSITIVITY PNEUMONITIS

The signs, symptoms, immunologic features, pulmonary function abnormalities, pathology,

TABLE 25.5. *Occupational hypersensitivity pneumonitides*

Disease	Exposure	Specific inhalant
Farmer's lung	Moldy hay	*Micropolyspora faeni*
		Thermoactinomyces vulgaris
Malt worker's disease	Fungal spores	*Aspergillus clavatus*
		Aspergillus fumigatus
Maple-bark stripper's disease	Moldy logs	*Cryptostroma corticale*
Wood-pulp worker's disease	Moldy logs	*Alternaria* species
Sequoiosis	Moldy redwood sawdust	*Graphium* species; *Aureobasidium pullulans*
Humidifier/air conditioner disease	Fungal spores	Thermophilic actinomycetes
		Naegleria gruberi
Bird breeder's disease	Avian dust	Avian serum
Bagassosis	Moldy sugarcane	*Thermoactinomyces vulgaris*
Mushroom worker's disease	Mushroom compost	*Micropolyspora faeni*
		Thermoactinomyces vulgaris
Suberosis	Moldy cork dust	*Penicillium frequetans*
Isocyanate disease	Isocyanates	Toluene diisocyanate
		Diphenylmethane diisocyanate

and laboratory findings of hypersensitivity pneumonitis are reviewed in Chapter 23. No matter what the etiologic agent, the presentation follows one of three patterns. In the acute form, patients have fever, chills, chest tightness, dyspnea without wheezing, and nonproductive cough 4 to 8 hours after exposure. The acute form resolves within 24 hours. In the chronic form, which results from prolonged low-level exposure, patients have mild coughing, dyspnea, fatigue, pulmonary fibrosis, and weight loss. There is also a subacute form, which presents as a clinical syndrome of productive cough, malaise, myalgias, dyspnea, and nodular infiltrates on chest film. Any form can lead to severe pulmonary fibrosis with irreversible change; thus, it is important to recognize this disease early so that significant irreversible lung damage does not occur.

A variety of organic dusts from fungal, bacterial, or serum protein sources in occupational settings have been identified as etiologic agents of hypersensitivity pneumonitis (79) (Table 25.5). Several chemicals, including anhydrides and isocyanates, as discussed previously, have been reported to cause hypersensitivity pneumonitis.

DIAGNOSIS

The diagnosis of OILD is not complex in the individual worker if symptoms appear at the workplace shortly after exposure to a well-recognized antigen. However, the diagnosis can be very difficult in patients whose symptoms occur many hours after exposure, for instance, late asthma from TMA. Because of the increasing importance of OILD, it has now become essential to evaluate patients with respiratory syndromes for a possible association between their present disease states, their pulmonary function test results, and their immunologic exposure in the work environment (80–82). It is being increasingly reported that rhinoconjunctivitis precedes occupational asthma in many cases (83,84).

In the case of the well-established OILD syndrome, a careful history and physical examination with corroborative immunology and spirometry will suffice (85). The history and physical examination findings in asthma and hypersensitivity pneumonitis are discussed in Chapters 22 and 23. A negative methacholine test can almost exclude occupational asthma (80).

Immunologic evaluations may provide important information about the cause of the respiratory disease. Skin tests, with antigens determined to be present in the environment, may detect IgE antibodies and suggest a causal relationship (86). Haptens may be coupled to carrier proteins, such as human serum albumin, and used in skin tests (78) or radioimmunoassays. In cases of interstitial lung disease, double gel immunodiffusion techniques may be used to determine the presence of precipitating antibody, which would indicate antibody production against antigens known to cause disease (79).

It may be necessary to attempt to reproduce the clinical features of asthma or interstitial lung disease by bronchial challenge, followed by careful observation of the worker. Challenge may be conducted by natural exposure of the patient to the work environment with preexposure and postexposure pulmonary functions, compared with similar studies on nonwork days. Another technique used for diagnosis of OILD is controlled bronchoprovocation in the laboratory with preexposure and postexposure pulmonary function measurements (27,86). It is important that the intensity of exposure not exceed that ordinarily encountered on the job and that appropriate personnel and equipment be available to treat respiratory abnormalities that may occur. Some advocate the use of peak flow monitoring, whereas others find it unreliable (87,88). Evaluating induced sputum eosinophils has been reported to be a potentially useful technique to diagnose occupational asthma (89).

If the analysis of OILD is not for an individual patient but rather for a group of workers afflicted with a respiratory illness, the approach is somewhat different. The initial approach to an epidemiologic evaluation of OILD is usually a cross-sectional survey using a well-designed questionnaire (90). The questionnaire should include a chronologic description of all past job exposures, symptoms, chemical exposures and levels, length of employment, and protective respiratory equipment used. Analysis of the survey can establish possible sources of exposure. All known information about the sources of exposure should be sought in the form of previously reported toxic or immunologic reactions. Ultimately, immunologic tests and challenges may be done selectively.

PROGNOSIS

Unfortunately, many workers with occupational asthma do not completely recover, even though they have been removed from exposure to a sensitizing agent (91–93). Prognostic factors that been examined include specific IgE, duration of symptoms, pulmonary function testing, and nonspecific bronchial hyperreactivity (BHR). An unfavorable prognosis has been reported to be associated with a persistent high level of specific IgE, long duration of symptoms (>1 to 2 years), abnormal pulmonary function test results, and a high degree of BHR (94). The obvious conclusion from these studies is that early diagnosis and removal from exposure are requisites for the goal of complete recovery. In workers who remain exposed after a diagnosis of occupational asthma is made, further deterioration of lung function and increase in BHR have been reported (95). It must be appreciated that life-threatening attacks and even deaths have been reported when exposure continued after diagnosis (1).

TREATMENT

The management of OILD consists of controlling the worker's exposure to the offending agent. This can be accomplished in various ways. Sometimes, the worker can be moved to another station; efficient dust and vapor extraction can be instituted; or the ventilation can be improved in other ways, so that a total job change is not required (96). Consultation with an industrial hygienist familiar with exposure levels may be helpful in this regard. It is important to remember that levels of exposure below the legal limits that are based on toxicity may still cause immunologic reactions. Facemasks of the filtering type are not especially efficient or well tolerated. Ideally, the working environment should be designed to limit concentration of potential sensitizers to safe levels. Unfortunately, this is impractical in many manufacturing processes, and even in a carefully monitored facility, recommended thresholds may be exceeded (97). Thus, avoidance may well entail retraining and reassigning an employee to another job.

Pharmacologic management of OILD is rarely helpful in the presence of continued exposure on a chronic basis. Certainly, in acute hypersensitivity pneumonitis, a short course of corticosteroids (as discussed in Chapter 23) is useful in conjunction with avoidance. However, chronic administration of steroids for occupational hypersensitivity pneumonitis is not recommended. Asthma resulting from contact with occupational exposures responds to therapeutic agents such as β-adrenergic receptor agonists, cromolyn, and steroids, as discussed in Chapter 22. As exposure continues, sensitivity may increase, making medication requirements prohibitive.

Immunotherapy has been used with various occupational allergens causing asthma, including treatment of laboratory animal workers, bakers, and oyster gatherers, with reported success. However, there are no double-blind placebo-controlled trials. Immunotherapy may be feasible in a limited number of patients, with certain occupational allergens of the same nature as the common inhalant allergens; however, it is difficult and hazardous with many agents that cause occupational immunologic asthma.

PREVENTION

The key principle in OILD is that prevention, rather than treatment, must be the goal. Such preventative measures as improved ventilation and adhering to threshold limits, as discussed under Treatment, would be helpful to this end. There should be efforts to educate individual workers and managers in high-risk industries so that affected workers can be recognized early. Right-to-know legislation should increase awareness of occupational asthma.

Currently, there are no preemployment screening criteria that have been shown to be useful in predicting the eventual appearance of OILD. There is conflicting evidence as to whether HLA studies are useful in predicting isocyanate asthma (70,71) or anhydride asthma (98,99). It is known that atopy is a predisposing factor to a worker developing IgE-mediated disease (60), but there is at least one conflicting study (100). Whether or not cigarette smoking is a risk factor for OILD is unclear.

Prospective studies, such as those of Zeiss, Baur, Newman, Taylor, and colleagues, of TMA workers may demonstrate that serial immunologic studies are useful in predicting which workers are likely to develop immunologically mediated diseases. At the first sign of occupational asthma, those workers then could be removed from the offending exposure and retrained before permanent illness develops. This approach has been studied in TMA-exposed employees.

Another prospective study of TMA workers has reported that decreasing the airborne levels will reduce disease prevalence (101). This may prove to be the best approach to preventing OILD from other agents. Already, medical surveillance has been reported to reduce cases of permanent occupational asthma in Germany (102). A cost-benefit analysis suggests that this is also the case in the United States (103).

REFERENCES

1. Venables KM, Chan-Yeung M. Occupational asthma. *Lancet* 1997;349:1465–1469.
2. Cartier A. Occupational asthma: what have we learned? *J Allergy Clin Immunol* 1998;102:90–95.
3. Grammer LC, Patterson R. Trimellitic anhydride. In: Rom WN, ed. *Environmental and occupational medicine.* 3rd ed. Philadelphia: Lippincott-Raven, 1998:1215–1220.
4. Mapp CE, Saetta M, Maesrelli P. Mechanisms and pathology of occupational asthma. *Eur Respir J,* 1994;7:544–554.
5. Perks WH, Burge PS, Rehahn M, et al. Work-related respiratory disease in employees leaving an electronic factory. *Thorax* 1979;34:19–22.
6. Bernstein IL. Occupational asthma. *Clin Chest Med* 1981;2:255–272.
7. Discher DP, Feinberg HC. Pilot study for development of an occupational disease surveillance method. HEW Publication (NIOSH) No. 75-162. 1975.
8. Cullinan P, Lowson D, Nieuwenhuijsen MJ, et al. Work related symptoms, sensitization, and estimated exposure in workers not previously exposed to laboratory rats. *Occup Environ Med* 1994;51:589–592.
9. Brooks SM. The evaluation of occupational airways disease in the laboratory and workplace. *J Allergy Clin Immunol* 1982;70:56–66.
10. Blanc P. Occupational asthma in a national disability survey. *Chest* 1987;92:613–617.
11. Blanc PD, Eisner MD, Israel L, et al. The association between occupation and asthma in general medical practice. *Chest* 1999;115:1259–1264.
12. Milton DK, Solomon GM, Rosiello RA, et al. Risk and incidence of asthma attributable to occupational exposure among HMO members. *Am J Ind Med* 1998;33:1–10.
13. Kogevinas M, Anto JM, Sunyer J, et al. Occupational asthma in Europe and other industrialized areas: a population-based study. *Lancet* 1999;353:1750–1754.
14. Jajosky RA, Harrison R, Reinisch F, et al. Surveillance of work-related asthma in selected U.S. states using surveillance guidelines for state health departments—California, Massachusetts, Michigan, and New Jersey, 1993–1995. *Morb Mortal Wkly Rep* 1999;48:1–20.
15. Office of the Federal Register National Archives and Records Administration. *Code of Federal Regulations 1900–1910.* Washington, DC: Federal Register, 2000.
16. Chan-Yeung M, Malo J-L. Aetiological agents in occupational asthma. *Eur Respir J* 1994;7:346–371.
17. Richman SI. Legal treatment of the asthmatic worker:

a major problem for the nineties. *J Occup Med* 1990;32:1027–1031.

18. Howard J. OSHA and the regulatory agencies. In Rom WN, ed. *Environ Occup Med* 3rd ed. Philadelphia: Lippincott-Raven, 1998:1671–1679.

19. Oliver LC. Occupational and environmental asthma: legal and ethical aspects of patient management. *Chest* 1990;98:220S–224S.

20. Engleberg AL, ed. *Guides to the evaluation of permanent impairment.* 3rd ed. Chicago: American Medical Association, 1988.

21. Miller A. Guidelines for the evaluation of impairment/disability in patients with asthma. *Am J Respir Crit Care Med* 1994;149:834–835.

22. Hamid QA, Minshall EM. Molecular pathology of allergic disease I: lower airway. *J Allergy Clin Immunol* 2000;105:20–36.

23. Leigh R, Hargreave FE. Occupational neutrophilic asthma. *Can Respir J* 1999;6:194–196.

24. Kay AB. Concepts of allergy and hypersensitivity. In: Kay AB, ed. *Allergy and allergic diseases.* Oxford: Blackwell Science, 1997:23–35.

25. Lemiere C, Malo J-L, Gautrin D. Nonsensitizing causes of occupational asthma. *Med Clin North Am* 1996;80:749–774.

26. Alberts WM, do Pico GA. Reactive airways dysfunction syndrome. *Chest* 1996;109:1618–1626.

27. Boschetto P, Fabbri LM, Zocca E, et al. Prednisone inhibits late asthmatic reactions and airway inflammation induced by toluene diisocyanate in sensitized subjects. *J Allergy Clin Immunol* 1987;80:261–267.

28. Cartier A, Malo J-L. Occupational challenge tests. In: Bernstein IL, Chan-Yeung M, Malo J-L, et al, eds. *Asthma in the workplace.* 2nd ed. New York: Marcel Dekker, 1998:211–234.

29. Maestrelli P, Occari P, Turato G, et al. Expression of interleukin (IL)-4 and IL-5 proteins in asthma induced by toluene diisocyanate (TDI). *Clin Exp Allergy* 1997;27:1292–1298.

30. Raulf-Heimsoth M, Baur X. Pathomechanisms and pathophysiology of isocyanate-induced diseases: summary of present knowledge. *Am J Ind Med* 1998; 34:137–143.

31. Grammer LC, Shaughnessy MA, Kabalin CS, et al. Immunologic aspects of isocyanate asthma: IL-1 beta, IL-3, IL-4, sIL2R, and sICAM-1. *Allergy Asthma Proc* 1998;19:301–305.

32. Bernstein DI, Bernstein IL. Occupational asthma. In: Middleton E Jr, Reed CE, Ellis EF, et al, eds. *Allergy: principles and practice.* 5th ed. St. Louis: Mosby–Year Book, 1998:963–980.

33. Colten HR, Polakoff PL, Weinstein SF, et al. Immediate hypersensitivity to hog trypsin resulting from industrial exposure. *N Engl J Med* 1975;292:1050–1053.

34. Lemiere C, Cartier A, Dolovich J, et al. Isolated late asthmatic reaction after exposure to a high-molecular-weight occupational agent, subtilisin. *Chest* 1996;110:823–824.

35. Slavin RG, Lewis GR. Hypersensitivity to enzyme additives in laundry detergent workers. *J Lab Clin Med* 1971;78:977–978.

36. Novey HS, Keenan WJ, Fairshter RD, et al. Pulmonary disease in workers exposed to papain: clinico-physiological and immunological studies. *Clin Allergy* 1980;10:721–731.

37. Gross NJ. Allergy to laboratory animals: epidemiologic, clinical and physiologic aspects and a trial of cromolyn in its management. *J Allergy Clin Immunol* 1980;66:158–165.

38. Hargreave FE, Pepys J. Allergic respiratory reactions in bird fanciers provoked by allergen inhalation provocation tests. *J Allergy Clin Immunol* 1972;50:157–173.

39. Bernstein DI, Gallagher JS, Bernstein IL. Meal worm asthma: clinical and immunologic studies. *J Allergy Clin Immunol* 1983;72:475–480.

40. Gibbons HL, Dillie JR, Cauley RG. Inhalant allergy to the screw worm fly. *Arch Environ Health* 1965;10:424–426.

41. Stevenson DD, Mathews KP. Occupational asthma following inhalation of moth particles. *J Allergy* 1967;39:274–283.

42. Lunn JA. Millworkers' asthma: allergic responses to the grain weevil (sitophilus granarius). *Br J Ind Med* 1966;23:149–152.

43. Wada S, Nishimoto Y, Nakashima T, et al. Clinical observation of bronchial asthma in workers who culture oysters. *Hiroshima J Med Sci* 1967;16:255–266.

44. Weytjens K, Cartier A, Malo J-L, et al. Aerosolized snow- crab allergens in a processing facility. *Allergy* 1999;54:892–893.

45. Slater JE. Continuing medical education: latex allergy. *J Allergy Clin Immunol* 1994;94:139–149.

46. Weytjens K, Labrecque M, Malo J-L, et al. Asthma to latex in a seamstress. *Allergy* 1999;54:290–291.

47. Blanco Carmona JG, Juste Picon S, Garces Sotillos M. Occupational asthma in bakeries caused by sensitivity to alpha-amylase. *Allergy* 1991;46:274–276.

48. Baur X, Sander I, Posch A, et al. Baker's asthma due to the enzyme xylanase-a new occupational allergen. *Clin Exp Allergy* 1998;28:1591–1593.

49. Cartier A, Malo J-L. Occupational asthma due to tea dust. *Thorax* 1990;45:203–206.

50. Lehrer SB. Bean hypersensitivity in coffee workers' asthma: a clinical and immunological appraisal. *Allergy Proc* 1990;11:65–66.

51. Lemiere C, Cartier A, Lehrer SB, et al. Occupational asthma caused by aromatic herbs. *Allergy* 1996;51:647–649.

52. Ferrer A, Torres A, Roca J, et al. Characteristics of patients with soybean dust-induced acute severe asthma requiring mechanical ventilation. *Eur Respir J* 1990;3:429–433.

53. Coombs RR, Hunter A, Jonas WE, et al. Detection of IgE (IgND) specific antibody (probably reagin) to castor bean allergen by the red cell linked antigen antiglobulin reaction. *Lancet* 1968;1:1115–1118.

54. Lagier F, Cartier A, Somer J, et al. Occupational asthma caused by guar gum. *J Allergy Clin Immunol* 1990;85:785–790.

55. Park HS, Nahm DH, Suh CH, et al. Occupational asthma and IgE sensitization to grain dust. *J Korean Med Sci* 1998;13:275–280.

56. Godnic-Cvar J, Gomzi M. Case report of occupational asthma due to palisander wood dust and bronchoprovocation challenge by inhalation of pure wood dust from a capsule. *Am J Ind Med* 1990;18:541–545.

57. Schroeckenstein DC, Meier-Davis S, Yunginger JW, et al. Allergens involved in occupational asthma caused by baby's breath (Gypsophila paniculata). *J Allergy Clin Immunol* 1990;86:189–193.

58. Chan-Yeung M. Immunologic and non-immunologic mechanisms in asthma due to western red cedar (Thuja plicata). *J Allergy Clin Immunol* 1982;70:32–37.

59. Gottlieb SJ, Garibaldi E, Hutcheson PS, et al. Occupational asthma to the slime mold *Dictyostelium discoideum. J Occup Med* 1993;35:1231–1235.

60. Brooks SM. Occupational and environmental asthma. In: Rom WN, ed. *Environmental and Occupational Medicine.* 3rd ed. Boston: Little, Brown, 1998:481–524.

61. Bernstein JA, Bernstein DI, Stauder T, et al. A cross-sectional survey of sensitization to *Aspergillus oryzae*-derived lactase in pharmaceutical workers. *J Allergy Clin Immunol* 1999;103:1153–1157.

62. Cromwell O, Pepys J, Parish WE, et al. Specific IgE antibodies to platinum salts in sensitized workers. *Clin Allergy* 1979;9:109–117.

63. Malo J-L, Cartier A, Doepner M, et al. Occupational asthma caused by nickel sulfate. *J Allergy Clin Immunol* 1982;69:55–59.

64. Banks DE. The respiratory effects of isocyanates. In: Rom WN, ed. *Environmental and Occupational Medicine.* 3rd ed. Boston: Little, Brown, 1998:537–564.

65. Saetta M, Maestrelli P, di Stefano A, et al. Effect of cessation of exposure to toluene diisocyanate (TDI) on bronchial mucosa of subjects with TDI-induced asthma. *Am Rev Respir Dis* 1992;145:169–174.

66. Grammer LC, Harris KE, Malo J-L, et al. The use of an immunoassay index for antibodies against isocyanate human protein conjugates and application to human isocyanate disease. *J Allergy Clin Immunol* 1990;86:94–98.

67. Tee RD, Cullinan P, Welch J, et al. Specific IgE to isocyanates: a useful diagnostic role in occupational asthma. *J Allergy Clin Immunol* 1998;101:709–715.

68. Walker CL, Grammer LC, Shaughnessy MA, et al. Diphenylmethan diisocyanate hypersensitivity pneumonitis: a serologic evaluation. *J Occup Med* 1989;31:315–319.

69. Patterson R, Nugent KM, Harris KE, et al. Case reports: immunologic hemorrhagic pneumonia caused by isocyanates. *Am Rev Respir Dis* 1990;141:225–230.

70. Mapp CE, Balboni A, Baricordi R, et al. Human leukocyte antigen associations in occupational asthma induced by isocyanates. *Am J Respir Crit Care Med* 1997;156:S139–S143.

71. Rihs HP, Barbalho-Krolls T, Huber H, et al. No evidence for the influence of HLA class II in alleles in isocyanate-induced asthma. *Am J Ind Med* 1997;32:522–527.

72. Dykewicz MS, Patterson R, Cugell DW, et al. Serum IgE and IgG to formaldehyde-human serum albumin: lack of relation to gaseous formaldehyde exposure and symptoms. *J Allergy Clin Immunol* 1991;87:48–57.

73. Chan-Yeung M, McMurren T, Catonio-Begley F, et al. Clinical aspects of allergic disease: occupational asthma in a technologist exposed to glutaraldehyde. *J Allergy Clin Immunol* 1993;91:974–978.

74. Lam S, Chan-Yeung M. Ethylenediamine-induced asthma. *Am Rev Respir Dis* 1980;121:151–155.

75. Blasco A, Joral A, Fuente R, et al. Bronchial asthma due to sensitization to chloramine T. *J Invest Allergol Clin Immunol* 1992;2:167–170.

76. Nilsson R, Nordlinder R, Wass U, et al. Asthma, rhinitis, and dermatitis in workers exposed to reactive dyes. *Br J Ind Med* 1993;50:65–70.

77. Weytjens K, Cartier A, Lemiere C, et al. Occupational asthma to diacrylate. *Allergy* 1999;54:289–290.

78. Vallieres M, Cockcroft DW, Taylor DM, et al. Dimethyl ethanolamine-induced asthma. *Am Rev Respir Dis* 1977;115:867–871.

79. Grammer LC. Occupational allergic alveolitis. *Ann Asthma Allergy* 1999;83:602–606.

80. Bernstein DI. Clinical assessment and management of occupational asthma. In: Bernstein IL, Chan-Yeung M, Malo J-L, et al, eds. *Asthma in the workplace.* New York: Marcel Dekker, 1999:145–158.

81. Chan-Yeung M. Assessment of asthma in the workplace. ACCP consensus statement. American College of Chest Physicians. *Chest* 1995;108:1084–1117.

82. Baur X, Huber H, Degens PO, et al. Relation between occupational asthma case history, bronchial methacholine challenge, and specific challenge test in patients with suspected occupational asthma. *Am J Ind Med* 1998;33:114–122.

83. Malo J-L, Lemiere C, Desjardins A, et al. Prevalence and intensity of rhinoconjunctivitis in subjects with occupational asthma. *Eur Respir J* 1997;10:1513–1515.

84. Piirilä P, Estlander T, Hytönen M, et al. Rhinitis caused by ninhydrin develops into occupational asthma. *European Respiratory Journal*, 1997;10:1918–1921.

85. Grammer LC, Patterson R. Immunologic evaluation of occupational asthma. In: Bernstein IL, Chan-Yeung M, Malo J-L, et al, eds. *Asthma in the workplace.* New York: Marcel Dekker, 1999:159–171.

86. Baur X, Stahlkopf H, Merget R. Prevention of occupational asthma including medical surveillance. *Am J Ind Med* 1998;34:632–639.

87. Quirce S, Contreras G, Dybuncio A, et al. Peak expiratory flow monitoring is not a reliable method for establishing the diagnosis of occupational asthma. *Am J Respir Crit Care Med* 1995;152:1100–1102.

88. Leroyer C, Perfetti L, Trudeau C, et al. Comparison of serial monitoring of peak expiratory flow and FEV_1 in the diagnosis of occupational asthma. *Am J Respir Crit Care Med* 1998;158:827–832.

89. Lemiere C, Pizzichini MM, Balkissoon R, et al. Diagnosing occupational asthma: Use of induced sputum. *Eur Respir J* 1999;13:482–488.

90. Smith AB, Castellan RM, Lewis D, et al. Guidelines for the epidemiologic assessment of occupational asthma. *J Allergy Clin Immunol* 1989;84:794–804.

91. Barker RD, Harris JM, Welch JA, et al. Occupational asthma caused by tetrachlorophthalic anhydride: a 12-year follow-up. *J Allergy Clin Immunol* 1998;101:717–719.

92. Park HS, Nahm DH. Prognostic factors for toluene diisocyanate-induced occupational asthma after removal from exposure. *Clin Exp Allergy* 1997;27:1145–1150.

93. Perfetti L, Cartier A, Ghezzo H. Follow-up of occupational asthma after removal from or diminution of exposure to the responsible agent: relevance of the length of the interval from cessation of exposure. *Chest* 1998;114:398–403.

94. Hudson P, Cartier A, Pineau L, et al. Follow-up of occupational asthma caused by crab and various agents. *J Allergy Clin Immunol* 1985;76:682–688.

95. Marabini A, Dimich-Ward H, Kwan SY, et al. Clinical and socioeconomic features of subjects with red cedar asthma: a follow-up study. *Chest* 1993;104:821–824.

96. Merget R, Schulte A, Gebler A, et al. Outcome of occupational asthma due to platinum salts after transferral to low-exposure areas. *Int Arch Occup Environ Health* 1999;72:33–39.

97. Diem JE. Five year longitudinal study of workers employed in a new toluene diisocyanate manufacturing plant. *Am Rev Respir Dis* 1982;126:420–428.

98. Young RP, Barker RD, Pile KD, et al. The association of HLA-DR3 with specific IgE to inhaled acid anhydrides. *Am J Respir Crit Care Med* 1995;151:219–221.

99. Nielsen J, Johnson U, Welinder H, et al. HLA and immune nonresponsiveness in workers exposed to organic acid anhydrides. *J Occup Environ Med* 1996;38:1087–1090.

100. Calverley AE, Rees D, Dowdeswell RJ. Allergy to complex salts of platinum in refinery workers: Prospective evaluations of IgE and Phadiatop[SC] status. *Clin Exp Allergy* 1999;29:703–711.

101. Grammer LC, Harris KE, Sonenthal KR, et al. A cross-sectional survey of 46 employees exposed to trimellitic anhydride. *Allergy Proc*, 1992;13:139–142.

102. Baur X, Stahlkopf H, Merget R. Prevention of occupational asthma including medical surveillance. *Am J Ind Med* 1998;34:632–639.

103. Phillips VL, Goodrich MA, Sullivan TJ. Health care worker disability due to latex allergy and asthma: a cost analysis. *Am J Public Health* 1999;89:1024–1028.

26

Controversial and Unproved Methods in Allergy Diagnosis and Treatment

Abba I. Terr

Department of Medicine, University of California San Francisco School of Medicine, San Francisco, California

Unconventional and unproved procedures, theories, and practices are often referred to as "complementary and alternative medicine" (1). Many of these practices are offered for patients with real or suspected allergy (2). They are especially popular today, even though there is no evidence that they are either alternative or complementary to rational scientifically based medical practice.

Accurate diagnosis and effective therapy of allergic disorders based on sound theory and clinical research can be accomplished efficiently, safely, and cost effectively. There is little if any justification today for an empirical approach to the allergic patient. However, the clinician who treats allergic patients must be sufficiently knowledgeable about both accepted and unproved techniques and theories in order to practice rationally and successfully.

DEFINITIONS

A number of terms have been used to describe different forms of medical practice (Table 26.1).

Standard practice is generally defined as the methods of diagnosis and treatment used by reputable physicians in a particular subspecialty or primary care practice. Standard practice usually involves a range of options. Procedures must be tailored to the individual patient. In general, physicians who are knowledgeable, trained, and experienced in allergy may prefer certain diagnostic and therapeutic methods while at the same time recognizing that other methods are acceptable.

Acceptable methods are based on, or consistent with, current scientifically established mechanisms of allergy. In addition, they have "stood the test of time" through a sufficient period of usage and an evaluation by properly conducted scientifically based clinical trials demonstrating efficacy and safety.

Experimental procedures are potentially new methods of practice arising from the results of scientific studies or from chance empiric observation. Experimental methods of diagnosis and treatment are those that are used in clinical trials on subjects who are informed of the experimental nature of the procedure, their potential risks, and their potential benefits. Subjects must give informed consent to participate in experimental trials.

Controversial methods refer to those procedures that lack scientific credibility and have not been shown to have clinical efficacy, even though they may be used by a few physicians in their practices. They are not used by most practicing allergists. Most of the controversial methods discussed in this chapter have been tested in clinical trials; the published results show either ineffectiveness or insufficient data to establish effectiveness. In some cases only anecdotal testimonies are available. The expression *unproved* is another term for procedures that are controversial, as defined above.

TABLE 26.1. *Terminology*

1. Standard Practice
2. Accepted Practice
3. Conventional (or unconventional) methods
4. Proven (or unproven) methods
5. Controversial methods
6. Experimental (investigational) procedures
7. Alternative medicine
8. Complementary medicine
9. Fraud
10. Quakery
11. Standard of care

TABLE 26.2. *Categories of inappropriate procedures*

Ineffective
Effective by misused
Effective but misinterpreted

The terms *alternative* and *complementary* are not appropriate because they tend to obscure the real issue of whether or not a particular procedure has been validated for clinical use by proper scientific scrutiny. The terms *fraud* and *quackery* generally equate to medical practices performed by those individuals who knowingly, deliberately, and deceitfully use unproven and controversial methods for profit. Many physicians who use controversial procedures in allergy practice, however, do so because they sincerely believe that these practices are worthwhile and are unwilling to accept evidence to the contrary.

Standard of care is terminology usually used in the course of litigation. The definition will vary according to jurisdiction.

UNCONVENTIONAL DIAGNOSTIC METHODS

Experienced allergists recognize that a thorough history and physical examination are essential for diagnosis. Laboratory testing is used selectively to supplement the history and physical findings, especially when objective measurement of a functional abnormality such as airway obstruction is desired, or when other diseases must be ruled out of consideration. Allergy tests such as skin-prick or intradermal tests, patch tests, or *in vitro* antibody tests are in fact tests for the presence of an immune response of a particular type [e.g., immunoglobulin E (IgE) antibody or cell-mediated immunity] to a specific allergen. These tests alone do not diagnose or necessarily predict an allergic disease, but they do assist the clinician in diagnosis when the results are correlated with the patient's history.

Inappropriate diagnostic tests fall into three categories (Table 26.2): (a) procedures of no possible diagnostic value under any circumstances; (b) procedures that are intrinsically capable of a valid measurement but not appropriate for use in the diagnosis of allergic disorders; and (c) procedures that are intrinsically capable of being used in allergy diagnosis but are not appropriate for general clinical use because of low sensitivity or specificity, lack of general availability, or expense. For example, the *in vitro* histamine release test has been widely used in allergy research, where it has been invaluable in furthering knowledge of disease, but it cannot be recommended for clinical use at this time. It may eventually be modified to assume a place in allergy practice in the future.

"Diagnostic" Procedures of No Value Under Any Circumstances

The procedures included in this category are not based on sound scientific principles, and they have not been shown by proper controlled clinical trials to be capable of assisting in diagnosis for any condition.

The Cytotoxic Test

This is also known as the leukocytotoxic test or Bryan test (3,4). It is the microscopic examination of an unstained wet mount of whole blood or buffy coat on a slide that had been previously coated with a dried food extract. Subjective impressions of swelling, vacuolation, crenation, or other changes in morphology of leukocytes indicate a "positive" test result, and this in turn is considered evidence of allergy to the food. The procedure has not been standardized for time of incubation, pH, osmolarity, temperature, or other conditions that may be responsible for the observed changes (4). Reproducibility of identifying unstained leukocyte morphologic changes has not been established. The procedure is advertised as a test for allergy to foods or drugs.

There are no known allergic diseases caused by leukocyte cytotoxicity from foods, either directly or immunologically. Some drugs do cause immunologically mediated cytotoxicity of leukocytes, but there have been no studies to show that this can be demonstrated *in vitro* by the Bryan test.

Several controlled clinical trials have reported that the cytotoxic test is not reproducible, and it does not correlate with any clinical evidence of food allergy (5,6).

The ALCAT Test

A recent modification of the cytotoxic test, the ALCAT (antigen leukocyte cellular antibody test) uses electronic hematology instrumentation and computerized data analysis to examine and monitor changes in cell volumes. Like the cytotoxic test, it also has been promoted as a screening procedure for diagnosing food allergy or intolerance in a host of conditions, including arthritis, urticaria, bronchitis, gastroenteritis, childhood hypereactivity, rhinitis, and atopic dermatitis. Results are used to recommend elimination diets for these diseases. There are no proper controlled trials to establish diagnostic efficacy (7).

Provocation–Neutralization

This is a procedure that is claimed by its proponents to diagnose "allergy" to foods, inhalant allergens, environmental chemicals, hormones, and microorganisms, such as *Candida albicans*.

The test is performed by giving the patient a test dose of an extract of one of these substances by either intracutaneous injection, subcutaneous injection, or by sublingual drop. The patient then records any subjective sensations appearing during the next 10 minutes. Any reported symptom constitutes a "positive" test result, that is, evidence for allergy to the substance. If the test is negative, it is repeated with higher concentrations of the substance until the patient reports a sensation or symptom. The patient is then given a lower concentration of the extract, and if fewer or no symptoms are reported, the reaction is said to be "neutralized" (8–15). The neutralizing dose is then used for therapy. When the test is performed by intradermal injection, increasing wheal diameter with increasing dose is considered corroborative evidence of a positive test result. In provocation–neutralization, the test result is graded as positive regardless of whether the reported sensations are the same as those in the patient's history. Some proponents measure change in pulse rate during the test, but there is disagreement about its significance.

Published reports of provocation–neutralization testing yield conflicting results (16). Studies have included subjects with varying clinical manifestations, different testing methods, and variable criteria for a positive test result. Many lack placebo controls, reflecting the absence of standardization and the subjective nature of provocation–neutralization.

Modern concepts of immunologic disease provide no rationale for the provocation of subjective symptoms and their immediate neutralization under the conditions used in this procedure (17). A placebo-controlled double-blind evaluation of provocation–neutralization for diagnosis of food allergy in 18 patients showed that symptoms were provoked with equal frequency by food extracts and by placebo (18), showing that results are based on suggestion (19). Furthermore, there is a potential danger of causing a local reaction in the mouth or even a systemic reaction (20) in a patient tested with an allergen to which there is a significant IgE sensitivity. The procedure is time consuming, because only a single concentration of a single allergen can be "tested" at one time.

In the United States, there are several environmental control units in which patients are subjected to airborne exposure to chemicals in testing booths (21). Unlike bronchial provocation testing in asthma, a positive test for environmental illness is designated by the appearance of self-reported symptoms only. There are no published reports of controlled studies of this method of testing.

Electrodermal Diagnosis

This procedure purports to measure changes in skin resistance after the patient is exposed to an allergen (22). The allergen extract, usually a food, is placed in a glass vial that is then put on a metal plate inserted into the electrical circuit between the skin and a galvanometer. A decrease in skin electrical resistance is said to be a positive test indicating allergy to the food.

This procedure is without any rational basis, and there have been no studies to support its use. Proponents use acupuncture points on the skin when performing this bizarre procedure, often referred to as electroacupuncture. A recent controlled study reported that it was incapable of detecting specific allergic sensitivities (23).

Applied Kinesiology

In this case, the muscle strength of a limb is measured before and after the patient is exposed to a test allergen (24). Exposure to the allergen, usually a food, is done by placing a glass vial of the allergen extract on the patient's skin, and an estimate of the muscle strength is made subjectively. A loss or weakening of muscle strength is considered a positive test result, indicating allergy to the tested food.

There is no scientific rationale to justify the belief that allergy to a food or to any other allergen changes the function of skeletal muscle, and the belief that any exposure to the allergen could occur through a glass vial on contact with the skin is clearly untenable.

Diagnostic Procedures Misused for Allergy "Diagnosis"

The procedures included in this category are ineffective for allergy diagnosis, although they may be useful for diagnosis of other medical conditions. They are considered under two categories: nonimmunologic tests and immunologic tests.

Nonimmunologic Tests that Are Inappropriate for Allergy Diagnosis

Certain procedures are valid diagnostic tests, although not for allergy. Those discussed here are the pulse test and quantification of chemicals in body fluids and tissues. These tests have been promoted for allergy diagnosis based on erroneous concepts of the pathogenesis of allergy.

Pulse Test

Measuring a change in pulse rate, either an increase or decrease, after a test substance is ingested or injected has been used by some as indication of allergy (25). A change in pulse rate occurs from a variety of physiologic conditions and in the course of many other diseases. There is no rationale or documentation that an increase or decrease in heart rate by itself can diagnose allergy.

Testing for Environmental Chemicals in the Body

A small number of physicians subscribe to the unsubstantiated belief that synthetic chemicals are toxic to the human immune system, resulting in "sensitivities" to numerous chemicals, foods, drugs, and other agents (26,27). Samples of whole blood, erythrocytes, serum, urine, fat, and hair are analyzed for the presence of a variety of environmental chemicals. The usual chemicals tested are organic solvents, other hydrocarbons, and pesticides. Analytical methods and instrumentation are available for quantifying almost any chemical at the level of parts per billion, and indeed many environmental chemicals are found at this low level in almost everyone because of the ubiquitous presence of these substances in today's environment. Under some circumstances, it may be appropriate to detect toxic quantities of a suspected chemical where poisoning is suspected, but the presence of such chemicals in the body, regardless of quantity, bears no relationship to allergic disease. The concept of an immunotoxic cause of allergic "sensitivity" is unproved.

Immunologic Tests that Are Inappropriate in Allergy Diagnosis

The immunologic pathogenesis of allergy is firmly established. The mechanisms of allergy caused by IgE antibodies, immune complexes, or cell-mediated hypersensitivity are described thoroughly elsewhere in this book. The clinical manifestations of diseases mediated in these ways and the appropriate immunologic tests for diagnosis are explained in detail. Some clinical laboratories provide valid tests for detecting certain antibodies, circulating immune complexes, and blood levels of lymphocyte subsets, immunoglobulins, and complement components, which they promote for use in allergy diagnosis, even though these tests are not appropriate for this purpose. It should be emphasized that the tests themselves may be highly sensitive and specific and the results valid, although they are irrelevant for the clinical evaluation of allergic disease.

Serum Immunoglobulin G Antibodies

Immunoglobulin G antibodies to atopic allergens such as foods or inhalants are not involved in the pathogenesis of atopic diseases. Although some allergists have speculated that delayed adverse reactions to foods may be caused by circulating immune complexes containing IgG or IgE antibodies to foods (28–30), this concept is unproved. In fact, IgG antibodies and postprandial circulating immune complexes to foods are probably normal phenomena and not indicative of disease (31). They are found in very low concentrations in serum compared with the quantity of antibody and immune complex required to evoke inflammation in serum sickness. Circulating IgG antibodies to the common injected allergens can usually be detected in the serum of patients receiving allergen immunotherapy (hyposensitization). Although referred to as "blocking antibodies," their protective role in injection therapy of atopic respiratory disease and Hymenoptera insect venom anaphylaxis is uncertain, so measurement of IgG antibodies or immune complexes has no diagnostic value in the management of atopic patients. In contrast, detecting IgG antibody to the relevant antigen may be diagnostically useful in serum sickness and in allergic bronchopulmonary aspergillosis.

Total Serum Immunoglobulin Concentrations

Quantifying the total serum concentrations of IgG, IgA, IgM, and IgE can be accomplished easily and accurately. Significant reductions of one or more of IgG, IgA, and IgM constitute the immunoglobulin deficiency diseases, wherein deficient antibody production leads to susceptibility to certain infections (32). Polyclonal increases in the serum concentrations of these immunoglobulins occur in certain chronic infections and autoimmune diseases. Monoclonal hyperproduction occurs in multiple myeloma and Waldenström macroglobulinemia. Alterations in the total serum concentration of these three immunoglobulins is not a feature of allergic disorders, even in diseases involving IgG antibodies, such as serum sickness. Conversely, serum IgE concentrations are generally higher in atopic patients than in nonatopic controls. Patients with allergic asthma have higher concentrations than those with allergic rhinitis, and in some patients with atopic dermatitis serum IgE is very high. However, the total serum IgE is not a useful "screen" for atopy, because a significant number of atopic patients have concentrations that fall within the range of nonatopic controls. Furthermore, the total concentration of any immunoglobulin gives no information about antibody specificity. Immunologic specificity is the cornerstone of allergy diagnosis. In allergic bronchopulmonary aspergillosis, the total serum IgE concentration has prognostic significance because it correlates with disease activity (33).

Lymphocyte Subset Counts

Monoclonal antibody technology has made it possible to obtain accurate counts of each of the many lymphocyte subsets that are identified by specific cell surface markers, termed clusters of differentiation. Quantifying lymphocyte subsets in blood by their cell surface markers is useful in the diagnosis of lymphocyte cellular immunodeficiencies and lymphocytic leukemias, but not in allergy. The "normal" range of circulating levels for many of the subsets of lymphocytes is wide and fluctuates considerably under usual circumstances.

Food Immune Complex Assay

Some commercial clinical laboratories offer tests that detect circulating immune complexes containing specific food antigens purportedly for the diagnosis of allergy to foods. The method involves a two-site recognition system in which a heterologous antibody to the food is bound to a solid-phase immunosorbent medium (34,35). When incubated with the test serum, the reagent antibody detects the antigen in the immune complex and immobilizes the complex, which is then detected and quantified by a labeled antiimmunoglobulin.

A portion of ingested food protein is normally absorbed intact through the gastrointestinal tract, permitting the formation of an immune response and low levels of circulating antibody to these food proteins (31–33). It has been suggested that certain allergic reactions may be caused by circulating immune complexes that contain food antigens complexed with IgE or IgG antibodies (34,35). Such immune complexes, however, are more likely to be a physiologic mechanism for clearing the food antigens from the circulation and not pathogenic (36).

To date there is no clinical evidence that circulating food immune complexes cause any form of human disease. Patients with IgA deficiency may have high circulating concentrations of immune complexes to bovine albumin, but the pathophysiologic role of these complexes is unknown (36,37). No support exists for the use of assays for food immune complexes in the diagnosis of allergic disease.

UNCONVENTIONAL TREATMENT METHODS

Effective management of the patient with allergic disease must be based on an accurate diagnosis. Once this is accomplished, the three principal forms of treatment are allergen avoidance, medications to reverse the symptoms and pathophys-iologic abnormalities, and allergen immunotherapy. Management of allergy, or any other disease, also must take into account the physical, emotional, and social conditions of the patient, and therefore the program must be individualized in each case. All forms of treatment, including allergen avoidance, are subject to undesired adverse effects. Monitoring the course of treatment for both efficacy and complications should be part of the overall program of management.

This section discusses specific forms of treatment that are ineffective or inappropriate for allergy. These methods are considered in two categories: (a) treatments that have not been shown to be effective for any disease, and (b) treatments that are not appropriate for allergy but may be effective in other conditions.

Treatment Methods of No Value

The modalities discussed in this section include some that are directed specifically toward allergy and others that are promoted for allergy and other chronic conditions. All of these are without any proven therapeutic effect, even though they may be widely used and in some cases may result in temporary symptomatic improvement or sense of well-being. Such placebo effect accompanies any therapeutic maneuver, whether effective or not.

Neutralization

Neutralization (also called symptom-relieving) therapy is an extension of provocation–neutralization testing (8,38–41). A set of treatment extracts consisting of allergens, foods, or chemicals at a concentration determined from the prior testing to neutralize symptoms is supplied to the patient for self-treatment. The patient injects or applies sublingually a certain small amount of these neutralizing extracts to either relieve or prevent symptoms from environmental exposure. They are also recommended for a continuous maintenance program. There is no rational mechanism based on current immunologic theory that could account for immediate symptom neutralization in this way. The published studies of this form of therapy are either anecdotal or inadequate, suggesting that any beneficial effect is based on suggestion (19). The treatment is usually prescribed for chemical and food hypersensitivity, not for allergic diseases.

Acupuncture

The ancient Chinese method of acupuncture has been used over the centuries to treat virtually every disease. It has become popular in Western culture in recent years, although modern medical science offers little theoretical support for its continued use. It is used exclusively by some practitioners and as an adjunct to medications, homeopathy, naturopathy, and psychotherapy by others. It is likely that a significant number of allergic patients in the United States have tried acupuncture at some time for relief of asthma, allergic rhinitis, and allergic dermatoses. It is also used by patients who have other symptoms or medical problems that they consider to be allergic. Although some patients report temporary benefit, there have been no reported studies documenting either symptomatic improvement or long-term alteration in the course of allergic disease (42).

Homeopathic Remedies

Homeopathy is an alternative form of "healing" based on treating "like with like," meaning that the causative agent of a disease is administered therapeutically in exceedingly small amounts. There is no scientific theory to support homeopathic practice, despite its popularity. Because this procedure has a superficial resemblance to immunotherapy or desensitization, it is not surprising that homeopathic practitioners offer their remedies in the treatment of allergy. Homeopathic remedies consist of extracts of a number of natural substances, including plants, animal products, and insects. These extracts are serially diluted through a process known as succussion, which is merely the violent shaking of a container of diluted extract. Homeopathists also prescribe "natural" hormones in the form of orally administered extracts of animal adrenal cortex, thyroid, thymus, pancreas, and spleen. There is no evidence that homeopathic remedies have

any therapeutic effect for any disease, including allergy.

Detoxification

Detoxification is the method of allergy treatment used by those who subscribe to the unfounded theory that an allergic state can be induced by toxic damage to the immune system from exposure to environmental chemicals (26,27). Supporters of this idea believe that certain lipid-soluble chemicals may be stored in body fat for long periods.

The method consists of exercise and sauna. High-dose niacin is given to induce erythema. Body fluids are replenished with water and electrolytes, and certain "essential" oils are consumed, presumably to help replace fat-soluble chemical contaminants. This procedure takes about 5 hours and is repeated daily for 20 to 30 days.

The theory of immunotoxicity as a cause of allergic disease is unproved and contrary to an extensive body of clinical experience. The concept that increased circulation, vasodilatation, and oral ingestion of vegetable oils can mobilize "toxins" from fat into sweat is unproved. Potential dangers of this detoxification program have not been adequately studied.

Injection of Food Extracts

A detailed description of the technique of allergen immunotherapy using inhalant allergens for allergic respiratory disease and for Hymenoptera venom anaphylaxis are found elsewhere in this book. This form of therapy has been shown to be effective in these IgE-mediated diseases. Anaphylaxis and urticaria also can occur as a result of IgE antibodies to foods. Some patients experience life-threatening anaphylactic reactions from ingestion of exceedingly minute amounts of the food allergen. Fatalities from food anaphylaxis have been reported most commonly in cases of peanut allergy. Peanut protein is found in a variety of foods, so that strict avoidance is difficult for even the most conscientious patient. Allergen immunotherapy to eliminate or reduce the anaphylactic sensitivity in IgE-mediated food allergy is currently undergoing investigational controlled clinical trials.

Nevertheless, some practitioners routinely prescribe food extract injections, often consisting of a combination of foods based on skin test results or patients' reports of intolerance to foods. This form of treatment must be considered unproved as to efficacy and potential danger until appropriate clinical trials have been conducted.

Urine Injections

The drinking of urine was an ancient healing practice. The modern medical literature contains a single paper on "urine therapy," published in 1947, in which intramuscular injections of the patient's own urine was recommended for a long list of symptoms and illnesses, including allergy (43). In recent years, a small number of medical and "alternative" practitioners have revived this bizarre procedure, claiming that urine contains unspecified chemicals produced by the patient during an allergic reaction and that injections of these chemicals inhibit or neutralize future allergic reactions. There is no scientific evidence to support autogenous urine injections, nor are there clinical reports that the treatment is effective.

The risk of injecting urine is potentially great, because soluble renal tubular and glomerular antigens are normally excreted in the urine. Repeated injections of these antigens could theoretically induce autoimmune nephritis.

Enzyme-potentiated Desensitization

A modification of conventional allergy immunotherapy consists of injecting an exceedingly low dose of allergen—the amount delivered in a standard skin-prick test—premixed with a very small quantity of β-glucuronidase as a single preseasonal intradermal injection for seasonal pollen allergies or every 2 to 6 months for patients with perennial symptoms. Only a few practitioners use this method. For unexplained reasons, they advise the patient to avoid common food allergens, food additives, and all medications for 3 days before and 3 weeks after each injection. They also must avoid allergen exposure for 1 to 2 days before and

after the injection and consume a special "EPD diet." It is recommended for not only atopic and anaphylactic diseases, but also for ulcerative colitis, irritable bowel syndrome, rheumatoid arthritis, migraine headaches, petit mal seizures, chronic fatigue syndrome, "immune dysfunction syndrome," food-induced depression and anxiety, and childhood hyperactivity.

Recent controlled short-term clinical trials claim to show improved symptoms of allergic rhinitis or asthma, but objective measures of disease activity are either absent or were not measured. No trial has compared enzyme potentiated desensitization treatment with the allergen alone or the enzyme alone. There is no information about possible chemical or biological alteration of the allergen when mixed with the enzyme (44,45).

Inappropriate Treatment Methods

The forms of therapy discussed below each have a specific role in the management of certain diseases, but not for the treatment of allergy.

Vitamin, Mineral, and Nutrient Supplementation

A variety of "supplements" have been recommended for patients with allergies to relieve symptoms or as a cure for the disease. Various incorrect theories have arisen to rationalize their use.

Deficiency of vitamins, minerals, or amino acids as a cause of allergy is the usual explanation, even though there is no scientific basis for such a statement, nor have there been controlled clinical trials demonstrating that replacement by dietary supplementation is efficacious for any allergic disease. Fortunately, most patients taking such supplements suffer no harm, although excessive intake of fat-soluble vitamins could result in toxicity. Proponents of therapy with antioxidants—such as vitamin C and E and glutathione—justify the practice by citing evidence that allergic inflammation generates free radicals that cause oxidative damage to tissues (46). Although it is true that toxic oxygen metabolites are activated during the course of certain inflammatory reactions, the kinetics and localization of these events and the normal activation of endogenous antioxidants make it unlikely that ingestion of these dietary supplements would be effective.

Diets

Avoidance is the only certain method for treating food allergy. Although any food has the potential for being allergenic, food allergy in adults is relatively uncommon, and in each case it is usually limited to one or at most a few foods. Food allergy is more common among allergic infants and small children. Except for rare instances in some infants, avoidance therapy does not require an extensive elimination diet, and adequate food substitutes are available.

Unfortunately, adherence to the unsubstantiated concept of multiple food allergies as a cause of vague subjective symptoms, behavioral problems, and emotional illness leads to the unnecessary restriction of large numbers of foods. The risk of nutritional deficiency is obvious, although in practice many patients abandon highly restrictive diets because of the lack of long-term benefit.

Proponents of the concept of multiple food allergies sometimes recommend a "rotary diversified diet," in which the patient rotates foods so that the same food is eaten only once every 4 to 5 days (47). To do this, it is necessary to keep extensive and accurate records, causing further unnecessary and time-consuming attention to diet and symptoms (48).

Environmental Chemical Avoidance

Allergists recommend a reasonable program of allergen avoidance for patients with respiratory allergy. Simple measures to reduce exposure to house dust and dust mite through the elimination of bedroom carpeting and special casings for the bedding are clinically effective and pose no undue hardship on the patient and family. Similar measures can be taken to reduce indoor air levels of mold spores and other allergens, efficiently and cheaply in most cases. Occupational exposure to proven workplace allergens and irritants,

such as animals, isocyanate fumes, acid anhydrides, wood dusts, and grain dusts, are mandatory for patients with documented occupational asthma or hypersensitivity pneumonitis caused by these agents.

In contrast, the concept of multiple food and chemical sensitivities discussed below carries with it a recommendation for extensive avoidance of environmental "chemicals." The recommendation to avoid any exposure, even minute amounts, of multiple chemicals (49–51), such as pesticides, organic solvents, vehicle exhaust fumes, gasoline fumes, household cleaners, glue and adhesives, new carpets, and many others, is an unproven "treatment" for a group of patients with multiple chronic vague symptoms who are diagnosed as having chemical sensitivity based on unproved diagnostic methods, primarily provocation–neutralization. There no proof that these drastic measures are helpful; on the contrary, there is evidence for significant psychologic harm (52).

Antifungal Medications

The unsubstantiated theories of "*Candida* hypersensitivity syndrome" and disease caused by indoor molds, both discussed below, have prompted some physicians to prescribe a treatment program of antifungal medications and a special "mold-free" diet. Nystatin is usually prescribed first in a powder form given in a minute dose orally, followed by ketoconazole if the desired effect is not achieved. Although these drugs are effective in the treatment of cutaneous and systemic candidiasis, their use in the unsubstantiated *Candida* syndrome cannot be justified, and a controlled clinical trial showed that nystatin did not differ from placebo in its effect on such patients (53).

Immunologic Manipulation

Allergic diseases affect a minority of the population exposed to allergens. Allergen avoidance prevents disease but without altering the underlying immunologically induced hypersensitive state. It is not currently possible to manipulate the immune system therapeutically in a way that will remove all of a patient's specific allergic sensitivities completely and predictably without also inhibiting other necessary immune functions. Allergen immunotherapy, discussed elsewhere in this book, does not achieve this goal, although it is clinically beneficial in most cases.

Immunologic manipulation through the use of immunosuppressive drugs, immunostimulating drugs, therapeutic monoclonal antibodies to certain components of the immune system, and immunoregulatory cytokines is now standard treatment for other diseases, particularly autoimmunity and cancer.

Therapeutic gammaglobulin injections are a standard treatment for documented IgG antibody deficiency, and they have proved effective for this purpose. Gammaglobulin injections also have been used empirically for other diseases. They are effective in idiopathic thrombocytopenic purpura and in Kawasaki disease, although the mechanism of efficacy is unknown. Gammaglobulin injections are being recommended by some practitioners for allergy, but until effectiveness is shown by proper double-blind studies, such treatment should be considered experimental.

CONTROVERSIAL THEORIES ABOUT ALLERGY

The clinical practice of allergy today is based on a foundation of firmly established immunologic and physiologic principles. These are thoroughly discussed elsewhere in this book. Some unconventional methods of diagnosis and treatment are based on conventional theories, others on unsubstantiated theories arising from empirical observations, and still others appear to lack any theoretical basis. Some of these unconventional theories are discussed in this section.

Allergic Toxemia

Allergic diseases are characterized by focal inflammation in certain target organs such as the bronchi in asthma; the nasal mucosa and conjunctivae in allergic rhinitis; the gastrointestinal mucosa in allergic gastroenteropathy; the skin in atopic dermatitis, urticaria, and allergic contact dermatitis; and the lung parenchyma in hypersensitivity pneumonitis. Multiple target organs are involved in systemic anaphylaxis and in serum sickness. During the course of illness, the allergic patient with localized disease may experience systemic symptoms such as fatigue or other focal symptoms (such as headache) in parts of the body not directly involved in the allergic inflammation. These collateral symptoms are sometimes explainable pathophysiologically, for example as secondary effects of hypoxemia and hyperventilation in asthma or from cranial and neck muscle tension because of excessive sneezing in rhinitis. Furthermore, it is possible that locally released inflammatory mediators and cytokines may produce systemic effects, although direct proof of this is lacking.

For a number of years, certain practitioners have proposed that a variety of systemic complaints, especially fatigue, drowsiness, weakness, body aching, nervousness, irritability, mental confusion or sluggishness, and poor memory in the absence of any clinical sign of allergic inflammation could in fact be caused by exposure to environmental allergens. The allergens most often implicated in this concept are foods, environmental chemicals, food additives, and drugs. This "syndrome" has been referred to as allergic toxemia, allergic tension fatigue syndrome (54), or cerebral allergy (55). The literature on this subject is largely anecdotal. No definitive controlled studies have yet shown the existence of such a syndrome (16). Although there are frequent claims of dramatic improvement with the elimination of certain foods or chemicals, these claims are not supported by scientific evidence.

An extension of the allergic toxemia concept is the proposal that allergy is the cause of certain psychiatric conditions. According to one theory, attention deficit disorder in children is caused by food coloring and preservatives (56). This concept was embraced by certain physicians and parents who recommended and used food additive–free diets for hyperactive children. Several controlled studies, however, do not support this concept (57). There are also reports claiming that ingestion of certain foods, particularly wheat, is a cause or contributing factor to adult schizophrenia (58,59). These studies are not definitive and have not been confirmed.

Idiopathic Environmental Intolerances (Multiple Chemical Sensitivities)

In recent years, a small group of physicians have promoted a practice based on the theory that a wide range of environmental chemicals cause a variety of physical and psychological illnesses; symptoms involving the musculoskeletal system, joints, and gastrointestinal tract; and a host of nonspecific complaints in patients who have no objective physical signs of disease. The same patients typically blame multiple food sensitivities as a cause of these symptoms.

The practice based on these ideas is known as clinical ecology (50,60,61), which postulates that these patients suffer from failure of the human species to adapt to synthetic chemicals (62). One theory proposes that symptoms represent an exhaustion of normal homeostasis, caused by ingestion of foods and inhalation of chemicals. Another theory proposes that common environmental substances are toxic to the human immune system (63). These and other clinical ecology theories rely on certain unique and unscientific concepts, such as a maximum total body load of antigen, masked food hypersensitivity, and a "spreading phenomenon," whereby the existence of one specific allergy induces others of different specificities.

This practice centers on a diagnosis of "environmental illness," also called multiple chemical sensitivities, ecologic illness, chemical hypersensitivity syndrome, total allergy syndrome, and 20th century disease. The recent term *idiopathic environmental intolerances* is the most accurate name because it does not include any of the proposed but unproved mechanisms (64). Patients with this diagnosis generally have a wide range of symptoms that are often compatible with conversion reactions, anxiety and depression, or psychosomatic illness. No specific physical findings or laboratory abnormality is required for diagnosis.

Because there is no characteristic history and no pathognomonic physical sign or laboratory test (17,65,66), the diagnosis usually follows the provocation–neutralization procedure described above. Some clinical ecologists also use measurement of serum immunoglobulins, complement components, blood level of lymphocyte subsets, and blood or tissue level of environmental chemicals as a supplement to provocation–neutralization testing. It is not clear, however, how these test results indicate the presence of environmental illness. The few published reports show a variable and often conflicting set of abnormalities of dubious clinical significance, because these reports lack proper controls or evidence of reproducibility (16).

The principal methods of treatment advocated by clinical ecologists are avoidance and neutralization therapy. Avoidance of foods believed to cause or aggravate illness is accomplished by a rotary diversified diet, which is based on the belief that multiple food "sensitivities" occur in this illness. Avoidance of all food additives, environmental synthetic chemicals, and even some natural chemicals is a feature of clinical ecology treatment, but the extent of avoidance varies with the enthusiasm of the patient and physician and not on scientific evidence of efficacy. Most commonly, patients eliminate scented household products, synthetic fabrics and plastics, and pesticides. They generally try to limit exposure to air pollutants, gasoline fumes, and vehicle exhaust fumes. In the United States, several isolated rural communities have been established for those patients deemed unsuitable for the urban environment.

Neutralization therapy with food and chemical extracts, megadose vitamin therapy, mineral or amino acid supplements, and antioxidants are commonly prescribed. Drug therapy is generally condemned as a form of chemical exposure, although oxygen, mineral salts, and antifungal drugs are frequently recommended for these patients. None of these forms of treatment—either singly or in combination—have been evaluated in properly controlled studies to determine efficacy or potential adverse effects.

Candida Hypersensitivity Syndrome

In recent years a claim has been made that "environmental illness" is caused by *Candida albicans* normally resident in the microflora of the gastrointestinal and female genitourinary mucous membranes. Many persons with no clinical evidence of *Candida* infection and no evidence of defective local or systemic immunity, pregnancy, diabetes mellitus, endocrine diseases, or medications known to cause opportunistic candidiasis are said to suffer an illness known as *Candida* hypersensitivity syndrome (67,68). Clinically, the syndrome is indistinguishable from environmental illness. *Candida albicans* also has been claimed to cause behavioral and emotional diseases and a variety of physical illnesses and symptomatic states. Individuals who have ever received antibiotics, corticosteroids, birth control pills, or have ever been pregnant, even in the remote past, are said to be susceptible to this syndrome. Diagnosis is made by history and not by diagnostic testing. The recommended treatment is avoidance of sugar, yeast, and mold in the diet, and the use of a rotary diversified diet. Nystatin, ketoconazole, caprylic acid, and vitamin and mineral supplements are recommended. This syndrome is reminiscent of the concept of autointoxication that was popular in the early 20th century. In the opinion of some practitioners in that era, the bacterial component of the normal intestinal flora was considered to cause numerous physical and psychologic disabilities (69).

Disease from Indoor Molds

Atmospheric mold sensitivity has recently replaced environmental chemical sensitivity as causing a variety of subjective complaints or illnesses in persons living in homes or working in buildings that have sustained water damage from flooding or excessive humidity, promoting indoor mold growth (70).

Fungi are a major component of the environment, and fungal spores are almost always present in the atmosphere. In contrast to well-recognized infectious and allergic diseases caused by molds, the diagnosis in these cases rests on the presence of low levels of antifungal IgG antibodies in serum that have not been shown to be different from those found in healthy persons. As in the case of environmental illness, a combined toxicity/hypersensitivity theory is often invoked.

One particular fungus, *Stachybotrys atra* (chartarum), has created considerable publicity because of the suspicion that *Stachybotrys* mycotoxin was the causative agent in cases of pulmonary hemorrhage/hemosiderosis in young infants living in water-damaged homes (71). The role of the mycotoxin in these cases has been called into question (72), but there remains unsubstantiated fear of the presence of any indoor mold spores as pathogenic. This unproved theory should not be confused with allergic diseases caused by fungal allergy, especially asthma, some cases of hypersensitivity pneumonitis, allergic bronchopulmonary aspergillosis, and allergic fungal sinusitis. These can be identified by localized symptomatology and objective physical findings, functional or imaging studies that confirm pathology, and the presence of the relevant immune response by the patient.

REMOTE PRACTICE OF ALLERGY

In allergy practice, the proper diagnosis and treatment for each patient is based on a thorough history and physical examination by a physician knowledgeable about allergic diseases. In many cases, testing for specific sensitivities by skin or *in vitro* tests and other laboratory tests, x-rays, and other diagnostic procedures may be indicated to supplement the findings from the history and physical examination. Accurate diagnoses and therapy require knowledge of the patient's current and past symptomatology and the associated physical findings. The results of allergy skin tests and *in vitro* tests for IgE antibodies do not distinguish whether the patient has current, present, or future symptomatic disease, and therefore test results alone reveal only potential, but not clinical, sensitivities. They therefore cannot be used alone as the basis for recommending drug therapy or allergy immunotherapy.

Unfortunately, because skin and *in vitro* testing for IgE antibody sensitivities are relatively easy to perform, some practitioners do in fact provide a diagnosis and recommend treatment based solely on these test results. This is known as the remote practice of allergy (73). It is clearly unacceptable, because allergic disease occurs through a complex interplay of constitutional, environmental, and allergic factors, all of which must be known to the treating physician to avoid unnecessary, inappropriate, and potentially dangerous treatment.

REFERENCES

1. Owen DK, Lewith G, Stephens CR. Can doctors respond to patients' increasing interest in complementary and alternative medicine? *BMJ* 2001;322:154.
2. Gershwin ME, Terr A. Introduction: alternative and complementary therapy for asthma. *Clin Rev Allergy Immunol* 1996;14:241.
3. Bryan WTK, Bryan M. The application of in vitro cytotoxic reactions to clinical diagnosis of food allergy. *Laryngoscope* 1960;70:810.
4. Bryan MP, Bryan WTK. Cytologic diagnosis of allergic disorders. *Otolaryngol Clin North Am* 1974;7:637
5. Lieberman P, Crawford L, Bjelland J, et al. Controlled study of the cytotoxic food test. *JAMA* 1974;231:728.
6. Lehman CW. The leukocytic food allergy test: a study of its reliability and reproducibility: effect of diet and sublingual food drops on this test. *Ann Allergy* 1980;45:150.
7. Potter PC, Mullineux J, Weinberg EG, et al. The ALCAT test-inappropriate in testing for food allergy in clinical practice [Letter]. *S Afr Med J* 1992;81:384.
8. Lee CH, Williams RI, Binkley EL. Provocative inhalant testing and treatment. *Arch Otolaryngol* 1969;90:81.
9. Lehman CW. A double-blind study of sublingual provocative food testing: a study of its efficacy. *Ann Allergy* 1980;45:144.
10. Draper LW. Food testing in allergy: intradermal provocative vs. deliberate feeding. *Arch Otolaryngol* 1972:95:169.
11. Crawford LV, Lieberman P, Harfi HA, et al. A double-blind study of subcutaneous food testing sponsored by the Food Committee of the American Academy of Allergy [Abstract]. *J Allergy Clin Immunol* 1976;57:236.
12. King DS. Can allergic exposure provoke psychological symptoms? A double-blind test. *Biol Psychiatry* 1981;16:3.
13. Willoughby JW. Provocative food test technique. *Ann Allergy* 1965;23:543.
14. Rinkel RH, Lee CH, Brown DW, et al. The diagnosis of food allergy. *Arch Otolaryngol* 1964;79:71.
15. Lee CH, William RI, Binkley EL. Provocative inhalation testing and treatment. *Arch Otolaryngol* 1969;90:173.
16. American College of Physicians. Position paper: clinical ecology. *Ann Intern Med* 1989;111:108.
17. Terr AI. Multiple chemical hypersensitivities: immunologic critique of clinical ecology theories and practice. *Occup Med* 1987;2:683.
18. Jewett DL, Fein G, Greenberg MH. A double-blind study of symptom provocation to determine food sensitivity. *N Engl J Med* 1990;323:429.
19. Ferguson A. Food sensitivity or self-deception? *N Engl J Med* 1990;323:476.
20. Green M. Sublingual provocative testing for food and FD and C dyes. *Ann Allergy* 1974;33:274.
21. Rea WJ, Peters DW, Smiley RE, et al. Recurrent environmentally triggered thrombophlebitis: a five-year follow-up. *Ann Allergy* 1977;38:245.
22. Tsuei JJ, Lehman CW, Lam FMK, et al. A food allergy study utilizing the EAV acupuncture technique. *Am J Acupuncture* 1984;12:105.
23. Lewith GT, Kenyon JF, Broomfield PP, et al. Is electrodermal testing as effective as skin prick tests for diagnosing allergies? A double blind, randomized block design study. *BMJ* 2001; 332:131.
24. Garrow JS. Kinesiology and food allergy. *Lancet* 1988;296:1573.
25. Coca A. *The pulse test.* New York: University Books, 1956.
26. Laseter JL, DeLeon IR, Rea WJ, et al. Chlorinated hydrocarbon pesticides in environmentally sensitive patients. *Clin Ecol* 1983;2:3.
27. Rousseaux CG. Immunologic responses that may follow exposure to chemicals. *Clin Ecol* 1987;5:33.
28. Paganelli R, Levinsky RJ, Brostoff J, et al. Immune complexes containing food proteins in normal and atopic subjects after oral challenge and effect of sodium cromoglycate on antigen absorption. *Lancet* 1979;1:1270.
29. Delire M, Cambiaso CL, Masson PL. Circulating immune complexes in infants fed on cow's milk. *Nature* 1978;272:632.
30. Paganelli R, Atherton DJ, Levinsky R. The differences between normal and milk allergic subjects in their immune response after milk ingestion. *Arch Dis Child* 1983;58:201.
31. Husby S, Oxelius V-A, Teisner B, et al. Humoral immunity to dietary antigens in healthy adults. Occurrence, isotype and IgG subclass distribution of serum antibodies to protein antigens. *Int Arch Allergy Appl Immunol* 1985;77:416.
32. Roberts RI, Stiehm R. Antibody (B cell) immunodeficiency disorders. In: Parslow TG, Stites DP, Terr AI, Imboden JB, eds. *Human immunology*, 10th ed. New York: Lange Medical Books, 2001:299.
33. Greenberger PA, Patterson R. Allergic bronchopulmonary aspergillosis and the evaluation of the patient with asthma. *J Allergy Clin Immunol* 1988; 81:646.
34. Haddad ZH, Vetter M, Friedman J. et al. Detection and kinetics of antigen-specific IgE and IgG immune complexes in food allergy. *Ann Allergy* 1983;51:255.
35. Leary HL, Halsey JF. An assay to measure antigen-specific immune complexes in food allergy patients. *J Allergy Clin Immunol* 1984;74:190.
36. Cunningham-Rundels C, Brandeis WE, Good RA, et al. Milk precipitins, circulating immune complexes and IgA deficiency. *Proc Natl Acad Sci U S A* 1978;75:3387.
37. Cunningham-Rundels C, Brandies WE, Good RA, et al. Bovine proteins and the formation of circulating immune complexes in selective IgA deficiency. *J Clin Invest* 1979;64:272.
38. Morris DL. Use of sublingual antigen in diagnosis and treatment of food allergy. *Ann Allergy* 1969;27:289.
39. Rea WJ, Podell RN, Williams ML, et al. Intracutaneous neutralization of food sensitivity: a double-blind evaluation. *Arch Otolaryngol* 1984;110:248.
40. Kailin EW, Collier R. "Relieving" therapy for antigen exposure [Letter]. *JAMA* 1971;217:78.
41. Golbert TM. Sublingual desensitization. *JAMA* 1971;217:1703.

42. Chanez P, Bousquet J, Godard P, et al. Controversial forms of treatment for asthma. *Clin Rev Allergy Immunol* 1996;14:247.
43. Plesch J. Urine therapy. *Med Press* 1947;218:128.
44. Cantani A, Ragno V, Monteleone MA, et al. Enzyme-potentiated desensitization in children with asthma and mite allergy: a double-blind study. *J Invest Allergology Clin Immunol* 6:270, 1996.
45. Astarita C, Scala G, Sproviero S, et al. Effects of enzyme-potentiated desensitization in the treatment of pollinosis: a double-blind placebo-controlled trial. *J Invest Allergol Clin Immunol* 1996;6:248.
46. Levine SA, Reinhardt JH. Biochemical-pathology initiated by free radicals, oxidant chemicals, and therapeutic drugs in the etiology of chemical hypersensitivity disease. *Orthomol Psychiatry* 1983;12:166.
47. Rinkel HJ. Food allergy: function and clinical application of the rotary diversified diet. *J Pediatr* 1948;32:266.
48. Terr AI. Editorial: clinical ecology. *J Allergy Clin Immunol* 1987;79:423.
49. Rea WJ, Bell IR, Suits CW et al. Food and chemical susceptibility after environmental chemical overexposure: case histories. *Ann Allergy* 1978;41:101.
50. Dickey LD. *Clinical ecology.* Springfield, IL: Charles C. Thomas, 1976.
51. Randolph TG. *Human ecology and susceptibility to the chemical environment.* Springfield, IL: Charles C. Thomas, 1962.
52. Brodsky CM. Allergic to everything: a medical subculture. *Psychosomatics* 1983;24:731.
53. Dismukes WE, Wade JS, Lee JY, et al. A randomized double-blind trial of nystatin therapy for the candidiasis hypersensitivity syndrome. *N Engl J Med* 1990;323:1717.
54. Speer F. The allergic tension-fatigue syndrome. *Pediatr Clin North Am* 1954;1:1029.
55. Miller JB. *Food allergy: provocative testing and injection therapy.* Springfield, IL: Charles C. Thomas, 1972.
56. Feingold B. *Why your child is hyperactive.* New York: Random House, 1975.
57. Consensus Conference. Defined diets and childhood hyperactivity. *JAMA* 1982;248:290.
58. Dohan FC, Grasberger JC. Relapsed schizophrenics: earlier discharge from the hospital after cereal-free, milk-free diet. *Am Psychiatry* 1973;130:685.
59. Singh MM, Na SR. Wheat gluten as a pathogenic factor in schizophrenia. *Science* 1976;191:401.
60. Bell IR. *Clinical ecology: a new medical approach to environmental illness.* Bolinas, CA: Common Knowledge Press, 1982.
61. Randolph TG, Moss RW. *An alternative approach to allergies.* New York: Lippincott and Cromwell, 1980.
62. Randolph TG. Sensitivity to petroleum including its derivatives and antecedents [Abstract]. *J Lab Clin Med* 1952;40:931.
63. Levin AS, Byers VS. Environmental illness: a disorder of immune regulation. *Occup Med* 1987;2:669.
64. American Academy of Allergy and Asthma Immunology. Position statement: idiopathic environmental intolerances. *J Allergy Clin Immunol* 1999;103:36.
65. Terr AI. Environmental illness: clinical review of 50 cases. *Arch Intern Med* 1986;146:145.
66. Terr AI. Clinical ecology in the workplace. *J Occup Med* 1989:31:257.
67. Truss CO. The role of *Candida albicans* in human illness. *J Orthomol Psychiatry* 1981;10:228.
68. Truss CO. Tissue injury induced by *Candida albicans*: mental and neurologic manifestations. *J Orthomol Psychiatry* 1978;7:17.
69. Bassler A. *Intestinal toxemia (autointoxication) biologically considered.* Philadelphia: FA Davis, 1930.
70. Johanning E, Landsbergis P, Gareis M, et al. Clinical experience and results of a sentinel health investigation related to indoor fungal exposure. *Environ Health Perspect* 1999;107(suppl 3):489.
71. Etzel RA, Montana E, Sorenson WG, et al. Acute pulmonary hemorrhage in infants associated with exposure to *Stachybotrys atra* and other fungi. *Arch Pediatr Adolesc Med* 1998;152:757.
72. Morbidity and Mortality Reports. Update: pulmonary hemorrhage/hemosiderosis among infants—Cleveland, Ohio, 1993–1996. *MMWR* 2000;49:180.
73. American Academy of Allergy and Immunology. Position statement: the remote practice of allergy. *J Allergy Clin Immunol* 1986;77:651.

27

Allergic Disorders and Pregnancy

Paul A. Greenberger

Division of Allergy-Immunology, Department of Medicine, Northwestern University
Medical School, Chicago, Illinois

Many of the major conditions the allergist-immunologist treats can occur in the context of gestation or in anticipation of pregnancy. Specific conditions include asthma, urticaria, angioedema, anaphylaxis, rhinitis, sinusitis, and nasal polyposis. Goals of managing gravidas should include effective control of underlying allergic-immunologic conditions, proper avoidance measures, limitation on medications to those considered appropriate for use during gestation, planning for possible allergic emergencies such as status asthmaticus or anaphylaxis and communication between the physician managing the allergic-immunologic conditions and the physician managing the pregnancy.

ASTHMA

Asthma occurs in 1% to 5.6% of pregnancies (1–3). In some cases, asthma has its onset during gestation and may be severe in that status asthmaticus occurs or wheezing dyspnea results in interrupted sleep, persistent coughing, and hypoxemia. The effects of ineffectively managed asthma on the gravida can be devastating in that maternal deaths may occur when there have been repeated episodes of severe asthma (4). Other untoward effects from asthma have included fetal loss (stillbirths or abortions), increased rate of preterm deliveries (<37 weeks' gestation), intrauterine growth retardation (<2,400 g), antepartum and postpartum hemorrhage, gestational hypertension, and preeclampsia (3–13).

Fortunately, not all studies reported all listed complications. Repeated episodes of status asthmaticus during gestation have resulted in hypoxemic effects on the fetus. Termination of a pregnancy has been deemed necessary because of life-threatening status asthmaticus (14). Conversely, with cooperation between the gravida and physician managing asthma and effective asthma management, there can be successful pregnancy outcomes (8–12,15–18). Prevention of status asthmaticus has been associated with pregnancy outcomes approaching that of the general population (8–12,15–18). Use of inhaled beclomethasone dipropionate (8,9,11) has been effective, as has prednisone (8–11), in managing even the most severe cases of asthma.

Acute exacerbations of asthma during pregnancy may result in more hospitalizations than in nonpregnant patients with asthma. For example, 65 (62%) of 105 pregnant women with acute asthma episodes who presented to the emergency department or ambulatory clinic were hospitalized (19). A criterion of postnebulization treatment forced expiratory volume in 1 second (FEV_1) of less than 70% was used in addition for gravidas who had to be admitted to the obstetric intensive care unit immediately (19). Cesarean delivery was required ultimately in 30% of cases (19). These findings are consistent with less respiratory reserve in gravidas with acute asthma episodes.

Gravidas with asthma may receive less than recommended treatment because they are pregnant. When a comparison was made of emergency department treatment, 51 gravidas were compared with 500 nonpregnant women with asthma (20). Presentation peak expiratory flow rate (PEFR) was comparable (51% vs. 53%) (20). However, corticosteroids were administered to 44% of gravidas compared with 66% of nonpregnant women (20). Hospitalization rates were similar (24% vs. 21%). Unexpectedly, upon discharge, oral corticosteroids were prescribed for 38% of gravidas and 64% of nonpregnant women with asthma (20). At the 2-week follow-up by telephone, asthma symptoms were reported by 35% of gravidas compared with 23% of nonpregnant women (20). Thus, pharmacotherapy was inadequate in that oral corticosteroids were less likely to be prescribed with continued asthma symptoms at 2 weeks after emergency department treatment.

PHYSIOLOGIC CHANGES DURING GESTATION

Pulmonary

Tidal volume increases during gestation, whereas the frequency of respiration is unchanged (2,21). This combination produces a 19% to 50% increase in minute ventilation by late pregnancy (22–24). Oxygen consumption increases 20% to 32%. The increase in minute ventilation produces a respiratory alkalosis attributable to increases in progesterone. These changes occur before significant uterine enlargement takes place. Arterial blood gas concentrations reflect a compensated respiratory alkalosis with pH ranging from 7.40 to 7.47 and partial pressure of carbon dioxide (Pco_2) from 25 to 32 mm Hg (24,25). The maternal partial pressure of oxygen (P_{o_2}) has been reported to be from 91 to 106 mm Hg (25). The near-term alveolar-arterial oxygen gradient is 14 mm Hg in the sitting position compared with 20 mm Hg in the supine position. An explanation for the larger alveolar-arterial oxygen gradient supine is decreased cardiac output because compression of the inferior vena cava by the uterus reduces venous return. In the third trimester, gravidas should try to avoid sleeping supine (24).

Total lung capacity is unchanged or reduced by 4% to 6%, and vital capacity is preserved in the absence of exacerbations of asthma. The gravida breathes at reduced lung volumes because residual volume and functional residual capacity are reduced. The diaphragm moves cephalad (21). As with the development of maternal hyperventilation, the residual volume and functional residual capacity decline before significant uterine enlargement occurs. The diaphragm flattens during gestation, and there is less negative intrathoracic pressure reported in some studies. One could speculate that early airway closure would occur if there were less negative intrathoracic pressure. Because during acute asthma episodes the patient with asthma generates large negative intrathoracic pressures to apply radial bronchodilating traction, any decline in ability to develop more negative inspiratory pressures would predispose gravidas with asthma to more sudden deteriorations because of airway closure.

Bronchial responsiveness to methacholine does not change to a large degree, although a statistically significant change has been reported with PC20 increasing from 0.35 to 0.72 mg/mL preconception to postpartum (26). In this study of gravidas with mild asthma, the FEV_1 improved by 150 mL and FEV_1 increased from 82% to 87% (26). The increase in serum progesterone concentration during gestation did not correlate with improvement in bronchial responsiveness (27). This observation suggests that factors other than progesterone contribute to changes in bronchial responsiveness, although progesterone relaxes smooth muscles of the uterus and gastrointestinal tract.

Other Physiologic Changes

Cardiac output increases 30% to 60% because of an increase in heart rate, yet stroke volume increases little (28). The decrease in systemic vascular resistance is accompanied by an increase in the heart rate from 10 to 20 beats/min. Uterine blood flow increases 10-fold, from 50 to 500 mL/min at term (25). The blood volume increases an average of 1,600 mL, and gravidas appear vasodilated as total body water expands by 1 to 5 L (25,28,29). Gravidas are sensitive to overzealous fluid administration. Although correcting any dehydration is indicated, injudicious fluid replacement has resulted in acute pulmonary edema with normal cardiac function. During the latter half of gestation, these changes become manifest because the gravida has increased preload (mild volume overload), increased chronotropy, and reduced afterload (28).

The maternal hemoglobulin concentration decreases, although during gestation there is a 20% to 40% increase in erythrocyte mass (28). Such an increase is offset by the even larger increase of plasma volume, resulting in relative anemia.

FETAL OXYGENATION

The vascular resistance of uterine vessels (progesterone effect) declines so that there can be the large increase in uterine blood flow (25). The fetus survives in a low-oxygen environment with little reserve oxygen stores, should the supply of oxygen-rich uterine blood be compromised. Animal and human studies demonstrate reduced fetal oxygenation if there is reduced uterine blood flow such as occurs with severe maternal hypotension, hypocarbia, or shock (25). Maternal hyperventilation can reduce venous return and shift the maternal oxyhemoglobin dissociation curve to the left. Modest declines in maternal oxygenation seem to be tolerated by the fetus, but substantial degrees of maternal hypoxemia can threaten fetal survival. Uterine vessels during gestation are dilated maximally based on experimental data primarily from pregnant sheep and some human studies. Uterine vessels do not vasodilate after β-adrenergic agonist stimulation, but do vasoconstrict from α-adrenergic agonists. Some obstetric anesthesiologists administer intravenous ephedrine 25 to 50 mg for hypotension during epidural anesthesia. The β-adrenergic effects of ephedrine result in increased cardiac output, which raises systolic pressure and maintains uterine perfusion. Subcutaneous epinephrine provides primarily β-adrenergic stimulation, whereas intravenous epinephrine results in both α- and β-adrenergic effects.

The fetal hemoglobin is 16.5 g/L and the oxygen pressure at which hemoglobin is 50% saturated is 22 mm Hg in the fetus, in contrast to 26 to 28 mm Hg in the gravida (25). Fetal umbilical venous PO_2 measurements at term average about 32 mm Hg, with PCO_2 49 mm Hg. When the gravida inspires 100% oxygen in the absence of acute asthma, fetal umbilical venous PO_2 increases to 40 mm Hg and PCO_2 to 48 mm Hg (30). For the fetus in distress, such changes can be important, but clearly the uteroplacental circulation is a large shunt. For the same incremental increases in arterial PO_2, the leftward shift of the fetal hemoglobin oxygen dissociation curve results in larger increases in fetal PO_2 than in maternal blood.

In summary, fetal oxygen delivery depends on many factors, but most critical are blood flow (maternal cardiac output) to the uterus, integrity of the placenta, and maternal arterial oxygen content.

EFFECTS OF PREGNANCY ON ASTHMA

For the individual gravida, it is not possible to predict the effects of pregnancy on asthma. Studies in the literature report varying degrees of improvement, deterioration, or no change in clinical course (31). In one review of nine studies involving 1,059 pregnancies, 49% of gravidas were unchanged in terms of severity of asthma, 29% improved, and 22% worsened (32). A prospective study of 198 pregnancies recorded similar results in that 40% of gravidas had no change in antiasthma medications, 42% required more medications, and 18% of gravidas required fewer medications (12). Similarly, using medication and symptom diary cards, during 366 gestations in 330 gravidas with mild or moderate asthma, asthma was unchanged in 33%, improved in 28%, and worsened in 35% (33).

Pregnancy in adolescents with asthma has been associated with many emergency department visits and hospitalizations for asthma (34). Accurate serial data were not available to compare preconception and gestational asthma events. Some adolescents with severe asthma may not benefit from antiinflammatory medications such as inhaled beclomethasone dipropionate because of their poor compliance with physician advice and medications (34). The combination of poverty, inadequate or no prenatal care, and limited education can complicate adolescent pregnancies (35).

PREGNANCY OUTCOMES IN THE GENERAL POPULATION

The mean birth weight from 1983 data from the National Center for Health Statistics was 3,370 g (9). The incidence of miscarriage was 11.8% to 13.8% in a study of women residents and wives of male residents (36). Preterm deliveries (<37 weeks' gestation) occurred in 6.0% to 6.5% of study gravidas in comparison with 9.6% in the general population (9). Intrauterine growth retardation (birth weight <2,500 g) occurred in 6.8% of gestations (9) in the general population and 5.3% to 5.8% of women residents or wives of male residents (36). The frequency of gravidas requiring cesarean deliveries was about 20%.

Adverse effects on the child's lung function (FEV_1 and maximal midexpiratory flow [MMEF]) have been demonstrated in 7- to 19-year-olds whose mothers smoked during their pregnancy or where another household member (but not the gravida) smoked during the pregnancy (37). Clearly, gravidas must not smoke during gestation for their own well-being and that of their children.

CHOICE OF THERAPY

Avoidance Measures

As in management of the nonpregnant patient with asthma, general avoidance measures as well as those specific to the individual are indicated. General avoidance measures include smoking cessation, minimal or no alcoholic beverages, cessation of illicit drug use, avoidance of tetracyclines (discoloration of infant's teeth), sulfonamides [glucose-6-phosphate dehydrogenase (G6PD) deficiency could cause hemolytic anemia], troleandomycin, and antibiotics such as clarithromycin and quinolones until safety data become available. Methotrexate is contraindicated. Individual avoidance measures relate to animals, birds, dust mites, cockroaches, and fungi that may be causing immunoglobulin E (IgE)-mediated asthma. Aspirin and nonsteroidal

antiinflammatory drugs should be withheld in the aspirin-intolerant gravida. Concomitant rhinitis, sinusitis, or nasal polyps should be treated.

Medications

It is preferable to recommend antiasthma medications for which established data from human pregnancies are available. Furthermore, inhaled drugs are favored as the potential drug dosage that would cross the placenta is reduced. Organogenesis in human pregnancies is relatively short (days 12–56) compared with animals. The time for fetal growth and development is much longer in humans, whereas it is shorter in animals. Drugs are infrequent causes of major congenital malformations (38). Congenital malformations occur in about 3% to 5% of pregnancies (38). Although a small number, up to 5%, are attributable to environmental factors such as drug effects, maternal infections, and radiation, 65% to 70% of malformations are from unknown factors. About 25% of major malformations are genetically related, and 3% are due to recognized chromosomal abnormalities.

Examples of teratogenic agents include ethanol, isotretinoin, phenytoin, carbamazepine, valproic acid, diethylstilbestrol (vaginal carcinoma), thalidomide, inorganic iodides, lithium carbonate, tetracycline, streptomycin, and some antineoplastic drugs that have not caused abortions earlier. Most antiasthma medications are considered appropriate for use in pregnancy. Specific drugs to avoid include troleandomycin, methotrexate, triamcinolone, inorganic iodides, and quinolones. The U.S. Food and Drug Administration classification system for drug administration during gestation must be considered in the context of drug advertising by manufacturers and is not an absolute prohibition on prescription of a drug during gestation, with the exception of a class X agent.

Human data on the use of most antiasthma medications are available and have not identified increased teratogenic risks for oral corticosteroids such as prednisone or methylprednisolone, or the intravenous preparations hydrocortisone or methylprednisolone (2,8–11,25,34). Experience with inhaled beclomethasone dipropionate has not identified fetal abnormalities in pregnancies where therapeutic dosages were used at conception or during the first trimester (8,9,11,34). Budesonide also has not been associated with harmful effects during conception and the first trimester (16). These corticosteroids are considered appropriate during gestation. Published experience from Northwestern University with prednisone, beclomethasone dipropionate, or both totals over 300 pregnancies without an increased risk of teratogenesis.

Another antiinflammatory drug, cromolyn, has not been associated with an increased risk of congenital malformations in a series of 296 cases (39) as well as during use in the United States since 1973 (2). Reports on the use of nedocromil, which blocks early and late allergic-induced bronchial reactions and has antieosinophil activity, in the first trimester are meager. However, animal studies have yielded negative results for teratogenicity. The most cautious view would be to withhold nedocromil and use one of the two inhaled corticosteroids mentioned with or without cromolyn.

Theophylline is considered appropriate for use during gestation, should it be required (2,15,25). The hepatic elimination clearance of theophylline has been shown to decrease in the third trimester by approximately 4% to 6% (40). Protein binding decreases in the second and third trimesters so more free theophylline is available for elimination. Furthermore, increased glomerular filtration rate increases renal clearance of theophylline during gestation. These changes offset reduced hepatic clearance (40). Overall, the last trimester may be associated with 10% increases in the theophylline serum concentrations. Aiming for maximal theophylline serum concentrations of 8 to 15 μg/mL should help reduce the likelihood of accumulations of theophylline during pregnancy. However, theophylline is not essential with moderate to high doses of beclomethasone dipropionate or budesonide.

Albuterol is used as a β_2-adrenergic agonist during gestation (17,41). Other drugs considered appropriate for human use include epinephrine (intramuscularly), terbutaline (orally), and ephedrine (32). The latter is rarely indicated, but is available without prescription or as a dietary aid. Albuterol, pirbuterol, and metaproterenol were listed as appropriate by the National Institutes of Health Working Group on Asthma and Pregnancy (2). Overuse must be avoided. The inhaled route should minimize drug delivered to the placenta. Salmeterol and formoterol may be appropriate, but safety data are not available from human gestations.

Ipratropium bromide by inhalation would appear to be appropriate during gestation because it is delivered topically and has minimal absorption. Whether it will be a useful adjunct for most gravidas with asthma is less convincing, but ipratropium bromide can be recommended. Without data in human gestations, the leukotriene antagonists should be avoided.

Influenza immunization is advisable for gravidas with persistent asthma. It is administered during the second or third trimester.

Allergen Immunotherapy

Allergen immunotherapy can be continued or initiated during pregnancy. The only recognized risk from this modality is the well-recognized risk of anaphylaxis. There are no data to suggest that gravidas are more likely to experience anaphylaxis from allergen immunotherapy. Data from the 121 pregnancies in 90 gravidas receiving allergen immunotherapy showed a low incidence of anaphylaxis (42). Immunotherapy should be administered with the usual precautions to avoid anaphylaxis or it should be withheld until postpartum. Anaphylaxis during gestation can cause abortions, as in beekeepers' wives who are stung (43), shock (44), or perinatal death (44). Allergen immunotherapy does not protect the fetus from subsequent development of atopic disorders (42,45).

As long as the gravida is not experiencing large local reactions or having systemic reactions, the dosage can be escalated to maintenance during the pregnancy.

ACUTE ASTHMA

As in managing the nonpregnant patient with asthma, acute asthma should be reversed as quickly and effectively as possible. Status asthmaticus has been associated with intrauterine growth retardation (8,9), stillbirths, maternal deaths, and additional untoward effects on the fetus such as cerebral palsy. The goal in treating acute asthma is to minimize maternal hypoxemia, hypocarbia, or respiratory acidosis and to maintain adequate oxygenation for the fetus.

β_2-adrenergic agonists (such as albuterol) are the drugs of choice for acute asthma. Alternatively, subcutaneous terbutaline or intramuscular epinephrine can be administered and repeated in 30 minutes (32). There are no reports of teratogenic effects from epinephrine or terbutaline. Some gravidas who do not respond to albuterol will respond to epinephrine given intramuscularly. The justification for epinephrine is as follows: (a) it is synthesized endogenously, (b) it is not teratogenic, (c) it is metabolized rapidly, (d) it is readily available, and (e) variables associated with drug delivery by inhalation do not have to be considered. When epinephrine is administered by the intramuscular route, its effects are primarily β-adrenergic stimulation. There is a fear that epinephrine will cause fetal loss by decreasing uterine blood flow. The use of intramuscular epinephrine (for acute asthma or anaphylaxis) increases cardiac output, which can maintain uterine perfusion. The adverse effects of acute asthma can be a serious threat to the gravida and fetus; therefore, effective control of acute asthma is necessary.

Inhaled β_2-adrenergic therapy with metaproterenol has not been associated with adverse effects and is considered acceptable therapy by some investigators (2).

When the gravida presents with moderate or severe acute wheezing dyspnea, oral corticosteroids should be administered with initial β_2-adrenergic agonists. For example, prednisone 40 to 60 mg orally is an appropriate dosage. Corticosteroids have a number of beneficial effects in acute asthma, although an effect in the first 6 hours may not be detectable.

When the gravida has not improved substantially after albuterol (or intramuscular epinephrine), status asthmaticus is present and hospitalization is indicated. Theophylline intravenously has not been found to be superior to intravenous methylprednisone and albuterol therapy

in hospitalized gravidas (19). The gravida should receive systemic corticosteroids as soon as possible.

When assessing a gravida in the emergency room, if hospitalization is required for status asthmaticus, an arterial blood gas measurement is indicated, as is supplemental oxygen administration. The physician managing the pregnancy should assess the gravida from the obstetric perspective. Some gravidas require fetal heart monitoring, for example, before discharge.

Excessive fluid replacement is not indicated, but volume depletion should be corrected. The gravida can develop acute pulmonary edema (noncardiac) from excessive crystalloid administration as she is volume expanded during gestation.

If the gravida can be discharged from the emergency room, a short course of oral corticosteroids should be given to prevent continued asthma symptoms and signs (47). Arrangements for an outpatient visit in 1 week is advised.

In the rare setting of acute respiratory failure during status asthmaticus, an emergency cesarean delivery may be necessary (14). If mechanical ventilation (48) is indicated, the physician managing asthma and the obstetrician must plan for when a cesarean delivery might be indicated.

PERSISTENT ASTHMA

Some types of persistent asthma during gestation are listed in Table 27.1. Should gravidas require daily medication, an allergy-immunology consultation is indicated to identify and address IgE-mediated triggers of asthma, to determine if allergic bronchopulmonary aspergillosis is present,

TABLE 27.1. *Types of persistent asthma during pregnancy*

Allergic[a]
Nonallergic[a]
Mixed[a]
Potentially fatal asthma
Malignant potentially fatal asthma
Adolescent asthma
Asthma and allergic bronchopulmonary aspergillosis
Aspirin-intolerant asthma

[a]Can be subdivided into mild persistent, moderate persistent, or severe persistent asthma.

and to provide expertise in the diagnosis and treatment of nasal polyps, rhinitis, or sinusitis. Avoidance measures are indicated to reduce bronchial hyperresponsiveness and the need for antiasthma medications.

The goals of management include maintaining a functional respiratory status, as well as minimizing wheezing dyspnea, nocturnal asthma, exercise intolerance, emergency department visits, status asthmaticus, and maternal fatalities or loss of the fetus.

Dyspnea can be sensed during gestation in the absence of asthma during the first two trimesters (49). A respiratory rate of more than 18 breaths/min has been considered a warning sign for pulmonary pathology complicating "dyspnea during pregnancy" (49).

Many gravidas can be managed effectively with inhaled beclomethasone dipropionate (2,9,11) or budesonide (16) and inhaled albuterol (2,17,33) for symptomatic relief (2,8,46). For severe persistent asthma, beclomethasone dipropionate (840 μg) or budesonide (800 μg) can be inhaled. Higher doses may produce systemic side effects. A proper inhalation technique is necessary and should be assessed periodically. Should asthma be managed ineffectively with avoidance measures and this combination of medications, cromolyn or theophylline can be considered. If the gravida has wheezing on examination or nocturnal asthma, however, a short course of prednisone may be indicated to relieve symptoms (25). If the gravida has improved after 1 week of prednisone, either the prednisone can be discontinued or it can be converted to alternate-day administration and tapered (8,9,11,25,46). The most effective antiasthma medications for chronic administration during gestation in order of efficacy are prednisone, inhaled beclomethasone dipropionate and budesonide, inhaled β-adrenergic agonists (albuterol or terbutaline), cromolyn, and theophylline. Theophylline is out of vogue and not considered antiinflammatory. In some gravidas with severe persistent asthma, bronchiectasis from allergic bronchopulmonary aspergillosis, or inhaled corticosteroid phobia, theophylline can be used. It is not teratogenic in humans.

For non–corticosteroid-requiring asthma, inhaled beclomethasone dipropionate or budesonide, cromolyn, or possibly theophylline are appropriate during gestation. If these drugs are ineffective because of worsening asthma such as from an upper respiratory infection, a short course of prednisone such as 40 mg daily for 5 to 7 days may be administered. Antibiotics can be prescribed for purulent rhinitis, bronchitis, or sinusitis. Erythromycin, azithromycin, ampicillin, amoxicillin, amoxicillin-clavulanate, or cephalosporins are appropriate antibiotics. There are no data supporting teratogenicity of penicillins or cephalosporins (50).

A summary of appropriate medications during gestation is listed in Table 27.2. These medications have been used throughout gestation without an increased risk of reported teratogenicity.

Essentially all patients can be managed successfully during gestation. Some patients with potentially fatal asthma are unmanageable because of noncompliance with physician advice, medications, or in keeping ambulatory clinical appointments. Such gravidas are considered to have malignant potentially fatal asthma. Long-acting methylprednisolone (80–120 mg intramuscularly) is of value to prevent repeated episodes of status asthmaticus or respiratory failure (51). This approach should be instituted

TABLE 27.2. *Appropriate therapy during gestation in the ambulatory patient*

Mild persistent asthma
  Inhaled beclomethasone dipropionate or budesonide
  Inhaled albuterol
  Inhaled cromolyn
  Theophylline (optional)

Moderate or severe persistent asthma
  Inhaled beclomethasone dipropionate or budesonide
  Prednisone (short daily course, then alternate day)
  Inhaled albuterol
  Theophylline (optional)
  Long-acting methylprednisolone (selected cases)

Rhinitis
  Chlorpheniramine
  Tripelennamine
  Diphenhydramine
  Intranasal beclomethasone dipropionate or
    budesonide
  Allergen immunotherapy for severe allergic rhinitis

Purulent rhinitis, bronchitis, sinusitis
  Erythromycin or azithromycin
  Amoxicillin or amoxicillin-clavulanate
  Cephalosporins
  Intranasal beclomethasone dipropionate or
    budesonide

to try to prevent fetal loss or maternal death in the nearly impossible to manage gravida. Adequate documentation in the medical record is needed. Psychologic, psychiatric, and social work evaluations may be obtained. Gravidas with malignant potentially fatal asthma, however, may refuse evaluation or necessary therapy. The serum glucose should be determined regularly because of hyperglycemia produced by long-acting methylprednisolone. Other antiasthma medications should be minimized to simplify the medication regimen.

LABOR AND DELIVERY

When asthma is controlled effectively, the gravida can participate in prepared childbirth methods such as Lamaze without limitation. Minute ventilation increases to as great as 20 L/min during labor and delivery (30). Should cesarean delivery be necessary, complications from anesthesia should not create difficulty if asthma is well controlled. When the gravida has used inhaled corticosteroids or oral corticosteroids during gestation, predelivery corticosteroid coverage should include 100 mg hydrocortisone intravenously every 8 hours until postpartum, and other medications can be used. Parenteral corticosteroids suppress any asthma that might complicate anesthesia required for cesarean delivery. The prior use of inhaled corticosteroids or alternate-day prednisone should not suppress the surge of adrenal corticosteroids associated with labor or during anesthesia.

When the gravida who requires regular moderate- to high-dose inhaled corticosteroids or daily or alternate-day prednisone plans to have a cesarean delivery, preoperative prednisone should be administered for 3 days before anesthesia. The gravida should be examined ideally 1 to 2 weeks before delivery to confirm stable respiratory status and satisfactory pulmonary function. In gravidas with persistent mild asthma whose antiasthma medications consisted of theophylline, cromolyn, or inhaled β_2-adrenergic agonists, additional preanesthetic therapy can consist of 5 days of inhaled corticosteroid.

When the gravida presents in labor in respiratory distress, emergency measures such as inhaled albuterol, intramuscular epinephrine, or subcutaneous terbutaline should be administered promptly. Intravenous corticosteroids should be administered without delay. Adequate oxygenation and fetal monitoring are essential.

RHINITIS DURING PREGNANCY

Intranasal obstruction and nasal secretions can be very troublesome during gestation and interfere with sleep. It has been estimated that 30% to 72% of gravidas experience symptoms of rhinitis during gestation (52). Nasal congestion during gestation can be influenced by (a) increased blood volume, (b) progesterone's effects causing smooth muscle relaxation of nasal vessels, and (c) estrogen's effects causing mucosal edema (53). Nasal biopsy results from symptom-free gravidas showed glandular hyperactivity manifested by swollen mitochondria and increased number of secretory granules (54). Special stains demonstrated increased metabolic activity, increased phagocytosis, and increased acid mucopolysaccharides, thought to be attributed to high concentrations of estrogens. Similar findings were present in gravidas with nasal symptoms. Additional findings included increased (a) goblet cell numbers in the nasal epithelium, (b) cholinergic nerve fibers around glands and vessels, and (c) vascularity and transfer of metabolites through cell membranes (54). Women using oral contraceptives but in whom no nasal symptoms had occurred have similar histopathologic and histochemical changes, as do symptom-free gravidas (55). Oral contraceptive use in women who developed nasal symptoms was associated with interepithelial cell edema, mucus gland hyperplasia, and proliferation of ground substance analogous to symptomatic gravidas (55). Serum concentrations of estradiol, progesterone, and vasoactive intestinal polypeptide did not differentiate symptomatic from asymptomatic gravidas (56). It has been estimated that in nonpregnant adults, 700 to 900 mL of nasal secretions are generated per day for proper conditioning of inspired air. In some gravidas, this volume may be even greater.

Nasal congestion that causes symptoms is likely to occur in the second and third trimesters

(52). The differential diagnosis for rhinitis of pregnancy includes allergic rhinitis, nonallergic rhinitis (including vasomotor rhinitis or nonallergic rhinitis with eosinophilia), nasal polyposis, and sinusitis or purulent rhinitis. Rhinitis medicamentosa may be present when there has been excessive use of topical decongestants.

Treatment of nasal symptoms during gestation necessitates an accurate diagnosis, effective pharmacotherapy, and in some cases avoidance measures. For example, smoking and illicit drugs should be discontinued, as should topical decongestants. Intranasal beclomethasone dipropionate or budesonide are valuable to relieve nasal obstruction. If large nasal polyps are present and topical corticosteroids are ineffective, a short course of prednisone should be prescribed. The blood glucose should be monitored because the gravida is prone to hyperglycemia.

Antihistamines help gravidas with milder degrees of allergic rhinitis and some nonallergic types of rhinitis occasionally. Long-term experience and the Collaborative Perinatal Project have demonstrated safety for chlorpheniramine (1,070 exposures), diphenhydramine (595 exposures), and tripelennamine (121 exposures) (57). There remain too few data to support use of brompheniramine, and surprisingly, in the Collaborative Perinatal Project, its use in 65 pregnancies was associated with an increased risk of congenital malformations (57).

Cetirizine and its parent, hydroxyzine, were not associated with teratogenic effects in 39 and 53 pregnancies, respectively (58). These preliminary data are of value because in the collaborative perinatal project, some concern was reported with hydroxyzine administration in the first trimester (57). First-trimester use of terfenadine, the parent compound of fexofenadine, in 65 pregnancies was not associated with teratogenic effects (59). The birth weights of terfenadine-exposed infants (3,335 g), however, were lower than in controls (3,499 g) (59). Astemizole, administered in the first trimester and for at least 16 weeks, was not associated with adverse pregnancy outcomes or teratogenic effects in 76 women compared with controls (60). These emerging data hopefully will be supported by additional evidence of a lack of teratogenic effects or adverse gestational effects. Because antihistamines are not truly essential during gestation, older antihistamines with years of experience should be tried first. For example, chlorpheniramine 2 to 4 mg at bedtime may be tolerated and may be useful therapeutically. Data on cetirizine have shown that it is not teratogenic (58). An approach is to avoid its first trimester use or use in women planning a pregnancy. Perhaps it can be used in the second and third trimester after explaining this information to the gravida.

I try not to prescribe pseudoephedrine to avoid potential α-adrenergic stimulation of uterine vessels, although this treatment has been recommended by others (2,53). Phenylpropanolamine in 726 exposures was associated with significantly greater risk of malformations (ear and eye), whereas this risk was not detected with pseudoephedrine (39 exposures) or phenylephrine (1,249 exposures) (57). Phenylpropanolamine is being removed from many nonproprietary medications, and pseudoephedrine is being used instead. Hopefully, there will be no adverse pregnancy outcomes because these medications are used without prescription (or perhaps with knowledge of an existing early pregnancy).

Intranasal cromolyn can be used for mild allergic rhinitis, based on experience with 296 gravidas with asthma (39). It has been recommended in an editorial as well (61). I favor the use of intranasal beclomethasone dipropionate or budesonide.

Antibiotics for infectious sinusitis or purulent rhinitis are listed in Table 27.2. Ampicillin, amoxicillin, amoxicillin-clavulanate, erythromycin, azithromycin, and cephalosporins are initial antibiotics, depending on the prior therapy of the gravida. Sulfonamides are contraindicated because of the possibility of G6PD deficiency in the fetus. Tetracyclines are contraindicated because of maternal fatty liver during gestation (third trimester) and staining of teeth in the infant. Human experience with clarithromycin is not available, so azithromycin should be used if it is indicated.

Allergen immunotherapy helps reduce the need for medications in cases of allergic rhinitis. This therapy can be continued in pregnancy and, if symptoms are severe and the gravida agrees, immunotherapy may be initiated during gestation. During immunotherapy in 121 pregnancies in 90 gravidas, 6 gravidas experienced anaphylaxis (42). No abortions or other adverse effects occurred (42). The decision to begin immunotherapy after delivery often is made for the purpose of convenience and ability of the woman to present for injections in a timely fashion. Severe allergic rhinitis symptoms during gestation can be treated with intranasal corticosteroids and antihistamines.

As stated earlier, the dose of allergen immunotherapy can be increased in the absence of large local reactions or systemic reactions. There is no evidence that the incidence of anaphylaxis from allergen immunotherapy (or skin testing) is greater during the time of gestation.

URTICARIA, ANGIOEDEMA, AND ANAPHYLAXIS

Urticaria or angioedema should be evaluated and treated during gestation with little change from the nongravid state. Causes for urticaria and angioedema include foods, medications, infections (viral), and underlying conditions such as collagen vascular disorders. Some episodes of urticaria are attributable to dermatographism or other physical urticarias, chronic (autoimmune) urticaria, or idiopathic acute urticaria. The differential diagnosis during gestation includes hereditary angioedema (HAE) (62,63), pruritic urticaria papules and plaques of pregnancy (PUPPP) (64), and herpes gestationis (65).

In the series of Frank et al. (63), there was an increased frequency of attacks of HAE in only 2 of 25 gestations. No acute episodes of HAE occurred during delivery. In contrast, Chappatte and deSwiet reported on the unpredictability of HAE during gestation and a maternal fatality (62). The concentration of C1 inhibitor declines in normal pregnancy because of increased plasma volume. Some gravidas have worsening clinical symptoms and create major management problems. Contraception is advisable as a rule. Stanozolol or danazol result in a fourfold to fivefold increase in the concentration of C1 inhibitor and C4. Although stanozolol has been administered during gestation without masculinizing fetal effects, or

fetal loss (62), its use is discouraged in gravidas with HAE. Contraception should be used if a woman is receiving attenuated androgens for HAE. Genetic counseling is advisable for women with HAE because it is an autosomal-dominant condition, although there is incomplete penetration.

For acute severe central episodes of HAE, rapid administration of intramuscular epinephrine has been used, but additional specific therapy will have to include stanozolol, 4 mg four times a day, and airway care measures (intubation or tracheostomy). Fresh frozen plasma also may be infused on an emergent basis in some situations. Although unavailable in the United States, a concentrate of C1 inhibitor for parenteral administration has proved effective, with onset of action in 30 to 60 minutes (66). Antifibrinolytic agents are considered unwise to use in pregnancy because of their potential thrombotic effects. Nevertheless, three pregnancies in one gravida occurred uneventfully despite use of ε-aminocaproic acid (66).

During gestation, no specific maintenance therapy is necessary in gravidas with peripheral HAE. Based on Frank's series of gravidas with peripheral or central (upper airway involvement) HAE, exacerbations during the time of tissue trauma, delivery did not occur (63). If an episode of upper airway obstruction occurs during a cesarean delivery, epinephrine, stanozolol, and intubation would be indicated. Use of C1 inhibitor concentrates, if available and of low risk, otherwise would be of value acutely.

The PUPPP syndrome occurs in the last trimester and begins on the abdomen with numerous extremely pruritic erythematous urticarial plaques and papules surrounded by pale halos (64,65). Topical corticosteroids are of value, and maternal or fetal complications are unlikely. Herpes gestationis consists of intense pruritus followed by lesions that may be bullous, papulovesicular, or pustular (65). Some gravidas develop tense grouped vesicles on the abdomen or extremity.

Pharmacologic treatment of chronic urticaria or angioedema often is required. Despite its long-term use, there are few data regarding the appropriateness of hydroxyzine in the first trimester, but preliminary data do not reveal teratogenic effects for its metabolite cetirizine (58). The established appropriateness of diphenhydramine, chlorpheniramine, or tripelennamine favors their use. Oral albuterol or terbutaline may be attempted for more difficult cases, but often prednisone 20 to 30 mg daily may be necessary to control moderate to severe urticaria or angioedema.

Anaphylaxis during gestation has been described after penicillin, cefotetan (67), Hymenoptera stings (43,68), oxytocin (69), diclofenac (70), phytomenadione (71), fentanyl (72), iron dextran (73,74), antisnakebite venom (75), latex (76), and even bupivacaine (77). The latter is unexpected based on current knowledge of local anesthetic reactions and may have been an untoward effect of 23 mL being used. Anaphylaxis during gestation has caused fetal distress, fetal encephalopathy, or fetal demise. Gravidas have experienced profound shock with reduced uterine blood flow during anaphylaxis in pregnancy as the fundamental insult to the fetus. As in other cases of anaphylaxis, prevention and emergency medications and therapy are needed. Epinephrine intramuscularly should be administered promptly. If the gravida is hypotensive, then usual resuscitative measures should be instituted to maintain blood pressure and the airway. Obstetric assistance should be obtained immediately should cesarean delivery be indicated.

VENOM IMMUNOTHERAPY

Venom immunotherapy is a highly efficacious form of therapy to prevent future episodes of Hymenoptera anaphylaxis. Graft (78) reported a successful pregnancy in a gravida treated with maintenance dosages of wasp and mixed vespid venoms. Subsequently the Committee on Insects of the American Academy of Allergy and Immunology reported 63 pregnancies in 26 gravidas with no definite systemic reactions (79). Five of 43 gestations resulted in spontaneous abortions, thought to be unrelated to stings or immunotherapy. One term infant (2.7%) had multiple congenital cardiovascular malformations; this incidence is within the range of expected congenital malformations. The use of venom immunotherapy appears appropriate (79). Other issues should

be discussed with the gravida, such as avoidance measures and personal use of epinephrine.

REFERENCES

1. deSwiet M. Diseases of the respiratory system. *Clin Obstet Gynecol* 1977;4:287–296.
2. National Institutes of Health, National Heart, Lung and Blood Institute Working Group on Asthma and Pregnancy, National Asthma Education Program, Management of Asthma during Pregnancy. Public Health Service, U.S. Department of Health and Human Services, NIH Publication No. 93-3279, 1993.
3. Alexander S, Dodds L, Armson BA. Perinatal outcomes in women with asthma during pregnancy. *Obstet Gynecol* 1998;92:435–440.
4. Gordon M, Niswander KR, Berendes H, et al. Fetal morbidity following potentially anoxigenic obstetric conditions: VII. Bronchial asthma. *Am J Obstet Gynecol* 1970;106:421–429.
5. Demissie K, Breckenridge MB, Rhoads GG. Infant and maternal outcomes in the pregnancies of asthmatic women. *Am J Respir Crit Care Med* 1998;158:1091–1095.
6. Schaefer G, Silverman F. Pregnancy complicated by asthma. *Am J Obstet Gynecol* 1961;82:182–191.
7. Bahna SL, Bjerkedal J. The course and outcome of pregnancy in women with bronchial asthma. *Acta Allergol* 1972;27:397–406.
8. Greenberger PA, Patterson R. The outcome of pregnancy complicated by severe asthma. *Allergy Proc* 1988;9:539–543.
9. Fitzsimmons R, Greenberger PA, Patterson R. Outcome of pregnancy in women requiring corticosteroids for severe asthma. *J Allergy Clin Immunol* 1986;78:349–353.
10. Schatz M, Patterson R, Zeitz S, et al. Corticosteroid therapy for the pregnant asthmatic patient. *JAMA* 1975;23:804–807.
11. Greenberger PA, Patterson R. Beclomethasone dipropionate for severe asthma during pregnancy. *Ann Intern Med* 1983;98:478–480.
12. Stenius-Aarniala B, Piirila P, Teramo K. Asthma and pregnancy: a prospective study of 198 pregnancies. *Thorax* 1988;43:12–18.
13. Perlow JH, Montgomery D, Morgan MA, et al. Severity of asthma and perinatal outcome. *Am J Obstet Gynecol* 1992;167:963–967.
14. Gelber M, Sidi Y, Gassner S, et al. Uncontrollable life-threatening status asthmaticus: an indication for termination of pregnant by caesarean section. *Respiration* 1984;46:320–322.
15. Stenius-Aarniala B, Riikonen S, Teramo K. Slow-release theophylline in pregnant asthmatics. *Chest* 1995;107:642–647.
16. Stenius-Aarniala BSM, Hedman J, Teramo KA. Acute asthma during pregnancy. *Thorax* 1996;51:411–414.
17. Greenberger PA, Beckman D. Albuterol use in early pregnancy. *J Allergy Clin Immunol* 1998;101(suppl):67.
18. Schatz M, Zeiger RS, Hoffman CP, et al. Perinatal outcomes in the pregnancies of asthmatic women: a prospective controlled analysis. *Am J Respir Crit Care Med* 1995;151:1170–1174.

19. Wendel PJ, Ramin SM, Barnett-Hamm C, et al. Asthma treatment in pregnancy: a randomized controlled study. *Am J Obstet Gynecol* 1996;175:150–154.

20. Cydulka RK, Emerman CL, Schreiber D, et al. Acute asthma among pregnant women presenting to the emergency department. *Am J Respir Crit Care Med* 1999; 160:887–892.

21. Gilroy RJ, Mangura BT, Lavietes MH. Rib cage and abdominal volume displacements during breathing in pregnancy. *Am Rev Respir Dis* 1988;137:668–672.

22. Alaily AB, Carrol KB. Pulmonary ventilation in pregnancy. *Br J Obstet Gynaecol* 1978;85:518–524.

23. Cugell DW, Frank NR, Gaensler EA, et al. Pulmonary function in pregnancy: 1. Serial observations in normal women. *Am Rev Tuberculosis* 1953;67:568–597.

24. Cousins L. Fetal oxygenation, assessment of fetal well-being, and obstetric management of the pregnant patient with asthma. *J Allergy Clin Immunol* 1999; 103(suppl):343–349.

25. Greenberger PA, Patterson R. Management of asthma during pregnancy. *N Engl J Med* 1985;312:897–902.

26. Juniper EF, Daniel EE, Roberts RS, et al. Improvement in airway responsiveness and asthma severity during pregnancy. *Am Rev Respir Dis* 1989;140:924–931.

27. Juniper EF, Daniel EE, Roberts RS, et al. Effect of pregnancy on airway responsiveness and asthma severity: relationship to serum progesterone. *Am Rev Respir Dis* 1991;143(suppl):78.

28. Sullivan JM, Ramanathan KB. Management of medical problems in pregnancy: severe cardiac disease. *N Engl J Med* 1985;313:304–309.

29. Clark SL, Cotton DB, Lee W, et al. Central hemodynamic assessment of normal term pregnancy. *Am J Obstet Gynecol* 1989; 161:1439–1442.

30. Wulf KH, Kunzel W, Lehmann V. Clinical aspects of placental gas exchange. In: Longo LD, Bartels H, eds. *Respiratory gas exchange and blood flow in the placenta.* DHEW Publication No. 73-361 (NIH). Bethesda, MD: Public Health Service, 1972:505.

31. Schatz M. Interrelationships between asthma and pregnancy: a literature review. *J Allergy Clin Immunol* 1999;103(suppl):330–336.

32. Turner ES, Greenberger PA, Patterson R. Management of the pregnant asthmatic patient. *Ann Intern Med* 1980;93:905–918.

33. Schatz M, Harden K, Forsythe A, et al. The course of asthma during pregnancy, postpartum, and with successive pregnancies: a prospective analysis. *J Allergy Clin Immunol* 1988;81:509–517.

34. Apter AJ, Greenberger PA, Patterson R. Outcomes of pregnancy in adolescents with severe asthma. *Arch Intern Med* 1989;149:2571–2575.

35. Shulman V, Adlerman E, Ewig JM, et al. Asthma in the pregnant adolescent: a review. *J Adolesc Health* 1996; 18:168–176.

36. Klebanoff MA, Shiono PH, Rhoads GG. Outcomes of pregnancy in a national sample of resident physicians. *N Engl J Med* 1990;323:1040–1045.

37. Li Y-F, Gilliland FD, Berhane K, et al. Effects of *in utero* and environmental tobacco smoke exposure on lung function in boys and girls with and without asthma. *Am J Respir Crit Care Med* 2000;162:2097–2104.

38. Finnell RH. Teratology: general considerations and principles. *J Allergy Clin Immunol* 1999;103(suppl):337–342.

39. Wilson J. Utilisation du cromolyglycate de sodium au cours de la grosse. *Acta Ther (Suppl)* 1982;8:45–51.

40. Frederiksen MC, Ruo TI, Chow MJ, et al. Theophylline pharmacokinetics in pregnancy. *Clin Pharmacol Ther* 1986;40:321–328.

41. Rosa F. Databases in the assessment of the effects of drugs during pregnancy. *J Allergy Clin Immunol* 1999; 103(suppl):360–361.

42. Metzger WJ, Turner E, Patterson R. The safety of immunotherapy during pregnancy. *J Allergy Clin Immunol* 1978;61:268–272.

43. Bousquet J, Miuller UR, Dreborg S, et al. Immunotherapy with hymenoptera venoms. Position paper of the Working Group on Immunotherapy of the European Academy of Allergy and Clinical Immunology. *Allergy* 1987;42:401–413.

44. Entman SS, Moise KJ. Anaphylaxis in pregnancy. *South Med J* 1984;77:402.

45. Settipane RA, Chafee FH, Settipane GA. Pollen immunotherapy during pregnancy: long-term follow-up of offsprings. *Allergy Proc* 1988;9:555–561.

46. Patterson R, Greenberger PA, Frederiksen MC. Asthma and pregnancy: responsibility of physicians and patients. *Ann Allergy* 1990;65:469–472.

47. Chapman KR, Verbeek PR, White JG, et al. Effect of a short course of prednisone in the prevention of early relapse after the emergency room treatment of acute asthma. *N Engl J Med* 1991;324:788–794.

48. Schreier L, Cutler RM, Saigal V. Respiratory failure in asthma during the third trimester: report of two cases. *Am J Obstet Gynecol* 1989; 160:80–81.

49. Tenholder MF, South-Paul JE. Dyspnea in pregnancy. *Chest* 1989;96:381–388.

50. American Medical Association. *Drug Evaluation Annual 1994, Department of Drugs, Division of Drugs and Toxicology*, 6th ed. Chicago: American Medical Association, 1993:1359.

51. Chandler MJ, Grammer LC, Patterson R. Noncompliance and prevarication in life-threatening adolescent asthma. *N Engl Regional Allergy Proc* 1986;7:367–370.

52. Bende M, Hallgarde V, Sjogren C. Occurrence of nasal congestion during pregnancy. *Am J Rhinol* 1989;3:217.

53. Schatz M, Zeiger RS. Diagnosis and management of rhinitis during pregnancy. *Allergy Proc* 1988;9:545–554.

54. Toppozada H, Michaels L, Toppozada M, et al. The human respiratory nasal mucosa in pregnancy: an electron microscopic and histochemical study. *J Laryngol Otol* 1982;96:613–626.

55. Toppozada H, Toppozada M, El-Ghazzawi I, et al. The human respiratory nasal mucosa in females using contraceptive pills. An ultramicroscopic and histochemical study. *J Laryngol Otol* 1984;98:43–51.

56. Bende M, Hallgarde M, Sjogren V, et al. Nasal congestion during pregnancy. *Clin Otolaryngol Allied Sci* 1989;14:385–387.

57. Heinonen OP, Sloan D, Shapiro S. *Birth defects and drugs in pregnancy.* Littleton, MA: PSG Publishing, 1977:1.

58. Einarson A, Bailey B, Jung G, et al. Prospective controlled study of hydroxyzine and cetirizine in pregnancy. *Ann Allergy Asthma Immunol* 1997;78:183–186.

59. Loebstein R, Lalkin A, Addis A, et al. Pregnancy outcome after gestational exposure to terfenadine: a multicenter, prospective controlled study. *J Allergy Clin Immunol* 1999;104:953–956.

60. Pastuszak A, Schick B, D'Alimonte D, et al. The safety of astemizole in pregnancy. *J Allergy Clin Immunol* 1996;98:748–750.
61. Schatz M, Petitti D. Antihistamines and pregnancy [Guest Editorial]. *Ann Allergy Asthma Immunol* 1997; 78:157–159.
62. Chappatte O, deSwiet M. Hereditary angioneurotic oedema and pregnancy: case reports and review of the literature. *Br J Obstet Gynaecol* 1988;95:938–942.
63. Frank MM, Gelfand JA, Atkinson JP. Hereditary angioedema: the clinical syndrome and its management. *Ann Intern Med* 1976;4:580–593.
64. Lawley T, Hertz K, Wade TR, et al. Pruritic urticarial papules and plaques of pregnancy. *JAMA* 1979;241: 1696–1699.
65. Smith A, Burkhart CG. Pruritus of pregnancy. *Cutis* 1984;34:486–488.
66. Bork K, Barnstedt S-E. Treatment of 193 episodes of laryngeal edema with C I inhibitor concentrate in patients with hereditary angioedema. *Arch Intern Med* 2001;161:714–718.
67. Bloomberg RJ. Cefotetan-induced anaphylaxis. *Am J Obstet Gynecol* 1988;159:125–126.
68. Habek D, Cerkez-Habek J, Jalsovec D. Anaphylactic shock in response in wasp sting in pregnancy. *Zentralbl Gynakol* 2000;122:393–394.
69. Kawarabayaski T, Narisawa Y, Nakamura K, et al. Anaphylactoid reaction to oxytocin during caesarean section. *Gynecol Obstet Invest* 1988;25:277–279.
70. Hadar A, Holcberg G, Mazor M. Anaphylactic shock after diclofenac sodium (Voltaren). *Harefuah* 2000; 138:211–212.
71. Anderson TH, Hindsholm KB, Fallingborg J. Severe complication to phytomenadione after intramuscular injection in woman in labor. *Acta Obstet Gynecol Scand* 1989;68:381–382.
72. Zucker-Pinchoff B, Ramanathan S. Anaphylactic reaction to epidural fentanyl. *Anesthesiology* 1989;71:599–601.
73. Sharpe O, Hall EG. Renal impairment, hypertension and encephalomacia in an infant surviving severe intrauterine anoxia. *Proc R Soc Med* 1953;46:1063.
74. Luciano R, Zuppa AA, Maragliano G, et al. Fetal encephalopathy after maternal anaphylaxis. Case report. *Biol Neonate* 1997;71:190–193.
75. Schatz M. Asthma and pregnancy. *J Asthma* 1990; 27:335–339.
76. Takamatsu I, Karasawa F, Kamei M, et al. A case of emergency caesarean section as a result of anaphylaxis to latex. *Masui* 1999;48:83–85.
77. Emmott RS. Recurrent anaphylactoid reaction during caesarean section [Letter]. *Anesthesiology* 1990; 45:62.
78. Graft DF. Venom immunotherapy during pregnancy. *Allergy Proc* 1988;9:563–565.
79. Schwartz HJ, Golden DBK, Lockey RF. Venom immunotherapy in the hymenoptera-allergic pregnant patient. *J Allergy Clin Immunol* 1990;85:709–712.

28

Management of Acute Severe Asthma

Thomas Corbridge and *Babak Mokhlesi

*Department of Medicine, Northwestern University Medical School, Medical Intensive Care Unit
Northwestern Memorial Hospital, Chicago, Illinois; *Division of Pulmonary and Critical Care,
Rush Medical College and Cook County Hospital, Chicago, Illinois*

Acute severe asthma (ASA), also called status asthmaticus, frequently represents failure of outpatient management—particularly in the subgroup of patients that depend on crisis-oriented management. These patients often reside in inner cities with low income, inadequate knowledge of asthma and its management, and no predetermined crisis plan (1). Physicians and nurses must address this problem, even in the acute care setting, to diminish the risk of repeated exacerbation. The importance of this intervention cannot be overstated. Acute asthma accounts for approximately 1.8 million emergency room visits, 460,000 hospitalizations, 25,000 episodes of respiratory failure requiring intubation, and 5,000 deaths each year in the United States (2–4). The total annual cost is $5 billion (2).

Asthma education is effective in the emergency room (5). Instruction takes time and may not be feasible for all patients; still, reallocation of resources to allow for education in the acute setting may be cost-effective in the long run. Follow-up appointments with an asthma specialist also are recommended to reduce further the risk of subsequent hospitalization (6).

This chapter reviews the more immediate concern of restoring the state of unlabored breathing. Fortunately this goal is achieved by medications alone in the majority of cases. Proven in this regard are β-agonist bronchodilators and systemic corticosteroids, with accumulating evidence supporting the use of anticholinergic bronchodilators. For a number of medications, including theophylline, magnesium sulfate, heliox, and leukotriene modifiers, efficacy is less clear (7). For patients requiring intubation and mechanical ventilation, a strategy that avoids excessive lung inflation, mainly through prolongation of exhalation time, decreases morbidity and mortality (7).

Insofar as it provides rationale for patient assessment, drug management, and ventilator strategy, the pathophysiology of acute asthma will be reviewed. Then the clinical presentation, differential diagnosis, physical examination, measurement of airflow rates, and laboratory testing will be discussed. Finally, there will be an overview of the specifics of drug management and recommendations for ventilator management.

PATHOPHYSIOLOGY OF ACUTE AIRFLOW OBSTRUCTION

The speed with which ASA develops varies considerably (8). In sudden asphyxic asthma, severe airflow obstruction develops in less than 3 hours. This type of asthma represents a relatively pure form of smooth muscle–mediated bronchospasm, with the potential for rapid improvement after bronchodilator therapy (9,10). There are more submucosal neutrophils and fewer airway secretions in sudden asphyxic asthma compared with attacks of slower progression (11,12). Triggers of sudden attacks include use of nonsteroidal antiinflammatory agents or β blockers in susceptible patients, allergen or irritant exposure, sulphites, or inhalation of crack cocaine or heroin (13–15). Respiratory track infection is not a significant trigger; commonly, no identifiable cause is found (16).

Attacks of slower onset are triggered by a variety of infectious, allergic, and nonspecific irritant exposures. They are characterized by progressive airway wall inflammation, accumulations of thick intraluminal mucus, and bronchospasm. Mucus plugs obstruct large and small airways and can be a striking finding at postmortem (17). They consist of sloughed epithelial cells, eosinophils, fibrin, and other serum components that have leaked through the denuded airway epithelium. Importantly, these attacks represent clear but often missed opportunities to increase antiinflammatory medications in the outpatient setting (18).

No matter the tempo, patients with ASA have critical airflow obstruction that interferes with emptying of alveolar gas. In severe cases it may take as long as 60 seconds for expiratory flow to cease. Of course, expiratory time is always shorter than this during spontaneous or assisted breathing. As a result, there is incomplete emptying of gas and dynamic lung hyperinflation (DHI). Fortunately, DHI is self-limiting because as lung volume increases so does lung elastic recoil pressure and airway diameter. These factors increase expiratory flow so that at a sufficiently large lung volume airflow is adequate to exhale the inspired breath.

At the end of exhalation, incomplete alveolar gas emptying elevates alveolar volume and pressure, a state referred to as auto–positive end-expiratory pressure (auto-PEEP) (19). Auto-PEEP represents a threshold pressure that must be overcome before inspiratory flow can occur. This, plus the fact that it is harder to fill a hyperinflated lung, increases the inspiratory work of breathing at a time when the diaphragm is placed in a mechanically disadvantageous position by DHI, and at a time when hypoperfusion and respiratory acidosis may further decrease diaphragm force generation (20). It is this potential imbalance between strength and load that predisposes to ventilatory failure.

Dead space (Vd) is defined as ventilated but not perfused lung units. It increases in acute asthma, presumably because of hypoperfusion of

hyperinflated lung. An increase in the dead space to tidal volume ratio (Vd/Vt) follows, favoring the development of hypercapnia:

$$P_{CO_2} = V_{CO_2} \times 0.863/V_a$$
$$= V_{CO_2} \times 0.863/[V_e \times (1 - V_d/V_t)]$$

where, P_{CO_2} is the partial pressure of carbon dioxide, V_{CO_2} is carbon dioxide production, V_a is alveolar ventilation, and V_e is minute ventilation.

However, V_e increases more than Vd/Vt in mild acute asthma, causing acute respiratory alkalosis. As the severity of airflow obstruction increases [particularly when the forced expiratory volume in 1 second (FEV_1) is less than 25% of predicted], the partial pressure of arterial carbon dioxide (Pa_{CO_2}) increases due to inadequate V_a (reflecting an increase in Vd/Vt and a decrease in V_e as the patient nears respiratory arrest).

Airway obstruction also decreases ventilation (V) relative to perfusion (Q), resulting in hypoxemia (21). Because this is not shunt (a V/Q of zero), supplementation of inspired oxygen readily corrects hypoxemia. Even when mechanical ventilation is required, hypoxemia is easily corrected; if not, other problems should be considered: pneumonia, aspiration, acute lobar atelectasis, or pneumothorax.

There is a rough correlation between severity of airflow obstruction as measured by FEV_1 or peak expiratory flow rate (PEFR) and hypoxemia (22,23). However, no cut-off value exists for either measurement that accurately predicts hypoxemia. Hypoxemia, which results from peripheral airway obstruction, may occur sooner and/or resolve later than airflow rates that mainly reflect large airway function (24,25).

Large swings in pleural pressure caused by breathing against obstructed airways are responsible for the circulatory changes in acute asthma. Blood return to the right heart decreases during expiration because of positive intrathoracic pressure, but during vigorous inspiration, intrathoracic pressure decreases and blood flow increases. This fills the right ventricle early in inspiration, shifting the intraventricular septum leftward. There is a conformational change in the left ventricle (LV) that causes diastolic dysfunction and incomplete LV filling. Large negative pleural pressures also impair LV emptying by increasing LV afterload (26,27). The net effect of these cyclical changes is to accentuate the normal inspiratory reduction in stroke volume, a phenomenon termed pulsus paradoxus (PP). The PP can be a valuable sign indicating asthma severity (28); however, the absence of a widened PP does not ensure a mild attack because PP decreases in the fatiguing asthmatic unable to generate significant swings in pleural pressure. Rarely, diastolic dysfunction and increased LV afterload cause pulmonary edema (29). Lung hyperinflation increases pulmonary vascular resistance and results in transient pulmonary hypertension (30,31).

TABLE 28.1. *Risk factors for fatal or near-fatal severe asthma*

Frequent emergency room visits
Frequent hospitalization
Intensive care unit admission
Intubation
Hypercapnia
Barotrauma
Psychiatric illness
Medical noncompliance
Illicit drug abuse
Low socioeconomic status
Inadequate access to medical care
Use of more than two canisters per month of inhaled β-agonist
Difficulty perceiving airflow obstruction
Comorbidities such as coronary artery disease
Sensitivity to *Alternaria* species

CLINICAL PRESENTATION, DIFFERENTIAL DIAGNOSIS, AND SEVERITY ASSESSMENT

Analysis of multiple factors, including the medical history, physical examination, objective measurement of airflow obstruction, initial response to therapy, arterial blood gases, and chest radiography are important to assess disease severity, risk of deterioration, and differential diagnosis. Multifactorial analysis is necessary because no single clinical measurement has been found to predict outcome reliably (32).

Risk Factors

Risk factors for death from ASA are listed in Table 28.1 (13,14,33–38).

Prior intubation is the greatest single predictor of subsequent asthma death (39). Other concerning features include symptoms of long duration, late arrival for care, extreme fatigue, abnormal mental status, and sleep deprivation. Deterioration despite optimal treatment, including the concurrent use of oral steroids, identifies high-risk patients who are unlikely to improve quickly.

Differential Diagnosis

"All that wheezes is not asthma" is a fitting clinical saw worth considering during the initial evaluation. In most cases, the history and physical examination will identify conditions that are mistaken for asthma. An extensive smoking history suggests chronic obstructive pulmonary disease and a more fixed form of expiratory airflow obstruction that may be associated with pulmonary hypertension and chronic respiratory acidosis. Congestive heart failure rarely causes airway hyperreactivity and wheeze, so-called cardiac asthma (40). The presence of an enlarged cardiac silhouette, vascular redistribution or a pulmonary edema pattern, and a left-sided third heart sound are clues to this diagnosis. Occasionally, distinguishing between congestive heart failure and asthma can be difficult because airflow obstruction rarely causes pulmonary edema through mechanisms specified above, and bronchodilators partially reverse cardiac asthma (41). Myocardial ischemia should be considered in older patients with risk factors for coronary artery disease. ASA may cause myocardial ischemia (myocardial oxygen supply/demand imbalance) by increasing LV afterload and tachycardia, and decreasing coronary blood flow and oxygenation (42).

Foreign body should be considered in very young and old patients, patients with altered mental status or neuromuscular disease, and when symptoms develop after eating or dental work. Localized wheeze and, rarely, asymmetric hyperinflation on chest radiography are clues to foreign body aspiration.

Upper airway obstruction from granulation tissue, tumor, laryngeal edema, or vocal cord dysfunction may mimic asthma. In contrast to asthma, upper airway (extrathoracic) obstruction flattens the inspiratory portion of the flow-volume loop, leaving the expiratory loop intact. An erratic flow-volume loop also suggests vocal cord dysfunction. When this condition is suspected, fiberoptic laryngoscopy is indicated to confirm paradoxical vocal cord movement. Significant response to helium-oxygen mixtures (heliox) suggests upper airway obstruction, although heliox response may occur in asthma and should not be used to distinguish upper from lower airway obstruction. Additional features suggesting upper airway obstruction include stridor, normal oxygenation, and resolution of airflow obstruction after intubation (43). In cases of suspected tracheal stenosis (e.g., from prior intubation), fiberoptic bronchoscopy or spiral computed tomography (CT) are the tests of choice.

Pneumonia complicating asthma is unusual, but it should be considered when there is fever, purulent sputum, localizing signs, and hypoxemia that does not correct with low-flow oxygen. Antibiotics are frequently prescribed for asthmatics with increased sputum production. However, sputum that looks purulent in asthma contains eosinophils, not polymorphonuclear leukocytes, and antibiotics are of no benefit in this setting (44). Antibiotics should be reserved for treatment of concurrent sinusitis, or when mycoplasmal or chlamydial infections are suspected. In *Pneumocystis carinii* pneumonia, airway hyperreactivity is common; however, this condition is rarely mistaken for ASA.

Wheezing occurs rarely in pulmonary embolism (45). When dyspnea is out of proportion to objective findings, particularly the PEFR, consider this diagnosis. Noninvasive lower extremity Doppler ultrasonographic examinations are helpful when they indicate thrombus; however, results of lower extremity Doppler studies are negative in 30% to 40% of patients with acute pulmonary embolism. Serial lower extremity Doppler studies provide an added sense of security, but the utility of this approach has not been validated in this setting. Ventilation-perfusion scans are difficult to interpret if there is airflow obstruction, but still may be diagnostic. In selected cases, a pulmonary embolism protocol CT scan or pulmonary angiogram may be required.

Physical Examination

The general appearance of the patient (posture, speech, positioning, and alertness) provides a quick guide to severity, response to therapy, and need for intubation. Patients assuming the upright position have a higher heart rate, respiratory rate, and pulsus paradoxus, and a significantly lower partial pressure of arterial oxygen (PaO_2) and PEFR than patients who are able to lie supine (46). Diaphoresis is associated with an even lower PEFR. Accessory muscle use and a widened PP indicate severe asthma; however, their absence does not exclude a severe attack (47).

Examination of the head and neck should focus on identifying barotrauma and upper airway obstruction. Prolongation of inspiration, stridor, and suprasternal retractions suggest upper airway obstruction. Tracheal deviation, asymmetric breath sounds, mediastinal crunch, and subcutaneous emphysema suggest pneumomediastinum or pneumothorax. Rarely, tracheal deviation is caused by atelectasis from mucus plugging, foreign body aspiration, or endobronchial tumor. The mouth and neck should be inspected for mass lesions or signs of previous surgery such as tracheostomy or thyroidectomy. The oropharynx should be inspected for signs of angioedema.

Chest auscultation reveals expiratory phase prolongation and wheeze. However, wheeze is not a reliable indicator of the severity of airflow obstruction (48). A silent chest indicates severe obstruction, with insufficient flow for wheezes to occur. In this situation, increasing wheeze signals improvement. Localized wheeze or crackles may represent mucus plugging and atelectasis, but should prompt consideration of pneumonia, pneumothorax, endobronchial lesions, or foreign body.

Tachycardia is common (49). Heart rate generally decreases in improving patients (although some improving patients remain tachycardic because of chronotropic effects of medications). The usual rhythm is sinus tachycardia. Supraventricular and ventricular arrhythmias occur, particularly in the elderly (50). As mentioned above, widened pulsus paradoxus is common. The finding of a third heart sound, jugular venous distention, or pedal edema suggests primary heart disease. Yet, ASA alone can cause examination and electrocardiographic findings of right heart strain and, less commonly, pulmonary edema (51). Jugular venous distention is a manifestation of dynamic hyperinflation, forceful exhalation, and tension pneumothorax.

Measurement of Airflow Obstruction

Measuring PEFR or FEV_1 helps assess the severity of airflow obstruction. A PEFR or FEV_1 less than 30% to 50% predicted or the patient's personal best (usually corresponding to a PEFR of <120 L/min and an FEV_1 of <1 L) suggests a severe exacerbation. Objective measurements are important because physician estimates of severity are often wrong—with errors equally distributed between over- and underestimates of the actual PEFR (52). In general, it is easier to measure PEFR than FEV_1, although this maneuver is still difficult for sick patients to perform. In severely dyspneic patients, peak flow determination is generously deferred because it rarely alters initial management and may worsen bronchospasm (53), even to the point of respiratory arrest (54).

Measurement of the change in PEFR or FEV_1 is one of the best ways to predict the need for hospitalization. Several studies have demonstrated that failure of initial therapy to improve expiratory flow after 30 minutes predicts a more severe course and need for hospitalization (55–58). Values before 30 minutes of treatment are not predictive (59).

Arterial Blood Gases

When FEV_1 is less than 1 L or PEFR is less than 120 L/min, arterial blood gas analysis is useful to assess the degree of hypoxemia and acid-base status. In the early stages of ASA, mild hypoxemia and respiratory alkalosis are common. As the severity of airflow obstruction increases, $PaCO_2$ increases due to inadequate Va. The presence of hypercapnia denotes severe disease; however, it alone is not an indication for intubation. Hypercapnic patients may respond to medications and not require intubation (60). Conversely, the absence of hypercapnia does not rule out impending respiratory arrest (61).

Patients who waste serum bicarbonate in response to persistent respiratory alkalosis develop a metabolic acidosis with a normal anion gap. Metabolic acidosis with an elevated anion gap reflects excess serum lactate, possibly secondary to increased work of breathing, tissue hypoxia, intracellular alkalosis, or decreased lactate clearance by the liver, which conceivably could develop from passive congestion of the liver in the setting of high intrathoracic pressures. Lactic acidosis is more common in men, severely obstructed patients (62,63), and patients receiving parenteral β agonists (64).

Repeat blood gas sampling is not necessary to determine clinical course. In most cases, valid judgments follow serial examinations with attention to patient posture, use of accessory muscles, diaphoresis, estimates of air movement during chest auscultation, pulse oximetry, and PEFR determinations. Patients who deteriorate on these grounds should be considered for intubation whether or not $PaCO_2$ is increasing. Conversely, patients who are more comfortable should not be intubated despite an elevated $PaCO_2$. In mechanically ventilated patients, serial blood gases help guide ventilator management.

Chest Radiography

Chest radiographs influence treatment in 1% to 5% of cases (65–67). In one study (68) that reported radiographic abnormalities in 34% of cases, the majority of findings were classified as focal parenchymal opacities or increased interstitial markings, common indicators of atelectasis in asthma. The available data suggest that radiography is indicated only when there are localizing signs or symptoms, concerns regarding barotrauma or pneumonia, or when it is not clear that asthma is the correct diagnosis. In mechanically ventilated patients, chest radiography confirms proper endotracheal tube position.

EMERGENCY DEPARTMENT MANAGEMENT

Patients demonstrating a good response to initial therapy may be discharged home with close follow-up. These patients should report no distress and have an essentially normal examination and an FEV_1 or PEFR of greater than or equal to 70% predicted or personal best (35). Observation for at least 60 minutes after the last dose of β-agonist helps ensure stability prior to discharge. Before discharge, patients should receive written medication instructions as well as a written plan of action to be followed in the event of deterioration. In general, patients should be discharged home on oral steroids. Mild cases with a complete response to bronchodilators may be considered for inhaled steroids alone. Most patients do well with oral steroids, particularly if they had not been optimally treated prior to the emergency room visit (69). An 8-day course of 40 mg/day prednisone is as efficacious and safe as an 8-day tapering schedule (70). Alternatively, a single dose of triamcinolone diacetate 40 mg intramuscularly also has been reported to be as effective as prednisone 40 mg/day for 5 days after treatment in the emergency room for asthma (71). Inhaled steroids should be started, continued, or increased, depending on the situation, while the patient is in the emergency room.

Patients in severe exacerbation (PEFR <50% predicted or personal best) who demonstrate a poor response to initial therapy (e.g., <10% increase in PEFR) or any patient who deteriorates during therapy should be admitted to an intensive care unit. Intensive care unit admission is also indicated for respiratory arrest, altered mental status, and cardiac disease (tachyarrhythmias, angina, or myocardial infarction).

An incomplete response to treatment may be defined as the persistence of shortness of breath and a PEFR or FEV_1 between 50% and 70% predicted (35). Patients in this group require ongoing treatment either in the emergency room or general medical ward. Physicians should err on the side of admission when there is a harmful home environment and when directly observed therapy is needed in noncompliant patients.

PHARMACOLOGIC THERAPY

Oxygen

Low-flow oxygen by nasal cannula is recommended to maintain arterial oxygen saturation greater than 90% (>95% in pregnancy and ischemic heart disease). This practice improves oxygen delivery to peripheral tissues such as respiratory muscles, reverses hypoxic pulmonary vasoconstriction, and may result in bronchodilation. Oxygen also protects against the decrease in PaO_2 resulting from β agonist–induced pulmonary vasodilation and increased blood flow to low V/Q units (72,73).

β agonists

Inhaled β agonists are indicated for immediate relief of smooth muscle–mediated bronchoconstriction. They should be given until there is either a clinical response or side effects limit further administration. In general, patients can be classified as albuterol responders (approximately two thirds of patients) or albuterol nonresponders (who may have a greater component of inflammation and airway architectural distortion). In the study by Rodrigo and Rodrigo, 67% of patients improved significantly and could be discharged from the emergency room after 2.4 mg albuterol (Fig. 28.1) (74). Half of the responders met discharge criteria after receiving only 12 puffs of albuterol. Similarly, Strauss and coworkers found that two thirds of patients with acute asthma could be discharged after three 2.5-mg doses of albuterol by nebulization every 20 minutes (75).

The optimal dose of albuterol has yet to be established. McFadden and colleagues compared two 5.0-mg treatments of albuterol by nebulization over 40 minutes with three 2.5-mg albuterol every 20 minutes in 160 emergency room patients (76). Peak expiratory flow rates improved in a dose-response fashion as the cumulative quantity of albuterol increased. A single treatment of

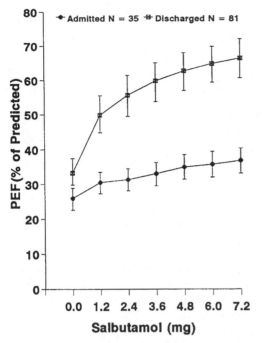

FIG. 28.1. Dose-response relationship to 4 puffs albuterol (400 μg) every 10 minutes in 116 acute asthmatics. Sixty-seven percent of patients obtained discharge criteria after administration of 2.4 mg albuterol within 1 hour; half the responders met discharge criteria after 12 puffs. Patients with a blunted cumulative dose-response relationship were hospitalized. (Reprinted from Rodrigo C, Rodrigo G. Therapeutic response patterns to high and cumulative doses of salbutamol in acute severe asthma. *Chest* 1998;113:593.)

5 mg albuterol achieved the same effect as two doses of 2.5 mg each, and 10 mg albuterol resulted in greater bronchodilation than did 7.5 mg. Overall, the 5-mg regimen increased peak flows more rapidly and to a greater extent than the standard 2.5-mg approach. Patients receiving 5 mg doses also reached discharge criteria quicker and left the emergency room with higher PEFRs. There was also a trend toward fewer hospitalizations in the high-dose group (25 of 80 patients, 31%) than in the lower dose group (37 of 80 patients, 46%) ($p = 0.06$). Emerman and colleagues compared the effects of 2.5 or 7.5 mg albuterol every 20 minutes in 160 acute asthmatics (77). There was no difference in improvement in FEV_1 or admission rates between groups. There is no difference between continuous and repeated dose administration

In general, albuterol should be used in a continuous or repetitive manner (both work equally well) (78) until there is a convincing clinical response or side effects limit further drug administration (Table 28.2) (79–82). Fortunately, high-dose inhaled β agonists are generally well tolerated. Tremor and tachycardia are common, but significant cardiovascular morbidity is not (83).

Albuterol is preferred over metaproterenol because its greater β_2 selectivity is associated with fewer side effects, and it has a longer duration of action (84,85). Some clinicians prefer metaproterenol or isoetharine for initial therapy because of their faster onset of action, despite the tendency of these drugs to increase side effects (86). Levalbuterol, the R-isomer of racemic albuterol, has been reported to have a slighter better safety profile than racemic albuterol. Although similar in efficacy, 1.25 mg levalbuterol has been shown to increase FEV_1 to a greater extent than 2.5 mg of racemic albuterol in stable patients with FEV_1 of less than or equal to 60% of predicted (87). Levalbuterol has not been studied adequately in ASA.

Long-acting β agonists are not indicated in the initial treatment of ASA because of their slow onset of action. The addition of salmeterol to albuterol in hospitalized asthmatics is safe and results in greater improvements in FEV_1 after 48 hours compared with placebo (88). Salmeterol maintenance therapy results in fewer exacerbations and exacerbations of lesser severity (89).

Metered-dose inhalers (MDIs) or hand-held nebulizers deliver inhaled β agonists equally well. Anywhere from 4 to 12 puffs by MDI with spacer achieves the same degree of bronchodilation as one 2.5-mg nebulized treatment of albuterol (90–93). MDIs with spacers carry the advantage of lesser cost and faster drug delivery times; hand-held nebulizers require fewer instructions, less supervision, and less coordination.

There is no advantage to parenteral delivery in the initial management of ASA, unless the patient is unable to comply with inhaled therapy (such as those with altered mental status or those in cardiopulmonary arrest) (94–96). After several

TABLE 28.2. *Drugs used in the initial treatment of acute asthma*

Standard therapies	
Albuterol	2.5 mg in 2.5 mL normal saline by nebulization every 15–20 min or 4–6 puffs by MDI with spacer every 10–20 min; for intubated patients, titrate to physiologic effect and side effects.
Epinephrine	0.3 mL of a 1:1,000 solution subcutaneously every 20 min three times. Use with caution in patients over age 40 and in patients with coronary artery disease.
Corticosteroids	Methylprednisolone 60 mg i.v. every 6 h or prednisone 40 mg orally every 6 h.
Anticholinergics	Ipratropium bromide 0.5 mg by nebulization every 20–60 min added to albuterol concentrate, or 4 puffs by MDI with spacer every 10–20 min.
Theophylline	5 mg/kg i.v. over 30 min loading dose in patients not on theophylline followed by 0.4 mg/kg/h i.v. maintenance dose. Check serum concentration within 6 h of loading dose. Watch for drug interactions and disease states that alter clearance.
Adjunctive therapies	
Magnesium sulfate	2 g i.v. over 20 min, repeat in 20 min (total dose 4 g unless hypomagnesemic).
Heliox	80:20 or 70:30 helium:oxygen mix by tight-fitting, non-rebreathing face mask. Higher helium concentrations are needed for maximal effect.

MDI, metered-dose inhaler; i.v., intravenously.

hours of inhaled β agonist (without a convincing response) subcutaneous epinephrine may be helpful (97). Known ischemic heart disease and age greater than 40 years are relative contraindications to parenteral therapy (98). Older patients without a history of recent myocardial infarction or angina tolerate subcutaneous epinephrine reasonably well.

Intravenous β agonists are not recommended, with the possible exception of patients in cardiac arrest. Several studies have demonstrated that inhaled drug results in greater improvement in airflow and less toxicity compared with intravenous administration (99–102).

Corticosteroids

Airway inflammation is important in most cases of ASA. Systemically administered corticosteroids are the most effective treatment of this inflammation, justifying their use in most cases. Corticosteroids should be given quickly in the emergency room to all but the mildest cases because antiinflammatory effects do not occur for hours. This delay explains the results of several studies demonstrating that corticosteroid use in the emergency room does not improve lung function over the first few hours and does not decrease hospitalization rates (103–105). In two studies to the contrary, methylprednisolone 125 mg intravenously on emergency room presentation decreased hospitalizations (106) and improved PEFR at 60 and 120 minutes compared with controls (107). Corticosteroids improve the

speed of acute asthma resolution, the number of relapses in the first week or two after treatment, and the risk of asthma death (108–113).

Whether there is a dose-response relationship to systemic steroids in ASA is not clear. In the meta-analysis by Rowe and colleagues, (108) doses lower than 30 mg of prednisone every six hours were less effective, but higher doses were no more effective. In another metaanalysis by Reid and colleagues, no therapeutic differences were identified among different doses of corticosteroids (60–80 mg/day of methylprednisolone vs. higher doses) in acute asthma requiring hospital admission (114). Emerman and Cydulka compared 500- and 100-mg doses of methylprednisolone in the emergency room, finding no benefit to higher dose therapy (115). Haskell and co-workers reported that patients receiving 125 mg intravenous methylprednisolone every 6 hours improved more rapidly than patients receiving 40 mg, although there was no difference in peak improvement (116). In this study, both 125- and 40-mg doses of methylprednisolone were superior to 15 mg every 6 hours in terms of the rate and absolute level of improvement. Bowler and colleagues found no difference between hydrocortisone 50 mg intravenously four times daily for 2 days, followed by low-dose oral prednisone and 200 or 500 mg of hydrocortisone, followed by higher doses of prednisone (117).

The recommendation by the expert panel from the National Institutes of Health is to deliver 120 to 180 mg/day of either prednisone, methylprednisolone, or prednisolone in three or four divided doses for 48 hours, then 60 to 80 mg/day until the PEFR reaches 70% of predicted or the patient's personal best (35). For adults, we recommend 40 to 60 mg of methylprednisolone (or its equivalent) every 6 hours by vein during initial management. Oral drug is as effective (118) but should be avoided in patients with gastrointestinal upset or in patients at risk for intubation.

Recent trials have demonstrated the benefit of inhaled corticosteroids in acute asthma. In children discharged from the emergency room, a short-term dose schedule of inhaled budesonide, starting at high dose and then tapered over 1 week, was reported to be as effective as a tapering course of oral prednisolone (119). Rodrigo and Rodrigo conducted a randomized, double-blind trial of the addition of flunisolide 1 mg versus placebo with 400 μg salbutamol every 10 minutes for 3 hours in 94 emergency room patients (120). They found that PEFR and FEV_1 were approximately 20% higher in the flunisolide group, beginning at 90 minutes. McFadden has suggested that this early benefit may stem from high-dose inhaled steroid-induced vasoconstriction, decreasing airway wall edema, vascular congestion, and plasma exudation (121). On the other hand, Guttman and colleagues found no benefit from the addition of beclomethasone dipropionate 7 mg every 8 hours by MDI with spacer to nebulized albuterol and systemic corticosteroid therapy (122). Similarly, these investigators also demonstrated that beclomethasone dipropionate (5 mg delivered by MDI) during the initial 4 hours of emergency room treatment did not confer added benefit to albuterol in adults with mild to moderately severe asthma (123). Overall, these data suggest that there is little benefit to the addition of inhaled steroids to high-dose β-adrenergic agonists and systemic corticosteroids in the management of acute asthma. Still, consideration should be given to the use of high-dose inhaled corticosteroids in refractory patients.

Ipratropium Bromide

Sufficient data support the use of ipratropium bromide, in combination with albuterol, in

acute asthma (124–134). Karpel and colleagues studied 384 patients randomized to receive nebulized albuterol 2.5 mg or albuterol 2.5 mg mixed with ipratropium 0.5 mg at entry and at 45 minutes (128). At 45 minutes, there were significantly more responders in the ipratropium group; however, the median change of FEV_1 from baseline did not differ between groups, and by 90 minutes there was no difference in the percentage of responders and median change in FEV_1 between groups. Additionally, there were no significant differences in the number of patients requiring additional emergency room or hospital treatment. Garrett and colleagues randomized 338 asthmatics to a single dose of nebulized ipratropium bromide 0.5 mg combined with albuterol 3.0 mg or albuterol 3.0 mg alone (129). Mean FEV_1 at 45 and 90 minutes was significantly higher with combined therapy. Lin and colleagues demonstrated that combination therapy resulted in greater improvement in PEFR than albuterol alone in 55 adult asthmatics (130). Results of a recent metaanalysis and a pooled analysis of three studies also demonstrate a modest benefit for combination therapy. In children, combination therapy decreases emergency room treatment time, albuterol dose requirements, and hospitalization rates (133,134).

To the contrary, Weber and colleagues reported the results of their prospective, randomized, double-blind, placebo-controlled trial of 67 patients receiving either a combination of albuterol plus ipratropium bromide or albuterol alone by continuous nebulization for a maximum of 3 hours (135). Primary outcome measures were improvement in PEFR, hospital admission rates, and length of stay in the emergency room. The direction of all three outcome measures favored combination therapy, but differences did not reach statistical significance. Fitzgerald and co-workers have reported similar results (136). In children, Ducharme and Davis did not demonstrate benefit from combination therapy in their study of nearly 300 asthmatics with mild to moderate acute asthma (137). Other small studies examining the addition of ipratropium bromide to β-adrenergic agonists in acute asthma have yielded mixed results (138,139).

The above studies demonstrating modest (or no) benefit to combination therapy generally used small doses of ipratropium bromide. Few trials have studied high and cumulative doses of both ipratropium bromide and albuterol. In one such study, Rodrigo and Rodrigo conducted a double-blind, randomized, prospective trial of albuterol and ipratropium bromide (120 μg of albuterol and 21 μg of ipratropium per puff, combined in one inhaler) versus albuterol (120 μg per puff) and placebo in 180 patients with acute asthma (140). Four puffs were administered through an MDI with a spacer every 10 minutes for 3 hours. Subjects who received combination therapy had 20.5% and 48.1% greater improvements in PEFR and FEV_1, respectively, compared with albuterol alone. The rate of hospitalization decreased significantly from 39% for albuterol and placebo to 20% for the combination therapy. Subgroup analysis showed that patients most likely to benefit from high doses of ipratropium bromide were those with FEV_1 less than 30% of predicted and symptoms for more than 24 hours prior to emergency room presentation.

Overall, the data suggest an advantage in maximal bronchodilation response when high doses of ipratropium bromide and albuterol are combined in the emergency treatment of asthma. Combination therapy is recommended in any patient who is extremely ill on first presentation or not responding quickly (e.g., within 30 minutes) to albuterol alone.

Theophylline

Several studies have demonstrated that theophylline does not improve the efficacy of maximal doses of β-adrenergic agonists in the first few hours of treatment, and that theophylline increases the incidence of tremor, nausea, anxiety, and tachyarrhythmias (141–146). A few studies have reported the benefit of theophylline in the management of ASA (147–149); in a study by Wrenn and colleagues, theophylline use in the emergency room resulted in fewer hospitalizations—even though airflow rates were not different from placebo (150). This finding raises the possibility that theophylline is not just a bronchodilator, and that it may benefit patients by improving respiratory muscle function or inflammation (151,152). Furthermore, results of

short-term studies do not exclude a delayed benefit from the early use of this drug. Theophylline may benefit patients after 24 hours of treatment (153–156).

On the whole, the available data do not allow for strong conclusions regarding the use of theophylline in acute asthma. Littenberg (157) analyzed 13 trials of theophylline use in the emergency room treatment of asthma and concluded that there was inadequate evidence to support or reject the use of theophylline in this setting. Little has changed over the years since this study was published to change this conclusion. Still there seems to be little benefit to using theophylline in most cases; we use it rarely when there is a poor response to β-adrenergic agonists, ipratropium bromide, and corticosteroids. Intravenous administration is preferred to limit oral intake in patients who may require intubation, although there is no difference in efficacy between intravenous and oral therapy. In patients not taking theophylline, the loading dose is 5 mg/kg (6 mg/kg aminophylline) by peripheral vein over 30 minutes followed by a continuous infusion of 0.4 mg/kg/h (0.5 mg/kg/h aminophylline). In patients on theophylline, serum concentrations should be checked on arrival to the emergency room before additional theophylline is given. If the concentration is within the therapeutic range, a continuous infusion may be started, or the oral preparation may be continued. Serum concentrations should be checked within 6 hours of intravenous loading to avoid toxic levels and to guide further dosing. We aim for levels between 8 and 12 μg/mL to avoid toxicity. Theophylline is safe in most cases if attention is directed to serum concentrations and to factors that increase them—and if it is discontinued in patients with tachyarrhythmias (158–160).

Magnesium Sulfate

Several prospective trials have failed to confirm a benefit to administering intravenous magnesium sulfate in acute asthmatics in the emergency room (161–164). Other prospective trials have reported benefit (165,166). In an attempt to shed further light on these results, three metaanalyses have been recently published (167–169).

However, they reach different conclusions as well. Rodrigo and colleagues reported that the addition of magnesium sulfate in moderate to severe exacerbations does not alter outcome (167). On the other hand, Alters and co-workers concluded that intravenous magnesium sulfate statistically improves spirometry (168). Rowe and others suggested that although the current evidence does not support the routine use of intravenous magnesium sulfate in all patients with acute asthma, magnesium may benefit patients who present with severe disease (169).

The notion that magnesium sulfate works better in severe disease is not new. In one study, 135 asthmatics were randomized to 2 g magnesium sulfate intravenously or placebo after 30 minutes and followed for 4 hours (170). Hospital admission rates and FEV_1 were no different between magnesium-treated patients and controls. On subgroup analysis, however, magnesium sulfate was reported to decrease admission rates and improve FEV_1 in patients with FEV_1 less than 25% predicted. Additional evidence supporting benefit in severe disease comes from a study of five mechanically ventilated asthmatics given magnesium (171). In this study, patients were given high doses of magnesium sulfate (10–20 g) over 1 hour, after which there was a significant decrease in peak airway pressure (43–32 cm H_2O) and in inspiratory flow resistance.

Of interest, magnesium sulfate also may be of greater benefit in premenopausal women because estrogen augments the bronchodilating effect of magnesium (172).

Nannini and colleagues recently evaluated the efficacy of inhaled magnesium sulfate (225 mg) versus normal saline as a vehicle for nebulized albuterol in a randomized, double-blind, controlled trial of 35 patients who presented to the emergency room (173). At 20 minutes, patients who received magnesium sulfate–albuterol had an absolute increase in PEFR of 134 ± 70 L/min versus 86 ± 64 L/min in the saline-albuterol group, a 57% greater percentage increase in PEFR.

Clearly additional data are needed to establish the role of magnesium in ASA. For now, routine use is not justified, with the possible exception of patients with severe disease and premenopausal women.

Heliox

Heliox is a gas consisting of 20% oxygen and 80% helium (30%:70% and 40%:60% mixtures are also available). As the percentage of helium decreases, so does the benefit of breathing this gas blend. Concentrations of helium of less than 60% are not effective, precluding its use in patients requiring significant supplemental oxygen. Heliox is slightly more viscous than air, but significantly less dense, resulting in a more than threefold increase in kinematic viscosity (the ratio of gas viscosity to gas density) compared with air. Theoretically, this property decreases the driving pressure required for gas flow by two mechanisms. First, for any level of turbulent flow, breathing low-density gas decreases the pressure gradient required for flow. Second, heliox decreases the Reynold number favoring conversion of turbulent flow to laminar flow (174). Heliox does not treat bronchospasm or airway wall inflammation.

Heliox promptly improves dyspnea, work of breathing, and arterial blood gas abnormalities in patients with upper airway obstruction (175). Benefits also have been reported in ASA. In adult asthmatics treated in the emergency room, a 20:80 mix increases PEFR and decreases pulsus paradoxus, suggesting improved airway resistance and work of breathing (176). Similar results also have been published in children (177). Other studies have failed to demonstrate a benefit (178,179). If heliox is effective, it may "buy time" for concurrent therapies to work, and thereby avert the need for intubation in some cases. Of theoretical concern is the potential for heliox to mask worsening airflow obstruction, so that there may be less time (and no margin for error) to control the airway.

Whether heliox augments the bronchodilator effect of inhaled β agonists compared with delivery in air is unclear. Data are available demonstrating a benefit to heliox as a driving gas (180), but there are also data to the contrary (181).

Other Medications

Leukotriene modifiers have been inadequately studied in acute asthma. In a preliminary report,

Silverman and colleagues demonstrated a trend toward fewer hospitalizations in patients who received zafirlukast 160 mg in addition to standard therapies (182). Regarding a number of other medications, including nitric oxide, furosemide, glucagon, lidocaine, surfactant, there are no compelling data to date to support their use (183).

MECHANICAL VENTILATION

Noninvasive Positive Pressure Ventilation

Noninvasive positive pressure ventilation (NPPV) by facemask is potentially useful in refractory patients who are not in need of immediate airway control. Supportive data are sparse, however, precluding strong conclusions. In one study (184) of 21 acute asthmatics with a mean PEFR of 144 L/min, nasal continuous positive airway pressure of 5 or 7.5 cm H_2O significantly decreased respiratory rate and dyspnea compared with placebo, presumably by helping to overcome the inspiratory threshold load created by auto-PEEP (185). In the largest study published to date (186), Meduri and colleagues reported their observational experience with NPPV during 17 episodes of ASA. In all but one patient (who subsequently required intubation), NPPV improved dyspnea. NPPV improved blood gases, heart rate, and respiratory rate, and only two patients required intubation. There were no NPPV-related complications.

Intubation

Respiratory arrest, patient deterioration with exhaustion, and changes in mental status all indicate the need for intubation. In breathing patients, the decision to intubate ultimately relies on the judgment of an experienced clinician as to whether a patient can safely maintain spontaneous respirations until bronchodilator/antiinflammatory therapy takes hold.

Once the decision to intubate has been made, the goal is to take rapid control of the patient's cardiopulmonary status. Oral intubation is preferred because it allows for placement of a large endotracheal tube—important to decrease airway resistance and facilitate removal of

tenacious mucus plugs. Nasal intubation is safe in most patients and may be preferred in an awake patient anticipated to be difficult to ventilate and intubate in the supine position (e.g., short, obese patients). Several problems are associated with nasal intubation, including the need for a smaller endotracheal tube and the higher incidence of nasal polyps and sinusitis in asthmatics.

Postintubation Hypotension

The time immediately following intubation can be extremely difficult for the patient with severe airflow obstruction, particularly because airflow obstruction may continue to deteriorate during the first 24 hours of mechanical ventilation, possibly due to irritant effects of tracheal cannulation. Considerable care must be taken to stabilize the patient during this period, including the thoughtful use of sedatives, paralytics, bronchodilators, intravenous fluids, and careful delivery of positive pressure ventilation.

Immediate concerns are hypotension and pneumothorax. Hypotension has been reported in 25% to 35% of patients following intubation (187). It occurs for several reasons. First, there is loss of vascular tone due to a direct effect of sedation and loss of sympathetic activity. Second, many patients are hypovolemic because of high insensible losses and decreased oral fluid intake during their exacerbation. Third, overzealous AMBU-bag ventilation can result in dangerous levels of DHI because adequate time is not provided for exhalation. When this occurs, the patient becomes difficult to ventilate. Breath sounds diminish, blood pressure decreases, and heart rate increases. A trial of hypopnea (2–3 breaths/min) or apnea in a preoxygenated patient may deflate the lung and demonstrate this pathophysiology. After 30 to 60 seconds of hypoventilation, intrathoracic pressure decreases, allowing for greater blood return to the right atrium. Blood pressure increases, heart rate decreases falls, and the inspired breath becomes easier to deliver.

Thus, a trial of hypopnea or apnea is diagnostic and therapeutic for DHI. If such a trial does not quickly restore cardiopulmonary stability, consideration should be given to tension pneumothorax. Tension pneumothoraces may have been responsible for more than 6% of deaths of patients who required mechanical ventilation for severe asthma (187). Hemodynamic improvement during a trial of apnea suggests DHI but does not completely exclude tension pneumothorax. Careful inspection of the chest radiograph is mandatory because there may not be significant lung collapse in the setting of DHI. When pneumothorax is present, the contralateral lung deserves close attention because unilateral pneumothorax causes preferential ventilation of the contralateral lung, increasing the risk of bilateral pneumothoraces. Management of this situation consists of hypoventilation, volume resuscitation, and chest tubes placed bilaterally.

Initial Ventilator Settings and Dynamic Hyperinflation

During mechanical ventilation, the expiratory time, tidal volume, and severity of airway obstruction determine the level of DHI. Because standard treatment for airway obstruction has usually been maximized in the intubated patient, expiratory time and tidal volume become important variables during ventilator management. Minute ventilation and inspiratory flow rates determine exhalation time (188,189). When minute ventilation is decreased, expiratory time is prolonged and there is less DHI. To avoid dangerous levels of DHI, initial minute ventilation should not exceed 115 mL/kg/min or approximately 8 L/m in a 70-kg patient (190). To achieve this minute ventilation, we recommend a respiratory rate of 12 to 14 breaths/min combined with a tidal volume of 7 to 8 mL/kg. The use of relatively low tidal volumes avoids excessive peak lung inflation, which may occur even when there is acceptably low minute ventilation.

Shortening the inspiratory time by use of a high inspiratory flow rate is another way to prolong expiratory time. We favor an inspiratory flow rate of 80 L/min, using a square flow pattern (i.e., a constant flow rate). High inspiratory flow rates increase peak airway pressure by elevating airway resistive pressure. Importantly, peak airway pressures per se do not correlate with morbidity or mortality. Rather it is the state of lung hyperinflation that predicts outcome. Any strategy that lowers peak airway pressure, such as use of a lower constant inspiratory flow rate or a decelerating flow regimen, will shorten expiratory time and worsen DHI.

There is no consensus as to which ventilator mode should be used in asthmatics. In paralyzed patients, synchronized intermittent mandatory ventilation (SIMV) and assist-controlled ventilation (AC) are equivalent. In patients triggering the ventilator, SIMV is generally preferred because of the unproven concern that minute ventilation will be higher during AC because each triggered breath receives a guaranteed tidal volume (191). Volume-controlled ventilation (VC) is recommended over pressure-controlled ventilation (PC) for several reasons, including staff familiarity with its use. PC offers the advantage of limiting peak airway pressure to a predetermined set value (e.g., 35 cm H_2O). However, during PC, tidal volume is inversely related to auto-PEEP and minute ventilation is not guaranteed. PC also requires a decelerating inspiratory flow pattern that is associated with longer inspiratory times and shorter Te.

Ventilator-applied PEEP is not recommended in sedated and paralyzed patients because it may increase lung volume if used excessively (192). In spontaneously breathing patients, small amounts of ventilator-applied PEEP (e.g., 5 cm H_2O) decrease inspiratory work of breathing by decreasing the pressure gradient required to overcome auto-PEEP.

Assessing Lung Inflation

Determination of the severity of DHI is central to risk assessment and adjustment of ventilator settings. Numerous methods have been proposed to measure DHI. The volume at end-inspiration, termed Vei, is determined by collecting all expired gas from total lung capacity (TLC) to functional residual capacity (FRC) during 40 to 60 seconds of apnea. A Vei of greater than 20 mL/kg has been correlated with barotrauma. Indeed, this is the only measure of DHI that has been shown to predict barotrauma (although it may underestimate the degree of air trapping if there are very slowly emptying air spaces). The utility of this measure is limited by the need for paralysis and the fact that most clinicians and respiratory therapists are unfamiliar with expiratory gas collection.

Surrogate measures of DHI include the single-breath plateau pressure (Pplat) and auto-PEEP. Pplat is an estimate of average end-inspiratory alveolar pressures that is easily determined by stopping flow at end-inspiration. Auto-PEEP is the lowest average alveolar pressure achieved during the respiratory cycle. It is obtained by measuring airway opening pressure during an end-expiratory hold maneuver. In the presence of auto-PEEP, airway opening pressure increases by the amount of auto-PEEP present. Persistence of expiratory gas flow at the beginning of inspiration (which can be detected by auscultation or monitoring of flow tracings) also demonstrates auto-PEEP.

Accurate measurement of Pplat and auto-PEEP requires patient–ventilator synchrony and no patient effort. Paralysis is generally not required for valid measurements. Unfortunately, both measures are problematic and neither has been validated as a predictor of complications. Pplat is affected by the entire respiratory system, including lung tissue and chest wall; thus, significant variations in DHI may occur from patient to patient at the same pressure. Obese patients, for example, have a higher Pplat than do thin patients for the same degree of DHI. Despite these limitations, extensive experience suggests that when Pplat is less than 30 cm H_2O, outcome is generally good.

Auto-PEEP may underestimate the severity of DHI (193). This is thought to occur when severe airway narrowing limits the communication between the alveolus and mouth so that during an end-exhalation hold maneuver airway opening pressure does not increase. In most cases, however, auto-PEEP of less than 15 cm H_2O appears to be acceptable.

Ventilator Adjustments

With the above considerations in mind, we offer an algorithm for the ventilator adjustments. This algorithm relies on Pplat as a measure of lung hyperinflation and arterial pH as a marker of ventilation. If initial ventilator settings result in Pplat of more than 30 cm H_2O, respiratory rate should be decreased until this goal is achieved. Hypercapnia may well ensue, but fortunately this is generally well tolerated, even with arterial P_{CO_2} values as high as 90 mm Hg, as long as a sudden increase in P_{CO_2} does not occur (194,195). Anoxic brain injury and myocardial dysfunction are contraindications to permissive hypercapnia because hypercapnia causes cerebral vasodilation, decreased myocardial contractility, and pulmonary vasoconstriction (196). Fortunately, lowering minute ventilation does not always cause the expected increase in P_{CO_2}, possibly because less DHI lowers dead space. If hypercapnia results in a blood pH of less than 7.20 (and respiratory rate cannot be increased because of the Pplat limit), we generally start a slow infusion of sodium bicarbonate, although this has not been shown to improve outcome (197). If Pplat is less than 30 cm H_2O and pH is less than 7.20, respiratory rate can be safely increased for the purpose of lowering $PaCO_2$ and elevating arterial pH until Pplat nears the threshold pressure. Commonly, patients can be ventilated to a pH of more than 7.20 with a Pplat of less than 30 cm H_2O, particularly as they improve and near extubation.

Sedation and Paralysis

Sedation is indicated to improve comfort, safety, and patient–ventilator synchrony (Table 28.3). This is particularly true when hypercapnia serves as a potent stimulus to respiratory drive. Some patients (such as those with sudden asphyxic asthma) may be ready for extubation within hours. In these patients, propofol is attractive because it can be rapidly titrated to a deep level of sedation and still allow reliable reversal of sedation quickly after discontinuation (198). Benzodiazepines, such as lorazepam and midazolam, are cheaper alternatives and also good choices for sedation of the intubated asthmatic patient (199). Time to awakening after discontinuation of these drugs is longer and less predictable than with propofol.

TABLE 28.3. *Sedatives used in ventilated asthmatics*

Agent	Dose	Cautions
Periintubation period		
Midazolam	1 mg i.v. slow push; repeat every 2–3 min as needed	Hypotension, respiratory depression
Ketamine	1–2 mg/kg i.v. at a rate of 0.5 mg/kg/min	Sympathomimetic effects, respiratory depression, mood changes, delirium
Propofol	60–80 mg/min i.v. initial infusion up to 2.0 mg/kg followed by an infusion of 5–10 mg/kg/h as needed	Respiratory depression
Sedation for protracted mechanical ventilation		
Lorazepam	1–5 mg/h i.v. continuous infusion or i.v. bolus as needed	Drug accumulation
Morphine sulfate	1–5 mg/h i.v. continuous infusion; avoid bolus	Ileus
Ketamine	0.1–0.5 mg/min i.v.	Sympathomimetic effects, delirium
Propofol	1–4.5 mg/kg/h i.v.	Seizures, hyperlipidemia

In order to provide the best combination of amnesia, sedation, analgesia, and suppression of respiratory drive, we recommend the addition of a narcotic (best given by continuous infusion) to either propofol or a benzodiazepine (200). Morphine and fentanyl are the two most commonly used narcotics. Fentanyl has a quicker onset of action and is slightly more expensive than morphine, although the magnitude of this difference is not large. Morphine has the theoretical disadvantage of histamine release and the potential to worsen bronchospasm.

Ketamine, an intravenous anesthetic with sedative, analgesic, and bronchodilating properties, is generally reserved for use in intubated patients with severe bronchospasm that precludes safe mechanical ventilation (201–203). Ketamine must be used with caution because of its sympathomimetic effects and ability to cause delirium.

When safe and effective mechanical ventilation cannot be achieved by sedation alone, consideration should be given to short-term muscle paralysis. Short- to intermediate-acting agents include atracurium, cis-atracurium, and vecuronium. Pancuronium is longer acting and the least expensive of the paralytics. Its vagolytic effects also may result in unwanted tachycardia. Pancuronium and atracurium both release histamine; but the clinical significance of this property is doubtful (204). In our intensive care unit we pre-fer cis-atracurium because it is essentially free of cardiovascular effects, does not release histamine, and does not require hepatic and renal function for clearance.

Paralytics may be given intermittently by bolus or continuous intravenous infusion. If a continuous infusion is used, a nerve stimulator should be used or the drug withheld every 4 to 6 hours to avoid drug accumulation and prolonged paralysis. Paralytic agents should be minimized whenever possible because of the risk of postparalytic myopathy (205–207). Acute myopathy is rare in patients paralyzed for less than 24 hours; thus, paralytics should be discontinued as soon as possible. Most patients with postparalytic myopathy recover completely, although some require several weeks of rehabilitation.

Administration of Bronchodilators During Mechanical Ventilation

Many questions remain regarding the optimal administration of inhaled bronchodilators during mechanical ventilation. In one study (208), only 2.9% of a radioactive aerosol delivered by nebulizer was deposited in the lungs of mechanically ventilated patients. Manthous and colleagues (209) compared the efficacy of albuterol delivered by MDI via a simple inspiratory adapter (no spacer) to nebulized albuterol in mechanically ventilated patients. Using the peak-to-pause pressure gradient at a constant inspiratory flow to measure airway resistance, they found no effect (and no side effects) from the administration of 100 puffs (9.0 mg) of albuterol; whereas albuterol delivered by nebulizer to a total dose of 2.5 mg reduced the inspiratory flow-resistive pressure by 18%. Increasing the nebulized dose to a total of 7.5 mg reduced airway resistance further in 8 of 10 patients, but caused side effects in half of the patients. If MDIs are used during mechanical ventilation, use of a spacing device on the inspiratory limb of the ventilator may significantly improve drug delivery (210). In either case (MDI with spacer or nebulizer), higher drug dosages are required and the dosage should be titrated to achieve a decrease in the peak-to-pause airway pressure gradient. When no measurable decrease in airway resistance occurs, other causes of elevated airway resistance such as a kinked or plugged endotracheal tube should be excluded. Bronchodilator nonresponders also should be considered for a drug holiday. In general, nebulizers should be placed close to the ventilator, and in-line humidifiers stopped during treatments. Inspiratory flow should be reduced to approximately 40 L/min during treatments to minimize turbulence, although this strategy has the potential to worsen lung hyperinflation and must be time-limited. Patient–ventilator synchrony is crucial to optimize drug delivery.

Other Considerations

Rarely, the above strategies are unable to stabilize the patient on the ventilator in these situations, and consideration should be given to the use of other therapies. Halothane and enflurane are general anesthetic bronchodilators that can acutely reduce Ppk and $PaCO_2$ (211,212). These agents are associated with myocardial depression, arterial vasodilation, and arrhythmias, and their benefit does not last after drug discontinuation. Heliox delivered through the ventilator circuit may decrease Ppk and $PaCO_2$ (213) However, safe use of heliox requires significant institutional expertise. Ventilator flow meters (which are gas density dependent) must be recalibrated during heliox to low-density gas, and a spirome-

ter should be placed on the expiratory port of the ventilator during heliox administration to measure tidal volume. Careful planning, including a trial of heliox use in a lung model, is mandatory prior to patient use.

Strategies to mobilize mucus, such as chest physiotherapy or treatment with mucolytics or expectorants, have not proved to be efficacious in controlled trials. Bronchoalveolar lavage, on the other hand, using either saline or acetylcysteine, may be useful in nonintubated patients (214–216). This procedure is theoretically risky because the bronchoscope increases expiratory airway resistance and may worsen auto-PEEP and bronchospasm.

Extubation

Although some patients with labile asthma respond to therapy within hours, more typically the patient will require 24 to 48 hours of bronchodilator/antiinflammatory therapy before they are ready for extubation. Patients should be considered for extubation when their PO_2 normalizes at a safe minute ventilation (i.e., a minute ventilation associated with a safe level of DHI), and their airway resistance is less than 20 cm H_2O. If pneumonia, central nervous system injury, or muscle weakness has not complicated the patient's course, progression to spontaneous breathing should be prompt. We extubate as soon as possible because the endotracheal tube itself may perpetuate bronchospasm. After extubation, close observation in the intensive care unit is recommended for an additional 12 to 24 hours. During this time clinicians can focus on safe transfer to the general medical ward and on maximizing outpatient management.

REFERENCES

1. Hanania NA, David-Wang A, Kesten S, et al. Factors associated with emergency department dependence of patients with asthma. *Chest* 1997;111:290–295.
2. Weiss KB. An economic evaluation of asthma in the United States. *N Engl J Med* 1992;326:862.
3. LeSon S, Gershwin, ME. Risk factors for asthmatic patients requiring intubation: a comprehensive review.*Allergol Immunopathol* 1995;23:235.
4. Asthma—United States, 1982–1992. *MMWR* 1995; 43:952.

5. Kelso TM, Self TH, Rumbak MJ, et al. Educational and long-term therapeutic intervention in the ED: effect on outcomes in adult indigent minority asthmatics. *Am J Emerg Med* 1995;13:632–637.

6. Zeigler RS, Heller S, Mellon MH, et al. Facilitated referral to asthma specialist reduces relapses in asthma emergency room visits. *J Allergy Clin Immunol* 1991;87:1160–1168.

7. Corbridge T, Hall JB. The assessment and management of status asthmaticus in adults. *Am J Respir Crit Care Med* 1995;151:1296–1316.

8. Picado C. Classification of severe asthma exacerbations: a proposal. *Eur Respir J* 1996;9:1775–1778.

9. Wasserfallen JB, Schaller MD, Feihl F, et al. Sudden asphyxic asthma: a distinct entity? *Am Rev Respir Dis* 1990;142:108.

10. Arnold AG, Lane DJ, Zapata E. The speed of onset and severity of acute severe asthma. *Br J Dis Chest* 1982;76:157.

11. Sur S, Crotty TB, Kephart GM, et al. Sudden-onset fatal asthma: a distinct clinical entity with few eosinophils and relatively more neutrophils in the airway submucosa. *Am Rev Respir Dis* 1993;148:713.

12. Ried LM. The presence or absence of bronchial mucus in fatal asthma. *J Allergy Clin Immunol* 1987;80:415.

13. Rome LA, Lippmann ML, Dalsey WC, et al. Prevalence of cocaine use and its impact on asthma exacerbation in an urban population. *Chest* 2000;117:1324–1329.

14. Cygan J, Trunsky M, Corbridge T. Inhaled heroin-induced status asthmaticus. *Chest* 2000;117:272–275.

15. Levenson T, Greenberger PA, Donoghue ER, Lifshultz BD. Asthma deaths confounded by substance abuse: an assessment of fatal asthma. *Chest* 1996;110:604–610.

16. Rodrigo G, Rodrigo C. Rapid-onset asthma attack: a prospective cohort study about characteristics and response to emergency department treatment. *Chest* 2000;118:1547.

17. Hogg JC. The pathology of asthma. *Clin Chest Med* 1984;5:567.

18. Petty TL. Treat status asthmaticus three days before it occurs. *J Intens Care Med* 1989;4:135.

19. Pepe PE, Marini JJ. Occult positive end-expiratory pressure in mechanically ventilated patients with airflow obstruction: the auto-PEEP effect. *Am Rev Respir Dis* 1982;126:166–170.

20. Yanos J, Wood LD, Davis K, et al. The effect of respiratory and lactic acidosis on diaphragm function. *Am Rev Respir Dis* 1993;147:616.

21. Rodriguez-Roisin R, Ballester E, Roca J, et al. Mechanisms of hypoxemia in patients with status asthmaticus requiring mechanical ventilation. *Am Rev Respir Dis* 1989;139:732.

22. Nowak RM, Tomlanovich MC, Sarker DD, et al. Arterial blood gases and pulmonary function testing in acute bronchial asthma: predicting patient outcomes. *JAMA* 1983;249:2043.

23. McFadden ER Jr, Lyons HA. Arterial-blood gas tension in asthma. *N Engl J Med* 1968;278:1027.

24. Ferrer A, Roca J, Wagner PD, et al. Airway obstruction and ventilation–perfusion relationships in acute severe asthma. *Am Rev Respir Dis* 1993;147:579.

25. Roca J, Ramis L, Rodriguez-Roisin R, et al. Serial relationships between ventilation perfusion inequality and spirometry in acute severe asthma requiring hospitalization. *Am Rev Respir Dis* 1988;137:1055.

26. Scharf S, Brown R, Saunders N, et al. Effects of normal and loaded spontaneous inspiration on cardiovascular function. *J Appl Physiol* 1979;47:582.

27. Scharf S, Brown R, Tow D, et al. Cardiac effects of increased lung volume and decreased pleural pressure. *J Appl Physiol* 1979;47:257.

28. Knowles G, Clark TJ. Pulsus paradoxus as a valuable sign indicating severity of asthma. *Lancet* 1973; 2:1356.

29. Stalcup SA, Mellins RB. Mechanical forces producing pulmonary edema in acute asthma. *N Engl J Med* 1977;297:592–596.

30. Permutt S, Wise RA. Mechanical interaction of respiration and circulation. In: Fishman A, ed. *Handbook of physiology.* Vol. 3. American Physiological Society. Baltimore: Williams & Wilkins, 1986:647.

31. Corbridge T, Hall JB. Pulmonary hypertension in status asthmaticus. In: Cosentino AM, Martin RJ, eds. *Cardiothoracic interrelationships in clinical practice.* Armonk, NY: Futura, 1997:137–156.

32. Rodrigo G, Rodrigo C. Assessment of the patient with acute asthma in the emergency department: a factor analytic study. *Chest* 1993;104:1325.

33. Greenberger PA, Patterson R. The diagnosis of potentially fatal asthma. *N Engl Regional Allergy Proc* 1988;9:147.

34. Lowenthal M, Patterson R, Greenberger PA. The application of an asthma severity index in patients with potentially fatal asthma. *Chest* 1993;104:1329.

35. *Guidelines for the diagnosis and management of asthma: Expert Panel Report II.* Bethesda, MD: National Institutes of Health, 1997.

36. Suissa S, Ernst P, Boivin JF, et al. A cohort analysis of excess mortality in asthma and the use of inhaled beta-agonists. *Am J Respir Crit Care Med* 1994;149:604.

37. Levnson T, Greenberger PA, Donoghue ER, et al. Asthma deaths confounded by substance abuse: an assessment of fatal asthma. *Chest* 1996;110:604.

38. Kikuchi Y, Okabe S, Tamura G, et al. Chemosensitivity and perception of dyspnea in patients with a history of near-fatal asthma. *N Engl J Med* 1994; 330:1329.

39. Rea HH, Scragg R, Jackson R, et al. A case-controlled study of deaths from asthma. *Thorax* 1986;41:833.

40. Fishman AP. Cardiac asthma—a fresh look at an old wheeze. *N Engl J Med* 1989;320:1346.

41. Cabanes LR, Weber SN, Matran R, et al. Bronchial hyperresponsiveness to methacholine in patients with impaired left ventricular function. *N Engl J Med* 1989;320:1317.

42. Scharf S. Mechanical cardiopulmonary interactions with asthma. *Clin Rev Allergy* 1985;3:487.

43. Baughman RP, Loudon RC. Stridor: differentiation from wheezing or upper airway noise. *Am Rev Respir Dis* 1989;139:1407.

44. Graham VAL, Knowles GK, Milton AF, et al. Routine antibiotics in hospital management of acute asthma. *Lancet* 1982;1:418.

45. Hall JB, Wood LDH. Management of the critically ill asthmatic patient. *Med Clin North Am* 1990;74:779.

46. Brenner BE, Abraham E, Simon RR. Position and diaphoresis in acute asthma. *Am J Med* 1983;74:1005.

47. Kelsen SG, Kelsen DP, Fleegler BF, et al. Emergency room assessment and treatment of patients with acute asthma. *Am J Med* 1978;64:622.

48. Shim CS, Williams MH. Relationship of wheezing to the severity of obstruction in asthma. *Arch Intern Med* 1983;143:890.

49. Grossman J. The occurrence of arrhythmias in hospitalized asthma patients. *J Allergy Clin Immunol* 1976;57:310.

50. Josephson GW, Kennedy HL, MacKenzie EJ. Cardiac dysrhythmias during the treatment of acute asthma: a comparison of two treatment regimens by a double blind protocol. *Chest* 1980;78:429.

51. Rebuck AS, Read J. Assessment and management of severe asthma. *Am J Med* 1971;51:788.

52. Shim CS, Williams MH Jr. Evaluation of the severity of asthma: patients versus physicians. *Am J Med* 1980;68:11.

53. Lim TK, Ang SM, Rossing TH, et al. The effects of deep inhalation on maximal expiratory flow during intensive treatment of spontaneous asthmatic episodes. *Am Rev Respir Dis* 1989;140:340.

54. Lemarchand P, Labrune S, Herer B, et al. Cardiorespiratory arrest following peak expiratory flow measurement during attack of asthma. *Chest* 1991;100:1168.

55. Banner AS, Shah RS, Addington WW. Rapid prediction of need for hospitalization in acute asthma. *JAMA* 1976;235:1337.

56. Fanta CH, Rossing TH, McFadden ER Jr. Emergency room treatment of asthma: relationships among therapeutic combinations, severity of obstruction and time course of response. *Am J Med* 1982;72:416.

57. Stein LM, Cole RP: Early administration of corticosteroids in emergency room treatment of acute asthma. *Ann Intern Med* 1990;112:822.

58. Rodrigo G, Rodrigo C. Early prediction of poor response in acute asthma patients in the emergency department. *Chest* 1998;114:1016–1021.

59. Martin TG, Elenbaas RM, Pingleton SH. Failure of peak expiratory flow rate to predict hospital admission in acute asthma. *Ann Emerg Med* 1982;11:466.

60. Mountain RD, Sahn S. Clinical features and outcome in patients with acute asthma presenting with hypercapnia. *Am Rev Respir Dis* 1988;138:535.

61. McFadden ER Jr, Lyons HA. Arterial-blood gas tension in asthma. *N Engl J Med* 1968;278:1027.

62. Appel D, Rubenstein R, Shrager K, et al. Lactic acidosis in severe asthma. *Am J Med* 1983;75:580.

63. Mountain RD, Heffner JE, Brackett NC. Acid-base disturbances in acute asthma. *Chest* 1990;98:651.

64. O'Connell MB, Iber C. Continuous intravenous terbutaline infusions for adult patients with status asthmaticus. *Ann Allergy* 1990;64:213.

65. Findley LJ, Sahn SA. The value of chest roentgenograms in acute asthma in adults. *Chest* 1980;5:535.

66. Zieverink SE, Harper AP, Holden RW, et al. Emergency room radiography of asthma: an efficacy study. *Radiology* 1982;145:27.

67. Sherman S, Skoney JA, Ravikrishnan KP. Routine chest radiographs in exacerbations of acute obstructive pulmonary disease. *Arch Intern Med* 1989;149:2493.

68. White CS, Cole RP, Lubetsky HW, et al. Acute asthma: admission chest radiography in hospitalized adult patients. *Chest* 1991;100:14.

69. Feil SB, Swartz MA, Glanz K, et al. Efficacy of short-term corticosteroid therapy in outpatient treatment of acute bronchial asthma. *Am J Med* 1983;75:259.

70. Cydulka RK, Emerman CL. A pilot study of steroid therapy after emergency department treatment of acute asthma: is a taper needed? *J Emerg Med* 1998;16:15–19.

71. Schuckman H, DeJulius DP, Blanda M, et al. Comparison of intramuscular triamcinolone and oral prednisone in the outpatient treatment of acute asthma: a randomized controlled trial. *Ann Emerg Med* 1998;31:333–338.

72. West JB. State of the art: ventilation–perfusion relationships. *Am Rev Respir Dis* 1977;116:919.

73. Ballester E, Reyes A, Roca J, et al. Ventilation–perfusion mismatching in acute severe asthma: effects of salbutamol and 100% oxygen. *Thorax* 1989;44:258.

74. Rodrigo C, Rodrigo G. Therapeutic response patterns to high and cumulative doses of salbutamol in acute severe asthma. *Chest* 1998;113:593.

75. Strauss L, Hejal R, Galan G, et al. Observations of the effects of aerosolized albuterol in acute asthma. *Am J Respir Crit Care Med* 1997;155:454.

76. McFadden ER Jr, Strauss L, Hejal R, et al. Comparison of two dosage regimens of albuterol in acute asthma. *Am J Med* 1998;105:12.

77. Emerman CL, Cydulka RK, McFadden ER. Comparison of 2.5 mg vs 7.5 mg of inhaled albuterol in the treatment of acute asthma. *Chest* 1999;115: 92.

78. Besbes-Ouanes L, Nouira S, Elatrous S, et al. Continuous versus intermittent nebulization of salbutamol in acute severe asthma: a randomized, controlled trial. *Ann Emerg Med* 2000;36:198.

79. Rossing TH, Fanta CH, McFadden ER. Effect of outpatient treatment of asthma with beta agonists on the response to sympathomimetics in an emergency room. *Am J Med* 1983;75:781.

80. Rudnitsky GS, Eberlein RS, Schoffstall JM, et al. Comparison of intermittent and continuously nebulized albuterol for treatment of asthma in an urban emergency department. *Ann Emerg Med* 1993;22:1842–1846.

81. Lin RY, Sauter D, Newman T, et al. Continuous versus intermittent albuterol nebulization in the treatment of acute asthma. *Ann Emerg Med* 1993;22:1847–1853.

82. Lipworth BJ, Clark RA, Dhillon DP, et al. Beta-adrenoceptor responses to high doses of inhaled salbutamol in patients with bronchial asthma. *Br J Clin Pharmacol* 1988;26:527–533.

83. Newhouse MT, Chapman KR, McCallum AL, et al. Cardiovascular safety of high doses of inhaled fenoterol and albuterol in acute severe asthma. *Chest* 1996;110:595.

84. Gern JE, Lemanske RF. Beta-adrenergic agonist therapy. *Immunol Allergy Clin North Am* 1993;13:839.

85. Paterson JW, Evans RJC, Prime FJ. Selectivity of bronchodilator action of salbutamol in asthmatic patients. *Br J Dis Chest* 1971;65:21.

86. Shrestha M, Gourlay S, Robertson S, et al. Isoetharine versus albuterol for acute asthma: greater immediate effect, but more side effects. *Am J Med* 1996;100:323.

87. Nelson H, Bensch G, Pleskow WW, et al. Improved bronchodilation with levalbuterol compared with racemic albuterol in patients with asthma. *J Allergy Clin Immunol* 1998;102:943.

88. Peters JI, Shelledy DC, Jones AP, et al. A randomized, placebo-controlled study to evaluate the role of salmeterol in the in-hospital management of asthma. *Chest* 2000;118:313.

89. Matz J, et al. *Allergy Clin Immunol* 2000;105(suppl): 162.

90. Idris AH, McDermott MF, Raucci JC, et al. Emergency department treatment of severe asthma: metered-dose inhaler plus holding chamber is equivalent in effectiveness to nebulizer. *Chest* 1993;103:665.

91. Colacone A, Afilalo M, Wolkove N, et al. A comparison of albuterol administered by metered dose inhaler (and holding chamber) or wet nebulizer in acute asthma. *Chest* 1993;104:835–841.

92. Kerem E, Levison H, Shuh S, et al. Efficacy of albuterol administered by nebulizer versus spacer device in children with acute asthma. *J Pediatr* 1993;123:313–317.

93. Rodrigo C, Rodrigo G. Salbutamol treatment of acute severe asthma in the ED: MDI vs hand-held nebulizer. *Am J Med* 1998;16:637.

94. Fanta CH, Rossing TH, McFadden ER. Treatment of acute asthma: is combination therapy with sympathomimetics and methylxanthines indicated? *Am J Med* 1986;80:5.

95. Uden DL, Goetz, DR, Kohen DP, et al. Comparison of nebulized terbutaline and subcutaneous epinephrine in the treatment of acute asthma. *Ann Emerg Med* 1985;14:229.

96. Becker AB, Nelson NA, Simons FER. Inhaled salbutamol (albuterol) vs injected epinephrine in the treatment of acute asthma in children. *J Pediatr* 1983;102:465.

97. Appel D, Karpel JP, Sherman M. Epinephrine improves expiratory airflow rates in patients with asthma who do not respond to inhaled metaproterenol sulfate. *J Allergy Clin Immunol* 1989;84:90.

98. Cydulka R, Davison R, Grammer L, et al. The use of epinephrine in the treatment of older adult asthmatics. *Ann Emerg Med* 1990;17:322.

99. Lawford P, Jones BMJ, Milledge JS. Comparison of intravenous and nebulised salbutamol in initial treatment of severe asthma. *BMJ* 1978;1:84.

100. Williams SJ, Winner SJ, Clark TJH. Comparison of inhaled and intravenous terbutaline in acute severe asthma. *Thorax* 1981;36:629.

101. Bloomfield P, Carmichael J, Petrie GR, et al. Comparison of salbutamol given intravenously and by intermittent positive-pressure breathing in life-threatening asthma. *BMJ* 1979;1:848.

102. Salmeron S, Brochard L, Mal H, et al. Nebulized versus intravenous albuterol in hypercapnic acute asthma: a multicenter, double-blind, randomized study. *Am J Respir Crit Care Med* 1994;149:1466.

103. McFadden ER Jr, Kiser R, deGroot WJ, et al. A controlled study of the effects of single doses of hydrocortisone on the resolution of acute attacks of asthma. *Am J Med* 1976;60:52.

104. Rodrigo G, Rodrigo C. Corticosteroids in the emergency department therapy of acute asthma: an evidence-based evaluation. *Chest* 1999;116:285.

105. Rodrigo C, Rodrigo G. Early administration of hydrocortisone in the emergency room treatment of acute asthma: a controlled clinical trial. *Respir Med* 1994;88:755.

106. Littenberg B, Gluck EH. A controlled trial of methylprednisolone in the emergency treatment of acute asthma. *N Engl J Med* 1986;314:150–152.

107. Lin RY, Pesola GR, Bakalchuk L, et al. Rapid improvement of peak flow in asthmatic patients treated with parenteral methylprednisolone in the emergency department: a randomized controlled study. *Ann Emerg Med* 1999;33:487.

108. Rowe BH, Keller JL, Oxman AD. Effectiveness of steroid therapy in acute exacerbations of asthma: a meta-analysis. *Am J Emerg Med* 1992;10:301.

109. Connett GJ, Warde C, Wooler E, et al. Prednisolone and salbutamol in the hospital treatment of acute asthma. *Arch Dis Child* 1994;70:170–173.

110. Fanta CH, Rossing TH, McFadden ER Jr. Glucocorticoids in acute asthma. A critical controlled trial. *Am J Med* 1983;74:845–851.

111. Scarfone RJ, Fuchs SM, Nager AL, et al. Controlled trial of oral prednisone in the emergency room treatment of children with acute asthma. *Pediatrics* 1993;2:513–518.

112. Chapman KR, Verbeek PR, White JG, et al. Effect of a short course of prednisone in the prevention of early relapse after the emergency room treatment of acute asthma. *N Engl J Med* 1991;324:788–794.

113. Benatar SR. Fatal asthma. *N Engl J Med* 1986;314:423.

114. Reid MR, Abramson M. Corticosteroids for acute severe asthma in hospitalized patients. *Cochrane Database System Review* 2000;2:CD001740.

115. Emerman CL, Cydulka RK. A randomized comparison of 100-mg vs 500-mg dose of methylprednisolone in the treatment of acute asthma. *Chest* 1995;107: 1559–1563.

116. Haskell RJ, Wong BM, Hansen JE. A double-blind, randomized clinical trial of methylprednisolone in status asthmaticus. *Arch Intern Med* 1983;143:1324–1327.

117. Bowler SD, Mitchell CA, Armstrong JG. Corticosteroids in acute severe asthma: effectiveness of low doses. *Thorax* 1992;47:584.

118. Engel T, Dirksen A, Frolund L. Methylprednisolone pulse therapy in acute sever asthma. A randomized, double-blind study. *Allergy* 1990;45:224.

119. Volovitz B, Bentur L, Finkelstein Y, et al. Effectiveness and safety of inhaled corticosteroids in controlling acute asthma attacks in children who were treated in the emergency department: a controlled comparative study with oral prednisone. *J Allergy Clin Immunol* 1998;102: 605.

120. Rodrigo G, Rodrigo C. Inhaled flunisolide for acute severe asthma. *Am J Respir Crit Care Med* 1998;157: 698.

121. McFadden ER Jr. Inhaled glucocorticoids in acute asthma. Therapeutic breakthrough or nonspecific effect. *Am J Respir Crit Care Med* 1998;157:677.

122. Guttman A, Afilalo M, Colacone A, et al. The effects of combined intravenous and inhaled steroids (beclomethasone dipropionate) for the emergency treatment of acute asthma. The Asthma ED Study Group. *Acad Emerg Med* 1997;4:100–106.

123. Afilalo M, Guttman A, Colacone A, et al. Efficacy of inhaled steroids (beclomethasone dipropionate) for treatment of mild to moderately severe asthma in the emergency department: a randomized clinical trial. *Ann Emerg Med* 1999;33:304.

124. Bryant DH. Nebulised ipratropium bromide in the treatment of acute asthma. *Chest* 1985;88:24.

125. Bryant DH, Rogers P. Effects of ipratropium bromide nebulizer solution with and without preservatives in the treatment of acute and stable asthma. *Chest* 1992;102:742.

126. Shuh S, Johnson DW, Callahan S, et al. Efficacy of frequent nebulized ipratropium bromide added to

frequent high-dose albuterol in severe childhood asthma. *J Pediatr* 1995;126:639–645.

127. Kelly HW, Murphy S. Should anticholinergics be used in acute severe asthma? *DICP Ann Pharmacother* 1990:24:409–414.

128. Karpel JP, Schacter EN, Fanta C, et al. A comparison of ipratropium and albuterol vs albuterol alone for treatment of acute asthma. *Chest* 1996;110:611.

129. Garrett JE, Town GI, Rodwell P, Kelly AM. Nebulized salbutamol with and without ipratropium bromide in the treatment of acute asthma. *J Allergy Clin Immunol* 1997;100:165–170.

130. Lin RY, Pesola GR, Bakalchuk L, et al. Superiority of ipratropium bromide plus albuterol over albuterol alone in the emergency department management of adult asthma: a randomized clinical trial. *Ann Emerg Med* 1998;31:208.

131. Stoodley RG, Aaron SD, Dales RE. The role of ipratropium bromide in the emergency management of acute asthma exacerbation: a meta-analysis of randomized clinical trials. *Ann Emerg Med* 1999; 34:8.

132. Lanes SF, Garrett JE, Wentworth CE 3rd, et al. The effect of adding ipratropium bromide to salbutamol in the treatment of acute asthma: a pooled analysis of three trials. *Chest* 1998;114:365.

133. Zorc JJ, Pusic MV, Ogborn CJ, et al. Ipratropium bromide added to asthma treatment in the pediatric emergency department. *Pediatrics* 1999;103:748.

134. Qureshi F, Pestian J, Davis P, et al. Effect of nebulized ipratropium on hospitalization rates of children with asthma. *N Engl J Med* 1998;339:1030.

135. Weber EJ, Levitt A, Covington JK, Gambrioli E. Effect of continuously nebulized ipratropium bromide plus albuterol on emergency department length of stay and hospital admission rates in patients with acute bronchospasm. *Chest* 1999;115:937.

136. Fitzgerald JM, Grunfeld A, Pare PD, et al., and the Canadian Combivent Study Group. The clinical efficacy of combination nebulized anticholinergic and adrenergic bronchodilators vs nebulized adrenergic bronchodilator alone in acute asthma. *Chest* 1997;111:311–315.

137. Ducharme FM, Davis GM. Randomized controlled trial of ipratropium bromide and frequent low doses of salbutamol in the management of mild and moderate acute pediatric asthma. *J Pediatr* 1998;133:479.

138. O'Driscoll BR, Taylor RJ, Horsley MG, et al. Nebulised salbutamol with and without ipratropium in acute airflow obstruction. *Lancet* 1989;1:1418–1420.

139. McFadden ER, El Sanadi N, Strauss L, et al. The influence of parasympatholytics on the resolution of acute attacks of asthma. *Am J Med* 1997;102:7–13.

140. Rodrigo GJ, Rodrigo C. First-line therapy for adult patients with acute severe asthma receiving a multiple-dose protocol of ipratropium bromide plus albuterol in the emergency department. *Am J Respir Crit Care Med* 2000;161:1862–1868.

141. Rodrigo C, Rodrigo G. Treatment of acute asthma: lack of therapeutic benefit and increase of the toxicity from aminophylline given in addition to high doses of salbutamol delivered by metered-dose inhaler with a spacer. *Chest* 1994;106:1071.

142. Murphy DG, McDermott MF, Rydman RJ, et al. Aminophylline in the treatment of acute asthma when beta two adrenergics and steroids are provided. *Arch Intern Med* 1993;153:1784–1788.

143. Siegel D, Sheppard D, Gelb A, et al. Aminophylline increases the toxicity but not the efficacy of an inhaled beta-adrenergic agonist in the treatment of acute exacerbations of asthma. *Am Rev Respir Dis* 1985;132:283–286.

144. Coleridge J, Cameron P, Epstein J, et al. Intravenous aminophylline confers no benefit in acute asthma treated with intravenous steroids and inhaled bronchodilators. *Aust N Z J Med* 1993;23:348–354.

145. Nuhoglu Y, Dai A, Barlan IB, et al. Efficacy of aminophylline in the treatment of acute asthma exacerbation in children. *Ann Allergy Asthma Immunol* 1998;80:395.

146. Vieira SE, Lotufo JP, Ejzenberg B, et al. Efficacy of IV aminophylline as a supplemental therapy in moderate broncho-obstructive crisis in infants and preschool children.*Pulm Pharmacol Ther* 2000;13:189.

147. Huang D, O'Brien RG, Harman E, et al. Does aminophylline benefit adults admitted to the hospital for an acute exacerbation of asthma? *Ann Intern Med* 1993;119:1155–1160.

148. Pierson WE, Bierman CW, Stamm SJ, et al. Double-blind trial of aminophylline in status asthmaticus. *Pediatrics* 1971;48:642–646.

149. Yung M, South M. Randomised controlled trial of aminophylline for severe acute asthma. *Arch Dis Child* 1998;79:405.

150. Wrenn K, Slovis CM, Murphy F, et al. Aminophylline therapy for acute bronchospastic disease in the emergency room. *Ann Intern Med* 1991;115:241–247.

151. Persson CGA. Xanthines as airway antiinflammatory drugs. *J Allergy Clin Immunol* 1988;81:615–617.

152. Pauwels RA. New aspects of the therapeutic potential of theophylline in asthma. *J Allergy Clin Immunol* 1989;83:548–553.

153. Evans WV, Monie RDH, Crimmins J, et al. Aminophylline, salbutamol and combined intravenous infusions in acute severe asthma. *Br J Dis Chest* 1980;74:385.

154. Pierson WE, Bierman CW, Stamm SJ, et al. Double-blind trial of aminophylline in status asthmaticus. *Pediatrics* 1971;48:642–646.

155. Kelly HW, Murphy S. Should we stop using theophylline for the treatment of the hospitalized patient with status asthmaticus. *DICP* 1989;23:995–998.

156. Milgrom H. Theophylline. *Immunol Allergy Clin North Am* 1993;13:819–838.

157. Littenberg B. Aminophylline in severe, acute asthma: a meta-analysis. *JAMA* 1988;259:1678–1684.

158. Weinberger M, Hendeles L. Slow-release theophylline: rationale and basis for product selection. *N Engl J Med* 1983;308:760–764.

159. Reynolds RJ, Buford JG, George RB. Treating asthma and COPD in patients with heart disease. *J Respir Dis* 1982;3:41–51.

160. George RB. Preventing arrhythmias in acute asthma. *J Respir Dis* 1991;12:545–561.

161. Green SM, Rothrock SG. Intravenous magnesium for acute asthma: failure to decrease emergency treatment duration or need for hospitalization. *Ann Emerg Med* 1992;21:260.

162. Tiffany BR, Berk W, Todd IK, et al. Magnesium bolus or infusion fails to improve expiratory flow in acute asthma exacerbations. *Chest* 1993;104:831.

163. Scarfone RJ, Loiselle JM, Joffe MD, et al. A randomized trial of magnesium in the emergency department treatment of children with asthma. *Ann Emerg Med* 2000;36:572.

164. Boonyavorakul C, Thakkinstian A, Charoenpan P. Intravenous magnesium sulfate in acute severe asthma. *Respirology* 2000;5:221.

165. Ciarallo L, Brousseau D, Reinert S. Higher-dose intravenous magnesium therapy for children with moderate to severe acute asthma. *Arch Pediatr Adolesc Med* 2000;154:979.

166. Gurkan F, Haspolat K, Bosnak M, et al. Intravenous magnesium sulphate in the management of moderate to severe acute asthmatic children nonresponding to conventional therapy. *Eur J Emerg Med* 1999;6:201.

167. Rodrigo G, Rodrigo C, Burschtin O. Efficacy of magnesium sulfate in acute adult asthma: a meta-analysis of randomized trials. *Am J Emerg Med* 2000;18:216–221.

168. Alters HJ, Koepsell TD, Hilty WM. Intravenous magnesium as an adjuvant in acute bronchospasm: a meta-analysis. *Ann Emerg Med* 2000;36:191.

169. Rowe BH, Bretzlaff JA, Bourdon C, et al. Intravenous magnesium sulfate treatment for acute asthma in the emergency department: a systematic review of the literature. *Ann Emerg Med* 2000;36:181.

170. Bloch H, Silverman R, Mancherje N, et al. Intravenous magnesium sulfate as an adjunct in the treatment of acute asthma. *Chest* 1995;107.1576.

171. Sydow M, Crozier TA, Zielmann S, et al. High-dose intravenous magnesium sulfate in the management of life-threatening status asthmaticus. *Intens Care Med* 1993;19:467.

172. Skobeloff EM, Spivey WH, McNamara RM. Estrogen alters the response of bronchial smooth muscle [Abstract]. *Ann Emerg Med* 1992;21:647.

173. Nannini LJ, Pendino JC, Corna RA, et al. Magnesium sulfate as a vehicle for nebulized salbutamol in acute asthma. *Am J Med* 2000;108:193–197.

174. Madison JM, Irwin RS. Heliox for asthma: a trial balloon. *Chest* 1995;107:597–598.

175. Curtis JL, Mahlmeister M, Fink JB, et al. Helium oxygen gas therapy: use and availability for the emergency treatment of inoperable airway obstruction. *Chest* 1986;90:455.

176. Manthous CA, Hall JB, Caputo ME, et al. The effect of heliox on pulsus paradoxus and peak flow in non-intubated patients with severe asthma. *Am J Respir Crit Care Med* 1995;151:310.

177. Kudukis TM, Manthous CA, Schmidt GA, et al. Inhaled helium-oxygen revisited: effect of inhaled helium-oxygen during the treatment of status asthmaticus in children. *J Pediatr* 1997;130:217–224.

178. Verbeek PR, Chopra A. Heliox does not improve FEV1 in acute asthma patients. *J Emerg Med* 1998;16:545–548.

179. Dorfman TA, Shipley ER, Burton JH, et al. Inhaled heliox does not benefit ED patients with moderate to severe ashtma. *Am J Emerg Med* 2000;18:495.

180. Melmed A, Hebb DB, Pohlman A, et al. The use of heliox as a vehicle for beta-agonist nebulization in patients with severe asthma [Abstract]. *Am J Respir Crit Care Med* 1995;151:269.

181. Henderson SO, Acharya P, Kilaghbian T, et al. Use of heliox-driven nebulizer therapy in the treatment of acute asthma. *Ann Emerg Med* 1999;33:141.

182. Silverman R, Miller C, Chen Y, et al. Zafirlukast reduces relapses and treatment failures after an acute asthma episode. *Chest* 1999;116(suppl):296.

183. Murray PT, Corbridge T. Pharmacotherapy of acute asthma. In: Hall, Corbridge, Rodrigo, et al., eds. *Acute asthma: assessment and management.* New York: McGraw-Hill, 2000:139–160.

184. Shivaram U, Miro AM, Cash ME, et al. Cardiopulmonary responses to continuous positive airway pressure in acute asthma. *J Crit Care* 1993;8:87.

185. Martin JG, Shore S, Engel LA. Effect of continuous positive airway pressure on respiratory mechanics and pattern of breathing in induced asthma. *Am Rev Respir Dis* 1982;126:812.

186. Meduri GU, Cook TR, Turner RE, et al. Noninvasive positive pressure ventilation in status asthmaticus. *Chest* 1996;110:767.

187. Tuxen D. Mechanical ventilation in asthma. In: Evans T, Hinds C, eds. *Recent advances in critical care,* 4th ed. London: Churchill Livingstone, 1996:165.

188. Tuxen DV, Williams TJ, Scheinkestel CD, et al. Use of a measurement of pulmonary hyperinflation to control the level of mechanical ventilation in patients with acute severe asthma. *Am Rev Respir Dis* 1992;146:1136.

189. Tuxen DV, Lane S. The effects of ventilatory pattern on hyperinflation, airway pressures, and circulation in mechanical ventilation of patients with severe air-flow obstruction. *Am Rev Respir Dis* 1987;136:872.

190. Williams TJ, Tuxen DV, Scheinkestel CD, et al. Risk factors for morbidity in mechanically ventilated patients with acute severe asthma. *Am Rev Respir Dis* 1992;146:607.

191. Marini JJ, Capps JS, Culver BH. The inspiratory work of breathing during assisted mechanical ventilation. *Chest* 1985;87:612.

192. Tuxen DV. Detrimental effects of positive end-expiratory pressure during controlled mechanical ventilation of patients with severe airflow obstruction. *Am Rev Respir Dis* 1989;140:5.

193. Leatherman JW, Ravenscraft SA. Low measured auto-positive end-expiratory pressure during mechanical ventilation of patients with severe asthma: hidden auto-positive end-expiratory pressure. *Crit Care Med* 1996;24:541.

194. Feihl F, Perret C. State of the art: permissive hypercapnia: how permissive should we be? *Am J Respir Crit Care Med* 1994;150:1722.

195. Darioli R, Perret C. Mechanical controlled hypoventilation in status asthmaticus. *Am Rev Respir Dis* 1984;129:385.

196. Tuxen DV. Permissive hypercapnic ventilation. *Am J Respir Crit Care Med* 1994;150:870.

197. Cooper DJ, Calles JB, Scheinkestel CD, et al. Does bicarbonate improve cardiac or respiratory function during respiratory acidosis and acute severe asthma—a prospective randomized study [Abstract]. *Am Rev Respir Dis* 1993;147:614.

198. Kress JP, O'Connor MF, Pohlman AS, et al. Sedation of critically ill patients during mechanical ventilation: a comparison of propofol and midazolam. *Am J Resp Crit Care Med* 1996;153:1012.

199. Pohlman A, Simpson K, Hall J. Continuous intravenous infusions of lorazepam vs. midazolam for sedation during mechanical ventilatory support: a prospective, randomized study. *Crit Care Med* 1994; 22:1241.

200. Murray MJ, DeRuyter ML, Harrison BA. Opioids and benzodiazepines. *Crit Care Clin* 1995;4:849.
201. Corseen G, Gutierrez J, Reves JG, et al. Ketamine in the anaesthetic management of asthmatic patients. *Anesth Analg* 1972;51:588.
202. Sarma VJ. Use of ketamine in acute severe asthma. *Acta Anaesthesiol Scand* 1992;36:106.
203. Rock MJ, Reyes de la Rocha S, L'Hommedieu ET. Use of ketamine in asthmatic children to treat respiratory failure refractory to conventional therapy. *Crit Care Med* 1986;14:514.
204. Caldwell JE, Lau M, Fisher DM. Atracurium versus vecuronium in asthmatic patients. A blinded, randomized comparison of advere events. *Anesthesiology* 1995;83:986.
205. Leatherman JW, Fluegel WL, David WS, et al. Muscle weakness in mechanically ventilated patients with severe asthma. *Am J Respir Crit Care Med* 1996;153:1686.
206. Behbehani NA, Al-Mane F, D'yachkova Y, et al. Myopathy following mechanical ventilation for acute severe asthma: the role of muscle relaxants and corticosteroids. *Chest* 1999;115:1627.
207. Douglass JA, Tuxen D, Horne M, et al. Myopathy in severe asthma. *Am Rev Respir Dis* 1992;146:517.
208. MacIntyre NR, Silver RM, Miller CW, etal. Aerosol delivery in intubated, mechanically ventilated patients. *Crit Care Med* 1985;13:81.
209. Manthous CA, Hall JB, Schmidt GA, et al. Metered-dose inhaler versus nebulized albuterol in mechanically ventilated patients. *Am Rev Respir Dis* 1993;148:1567.
210. Manthous CA, Hall JB. Update on using therapeutic aerosols in mechanically ventilated patients. *J Crit Illness* 1996;11:457.
211. Saulnier FF, Durocher AV, Deturck RA, et al. Respiratory and hemodynamic effects of halothane in status asthmaticus. *Intens Care Med* 1990;16:104.
212. Echeverria M, Gelb AW, Wexler HR, et al. Enflurane and halothane in status asthmaticus. *Chest* 1986;89:153.
213. Gluck EH, Onorato DJ, Castriotta R. Helium-oxygen mixtures in intubated patients with status asthmaticus and respiratory acidosis. *Chest* 1990;98:693.
214. Smith DL, Deshazo RD. Bronchoalveolar lavage in asthma. State of the art. *Am Rev Respir Dis* 1993;148:523–532.
215. Millman M, Millman FM, Goldstein IM, et al. Use of acetylcysteine in bronchial asthma—another look. *Ann Allergy* 1985;54:294.
216. Lang DM, Simon RA, Mathison DA, et al. Safety and possible efficacy of fiberoptic bronchoscopy with lavage in the management of refractory asthma with mucous impaction. *Ann Allergy* 1991;67:324–330.

29

Radiologic Evaluation of Allergic and Related Diseases of the Upper Airway

Michelle J. Naidich and *Eric J. Russell

*Department of Radiology, Northwestern University Medical School,
Northwestern Memorial Hospital, Chicago, Illinois; *Department of Radiology,
Neurosurgery, and Otolaryngology, Northwestern University, Department of Radiology,
Northwestern Memorial Hospital, Chicago, Illinois*

ANATOMY

The complex anatomy, and the terminology used to describe the anatomy of the paranasal sinuses and nasal cavity, is best approached by first reviewing the normal drainage pattern of sinonasal secretions. Functional anatomy is intimately related to the pathophysiology of sinus inflammatory disease, and understanding it is critical in the planning of functional endoscopic sinus surgery (FESS).

The osteomeatal complex comprises the primary functional drainage unit for the anterior paranasal sinuses. This region encompasses the maxillary and anterior and middle ethmoid sinus ostia, frontonasal recess, ethmoidal infundibulum, uncinate process, ethmoid bulla, semilunar hiatus, and middle meatus.

Within the maxillary sinus, mucous secretions, trapped dust particles, and inflammatory cells are propelled in a circumferential fashion by mucoperiosteal ciliated epithelium, and directed superomedially toward the natural ostium of the antrum. Extending from the ostium is an aerated channel called the infundibulum, which is bordered by the inferomedial orbital wall laterally and by the uncinate process medially. The uncinate process arises as an extension from the lateral wall of the nasal cavity behind the nasolacrimal fossa (Fig. 29.1). Secretions passing through the infundibulum reach the semilunar hiatus, a region just beyond the tip of the uncinate process and below the ethmoid bulla, which in turn opens into the middle meatus. The ethmoid bulla is defined as the largest anteroinferior ethmoid air cell. It receives secretions from the middle ethmoid air cells and itself drains into the semilunar hiatus. The anterior ethmoid air cells have individual ostia that open into the infundibulum. The frontal sinus drains through the frontonasal recess, into the infundibulum and middle meatus. Secretions from the middle meatus drain posteriorly through the posterior nasal choanae into the nasopharynx (1,2).

Within the nasal cavity there are typically three paired sets of bony projections (the superior, middle, and inferior nasal turbinates) that arise from the lateral nasal wall. The middle meatus is the air space lateral to the middle nasal turbinate. The middle nasal turbinate has a vertical plate (lamella) that attaches to the cribriform plate, and a lateral lamella, which is a small projection of bone extending lateral to this vertical attachment to the roof of the ethmoid air cells (fovea ethmoidalis). This segment is susceptible to injury during sinus surgery. There is also a horizontal attachment of the middle turbinate to the lamina papyracea (medial orbital wall) called the basal lamella. The basal lamella is the bony plate that separates the anterior and middle ethmoid air cells from the posterior ethmoid cells. The

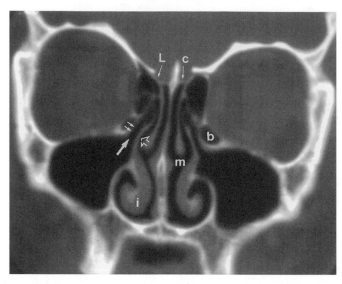

FIG. 29.1. Normal coronal computed tomogram through the region of the osteomeatal complex. The maxillary sinus drains through its ostium (*solid arrow*) into the infundibulum (*small double arrows*). The infundibulum is bordered by the medial orbital floor, the ethmoid bulla (*b*), and the uncinate process (*open arrow*). Both the inferior (*i*) and middle (*m*) turbinates are seen. The middle turbinate has a vertical attachment to the cribriform plate (*c*). The segment of bone lateral to this vertical attachment is called the lateral lamella (*L*).

superior meatus is the region lateral to the superior turbinate. It receives secretions from the posterior ethmoid cells and the sphenoid sinuses via the sphenoethmoidal recesses (Fig. 29.2). This distinct functional region is sometimes called the posterior osteomeatal unit. The inferior meatus, which lies lateral to the inferior turbinate, does not serve as a drainage passageway for sinus secretions, but receives drainage of tears from the nasolacrimal sac and duct (1–3).

The nasal cavity is divided vertically by the nasal septum. The anterior part of the septum is cartilaginous (quadrangular cartilage), and the bony posterior portion is made up of the vomer inferiorly and the perpendicular plate of the ethmoid bone superiorly. The nasal cavity communicates posteriorly with the nasopharynx via the posterior nasal choanae. The floor of the nasal cavity consists of the hard palate (anteriorly) and the soft palate (posteriorly) (1–3).

ANATOMIC VARIANTS

Earwaker (4) analyzed the computed tomography (CT) scans of 800 patients who were referred for evaluation prior to FESS. He found that only

57 of these 800 patients had no anatomic variants. Of the described 52 types of anatomic variants, 93% of the patients had one or more variants. Although these variants are frequently of no clinical significance, in some circumstances they may predispose to obstruction of the normal pathways of mucous drainage, or they may serve to increase the risk of complications associated with FESS. Consequently, familiarity with some of the more common variants is important.

Several variations in the anatomy of the nasal cavity can result in narrowing of the middle meatus and predispose to obstruction to drainage of the ipsilateral maxillary, ethmoidal, and frontal sinuses. For example, the nasal septum may be severely deviated toward one side, narrowing the ipsilateral osteomeatal complex. Similarly, a bony nasal septal spur may compromise the middle meatus. Normally, the middle turbinates are convex medially. Paradoxic middle turbinate is a term referring to a reversal of this curvature, so that convexity is directed laterally toward the nasal wall. The middle meatus is narrowed, which may predispose to sinus obstruction when associated with mucosa inflammation or edema. Earwaker (4) found in his series that 94% of the

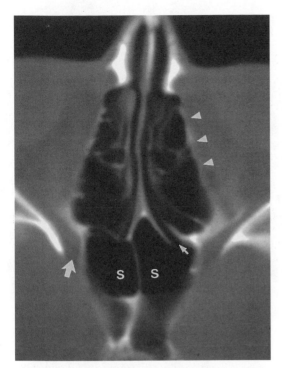

FIG. 29.2. Normal axial computed tomogram through the sphenoid sinus ostia. The posterior ethmoid air cells and the sphenoid sinuses (*S*) drain through the sphenoethmoidal recess (*small arrow*) into the superior meatus. The lamina papyracea (*arrowheads*) is the thin bony separation that makes up the lateral wall of the ethmoid sinuses and the medial wall of the orbit. Note the close proximity of the superior orbital fissure (*large arrow*) to the sphenoid sinus wall.

cases of large paradoxic middle turbinates had associated ipsilateral nasal septal deviation. A concha bullosa is a middle turbinate that is aerated from the ethmoidal cells (Fig. 29.3). Various studies use different degrees of pneumatization to define a concha bullosa; consequently, the reported prevalence ranges from 4% to 80% (5). When large, and some are quite large, the concha bullosa may obstruct the middle meatus. Also, because it is lined by secretory mucoperiosteum, the concha bullosa is prone to the same sinus disease processes as other air cells (2).

A Haller cell is an air cell that lies below the ethmoid bulla, within the superomedial maxillary antrum, along the inferior medial margin of the orbit (Fig. 29.4). A large Haller cell may narrow the maxillary sinus ostium or the infundibulum, depending on its specific position along the

sinus margin. Agger nasi cells are the most anterior ethmoidal air cells, located anterior, lateral, and inferior to the frontal recess. These cells are in, or adjacent to, the nasal bones, and may anatomically narrow the frontal sinus outlet (1,6). These cells also are important surgical landmarks for the position of the frontal-nasal recess.

Variations in the uncinate process can contribute to obstruction of the infundibulum. The free margin of the uncinate may be pneumatized and thereby expanded. The orientation of the uncinate process may be vertical, horizontal or anywhere in between. Occasionally, the tip of the uncinate process is laterally deviated and adherent to the adjacent orbital wall, a situation called atelectatic uncinate. Associated findings may include ipsilateral hypoplastic maxillary sinus and a low-lying orbital floor (4). This variant also may contribute to infundibular obstruction.

Variations in the degree of pneumatization of the sphenoid sinus are particularly important in increasing the risk of surgical mishap. The internal carotid artery runs lateral to the lateral sinus wall, and if medially displaced, may bulge into the sinus lumen, with the possibility of injury during sinus surgery, which may lead to fatal hemorrhage or pseudoaneurysm formation (Fig. 29.5). Onodi cells are posterior ethmoid air cells that have pneumatized the anterior sphenoid bone. They lie in proximity to the orbital apex, optic canal, and optic nerves. This variant therefore increases the risk of injury to these structures during endoscopic surgery. The anterior clinoid processes (and the optic struts) normally form the lateral wall of the optic canal. Clinoid pneumatization can therefore expose the optic nerve to surgical damage during sphenoid sinus surgery. Also, an asymmetric low-lying ethmoid roof increases the chances of inadvertent breech by the unsuspecting surgeon; this may result in damage to the anterior ethmoidal artery with the risk of intracranial hemorrhage (2,4,6,7).

IMAGING TECHNIQUE

Full radiographic imaging of the sinuses is usually reserved for those patients with clinical signs and symptoms of sinusitis who have failed standard antibiotic treatment (chronic sinusitis) or who have recurrent episodes of sinusitis, and are

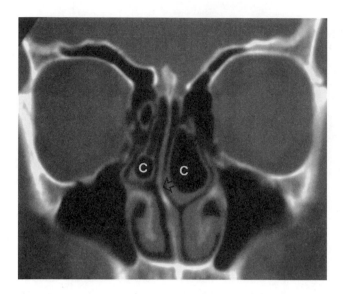

FIG. 29.3. Coronal computed tomogram demonstrating bilateral, left larger than right, concha bullosa (*C*) of the middle turbinates. The nasal septum is deviated to the right (*open black arrow*).

potentially surgical candidates. Anatomic causes and underlying disease processes can be visualized, and the feasibility and risk of surgery can be evaluated. Additionally, any patient with a suspected complication of sinusitis or a presumed surgical complication should be imaged.

Standard radiography, while being fast and relatively cheap, is only able to reliably evaluate the lower third of the nasal cavity, and the maxillary, frontal, sphenoid, and posterior ethmoid sinuses.

The anterior ethmoid cells, the upper two thirds of the nasal cavity, the middle meatus, and the frontal recess are often obscured by overlying structures. Consequently, cross-sectional imaging modalities, which eliminate the overlap of adjacent structures, are usually more definitive (2,6).

Computed tomography is the imaging modality of choice for routine evaluation of the sinuses. When performed for preoperative evaluation of

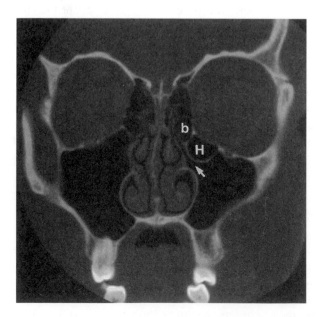

FIG. 29.4. Coronal computed tomogram of a Haller cell (*H*). It is positioned along the inferior medial margin of the orbit and below the ethmoid bulla (*b*). The infundibulum (*arrow*) has a more medial position as a result of the presence of the Haller cell.

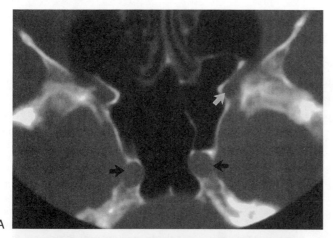

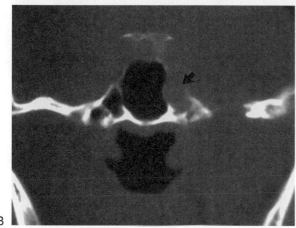

FIG. 29.5. Axial **(A)** and coronal **(B)** computed tomography images demonstrate medial bulging of the internal carotid arteries (*black arrows*) into the sphenoid sinus; the arteries are susceptible to injury during surgery in this location. The superior orbital fissure is again seen (*white arrow*).

fixed sinus obstructive disease, some clinicians recommend preimaging patient preparation consisting of a course of antibiotics to eliminate any acute (transient) mucoperiosteal disease. This is followed by sympathomimetic spray just prior to the scan to minimize reversible congestion and mucous (1,6,8). In theory, this will allow for optimal delineation of the chronic nonreversible sinus disease that should be the target of operative intervention.

Coronal and axial imaging is preferred prior to FESS (6,8). The coronal plane optimally visualizes the osteomeatal unit and corresponds to the surgeon's orientation during endoscopy. The patient is preferably placed prone on the table and the neck is hyperextended. If the patient is unable to tolerate the prone position, the scan may be performed supine with the neck hanging back. Prone images permit fluid to fall away from

the sinus ostium and infundibulum, for a better assessment of these regions. Images are obtained and displayed at both wide "bone" windows and narrow "soft tissue" windows. This is facilitated by soft copy viewing. Transverse axial views are best for evaluation of the posterior wall of the frontal sinus (important to evaluate for bony dehiscence prior to mucosal stripping), and the sphenoid sinus margins and ostia. A standard screening examination, or "limited" sinus examination, can be performed as a screening procedure in patients with clinical signs that are inconclusive for sinusitis. The coronal-only imaging technique is meant to minimize radiation dose and expense. If the patient cannot tolerate hyperextension of the neck, helical or thin overlapped transverse axial images may be obtained, and computer reformatting can be performed to provide images in the coronal or sagittal planes.

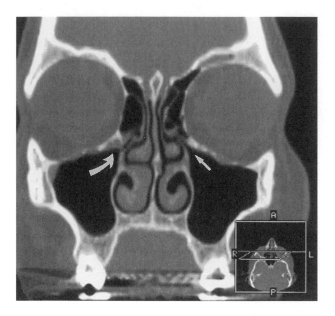

FIG. 29.6. This is a reformatted coronal image. The patient was scanned using helical technique in the axial plane. The volumetric data acquired were then used to create coronal images. The small box on the lower right-hand side indicates the plane at which this image was created. The patent maxillary ostium and infundibulum is clearly seen on the left (*white arrow*). The ostium and infundibulum on the right (*curved arrow*) are not in plane and consequently not as well seen.

With the advent of helical CT scanning, several of the difficulties with patient positioning have been eliminated, and there are opportunities for reducing radiation dose and examination time. This technology allows for rapid acquisition of volumetric data that subsequently can be reformatted at narrow increments in any plane chosen, providing orthogonal reformatted images instead of a second set of direct images, further reducing the examination time and radiation dose. Consequently, the imaging time for the helical technique is faster than with the conventional methods. Although these reformats at the present time are not quite as good as the direct scans, they are a viable alternative (Fig. 29.6). As the technology of helical scanning progresses, the quality of the reformatted images will certainly improve (9,10).

An advantage of magnetic resonance imaging (MRI) over CT scans is the lack of ionizing radiation, and improved soft tissue contrast. In addition, the extensive artifact from dental hardware that may occur on CT is often less problematic with MRI. However, upon directly comparing visualization of the various anatomic structures using both of these imaging techniques, it is clear that the bone detail necessary for evaluating the paranasal sinuses is superior on CT, whereas intraorbital and intracranial contents are better

demonstrated on MRI. Consequently, MRI is the technique of choice for evaluating the complications of sinusitis, spread of neoplastic processes, and postoperative complications, not as the primary modality for evaluating simple inflammatory disease (11).

SINUSITIS

Sinusitis often occurs following an upper respiratory tract infection. The respiratory infection causes mucoperiosteal congestion. At the ostia, there is apposition of mucosal surfaces with obstruction of normal mucociliary clearance, resulting in retention of secretions and stasis. These static secretions provide a medium for bacterial superinfection. Clinically, sinusitis may be classified as acute, recurrent acute, subacute, and chronic (12). These clinical categories do not have well-defined imaging correlates. Bhattacharyya et al. (13) examined the relationship of patients' symptoms and CT findings in 221 subjects. These patients filled out a clinical questionnaire that assessed the severity of their symptoms prior to undergoing CT. Thirty-four percent of these patients had a normal CT scan. There was no significant correlation between the subset of patients with "positive" and "very positive" CT findings and the severity of

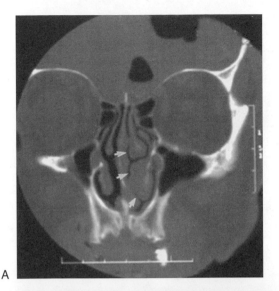

A

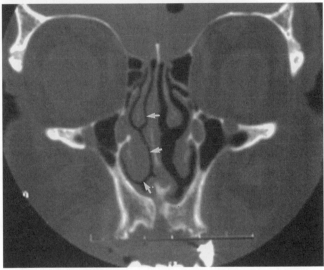

B

FIG. 29.7. Two coronal computed tomography images of the same patient shown in Fig. 29.6 obtained the same day. The first examination **(A)** was performed at 4 PM and the second study **(B)** at 7 PM. There is congestion of the nasal turbinates on the left initially. Later in the same day the congestion is on the right; this is the normal cyclic pattern of congestion of the turbinates (nasal cycle).

their symptoms. Furthermore, the subgroup of patients reporting facial pain as their primary symptom had less impressive imaging findings overall than the patients without facial pain.

It has been noted that the mucoperiosteum lining the nasal turbinates, nasal septum, and ethmoid air cells demonstrates normal cyclic congestion (Fig. 29.7) over each 6-hour period (14). Consequently, mild 1- to 2-mm ethmoid air cell mucoperiosteal thickening may not represent an infectious process but rather transient congestion. It is not surprising that a prospective study performed by Rak et al. (15) showed that 69% of

a group of patients undergoing brain MRI for unrelated reasons demonstrated minimal (1–2 mm) ethmoid mucosal thickening. Sixty-three percent of these patients did not report any symptoms of sinusitis. In fact, only when the mucosal thickening was 4 mm or greater was there significant correlation to symptoms of sinusitis.

The best imaging correlate for acute sinusitis is the air-fluid level, although fluid may accumulate without infection. Transient osteal obstruction may lead to sterile fluid accumulation. Hemorrhage into the sinuses or even tears may accumulate (Fig. 29.8). Acute infection is a

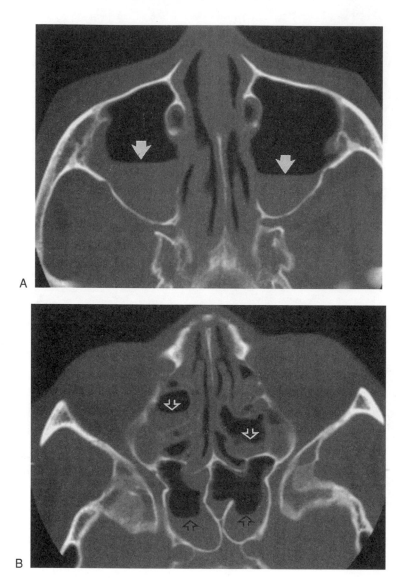

FIG. 29.8. Axial images demonstrate air-fluid levels (*white arrows*) in the maxillary sinuses bilaterally **(A)**, as well as the ethmoid air cells (*white open arrows*) and sphenoid sinuses (*black open arrows*) **(B)** in a patient with acute sinusitis. A coronal image **(C)** from the same patient was obtained with the patient in a supine head-hanging position. The air-fluid levels in the ethmoid and maxillary sinuses are again seen layering in the dependent portions of the sinus cavities. A coronal computed tomogram **(D)** obtained from a different patient in a prone position shows similar maxillary sinus air-fluid levels, but this patient had epistaxis, not acute sinusitis, and the fluid is blood, not secretions.

clinical diagnosis; imaging can support this impression (16). Consequently, sinus images may be interpreted descriptively, without necessarily drawing conclusions regarding the patient's clinical status.

Five major patterns of obstructive and inflammatory change within the nasal cavity and paranasal sinuses have been described (17). These patterns are (a) infundibular, (b) osteomeatal, (c) sphenoethmoidal, (d) sinonasal polyposis, and (e) sporadic (or unclassifiable). The first three patterns correspond to obstruction of known drainage routes with predictable patterns of paranasal sinus involvement (Fig. 29.9).

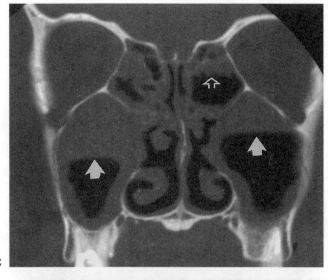

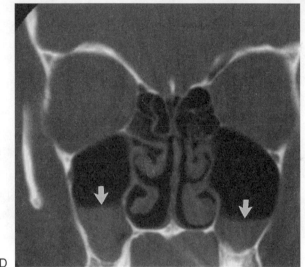

FIG. 29.8. *Continued.*

Sinonasal polyposis is discussed further below. The sporadic category is reserved for mucoperiosteal thickening or other sinus disease without focal obstruction of the drainage pathways. The degree of mucoperiosteal thickening can be graded as mild (<5 mm), moderate (5–10 mm), and severe (>10 mm) (16). The location of mucoperiosteal thickening is also important. It is obvious that a patient with a mild degree of thickening in the region of the infundibulum is more likely to suffer from obstructive sinusitis than a patient with moderate thickening

involving the inferior aspect of the maxillary antrum.

Chronic sinusitis is difficult to define on a single imaging study. Certainly, if a series of examinations demonstrates persistent mucoperiosteal thickening in a symptomatic patient, the diagnosis of chronic sinusitis is likely. Chronic infection can be associated with reactive bony sclerosis and thickening of the walls of the sinus.

On CT scans, chronic inspissated secretions appear as focal central areas of higher attenuation, with more peripheral low attenuation within

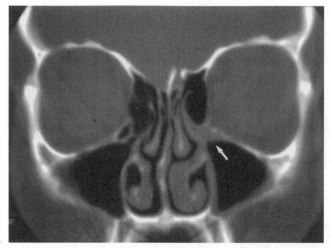

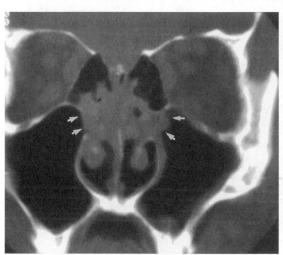

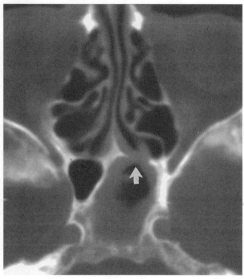

FIG. 29.9. A: A coronal computed tomogram (CT) showing isolated obstruction of the infundibulum on the left (*arrow*). **B:** A coronal CT from a different patient with bilateral obstruction of the osteomeatal complexes due to polyposis. **C:** An axial CT from a third patient with obstruction of the left sphenoid ostium and accumulation of secretions within the sinus cavity.

A

B

C

edematous mucoperiosteum. This finding also raises the possibility of fungal sinusitis (6). The MRI appearance of the soft tissue contents within the sinus cavity is variable, dependent on the proportion of water and protein contents within the secretions. Normal sinus secretions contain 95% water and 5% solid materials, predominately glycomucoproteins. On MRI, the appearance of normal secretions reflects water content; long T1 and T2 relaxation times result in low signal on T1-weighted images, and bright signal on T2-weighted images. With chronic obstruction, there is continuous secretory activity and resorption of water. There are also mucosal changes resulting in an increased number of glycomucoprotein-producing goblet cells. As a result, the overall water content of the secretions is decreased, and the protein concentration and viscosity is increased. At first these changes are reflected in shortening of the T1 relaxation time, causing the secretions to become bright on T1-weighted images. T2 relaxation time is not noticeably affected until the protein concentration is greater than 25%. At this protein concentration, there is cross-linking of the protein molecules, which increases the viscosity of the secretions. This further decreases the T2 relaxation time, and diminished macromolecular motion is also reflected by decreased signal intensity. Eventually, as the secretions become completely dessicated, there is elimination of free water, resulting in marked hypointensity on both sequences. As a result, the sinus may appear as a signal "void" on imaging. Consequently, a chronically obstructed sinus cavity may be falsely interpreted as aerated because the contents look completely devoid of signal (18,19). Fungal sinusitis may have a similar imaging appearance.

Complications of Sinusitis

Mucocele

A complication of chronic sinusitis, a mucocele is an obstructed, completely airless, and expanded sinus, formed by long-standing outlet obstruction (Fig. 29.10). The accumulation of fluid under pressure results in sinus wall remodeling. In fact, it is the most common expansile lesion of the sinuses. Mucoceles are typically solitary, although multiple lesions may occur. Mucoceles most commonly occur in the frontal sinuses (60%–65%), where they may erode into the orbit, resulting in proptosis. The ethmoid sinuses are the second most commonly involved area (20%–25%) followed by the maxillary and rarely the sphenoid sinuses (20). Initially, the appearance of a mucocele may be indistinguishable from a completely opacified sinus due to acute sinusitis. However, with time, there is expansion of the sinus cavity and bony remodeling. Focal lytic changes also may occur, resulting in wall dehiscence. Sinus contents may bulge through bony defects into adjacent regions, and these destructive bony changes may mimic sinus malignancy. The MRI appearance of a mucocele depends on the relative water and protein concentration of its contents. The mucocele may resemble a neoplasm, but generally the T1 and T2 patterns suggest the diagnosis of proteinaceous fluid. With the administration of gadolinium, an MRI contrast agent, a mucocele typically demonstrates thin, regular peripheral enhancement of the mucoperiosteal lining, whereas a neoplasm rarely has a cystic appearance (21,22).

Sinonasal Polyps and Retention Cysts

If there is obstruction of a solitary mucous gland duct and not the whole sinus cavity, a mucous retention cyst arises. This is a homogenous, dome-shaped lesion, with a very thin wall that easily ruptures if the sinus is entered surgically. It rarely fills the entire sinus cavity and does not cause the sinus expansion associated with mucoceles (Fig. 29.11). On MRI, retention cysts have a characteristic morphology, with the fluid contents very bright on T2-weighted images (23). Another complication of chronic sinusitis is the development of sinus polyps. Polyps develop as the result of mucoperiosteal hyperplasia, with abnormal accumulation of submucosal fluid. These lesions are usually solitary and appear as abnormal rounded soft tissue masses, similar to retention cysts. However, polyps are generally not as bright on T2-weighted imaging. Polyps are of little clinical concern unless they cause obstruction of a drainage pathway. When a solitary polyp arises in the maxillary antrum and extends through the middle meatus (between the middle turbinate and the lateral wall of the nasal cavity) posteriorly into the choana, it is called an antrochoanal polyp. The antrochoanal polyp may protrude into the nasopharynx and mimic a mass originating in the oropharynx or nasopharynx. It also may cause obstruction of these air passageways. Much less common is a sphenochoanal polyp, which originates in the sphenoid sinus, protrudes through the sphenoethmoid recess into the nasopharynx, and eventually herniates through the choana. Surgery requires resecting not only the protruding portion of the polyp, but also the sinus component in order to prevent reoccurrence; therefore, definition of the exact origin of these lesions by imaging is imperative (24).

Intracranial Complications of Sinusitis

The incidence of intracranial complications from sinusitis has markedly decreased in recent decades, due to improved management of these cases and imaging guidance of treatment planning. A range of complications may occur (Figs. 29.12 and 29.13), including meningitis, epidural abscess, subdural empyema, brain abscess, cortical venous thrombosis, and venous sinus thrombosis (6,25). Gallagher et al. (26) conducted a chart review for a 5-year period

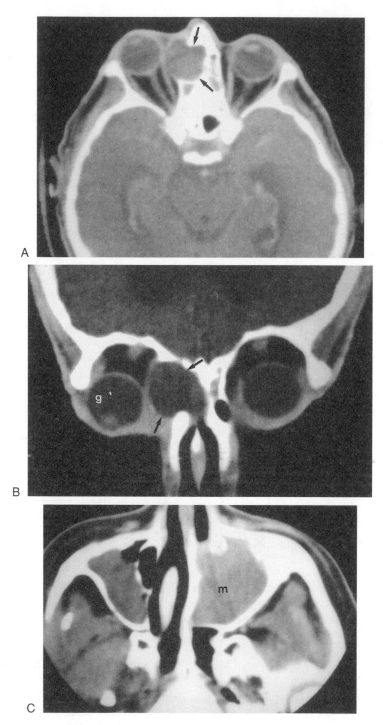

FIG. 29.10. Three examples of mucoceles. An axial **(A)** and a coronal **(B)** computed tomography (CT) image from a patient with a right ethmoid mucocele (*black arrows*). The ethmoid air cell is completely filled with abnormal soft tissue. There is absence of the lateral bony wall and bulging of the mucocele into the orbit. The globe (*g*) is displaced inferolaterally. The second patient has a left maxillary sinus mucocele (*m*). The axial CT **(C)** shows complete opacification of the left maxillary sinus and near complete opacification of the right.   (*Legend continues*)

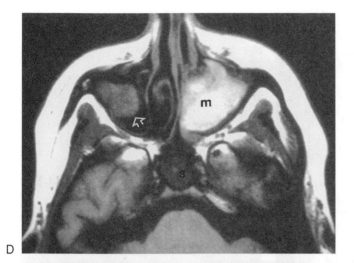

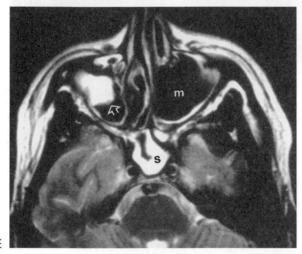

FIG. 29.10. (*Legend "continued" from A–C*) The attenuation of the sinus contents on the left is greater than on the right, consistent with inspissated secretions within the mucocele. This is confirmed on axial magnetic resonance imaging, where the inspissated secretions within the mucocele on the left are bright on the T1-weighted image **(D)** and dark on the T2-weighted image **(E)**. Notice that looking at the T2-weighted image alone, the left maxillary sinus could be mistakenly interpreted as aerated.   (*Legend "continues"*)

of all patients admitted to their institution with one of the above diagnoses. They found that 15 of 176 patients had 22 intracranial complications of sinusitis. The incidence of complications among this group was as follows: epidural abscess, 23%; subdural empyema, 18%; meningitis, 18%; cerebral abscess, 14%; superior sagittal sinus thrombosis, 9%; cavernous sinus thrombosis, 9%; and osteomyelitis, 9%. Intracranial spread can be secondary to direct communication with the intracranial contents via anatomic pathways. These pathways may arise from congenital or traumatic dehiscences, bone erosion, or through normal foramina such as the cribriform plate. Alternatively, the diploic bone of the sinus wall has draining veins that connect to intracranial veins and draining venous sinuses. These

routes may permit the spread of infection without obvious bone destruction. Such spread also may give rise to orbital complications (Fig. 29.14) such as preseptal cellulititis, postseptal cellulititis, and subperiosteal (subperiorbital)/orbital abscesses (25).

Complications of Functional Endoscopic Sinus Surgery

The anatomy of the nasal cavity and ethmoid labyrinth is extremely complex and variable. Endoscopy provides a two-dimensional view of three-dimensional anatomy. Conventional cross-sectional imaging and, more recently, intraoperative framed and frameless stereotaxically guided techniques can help avoid complications.

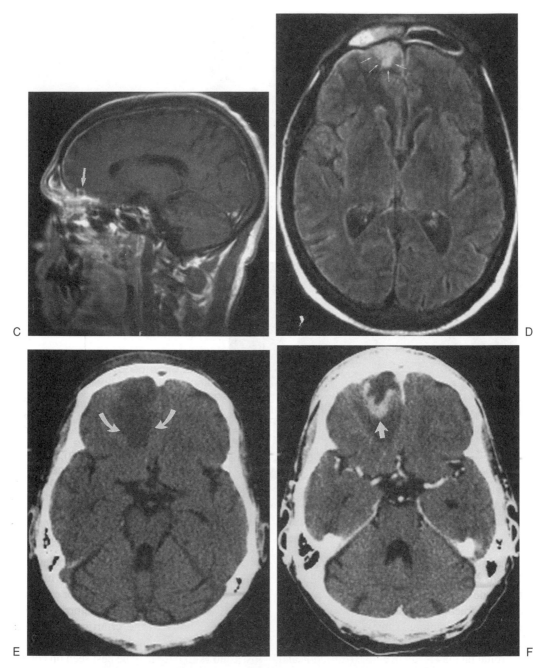

FIG. 29.12. (*Legend "continued" from A, B*) Magnetic resonance imaging performed the next day confirmed the presence of a small right frontal lobe ring-enhancing lesion (**C**, sagittal postcontrast T1-weighted image) felt to represent an intracranial abscess secondary to intracranial spread from the sinus infection. There is surrounding edema or cerebritis (*small white arrows*) on the axial FLAIR image (**D**). Repeat noncontrast (**E**) and postcontrast (**F**) CT of the brain obtained 10 days later showed interval growth of the intracranial abscess (*short arrow*) and surrounding abnormal low-attenuation edema/cerebritis (*curved arrows*) despite intravenous antibiotics.

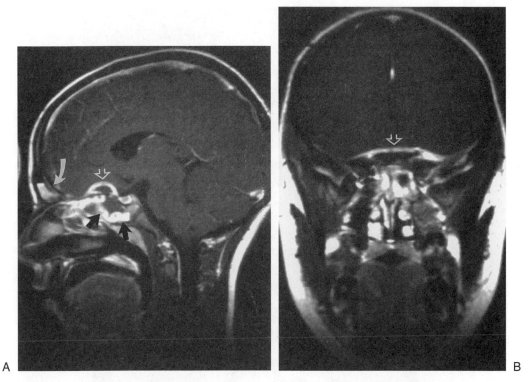

FIG. 29.13. Sagittal **(A)** and coronal **(B)** postcontrast T1-weighted images from a child with an epidural abscess as the result of intracranial spread from a sinus infection. The abscess is seen as a ring-enhancing lesion (*open white arrow*) in the epidural space. There is sinusitis involving the frontal (*curved white arrow*) and sphenoid (*black arrows*) sinuses.

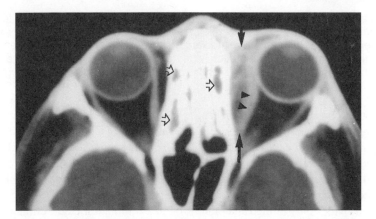

FIG. 29.14. Axial postcontrast computed tomography scan from a patient with left orbital cellulitis due to spread from adjacent ethmoid sinusitis. A medial subperiosteal abscess (*large black arrows*) seen adjacent to the lamina papyracea is displacing the medial rectus muscle (*arrowheads*). The infection has not spread intraconally. The visualized ethmoid air cells are opacified (*open black arrows*).

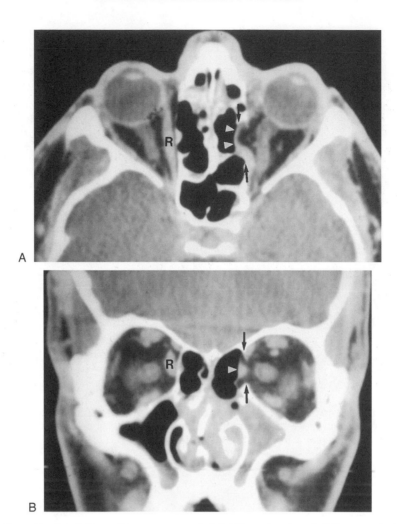

FIG. 29.15. Complications from sinus surgery. Axial **(A)** and coronal **(B)** computed tomography (CT) images from a patient who experienced left medial rectus palsy following sinus surgery. There has been inadvertent resection of the left medial orbital wall (*black arrows*). The left medial rectus muscle is seen herniating through the defect (*white arrowhead*) into the adjacent ethmoid air cell. The normal position of the medial rectus muscle is seen on the right (*R*).   (*Legend continues*)

plate. Patients may present with rhinorrhea, recurrent meningitis, or, rarely, meningoencephalocele. Symptoms may occur immediately or may be delayed up to 2 years after the operative procedure (7,16). A radionuclide cisternogram may be performed to confirm the presence of the leak, but this test provides only limited anatomic information concerning the exact location of the leak. A CT cisternogram is a procedure whereby contrast is placed into the subarachnoid space (via a lumbar puncture) and a CT is performed to demonstrate contrast leaking through a defect into the sinus. The reported sensitivity of CT cisternography to CSF leaks (of all causes) is 36% to 81%. Although CT cisternography may be used to anatomically localize the site of injury such as a break in a bone, the sensitivity is diminished if the patient is not actively leaking CSF at the time of the examination. Some clinicians advocate the use of MRI to localize the site of CSF leakage. T2-weighted images provide excellent contrast between the CSF and bone–air interface. Continuity of high T2 signal CSF from the intracranial subarachnoid space through a bone defect

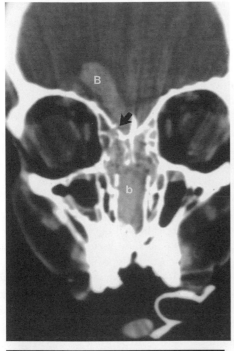

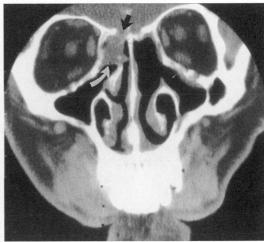

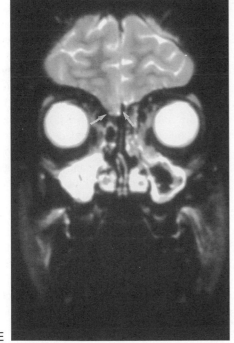

FIG. 29.15. (*Legend "continued" from A, B*) A coronal CT **(C)** from a different patient demonstrates an intracranial hemorrhage (*B*) as a result of injury to the fovea ethmoidalis (*black arrow*). Blood (*b*) is also filling the sinus and nasal cavities. A coronal CT **(D)** from another postoperative patient who suffered a similar injury shows abnormal soft tissue density (*curved white arrow*) adjacent to an apparent discontinuity of the bony fovea ethmoidalis and cribriform plate (*black arrow*). A coronal T2-weighted magnetic resonance image **(E)** illustrates this soft tissue density to be brain parenchyma herniating through the bone defect (*white arrows*). This is called a postoperative encephalocele.

into extracranial sites can sometimes be identified (28). One drawback is that the CSF may be obscured by sinus mucosal thickening and fluid.

Association of Allergy, Sinusitis, and Polyposis

The exact relationship between allergy and sinusitis has not been determined. It is thought that in response to an inhaled allergen, an immunoglobulin E (IgE)-mediated (type 1 hypersensitivity) response occurs within the nasal mucosa. Nasal mucosal edema results in obstruction of the sinus ostia, decreased ciliary action, and increased mucus production with subsequent sinusitis. One study showed that those patients with CT findings of extensive sinus disease had more markers of allergy. Specifically, this group had a much higher prevalence of IgE antibodies to common inhalant allergens than the group of patients with limited sinus disease (29). Pelikan et al. (30) performed a study attempting to prove a direct causal relationship between the type I hypersensitivity reaction and sinusitis. Seventy-three nasal provocation tests were performed in 37 patients with a history of chronic sinusitis. These patients then underwent rhinomanometry and maxillary sinus radiographs. There were 41 positive results of the nasal provocation tests, of which 32 demonstrated radiographic signs of increase in mucosal edema or sinus opacification, as well as clinical symptoms. However, 5 cases demonstrated radiographic changes within the maxillary sinuses with a negative nasal response. Pelikan suggested that in these cases, the IgE-mediated response occurred not at the level of the nasal mucosa but within the sinus itself.

Sinonasal polyposis is the term used to describe extensive polyp disease. As with sinusitis, there is debate concerning the relationship of polyposis with allergy. It has been noted that approximately 25% of patients with allergic rhinitis have nasal polyps (6). Perkins et al. (31) designed a study that searched for markers of allergic disease in those patients with sinonasal polyposis, compared with patients without polyps who had known allergic rhinitis, nonallergic rhinitis, and no rhinitis. The study found a subgroup of patients with polyps who had markers indicating allergic disease (similar markers were seen in an allergic rhinitis control group). There was also a group of patients with sinonasal polyposis that had no evidence of allergic disease. Consequently, it was concluded that there is no causal relationship between allergy (positive skin tests, family history of atopy, eosinophils in nasal secretions or in nasal polyps) and polyps. It has been reported that 46% of patients with allergic rhinitis have clinical and radiologic evidence of sinonasal polyposis (32). It also has been reported that the incidence of asthma in patients with polyps is 20%, and that up to 32% of the asthmatic patients have nasal polyps. The triad of aspirin intolerance, nasal polyposis, and bronchial asthma is well documented (33).

Regardless of the etiologic factors, the imaging appearance of polyposis is quite dramatic (Fig. 29.16). Rounded masses are seen filling the nasal cavities (unilateral or bilateral), often extending into and filling the adjacent sinuses. The involved ostia are typically enlarged (in 89% of patients). There is expansion of the nasal cavity and involved sinuses. The lateral walls of the ethmoid sinus often bulge laterally. The bony walls may be thinned and at times appear eroded, making the possibility of a malignant mass a differential consideration. On CT, the soft tissue contents within the sinus cavity may have central high-attenuation material surrounded by peripheral low attenuation. On MRI, the appearance of the contents will be mixed, depending on the relative free water and protein concentration. Following administration of contrast, however, the polypoid mucosa does not enhance homogenously as would malignancy (6,32).

Polypoid ethmoid mucocele is a process that involves bilaterally all the ethmoid cells, with diffuse expansion of the sinus. Its appearance is similar to the diffuse sinus abnormality seen with polyposis, except that the polypoid mucocele preserves the ethmoid septa and lamina papyracea. The polypoid ethmoid mucocele also has been associated with allergy (23,34).

Fungal Sinusitis

Fungal sinusitis can be divided into four categories. Acute or fulminant invasive fungal sinusitis is a rapidly progressive disease seen in the immunocompromised host. Chronic or indolent

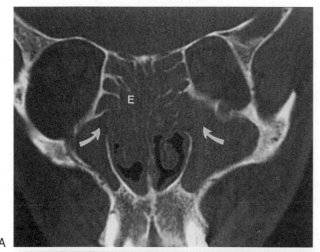

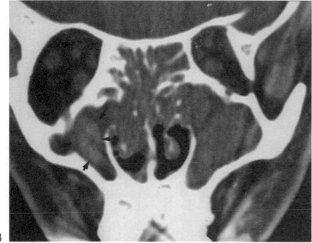

FIG. 29.16. Coronal computed tomography images viewed at a wide/bone window **(A)** and a narrow/soft tissue window **(B)** in a patient with sinonasal polyposis. There is complete opacification of bilateral ethmoid and maxillary sinuses. The maxillary ostia are expanded bilaterally (*curved white arrows*). The ethmoid septa (*E*) are partially eroded. Soft tissue windows suggest central high attenuation of the proteinaceous secretions (*small black arrows*) in the maxillary sinus.

invasive fungal sinusitis occurs in an immunocompetent patient; the fungus proliferates in the sinus cavity and penetrates the mucus. A mycetoma or fungal ball is also seen in immunocompetent nonatopic individuals; the fungus is found in the secretions without penetration of the mucosa. Lastly, allergic fungal sinusitis occurs when the fungi colonize the sinus of an atopic immunocompetent host and act as an allergen, eliciting an immune response. This response is both IgE mediated (type I hypersensitivity) and immune complex (type III reaction) mediated. The inflammation results in obstruction of the sinus, stasis of secretions, and further fungal proliferation. The diagnostic criteria for fungal sinusitis are as follows: the presence of allergic mucin at endoscopy; identification of fungal hyphae within

the allergic mucin; absence of fungal invasion of the submucosa, blood vessels, or bone; immunocompetency; and radiologic confirmation (35–37).

Computed tomographic findings in allergic fungal sinusitis are nonspecific. The air-fluid levels associated with acute bacterial sinusitis are less common in fungal sinusitis; in fact, the absence of fluid levels is suggestive of fungal disease. There is often complete opacification of the involved sinus. In a study performed by Mukherji et al. (36), 98% of patients with allergic fungal sinusitis had complete opacification of one sinus on CT. In this same study it was noted that 96% of the patients had more than one sinus involved by the disease process. If more than one sinus is involved, it may difficult to distinguish fungal sinusitis from sinonasal polyposis. Furthermore, cases of polyposis may be superinfected by fungi. The secretions in fungal sinusitis may demonstrate areas of high CT attenuation (Fig. 29.17). This is felt to be secondary to the presence of calcium, heavy metals (iron and manganese), and inspissated secretions (36,38). A similar appearance may occur with the inspissated secretions in chronic bacterial sinusitis. However, one study (39) demonstrated that the calcifications seen in fungal sinusitis are more commonly central in location and more likely to be punctate in morphology. The calcifications in nonfungal sinusitis are more likely at the periphery (near the wall) of the sinus. Nonfungal calcifications are often smoothly marginated with a round or eggshell appearance. Unfortunately, calcifications that are noted to be nodular or linear in shape can be seen with either process.

On MRI, the T1 signal of the secretions in fungal sinusitis is isointense or hypointense. As a result of the presence of calcification or paramagnetic ions within the inspissated secretions, T2-weighted images show a markedly low signal and often a signal void (38).

A mycetoma, or fungus ball, may resemble a calcification or concretion within an opacified sinus. Bony erosion does not usually occur. MRI shows intermediate T1-weighted signal and hypointense T2-weighted signal.

Fungal sinusitis may cause areas of bone erosion from pressure remodeling (36,38). Often it is this aggressive nature that identifies the sinus process as more complicated than bacterial/inflammatory disease. Silverman et al. (40) noted that in some cases there is loss of the normal periantral fat planes as fungal sinusitis spreads via perivascular channels outside the sinus lumen. This occurs prior to bone destruction, and may be an early sign of an invasive process. Invasive fungal sinusitis demonstrates an enhancing mass with bone erosion that extends beyond the sinus walls to involve the superficial soft tissues, orbit, or intracranial contents.

OTHER SINONASAL MASSES

As has already been implied, definitive diagnosis of sinonasal pathology is difficult—many processes demonstrate nearly identical imaging features. Imaging of sinonasal neoplasms is no exception, although some generalizations can be made. On MRI, tumors most often are intermediate in signal intensity on T2-weighted images. Hydrated secretions and hypertrophic mucosa are generally more hyperintense on T2-weighted imaging. This assumes that the secretions are not inspissated. Neoplasms often demonstrate homogenous enhancement, but sinusitis does not; this is a key finding. Normal mucosa also enhances, but an obstructed sinus demonstrates more peripheral mucosal enhancement with central low signal intensity. However, in a small sinus cavity where the walls are apposed, the appearance of sinusitis may still suggest a solid lesion (16). The problem with using bone destruction and extension to surrounding structures as a distinguishing feature is apparent, because this may be seen in aggressive nonneoplastic processes as well.

Inverted papilloma is an epithelial tumor that occurs in individuals 50 to 70 years of age. This tumor is unusual in that the epithelium grows (inverts) into the underlying stroma, rather than growing exophytically. It is usually a unilateral mass that arises from the lateral nasal wall adjacent to the middle turbinate, and commonly extends into the maxillary sinus. The tumor is primarily of soft tissue density on CT, and may have a lobulated surface with foci of calcification. There may be associated bony destruction. The MR appearance is nonspecific. The inverted papilloma commonly recurs following local resection. There is an association between inverted papilloma and malignancy; the prevalence ranges from 2% to 56%. The malignancy may arise directly from the inverted papilloma, adjacent to the papilloma (synchronous tumor) or in the same anatomic site as a previously resected papilloma (metachronous tumor) (41–44).

Juvenile angiofibroma begins as a unilateral mass that arises in the nasal vault, near the choana and sphenomaxillary fissure. This tumor presents in the second decade of life in men, often with epistaxis or nasal obstruction. Although histologically benign, it is locally aggressive. It commonly extends into and widens and destroys the pterygopalatine fossa and the pterygoid plates as

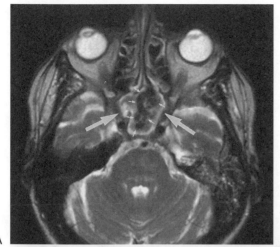

A

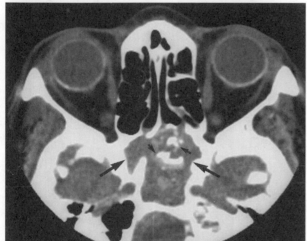

B

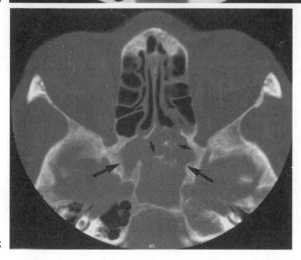

C

FIG. 29.17. A T2-weighted image from a brain magnetic resonance image **(A)** shows opacification of the sphenoid sinus (*large white arrows*). The majority of the secretions are isointense, but centrally there are serpiginous, linear areas of signal void (*small white arrows*). A computed tomographic examination of the sinuses was subsequently obtained (**B**, narrow/soft tissue window and **C**, wide/bone window). The sphenoid sinus (*large black arrows*) is completely opacified with central areas of linear calcification (*small black arrows*). Pathology confirmed fungal sinusitis.

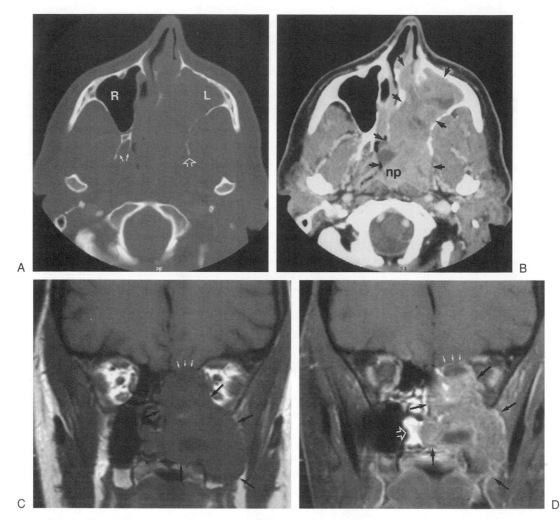

FIG. 29.18. Imaging studies from a patient with sinonasal undifferentiated carcinoma. An axial computed tomography (CT) image displayed at a wide/bone window **(A)** shows a normally aerated right maxillary sinus (*R*). The left maxillary sinus (*L*) is completely opacified by a mass that also completely fills the adjacent nasal cavity and extends back toward the nasopharynx. There is destruction of the medial wall of the left maxillary sinus. The normal pterygoid plates are seen on the right (*small white arrows*). On the left only a portion of the lateral pterygoid plate remains (*open white arrow*), the medial plate has been eroded by tumor. The corresponding postcontrast CT image displayed at a narrow/soft tissue window **(B)** shows this fairly homogenously enhancing mass (*small black arrows*). Note that the mass extends into and nearly completely fills the nasopharynx (*np*). A noncontrast T1-weighted coronal magnetic resonance image **(C)** shows the isointense mass (*black arrows*) filling the left maxillary sinus, nasal cavity, and ethmoid air cells. It is difficult to clearly demarcate a separation between the mass and the intracranial structures, suggesting that the mass has spread superiorly through the fovea ethmoidalis (*small white arrows*). The corresponding postcontrast T1-weighted image **(D)** shows the enhancing mass (*black arrows*). The normal, avidly enhancing mucosa in the right nasal cavity (*open white arrow*) can easily be distinguished from the less intensely enhancing tumor. The bony boundary between the mass and the intracranial contents is breached (*small white arrows*).

it extends into the nasopharynx. The characteristic location, often with destruction of the posterolateral wall of the maxillary sinus, is one of the few specific features that can be identified on CT. In addition, the tumor is highly vascular and will show intense enhancement and vascular flow on MRI and MR angiography (45).

Malignancies of the nasal cavity and paranasal sinuses are rare. When they do occur they most often involve the maxillary sinus, then the ethmoid sinuses, and finally the nasal cavity. Eighty percent of all sinus malignancies are squamous cell carcinoma (16). Nonspecific CT findings include bone erosion and extension of disease beyond the sinus or nasal cavity. MRI shows a homogenously enhancing soft tissue mass with surrounding inflammatory tissue and obstructed secretions.

Other neoplasms that occur in this region with variable frequency are lymphoma, adenoid cystic carcinoma, adenocarcinoma, plasmacytoma, and metastases (most commonly from renal cell carcinoma). There are no imaging findings specific to these neoplastic processes (Fig. 29.18). Olfactory neuroblastoma, also known as esthesioneuroblastoma, is a neural crest tumor that arises from the olfactory epithelium of the nasal cavity. There is a bimodal age distribution affecting teenagers and individuals in their sixth decade of life. The imaging findings are not unique other than the characteristic location of this tumor in the superior aspect of the nasal cavity, adjacent to the cribriform plate (46,47). Melanoma of the nasal and paranasal sinus mucosa has a unique MRI appearance that may suggest the diagnosis. Melanotic tumors are hyperintense on T1-weighted images and hypointense on T2-weighted images (16).

CONCLUSION

The intricate anatomy of the paranasal sinuses makes interpreting sinus examinations a challenge. Imaging examinations are designed not only to recognize acute disease processes, but also to identify any anatomic variations that may be causative factors. Furthermore, imaging helps map out a course of action for the surgeons and helps to identify potential areas at risk for complications. Although sinusitis is essentially a clinical diagnosis, there are some imaging correlates. In addition, the complications from the natural progression of the primary disease process or from surgery are best diagnosed by imaging studies. The exact relationship of allergy to the various inflammatory disease processes affecting the sinus remains unclear. Inflammatory disease processes can have a nearly identical appearance to the more aggressive fungal and malignant entities; therefore, close attention to the imaging findings is required in order to differentiate these processes.

REFERENCES

1. Babbel RW, Harnsberger HR. A contemporary look at the imaging issues of sinusitis: sinonasal anatomy, physiology and computed tomography technique. *Semin Ultrasound CT MR* 1991;12:526–540.
2. Zinreich J. Imaging of inflammatory sinus disease. *Otolaryngol Clin North Am* 1993;26.535–547.
3. Davis WE, Templer J, Parsons DS. Anatomy of the paranasal sinuses. *Otolaryngol Clin North Am* 1996;29:57–74.
4. Earwaker J. Anatomic variants in sinonasal CT. *Radiographics* 1993;13:381–415.
5. Laine FJ, Smoker WRK. The osteomeatal unit and endoscopic surgery: anatomy, variations, and imaging findings in inflammatory diseases. *AJR* 1992;159:849–857.
6. Yousem DM. Imaging of sinonasal inflammatory disease. *Radiology* 1993;188:303–314.
7. Rao VM, El-Noueam K. Sinonasal imaging anatomy and pathology. *Radiol Clin North Am* 1998;36:921–939.
8. Nelson KL. CT of sinonasal inflammatory disease. *Imaging Decisions* 1994:26–38.
9. Klevansky A. The efficacy of multiplanar reconstructions of helical CT of the paranasal sinuses. *AJR* 1999;173:493–495.
10. Suojanen JN, Regan F. Spiral CT scanning of the paranasal sinuses. *Am J Neuroradiol* 1995;16:787–789.
11. Hahnel S, Ertl-Wagner B, Tasman A, et al. Relative value of MR imaging as compared with CT in the diagnosis of inflammatory paranasal sinus disease. *Radiology* 1999; 210:171–176.
12. Shapiro G, Rachelefsky G. Introduction and definition of sinusitis. *J Allergy Clin Immunol* 1992;90:417–418.
13. Bhattacharyya T, Piccirillo J, Wippold FJ. Relationship between patient based descriptions of sinusitis and paranasal sinus computed tomographic findings. *Arch Otolaryngol Head Neck Surg* 1997;123:1189–1192.
14. Zinreich SJ, Kennedy DW, Kumar AJ, et al. MR imaging of the normal nasal cycle: comparison with sinus pathology. *J Comput Assist Tomogr* 1988;12:1014–1019.
15. Rak KM, Newell JD, Yakes WF, et al. Paranasal sinuses on MR images of the brain: significance of mucosal thickening. *Am J Neuroradiol* 1990;11:1211–1214.
16. Hudgins PA. Sinonasal imaging. *Neuroimag Clin North Am* 1996;6:319–331.

17. Babbel RW, Harnsberger HR. Recurring patterns of inflammatory sinonasal disease demonstrated on screening sinus CT. *Am J Neuroradiol* 1992;13:903–912.

18. Som PM, Dillon WP, Fullerton GD, et al. Chronically obstructed sinonasal secretions: observations on T1 and T2 shortening. *Radiology* 1989;172:515–520.

19. Dillon WP, Som PM, Fullerton GD. Hypointense MR signal in chronically inspissated sinonasal secretions. *Radiology* 1990;174:73–78.

20. Weissman JL, Curtin HD, Eibling DE. Double mucocele of the paranasal sinuses. *Am J Neuroradiol* 1994;15:1263–1264.

21. Lanziero CF, Shah M, Krauss D, et al. Use of gadolinium-enhanced MR imaging for differentiating mucocele from neoplasms in the paranasal sinuses. *Radiology* 1991;179;425–428.

22. VanTassel P, Lee Y, Jing B, et al. Mucoceles of the paranasal sinuses: MR imaging with CT correlation. *AJR* 1989;153:407–412.

23. Som PM, Shugar JM. CT classification of ethmoid mucoceles. *J Comput Assist Tomogr* 1980;4:199–203.

24. Weissman JL, Tabor EK, Curtin HD. Sphenochoanal polyps: evaluation with CT and MR imaging. *Radiology* 1991;178:145–148.

25. Wegenmann M, Naclerio RM. Complications of sinusitis. *J Allergy Clin Immunol* 1992;90:552–554.

26. Gallagher RM, Gross CW, Phillips CD. Suppurative intracranial complications of sinusitis. *Laryngoscope* 1998;108(Part 1):1635–1642.

27. Hudgins PA, Browning DG, Gallups J, et al. Endoscopic paranasal sinus surgery: radiographic evaluation of severe complications. *Am J Neuroradiol* 1992;14:1161–1167.

28. Stafford DB, Brennan P, Toland J, et al. Magnetic resonance imaging in the evaluation of cerebrospinal fluid fistula. *Clin Radiol* 1996;51:837–841.

29. Phillips CD, Platts-Mills TAE. Chronic sinusitis: relationship between CT findings and clinical history of asthma, allergy, eosinophilia and infection. *AJR* 1995;164:185–187.

30. Pelikan Z, Pelikan-Filipek M. Role of nasal allergy in chronic maxillary sinusitis—diagnostic value of nasal challenge with allergen. *J Allergy Clin Immunol* 1990;56:484–491.

31. Perkins JA, Blakeslee DB, Andrade P. Nasal polyps: a manifestation of allergy? *Otolaryngol Head Neck Surg* 1989;101:641–645.

32. Drutman J, Babbel RW, Harnsberger JR, et al. Sinonasal polyposis. *Semin Ultrasound CT MR* 1991;12;561–574.

33. Slavin RG. Nasal polyps and sinusitis. *JAMA* 1997; 278:1849–1854.

34. Jacobs M, Som PM. The ethmoidal "polypoid mucocele." *J Comput Assist Tomogr* 1982;6:721–724.

35. Kupferberg SB, Bentill JP, Kuhn FA. Prognosis for allergic fungal sinusitis. *Otolaryngol Head Neck Surg* 1997;117:35–41.

36. Mukherji SK, Figueroa RE, Ginsberg LE, et al. Allergic fungal sinusitis: CT findings. *Radiology* 1998;207:417–422.

37. Corey JP, Delsupehe KG, Ferguson BJ. Allergic fungal sinusitis: allergic, infectious, or both? *Otolaryngol Head Neck Surg* 1995;113:110–119.

38. Zinreich SJ, Kennedy DW, Malat J, et al. Fungal sinusitis: diagnosis with CT and MR imaging. *Radiology* 1988;169:439–444.

39. Yoon JH, Na DG, Byun HS, et al. Calcification in chronic maxillary sinusitis: comparison of CT findings with histopathologic results. *Am J Neuroradiol* 1999;20:571–574.

40. Silverman CS, Mancuso AA. Periantral soft tissue infiltration and it relevance to early detection of invasive fungal sinusitis: CT and MR findings. *Am J Neuroradiol* 1998;19:321–325.

41. Woodruff WW, Vrabec DP. Inverted papilloma of the nasal vault and paranasal sinuses: spectrum of CT findings. *AJR* 1994;162:419–423.

42. Dammann F, Pereira P, Laniado M, et al. Inverted papilloma of the nasal cavity and the paranasal sinuses: using CT for primary diagnosis and follow-up. *AJR* 1999;172:543–548.

43. Yousem DM, Fellows DW, Kennedy DW, et al. Inverted papilloma: evaluation with MR imaging. *Radiology* 1992;185:501–505.

44. Som PM, Lawson W, Lidov MW. Simulated aggressive skull base erosion in response to benign sinonasal disease. *Radiology* 1991;180:755–759.

45. Albery SM, Chaljub G, Cho NL, et al. MR imaging of nasal masses. *Radiographics* 1995;15:1311–1327.

46. Hurst RW, Erickson S, Cail WS, et al. Computed tomographic features of esthesioneuroblastoma. *Neuroradiology* 1989;31:253–257.

47. Li C, Yousem DM, Hayden RE, et al. Olfactory neuroblastoma: MR evaluation. *Am J Neuroradiol* 1993;14:1167–1171.

30

Radiologic Evaluation of Allergic and Related Diseases of the Lower Airway

Thomas Grant

Department of Radiology, Northwestern University Medical School
and Northwestern Memorial Hospital, Chicago, Illinois

The radiographic appearance of thoracic manifestations of systemic immunologic disorders comprises a variety of abnormalities that are influenced by the pathophysiologic characteristics of the underlying disease. These disorders include collagen vascular diseases and the systemic vasculitides. The clinician must also be familiar with the diseases in this category, a diverse group with eosinophilic lung disease, including Churg-Strauss syndrome, Wegener granulomatosis, bronchocentric granulomatosis, allergic bronchopulmonary aspergillosis (ABPA), eosinophilic lung disease (Loffler syndrome), chronic and acute eosinophilic pneumonia, hypereosinophilic syndrome, drug hypersensitivity, and asthma.

Immunologic diseases of the lungs can manifest radiographically as diffuse or focal pulmonary parenchymal and airway disease (1,2). In earlier stages of the disease the lung radiographs may be normal. Although chest radiographs are usually abnormal in advanced disease, characterization is frequently impossible. Thin section computed tomography (CT) has become the most important imaging procedure in the diagnosis of immunologic lung disease.

COMPUTED TOMOGRAPHY

Due to the limitations of standard chest X-rays, CT is the imaging procedure of choice for the evaluation of suspected immunologic lung disease. CT has the advantage of cross-sectional image orientation and high contrast resolution that makes it ideal for detecting, characterizing and distinguishing among diseases of the lungs, mediastinum and pleura. Most CT scanners are spiral and acquire a volumetric data set. It is a technique in which continuous rotation of the x-ray tube and data acquisition are coupled with continuous movement of the patient through the gantry. Today's CT scanners have either single or more advanced multi-detectors that can image the entire thorax in 10 to 20 seconds. The width of the x-ray beam is called collimation and determines this section thickness.

High-resolution CT (HRCT) involves obtaining narrow (<2 mL) collimation, a small field of view, and a high spatial frequency reconstruction algorithm to obtain detailed images. By using a very thin section, structural superimposition within the section of thickness is reduced, permitting optimal evaluation of lung detail. HRCT can detect immunologic lung disease at an early and potentially treatable stage. HRCT is also valuable in detecting interstitial disease, differentiating acute from chronic disease and optimizing the site for bronchoscopic or open lung biopsy (3–5).

The use of intravenous contrast is frequently unnecessary for chest CT examinations, particularly for evaluating pulmonary nodules or interstitial lung disease. Contrast can help to distinguish lymph nodes from pulmonary vessels, characterize pleural disease, demonstrate vascular components of an arterial venous malformation, and detect pulmonary emboli.

Intravenous contrast should be avoided in patients with a creatinine level above 2.0 mg/dL, in patients with multiple myeloma, and in patients with suspected pheochromocytoma. Low osmotic contrast is now preferred because it has fewer side effects and should be used in patients with previous anaphylactoid reactions to radiocontrast media. Corticosteroid pretreatment supplemented with antihistamine, diminishes the risk of adverse reactions.

COMPUTED TOMOGRAPHY ANATOMY

The lung is composed of lobes, segments, subsegments, and secondary lobules and acini (6,7). Each level contains an airway and a pulmonary artery that act as a supporting structure, the peribronchovascular interstitium. The airway are a branching series of 20 generations that leads to the alveoli.

The secondary pulmonary lobule is the smallest unit of lung structure marginated by connective tissue septa (8). These lobules measure 1 to 2.5 centimeters in size and are supplied by a small bronchial and pulmonary artery. The secondary lobule can be identified in both normal and abnormal lungs, but in patients with interstitial lung diseases there are characteristic changes on thin-section CT.

There are patterns of abnormality on HRCT that help to define acute and chronic infiltrative lung diseases (Tables 30.1 and 30.2).

Reticular opacities result from thickening of the pulmonary interstitium by fluid, fibrosis, or other materials. A fine reticular pattern can be seen with fibrosis (Fig. 30.1). In idiopathic pulmonary fibrosis and fibrosing alveolitis associated with collagen vascular disease, this pattern is most often observed peripherally at the lung bases (3,5). In chronic hypersensitivity pneumonitis the fibrosis is usually most severe in the mid-lung zones (9,10). Cysts or rounded air-containing nodules are present in a number of acute and chronic infiltrative diseases. Nodules in centrilobular distribution can be

seen in hypersensitivity pneumonitis and bronchiolitis obliterans with organizing pneumonia (BOOP) (3).

Ground-glass attenuation is characterized by the presence of hazy increased attenuation of lung without obscuration of the underlying bronchial or vascular anatomy. If the vessels are obscured, the term *consolidation* is used. Ground-glass attenuation can result from interstitial thickening, air space filling, or both. Although ground-glass attenuation is nonspecific, it usually indicates the presence of an active, potentially treatable disease. Areas of ground-glass attenuation in patients with chronic infiltrative lung disease are commonly caused by hypersensitivity pneumonitis, collagen vascular diseases, and idiopathic pulmonary fibrosis (3,5).

RADIOLOGIC FINDINGS IN IMMUNOLOGIC LUNG DISEASE

Churg-Strauss Syndrome

Churg-Strauss syndrome is an allergic angiitis and granulomatosis necrotizing vasculitis that occurs almost exclusively in patients with asthma (11–13). The syndrome is most commonly seen in patients 30 to 50 years of age and has no gender predilection. Patients are typically asthmatic and present with eosinophilia, fever, and allergic rhinitis. Findings of chest radiography are usually abnormal and most often consist of patchy nonsegmental areas of consolidation with no zonal predominance. The areas of consolidation may have peripheral distribution and are often transient (Fig. 30.2). Nodules may occur, but cavitation is rare. A pleural effusion is present in approximately 30% of patients.

Recent reports on the CT findings of Churg-Strauss syndrome include areas of consolidation or ground-glass attenuation. Nodules, bronchial wall thickening, and bronchiectasis are common with both Churg-Strauss syndrome and allergic bronchopulmonary aspergillosis. Other less common findings include pulmonary nodules, interlobular septal thickening, and bronchial wall thickening (12).

TABLE 30.1. *Common computed tomographic (CT) features of immunologic lung diseases*

CT finding	ABPA	Hypersensitivity pneumonitis (HP)	Churg-Strauss syndrome	Wegener granulomatosis	Eosinophilic pneumonia (EP)	Asthma
Ground-glass opacities		Acute		Present with cytotoxic drug treatment		
Consolidating/air trappings			Consolidation		Consolidation	Air trappings
Irregular linear opacities		Chronic		Common		
Nodules	Centrilobular		0.5–3.0 cm in diameter	Common/cavitation		
Distribution	Central	Mid and lower lung	Peripheral		Upper lobe peripheral in chronic EP Chronic EP	
Honeycombing fibrosis	Late stage (for ABPA)	Late stages chronic HP		Late		
Bronchial abnormality	Bronchiectasis, mucoid impaction	Bronchiectasis in chronic HP	Wall thickening	Focal and diffuse narrowing		Bronchial wall thickening

ABPA, allergic bronchopulmonary aspergillosis.

TABLE 30.2. *Computed tomographic (CT) appearance of immunologic/eosinophilic lung disease*

Disease	CT appearance
Wegener granulomatosis	Multiple nodules or masses with or without cavitation, peripheral wedge-shaped areas of consolidation
Asthma	Air trapping on expiratory HRCT, bronchial wall thickening
Bronchocentric granulomatosis	Bronchiectasis, atelectasis, peripheral consolidation, ground-glass attenuation
Chronic eosinophilic pneumonia	Patchy unilateral or bilateral airspace consolidation, predominantly peripheral distribution, areas of ground-glass attenuation predominantly in the middle and upper lung zones
Acute eosinophilic pneumonia	Ground-glass attenuation, diffuse areas of ground-glass attenuation, defined nodules, smooth interlobular septal thickening
Churg-Strauss syndrome	Airspace consolidation, areas of ground-glass attenuation, peripheral predominance or random distribution, nodules, bronchial wall thickening or dilatation, interlobular septal thickening
ABPA	Bronchiectasis, mucous plugging, atelectasis, peripheral airspace consolidation or ground-glass attenuation
Simple pulmonary eosinophilia	Patchy unilateral or bilateral airspace consolidation, predominantly peripheral distribution, areas of ground-glass attenuation predominantly in the middle and upper lung zones, usually transient and migratory
Drug-induced eosinophilic pneumonia	Areas of ground-glass attenuation, airspace consolidation, nodules, irregular lines
Hypereosinophilic syndrome	Patchy areas of consolidation of nodules with or without pleural effusion

HRCT, high-resolution computed tomography; ABPA, allergic bronchopulmonary aspergillosis.

Bronchocentric Granulomatosis

Bronchocentric granulomatosis involves the bronchi and bronchioles. This entity can be classified into those patients with asthma and those without (13,14). About one third to one half of patients with bronchocentric granulomatosis are asthmatic with underlying ABPA. Pathologically it is characterized by thick-walled ectatic bronchi and bronchioles containing viscous material. CT may show evidence of mucoid impaction with branching opacities suggesting ABPA (1). Occasionally, it manifests as multiple or solitary nodules, masses, or ill-defined areas of consolidation, most often in the upper lobes.

Wegener Granulomatosis

Wegener granulomatosis is a systemic autoimmune disease characterized by a granulomatous vasculitis of the upper and lower respiratory tracts. The histologic features are a necrotizing

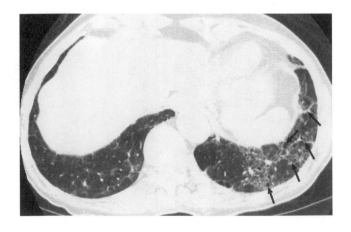

FIG. 30.1. A 70-year-old man with dyspnea and restrictive lung disease. High-resolution computed tomography demonstrates disruption of the underlying lung architecture, with a honeycomb pattern of thick irregular basilar septal lines (*arrowhead*) surrounding small cystic air spaces. (*arrows*).

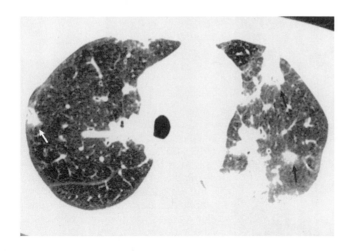

FIG. 30.2. Churg-Strauss syndrome. Computed tomography demonstrates irregular areas of consolidation (*arrows*) in this 57-year-old woman with previous episodes of eosinophilic pneumonia. An open lung biopsy revealed a necrotizing vasculitis.

vasculitis of small arteries and veins and granuloma formation. The clinical triad of classical Wegener granulomatosis is pulmonary disease, febrile sinusitis, and glomerulonephritis (2,15). A limited form of Wegener granulomatosis can be confined to the lungs. It is a disease that predominantly affects male patients.

The imaging findings in most patients are multiple nodules or irregularly marginated masses with no zonal predominance. The nodules or masses are usually multiple but can be solitary in approximately 25% of cases. Cavitation of the nodules occurs in approximately 50% of cases. The cavities usually have irregular, thick walls (2). After treatment, the nodules or cavities may resolve completely or result in a scar. On CT, the nodules typically have irregular margins and often have a peribronchovascular distribution (Fig. 30.3). Peripheral, wedge-shaped areas of consolidation representing an infarct may be present.

A localized or diffuse area of air space consolidation may be present. These areas usually represent pulmonary hemorrhage, and present as bilateral air space opacities. Involvement of the trachea or bronchial walls usually consists of mucosal or submucosal granulomatosis thickening. CT may show smooth nodular thickening of the tracheobronchial wall. If the thickening becomes severe, narrowing of the lumen and eventually calcification also may occur (1,2).

Allergic Bronchopulmonary Aspergillosis

The primary radiographic presentation of ABPA on CT is the presence of severe bronchiectasis. The presence of bronchial dilatation, bronchial wall thickening, and centrilobular nodules in an asthmatic patient should strongly suggest the diagnosis of an ABPA (13,14,16). The diagnosis is even more likely if the bronchial dilatation is moderate to severe, affects three or more lobes, and involves the central bronchi (Fig. 30.4). If bronchial dilatation is present in asthmatic patients without ABPA, it is most often mild and has an upper lobe distribution.

Other findings include mucoid plugging involving the dilated ectatic bronchi. Several studies have concluded that HRCT is highly suggestive of ABPA when the classic findings are present (16).

Asthma

Asthma is a disease of the airways that is characterized by an increased responsiveness of the tracheobronchial tree to a multiplicity of stimuli (17). Thin-section CT findings have been assessed in several studies and include bronchial wall thickening, bronchial dilation, emphysema, and air-trapping (18). Thin-section CT performed on expiration is helpful to determine the amount of air trapping (Fig. 30.5). Asthmatic patients with an FEV_1 of less than 60% of

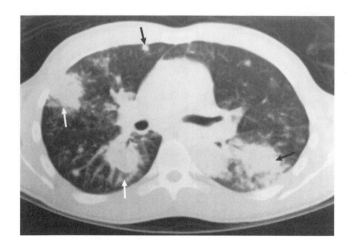

FIG. 30.3. Wegener granulomatosis in a 61-year-old man who presented with chronic cough, malaise, and weight loss. Computed tomography demonstrates bilateral irregular masses (*arrows*) and nodules in the mid-lung (*arrowhead*).

predicted value more frequently had bronchial wall thickening and a lower bronchial arterial diameter ratio than did patients with airflow or mild airflow obstruction. The use of inspiratory and expiratory thin-section CT is of value in distinguishing asthmatic patients with normal to mild airflow obstruction from healthy subjects (18).

Hypersensitivity Pneumonitis

Hypersensitivity pneumonitis, also known as extrinsic allergic alveolitis, is an inflammatory lung disease caused by inhalation of airborne organic particulate matter (10,13). Causative factors are numerous and include bacteria, fungi, avian proteins, wood dusts, and chemicals.

Acute hypersensitivity pneumonitis occurs after intense exposure to antigens. The radiographic manifestations have not been studied until recently. Chest radiographs are often normal in patients with mild symptoms. Thin-section CT can be useful in patients with suspected hypersensitivity pneumonitis with normal chest radiographs. Half of patients with normal chest radiographs have characteristic findings of centrilobular, ground-glass and nodular opacities on CT (Fig. 30.6). These findings are most typical in the middle to lower lung fields (19, 20).

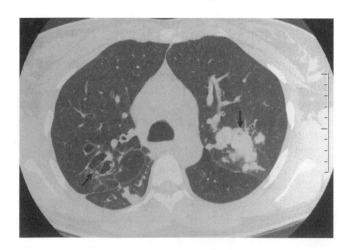

FIG. 30.4. Allergic bronchopulmonary aspergillosis in a 44-year-old man with asthma and eosinophilia. High-resolution computed tomography demonstrates extensive central bronchiectasis (*arrow*) and tubular densities (*arrowhead*) consistent with mucoid impaction.

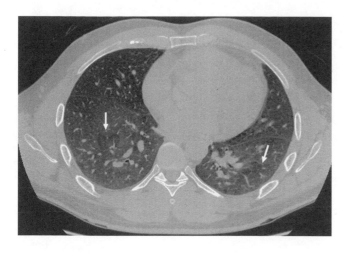

FIG. 30.5. Asthma in a 29-year-old man. Expiratory high resolution computed tomography demonstrates areas of air trapping (*arrows*).

Chronic hypersensitivity pneumonitis occurs after long-standing exposure to an offending antigen and can result in chronic pulmonary fibrosis (Fig. 30.7). In chronic hypersensitivity pneumonitis the chest radiograph most commonly reveals mild middle to upper lobe fibrosis (10,21). CT findings include small nodules, irregular linear opacities, traction bronchiectasis, architectural distortion, and honeycombing.

Acute Eosinophilic Pneumonia

Acute eosinophilic pneumonia is idiopathic disease in which acute upper respiratory failure is accompanied by markedly elevated levels of eosinophilia in fluid recovered from bronchoalveolar lavage (13,21). Peripheral blood eosinophilia is rarely present.

Patients with acute eosinophilic pneumonia present with fever and acute respiratory failure, and have radiographic signs consistent with pulmonary edema (22). These findings are in contrast to those of chronic eosinophilic pneumonia in which pulmonary infiltrates are peripheral in distribution. In addition, pleural effusions are common.

Chronic Eosinophilic Pneumonia

Chronic eosinophilic pneumonia is an idiopathic condition characterized histologically by

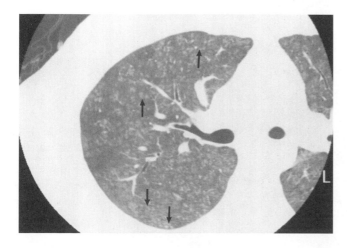

FIG. 30.6. Acute hypersensitivity pneumonitis in a 30-year-old woman with acute dyspnea, hypoxemia, and chills after cleaning her attic. High-resolution computed tomography shows numerous centrilobular nodules (*arrows*). The radiologic and clinical findings resolved 5 days after starting corticosteroid therapy.

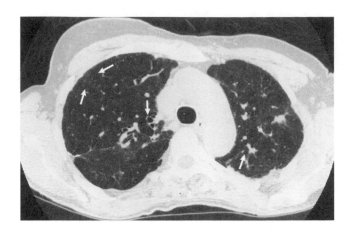

FIG. 30.7. Chronic hypersensitivity pneumonitis in a 52-year-old man with progressive dyspnea. Computed tomography shows nodules, linear opacities, centrilobular nodules (*arrowheads*), and bronchiectasis (*arrows*).

filling of the air spaces with eosinophils and macrophages and associated mild interstitial pneumonia. The patients are most often middle-aged women who present with at least 1 month of cough, fever, weight loss, and dyspnea (20,23).

The classic radiographic findings of chronic eosinophilic pneumonia consist of peripheral, nonsegmental areas of consolidation involving mainly the upper lobes. However, this pattern is only present in 50% of cases. The remaining cases show radiographic findings that are nonspecific and consist of unilateral or patchy bilateral consolidation.

On HRCT a peripheral distribution of consolidation is often present even when it is not apparent on chest radiographs (Fig. 30.8). The combination of peripheral consolidation and peripheral blood eosinophilia is virtually diagnostic of chronic eosinophilic pneumonia (23).

Drug-induced Lung Disease

Pulmonary drug hypersensitivity is increasingly being diagnosed as a cause of acute and chronic lung disease (24). Numerous agents including cytotoxic and noncytotoxic drugs have the potential to cause pulmonary disturbances. The clinical and radiologic manifestation of these drugs generally reflect the underlying histopathologic processes. These manifestations include diffuse

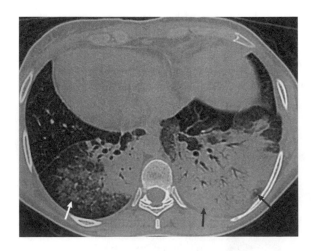

FIG. 30.8. Chronic eosinophilic pneumonia in a 60-year-old man. Transverse thin-section computed tomography demonstrates extensive areas of air space consolidation (*arrows*) and ground-glass attenuation (*arrowhead*) involving mainly the peripheral lung region.

alveolar damage, BOOP, eosinophilic pneumonia, and pulmonary hemorrhage (13,25). Radiographic manifestation on CT includes diffuse areas of ground-glass opacity, diffuse areas of heterogenous opacity, and, in the later stages, fibrosis, especially in a basilar distribution. BOOP, which is commonly caused by cytotoxic drugs, appears on radiographs as heterogenous and homogenous peripheral opacities and on CT as poorly defined nodules and consolidation (25).

The prevalence of drug-induced pulmonary hypersensitivity or toxicity is increasing, and more than 100 drugs are now known to cause injury. Because of its progressive nature, early recognition is important. The diagnosis of pulmonary drug toxicity should be considered in any patient with drug therapy who presents with new progressive respiratory complaints.

Idiopathic Hypereosinophilic Syndrome

The idiopathic hypereosinophilic syndrome is a rare and often fatal disorder characterized by elevated blood eosinophil levels ($>1,500/\mu$L) for more than 6 months. This syndrome is characterized by the absence of parasitic or other causes of secondary hypereosinophilia (13). Cardiac involvement, including endocardial fibrosis and restrictive cardiomyopathy, is one of the major complications of this entity. Pulmonary involvement occurs in up to 40% of patients, and typically presents on radiography as interstitial, nonlobar opacities (26,27). Typical CT finding are patchy areas of air space consolidation, nodules, diffuse areas with ground-glass attenuation, interlobular septal thickening, thickening of the bronchovascular bundles, bronchial wall thickening, and a random distribution (24).

REFERENCES

1. Mayberry JP, Primack SL, Muller NL. Thoracic manifestations of systemic autoimmune diseases: radiographic and high resolution CT findings. *Radiographics* 2000;20:1623–1635.
2. Frazier AA, Roado-de-Christenson, Galvin Jr. Pulmonary angiitis and granulomatosis: radiologic–pathologic correlation. *Radiographics* 1998;18:687–710.
3. Nishimura K, Izumi T, Kitaichi M, et al. The accuracy of high-resolution computed tomography in diffuse infiltrative lung disease. *Chest* 1993;104:1149–1155.
4. Swensen SJ, Aughenbaugh GL, Myers JL. Diffuse lung disease: diagnostic accuracy of CT in patients undergoing surgical biopsy the lung. *Radiology* 1997;205:229–234.
5. Itoh H, Murata K, Konishi J, et al. Diffuse lung disease: pathologic basis for the high-resolution computed tomography findings. *J Thorac Imaging* 1993;8:176–188.
6. Kuhn C III. Normal anatomy and histology. In: Thurlbeck WM, Churg AM, eds. *Pathology of the lung,* 2nd ed. New York: Thieme, 1995:1–36.
7. Miller WS. *The lung,* 2nd ed. Springfield, IL: Charles C. Thomas, 1950.
8. Heitzman ER, Markarian B, Berger I, et al. The secondary pulmonary lobule: a practical concept for interpretation of chest radiographs. *Radiology* 1969;93:507–512.
9. Mayo JR, Muller NL, Road J, et al. Chronic eosinophilic pneumonia: CT finding in six cases. *AJR* 1989;153:727–730.
10. Matar DL, Page McAdams H, Sporn TA. Hypersensitivity pneumonitis. *AJR* 2000;174:1061–1066.
11. Bushman DL, Waldron JA, Talmadge EK. Churg-Strauss pulmonary vasculitis high resolution computed tomography scanning and pathologic findings. *Am Rev Respir Dis* 1990;142:458–461.
12. Worthy SA, Muller NL, Hansell DM, et al. Churg-Strauss syndrome: the spectrum of pulmonary CT findings in 17 patients. *AJR* 1998;170:297–300.
13. Allen JN, Davis BW. Eosinophic lung diseases. *Am J Respir Crit Care Med* 1994;150:1423–1438.
14. Sulavik SB. Bronchocentric granulomatosis and allergic bronchopulmonary aspergillosis. *Clin Chest Med* 1988;9:609–621.
15. Aderelo DR, Gamsu G, Lynch D. Thoracic manifestations of Wegener granulomatosis: diagnosis and course. *Radiology* 1990;174:703–709.
16. Angus RM, Davies ML, Cowan MD, et al. Computed tomographic scanning of the lung in patients with allergic bronchopulmonary aspergillosis and in asthmatic patients with a positive skin test to *Aspergillus fumigatus. Thorax* 1994;49:586–589.
17. Newman RB, Lynch DA, Newman LS, et al. Quantitative computed tomography detects air trapping due to asthma. *Chest* 1994;160:105–109.
18. Chan SP, Muller NL, Worthy SA. Airway obstruction in a asthmatic and healthy individuals: inspiratory and expiratory thin-section CT findings. *Radiology* 1997;203:361–367.
19. Nansell DM, Wells AU, Padley SP, et al. Hypersensitivity pneumonitis: correlation of individual CT patterns with functional abnormalities. *Radiology* 1996;199:123–128.
20. Lynch DA, Newell DJ, Logan PM, et al. Can CT distinguish hypersensitivity pneumonitis from idiopathic fibrosis? *AJR* 1995;165:807–811.
21. King MA, Dope-Harman AJ, Allen JN, et al. Acute eosinophilic pneumonia: radiologic and clinical features. *Radiology* 1997;203:715–719.
22. Ebara H, Ikezoe J, Johkoh T, et al. Chronic eosinophilic

TABLE 31.1. *Common plants of the Euphorbiaceae family*

Genus and species	Common name
Hevea brasiliensis	Rubber tree
Euphorbia pulcherrima	Poinsettia
Euphorbia splendens	Crown of thorns
Manikot esculenta	Tapioca
Acalypha wilkesiana	Jacob's coat
Ricinus communis	Castor bean
Acalypha hispida	Chenile plant

of latex from a particular tree is dependent on the season, frequency of tapping the tree, age of the tree, hormone treatments such as ethepon to enhance the NRL yield, and other factors. Pressure to produce more NRL products with the introduction of universal medical precautions led to a marked reduction in storage time from 6 months to as low as a few weeks (personal communication, Paul Caccioli, PhD, 1995). In addition, more frequent tapping of trees and the use of yield-enhancing chemicals may have adversely enhanced the allergen content of NRL. These latter two procedures are known to induce production of defense proteins (see Natural Rubber Latex Allergens), which may have had the inadvertent consequence of disproportionately producing more allergenic proteins. This may have resulted in a high allergen content of finished products in the past decades. Scientific experiments to confirm that these known effects of chemicals and tapping frequency actually result in higher allergen content of a finished NRL product have not been accomplished to date.

The actual manufacturing process has numerous steps that may affect the final NRL allergen content of a finished product. During a dipped manufacturing process, specific formers (e.g., porcelain hand forms) are coated with a coagulant, such as calcium carbonate, and are then dipped into liquid NRL for a specific length of time to produce a product of the correct thickness. Multiple chemical accelerators and antioxidants are added to the NRL to ensure the correct consistency to produce a satisfactory finished product. Heating, coupled with the chemical accelerators, converts the liquid film of NRL into a solid layer coating the porcelain former, but with incomplete cross-linking of the polyisoprene. Subsequently, the NRL gloves are leached (washed) to remove proteins and residual chemicals. This leaching is incomplete and results in persistent levels of protein and chemicals that may lead to adverse health effects in people who contact the finished product. The gloves are then sulfur heat vulcanized at a relatively low temperature (100°C) compared with coagulated rubber products, to complete the cross-linking. Often, a slurry of cornstarch powder is applied to reduce the tackiness of the gloves. In other cases, halogenation with chlorine may be used to produce powder-free products. The cornstarch powder rarely causes allergic reactions alone but may efficiently promote protein adherence. The source of protein comes not only from the product itself but also from the cornstarch slurry baths that may be contaminated with excess protein from the NRL products that pass through them. This powder, when dry, may aerosolize, with subsequent induction of allergic symptoms in hypersensitive subjects (37–52). In the late 1980s and 1990s, allergen content of NRL gloves was markedly different among manufacturers but is likely due to multiple factors (9,53). Today, the least allergen release is found in nonpowdered, chlorinated, or highly washed gloves (38–47).

TABLE 31.2. *Composition of natural rubber latex*

Component	Fresh latex (%)	Acid coagulation (%)	Centrifugation (%)
Cis-1,4-polyisoprene	25–45	93.5	60
Protein	1–2	2.0	1.0
Amino acids	0.4	—	—
Carbohydrate	1–2	0.5	0.2
Lipids	1–1.5	3.5	2.0
Inorganic constituent	0.4–0.6	0.2	0.4
Water	—	0.3	36
Ammonia	—	—	0.2–0.7

Aeroallergen levels relate to the use of cornstarch powder carrying allergen into the air.

CLINICAL REACTIONS TO NATURAL RUBBER LATEX

Clinical reactions to NRL can be divided into irritant contact reactions and immunologic reactions, of which type IV cell-mediated contact dermatitis and type I immunoglobulin E (IgE)-mediated reactions are subsets. The most common reaction to NRL is irritant dermatitis. This is most often seen in health care workers and other individuals wearing NRL gloves frequently (9–11,21–32). More than 30% of health care workers may report irritant reactions of the hands. Frequent handwashing, multiple glove changes, glove powder, and failure to dry the skin completely may contribute to this common dermatitis. Irritant dermatitis can easily be recognized by the dry, cracked skin surface, itching, and erythema that are *not* accompanied by vesicles, blistering, or weeping of the skin. In addition, the dermatitis appears only in the area where contact with the NRL product occurs (54). This dermatitis may respond to cotton glove liners, reduction of powder use, thorough hand drying, nonpetroleum-based barrier creams that do not cause NRL to degrade, and moisturizers.

Contact dermatitis, a type IV immunologic reaction, may have a distinctly different presentation compared with irritant dermatitis (54). The onset of reaction may occur after hours of contact and is often accompanied by intense itching, erythema, blistering, and weeping skin that extends beyond the site of contact with the offending NRL product. These occur because lymphocytes and Langerhans cells may "home" to remote sites away from the site of contact but are activated upon contact with the offending allergen. Chronic contact dermatitis may be difficult to distinguish from irritant dermatitis. A diagnosis is confirmed with delayed hypersensitivity patch testing with chemicals retained in finished rubber products. Thiuram and mercaptobenzothiazole chemicals appear to be the most frequent cause of contact dermatitis diagnosed by patch testing. Recent studies suggest that some NRL proteins may be capable of inducing a type IV contact dermatitis in addition to their propensity to induce type I IgE-mediated reactions.

Regardless of the etiology of the dermatitis, it often precedes and is a risk factor for the development of type I IgE-mediated NRL allergy to proteins in individuals who directly contact NRL in their daily activities or work. Interestingly, dermatitis is rarely observed in other populations at high risk, such as spina bifida patients. Although the mechanism for how the dermatitis may predispose to the development of NRL allergy is not confirmed, it is speculated that the dermatitis may enhance penetration of proteins through the epidermis, resulting in access to the immune system and subsequent development of NRL-specific IgE.

Type I IgE-mediated NRL allergy to proteins retained in finished rubber products may result in local or generalized urticaria, angioedema, rhinitis, conjunctivitis, asthma, anaphylaxis, and rarely death. The unique aspect of NRL is the broad spectrum of disease that may be induced with wide variability among affected subjects. Some individuals develop only local contact urticaria, whereas others develop asthma with no other symptoms, and still others develop anaphylaxis alone. Predicting who will progress from local urticaria to life-threatening disease is currently not possible. This inability to predict accurately the outcome of each individual requires a uniform and aggressive approach to therapy and avoidance in all affected subjects (54).

EPIDEMIOLOGY

Considerable concern and confusion have been raised about the prevalence of NRL allergy in the general population. A modestly high prevalence of NRL allergy would be a cause for concern because of the risks this would present to millions of people with even casual contact with NRL, especially routine medical care. This clearly has not been the case because clinical allergic reactions to NRL in the general population remain exceedingly unusual. Thus, it is important that only clinically allergic individuals and those at risk for reactions are identified. This requires that a clear definition of NRL allergy be agreed on. The presence of circulating IgE in the serum alone is not sufficient to make a diagnosis of NRL allergy. Medical history and physical examination, coupled with laboratory confirmation, are necessary to confirm a diagnosis when possible. Insufficiently sensitive and specific diagnostic reagents have hindered this endeavor. This may lead to some cases of NRL allergy remaining undiagnosed while some others may be overdiagnosed. The clinician must use clinical judgment when the tests are asynchronous to the history and examination.

In the daily activities of medicine, clinicians infrequently find symptoms of latex allergy in their general practice with patients. One study confirmed that skin tests are positive in less than 1% of a randomly selected population of children. Even more important, all the skin test–reactive children in this study had no discernible clinical history of allergic reactions to NRL (33). A second study of more than 3,000 selected (seen in clinic for a medical problem) subjects who underwent skin testing for NRL allergy in an allergy/dermatology clinic in Finland showed a skin test reactivity rate of about 1.1% (55). A smaller case series in children showed reactivity to NRL in about 3% of the population by skin test (34). Unfortunately, the sample size of the study is too small to draw conclusions. In contrast, two blood donor studies using serologic testing alone found circulating anti-NRL IgE antibodies in 6% of the population (56,57). Given the current sensitivity and specificity of available serologic testing, without confirmatory medical histories or skin tests, standard statistical calculation confirms that the rate of false-positive serum test results is significant in populations in which there is a low prevalence of disease. In fact, screening the general population for NRL allergy by a blood test is not recommended for this reason (58).

Patients with spina bifida are at high risk for latex allergy. In one study, 68% of children with spina bifida had positive skin test results, with one of every eight experiencing anaphylaxis in the operating room during the induction of anesthesia during a single year (8). These individuals present with a unique set of circumstances that gives insight about risk factors for NRL allergy. Most patients with spina bifida undergo at least two operations (spinal defect repair and ventriculoperitoneal shunt for hydrocephalus associated with an Arnold-Chiari malformation) in the first 2 weeks of life. Neurosurgical, orthopedic, and urologic operations are common owing to complications from paraplegia, neurogenic bladder, and hydrocephalus. Poor bladder and bowel function lead to a need for repetitive bladder catheterization and manual rectal disimpaction. In fact, the highest risk factor for development of NRL-induced anaphylaxis in the operating room in one study of spina bifida patients was the need for daily rectal disimpaction. The implication of this was that NRL gloves would often contact mucosal surfaces. Some studies suggest this population may be highly atopic as well (8). A neural immune mechanism predisposing to the development of allergy has been postulated. However, spinal cord–injured patients are not at risk for NRL allergy (16). Because the actual routes of exposure are multiple (skin, bladder, neural, peritoneal, mucosal) and timing of the development of NRL allergy in this population is variable, it is recommended that these patients be handled with no direct contact to NRL from the time they are born. This includes contact with consumer as well as medical NRL products, especially those products made by a dipped method. The routine handling of patients with spina bifida has now led to safe management of these patients' medical care.

Although the prevalence rate of NRL allergy in health care workers is considerably higher in many studies than that in the general population, it has not been as high as was seen in the initial studies of the spina bifida population. Although a sampling bias may be involved in many published studies, some clear and accurate trends occurred. In 1987, about 3% of health care workers in Finland were found to have NRL allergy (9). By 1993, the prevalence was as high as 10% in France (30). Meanwhile, as many as 17% of health care workers in one hospital in the United States were found to be sensitive by 1994 (32). It is staggering to consider the shear volume of subjects who potentially would be affected at this prevalence rate. This is so critical because even the loss of one health care worker to a hospital or clinic is fraught with tremendous replacement cost, without mention of the personal implications to the affected worker (36). From the mid-1980s to the present, the sales and use of NRL *examination gloves* has risen almost 100-fold, whereas *surgical glove* use has risen a modest twofold (54). An incident study performed in Canada demonstrated that the use of NRL gloves in dental students accounted for a conversion from a prevalence of 0% at the outset of school to 10% by the fourth year of school (23).

Other groups at risk for latex allergy include housekeepers (59), greenhouse workers (14), and NRL workers in such businesses as tire plants and doll manufacturing (50). Premature infants and patients that require multiple surgical procedures appear to be at risk for NRL allergy as well. A common theme is that there is frequent contact with NRL in these settings by skin, mucous membrane, or inhalation.

DIAGNOSTIC TESTING FOR NATURAL RUBBER LATEX ALLERGY

Testing for NRL allergy has been hindered in the United States by lack of a standard reagent approved by the FDA (60–71). Despite a multicenter skin test study that confirmed one nonammoniated reagent to be reliable and safe, no licensed product has been forthcoming. In contrast, Europe and Canada have used NRL reagents for close to a decade. These reagents include Bencard (Canada), which is no longer available, Stallergenes (France), and Lofarma (Italy). The latter two products are ammoniated NRL extracts. In Finland, a finished product (high-allergen NRL glove) used as a source material has undergone skin testing with high reliability as well (9,10). Unfortunately, a standard finished product for such testing is not available to the clinician. Attempts to use finished materials in an office practice of allergy may result in false-negative reactions because the source product is low in allergen or even, in contrast, led to adverse reactions because of excessively high allergen content. To combat the latter problem, most practicing allergists have used sequential multiple dilutions to avoid the risk for systemic reactions. Initial reports of adverse reactions to skin testing may have slowed the enthusiasm for skin testing (60). A recent study from the Mayo Clinic demonstrated that adverse reactions to skin testing for NRL allergy are more frequent than in diagnostic skin testing for common environmental allergens. The rate of systemic reaction for NRL skin testing at the Mayo Clinic was 152 to 200 per 10,000 skin tests (72). This elevated rate can be expected because NRL allergen is known to result in life-threatening anaphylactic reactions in sensitized patients, whereas common environmental allergens rarely result in anaphylaxis. This risk should not deter the release and use of NRL skin test reagents. Inability to confirm a diagnosis of NRL allergy because of unavailability of skin testing reagents may present more risk to a patient who would continue NRL exposures (e.g., health care work) that result in life-threatening reactions or asthma.

The second available method to detect NRL-specific IgE is serologic testing. The three commercially available tests include the CAP radioallergosorbent test (RAST) FEIA from Pharmacia UpJohn, AlaSTAT from Diagnostics Products Corporation (DPC), and HY-TEC-EIA from HYTEC. The sensitivity of the CAP and AlaSTAT are similar, with about 25% false-negative test result rates. The HY-TEC has a 27% false-positive result rate (63). These tests are very useful when coupled to a medical history but do not demonstrate complete diagnostic reliability. Serologic testing in some research centers with Clinical Laboratories Improvement Act (CLIA)-approved laboratories has shown high sensitivity and specificity as well. Research findings indicate that specific challenges by glove provocation, hooded exposure chamber, and nasal provocation may result in improved diagnostic sensitivity. Currently, these are impractical given the lack of standard reagents or gloves for such challenges. The clinician must use judgment in discerning the proper diagnosis and therapy of a patient with a positive history and negative serologic test because 25% of subjects with NRL allergy have negative serum test results. Other research tests, including flow cytometry, cell proliferation, and patch testing, have been helpful but not available to the practicing clinician.

NATURAL RUBBER LATEX ALLERGENS

Field NRL contains about 1% to 2% protein. The protein content varies according to clonal origin of the rubber plants, climatic factors, soil types, and the fertilizers used for the NRL cultivation. The optimal temperature for growth of the rubber tree is between 20° and 28°C under humid conditions, where it is constantly exposed to a variety of microorganisms and insects. As a defense mechanism against the invading agents as well as protection from the damage inflicted during regular tapping, these plants carry a unique wound-sealing property (1–4). NRL contains a number of defense-related proteins that are involved in biosynthesis of polyisoprenes and coagulation of latex. These proteins may act as allergens responsible for the clinical type I IgE-mediated reactions. In addition, because of the cross-reactivity of some of these latex allergens with allergens from other sources, considerable overlapping of the clinical and immunologic symptoms, such as latex-fruit allergy and latex-mold allergy, also occurs (73). The actual number of proteins in latex has been reported to be more than 200, and hevein and hevamine constitute the majority of the proteins (74–76). The latex also contains lipids, carbohydrate, and inorganic constituents, such as potassium, manganese, calcium, sodium, zinc, copper, and iron (8). Most of the proteins present in NRL could also be detected in the finished latex products in natural or altered configuration (1). Chemical treatment of NRL, such as treatment with ammonia, increases the formation of protein fragments and components. In nonammoniated latex, more than 240 separate proteins or peptide fragments have been identified by two-dimensional gel electrophoresis. However, only 25% of these proteins showed IgE binding with sera from latex-allergic patients (77).

In earlier studies, IgE antibody against latex allergens was demonstrated with crude latex proteins or extracts from gloves or other latex products. The analysis of NRL proteins in SDS PAGE demonstrated a wide range of peptides with molecular masses of 5 to 200 kDa (78). The allergens of molecular sizes 11, 14, 18, 24, 27, 35, 66, and 100 kDa have been found to be significant in latex allergy (79,80). Several latex proteins in different molecular weight ranges also exhibited specificity either for IgE from allergic health care workers or for spina bifida patients by immunoblot (81,82).

To develop specific and sensitive immunodiagnosis of latex allergy, it is essential to have pure and standardized allergens. With advances in protein purification and molecular biology techniques, a number of latex proteins have been isolated, cloned, and purified to homogeneity (83). Based on their IgE-binding properties, the Allergen Nomenclature Subcommittee of IUIS has accepted 11 of them as latex allergens (*ftp:// biobase.dk/pub/who-iuis/allergen.list*). Subcellular localization, sequence similarity searches, and functional properties of these allergens are listed in Tables 31.3 and 31.4.

BIOLOGIC PROPERTIES OF LATEX ALLERGENS

Centrifugation of NRL, frequently performed to concentrate the isoprene particles, results in separation of NRL into three distinct layers. The bottom fraction contains lutoids or organelles of the latex. The center fraction or C serum contains many water-soluble proteins, and the top layer is rich in rubber particles. These rubber particles have distinct sizes with varying quantities of membrane-bound allergens. For example, *Hev b 1* is mainly found on large particles more than 350 nm in diameter, whereas *Hev b 3* is found on small particles less than 70 nm in diameter. Different allergens concentrate in these various layers.

Polyisoprene Elongation and Latex Coagulation

The first well-characterized NRL allergen, rubber elongation factor (REF, *Hev b 1*), allows the enzyme prenyltransferase to elongate the polyisoprene chains by adding several thousands of isoprene subunits (84,85). REF is tightly bound to large rubber particles in the interface between the aqueous layer and the insoluble upper layer, which consists of polyisoprene molecules. *Hev b 3*, another REF homologue present on the surface of the small rubber particles, plays a

TABLE 31.3. *Identification and characterization of* Hevea *species latex allergens*

Latex allergen/identification	Functional properties/homology	Subcellular localization
Rubber elongation factor/*Hev b 1*	Involved in biosynthesis of polyisoprene and rubber elongation	Tightly associated with large rubber particles
Endo-1,3-b glucosidase/*Hev b 2*	Involved in defense against fungus/homology to pathogenesis related protein, class II	Lutoids (bottom fraction)
Hev b 3	Involved in biosynthesis of polyisoprene	Tightly associated with small rubber particles
Hev b 4	Components of microhelix protein	Lutoids (bottom fraction)
Hev b 5	Function unknown/homology to kiwi fruit protein pKIWI501	Cytoplasm (aqueous layer)
Provein/*Hev b 6.01*	Two-domain protein that is processed into N-terminal, hevein, and C-terminal domain	Lutoids (bottom fraction)
Hevein/*Hev 6.02*	Involved on coagulation of latex/homology to several chitin-binding proteins	Lutoids (bottom fraction)
C domain of prohevein	Homology to wound-inducible protein (e.g., WINI of potato)	Lutoids (bottom fraction)
Patatin-like protein/*Hev b 7*	Esterase activity/homology to storage protein of Solanaceae	Cytoplasm (aqueous layer)
Profilin/*Hev b 8*	Cytoskeleton actin-binding protein, involved in signal transduction/homology to profilins from other sources	Cytoplasm (aqueous layer)
Enolase/*Hev b 9*	High-sequence homology to enolases from *Ricinus communis,* tomato, and *Cladosporium* species	Cytoplasm (aqueous layer)
Manganese superoxide dismutase (MnSOD)/*Hev b 10*	Protection from reactive oxygen/homology to MnSODs from *Aspergillus* species, *Escherichia coli,* and human	Mitochondria
Class 1 chitinase/*Hev b 11*	Degrade chitin, involved in plant pathogen interaction/shared homology with N-terminal hevein domain and chitinases from other sources	Lutoids (bottom fraction)

role in synthesis of long-chain polyisoprene (86). Hevein (*Hev b 6.02*) is one of the most abundant proteins in the lutoid fraction of *Hevea* species latex (87). Hevein is released from the cells when the plant is damaged and interacts with the glycoprotein receptors on the sacs around the rubber particles, resulting in the coagulation of latex (88). The cytosolic protein, *Hev b 7*, with esterase activity inhibits the rubber biosynthesis by restricting the incorporation of isoprenyl diphosphate (89).

Plant-defense–related Function

The latex allergen, *Hev b 2*, with β-1,3-glucanase property, catalyzes the hydrolytic cleavage of polymers of β-1,3-glucans, the essential cell wall component of most fungi. Hence, this protein appears to be involved in plant protection against fungal infection by degrading the cell walls of fungal pathogens (90,91). Chitinases are proteins

common in a wide variety of seed-producing plants. The recently characterized latex allergen, *Hev b 11*, shows endochitinase activity and may be involved in hydrolytic cleavage of chitin, the major structural component of the cell wall of many fungi as well as the exoskeleton of insects. The cross-reactivity among the class 1 endochitinases from avocado, banana, chestnut, and latex has been associated with latex-fruit syndrome (91–93). Hevamine, a basic protein from the lutoid fraction, functions as a defense-related bifunctional enzyme with chitinase and lysozyme activity (94). Hevamine catalyzes the cleavage of β-1,4-glycosidic bonds of chitin and the sugar moieties of the cell surface peptidoglycans (95).

Common Enzymes and Structural Proteins of *Hevea* Species Latex

The proline-rich *Hev b 5* with a predominantly random secondary structure shows a 46% amino

TABLE 31.4. *Immunologic characterization of* Hevea brasiliensis *latex allergens*

Allergens	Molecular weight (kDa)	PI	Accession number	Number of sensitized individuals (%)	Methods	Significance as allergens (References)
Hev b 1	14.6	4.9	X56535	81 (SB)	ELISA	Major (39)
				50 (HCW)	ELISA	
Hev b 2	36	9.5	U22147	20–61 (HCW)	ELISA	Major (36)
				54 (SB)	ELISA	
Hev b 3	23	4.8	AF-051317	80 (SB)	Immunoblot	Major (13,40,41)
			AJ223388	76 (SB)	ELISA	
				20 (HCW)	ELISA	
Hev b 4	50–57	4.5	NA	65 (HCW)	ELISA, RAST	Major (36)
				77 (SB)		
Hev b 5	16	3.5	U51361	92 (HCW)	RAST	Major (28,29)
			U42640	56 (SB)	RAST	
Hev b 6.01	20	5.6	M36986	84 (HCW)	ELISA	Major (46)
				48 (SB)	ELISA	
Hev b 6.02	4.7	4.9		88 (HCW)	ELISA	Major
				56 (SB)	ELISA	
Hev b 6.03	14	6.4–7.4		40 (HCW)	ELISA	Major
				28 (SB)	ELISA	
Hev b 7	42.9	4.8	AJ220388	22 (HCW)	Immunoblot	Minor (15,47,48)
				11 (HCW)	ELISA	
Hev b 8	13.9	4.9	Y15402	35 (HCW)	SPT	Minor (30)
				100 (SB)	SPT	
Hev b 9	47.7	5.6	AJ132580	Pooled HCW	Immunoblot	Minor (7)
Hev b 10	22.9	6.3	L11707	Pooled HCW	Immunoblot	Minor (7)
			AJ249148			
Hev b 11	33	5.1	AJ238579	Pooled HCW	Immunoblot	Minor (7,56)

SB, patients with spina bifida; HCW, health care worker; ELISA, enzyme-linked immunosorbent assay; RAST, radioallergosorbent test; SPT, skin-prick test.

acid sequence homology to an acidic protein from kiwi (96,97). The latex profilin *Hev b 8* is the actin-binding protein and appears to involve in the organization of actin network of the plant cytoskeleton (98). The latex enolase *Hev b 9* is a key enzyme of the glycolytic pathway, and *Hev b 10* with manganese-superoxide dismutase (Mn-SOD) activity protects the plant against highly toxic oxygen radical produced during the phagocytic processing of foreign organisms (83).

Immunologic Evaluation of Latex Allergens in Health Care Workers and Spinal Bifida Patients

The immune responses in latex-sensitized patients have recently been evaluated using purified recombinant allergens. The results of these studies confirm the specificity and reliability of purified allergens in the immunodiagnosis of latex allergy. The identified NRL allergens have been classified as minor and major allergens, depending on the frequency of reactivity with IgE from

sera of various groups of latex-allergic patients (Table 31.4).

Hev b 1 (Rubber Elongation Factor)

REF has been cloned and purified as a 137–amino acid protein. However, the native counterpart appears as a tetramer of molecular mass of 58 kDa (99–102). *Hev b 1* is a major allergen reacting with 81% of latex-sensitized spina bifida patients and 50% of health care workers (103). In a multicenter study using RAST and enzyme-linked immunosorbent assay (ELISA), 13% to 32% of health care workers and 52% to 100% of spina bifida patients with latex allergy showed strong IgE binding with *Hev b 1* (104).

Hev b 2

Hev b 2 is a basic β-1.3-gluanase isolated from the bottom fraction (B serum) containing lutoids of NRL exhibits strong IgE binding with NRL sensitized spina bifida patients and health care workers (105,106). Depending on the method used, the reactivity varied from 20% to 61% of latex-allergic patients (104). Recombinant *Hev b 2* overexpressed in a prokaryotic expression system failed to react with IgE from sera of latex-allergic patients (83). The reason for the nonreactivity of recombinant *Hev b 2* may result from the lack of glycosylation and posttranslational modifications compared with the native protein.

Hev b 3

The *Hev b 3* protein is associated with the small rubber particles in latex and demonstrates a strong IgE-binding reactivity in spina bifida patients with latex allergy (107–109). The reactivity of *Hev b 3* with serum IgE in health care workers is less frequent and weaker than in spina bifida patients (108,109). The amino acid sequence comparison of *Hev b 3* demonstrated 47% sequence homology with another major allergen, *Hev b 1*, a component of large rubber particles (108). In ELISA inhibition, *Hev b 1* preincubated latex-allergic sera exhibited more than 80% inhibition in IgE binding to the solid-phase–coated *Hev b 3*, indicating the presence of similar conformation in these proteins (110). Recombinant *Hev b 3* cloned and expressed in bacterial system exhibited specific binding to latex spina bifida patients (111).

Hev b 4

Hev b 4 has been reported by Sunderasen and colleagues as a microhelix component of latex that is purified using the conventional method (105). It is an acidic protein and, under reducing condition, appeared as broad band of about 50 to 57 kDa. Although this allergen detected significant IgE in 65% of health care workers, only 14% of these patients showed peripheral blood mononuclear cell (PBMC) stimulation to *Hev b 4* (104,112). This allergen has yet to be cloned and expressed.

Hev b 5

The molecular cloning and expression of *Hev b 5* has been reported independently by two investigators (96,97). This acidic protein is a major allergen with strong IgE-binding reactivity in both health care workers and spina bifida patients. In RAST assay, 92% of health care workers and 56% of spina bifida patients showed IgE binding with recombinant *Hev b 5*. *In vivo* IgE-binding property of *Hev b 5* is evident from its strong histamine release from basophils in latex-allergic patients (96,112).

Hev b 6 (Prohevein)

Hev b 6 shows strong reactivity with IgE in health care workers and spina bifida patients with latex allergy (104). In immunoblot and ELISA, the 43–amino acid N domain of prohevein appeared to exhibit IgE binding with a significantly higher number of latex-sensitized patients, compared with the 144–amino acid C domain of *Hev b 6*. The results of skin test reactions correlated well with the *in vitro* IgE to latex allergens (82,113,114). Epitope mapping of the prohevein molecule revealed more IgE-binding regions near the N-terminal end of the protein (114).

Hev b 7

Hev b 7, a patatin-like protein, showed IgE-binding reactivity with 23% of health care workers with latex allergy (115–117). Although both health care workers and spina bifida patients exhibited IgE binding with *Hev b 7*, this allergen recognized only a small group of patients, for whom IgE antibody against other major latex allergens could not be detected (112).

Hev b 8 (Profilin)

Profilins are actin-binding proteins involved in the formation of actin network of plant exoskeleton. The purified latex profilin, when used in skin-prick testing, showed positive reactions in all the 24 spina bifida patients and in 6 of 17 health care workers with latex allergy. The latex-derived profilin shows cross-reactivity with IgE from 36 patients with ragweed allergy (98).

Hev b 9 (Enolase)

Hev b 9 is a component present in the aqueous layer of NRL (75,83). A high degree of cross-reactivity can be expected because of the homology of enolases present in different organisms (*Cladosporium* species) and plants (tomato). However, preliminary studies in our laboratory of 26 health care workers with latex allergy failed to show IgE binding with the recombinant latex and fungal enolases (unpublished results).

Hev b 10 (Manganese Superoxide Dismutase)

This highly conserved enzyme (Mn-SOD) has been reported in a number of fungi, bacteria, and humans (75,83). Although Mn-SOD from the fungus *Aspergillus fumigatus* demonstrated significant IgE binding with sera in patients with allergic aspergillosis, only 1 of 26 latex-allergic patients demonstrated IgE antibody binding with latex Mn-SOD (unpublished results). This limited study indicates that despite the sequence similarities with Mn-SOD from other sources, such as mold, the NRL-derived Mn-SOD had only low levels of cross-allergenicity.

Hev b 11 (Endochitinase)

Chitinases and lysozymes constitute about 25% of the proteins in the lutoid fraction of NRL. This type 1 chitinase shares homology with N-terminal hevein domain and also shares epitopes with chitinases from avocado and banana (92,93). The cross-reactivity and immune responses of *Hev b 11* in allergic reaction have not been fully elucidated; hence, it is designated as a minor allergen in latex allergy.

HEVEA LATEX ALLERGENS NOT INCLUDED IN IUIS ALLERGEN LIST

Hevamine is one of the most abundant proteins isolated from the lutoids of *Hevea* species latex. This 30-kDa protein exhibits extensive sequence homology with chitinase and lysozymes from various sources (75,83). Purified hevamine demonstrated IgE reactivity with only 1 in 29 latex-allergic sera tested and hence are not con-sidered as an important allergen in inducing latex allergy (83). Type II chitinase is a 30-kDa acidic protein with high sequence homology to class 1 chitinase within the catalytic domain. The lack of a hevein-like domain near the N-terminal region of the protein may be responsible for its minimal allergenicity in latex-allergic patients. Several other latex allergens have been identified by two-dimensional immunoblotting and microsequencing (75). These proteins with sequence similarities to spinach, rice, and tomato triose phosphate isomerases and several proteosane subunits are yet to be purified and characterized for their role in latex allergy. Two-dimensional immunoblot demonstrates more than 200 peptides, with more than 50 spots demonstrating immune reactivity with IgE.

CO-SENSITIZATION AND CROSS-REACTIVITY OF LATEX ALLERGENS

Latex proteins exhibit strong cross-reactivity with a number of proteins from different fruits, vegetables, and grains (118,119). This widespread cross-reactivity among various plant proteins may be due to the presence of common T- and B-cell epitopes in them. Although extensive work has been carried out to identify the proteins involved in latex allergy, not much information is available on the cross-reactivity of latex allergens with proteins from other sources.

In a recent study, Beezhold and associates demonstrated the co-sensitization between latex and various foods by skin-prick testing (120). Of the 47 latex-sensitized patients used in this study, 53% exhibited positive skin-prick reaction to avocado, followed by 40% with potato, banana (38%), tomato (28%), chestnut (28%), and kiwi (17%). Cross-reactive allergens in banana appear in several molecular weight ranges between 23 and 47 kDa and in avocado between 27 and 91 kDa (121–123). Akasawa and colleagues identified an avocado chitinase as one of the cross-reacting proteins using sera from latex-allergic patients (124). Fourteen of 22 patients reacted to the 30-kDa avocado chitinase. Yagami and co-workers proposed that the pathogenesis-related latex proteins such as chitinase and

β-1,3-glucanase are potential cross-reacting proteins because they are common in different plant families and have comparable amino acid sequences and immunologic properties (91). In a recent study, Blanco and colleagues showed that chestnut and avocado type 1 chitinases with N-terminal hevein-like domain are the major allergens that cross-react with latex and suggested that type 1 chitinases are the pan allergens responsible for the latex-fruit syndrome (119). The cross-reactivity between fruits, pollen, and latex is also attributed to the highly conserved plant allergen profilin identified in all these different species (30).

As an example of polysensitization due to presence of cross-reactive proteins, mice immunized with timothy grass pollen extract alone, without subsequent exposure to latex, exhibited IgE reactivity to NRL allergens (125). These results demonstrated a mutual boosting effect of pollen and latex sensitization *in vivo*, which may be seen also in polysensitized plant allergic patients.

ANIMAL MODELS OF LATEX ALLERGY

Our murine model of latex hypersensitivity has provided several clues to the immunologic mechanisms in latex allergy. The model developed in two inbred strains of mice, C57BL/6 and BALB/c, typically mimics the disease condition with high serum IgE and increased eosinophilia in peripheral blood and lungs (126). Both strains showed significant increase in the cytokines interleukin-4 (IL-4) and IL-5 in sera without detectable interferon-γ (IFN-γ) level. This study confirmed that mice stimulated with latex proteins develop a predominantly T_H2 cytokine response. The histology of the lung and peritoneum reveals that the C57BL/6 mice were more resistant to inflammation, indicating that the response is species specific. In our rabbit model of NRL allergy, the animals were sensitized subcutaneously and intratracheally with antigens from ammoniated and nonammoniated Malaysian and Indian rubber tree sap (127). The results indicated that eosinophils and IgE antibodies play a major role in the immunopathogenesis of latex-induced allergy and anaphylaxis. A wide range

of inflammatory responses in rabbits immunized by subcutaneous route without intratracheal exposure suggests that NRL may pose a risk for a subsequent systemic reaction.

In another study, latex-immunized mice evaluated by body plethysmography exhibited a significant change in pulmonary conductance (G_L) and compliance (C_{dyn}) consistent with an asthma-like response. The latex-allergic response in this study is unique in that the direct challenge with latex antigen itself resulted in a significant airway response (128).

In our study with IL-4 knockout and wild-type BALB/c mice, the intranasal challenge with latex proteins resulted in elevated levels of IgE and peripheral and lung eosinophils in the wild-type animals compared with the IL-4 knockout group (129). On the other hand, the presence of airway resistance and comparable lung histology in both the wild-type and IL-4 knockout animals suggest that in addition to IgE antibody and eosinophils, other mediators, such as chemokines, may play a role in latex allergy.

CELL-MEDIATED IMMUNE RESPONSES IN LATEX-SENSITIZED PATIENTS

Although a substantial amount of work has been carried out on the characterization, purification, and cloning of latex allergens, not much information on the underlying T-cell responses in latex-sensitized patients is available. The accumulated data from animal models suggest that the nature of sensitization in patients may be solely dependent on the type of antibody production and the pattern of cytokine expression by allergen-specific T lymphocytes (126–129). The studies using crude ammoniated latex, non-ammoniated latex cytosol, and extracts demonstrated enhanced lymphoproliferative responses in latex sensitized patients (130). The distinct serologic patterns of patients against purified allergens were also reflected in their cell-mediated immune responses against these allergens. The monoclonal antibody affinity purified *Hev b 3* exhibited proliferative responses in spina bifida patients, but not in health care workers (81). On the other hand, significant stimulation of PBMCs from latex-sensitized health care workers has been detected with a 30-kDa latex protein purified by high-performance liquid chromatography and gel chromatography (131,132). In another study, purified *Hev b 1* induced lymphoproliferation in 52% of latex-allergic patients, compared with 25% of latex-exposed healthy subjects, suggesting that *Hev b 1* is a relevant allergen in health care workers (133).

In a recent study using six recombinant allergens, we found strong PBMC stimulation in 57% of health care workers with latex allergy against *Hev b 1*, but no correlation could be demonstrated between PBMC stimulation and high *Hev b 1*-specific IgE in serum (112). Whereas, *Hev b 2* showed stimulation in 56% patients, with more than 70% correlation between stimulation index and specific serum IgE binding (112). The other latex allergens, *Hev b 3*, *Hev b 4*, and *Hev b 7*, showed stimulation in the range of 14% to 25% without significant correlation between stimulation index and serum IgE levels in these patients. In a separate study, recombinant *Hev b 5* demonstrated T-cell stimulation in five of six health care workers with latex allergy (134). A detailed study on *Hev b 3*–specific T-cell clones from latex-sensitized spina bifida patients demonstrated a predominantly T_H2-like subset with a high level of IL-4 and IL-5 cytokine, consequently leading to IgE production and eosinophilia in patients (135).

EPITOPES OF LATEX ALLERGENS

Epitopes are defined as the sites or regions of an allergen that interact with T and B cells of immune system. The allergen interacts with the IgE as the B-cell epitope, whereas it is presented to the T cell after ingestion and processing by the antigen-presenting cell as linear peptide fragment in association with a class II major histocompatibility complex (MHC) molecule. T-cell epitopes of several known allergens are presented to the T-cell receptor in the context of a single human leukocyte antigen (HLA) molecule, such as DR, DQ, or DP (136). *In vitro* study conducted using overlapping synthetic peptides of latex allergen *Hev b 1* demonstrated that B lymphocytes of patients recognized several epitopes within the same allergen (137) (Table 31.5). As for the immunodominant T-cell epitope of *Hev b 1* in the amino acid region of 91-109, a strong HLA-DR4Dw4 (DRB1∗04010)–binding motif was predicted using a computer algorithm (138). Similarly, a major T-cell epitope of *Hev b 3* representing amino acid residues 103 to 114 carried an HLA-DR–binding motif (YSTS), indicating

TABLE 31.5. *Immunodominant epitopes of latex allergens in health care workers (HCW) and patients with spina bifida (SB)*

Allergens	T-cell epitopes/source	Immunoglobulin E epitopes/source	References
Hev b 1, 137 amino acids (aa)		30–49, 46–64, 121–137/HCW	137
		2–11, 16–25, 36–55, 61–70	110
	31–49, 91–109/PBMC	65–74, 90–108/HCW and SB	138
Hev b 3, 208 aa	10–24, 13–27, 48–59, 55–69,		135
	100–114, 103–114, 147–169,	2–17, 29–38, 41–50, 60–69,	110
	160–171, 178–189/SB-specific	85–94, 103–112, 118–127,	
	T-cell clones	138–147, 159–168, 179–188/ HCW and SB	
Hev b 5	46–65, 109–128/HCW-specific		134
	T-cell lines	15–22, 28–32, 50–56, 76–81,	139
		90–95,132–139/HCW	
Hev b 6		N-domain 13–24, 29–36	140
		C domain 62–69, 74–81	
		134–139, 164–171/HCW	114
		N-domain 19–24, 25–37	
		C domain 60–66, 76–79, 79–82,	
		82–96, 98–103, 164–172/HCW and SB	

PBMC, peripheral blood mononuclear cell

that the presentation of this peptide is HLA-DR restricted (135). The T-cell epitopes are linear and class II MHC restricted, whereas B-cell epitopes are either conformational or linear (136).

For *Hev b 5*, six IgE-binding regions were located throughout the molecule (139). Two epitopes (2 and 4) had common amino acid sequences of KTEEP, whereas epitopes 3 and 5 had a similar sequence of EEXXA, where X may be P, T, or K. In a separate study, murine B-cell epitopes of *Hev b 5* were located within a common motif of KXEE or KEXE, where X may be empty, threonine, or alanine (140).

In two separate studies, linear and conformational epitopes of prohevein have been identified; in both the studies, two linear epitopes were detected in the N-terminal region of *Hev b 6* (114,141). B-cell epitopes of *Hev b 6* specific for IgE antibody with sera from either latex-sensitized spina bifida patients or health care workers or common for both patients groups were reported. The IgE-binding epitopes of *Hev b 1* and *Hev b 3* were studied with sera from both health care workers and spina bifida patients with latex allergy (110). Of the eight epitopes of *Hev b 1* that reacted with sera from the spina bifida patients, only three near the C-terminal end showed binding with the sera of health care workers. For *Hev b 3*, however, common epitopes for spina bifida patients and health care workers were identified near the C-terminal region of the protein (110).

IMMUNOTHERAPY AND VACCINATION IN LATEX ALLERGY

Latex allergy has emerged as a potentially devastating disease with serious adverse outcomes. To reduce latex sensitization, the only immediate measure is the avoidance of latex products and exposure to latex allergens. Given the ubiquity of latex in the environment and the cost-effectiveness of latex products, complete avoidance may be an impossible proposition. Hence, as an alternative measure, immunotherapy has been attempted to reduce the disease severity and improve the quality of life of allergic individuals. The first oral latex desensitization was carried out in three health care workers, in whom nonammo-

niated latex extract was administered at 1 mg of proteins two to three times daily (142). After the treatment, participants were able to return to their jobs without undue symptoms.

The major drawback of these immunotherapeutic trials is the use of a crude aqueous mixture containing both allergenic and nonallergenic components. In another study, immunotherapy was carried out in a latex-sensitized hospital worker using ammoniated latex extract (143). There was steady improvement of the clinical symptoms in the subject without a significant change in lymphocyte subpopulation and serum immunoglobulin levels. Despite the success of these initial uncontrolled trials, immunotherapy of latex allergy is not advisable with the currently available allergen preparations. There is a need for the pharmacologic-grade recombinant allergens with immunologic properties comparable to the natural allergens for specific immunotherapy.

Allergen-specific therapy appears feasible in the near future because of the availability of an increasing number of functional latex allergens. The allergen-specific therapy may aim at prevention of allergy, induction of tolerance, or modification of ongoing immune responses (144–146). In an approach to induce T-cell nonresponsiveness in patients, strategies have been directed at synthetic peptides representing major T-cell epitopes administered to induce T-cell tolerance and anergy. The establishment of a patient's IgE reactivity profile (allergogram) with recombinant allergens may be of value in selecting the components against which a substantial IgE response is mounted. Another approach may use allergen fragments with disrupted conformational epitopes but intact T-cell epitopes. Although allergen-based therapy is effective, it may have undesirable side effects of anaphylaxis because of the presence of both IgE binding as well as T-cell epitopes in the whole allergen.

With the available immunodominant epitopes of several major latex allergens in hand, an attempt to use T-cell epitopes as multiple peptides or recombinant polypeptide hypoallergenic variants for immune modulation of the NRL allergic reaction is desirable. More recent approaches, such as modification of allergens by manipulating allergen encoding cyclic DNA (cDNA), or gene immunotherapy using cDNA encoding relevant allergens (naked DNA therapy), and modulation of the T_H2-type reaction to T_H1 by bacterial CpG DNA may also find application in immune intervention of NRL-allergic reactions.

The first study of DNA vaccination for latex allergy was attempted in mice using gene encoding the major latex allergen *Hev b 5* (147). The widespread appearance of *Hev b 5* transcript in immune and nonimmune tissues indicates that the careful selection of immunization protocols is necessary for controlling the expression of the allergen in specific target tissues.

MANAGEMENT OF THE PATIENT WITH NATURAL RUBBER LATEX ALLERGY

Successful management of the NRL-allergic patient is critical to avoid untoward allergic reactions and occupational asthma (148–154). Avoiding contact with NRL products has remained the mainstay of therapy (Table 31.6). Whether a latex-free environment is possible depends on a strict definition. However, it is more practical to speak about a latex-safe environment. Some concern has been raised about patients developing excessive vigilance and phobic reactions when in

TABLE 31.6. *Latex avoidance precautions in the hospital and clinical setting in patients with documented or suspected latex allergy*

Use nonlatex gloves only.
Provide allergy band or alert to patient.
Label door to room as needing "latex-safe precautions."
Check that all medical devices are labeled for their latex content.
Latex products should not contact skin or mucosal surfaces of patient (no respiratory source).
Do not use inline intravenous valves (this does not refer to injector ports).
Consider injecting medication using stopcock devices instead of injector ports or tubing.
Operating room—schedule as the first case of the day if powdered gloves in prior use in operating room.
Medication from multidose vials—take top off or change needle after drawing up medication.
Premedication—not necessary when strict latex avoidance precautions are used.
Ideal—all latex glove use in hospital should be powder free and low in allergen.
Ban powdered latex products manufactured by dipping process from building (e.g., balloons).

close proximity to NRL products after stringent warnings to adhere to a latex-free environment. A safe environment is one in which there is no NRL direct skin, mucous membrane, or aeroallergen contact by a person with NRL allergy. Currently, NRL products made by a dipping method with a powder-donning lubricant are the most likely to result in serious reactions from either direct contact or aeroallergen inhalation. A few common examples of these include gloves, balloons, and rubber bands. Dust from grinding NRL in a doll-manufacturing plant is an uncommon but predictable problem. In the past, it was highly unlikely that rubber products made after coagulation and extreme processing would induce reactions without direct skin or mucous membrane contact. It has been strongly advocated that long lists of rubber products, without designated allergen content or risk for reactivity, be furnished to patients with examples of alternative products that do not contain NRL. In the future, it makes sense to stratify the risks associated with these products in order to allow a patient to have a rational and safe approach to avoidance measures. This will require refinement of the current labeling of NRL medical products that stratifies the labeling of the product into low- and high-allergen risks. Although NRL medical devices are labeled with content and warnings, no stratification of risk has been made to date. An NRL product heat vulcanized at 600°C for 1 hour will have considerably less allergen content than a product heat vulcanized at 100°C for a few minutes.

Latex-safe precautions in the operating room have allowed uncomplicated anesthesia for most patients with NRL allergy. Premedication with antihistamines and corticosteroids is unnecessary and not likely to improve the outcome of the patient. Occasionally, latex-safe precautions have failed to prevent an allergic reaction in some individuals. However, it is not clear whether the institution reporting the reaction was actually using latex avoidance. Clearly, some of those institutions were still using powdered latex gloves except during an individual case. Because the level of aeroallergen in operating rooms declines when there is no activity, it has been suggested that a strategy of operating on latex-allergic patients as the first case of the day to avoid aeroallergen exposure is safe. A prospective study demonstrated that NRL aeroallergen could be detected in the operating rooms even when no surgery was being performed in that room, albeit at lower levels than on surgery days (42). Presumably, residual allergen from prior glove use or recirculation from ventilation systems may be the cause of these reactions. Thus, avoidance of NRL allergen must include a complete institutional buying change to powder-free gloves that do not release NRL aeroallergen. Many institutions have been unsuccessful in adopting such a policy because of price constraints and individual preference of workers for specific glove types. Placing NRL-allergic patients' needs first for safety purposes will require these changes in health care.

In addition to the operating room, safe care for NRL patients in an ambulance, emergency room, laboratory, radiology department, general ward, intensive care unit, postanesthesia care unit, and clinic is required. Medical literature repeatedly demonstrates that powdered NRL gloves are the major contributors of transferable allergen. Strict avoidance of the use of powdered NRL gloves is necessary in all these areas because it is impossible to predict when an NRL-allergic patient may present for care. Not only should the patient wear proper identification about the NRL allergy, but also the room or area where they are cared for should be clearly marked to prevent accidental exposure, for example, by bringing a powdered NRL balloon into the room. Policies and procedures for caring for such patients are necessary. Central purchasing should control ordering practices and maintain lists of alternative substitute products. Fortunately, mandatory content and warning labels on packaging of medical devices has made central lists of NRL-containing products unnecessary and cumbersome. Consumer products are not labeled at present, and some vigilance is necessary to avoid accidental exposures. With these measures, NRL allergy will diminish in frequency and severity in the future.

REFERENCES

1. Nutter AF. Contact urticaria to rubber. *Br J Dermatol* 1979;101:597–598.

2. Slater J. Rubber anaphylaxis. *N Engl J Med* 1989; 17:1126–1130.

3. Sussman G, Tarlo S, Dolovich J. The spectrum of IgE-mediated responses to latex. *JAMA* 1991;265:2844–2847.

4. Turjanmaa K, Alenius H, Makinen-Kiljunen S, et al. Natural rubber latex allergy. *Allergy* 1996;51:593–602.

5. Gazeley KF, Gorton ADT, Pendle TD. Technological processings of natural rubber latex. In: Roberts AD, ed. *Natural rubber science and technology.* Oxford, UK: Oxford University Press, 1988.

6. Archer BL, Barnard D, Cockbain EG, et al. Structure, composition and biochemistry of Hevea latex. In: Bateman L, ed. *The chemistry and physics of rubber-like substances.* New York: John Wiley, 1963:41.

7. Ownby D, Tomlanovich M, Sammons N, et al. Anaphylaxis associated with latex allergy during barium enema examinations. *AJR Am J Roentgenol* 1991;156:903–908.

8. Kelly KJ, Pearson ML, Kurup VP, et al. Anaphylactic reactions in patients with spina bifida during general anesthesia: epidemiologic features, risk factors, and latex hypersensitivity. *J Allergy Clin Immunol* 1994;94(1):53–61.

9. Turjanmaa K. Incidence of immediate allergy to latex gloves in hospital personnel. *Contact Dermatitis* 1987; 17:270–275.

10. Turjanmaa K, Laurila K, Makinen-Kiljunen S, et al. Rubber contact urticaria. *Contact Dermatitis* 1988; 19:362–367.

11. Salkie M. The prevalence of atopy and hypersensitivity to latex in medical laboratory technologists. *Arch Pathol Lab Med* 1993;117:897–899.

12. Axelsson IGK, Eriksson M, Wrangsjo K. Anaphylaxis and angioedema due to rubber allergy in children. *Acta Paediatr Scand* 1988;77:314–316.

13. Bascom R, Baser M, Thomas R, et al. Elevated serum IgE, eosinophilia, and lung function in rubber workers. *Arch Environ Health* 1990;45:15–19.

14. Carrillo T, Blanco C, Quiralte J, et al. Prevalence of latex allergy among greenhouse workers. *J Allergy Clin Immunol* 1995;96(5):699–701.

15. Chiu A, Kelly KJ, Thomason J, et al. Recurrent vaginitis as a manifestation of inhaled latex allergy. *Allergy* 1999;54:183–190.

16. Konz KR, Chia JK, Kurup VP, et al. Comparison of latex hypersensitivity among patients with neurologic defects. *J Allergy Clin Immunol* 1995;95(5):950–954.

17. Feczko PJ, Simms SM, Bakirci N. Fatal hypersensitivity during a barium enema. *AJR Am J Roentgenol* 1989;153:275–276.

18. Swartz J, Braude B, Gilmour R, et al. Intraoperative anaphylaxis to latex. *Can J Anaesth* 1990;37:589–592.

19. Kelly KJ, Setlock M, Davis JP. Anaphylactic reactions during general anesthesia among pediatric patients. *MMWR Morb Mortal Wkly Rep* 1991;40(26):437.

20. Gold M, Swartz J, Braude B, Dolovich J, et al. Intraoperative anaphylaxis: an association with latex sensitivity. *J Allergy Clin Immunol* 1991;87:662–666.

21. Katelaris CH, Widmer RP, Lazarus RM. Prevalence of latex allergy in a dental school. *Med J Aust* 1996; 164:711–714.

22. Safadi GS, Safadi TJ, Terezhalmy GT, et al. Latex hypersensitivity: its prevalence among dental professionals *J Am Dent Assoc* 1996;127:83–88.

23. Tarlo S, Sussman G, Holness D. Latex sensitivity in dental students and staff: a cross-sectional study. *J Allergy Clin Immunol* 1997;99:396–401.

24. Kelly KJ, Walsh-Kelly CM. Latex allergy: a patient and health care system emergency. *Ann Emerg Med* 1998;32(6):723–729.

25. Liss GM, Sussman GL, Deal K, et al. Latex allergy: epidemiological study of 1351 hospital workers. *Occup Environ Med* 1997;54:335–342.

26. Safidi GS, Corey EC, Taylor JS, et al. Latex hypersensitivity in emergency medical service providers. *Ann Allergy Asthma Immunol* 1996;77:39–42.

27. Mace S, Sussman G, Stark DF, et al. Latex allergy in operating room nurses. *J Allergy Clin Immunol* 1996;97:558.

28. Hunt LW, Fransway AF, Reed CE, et al. An epidemic of occupational allergy to latex involving health care workers. *J Occup Environ Med* 1995;37(10):1204–1209.

29. Sussman GL, Liss GM, Deal K, et al. Incidence of latex sensitization among latex glove users. *J Allergy Clin Immunol* 1998;101(2)(1):171–178.

30. Lagier F, Vervloet D, Lhermet I, et al. Prevalence of latex allergy in operating room nurses. *J Allergy Clin Immunol* 1993;90(3):319–322.

31. Brown RH, Schauble JF, Hamilton RG. Prevalence of latex allergy among anesthesiologists. *Anesthesiology* 1998;89(2):292–299.

32. Yassin MS, Lierl MB, Fischer TJ, et al. Latex allergy in hospital employees. *Ann Allergy* 1994;72:245–249.

33. Bernardini R, Novembre E, Inhargiola A, et al. Prevalence and risk factors of latex sensitization in an unselected pediatric population. *J Allergy Clin Immunol* 1998;101:621–625.

34. Shield S, Blaiss M. Prevalence of latex sensitivity in children evaluated for inhalant allergy. *Allergy Proc* 1992;13:129–130.

35. *NIOSH alert: preventing allergic reactions to natural rubber latex in the workplace*. DHHS Publication No. 97-135, 1997(6):1–11.

36. Cameron M. Cost implications of allergy and recent Canadian research findings. *Eur J Surg* 1997;163 [Suppl 579]:47–48.

37. Federal Register. *Natural rubber-containing medical devices: user Labeling*. Vol. 62, No. 189. Washington, D.C.: September 30, 1997:52021–51030.

38. Baur X, Ammon J, Chen Z, et al. Health risk in hospitals through airborne allergens for patients presensitized to latex. *Lancet* 1993;342:1148–1150.

39. Swanson MC, Bubak ME, Hunt LW, et al. Quantification of occupational latex aeroallergens in a medical center. *J Allergy Clin Immunol* 1994;94(3):445–551.

40. Tomazic VJ, Shampaine EL, Lamanna A, et al. Cornstarch powder on latex products is an allergen carrier. *J Allergy Clin Immunol* 1994;93:751–758.

41. Tarlo SM, Sussman G, Contala A, et al. Control of airborne latex by use of powder-free latex gloves. *J Allergy Clin Immunol* 1994;93:985–989.

42. Heilman DK, Jones RT, Swanson MC, et al. A prospective, controlled study showing that rubber gloves are the major contributor to latex aeroallergen levels in the operating room. *J Allergy Clin Immunol* 1996;98(2):325–330.

43. Allmers H, Brehler R, Chen Z, et al. Reduction of latex aeroallergens and latex-specific IgE antibodies in sensitized workers after removal of powdered natural rubber latex gloves in a hospital. *J Allergy Clin Immunol* 1998;102(5):841–846.

44. Brehler R, Kolling R, Webb M, et al. Glove powder: a risk factor for the development of latex allergy? *Eur J Surg* 1997;[Suppl 579]:23–25.

45. Baur X, Chen Z, Allmers H. Can a threshold limit value for natural rubber latex airborne allergens be defined? *J Allergy Clin Immunol* 1998;101:24–27.

46. Charous BL, Schuenemann PJ, Swanson MC. Passive dispersion of latex aeroallergen in a health care facility. *Ann Allergy Asthma Immunol* 2000;85:285–290.

47. Swanson MC, Olson DW. Latex allergen affinity for starch powders applied to natural rubber gloves and released as an aerosol: from dust to don. *Can J Allergy Clin Immunol* 2000;5(8):328–335.

48. Voelker R. Latex-induced asthma among health care workers. *JAMA* 1995;273(10):764.

49. Vandenplas O, Delwiche JP, Evrared G, et al. Prevalence of occupational asthma due to latex among hospital personnel. *Am J Respir Crit Care Med* 1995;151:54–60.

50. Orfan NA, Reed R, Dykewicz MS, et al. Occupational asthma in a latex doll manufacturing plant. *J Allergy Clin Immunol* 1994;94(5):826–830.

51. Tarlo SM, Wong L, Roos J, et al. Occupational asthma caused by latex in a surgical glove manufacturing plant. *J Allergy Clin Immunol* 1990;85:626–631.

52. Brugnami G, Marabini A, Siracuse A, et al. Work-related late asthmatic response induced by latex allergy. *J Allergy Clin Immunol* 1995;96(4):457–464.

53. Jones RT, Scheppmann DL, Heilman KD, et al. Prospective study of extractable latex allergen contents of disposable medical gloves. *Ann Allergy* 1994;73:321–325.

54. Kelly KJ. Latex allergy. [Kelly, KJ, CD Rom ed]. *Creative educational opportunities*. Hartland, 1998.

55. Ylitalo L, Turjanmaa K, Palosuo T, et al. Natural rubber latex allergy in children who had not undergone surgery and children who had undergone multiple operations. *J Allergy Clin Immunol* 1997;100(5):606–612.

56. Ownby DR, Ownby HE, McCullough J, et al. The prevalence of anti-latex IgE antibodies in 1000 volunteer blood donors. *J Allergy Clin Immunol* 1996; 97(6):1188–1192.

57. Saxon A, Ownby D, Huard T, et al. Prevalence of IgE to natural rubber latex in unselected blood donors and performance characteristics of AlaSTAT testing. *Ann Allergy Asthma Immunol* 2000;84:199–206.

58. Liss GM, Sussman GL. Latex sensitization: occupational versus general population prevalence rates. *Am J Ind Med* 1999;35:196–200.

59. Sussman GL, Lem D, Liss G, et al. Latex allergy in housekeeping personnel. *Ann Allergy Asthma Immunol* 1995;74:415–418.

60. Kelly KJ, Kurup VP, Reijula K, et al. The diagnosis of natural rubber latex allergy. *J Allergy Clin Immunol* 1994;93(5):813–816.

61. Yunginger JW. Diagnostic skin testing for natural rubber latex allergy. *J Allergy Clin Immunol* 1998;102:351–352.

62. Hamilton RG, Adkinson F, and the Multicenter Latex Skin Testing Study Task Force. Diagnosis of natural rubber latex allergy: multicenter latex skin testing efficacy study. *J Allergy Clin Immunol* 1998;102:482–490.

63. Hamilton RG, Biagini RE, Krieg EF, and the Multi-Center Latex Skin Testing Study Task Force. Diagnostic performance of FDA-cleared serological assays for

natural rubber latex-specific IgE antibody. *J Allergy Clin Immunol* 1999;103:925–930.

64. Fink JN, Kelly KJ, Elms N, et al. Comparative studies of latex extracts used in skin testing. *Ann Allergy Asthma Immunol* 1996;76:149–152.

65. Hamilton RG, Adkinson NF. Natural rubber latex skin testing reagents: safety and diagnostic accuracy of non-ammoniated latex, ammoniated latex, and latex rubber glove extracts. *J Allergy Clin Immunol* 1996;98:872–883.

66. Hamilton GR, Adkinson NF. Validation of the latex glove provocation procedure in latex-allergic subjects. *Ann Allergy Asthma Immunol* 1997;79:266–272.

67. Kelly KJ, Kurup VP, Zacharisen MC, et al. Skin and serologic testing in the diagnosis of latex allergy. *J Allergy Clin Immunol* 1993;91:1140–1145.

68. Ownby D, Magera B, Williams PB. A blinded, multi-center evaluation of two commercial in vitro tests for latex-specific IgE antibodies. *Ann Allergy Asthma Immunol* 2000;84:193–196.

69. Ownby D, McCullough J. Testing for latex allergy. *J Clin Immunoassay* 1993;16:109–113.

70. Laoprasert N, Swanson MC, Jones RT, et al. Inhalation challenge testing of latex-sensitive health care workers and the effectiveness of laminar flow HEPA-filtered helmets reducing rhinoconjunctival and asthmatic reactions. *J Allergy Clin Immunol* 1998;102(6):998–1004.

71. Slater J, Mostello L. Routine testing for latex allergy in patients with spina bifida is not recommended. *Anesthesiology* 1992;74:391.

72. Valyasevi MA, Maddox DE, Li JT. Systemic reactions to allergy skin tests. *Ann Allergy Asthma Immunol* 1999;83:132–136.

73. Sanchez-Monge R, Blanco C, Diaz-Perales A, et al. Isolation and characterization of major banana allergens: identification as fruit class I chitinases. *Clin Exp Allergy* 1999;29:673–680.

74. Kurup VP, Alenius H, Kelly KJ, et al. A two-dimensional electrophoretic analysis of latex particles reacting with IgE and IgG antibodies from patients with latex allergy. *Int Arch Allergy Immunol* 1996;109:58–67.

75. Posch A, Chen Z, Wheeler C, et al. Characterization and identification of latex allergens by two-dimensional electrophoresis and protein microsequencing. *J Allergy Clin Immunol* 1997;99:385–395.

76. Subramaniam A. The chemistry of natural rubber latex. In: Fink JN, ed. *Immunology and allergy clinics of North America*. Philadelphia: WB Saunders, 1995:1–20.

77. Alenius H, Kurup V, Kelly K, et al. Latex allergy: frequent occurrence of IgE antibodies to a cluster of 11 latex proteins in patients with spina bifida and histories of anaphylaxis. *J Lab Clin Med* 1994;123:712–720.

78. Makinen-Kiljunen S, Turjanmaa K, Palosuo T, et al. Characterization of latex antigens and allergens in surgical gloves and natural rubber by immunoelectrophoretic methods. *J Allergy Clin Immunol* 1992;90:230–235.

79. Chambeyron C, Dry J, Leynadier F, et al. Study of the allergic fractions of latex. *Allergy* 1992;47:92–97.

80. Lu L-J, Kurup VP, Fink JN, et al. Comparison of latex antigens from surgical gloves, ammoniated and nonammoniated latex: effect of ammonia treatment on natural rubber latex proteins. *J Lab Clin Med* 1995;126:161–168.

81. Lu L-J, Kurup VP, Hoffman DR, et al. Characterization

of a major latex allergen associated with hypersensitivity in spina bifida patients. *J Immunol* 1995;155:2721–2728.

82. Alenius H, Reunala T, Turjanmaa K, et al. Surgical glove latex glove allergy: characterization of rubber protein allergens by immunoblotting. *Int Arch Allergy Appl Immunol* 1991;96:376–380.

83. Breiteneder H. The allergens of *Hevea brasiliensis*. *ACI Int* 1998;10:101–109.

84. Dennis MS, Light DR. Rubber elongation factor from *Hevea brasiliensis*: identification, characterization, and role in rubber biosynthesis. *J Biol Chem* 1989;264:18608–18617.

85. Dennis MS, Henzel WJ, Bell J, et al. Amino acid sequence of rubber elongation factor protein associated with rubber particles in *Hevea* latex. *J Biol Chem* 1989;264:18618–18626.

86. Oh SK, Kang H, Shin DH, et al. Isolation, characterization, and functional analysis of a novel cDNA clone encoding a small rubber particle protein from *Hevea brasiliensis*. *J Biol Chem* 1999;274:17132–17138.

87. Broekaert W, Lee HI, Kush A, et al. Wound-induced accumulation of mRNA containing a hevein sequence in laticifers of rubber tree (*Hevea brasiliensis*). *Proc Natl Acad Sci USA* 1990;87:7633–7637.

88. Gidrol X, Chrestin H, Tan H-L, et al. Hevein, a lectin-like protein from *Hevea brasiliensis* (rubber tree) is involved in the coagulation of latex. *J Biol Chem* 1994;269:9278–9283.

89. Yusof F, Audley BG, Ward MA, et al. Purification and characterization of an inhibitor of rubber biosynthesis from C-serum of *Hevea brasiliensis* latex. *J Rubber Res* 1998;1:95–110.

90. Breton F, Coupé M, Sanier C, et al. Demonstration of beta-1,3-glucanase activities in lutoids of *Hevea brasiliensis* latex. *J Nat Rubber Res* 1995;10:37–45.

91. Yagami T, Sato M, Nakamura A, et al. Plant defense-related enzymes as latex antigens. *J Allergy Clin Immunol* 1998;101:379–385.

92. Graham LS, Sticklen MB. Plant chitinases. *Can J Bot* 1994;72:1057–1083.

93. Posch A, Wheeler CH, Chen Z, et al. Class I endochitinase containing a hevein domain is the causative allergen in latex-associated avocado allergy. *Clin Exp Allergy* 1999;29:667–672.

94. Terwissccha van Scheltinga T, Kalk AC, et al. Crystal structures of hevamine, a plant defense protein with chitinase and lysozyme activity, and its complex with an inhibitor. *Structure* 1994;2:1181–1189.

95. Bokma E, van Koningsveld GA, Jeronimus-Stratingh M, et al. Hevamine, a chitinase from the rubber tree *Hevea brasiliensis*, cleaves peptidoglycan between the C-1 of *N*-acetylglucosamine and C-4 of *N*-acetylmuramic acid and therefore is not a lysozyme. *FEBS Lett* 1997;411:161–163.

96. Slater JE, Vedvick T, Arthur-Smith A, et al. Identification, cloning, and sequence of a major allergen (Hev b 5) from natural rubber latex (*Hevea brasiliensis*). *J Biol Chem* 1996;271:25394–25399.

97. Akasawa A, Hsieh LS, Martin BM, et al. A novel acidic allergen, Hev b 5, in latex: purification, cloning and characterization. *J Biol Chem* 1996;271:25389–25393.

98. Vallier P, Balland S, Harf R, et al. Identification of profilin as an IgE-binding component in latex from *Hevea*

brasiliensis: clinical implications. *Clin Exp Allergy* 1995;25:332–339.

99. Czuppon AB, Chen Z, Rennert S, et al. The rubber elongation factor of rubber trees (*Hevea brasiliensis*) is the major allergen in latex. *J Allergy Clin Immunol* 1993;92:690–697.

100. Alenius H, Kalkkinen N, Yip E, et al. Significance of rubber elongation factor as a latex allergen. *Int Arch Allergy Immunol* 1996;109:362–368.

101. Tomazic VJ, Withrow TJ, Hamilton RG. Characterization of the allergen(s) in latex protein extracts. *J Allergy Clin Immunol* 1995;96:635–642.

102. Attanyaka DP, Kekwick RG, Franklin FC. Molecular cloning and nucleotide sequencing of the rubber elongation factor gene from *Hevea brasiliensis*. *Plant Mol Biol* 1991;16:1079–1081.

103. Chen ZP, Cremer R, Posch A, et al. On the allergenicity of Hev b 1 among health care workers and patients with spina bifida allergic to natural rubber latex. *J Allergy Clin Immunol* 1997;100:684–693.

104. Kurup VP, Yeang HY, Sussman GL, et al. Detection of immunoglobulin antibodies in the sera of patients using purified latex allergens. *Clin Exp Allergy* 1999;30:359–369.

105. Sunderasan E, Hamzah S, Hamid S, et al. Latex B-serum beta-1,3-glucanase (Hev b 2) and a component of the microhelix (Hev b 4) are major latex allergens. *J Nat Rubb Res* 1996;10:82–99.

106. Chye ML, Cheung KY. Beta-1,3-glucanase is highly-expressed in lactifers of *Hevea brasiliensis*. *Plant Mol Biol* 1995;29:397–402.

107. Yeang HY, Cheong KF, Sunderasan E, et al. The 14.6 kd rubber elongation factor (Hev b 1) and 24 kd (Hev b 3) rubber particle proteins are recognized by IgE from patients with spina bifida and latex allergy. *J Allergy Clin Immunol* 1996;98:628–639.

108. Alenius H, Kalkkinen N, Lukka M, et al. Purification and partial amino acid sequencing of a 27-kD natural rubber allergen recognized by latex-allergic children with spina bifida. *Int Arch Allergy Immunol* 1995;106:258–262.

109. Alenius H, Palosuo T, Kelly K, et al. IgE reactivity to 14-kD and 27-kD natural rubber proteins in latex-allergic children with spina bifida and other congential anomalies. *Int Arch Allergy Immunol* 1993;102:61–66.

110. Banerjee B, Kanitpong K, Fink JN, et al. Unique and shared IgE epitopes of Hev b 1 and Hev b 3 in latex allergy. *Mol Immunol* 2000;37:789–798.

111. Wagner B, Krebitz M, Buck D, et al. Cloning, expression, and characterization of recombinant Hev b 3, a *Hevea brasiliensis* protein associated with latex allergy in patients with spina bifida. *J Allergy Clin Immunol* 1999;104:1084–1092.

112. Johnson BD, Kurup VP, Sussman GL, et al. Purified and recombinant latex proteins stimulate peripheral blood lymphocytes of latex allergic patients. *Int Arch Allergy Immunol* 1999;120:270–279.

113. Alenius H, Kalkkinen N, Reunala T, et al. The main IgE binding epitopes of a major latex allergens, prohevein is present in its 43 amino acid fragment hevein. *J Immunol* 1996;156:1618–1625.

114. Banerjee B, Wang X, Kelly KJ, et al. IgE from latex-allergic patients binds to cloned and expressed b cell epitopes of prohevein. *J Immunol* 1997;159:5724–5732.

115. Kostyal DA, Hickey V, Noti JD, et al. Cloning and characterization of a latex allergen (Hev b 7): homology to patatin, a plant PLA2. *Clin Exp Immunol* 1998;112:355–362.

116. Beezhold DH, Sussman GL, Kostyal DA, et al. Identification of a 46-kD latex protein allergen in health care workers. *Clin Exp Immunol* 1994;98:408–413.

117. Sowka S, Wagner S, Krebitz M, et al. cDNA cloning of the 43-kDa latex allergen Hev b 7 with sequence similarity to patatins and its expression in the yeast *Pichia pastoris*. *Eur J Biochem* 1998;255:213–219.

118. Brehler R, Theissen U, Mohr C, et al. "Latex-fruit syndrome." Frequency of cross-reacting IgE antibodies. *Allergy* 1997;52:404–410.

119. Blanco C, Carrillo T, Castillo R, et al. Latex allergy: clinical features and cross reactivity with fruits. *Ann Allergy* 1994;73:309–314.

120. Beezhold DH, Sussman GL, Liss GM, et al. Latex allergy can induce clinical reactions to specific foods. *Clin Exp Immunol* 1996;26:416–422.

121. Lavaud F, Prevost A, Cossart C, et al. Allergy to latex avocado, pear, and banana: evidence for a 30 kd antigen in immunoblotting. *J Allergy Clin Immunol* 1995;95:557–564.

122. Alroth M, Alenius H, Turjanmaa K, et al. Cross-reacting allergens in natural rubber latex and avocado. *J Allergy Clin Immunol* 1995;96:167–173.

123. Alenius H, Makinen-Kiljunenen S, Alroth M, et al. Crossreactivity between allergens in natural rubber latex and banana studied by immunoblot inhibition. *Clin Exp Allergy* 1996;26:341–348.

124. Akasawa A, Hsieh L, Tanaka K, et al. Identification and characterization of avocado chitinase with cross-reactivity to a latex protein. *J Allergy Clin Immunol* 1996;97:321.

125. Mahler V, Diepgen TL, Kubeta O, et al. Mutual boosting effects of sensitization with timothy grass pollen and latex glove extract on IgE antibody responses in a mouse model. *J Invest Dermatol* 2000;114:1039–1043.

126. Kurup VP, Kumar A, Choi H, et al. Latex antigens induce IgE and eosinophils in mice. *Int Arch Allergy Immunol* 1994;103:370–377.

127. Reijula KE, Kelly KJ, Kurup VP, et al. Latex-induced dermal and pulmonary hypersensitivity in rabbits. *J Allergy Clin Immunol* 1994;94:891–902.

128. Thakker JC, Xia J-Q, Rickaby DA, et al. A murine model of latex allergy induced airway hypersensitivity. *Lung* 1999;177:89–100.

129. Xia J-Q, Rickaby DA, Kelly KJ, et al. Immune response and airway reactivity in wild and IL-4 knockout mice exposed to latex allergens. *Int Arch Allergy Immunol* 1999;118:23–29.

130. Murali PS, Kelly KJ, Fink JN, et al. Investigations into the cellular immune responses in latex allergy. *J Lab Clin Med* 1994;124:638–643.

131. Turjanmaa K, Rasanen L, Lehto M, et al. Basophil histamine release and lymphocyte proliferation tests in latex contact urticaria. *Allergy* 1989;44:181–186.

132. Fink JN, Kelly KJ. Latex hypersensitivity: an emerging problem. *ACI Int* 1994;6:4–6.

133. Raulf-Heismoth M, Chen Z, Libers V, et al. Lymphocyte proliferation response to extracts from different latex materials and to the purified latex allergen Hev b 1

(rubber elongation factor). *J Allergy Clin Immunol* 1996;98:640–651.

134. de Silva HD, Sutherland MF, Suphioglu C, et al. Human T-cell epitopes of the latex allergen Hev b 5 in health care workers. *J Allergy Clin Immunol* 2000;105:1017–1024.

135. Bohle B, Wagner B, Vollmann U, et al. Characterization of T cell responses to Hev b 3, an allergen associated with latex allergy in spina bifida patients. *J Immunol* 2000;164:4393–4398.

136. Kurup VP, Banerjee B. Fungal allergens and peptide epitopes. *Peptides* 2000;21:589–599.

137. Chen Z, vanKampen V, Raulf-Heimsoth M, et al. Allergenic and antigenic determinants of latex allergen Hev b 1: peptide mapping of epitopes recognized by human, murine and rabbit antibodies. *Clin Exp Allergy* 1996;26:406–415.

138. Raulf-Heimsoth M, Chen Z, Liebers V, et al. Lymphocyte proliferation response to extracts from different latex materials and to the purified latex allergen Hev b 1 (rubber elongation factor). *J Allergy Clin Immunol* 1996;98:640–651.

139. Beezhold DH, Hickey VL, Slater JE, et al. Human IgE-binding epitopes of the latex allergen Hev b 5. *J Allergy Clin Immunol* 1999;103:1166–1172.

140. Slater JE, Paupore EJ, O'Hehir RE. Murine B-cell and T-cell epitopes of the allergen Hev b 5 from natural rubber latex. *Mol Immunol* 1999;36:135–143.

141. Beezhold DH, Kostyal DA, Sussman GL. IgE epitope analysis of the hevein preprotein: a major latex allergen. *Clin Exp Immunol* 1997;108:114–121.

142. Toci G, Shah S, Al-Faqih A, et al. Oral latex desensitization of healthcare workers. *J Allergy Clin Immunol* 1998;101:S161(abst).

143. Pereira C, Lourenco R, Rico P, et al. Specific immunotherapy for occupational latex allergy. *Allergy* 1999;54:291–293.

144. Norman PS. Clinical and immunologic effects of component peptides in ALLERVAX CAT. *Int Arch Allergy Immunol* 1997;113:224–226.

145. Valenta R, Kraft D. Recombinant allergens for diagnosis and therapy of allergic disease. *Curr Opin Immunol* 1995;7:751–756.

146. Valenta R, Steinberger P, Duchene M, et al. Immunological and structural similarities among allergens: prerequisite for a specific and component-based therapy of allergy. *Immunol Cell Biol* 1996;74:187–194.

147. Slater J, Colberg-Poley A. A DNA vaccine for allergen immunotherapy using the latex allergen Hev b 5. *Arb Paul Ehrlich Inst Bundesamt Sera Impfstoffe Frankf A M.* 1997;91:230.

148. Anonymous. Task force on allergic reactions to latex. American Academy of Allergy and Immunology: committee report. *J Allergy Clin Immunol* 1993;92 (1 Pt. 1):16–18.

149. Hunt LW, Boone-Orke JL, Fransway AF, et al. A medical-center-wide multi disciplinary approach to the problem of natural rubber latex allergy. *J Occup Environ Med* 1996;38(8):765–770.

150. Vandenplas O, Delwiche JP, Depelchin S, et al. Latex gloves with a lower protein content reduce bronchial reactions in subjects with occupational asthma caused by latex. *Am J Respir Crit Care Med* 1995;151:887–981.

151. Hamilton RG, Abmli D, Brown RH. Impact of personal avoidance practices on health care workers sensitized to natural rubber latex. *J Allergy Clin Immunol* 2000;105(4):839–841.

152. Kelly KJ, Sussman G, Fink JN. Stop the sensitization. *J Allergy Clin Immunol* 1996;98(1):857–858.

153. Schwartz HJ. Latex: a potential hidden "food" allergen in fast food restaurants. *J Allergy Immunol* 1995; 95(1):139–140.

154. Kelly KJ. Latex allergy: where do we go from here? *Can J Allergy Clin Immunol* 2000;5(8):337–340.

32

Physiologic Assessment of Asthma and other Allergic Lung Diseases

Paul A. Greenberger

Division of Allergy-Immunology, Department of Medicine, Northwestern University
Medical School, Chicago, Illinois

Physiologic assessment of asthma or hypersensitivity pneumonitis is necessary in addition to recording signs and symptoms, response to pharmacotherapy, or avoidance measures and determining overall success with management. Dyspnea may not be recognized by some patients with asthma, and these "poor perceivers" may experience acute severe asthma episodes that may be fatal (1). More commonly, patients tolerate or acclimate to decreases in expiratory flow rates. Obtaining spirometry on the initial assessment of a patient with asthma or possible asthma was recommended by the Expert Panel Report 2 of the National Asthma Education and Prevention Program of the National Institutes of Health (2). Subsequent measurements are obtained after treatment to demonstrate expected improvement and then "at least every 1 to 2 years" (2). It is often necessary to obtain spirometric values more frequently, depending on the clinical response and severity of asthma. Spirometry may identify unrecognized decreases in forced expiratory volume in 1 second (FEV_1); the FEV_1-to-forced vital capacity (FVC) ratio (FEV_1/FVC); or the forced expiratory flow, midexpiratory phase ($FEF_{25\%-75\%}$; formerly the MMEF) despite complete symptom control. For some patients, additional therapy will be indicated. Alternatively, some patients with asthma have coexisting chronic obstructive pulmonary disease (COPD; usually having smoked more

than 40 pack-years of cigarettes) or, in the absence of smoking or other causes, irreversible asthma (3).

Spirometric results should be considered in terms of accepted parameters and test performance. For example, poor effort (manifested by decreased peak expiratory flow rate [PEFR]), coughing or hesitation during the expiratory effort, or failure to inspire fully to total lung capacity should be assessed during the spirometric procedure (4). It should be observed whether the patient has used correct technique. In addition, a poor seal around the mouthpiece will result in decreased results from air leakage into the environment. Some spirometers require frequent calibration.

INITIAL INTERPRETATION OF SPIROMETRIC VALUES

The American Thoracic Society (ATS) has published recommendations for interpretation of spirometry (5,6); in adults, a bronchodilator response consists of an improvement in FEV_1 or FVC of 12% with an absolute change of 200 mL (5,6). The FEV_1 is the gold standard because a change in FVC might be from longer time of expiration. If one uses a volume response of the FVC, it is necessary to have determined that the expiratory time was the same before and after bronchodilator use.

The ATS designations for degree of airflow obstruction (5) are as follows:

Mild	FEV_1 >70% but <100% predicted
Moderate	FEV_1 60% to 69% predicted
Moderately severe	FEV_1 50% to 59% predicted
Severe	FEV_1 34% to 49% predicted
Very severe	FEV_1 <34% predicted

Patients with asthma on average have increased loss of FEV_1 over time as compared with patients without asthma (3,7–9). For example, the annual declines of FEV_1 in patients with asthma compared with patients without asthma have been reported to be 24 mL/year versus 6 mL/year (7), 50 mL/year versus 35 mL/year (8), and 38 mL/year versus 22 mL/year (9). Nonsmokers lose FEV_1 at a rate of 20 to 30 mL/year (6). Cigarette smokers lose about 45 mL/year, with some more susceptible patients losing as much as 60 mL/year (6). Patients with irreversible asthma had deteriorations of FEV_1 of more than 90 mL/year despite intensive treatment (3). Because preservation of lung function should be one goal of management of patients with asthma, recording of spirometric measurements should be part of the patient's medical record. Comparison with previous annual or biannual FEV_1 values should be performed. Causes of excessive loss of FEV_1 should be investigated.

RESPIRATORY IMPAIRMENT AND DISABILITY FROM ASTHMA

Respiratory impairment is "a functional abnormality resulting from a medical condition ... that persists after appropriate therapy is permanent" (10). Disability "is a term used to indicate the total effect of impairment on the patient's life. It is affected by diverse factors such as age, sex, education, economic and social environment, and the energy requirement of the occupation." (10). Total impairment and disability "in a subject with asthma is defined as asthma that cannot be controlled adequately; despite maximal treatment, including >20 mg oral prednisone per day, the FEV_1 remains below 50% of predicted" (10). The Social Security Administration critical values for disability from asthma are an FEV_1 of 1.0 L in patients of height 60 inches or less without shoes, to up to 1.6 L in patients taller than 72 inches (11). These maximal values were after treatment of wheezing or bronchospasm (11). Also, a person may be disabled from asthma if there are episodes of severe attacks "in spite of prescribed treatment, occurring at least once every 2 months or on an average of at least 6 times a year, and prolonged expiration with wheezing or rhonchi on physical examination between attacks" (11). Fortunately, nearly all patients with asthma, even those with destructive lung diseases such as allergic bronchopulmonary aspergillosis (ABPA) or irreversible asthma, will not deteriorate to the severe level needed for disability if they are recognized and treated appropriately.

FLOW-VOLUME LOOP

Ideally, the patient should perform three forced expiratory maneuvers with a maximal inspiration to total lung capacity. There should be agreement of FVC within 5% for the best two efforts (6). The largest FEV_1 and FVC should be used, even if they come from different efforts (6). The vital capacity (VC) may be the FVC or the slow or relaxed VC, whereby the patient expires more slowly. Some patients with severe asthma have more ready airway collapsibility in that the FVC-to-slow VC ratio was 88%, compared with 97% in those with less severe asthma (12). The difference was associated with eosinophil presence in bronchial biopsy specimens but was not explained by differences in neutrophils (12). In the example in Table 32.1, there is a 1.2-L difference between the FVC and slow or relaxed VC.

The patterns of the expiratory curve and inspiratory loop should be examined. Obstruction on expiration produces a "scooping-out" pattern or one that is concave upward in appearance (Fig. 32.1). The expiratory curve shows that there is an initial increase to a maximal flow rate, which is designated as the PEFR, and that in the first second, at least 80% of the VC should be reached. It can be reduced in asthma depending on

TABLE 32.1. *Pulmonary function tests in a 19-year-old man with acute severe asthma*

| | May 1 | | June 16 | |
	Pre-albuterol measured (% predicted)	Post-albuterol measured (%)	Pre-albuterol measured (%)	Post-albuterol measured (%)
FVC (L)	1.85 (34)	1.71 (31)	4.87 (89)	4.82 (88)
FEV$_1$ (L)	0.85 (19)	0.77 (17)	4.23 (95)	4.44 (100)
FEV$_1$/FVC	46	45	87	92
VC—slow (L)	3.09 (57)		4.78 (87)	
FRC (L)	5.12 (134)		4.00 (105)	
RV (L)	4.19 (253)		3.07 (186)	
TLC (L)	7.28 (102)		7.86 (110)	

FVC, forced vital capacity; L, Liter; FEV$_1$, forced expiratory volume in 1 second; VC, vital capacity; FRC, functional residual capacity; RV, residual volume; TLC, total lung capacity

severity. Obstruction is present when the FEV$_1$/FVC is decreased (<80%) even if the FVC is normal. As airway obstruction in asthma worsens, the FVC is reduced, and the FEV$_1$/FVC is decreased even more (Table 32.1).

There should not be any major limitation of inspiratory flow in uncomplicated asthma, although it is recognized on the flow-volume loop that peak inspiratory flow rates are typically less than expiratory flow rates. There may be modest decreases of inspiratory flow in some patients with asthma, but not to the extent seen if a patient has a respiratory muscle myopathy that accompanies prolonged high-dose systemic corticosteroid use or systemic corticosteroid combined with muscle relaxants in previously mechanically

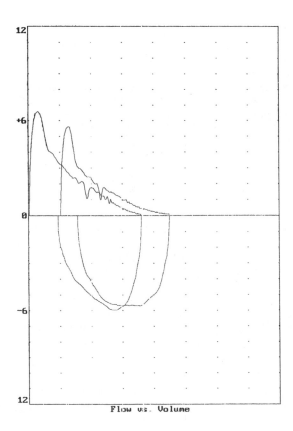

Flow vs. Volume

FIG. 32.1. Flow-volume loops in a 46-year-old man with severe persistent asthma. Inspiratory flow (to the *lower quadrant*) is unimpaired. The expiratory flow tracing (*upper quadrant*) shows a reduced peak flow, reduced forced vital capacity, and flattened expiratory curve consistent with obstruction.

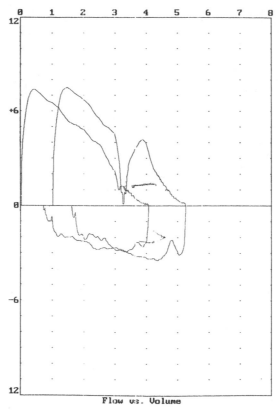

FIG. 32.2. Flow-volume loops in a 35-year-old woman with allergic (dust mite) and nonallergic rhinitis, postnasal drainage from both conditions, gastroesophageal reflux disease (GERD), and a nonproductive cough. The patient reported acute wheezing after an upper respiratory infection and felt that inhaled fluticasone into the airways helped reduce the cough. The current tracing demonstrates a flattened inspiratory curve (*lower quadrant*) and one adequate expiratory tracing in the upper quadrant. Notice the dip in the expiratory tracing when the patient did not complete the forced vital capacity maneuver without stopping. Her baseline and postalbuterol expiratory flows were as follows:

Measure	Before albuterol	After albuterol	Percentage change
FEV_1	3.19 L (91%)	3.46 L (99%)	8.5
FVC	4.51 L (101%)	4.45 L (100%)	−2.4
FEV_1/FVC	71%	78%	

The patient's peak expiratory flow rate (PEFR) was 7.2 L/sec (432 L/min), which is unimpaired. She has a curve consistent with extrathoracic obstruction, thought attributable to postnasal drainage and effects of GERD on the larynx. She may have a component of asthma as well based on the history of wheezing in the setting of an upper respiratory infection and response to fluticasone.

ventilated patients. If there is a flattened inspiratory loop, causes of extrathoracic obstruction should be considered unless the patient has a restrictive disorder. Some patients with or without asthma may have vocal cord dysfunction (VCD) (13,14), which is illustrated in Figure 32.2. To help in diagnosis, if such patients are asked to phonate "e" for as long as possible, they may say "e" for less than 3 seconds and, on spirometry, produce a reduced VC measurement. If the patient can be distracted or retaught, they may produce an "e" sound for up to 10 seconds, consistent with absence of a structural restriction, and if they then perform the spirometry with a large

VC maneuver, a true assessment of the VC will be demonstrated. This is termed *extrathoracic, variable obstruction* of VCD. Some patients with VCD or with factitious or malingering asthma will not inspire to total lung capacity and appear on spirometric testing to have restrictive lung disease. Such patients may also have self-induced arterial hypoxemia from breath-holding or self-induced reductions in their tidal breathing (13).

A restrictive condition produces a reduction in VC, as can obstruction. Full pulmonary function tests are required and demonstrate the key finding of reduced total lung capacity (6). In addition, there is reduced residual volume (RV; air in lung at the end of a maximal expiratory effort) and functional residual capacity (FRC; air in lung at the end of a tidal expiration). In restriction, the FEV_1/FVC is normal or increased in the presence of a reduced VC. In contrast, in acute asthma (Table 32.1), the VC is reduced from airways obstruction, and there is marked gas trapping with increases in RV and FRC.

If there is a flattened or reduced inspiratory flow pattern and there is reduced PEFR, FEV_1, FVC, and FEV_1/FVC, a combined defect consisting of restriction and obstruction likely may be present. Good effort during inspiration and expiration must be ensured, but some patients with asthma also have causes of restriction such as obesity or parenchymal pulmonary disease. This pattern can be consistent with a fixed restrictive defect if the FEV_1/FVC is not reduced. The tracing of the expiratory flow curve is helpful in characterizing the defect further.

ACUTE ASTHMA

Acute Severe Asthma

Hyperinflation

Hyperinflation of lung volumes accompanies airway obstruction and reduced expiratory flow rates in acute severe asthma (Table 32.1). Although asthma is characterized by responsiveness to bronchodilators, patients with acute severe asthma may not respond to albuterol, as in the case in Table 32.1. At the time of presentation on May 1, the patient had markedly elevated RV (253%) and FRC (134%). The FVC was 1.85 L (34%), but a slow VC was 3.09 L (57%), demonstrating the effect of a force effort on airway collapsibility. There was no bronchodilator effect of inhaled albuterol; in fact, a modest decrease occurred, consistent with bronchial hypersensitivity, even to a metered-dose inhaler treatment. The patient received prednisone daily for a week, then on alternate days, in addition to an inhaled corticosteroid and albuterol. He was symptom free in 1 week. The tests were repeated on June 16, when the patient's prednisone dose was still at 35 mg on alternate days. The RV was still increased at 1.86 L (186%), but the FRC was within normal limits. There had been a large increase in FVC to 4.87 L (89%) and in FEV_1 to 4.23 L (95%), and the PEFR improved from 166 to 654 L/minute. There was no bronchodilator effect, however, because the bronchi were now fully patent. Some points are that (a) asthma should not be overlooked if there is no bronchodilator response, especially if the patient is either very ill or with normal range FEV_1 (in this case, a 3-L change in VC and FEV_1 had occurred); (b) the hyperinflation of lung volumes persists for 6 weeks after acute severe asthma, meaning that the patient is not at optimal lung function even if symptom free with normal FEV_1 and FVC; (c) this patient had presented to an ambulatory clinic despite having an FEV_1 of 19% of predicted and a PEFR of 166 L/minute (29%).

Total lung capacity increases during acute severe asthma as the lung elastic recoil properties decrease (14), somewhat analogous to the recoil of the lung changing from that of a normal slinky toy to a broken one. The loss of lung elastic recoil is accompanied with increased outward recoil of the chest wall (14). Inspiratory pressures increase as the dyspneic patient applies additional radial traction to bronchi to maintain airway patency. This negative pressure generated by inspiratory muscles, however, is associated with airway collapsibility on expiration, so that air enters on inspiration but is trapped in the lung during expiration. The FRC and RV increase proportionately more than the total lung capacity, as in the example in Table 32.1 and in the literature (15). For example, in 22 patients presenting with acute severe asthma in which the initial FEV_1 was 30% of predicted, the initial FRC was about 200% of predicted, and RV was 300% to 450% of predicted (15). The patients who had retractions of the sternocleidomastoid muscle had the highest FRC and RV values (15).

Pulsus Paradoxus

Pulsus paradoxus is present in some patients with acute severe asthma and is identified by use of the sphygmomanometer with measurements during inspiration. There should be an inspiratory fall of at least 10 mm Hg. There are different methods for detection of pulsus paradoxus, and many relate to the setting of cardiac tamponade, in which there is little tachypnea or dyspnea. When the patient with acute severe asthma is assessed, the measurement can be carried out as follows: inflate the sphygmomanometer slightly above the level of systolic pressure at which point no Korotkoff sounds are heard. Then note during inspiration whether the Korotkoff sounds disappear as the systolic pressure reading is decreased quickly by 10 mm Hg. If there are no Korotkoff sounds heard during that new lower systolic blood pressure, a pulsus paradoxus is present. It will not be possible to have the patient inspire slowly as during cardiac tamponade. Thus, a patient with asthma may have a 10-mm Hg inspiratory fall at the systolic blood pressure and then at successively lower systolic pressures until there is no disappearance of Korotkoff sounds with inspiration. Some patients with acute asthma have pulsus paradoxus of 50 to 60 mm Hg because at each level of systolic blood pressure from 150 to between 90 and 100 mm Hg, there was a separate disappearance of Korotkoff sounds during inspiration over each 10-mm Hg drop. In a series of 76 patients with acute asthma, the 34 patients with pulsus paradoxus had a mean FEV_1 of 0.54 L, compared with 0.88 L for patients without pulsus paradoxus (16). Similarly, the FVC values were 1.17 L versus 1.82 L (16), indicating worse respiratory status. Experimentally, normal volunteers were asked to breathe through a resistance circuit in an attempt to produce pulsus paradoxus (16). Pulsus paradoxus occurred within 5 minutes when there was marked airway obstruction to FEV_1 of 0.60 L and FRC of 154% to 178% of predicted (16). It took the combination of increased lung volumes and marked airway obstruction to generate pulsus paradoxus.

Arterial Blood Gases and Ventilation-Perfusion Inequalities

Four stages of arterial blood gas patterns are presented in Table 22.14 in Chapter 22. The patients who are obstructed enough to develop pulsus paradoxus have the stage IV pattern of acute respiratory acidosis. Specifically, the mean PO_2 was 64 mm Hg, and the PCO_2 was 49 mm Hg (16). Patients without pulsus paradoxus in the same study had a PO_2 of 68 mm Hg and PCO_2 of 41 mm Hg. The primary physiologic explanation for arterial hypoxemia in acute asthma is ventilation-perfusion ($\dot{V}/\dot{Q}$) inequality (17). There is continued perfusion of very poorly ventilated alveoli resulting in low $\dot{V}/\dot{Q}$ ratios. In a study of eight patients mechanically ventilated for status asthmaticus, the mean PO_2 increased from 95 to 446 mm Hg after increasing the inspired air concentration to 100% (17). This change is consistent with $\dot{V}/\dot{Q}$ inequality, not a shunt. It was determined that on average, 27% of pulmonary blood flow perfused very low $\dot{V}/\dot{Q}$ units, whereas in normal subjects, such very low $\dot{V}/\dot{Q}$ units do not even exist (17). Only two patients had evidence of perfusion of very high $\dot{V}/\dot{Q}$ units, and these patients also had 21% and 46% of their pulmonary perfusion using low $\dot{V}/\dot{Q}$ units (17).

Diffusing Capacity

In patients with status asthmaticus, after treatment to the point at which pulmonary function tests can be performed, diffusing capacity is preserved or even increased (17,18). Low diffusing capacity is consistent with COPD, interstitial lung disease, pulmonary vascular disease, and anemia but not asthma. In patients with asthma without status asthmaticus, the diffusing capacity should not be decreased either.

Exercise-induced Asthma

A decline in FEV_1 or PEFR shortly after onset or cessation of exercise is consistent with exercise-induced asthma and occurs in the absence of other evidence of asthma in some patients. It also occurs in the presence of persistent asthma. There remains controversy as to what level of reduction of spirometry is needed (19). A 15% decline in FEV_1 or PEFR is a generally accepted value (2,20). However, a 20% reduction in FEV_1 in patients with known asthma has also been used (21), as has 10%. The spirometry returns to baseline within 60 minutes in nearly all cases and is not associated with a late bronchoconstrictive response. Nonspecific bronchial hyperresponsiveness does not accompany isolated exercise-induced asthma. Thus, some physicians prefer the term *exercise-induced bronchospasm*. In addition, unrecognized declines in PEFR or FEV_1 have been reported in highly conditioned athletes or military recruits (22) who would appear to meet criteria for exercise-induced asthma. The athlete can have increased FVC and decreased FEV_1/FVC on that basis. This observation is one reason for the controversy about the definition of exercise-induced asthma (19).

If the patient repeats the exercise within 40 minutes of the first episode of bronchoconstriction, there will be a reduced bronchoconstrictive response to exercise (20). Thus, some patients with asthma are able to "run through" their dyspnea. Exercise-induced asthma can also be produced by hyperventilation with frigid cold air (23). The mechanism of exercise-induced asthma is that of hyperventilation from exercise causing a heat flux of airway cooling followed by rewarming (23). The rewarming is attributable to increases in bronchial blood flow. The local hyperemia and airway wall vascular leakage participate in airways obstruction. Additional discussion of exercise-induced asthma and treatment options can be found in Chapter 22.

PERSISTENT ASTHMA

Spirometry

The National Asthma Education and Prevention Program Expert Panel Report 2 suggested that spirometric tests be performed initially, after treatment when symptoms have stabilized, and at least every 1 to 2 years (2). It may be necessary to obtain much more frequent determinations

depending on the severity of the patient's asthma, especially if the patient is a poor perceiver of symptoms. In adult patients who had moderate to severe asthma with FEV_1 66% of predicted, there was no correlation between a perceived level of airway obstruction (0 to 4 point scale) and FEV_1 (24). It was determined that using an FEV_1 percentage threshold of 60%, 31% of patients overestimated their own airway obstruction, and 17% underestimated it (24).

Peak Expiratory Flow Rates

Measurement of PEFR can be useful in individual patients who then identify the ranges of their PEFR over time. In patients who have anxiety or who hyperperceive their sensation of dyspnea, use of home peak flowmeters may be of value to the patient and physician. Nevertheless, when patients with moderate to severe asthma were asked to record their PEFR twice daily for 1 year, fabricated results were common (25).

Airway Hyperresponsiveness

Patients with asthma have airway hyperresponsiveness to a variety of stimuli, such as histamine, methacholine, and leukotriene D4 (26). Bronchial hyperresponsiveness is present in nearly all patients with asthma who have a 20% decline in FEV_1 from baseline (postdiluent) (27). During bronchial hyperresponsiveness testing, the patient's asthma should be stable and the FEV_1 more than 65% of predicted and not less than 1.5 L. The recommended times to withhold asthma medications have been published by the American Thoracic Society, such as 48 hours for salmeterol and formoterol and 8 hours for albuterol (28). The classic challenge protocol uses five breaths to total lung capacity from a dosimeter and nebulizer system (28,29). Very dilute concentrations of methacholine are used, and serial spirometric measurements are performed every 5 minutes until there has been a 20% decline in FEV_1. This target level should be calculated once the baseline, postdiluent FEV_1 is recorded. The initial dose of methacholine is 0.075 mg/mL, followed by 0.15 mg/mL, 0.31 mg/mL, 0.625 mg/mL, 1.25 mg/mL, 2.5 mg/mL, 5 mg/mL,

10 mg/mL, and 25 mg/mL (29). A modification of the protocol has been suggested, consisting of diluent, 0.0625 mg/mL, 0.25 mg/mL, 1 mg/mL, 4 mg/mL, and 16 mg/mL (28). After the five inhalations, which should be completed within 2 minutes, the patient waits 30 seconds and then performs three FVC maneuvers. Another protocol (American Thoracic Society) is that of a 2-minute inhalation from the nebulizer, with the previously described modified dosing schedule in which the patient takes tidal but not maximal inspirations during the methacholine inhalation (28). The FEV_1 data (percentage decrease from postdiluent FEV_1) are plotted against the log of the concentrations of methacholine. The PC_{20} is determined using the following formula:

$$PC_{20} = \text{antilog} \log C_1$$
$$+ \frac{(20 - R_1)(\log C_2 - \log C_1)}{(R_2 - R_1)}$$

where C_1 is the concentration of methacholine preceding the challenge that resulted in at least a decline in FEV_1 of 20%, and C_2 is the concentration causing the 20% decline of FEV_1. R_1 is the response of FEV_1 in percentage change caused by C_1 and R_2 is the percentage change in FEV_1 caused by C_2 (27.)

Nearly all patients with asthma have a PC_{20} of 8 mg/mL or less of methacholine. It is important to recall that methacholine hyperresponsiveness is sensitive for asthma but is a nonspecific finding (see Table 22.2 in Chapter 22).

Even though the cause of bronchial hyperresponsiveness in asthma remains unknown, decreases in methacholine hyperresponsiveness (but not resolution of it) occur with treatment with inhaled corticosteroids (30).

Excessive Bronchoconstriction

The airways of patients with asthma respond with excessive ease of bronchoconstriction in the setting of methacholine challenge, and this hypersensitivity is designated as the PC_{20} (31). In addition, the decline in FVC is excessive in patients with asthma (31). For example, during analysis of methacholine bronchoprovocation procedures, the end point occurs when the FEV_1 has decreased by 20%. In 146 patients with mild asthma and a mean PC_{20} of 3.3 mg/mL, there was a modest decline in FVC of 13.2% (31). Some patients were found to have a pattern of reduced FVC accounting for the reduced FEV_1, and others had an obstructive pattern of reduced FEV_1/FVC. There was a correlation ($\gamma = 0.55$) between percentage decrease in FVC at the PC_{20} and number of oral corticosteroid prescriptions written in the previous month (31). In contrast, there was no correlation between oral corticosteroids and PC_{20}, nor between PC_{20} and percentage decrease in FVC (31). Thus, in patients with asthma, especially those patients requiring oral corticosteroids, there is excessive bronchoconstriction to methacholine (as well as bronchial hypersensitivity).

Small Airways Obstruction

Small airways obstruction is present in patients with episodes of acute asthma and in the setting of persistent asthma. Various attempts have been made to identify the small airways that have an internal diameter of less than 3 mm. Much of the airways resistance is attributable to small airways and obstruction in asthma, and it is present in patients with normal FEV_1 measurements. $FEF_{25\%-75\%}$ formerly was proposed as a test of small airways obstruction because early effects of smoking occur in the small airways. However, according to the American Thoracic Society guidelines, $FEF_{25\%-75\%}$ and the instantaneous flows should not be used to diagnose small airways disease should not be graded regarding severity when the FEV_1 and FEV_1/FVC are within the normal range (5). Their role is "to confirm the presence of airway obstruction in the presence of a borderline FEV_1/FVC" (5). One limitation of the $FEF_{25\%-75\%}$ is that it is highly variable and is affected if, during successive FVC maneuvers, the time of the VC varies. If one is to use $FEF_{25\%-75\%}$ and $FEF_{75\%}$ as indicators of small airways obstruction, it should be when the FEV_1/FVC or FEV_1 is reduced.

HYPERSENSITIVITY PNEUMONITIS

The primary finding of hypersensitivity pneumonitis is restriction with a reduction in diffusing capacity. As stated, a reduction in total lung capacity is the initial evidence for restriction. With the spirometric values, the VC is reduced with normal or increased FEV_1/FVC. One should not diagnose restriction using the VC in the presence of obstruction as in asthma, the VC and the FEV_1/FVC are reduced.

If a patient with hypersensitivity pneumonitis is exposed to the causative organic antigen, there can be a restrictive respiratory response beginning by 4 to 6 hours and lasting up to 18 hours (see Chapter 23). If measured, the diffusing capacity for carbon monoxide will be reduced markedly. In the case of acute avian hypersensitivity pneumonitis, the acute response can be obstructive, restrictive, or have evidence for both (32). In subacute avian hypersensitivity pneumonitis, 4 hours after exposure, obstruction or restriction similarly occurs (32). In chronic avian hypersensitivity pneumonitis, there can be reductions in diffusing capacity as well as obstruction or restriction. End-stage pulmonary fibrosis with severe restrictive defects and arterial hypoxemia can occur (33).

The American Thoracic Society recommendations for degree of restriction using the VC measurement from spirometry require that the FEV_1/FVC not be reduced (5). They are as follows:

Mild	VC is 70% to the lower limit of normal predicted percentage.
Moderate	VC is 60% to 69%.
Moderately severe	VC is 50% to 59%.
Severe	VC is 34% to 49%.
Very severe	VC is less than 34%.

REFERENCES

1. Banzett RB, Dempsey JA, O'Donnell DE, et al. Symptom perception and respiratory sensation in asthma. *Am J Respir Crit Care Med* 2000;162:1178–1182.
2. National Asthma Education and Prevention Program. *Expert Panel Report 2: guidelines for the diagnosis and management of asthma: clinical practice guidelines.* National Institutes of Health, National Heart, Lung and Blood Institute, NIH Publication No. 97-4051, April 1997.
3. Bachman KS, Greenberger PA, Patterson R. Airways obstruction in patients with long-term asthma consistent with "irreversible asthma." *Chest* 1997;112:1234–1240.
4. American Thoracic Society Medical Section of the American Lung Association. Standardization of spirom-

etry: 1994 update. *Am J Respir Crit Care Med* 1995;152:1107–1136.
5. American Thoracic Society Medical Section of the American Lung Association. Lung function testing: selection of reference values and interpretative strategies. *Am Rev Respir Dis* 1991;144:1202–1218.
6. Crapo RO. Pulmonary-function testing. *N Engl J Med* 1994;331:25–30.
7. Schacter EN, Doyle CA, Beck GJ. A prospective study of asthma in a rural community. *Chest* 1984;85:623–630.
8. Peat JK, Woolcock AJ, Cullen K. Rate of decline of lung function in subjects with asthma. *Eur J Respir Dis* 1987;70:171–179.
9. Lange P, Parner J, Vestbo J, et al. A 15-year follow-up study of ventilatory function in adults with asthma. *N Engl J Med* 1998;339:1194–1200.
10. American Thoracic Society Medical Section of the American Lung Association. Guidelines for the evaluation of impairment/disability in patients with asthma. *Am Rev Respir Dis* 1993;147:1056–1061.
11. Department of Health & Human Services. *Disability evaluation under Social Security.* U.S. Department of Health and Human Services, Social Security Administration, SSA Publication No. 05-10089, Feburary 1986.
12. Wenzel SE, Schwartz LB, Langmack EL, et al. Evidence that severe asthma can be divided pathologically into two inflammatory subtypes with distinct physiologic and clinical characteristics. *Am J Respir Crit Care Med* 1999;160:1001–1008.
13. McGrath KG, Greenberger PA, Patterson R, et al. Factitious allergic disease: multiple factitious illness and familial Munchausen's stridor. *Immunol Allergy Pract* 1984;6:263–271.
14. Peress L, Sybrecht G, Macklem PT. The mechanism of increase in total lung capacity during acute asthma. *Am J Med* 1976;61:165–169.
15. McFadden Jr ER, Kiser R, DeGroot WJ. Acute bronchial asthma: Relations between clinical and physiologic manifestations. *N Engl J Med* 1973;288:221–225.
16. Rebuck AS, Pengelly LD. Development of pulsus paradoxus in the presence of airways obstruction. *N Engl J Med* 1973;288:66–69.
17. Rodriguez-Roisin R, Ballester E, Roca J, et al. Mechanisms of hypoxemia in patients with status asthmaticus requiring mechanical ventilation. *Am Rev Respir Dis* 1989;139:732–739.
18. American Thoracic Society. Proceedings of the ATS Workshop on Refractory Asthma: current understanding, recommendations, and unanswered questions. *Am J Respir Crit Care Med* 2000;162:2341–2351.
19. Weiler JM. What exactly is exercise-induced asthma? *Allergy Asthma Proc* 1997;18:311–312.
20. McFadden Jr ER, Gilbert IA. Current concepts: exercise-induced asthma. *N Engl J Med* 1994;330:1362–1367.
21. Leff JA, Busse WW, Pearlman D, et al. Montelukast, a leukotriene-receptor antagonist, for the treatment of mild asthma and exercise-induced bronchoconstriction. *N Engl J Med* 1998;339:147–152.
22. Sonna LA, Angel KC, Sharp MA, et al. The prevalence of exercise-induced bronchospasm among US Army recruits and its effects on physical performance. *Chest* 2001;119:1676–1684.
23. McFadden Jr ER, Nelson JA, Skowronski ME, et al. Thermally induced asthma and airway drying. *Am J Respir Crit Care Med* 1999;160:221–226.
24. Teeter JG, Bleecker ER. Relationship between airway

obstruction and respiratory symptoms in adult asthmatics. *Chest* 1998;113:272–277.

25. Cote J, Cartier A, Malo J-L, et al. Compliance with peak expiratory flow monitoring in home management of asthma. *Chest* 1998;113:968–972.

26. Greenberger PA, Smith LJ, Patterson R, et al. Comparison of cutaneous and bronchial reactivity to leukotriene D_4 in humans. *J Lab Clin Med* 1986;108:70–75.

27. Wanger JS, Ikle DN, Irvin CG. Airway responses to a diluent used in the methacholine challenge test. *Ann Allergy Asthma Immunol* 2001;86:277–282.

28. American Thoracic Society. Guidelines for methacholine and exercise challenge testing–1999. *Am J Respir Crit Care Med* 2000;161:309–329.

29. Chai H, Farr RS, Froehlich LA, et al. Standardization of bronchial inhalation challenge procedures. *J Allergy Clin Immunol* 1975;56:323–327.

30. Holgate ST. Therapeutic options for persistent asthma. *JAMA* 2001;285:2637–2640.

31. Gibbons WJ, Sharma A, Lougheed D, et al. Detection of excessive bronchoconstriction in asthma. *Am J Respir Crit Care Med* 1996;153:582–589.

32. Fink JN, Sosman AJ, Barboriak JJ, et al. Pigeon breeder's disease: a clinical study of a hypersensitivity pneumonitis. *Ann Intern Med* 1968;68:1205–1219.

33. Greenberger PA, Pien LC, Patterson R, et al. End-stage lung and ultimately fatal disease in a bird fancier. *Am J Med* 1989;86:119–122.

33

Evaluation of Eosinophilia

Carla Irani and Andrea J. Apter

Division of Pulmonary, Allergy, Critical Care Medicine,
Hospital of the University of Pennsylvania, Philadelphia, Pennsylvania

Eosinophilia is defined in this chapter as the presence of excess numbers of eosinophils in the blood or tissues. There are varied definitions of what constitutes an excess number of these cells in the circulation (1–3), but more than 400 cells/μL of blood would be considered excessive. Eosinophilia is associated with allergic, parasitic, and neoplastic disorders, but the disease process for some, such as the idiopathic hypereosinophilic syndrome (HES), is not understood fully. This chapter focuses on the diagnosis and management of disorders characterized by eosinophilia.

EOSINOPHILS IN THE BLOOD

Wharton Jones is believed to have been the first scientist to recognize the eosinophil in unstained preparations of peripheral blood in 1876 (4). Paul Ehrlich gave the cell the name *eosinophil* in 1879 because of the intense staining of its granules with the acidic aniline dyes like eosin (5). The staining procedures he developed allowed the cell to be recognized and studied.

The eosinophil count can be estimated by multiplying the percentage of eosinophils from the differential white blood cell count by the total number of white blood cells. Normally, 1% to 3% of blood leukocytes are eosinophils. A manual differential should be obtained if eosinophilia is suspected (3,6). For example, in our institution, if the percentage on the automated differential is 20% or greater, the blood smear will be examined manually. Various conditions may influence

the eosinophil count. In patients with leukopenia, the percentages of eosinophils may be increased, but not their absolute number. This has been called *pseudoeosinophilia* (6). The number of eosinophils in the blood has a diurnal variation, being highest at night (3,5) and falling in the morning when endogenous glucocorticoid levels increase (3). Exogenous glucocorticoids, endogenous glucocorticoid production, stress, and some bacterial and viral infections (3,7,8) may suppress eosinophil counts. Thus, a condition promoting eosinophilia could be masked if it occurred in the presence of such events.

EOSINOPHILS IN THE TISSUES

Eosinophils are present in only small numbers in the circulation; they are primarily tissue-dwelling cells, with more than a hundred times as many in the tissues compared with the circulation (3,9). Under normal circumstances, eosinophils are found almost exclusively in the circulation and the gastrointestinal mucosa (2). However, in disease, they can accumulate in any tissue, particularly in the tissues interfacing with the environment, such as the respiratory (e.g., asthma, nasal polyps, and nonallergic rhinitis with eosinophilia), skin (eosinophilic cellulitis, or Well's syndrome), eosinophilic fasciitis (Shulman's syndrome), and gastrointestinal and lower genitourinary systems (9), suggesting a role in host defense.

The usual lifespan of the eosinophil in the circulation is about 4 days, but eosinophils survive for weeks within tissues (2,9). Thus, blood eosinophil numbers do not necessarily reflect the extent of eosinophil involvement in affected tissues in various diseases (2,3). Prolonged eosinophilia, such as in the idiopathic HES, has been associated with organ damage, particularly cardiac (3).

Routine eosin staining of eosinophils may underestimate eosinophil numbers. Immunofluorescent stains with monoclonal antibodies directed against the cationic proteins from the granules are used to detect eosinophils in the tissues. It is important to recognize that degranulation, cytolysis, apoptosis, and necrosis alter the morphology of the eosinophil and its granules and, thus, staining properties (3).

MORPHOLOGY AND DEVELOPMENT OF EOSINOPHILS

In order to better understand the diagnosis and management of conditions characterized by eosinophilia, we present a brief synopsis of the morphology, development, and recruitment into tissue of the eosinophil. Figure 33.1 illustrates some of these concepts. Eosinophils are bone marrow–derived granulocyte leukocytes arising from $CD34^+$ hematopoietic progenitor cells (10). The cytokines granulocyte-macrophage colony-stimulating factor (GM-CSF), interleukin-3 (IL-3), and IL-5, are associated with promoting their growth and differentiation in the bone marrow (11,12). Of these, the actions of IL-5 are most specific for eosinophils. For example, IL-5 stimulates synthesis of granule proteins (10). IL-5 and the chemokine eotaxin promote release of eosinophils into the circulation and chemotaxis (2,10,13).

Eosinophils exit the circulation and migrate to mucosal surfaces: lung, gut, lower genitourinary tract (2,14). This migration is mediated by adhesion molecules on endothelial and eosinophil surfaces. Through binding of P-selectin glycoprotein ligand 1 on eosinophils with P-selectin on endothelial cells, rolling and margination of eosinophils occurs (12,15). The eosinophil is tethered to the endothelial wall by the binding of very late antigen-4 (VLA-4) on eosinophils to vascular cell adhesion molecule-1 (VCAM-1) (12). Similarly, β_1 and β_2 integrins

on eosinophils bind to intercellular cell adhesion molecule (ICAM) on endothelial cells (10,11). With the binding of integrins and their ligands, the rolling stops, and the eosinophil adheres more firmly to the endothelium and then migrates out of the vascular compartment. The migration of eosinophils into the tissues is controlled by chemoattractants. These include platelet-activating factor, complement components (C3a and C5a), and chemokines. The most important chemokine is eotaxin, which acts by binding to its receptor CCR3. Its chemoattractive effect is augmented by IL-5. Once eosinophils migrate into inflamed tissue, they are activated by many stimuli, including receptors for immunoglobulin A (IgA) and IgG, and cytokines, including IL-3, IL-5, and GM-CSF. IL-3, IL-5, and GM-CSF prolong survival of eosinophils and inhibit apoptosis (2,10,11).

As a result of secretion of chemokines, cytokines, growth factors, and toxic cationic granule proteins, eosinophils perform many functions: immunoregulatory, remodeling and repair, and protection from foreign invaders (14). Mature eosinophils produce their toxic and inflammatory effects by the release of mediators stored in their specific granules. The crystalloid core of these granules is composed of cationic major basic protein (MBP); the matrix contains eosinophil cationic protein, eosinophil-derived neurotoxin, and eosinophil peroxidase. These proteins are responsible for direct cytotoxic effects in part by producing hydrogen peroxide and halide acids generated by eosinophil peroxidase (2). Eosinophil cationic protein can disrupt membranes by causing pore formation that facilitates the entry of other toxic molecules. In the respiratory epithelium, activated eosinophil granule products can impair cilia beating and increase vascular permeability. MBP increases smooth muscle reactivity by acting on the epithelium and by antagonizing M2 muscarinic receptor function (10,16). Eosinophil granule proteins trigger degranulation of mast cells and basophils and amplify the inflammatory cascade by promoting release of chemotactants such as eotaxin, RANTES, and platelet-activating factor.

Eosinophilia can result from an excess of IL-5, an inhibition of apoptosis caused by IL-5 or other factors (14,17,18), or any mechanism

Selective Eosinophil Tissue Accumulation in Asthma
A Multi-Step Process

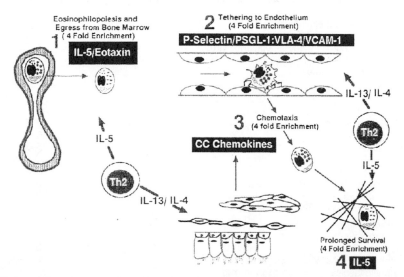

FIG. 33.1. Schematic representation of multistep paradigm of eosinophil recruitment into tissue, illustrating that selective accumulation of eosinophils occurs as sequential and cumulative approximately fourfold increases, in eosinophils compared with neutrophils, at several stages in the life cycle of the cell, with each step under separate molecular control, influenced either directly or indirectly by T$_H$2 cytokine production. The first step involves hematopoiesis and bone marrow egress mediated by interleukin-5 (IL-5) and chemotactic signals; the second step is through IL-4 and IL-13 upregulation of P-selectin and vascular cell adhesion molecule-1 (VCAM-1) on vascular endothelium; the third step involves selective chemotaxis under the influence of CC chemokines generated by IL-4– and IL-13– stimulated epithelial, fibroblast, and smooth muscle cells; and the fourth step is prolonged survival, again mediated by IL-5. PSGL, P-selective glycoprotein ligand; VLA, very late antigen. (From Wardlaw AJ. Molecular basis for selective eosinophil trafficking in asthma: a multistep paradigm. *J Allergy Clin Immunol* 1999;104:917–926, with permission.

causing an imbalance of the processes described previously. Current and new therapies for eosinophil-mediated disease interfere with these imbalances.

DIFFERENTIAL DIAGNOSIS OF EOSINOPHILIA

Table 33.1 displays the differential diagnosis of eosinophilia in blood and tissues. The diagnoses can be categorized as atopic, infectious, drug-induced, vasculitic, tissue-associated inflammatory, and neoplastic. It is beyond the scope of this chapter to discuss all causes of eosinophilia in detail, but Table 33.1 contains references for each. These references include the original description of disease, a review of the clinical presentation, or an update on the possible immunopathogenic mechanisms involved. Below there is a review of

some of the causes of eosinophilic infiltration of blood and tissues most pertinent to the allergist-immunologist and not covered in other chapters. Topics include helminthic infections, drugs, idiopathic HES, and the Churg-Strauss syndrome (CSS). Examples of tissue-specific eosinophilic conditions of the lung, gut, and lower genitourinary tract: eosinophilic pneumonias, gastroenteritis, and cystitis, are described.

Infections and Eosinophilia: Helminthic Diseases

In developing countries, helminthic diseases are the most common cause of eosinophilia, whereas in developed countries, atopic diseases are most common. Infections with bacteria and most viruses are generally associated with eosinopenia. However, it has been established

TABLE 33.1. *Diseases most frequently associated with eosinophilia of blood or tissues*

Disease	Reference(s)
Infectious	
Parasitic infections (helminths)	23, 61–63
Fungal (aspergillosis, coccidiomycosis)	64–66
Retroviral (e.g., human immunodeficiency virus)	67–70
Chronic tuberculosis	71
Pneumocystis carinii infection	72
Respiratory	
Asthma	73–81, 99
Allergic rhinitis	82
Nonallergic rhinitis with eosinophilia syndrome	83–85
Nasal polyposis	86
Chronic sinusitis	86–89
Allergic bronchopulmonary aspergillosis	See Chapter 24
Allergic fungal sinusitis	90–92
Acute eosinophilic pneumonia (drugs, parasites, other)	50, 54, 93, 94, 97
Chronic eosinophilic pneumonia	50, 52, 54
Eosinophilic granuloma (histiocytosis X)	50, 95, 96
Dermatologic	
Atopic dermatitis	100–102
Eosinophilic panniculitis	103
Eosinophilic cellulitis (Well's syndrome)	104–106
Eosinophilic fasciitis (Shulman's syndrome)	2, 107
Chronic urticaria and angioedema	108–110
Eosinophilic folliculitis	111–113
Vasculitic	
Churg-Strauss syndrome	49, 114
Eosinophilic vasculitis	115–116
Hematologic and neoplastic	
Hypereosinophilic syndrome	36, 37, 40
Leukemia	43, 59, 117, 118
Lymphoma (Hodgkin, non-Hodgkin)	119–12
Sézary syndrome	40, 122
Solid tumors (e.g., cervical tumors; large cell carcinoma of the lung; squamous cell carcinoma of skin, penis, vagina; adenocarcinoma of gastrointestinal tract; transitional cell bladder carcinoma; breast)	2, 123–125
Mastocytosis	126–129
Gastrointestinal	
Eosinophilic gastroenteritis	58, 98, 130–131
Inflammatory bowel disease	3, 132–133
Cardiac (see hypereosinophilic syndrome)	
Renal	
Eosinophilic cystitis	59
Immunologic	
Omenn's syndrome	134–136
Hyper-IgE syndrome	137
Transplant rejection	138–140
Endocrine	
Hypoadrenalism	3, 141

recently that respiratory syncytial virus stimulates endothelial cells to produce eosinophil chemoattractants and activates eosinophils (10). These findings may explain in part how viral infections trigger asthma exacerbations.

Parasitic, particularly helminthic infections are associated with eosinophilia. Helminths generate T_H2 responses and cause IL-5 production (2,3). Recent reports indicate that helminthic infection results in endothelial expression of eotaxin and RANTES, which promote eosinophil recruitment (19).

Helminthic diseases causing eosinophilia include strongyloidiasis, ascariasis, hookworm infection, schistosomiasis, trichinosis, filariasis, *Toxocara canis* infection causing visceral larva migrans, cysticercosis, and echinococcosis. With the exception of *Isospora belli* and *Dientamoeba fragilis*, protozoan infections do not elicit eosinophilia. Giardia does not cause eosinophilia.

In parasitic infections associated with eosinophilia, the level of peripheral blood eosinophilia may be modest or even nonexistent if the infection is well contained in tissues such as in an echinococcal cyst. The levels of peripheral eosinophilia may fluctuate as these cysts leak or adult filiaria migrate. Blood eosinophil levels tend to parallel the extent of tissue involvement and may be very marked as, for example, in disseminated *Strongyloides* species infection.

It is particularly important to diagnose *Strongyloides* species infection, which sometimes may be dormant and unrecognized in a patient for years. Potentially fatal dissemination of this helminth can occur if the patient becomes immunosuppressed or receives corticosteroids, which is also the treatment for many other eosinophilic conditions (20–22). Serial stool examinations with appropriate serologic tests are the initial diagnostic tests for many helminthic infections (23) (Fig. 33.2). For strongyloidiasis, if these tests are negative, examination of duodenojejunal aspirate or tissue biopsy or the Enterotest string method should be considered.

Drug Reactions Associated with Eosinophilia

Table 33.2 displays drugs most commonly associated with eosinophilia of blood and tissues as an adverse reaction. Among the drugs most frequently reported are nitrofurantoin, minocycline, and nonsteroidal antiinflammatory agents. Although numerous drugs have been cited, in many cases, these citations are based on case reports, as is evident from those provided in Table 33.2, making the associations difficult to interpret. When information is based on case reports, it is not clear how often eosinophilia occurs in all of the patients who take the drug. Furthermore, it is possible that a case report can describe a true association between the drug and eosinophilia, or temporally associated but

causally unrelated events, such as an association between eosinophilia and the underlying disease. For example, inhaled beclomethasone and cromolyn, prescribed for asthma, a disease associated with eosinophilia, have both been associated with eosinophilia in case reports (24–26). Asthma and associated eosinophilia may wax and wane as part of the disease course, and this may be incidental to whether a drug is taken. In contrast, doses of systemic steroids for asthma may have been reduced when inhaled steroids were added, resulting in an increase in peripheral blood eosinophilia. Thus, the true association may be between the extent of eosinophilia and the underlying asthma, and not the drug used for treatment. Indeed, the recent association between leukotriene antagonists and eosinophilia in asthma patients appears to result from unmasking of underlying CSS rather than a direct association between leukotriene antagonists and eosinophilia (27,28).

When taking a history for possible therapeutic agents associated with eosinophilia, inquiry about the use of agents used in complementary and alternative medicine and over-the-counter preparations should be made. For example, contaminated L-tryptophan and rapeseed oil were associated with the eosinophilia-myalgia syndrome (29,30). Patients should also be asked about the use of illicit drugs because cocaine and heroin use is sometimes associated with eosinophilia. The mechanisms by which a drug might cause eosinophilia have not been studied extensively, but some investigators have associated drug-induced eosinophilia with increased IL-5 production (31,32). The eosinophilia usually resolves with discontinuation of the drug (2).

Idiopathic Hypereosinophilic Syndrome

Idiopathic HES was described first in 1968 by Hardy and Anderson (33) and further characterized in several excellent more recent reviews (3,34–36). It is a diagnosis of exclusion, characterized by eosinophilia and damage to heart, lungs, skin, and other organs infiltrated with eosinophils (36,37). In 1975, Chusid and colleagues (34) proposed diagnostic criteria that still are used today: (a) blood eosinophilia

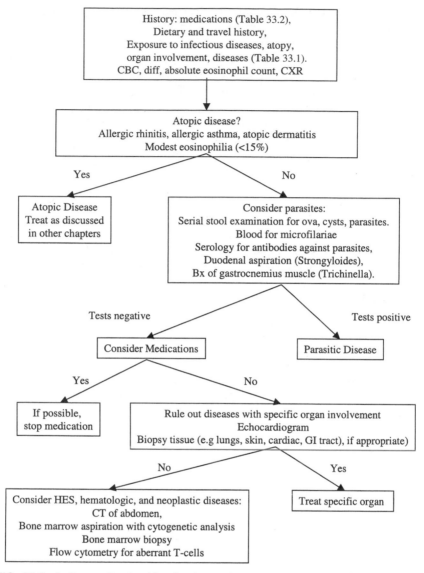

FIG. 33.2. A diagnostic algorithm for the evaluation of a patient with eosinophilia.

greater than 1500/μL persisting for more than 6 months; (b) exclusion of diseases associated with eosinophilia-like parasitic infections, allergic diseases, or medications; and (c) organ involvement.

The role of the eosinophil in the pathogenesis of HES is not clear. Some patients with persistent eosinophilia do not develop organ damage. In addition, the degree or duration of eosinophilia does not predict the severity of cardiac involvement, the organ most frequently and often severely in-

volved in HES. When damage occurs, it is the same as would occur with eosinophilic infiltration of the tissue in other eosinophil-related diseases, such as tropical endomyocardial fibrosis (36).

Recently, clonal expansions of abnormal T cells (CD3$^-$, CD4$^+$, CD8$^-$ and CD3$^+$, CD4$^-$, CD8$^-$) have been described in several patients with HES (38–40). Overproduction of IL-5 has been observed in almost all reports in which IL-5 has been measured and the patient has not already

TABLE 33.2. *Drug-induced reactions most commonly associated with eosinophilia of blood or tissues*

Drug	Clinical manifestations	References
Antiinfectious		
Penicillin, ampicillin	AIN, D, EP	50, 142–144
Sulfonamides	AIN, E, EP	50, 145
Tetracyclines	EP, E, E&H	146–148
Vancomycin	AIN	149
Quinolones	AIN	150
Ethambutol	E, EP, D	151–152
Pyrimethamine	EP	153
Didanosine	E	154
Pentamidine (inhaled)	EP	50
Nitrofurantoin	E, EP	50, 98, 155
Anticonvulsants and neuromuscular agents		
Phenytoin	AIN, D, E, EP, GV	156, 157
Carbamazepine	AIN, D, E, EP	144, 152, 158, 159
Phenobarbital	E	160
Valproic acid	E	161
Ethosuximide	E	161
Dantrolene	Pleural effusion, E	162
Antiinflammatory		
Nonsteroidal antiinflammatory drugs[a]	AIN, E, EP, EC, V	50, 79, 98, 144, 163–165
Methotrexate	E, EP	98, 166
Dapsone	EP	50, 167
Gold	E, EP	168, 169
Allopurinol	AIN, E	170
Cardiovascular		
Diltiazem	E	171
Captopril	AIN, E, EP	50, 172, 173
Mexiletine	E	174
Warfarin	AIN, E	175, 176
Gastrointestinal		
Omeprazole, lanzoprazole	AIN, E	177, 178
Cimetidine	AIN, EP	
Ranitidine	E, EP, M	179–181
Mesalazine	E, EP	182
Hypoglycemic		
Chlorpropamide	EP	50
Tolazamide	EP	50
Antidepressant and antipsychotic		
Triazolam	AIN	183
Imipramine, desipramine	E, EP	184–185
Venlafaxine	EP	186
Trazodone	E, EP	187
Clozapine	E	188
Antitumor and immune modulating		
Bleomycin	EP	189
Tamoxifen	EP	98
Pacliltaxel	D, EP	190–191
2-Chlorodeoxyadenosine	E	192
IL-3	E	193
IL-2	E, M	194–196
GM-CSF	E, EP	50, 197
Bicalutamide		198
Miscellaneous		
Radiographic contrast	EP	199
Cocaine, heroin	EP	50, 200
Halothane	E&H	201
L-Tryptophan	E, mylagia	202, 203
Rapeseed oil	E, EP, myalgia	29

[a]Acetaminophen, aspirin, diclofenac, ibuprofen, naproxen, paraaminosalicylic acid, piroxicam, sulindac tolfenamic acid.

AIN, acute interstitial nephritis; D, dermatitis; E, peripheral blood eosinophilia; EP, eosinophilic pneumonia; EC, eosinophilic colitis; EM, eosinphilic meningitis; E&H, eosinophilia and hepatitis; GV, granulomatous vasculitis; M, myocarditis; IL, interleukin; GM-CSF, granulocyte-macrophage colony-stimulating factor.

received corticosteroids (39–41). In one patient, eosinophils expressing the *Bcl-2* gene, whose products inhibit apoptosis, have been described (42). Recently, Means-Markwell and colleagues (37) reported a patient with activated T cells expressing markers for natural killer cells (CD16 and CD56). Together, these findings indicate that there is likely more than one mechanism responsible for the HES phenotype. It is not clear from this information whether those patients with clones of abnormal T cells will progress to T-cell neoplasia (40,43).

HES is more common in men, with a male-to-female ratio of 9:1 (34). It usually presents between the ages of 20 and 50 years and is rare in childhood. Presenting symptoms are often insidious and may be respiratory, cardiac, neurologic, or constitutional, such as low-grade fever, fatigue, myalgias, angioedema, or other skin rashes. Sweating and pruritus are common. Some patients may have abdominal discomfort, flushing, or alcohol intolerance. Weight loss is unusual, and patients do not have increased infections or anergy.

In HES, total leukocyte counts are usually less than 25,000/μL, with 30% to 70% of the total leukocyte count being eosinophils (36). Some patients may develop very high white blood cell counts (>90,000/μL), which is associated with a poor prognosis (36). Examination of the bone marrow reveals increased numbers of eosinophils, often 30% to 60% of marrow cells. There are increased numbers of early forms compared with normal bone marrow, but blast forms are not usually present (36). When blast forms are present in the blood or make up more than 10% of the eosinophils in the marrow, the diagnosis is eosinophilic leukemia. In addition to eosinophilia, neutrophilia is common in HES. Anemia and basophilia have been described. The clinical spectrum of hematologic findings ranges from very mild abnormalities to signs and symptoms typical of a myeloproliferative disease, such as abnormal leukocyte alkaline phosphatase levels, anemia, splenomegaly (in 43% of HES patients), cytogenetic abnormalities, and myelodysplasia. Patients with these latter findings are less likely to respond to corticosteroids and may require cytotoxic agents.

Cardiac manifestations are common in HES and are present in about 58% of patients (36). Cardiac damage is thought to progress through three stages: acute necrosis, the development of endocardial thrombi, and endocardial fibrosis (36,44). The first acute stage is frequently clinically silent, although histologically, damage to the endocardium, necrosis, and eosinophilic infiltration of myocardium with eosinophil degranulation products and microabscesses are present. It is hypothesized that treatment in the first stage with corticosteroids will prevent progression to the other nonreversible stages (36). The second stage is characterized by thrombi in either ventricle and occasionally in the atrium. In the third stage, fibrosis may lead to entrapment of the chordae tendineae and resultant mitral or tricuspid valve insufficiency or a restrictive cardiomyopathy. Clinically, patients may present with dyspnea, chest pain, or congestive heart failure. Murmurs of mitral regurgitation can be heard. Because the heart is the most common site of organ involvement and because the first stage may be clinically silent, an electrocardiogram and echocardiogram must be obtained if HES is under consideration. Serial echocardiograms should be used to monitor cardiac involvement in patients in whom HES is a diagnostic possibility and those with established disease.

Skin involvement affects 56% (36), with the most common cutaneous manifestations erythroderma, urticarial plaques, angioedema, pruritic papules and nodules (36,40). Patients who have urticaria or angioedema as skin manifestations tend to have a better prognosis; they are more likely to have no cardiac or neurologic manifestations (36). Biopsy specimens of the papular and nodular lesions are characterized by perivascular infiltrates of eosinophils, neutrophils, and mononuclear cells without evidence of vasculitis (36).

Neurologic involvement occurs in 54% of cases and has three forms: thromboembolic disease resulting from thrombotic cardiac disease, primary central nervous system dysfunction (36), and peripheral neuropathy. Clinically, patients who present with thromboembolic events have had strokes or transient ischemic attacks. Visual symptoms, occurring in 23% of patients, are also attributed to microemboli or possibly local thrombi. The most frequent visual abnormality is blurred vision. Central nervous system dysfunction is manifested as gait disturbances, behavioral changes, memory loss, or upper motor neuron signs such as increased muscle tone. Peripheral neuropathy may be expressed as mononeuritis multiplex with symmetric or asymmetric sensory deficits or painful paresthesias, or as motor neuropathies.

Pulmonary involvement occurs in 49% of HES patients, with the most frequent presentation a nonproductive cough (36). The chest radiograph in most patients is clear. Pulmonary involvement is believed to occur as a secondary manifestation of congestive heart failure or of embolic events originating from right ventricular thrombi or by primary infiltration of the lung by eosinophils. Thus, chest radiographs may show evidence of congestive heart failure, pleural effusions, or infiltrates. Interestingly, asthma does not occur more frequently in HES than in the general population (36).

About 20% of HES patients have gastrointestinal tract involvement. Diarrhea is the most frequent sign. Eosinophilic gastritis, enterocolitis, colitis, pancreatitis, hepatitis, and the Budd-Chiari syndrome all have been described (36). Rheumatologic symptoms include arthralgias, joint effusions, arthritis, Raynaud phenomenon, and digital necrosis.

When HES was first described, the prognosis was poor with a 3-year survival rate of 12% (34). Most deaths were cardiovascular. Today, if cardiovascular complications, including congestive heart failure, valvular disease, and arrhythmias, can be prevented or managed successfully, the prognosis is much better. In 1989, 40 HES patients from France were reported to have an 80% survival rate at 5 years and a 42% survival rate at 10 to15 years (36). Treatment begins with corticosteroids (usually prednisone, 1 mg/kg/day for several weeks and then on alternate days). Hydroxyurea (1 to 2 g/day) (37) is used for patients who do not respond adequately to corticosteroids. Vincristine (1.5 to 2.0 mg at 2-week intervals) may be used instead of hydroxyurea to induce a more rapid response (36). Interferon-α

administered subcutaneously in several dosage regimens has also been reported to be effective (38,40).

Churg-Strauss Syndrome

The major vasculitis associated with eosinophilia is CSS, also called *allergic angiitis* and *granulomatosis*. It was first described in 1951 (44,45). The syndrome is characterized by a necrotizing vasculitis in patients with asthma and eosinophilia. Diagnostic criteria formulated by the American College of Rheumatology, yielding a sensitivity of 85% and a specificity of 99.7%, are generally followed (46). For a diagnosis of CSS, four of the following six criteria must be satisfied: asthma, peripheral eosinophilia (>10%), mononeuropathy or polyneuropathy, nonfixed pulmonary infiltrates, paranasal sinus abnormality, and extravascular eosinophils in a blood vessel on biopsy (45,46).

The true incidence of CSS is unknown. Because it is relatively rare and therefore not readily recognized, the diagnosis may be missed. In addition, some cases initially treated as asthma, the prodrome of CSS, may be controlled by corticosteroid therapy for asthma and any progression to vasculitis not recognized until steroids are tapered (27,28). The mean age of onset is 38 years; men are affected slightly more frequently than women (47). Typically, asthma or rhinitis precedes the development of the other manifestations by a mean of 8.9 ± 10.9 years (48) and may present as new "allergies" in a patient without an allergic family history (44,47,49). Eosinophilia is observed, and then the vasculitis phase develops (50). This phase, which is often accompanied by constitutional symptoms, such as fever, malaise, and weight loss, typically begins years after asthma is diagnosed but sometimes occurs within months of the diagnosis of asthma.

The distribution of organ involvement is enumerated in Table 33.3. Virtually all patients have pulmonary involvement as asthma or bilateral migratory pulmonary infiltrates (48). Upper respiratory involvement is manifested by rhinitis and/or sinusitis. Mononeuritis multiplex is the most common form of neurologic involvement

TABLE 33.3. *Distribution of clinical manifestations in Churg-Strauss syndrome*

Organ system	Frequency (percentage of patients)
Lung[a]	100
Hematologic (eosinophilia)[a]	100
Peripheral nervous system[a]	80
Upper respiratory[a]	60–80
Skin	50–55
Cardiac	33[b]
Gastrointestinal tract	33–48
Renal	26–55
Musculoskeletal	21–40

[a]Part of the Diagnostic Criteria.
[b]By autopsy, up to 66% (48).
Data were summarized from Guillevin L, Cohen P, Gayraud M, et al. Churg-Strauss syndrome: clinical study and long-term follow-up of 96 patients. *Medicine* 1999;78:26–37; and Rochester CL. The eosinophilic pneumonias. In: Fishman AP (ed-in-chief). *Fishman's pulmonary diseases and disorders.* New York: McGraw-Hill, 1998:1133–1150.

(47,48). Typical dermatologic findings include palpable purpura, nodules, erythematous papules, and urticaria (47,48). Clinically, cardiac manifestations include congestive heart failure, pericarditis, pericardial effusions, and dysrhythmias. In one review, only about one third of patients had clinical cardiac disease, but almost two thirds were found to have findings at autopsy, including fibrosis, myocarditis, pericarditis, and eosinophilic granulomas in the pericardium (47). The most common gastrointestinal symptoms are abdominal pain, nausea or vomiting, diarrhea, and hematochezia. Ulcers and bowel perforation have been reported infrequently. Proteinuria is the most common manifestation of renal disease associated with CSS. Renal disease in CSS is less severe than in other related vasculitides, such as polyarteritis nodosa and Wegener granulomatosis (47,48). Myalgias and arthralgias are the most common musculoskeletal symptoms; however, true arthritis is rare (3,47).

Laboratory studies are most notable for fluctuating peripheral blood eosinophilia, with peaks ranging from 20% to 90% of the differential white blood cell count. Perinuclear antineutrophil cytoplasmic antibodies directed against myeloperoxidase occur in 50% to 70% of patients (48,49). The erythrocyte sedimentation rate is frequently elevated, with a mean of 52.7 ± 32.6 in one series of patients (48). Biopsy of involved tissues is characterized by necrotizing vasculitis of the small arteries and veins, eosinophils, and extravascular granulomas.

Without treatment, the prognosis is poor with 50% dying within 3 months of the onset of vasculitis (49). With treatment, 5-year survival has improved to more than 75% (48). Therapy begins with prednisone at approximately 40–60 mg/day. Cyclophosphamide is added if the response is inadequate. Some investigators believe that the early use of cyclophosphamide (Cytoxan) prevents irreversible organ damage (47). The patients at risk for a poor outcome are those with myocardial involvement, proteinuria (>1 g/day), severe gastrointestinal symptoms (intestinal bleeding, perforation, pancreatitis, or requiring laparotomy), or a short duration of asthma before the presentation of the vasculitic phase (48).

Eosinophilic Pneumonias

The eosinophilic pneumonias are a group of disorders characterized by blood or tissue eosinophilia and pulmonary infiltrates. In 1952, Reeder and Goodrich introduced the term *pulmonary infiltrates with eosinophilia* (PIE) for diseases with peripheral blood eosinophilia *and* pulmonary infiltrates (51). One of these, allergic bronchopulmonary aspergillosis, is discussed in Chapter 24. Drug-induced PIE was discussed previously and in Table 33.1. Löffler's syndrome, also a PIE syndrome, is described later. In 1969, Liebow and Carrington broadened the diseases that had been included in the PIE group by defining *eosinophilic pneumonias* (52). This term was intended to describe the more inclusive category of pulmonary diseases characterized by eosinophilic infiltrates with or without peripheral blood eosinophilia. Later, other related syndromes, such as acute eosinophilic pneumonia, were described. CSS, the only eosinophilic pneumonia with extrapulmonary involvement, first described about the same time as Reeder's report, was also included in this group of pulmonary diseases in which the eosinophil is thought to play a role in the pathogenesis. There are four eosinophilic pneumonias not discussed earlier: tropical pulmonary eosinophilia, Löffler syndrome, and chronic and acute eosinophilic pneumonia. Excellent reviews (45,49) provide further details and a description of several others for which space does not allow inclusion here.

Tropical pulmonary eosinophilia is caused by filarial infection. Löffler syndrome, or simple pulmonary eosinophilia, is characterized by fleeting migratory infiltrates, peripheral blood eosinophilia, and low-grade fever, dry cough, and dyspnea (45,49). There is no age predominance. Most patients with Löffler syndrome have either a parasitic infection or drug reaction, although no cause can be found in about one third of cases. The condition resolves spontaneously.

Chronic eosinophilic pneumonia has an insidious onset. Its symptoms include cough, fever, dyspnea, and weight loss. Women are affected twice as often as men (45,53). Patients are generally at least 30 years of age (6,54), and many have a history of atopy. Sputum production and wheezing are infrequent. Occasionally, hemoptysis is observed. The course is chronic, with the time from symptoms to diagnosis about 7 months. Blood eosinophilia is present in about 90%, but its absence does not exclude the diagnosis (55). The chest radiograph reveals progressive peripheral dense infiltrates, which resemble a "photographic negative of pulmonary edema" (53,55,56). This classic radiologic finding occurs in less than half of patients. Other radiographic findings may include nodular infiltrates, atelectasis, unilateral or bilateral involvement, cavitation, and pleural effusion. High-resolution computed tomography scans of the chest may identify peripheral infiltrates not evident on the radiograph and may also reveal mediastinal adenopathy. Pulmonary function tests may present a restrictive or normal pattern of lung volumes (45). The diffusing capacity is frequently reduced. Examination of the tissue reveals a predominantly eosinophilic infiltrate involving the alveoli and interstitium. Interstitial fibrosis, bronchiolitis, and bronchiolitis obliterans can be present, and occasionally, eosinophilic microabscesses and noncaseating granulomas are observed. Necrosis is rare. Infiltrates resolve rapidly with moderate-dose corticosteroid therapy, but therapy is often necessary for at least 6 months to resolve the impaired diffusing capacity and volume restriction (56). Although the prognosis is excellent, 34% experience recurrent episodes requiring low-dose alternate-day corticosteroids (45,55).

Acute eosinophilic pneumonia is an acute febrile illness characterized by hypoxemia and respiratory failure. Its course is precipitous, typically developing over a 5-day period. There is no predilection of gender. It is a diagnosis of exclusion; hypersensitivity reactions, reactions to medications and toxins, and infectious etiologies must be ruled out. Diffuse alveolar or alveolar-interstitial infiltrates are present on chest radiograph. Pulmonary function testing reveals diminished lung volumes and diffusing capacity. More than 25% of the inflammatory cells in the bronchoalveolar lavage fluid are eosinophils, although blood eosinophilia is unusual. Histopathology is characterized by diffuse acute and organizing alveolar damage with marked interstitial eosinophil infiltrates. Granulomas and vasculitis have not been observed, but the pathogenesis is not well understood. The treatment is high-dose corticosteroids. Recurrence is rare. In patients who present with a viral syndrome progressing to acute respiratory distress syndrome in 3 to 5 days, this diagnosis should be entertained and a bronchoalveolar lavage performed (45).

Eosinophilic Gastroenteritis

Eosinophilic gastroenteritis is a rare disorder that is characterized by abdominal discomfort, peripheral blood eosinophilia, and eosinophilic infiltration of the bowel wall (57). Although there are no standards for diagnosis, and although eosinophils are normally found in the gastrointestinal mucosa, the diagnosis is made by pathologic examination of a biopsy specimen showing extensive eosinophilic infiltration of the mucosa, the muscular layer, or the subserosa. The peak age of onset is the third decade, although it can occur in children. In children, food allergy may contribute, but it is rarely important in adults. Symptoms include nausea, abdominal pain, vomiting, diarrhea, weight loss, anemia, protein-losing enteropathy, and intestinal perforation. Corticosteroids provide symptomatic relief, as does oral cromolyn sodium. It must be appreciated that eosinophils can be present in a variety of gastrointestinal diseases, including irritable bowel syndrome and inflammatory bowel disease. Because of the rarity of the disease and

TABLE 33.4. *Currently available and potential therapy for reducing eosinophil numbers or their activity*

Drug	Mechanism	References
Currently available		
Corticosteroids	Promote eosinophil apoptosis	2, 60, 204
	Suppress transcription of IL-3, IL-4, IL-5, GM-CSF	
Hydroxyurea	Myelosuppression	2
Vincristine	Myelosuppression	2
Interferon-α	Inhibits eosinophil degranulation and effector function, induces apoptosis	38, 40, 60
Cyclosporine, tacrolimus	Suppress transcription of IL-5, GM-CSF through inhibition of T-cell function	2, 60, 205
Leukotriene modifiers	Inhibit generation of LTB4 and LTC4, LTD4, LTE4	2, 206, 207
	Interfere with eosinophil infiltration in the late phase and chemotaxis	
	Inhibit vascular permeability and muscle contraction from leukotriene products of eosinophils	
Cromolyn, nedocromil	Inhibit effector function of eosinophils (e.g., antibody-dependent cellular cytotoxicity)	2, 60
Cetirizine	Decreases eosinophil chemotaxis	60
PUVA	Unknown	208, 209
Potential therapy currently under investigation		
Anti–IL-5	Decreases eosinophil recruitment, activation, and survival	60, 210
IL-5 receptor blocker	Decreases eosinophil activation and survival	60
Eotaxin antagonist	Decreases eosinophil infiltration	211
Anti–IL-13	Blocks eotaxin secretion and eosinophil recruitment	60
CCRC receptor antagonist	Blocks chemotactic response of eosinophils to chemokines	117, 211, 212
Very late antigen 4 inhibitor	Blocks eosinophil adhesion and infiltration	60
Phosphodiesterase inhibitors (PDE4 inhibitor)	Inhibit intracellular signaling through increasing cAMP and reduce eosinophil infiltration	2, 60, 213
Nitric oxide inhibitors	Inhibit eosinophil recruitment and survival	60
Tryptase inhibitors	Inhibit eosinophil recruitment	60
Tyrosine kinase inhibitors (e.g., syk and lyn kinase)	Inhibit signaling through IgE receptor on mast cells leading to inhibition of degranulation and reduced eosinophil infiltration, inhibit eosinophil activation and survival	60
MAP kinase inhibitors	Reduced T_H2 cytokines, increase eosinophil apoptosis	60

PUVA, __; GM-CSF, granulocyte-macrophage colony-stimulating factor; MAP, __; CCRC, __; cAMP, cyclic adenosine monophosphate.

the lack of diagnostic standards, there is still much to be learned about this disease and of the role of the eosinophil in its pathogenesis (57).

Eosinophilic Cystitis

Eosinophilic cystitis is a rare disease characterized by urinary frequency (present in 67%), hematuria (68%), suprapubic pain (49%), and urinary retention (10%) (58). It is distributed equally between males and females but is most common in children, boys being more commonly affected. Peripheral eosinophilia is present in 43% (58). Cystoscopy reveals hyperemic mucosa with areas of elevation and nodularity. Biopsy is characterized by eosinophilic infiltrate, mucosal edema, and muscle necrosis. This inflammatory pattern may progress to chronic inflammation and fibrosis of the bladder mucosa and muscularis. The treatment is radical transurethral resection of the bladder lesions and treatment with corticosteroids, which promotes resolution.

Most patients experience spontaneous resolution, but recurrences are frequent.

EVALUATION OF THE PATIENT WITH EOSINOPHILIA

An approach to the evaluation of a patient with eosinophilia is depicted in Fig. 33.2. Most important is the history, with careful attention to travel and dietary history. Medications including over-the-counter and complementary medicine preparations must be considered and any nonessential medications discontinued. A history consistent with atopy should be sought, with the caveat that atopy causes only a modest increase in peripheral eosinophil count (<15%). If parasitic disease remains a consideration, examination of the stool and serologic tests should be ordered. Evidence of tissue infiltration should be sought. An echocardiogram and chest radiograph should be obtained. If the etiology remains unclear or the degree of eosinophilia is substantial, further examination for lymphoproliferative disease and the hypereosinophilic syndrome should be pursued. Additional tests necessary would include screening for autoantibodies, computed tomography of the abdomen, bone marrow aspiration with cytogenetic analysis, and bone marrow biopsy. Finally, flow cytometry for the detection of aberrant populations of T lymphocytes may be obtained, although the clinical implications are not fully understood at this point (40,59). Patients with persistent eosinophilia without a clear etiology should be monitored with physical examination and echocardiography for evidence of cardiac damage, including thrombi and endomyocardial fibrosis (3).

Current and potential therapies for eosinophilia and their mechanisms of action are described in Table 33.4 and in excellent review articles (2,60). Currently, corticosteroid treatment is the first line of approach, but as can be seen by the length of Table 33.4, significant advances in therapy are expected in the next few years.

CONCLUSION

Our understanding of the biology of the eosinophil is increasing rapidly, making it likely that important clinical advances in recognizing and treating eosinophil-mediated diseases will occur in the coming years.

ACKNOWLEDGMENTS

We gratefully acknowledge the critical reviews and suggestions of Drs. Burton Zweiman, Jay Hess, Arnold Levinson, and Anita Gewurz.

REFERENCES

1. Holland SM, Gallin JI. Disorders of granulocytes and monocytes. In: Fauci AS, Braunwald E, Isselbacher KJ, et al, eds. *Harrison's principles of internal medicine.* 14th ed. New York: McGraw Hill, 1998:351–359.
2. Rothenburg ME. Eosinophilia. *N Engl J Med* 1998; 338:1592–1600.
3. Weller PF. Eosinophilia. In: Rich RR, ed-in-chief. *Clinical immunology: principles and practice.* St. Louis: Mosby–Year Book, 1996;1022–1031.
4. Gleich GJ, Adolphson CR. The eosinophilic leukocyte: structure and function. *Adv Immunol* 1986;39:177–253.
5. Wardlaw AJ, Moqbel RM, Kay AB. Eosinophils and the allergic inflammatory response. In: Kay AB, ed. *Allergy and allergic diseases.* London: Blackwell, 1997:171–188.
6. Lim KG, Weller PF. Eosinophilia and eosinophil-related disorders. In: Middleton E Jr, Reed CE, Ellis EF, et al, eds. *Allergy, principles and practice.* 5th ed. St. Louis: Mosby, 1998:783–798.
7. Malathi A. Evaluation of anxiety status in medical students prior to examination stress. *Ind J Physiol Pharmacol* 1992;36:121–122.
8. Bass DA, Gonwa TA, Szejda P, et al. Eosinopenia of acute infection: production of eosinopenia by chemotactic factors of acute inflammation. *J Clin Invest* 1980;65:1265–1271.
9. Weller PF. The immunobiology of eosinophils. *N Eng J Med* 1991;324:1110–1118.
10. Gleich GJ. Mechanisms of eosinophil-associated inflammation. *J Allergy Clin Immunol* 2000;105:651–663.
11. Weller PF. Human eosinophils. *J Allergy Clin Immunol* 1997;100:283–287.
12. Wardlaw AJ. Molecular basis for selective eosinophil trafficking in asthma: a multistep paradigm. *J Allergy Clin Immunol* 1999;104:917–926.
13. Collins PD, Marleau S, Griffiths-Johnson DA, et al. Cooperation between interleukin-5 and the chemokine eotaxin to induce eosinophil accumulation in vivo. *J Exp Med* 1995;182:1169–1174.
14. Erjefalt JS, Persson CGA. New aspects of degranulation and fates of airway mucosal eosinophils. *Am J Respir Crit Care Med* 2000;161:2074–2085.
15. Resnick MB, Weller PF. Mechanisms of eosinophil recruitment. *Am Rev Respir Cell Mol Biol* 1993;8:349–355.
16. Jacoby DB, Gleich GJ, Fryer AD. Human eosinophil major basic protein is an endogenous allosteric

antagonist at the inhibitory muscarinic M2 receptor. *J Clin Invest* 1993;91:1314–1318.

17. Plotz SB, Dibbert B, Abeck D, et al. Bcl-2 expression by eosinophils in a patient with hypereosinophilia. *J Allergy Clin Immunol* 1998;102:1037–1040.

18. Simon HU, Yousefi S, Schranz C, et al. Direct demonstration of delayed eosinophil apoptosis as a mechanism causing tissue eosinophilia. *J Immunol* 1997;158:3902–3908.

19. Cooper PJ, Beck LA, Espinel I, et al. Eotaxin and RANTES expression by the dermal endothelium is associated with eosinophil infiltration after ivermectin treatment of onchocerciasis. *Clin Immunol* 2000;95:51–61.

20. Genta RM, Douce RW, Walzer PD. Diagnostic implications of parasite-specific immune responses in immunocompromised patients with strongyloidiasis. *J Clin Microbiol* 1986;23:1099–1103.

21. Genta RM, Miles P, Fields K. Opportunistic *Strongyloides stercoralis* infection in lymphoma patients: report of a case and review of the literature. *Cancer* 1989;63:1407–1411.

22. Thomas MC, Costello SA. Disseminated strongyloidiasis arising from a single dose of dexamethasone before stereotactic radiosurgery. *Int J Clin Pract* 1998;52:520–521.

23. Weller PF. Eosinophilia in travelers: travel medicine. *Med Clin North Am* 1992;76:1413–1432.

24. Klotz LR, Klotz SD, Moeller RK. The use of beclomethasone dipropionate inhaler complicated by the development of an eosinophilic pneumonia reaction. *Ann Allergy* 1977;39:133–136.

25. Mollura JL, Bernstein R, Fine SR, et al. Pulmonary eosinophilia in a patient receiving beclomethasone dipropionate aerosol. *Ann Allergy* 1979;42:326–329.

26. Lobel H, Machtey I, Eldror MY. Pulmonary infiltrates with eosinophilia in an asthmatic patient treated with disodium cromoglycate. *Lancet* 1972;1:1032.

27. Wechsler ME, Garpestad E, Flier SR, et al. Pulmonary infiltrates, eosinophilia, and cardiomyopathy following corticosteroid withdrawal in patients with asthma receiving zafirlukast. *JAMA* 1998;279(6):455–457.

28. Wechsler ME, Finn D, Gunawardena D, et al. Churg-Strauss syndrome in patients receiving montelukast as treatment for asthma. *Chest* 2000;117(3):708–713.

29. Kaufman LD, Gruber BL, Gregersen PK. Clinical follow-up and immunogenetic studies of 32 patients with eosinophilia-myalgia syndrome. *Lancet* 1991;337:1071–1074.

30. Sternberg EM. Pathogenesis of L-tryptophan eosinophilia myalgia syndrome. *Adv Exp Med Biol* 1996;398:325–330.

31. Mikami C, Ochiai K, Kagami M, et al. In vitro interleukin-5 (IL-5) production by peripheral blood mononuclear cells from patients with drug hypersensitivity. *J Dermatol* 1996;23:379–381.

32. Mikami C, Ochiai K, Umemiya K, et al. Eosinophil activation and in situ interleukin-5 production by mononuclear cells in skin lesions of patients with drug hypersensitivity. *J Dermatol* 1999;26:633–639.

33. Hardy WR, Anderson RE. The hypereosinophilic syndrome. *Ann Intern Med* 1968;68:1220–1229.

34. Chusid MJ, Dale DC, West BC, et al. The hypereosinophilic syndrome: analysis of fourteen cases with review of the literature. *Medicine* 1975;54:1–27.

35. Fauci AS, Harley JB, Roberts WC, et al. NIH Conference. The idiopathic hypereosinophilic syndrome: clinical, pathophysiologic, and therapeutic considerations. *Ann Intern Med* 1982;97:78–92.

36. Weller PF, Bubley GJ. The idopathic hypereosinophilic syndrome. *Blood* 1994;83:2759–2779.

37. Means-Markwell M, Burgess T, DeKeratry D, et al. Eosinophilia with aberrant T cells and elevated serum levels of interleukin-2 and interleukin-15. *N Eng J Med* 2000;342:1568–1571.

38. Cogan E, Schandene L, Crusiaux A, et al. Brief report: clonal proliferation of type 2 helper cells in a man with the hypereosinophilic syndrome. *N Engl J Med* 1994;330:535–538.

39. Brugnoni D, Airo P, Rossi G, et al. A case of hypereosinophilic syndrome is associated with the expansion of CD3−CD4+ T-cell population able to secrete large amounts of interleukin-5. *Blood* 1996;87:1416–1422.

40. Simon H-U, Plotz GB, Dummer R, et al. Abnormal clones of T cells producing interleukin-5 in idopathic eosinophilia. *N Eng J Med* 1999;341:1112–1120.

41. Owen WF, Rothenberg ME, Petersen J et al. Interleukin 5 and phenotypically altered eosinophils in the blood of patients with the idiopathic hypereosinophilic syndrome. *J Exp Med* 1989;170:343–348.

42. Plotz SG, Dibbert B, Abeck D, et al. Bcl-2 expression by eosinophils in a patient with hypereosinophilia. *J Allergy Clin Immunol* 1998;102:1037–1040.

43. Bain BJ. Eosinophilia: idiopathic or not? *N Engl J Med* 1999;34:1141–1142.

44. Churg J, Strauss L. Allergic granulomatosis, allergic angiitis and periarteritis nodosa. *Am J Pathol* 1951;27:277–301.

45. Allen JN, Davis WB. Eosinophilic lung diseases. *Am J Respir Crit Care Med* 1994;150:1423–1438.

46. Masi AT, Hunder GG, Lie JT, et al. The American College of Rheumatology 1990 criteria for the classification of the Churg-Strauss syndrome (allergic granulomatosis and angiitis). *Arthritis Rheum* 1990;33:1094–1100.

47. Hellmann DB, Stone JH. Small and medium vessel primary vasculitis. In: Rich RR, Fleisher TA, Shearer WT, et al., eds. *Clinical immunology, principles and practice*, 2nd Edition. London: Mosby:2001:67.1–67.24.

48. Guillevin L, Cohen P, Gayraud M, et al. Churg-Strauss syndrome: clinical study and long-term follow-up of 96 patients. *Medicine* 1999;78:26–37.

49. Rochester CL. The eosinophilic pneumonias. In: Fishman AP, ed-in-chief. *Fishman's pulmonary diseases and disorders*. New York: McGraw-Hill, 1998:1133–1150.

50. Lanham J, Elkon K, Pusey C, et al. Systemic vasculitis with asthma and eosinophilia: a clinical approach to the Churg-Strauss syndrome. *Medicine* (Baltimore) 1995;63:65–81.

51. Reeder WH, Goodrich BE. Pulmonary infiltration with eosinophilia (PIE syndrome). *Ann Intern Med* 1952;36:1217–1240.

52. Liebow AA, Carrington CB. The eosinophilic pneumonias. *Medicine* 1969;48:251–285.

53. Hayakawa H, Sato A, Toyoshima M, et al. A clinical study of idiopathic eosinophilic pneumonia. *Chest* 1994;105;1462–1466.

54. Oermann CM, Panesar KS, Langston C, et al. Pulmonary infiltrates with eosinophilia syndromes in children. *J Pediatr* 2000;136:351–358.

55. Jederlinic PJ, Sicilian L, Gaensler EA. Chronic

eosinophilic pneumonia: a report of 19 cases and a review of the literature. *Medicine* 1988;67:154–162.

56. Carrington CB, Addington WW, Goff AM, et al. Chronic eosinophilic pneumonia. *N Engl J Med* 1969;280:787–798.

57. Kelly KJ. Eosinophilic gastroenteritis. *Pediatr Gastroenterol Nutr* 2000;30[Suppl]:S28–S35.

58. van den Ouden D. Diagnosis and management of eosinophilic cystitis: a pooled analysis of 135 cases. *Eur Urol* 2000;37:386–394.

59. Bain BJ. Hypereosinophilia. *Curr Opin Hematol* 2000;7:21–25.

60. Barnes PJ. New directions in allergic diseases: mechanism-based anti-inflammatory therapies. *J Allergy Clin Immunol* 2000;106:5–16.

61. Wolfe MS. Eosinophilia in the returning traveler. *Med Clin North Am* 1999;83:1019–1032, vii.

62. Meeusen EN, Balic A. Do eosinophils have a role in the killing of helminth parasites? *Parasitol Today* 2000;16:95–101.

63. Ong RK, Doyle RL. Tropical pulmonary eosinophilia. *Chest* 1998;113:1673–1679.

64. Lombard CM, Tazelaar HD, Krasne DL. Pulmonary eosinophilia in coccidioidal infections. *Chest* 1987;91:734–736.

65. Schermoly MJ, Hinthorn DR. Eosinophilia in coccidioidomycosis. *Arch Intern Med* 1988;148:895–896.

66. Harley WB, Blaser MJ. Disseminated coccidioidomycosis associated with extreme eosinophilia. *Clin Infect Dis* 1994;18:627–629.

67. Sanchez-Borges M, Orozco A, Di Biagio E, et al. Eosinophilia in early-stage human immunodeficiency virus infection. *J Allergy Clin Immunol* 1993;92:494–495.

68. Cohen AJ, Steigbigel RT. Eosinophilia in patients infected with human immunodeficiency virus. *J Infect Dis* 1996;174:615–618.

69. Pagnelli R, Scala E, Mezzaroma I, et al. Immunologic aspects of hyperimmunolglobulinemia E-like syndrome in patients with AIDS. *J Allergy Clin Immunol* 1995;95:995–1003.

70. Tietz A, Sponagel L, Erb P, et al. Eosinophilia in patients infected with the human immunodeficiency virus. *Eur J Clin Microbiol Infect Dis* 1997;16:675–677.

71. Riantawan P, Bangpattanasiri K, Chaowalit P, et al. Etiology and clinical implications of eosinophilic pleural effusions. *Southeast Asian J Trop Med Public Health* 1998;29:655–659.

72. Fleury-Feith J, Van Nhieu JT, Picard C, et al. Bronchoalveolar lavage eosinophilia associated with *Pneumocystis carinii* pneumonitis in AIDS patients: comparative study with non-AIDS patients. *Chest* 1989;95:1198–1201.

73. Ellis AG. The pathological anatomy of bronchial asthma. *Am J Med Sci* 1908;1136:407.

74. Gleich GJ. The eosinophil and bronchial asthma: current understanding. *J Allergy Clin Immunol* 1990;85:422–436.

75. Wild JS, Sigounas A, Sur N, et al. IFN-gamma-inducing factor (IL-18) increases allergic sensitization, serum IgE, Th2 cytokines and airway eosinophilia I: a mouse model of allergic asthma. *J Immunol* 2000;164:2701–2710.

76. Shirota H, Sano K, Kikuchi T, et al. Regulation of T-helper type 2 cell and airway eosinophilia by transmucosal coadministration of antigen and oligodeoxy-nucleotides containing CpG motifs. *Am J Respir Cell Mol Biol* 2000;2:176–182.

77. Mould AW, Ramsay AJ, Matthaei KI, et al. The effect of IL-5 and eotaxin expression in the lung on eosinophil trafficking and degranulation and the induction of bronchial hyperreactivity. *J Immunol* 2000;164:2142–2150.

78. Zeibecoglou K, Ying S, Yamada T, et al. Increased mature and immature CCR3 messenger RNA+ eosinophils in bone marrow from patients with atopic asthma compared with atopic and nonatopic control subjects. *J Allergy Clin Immunol* 1999;103(1 Pt. 1):99–106.

79. Szczeklik A, Sladek K, Dworski R, et al. Bronchial aspirin challenge causes specific eicosanoid response in aspirin-sensitive asthmatics. *Am J Respir Crit Care Med* 1996;154:1608–1614.

80. Bousquet J, Chanez P, Lacost JY, et al. Eosinophilic inflammation in asthma. *N Engl J Med* 1990;323:1033–1039.

81. Jatakanon A, Lim S, Barnes PJ. Changes in sputum eosinophils predict loss of asthma control. *Am J Respir Crit Care Med* 2000;161:64–72.

82. Baraniuk JN. Pathogenesis of allergic rhinitis. *J Allergy Clin Immunol* 1997;99:S763–S772.

83. Leone C, Teodoro C, Pelucchi A, et al. Bronchial responsiveness and airway inflammation in patients with nonallergic rhinitis with eosinophilia syndrome. *J Allergy Clin Immunol* 1997;100(6 Pt. 1):775–780.

84. Jacobs RL, Freedman PM, Boswell RN. Nonallergic rhinitis with eosinophilia (NARES syndrome): clinical and immunologic presentation. *J Allergy Clin Immunol* 1981;67:253–262.

85. Moneret-Vautrin DA, Hsieh V, Wayoff M, et al. Nonallergic rhinitis with eosinophilia syndrome a precursor of the triad: nasal polyposis, intrinsic asthma, and intolerance to aspirin. *Ann Allergy* 1990;64:513–518.

86. Hamilos DL, Leung DY, Huston DP, et al. GM-CSF, IL-5 and RANTES immunoreactivity and mRNA expression in chronic hyperplastic sinusitis with nasal polyposis (NP). *Clin Exp Allergy* 1998;28:1145–1152.

87. Newman LJ, Platts-Mills TAE, Phillips CD, et al. Chronic sinusitis. *JAMA* 1994;271:363–367.

88. Hoover GE, Newman LJ, Platts-Mills TA, et al. Chronic sinusitis: risk factors for extensive disease. *J Allergy Clin Immunol* 1997;100:185–191.

89. Baroody FM, Hughes CA, McDowell P, et al. Eosinophilia in chronic childhood sinusitis. *Arch Otolaryngol Head Neck Surg* 1995;121:1396–1402.

90. Schwartz HJ. Allergic fungal sinusitis: experience in an ambulatory allergy practice. *Ann Allergy Asthma Immunol* 1996;77:500–502.

91. Ponikau JU, Sherris DA, Kern EB, et al. The diagnosis and incidence of allergic fungal sinusitis. *Mayo Clin Proc* 1999;74(9):877–884.

92. Feger TA, Rupp NT, Kuhn FA, et al. Local and systemic eosinophil activation in allergic fungal sinusitis. *Ann Allergy Asthma Immunol* 1997;79:221–225.

93. Taniguchi H, Kadota J, Fujii T, et al. Activation of lymphocytes and increased interleukin-5 levels in bronchoalveolar lavage fluid in acute eosinophilic pneumonia. *Eur Respir J* 1999;13:217–220.

94. Oermann CM, Panesar KS, Langston C, et al. Pulmonary infiltrates with eosinophilia syndromes in children. *J Pediatr* 2000;136:351–358.

95. Murin S, Bilello KS, Matthay R. Other smoking-affected pulmonary diseases. *Clin Chest Med* 2000;21: 121–137, ix.

96. Vassallo R, Ryu JH, Colby TV, et al. Pulmonary Langerhans'-cell histiocytosis. *N Engl J Med* 2000; 342:1969–1977.

97. Allen JN, Davis WB, Pacht ER. Diagnostic significance of increased bronchoalveolar lavage fluid eosinophils. *Am Rev Respir Dis* 1990;142:642–647.

98. Hogan MB, Piktel D, Landreth KS. IL-5 production by bone marrow stromal cells: implications for eosinophilia associated with asthma. *J Allergy Clin Immunol* 2000;106:329–336.

99. Rajakumar K, Hogan MB, Wilson NW. Failure to thrive and two weeks of persistent vomiting in an 11-month-old infant. *Ann Allergy Asthma Immunol* 2000;85:349–352.

100. Leiferman KM. Eosinophils in atopic dermatitis. *J Allergy Clin Immunol* 1994;94:1310–1317.

101. Taha RA, Minshall EM, Leung DY, et al. Evidence for increased expression of eotaxin and monocyte chemotactic protein-4 in atopic dermatitis. *J Allergy Clin Immunol* 2000;105:1002–1007.

102. Akdis CA, Akdis M, Simon HU, et al. Regulation of allergic inflammation by skin- homing T cells in allergic eczema. *Int Arch Allergy Immunol* 1999;118:140–144.

103. Adame J, Cohen PR. Eosinophilic panniculitis: diagnostic considerations and evaluation. *J Am Acad Dermatol* 1996;34:229–234.

104. Aberer W, Konrad K, Wolff K. Wells' syndrome is a distinctive disease entity and not a histologic diagnosis. *J Am Acad Dermatol* 1988;18:105–114.

105. Wells GC, GC, Smith NP. Eosinophilic cellulitis. *Br J Dermatol* 1979;100:101–109.

106. Espana A, Sanz ML, Sola J, et al. Wells' syndrome (eosinophilic cellulitis): correlation between clinical activity, eosinophil levels, eosinophil cation protein and interleukin-5. *Br J Dermatol* 1999;140:127–130.

107. Doyle JA, Ginsburg WW. Eosinophilic fasciitis. *Med Clin North Am* 1989;73:1157–1166.

108. McEvoy MT, Peterson EA, Kobza-Black A, et al. Immunohistological comparison of granulated cell proteins in induced immediate urticarial dermographism and delayed pressure urticaria lesions. *Br J Dermatol* 1995;133:853–860.

109. Gleich GJ, Schroeter AL, Marcoux JP, et al. Episodic angioedema associated with eosinophilia. *N Engl J Med* 1984;310:1621–1626.

110. Sabroe RA, Poon E, Orchard GE, et al. Cutaneous inflammatory cell infiltrate in chronic idiopathic urticaria: comparison of patients with and without anti-FcepsilonRI or anti-IgE autoantibodies. *J Allergy Clin Immunol* 1999;103:484–493.

111. Bull RH, Harland CA, Fallowfield ME, et al. Eosinophilic folliculitis: a self-limiting illness in patients being treated for haematological malignancy. *Br J Dermatol* 1993;129:178–182.

112. McCalmont TH, Altemus D, Maurer T, et al. Eosinophilic folliculitis. *Am J Dermatopathol* 1995;17: 439–446.

113. Fearfield LA, Rowe A, Francis N, et al. Itchy folliculitis and human immunodeficiency virus infection: clinico-pathological and immunological features, pathogenesis and treatment. *Br J Dermatol* 1999;141:3–11.

114. Schnabel A, Csernok E, Braun J, et al. Inflammatory cells and cellular activation in the lower respiratory tract in Churg-Strauss syndrome. *Thorax* 1999;54:771–778.

115. Chen KR, Su WPD, Pittelkow MR, et al. Eosinophilic vasculitis in connective tissue disease. *J Am Acad Dermatol* 1996;35:173–182.

116. Koarada S, Tada Y, Aihara S, et al. Polyangiitis overlap syndrome with eosinophilia associated with an elevated serum level of major basic protein. *Intern Med* 1999;38:739–743.

117. Zimmermann N, Daugherty BL, Stark JM, et al. Molecular analysis of CCR-3 events in eosinophilic cells. *J Immunol* 2000;164:1055–1064.

118. Haferlach T, Winkemann M, Loffler H, et al. The abnormal eosinophils are part of the leukemic cell population in acute myelomonocytic leukemia with abnormal eosinophils (AML M4Eo) and carry the pericentric inversion 16: a combination of May-Grunwald-Giemsa staining and fluorescence in situ hybridization. *Blood* 1996;87:2459–2463.

119. Von Wasielewski R, Seth S, Franklin J, et al. Tissue eosinophilia correlates strongly with poor prognosis in nodular sclerosing Hodgkin's disease, allowing for known prognostic factors. *Blood* 2000;95:1207–1213.

120. Navarro-Roman L, Medieros J, Kingma DW, et al. Malignant lymphomas of B-cell lineage with marked tissue eosinophilia. *Am J Surg Pathol* 1994;18:347–356.

121. Enblad G, Sundstrom C, Glimelius B. Infiltration of eosinophils in Hodgkin's disease involved lymph nodes predicts prognosis. *Hematol Oncol* 1993;11:187–193.

122. Borish L, Dishuck J, Cox L, et al. Sézary syndrome with elevated serum IgE and hypereosinophilia: role of dysregulated cytokine production. *J Allergy Clin Immunol* 1993;92:123–131.

123. Ali S, Kaur J, Patel KD. Intercellular cell adhesion molecule-1, vascular cell adhesion molecule-1, and regulated on activation normal T cell expressed and secreted are expressed by human breast carcinoma cells and support eosinophil adhesion and activation. *Am J Pathol* 2000;157:313–321.

124. Fernandez-Acenero MJ, Galindo-Gallego M, Sanz J, et al. Prognostic influence of tumor-associated eosinophilic infiltrate in colorectal carcinoma. *Cancer* 2000;88:1544–1548.

125. Samoszuk M. Eosinophils and human cancer. *Histol Histopathol* 1997;12:807–812.

126. Yam LT, Yam CF, Li CY. Eosinophilia in systemic mastocytosis. *Am J Clin Pathol* 1978;73:48–54.

127. McElroy EA Jr, Phyliky RL, Li CY. Systemic mast cell disease associated with the hypereosinophilic syndrome. *Mayo Clin Proc* 1998;73:47–50.

128. Stern RL, Manders SM, Buttress SH, et al. Urticaria pigmentosa presenting with massive peripheral eosinophilia. *Pediatr Dermatol* 1997;14:284–286.

129. Miranza RN, Esparza AR, Sanbandam S, et al. Systemic mast cell disease presenting with peripheral blood eosinophilia. *Hum Pathol* 1994;25:727–730.

130. Talley NJ, Shorter RG, Phillips SF, et al. Eosinophilic gastroenteritis: a clinicopathological study of patients with disease of the mucosa, muscle layer, and subserosal tissues. *Gut* 1990;31:54–58.

131. Scully RE, Mark EJ, McNeely WF, et al, eds. Case 20: 1992. *N Engl J Med* 1992;326:1342–1349.

132. Winterkamp S, Raithel M, Hahn EG. Secretion and tissue content of eosinophil cationic protein in Crohn's disease. *J Clin Gastroenterol* 2000;30:170–175.

133. Saitoh O, Kojima K, Sugi K, et al. Fecal eosinophil granule-derived proteins reflect disease activity in inflammatory bowel disease. *Am J Gastroenterol* 1999;94:3513–3520.

134. Businco L, Di Frazio A, Ziruolo MG, et al. Clinical and immunologic findings in four infants with Omenn's syndrome: a form of severe combined immunodeficiency with phenotypically normal T cells, elevated IgE, and eosinophilia. *Clin Immunol Immunopathol* 1987;44:123–133.

135. Wada T, Takei K, Kudo M, et al. Characterization of immune function and analysis of RAG gene mutations in Omenn syndrome and related disorders. *Clin Exp Immunol* 2000;119:148–155.

136. Dams ET, Mascart-Lemone F, Schandene L, et al. An unusual case of severe combined immunodeficiency with hypereosinophilia. *J Intern Med* 1997;242:267–269.

137. Buckley RH, Wray BB, Belmaker EZ. Extreme hyper-immunoglobulinemia E and undue susceptibility to infection. *Pediatrics* 1972;49:59–70.

138. Braun MY, Desalle F, Le Moine A, et al. IL-5 and eosinophils mediate the rejection of fully histoin-compatible vascularized cardiac allografts: regulatory role of alloreactive CD8(+) T lymphocytes and IFN-gamma. *Eur J Immunol* 2000;30:1290–1296.

139. Macdonald FI, Ashraf S, Picton M, et al. Banff criteria as predictors of outcome following acute renal allograft rejection. *Nephrol Dial Transplant* 1999;14:1692–1697.

140. de Groen PC, Kephart GM, Gleich GJ, et al. The eosinophil as an effector cell of the immune response during hepatic allograft rejection. *Hepatology* 1994;20:654–662.

141. Angelis M, Yu M, Takanishi D, et al. Eosinophilia as a marker of adrenal insufficiency in the surgical intensive care. *J Am Coll Surg* 1996;183:589–596.

142. Saxon A, Beall G, Rohr A, et al. Immediate hypersensitivity reactions to beta- lactams antibiotics. *Ann Intern Med* 1987;107:204–215.

143. Poe RH, Condemi JJ, Weinstein S, et al. Adult respiratory distress syndrome related to ampicillin sensitivity. *Chest* 1980;77:449–451.

144. Hawkins EP, Berry, Silva FG. Acute tubulointerstitial nephritis in children: clinical morphologic, and lectin studies. *Am J Kidney Dis* 1989;14:466–471.

145. Feigenberg DS, Weiss H, Kirshman H. Migratory pneumonia and eosinophilia associated with sulfonamide administration. *Arch Intern Med* 1967;120:85–89.

146. Sitbon O, Bidel N, Dussopt C, et al. Minocycline pneumonitis and eosinophilia. *Arch Intern Med* 1994;154:1633–1640.

147. MacNeil M, Haase D, Tremaine R, et al. Fever, lymphadenopathy, eosinophilia, lymphocytosis, hepatitis, and dermatitis: a severe adverse reaction to minocycline. *J Am Acad Dermatol* 1997;36:347–350.

148. Ho D, Tashkin DP, Bein ME, et al. Pulmonary infiltrates with eosinophilia associated with tetracycline. *Chest* 1979;76:33–36.

149. Wai A, Lo A, Abdo A, et al. Vancomycin-induced acute interstitial nephritis. *Ann Pharmacother* 1998;32:1160–1164.

150. Rastogi S, Atkinson JL, McCarthy JT. Allergic nephropathy associated with ciprofloxacin. *Mayo Clin Proc* 1990;65:987–989.

151. Wong PC, Yew WW, Wong CF, et al. Ethambutol-induced pulmonary infiltrates with eosinophilia and skin involvement. *Eur Respir J* 1995;8:866–868.

152. Takami A, Nakao S, Asakura H, et al. Pneumonitis and eosinophilia induced by ethambutol. *J Allergy Clin Immunol* 1997;100:712–713.

153. Davidson AC, Bateman C, Shovlin C, et al. Pulmonary toxicity of malaria prophylaxis. *Br Med J* 1988;297:1240–1241.

154. Lor E, Liu Y. Didanosine-associated eosinophilia with acute thrombocytopenia. *Ann Pharmacother* 1993;27:23–24.

155. Taskinen E, Tukiainen P, Sovijarvi AR. Nitrofurantoin-induced alterations in pulmonary tissue: a report on five patients with acute or subacute reactions. *Acta Pathol Microbiol Scand A Pathol* 1977;85:713–720.

156. Gaffey C, Chun B, Harvey J, et al. Phenytoin-induced systemic granulomatous vasculitis. *Arch Pathol Lab Med* 1986;10:131–135.

157. Mahatma M, Haponik EF, Nelson S, et al. Phenytoin-induced acute respiratory failure with pulmonary eosinophila. *Am J Med* 1989;87:93–94.

158. Cullinan SA, Bower GC. Acute pulmonary hypersensitivity to carbamazepine. *Chest* 1975;68:580–581.

159. Mizoguchi S, Setoyama M, Higashi Y, et al. Eosinophilic pustular folliculitis induced by carbamazepine. *J Am Acad Dermatol* 1998;38:641–643.

160. Gonzales FJ, Carvajal MJ, del Pozo V, et al. Erythema multiforme to phenobarbital: involvement of eosinophils and T cells expressing the skin homing receptor. *J Allergy Clin Immunol* 1997;100:135–137.

161. Conilleau V, Dompmartin A, Verneuil L, et al. Hypersensitivity syndrome due to two anticonvulsants drugs. *Contact Dermatitis* 1999;41:141–144.

162. Mahoney JM, Bachtel MD. Pleural effusion associated with chronic dantrolene administration. *Ann Pharmacother* 1994;28:587–589.

163. Buscaglia AJ, Cowden FE, Brill H. Pulmonary infiltrates associated with naproxen. *JAMA* 1984;251:65–66.

164. Goodwin SD, Glenny RW. Nonsteroidal anti-inflammatory drug-associated pulmonary infiltrates with eosinophilia. *Arch Intern Med* 1992;152:1521–1524.

165. Rich MW, Thomas RA. A case of eosinophilic pneumonia and vasculitis induced by diflunisal. *Chest* 1997;111:1767–1769.

166. Bruyn G, Velthuysen E, Joosten P, et al. Pancytopenia related eosinophilia in rheumatoid arthritis: a specific methotrexate phenomenon. *J Rheumatol* 1995;22:1373–1376.

167. Mok CC, Lau CS, Wong R. Toxicities of dapsone in the treatment of cutaneous manifestations of rheumatic diseases. *J Rheumatol* 1998;25:1246–1247.

168. Tomioka H, King TE Jr. Gold-induced pulmonary disease: clinical features, outcome, and differentiation from rheumatoid lung disease. *Am J Respir Crit Care Med* 1997;155:1011–1020.

169. Davis P, Hughes GRV. Significance of eosinophilia during gold therapy. *Arthritis Rheum* 1974;17:963–968.

170. Fam J, Lewtas J, Stein J. Desensitization to allopurinol in patients with gout and cutaneous reactions. *Am J Med* 1992;93:299–302.

171. Dominguez E, Hamill R. Drug-induced fever due to diltiazem. *Arch Intern Med* 1991;151:1869–1870.

172. Steinman TI, Silva P. Acute renal failure, skin rash, and eosinophilia associated with captopril therapy. *Am J Med* 1983;75:154–156.

173. Schatz PL, Mesolgites D, Hyun J, et al. Captopril-induced hypersensitivity lung disease. *Chest* 1989; 95:685–687.

174. Higa K, Hirata K, Dan K. Mexiletine-induced severe skin eruption, fever, eosinophilia, atypical lymphocytosis, and liver dysfunction. *Pain* 1997;73:97–99.

175. Hall D, Link K. Eosinophilia associated with Coumadin. *N Engl J Med* 1981;304:732–733.

176. Volpi A, Ferrario GM, Giordano F, et al. Acute renal failure due to hypersensitivity interstitial nephritis induced by warfarin sodium. *Nephron* 1989;52(2):196.

177. d'Adamo G, Spinelli C, Forte F, et al. Omeprazole-induced acute interstitial nephritis. *Renal Failure* 1997;19:171–175.

178. Smith JD, Chang KL, Gums JG. Possible lansoprazole-induced eosinophilic syndrome. *Ann Pharmacother* 1998;32:196–200.

179. Kendell KR, Day JD, Hruban RH, et al. Intimate association of eosinophils to collagen bundles in eosinophilic myocarditis and ranitidine-induced hypersensitivity myocarditis. *Arch Pathol Lab Med* 1995;119:1154–1160.

180. Andreu V, Bataller R, Caballeria J, et al. Acute eosinophilic pneumonia associated with ranitidine. *J Clin Gastroenterol* 1996;23:160–162.

181. Gafter U, Zevin D, Komlos L, et al. Thrombocytopenia associated with hypersensitivity to ranitidine: possible cross-reactivity with cimetidine. *Am J Gastroenterol* 1989;84:560–562.

182. Tanigawa K, Sugiyama K, Matsuyama H, et al. Mesalazine-induced eosinophilic pneumonia. *Respiration* 1999;66:69–72.

183. Makino H, Haramato T, Sasaki T, et al. Massive eosinophilic infiltration in a patient with the nephritic syndrome and drug-induced interstitial nephritis. *Am J Kidney Dis* 1995;26:62–67.

184. Cutler NR, Anderson DJ. Proven asymptomatic eosinophilia with imipramine. *Am J Psychiatry* 1977; 134:1296–1297.

185. Panuska JR, King TR, Korenblat PE, et al. Hypersensitivity reaction to desipramine. *J Allergy Clin Immunol* 1987;80:18–23.

186. Fleisch MC, Blauer F, Gubler JG, et al. Eosinophilic pneumonia and respiratory failure associated with venlafaxine treatment. *Eur Respir J* 2000;15:205–208.

187. Salerno SM, Strong JS, Roth BJ, et al. Eosinophilic pneumonia and respiratory failure associated with a trazodone overdose. *Am J Resp Crit Care Med* 1995;152:2170–2172.

188. Banov MD, Tohen M, Friedberg J. High risk of eosinophilia in women treated with clozapine. *J Clin Psychiatry* 1993;54:466–469.

189. White DA, Kris MG, Stover DE. Bronchoalveolar lavage cell populations in bleomycin lung toxicity. *Thorax* 1987;42:551–552.

190. Weiss R, Donehower R, Wiernik P, et al. Hypersensitivity reactions from Taxol. *J Clin Oncol* 1990;8:1263–1268.

191. Saville MW, Lietzau J, Pluda JM, et al. Treatment of HIV-associated Kaposi's sarcoma with paclitaxel. *Lancet* 1995;346:26–28.

192. Rutella S, Sica S, Rumi C, et al. Hypereosinophilia during 2-chlorodeoxyadenosine treatment for hairy cell leukemia. *Br J Haematol* 1996;92:426–428.

193. Aglietta M, Sanavio F, Stacchini A, et al. Interleukin-3 in vivo: kinetic of response of target cells. *Blood* 1993;82:2054–2061.

194. MacDonald D, Gordon AA, Kajitani H, et al. Interleukin-2 treatment-associated eosinophilia is mediated by interleukin-5 production. *Br J Haematol* 1990;76:168–173.

195. Schuchter LM, Hendricks CB, Holland KH, et al. Eosinophilic myocarditis associated with high-dose interleukin-2 therapy. *Am J Med* 1990;88:439–440.

196. Rodgers S, Rees RC, Hancock BW. Changes in the phenotypic characteristics of eosinophils from patients receiving recombinant human interleukin-2 (rhIL-2) therapy. *Br J Haematol* 1994;86:746–753.

197. Donhuijsen K, Haedicke C, Hattenberger, et al. Granulocyte-macrophage colony-stimulating factor-related eosinophilia and Loeffler's endocarditis. *Blood* 1992;79:2798.

198. Wong PW, Macris N, DiFabrizio L, et al. Eosinophilic lung disease induced by bicalutamide: a case report and review of the medical literature. *Chest* 1998;113:548–550.

199. Jennings CA, Deveikis J, Azumi N, et al. Eosinophilic pneumonia associated reaction to radiographic contrast medium. *South Med J* 1991;84:92–95.

200. Nadeem S, Nasir N, Israel RH. Loeffler's syndrome secondary to crack cocaine. *Chest* 1994;105:1599–1600.

201. Bond GR. Hepatitis, rash and eosinophilia following trichloroethylene exposure: a case report and speculation on mechanistic similarity to halothane induced hepatitis. *Clin Toxicol* 1996;34:461–466.

202. Hertzman PA, Blevins WL, Mayer J, et al. Association of the eosinophilia-myalgia syndrome with the ingestion of tryptophan. *N Engl J Med* 1990;322:869–973.

203. Hertzman PA, Clauw DJ, Kaufman LD, et al. The eosinophilia-myalgia syndrome: status of 205 patients and results of treatment 2 years after onset. *Ann Intern Med* 1995;122:851–855.

204. Kankaanranta H, Lindsay MA, Giembycz MA, et al. Delayed eosinophil apoptosis in asthma. *J Allergy Clin Immunol* 2000;106:77–83.

205. Sano T, Nakamura Y, Matsunaga Y, et al. FK506 and cyclosporin A inhibit granulocyte/macrophage colony-stimulating factor production by mononuclear cells in asthma. *Eur Respir J* 1995;8:1473–1478.

206. Lee E, Robertson T, Smith J, et al. Leukotriene receptor antagonists and synthesis inhibitors reverse survival in eosinophils of asthmatic individuals. *Am J Respir Crit Care Med* 2000;161:1881–1886.

207. Pizzichini E, Leff JA, Reiss TF, et al. Montelukast reduces airway eosinophilic inflammation in asthma: a randomized, controlled trial. *Eur Respir J* 1999; 14(1):12–18.

208. Newton JA, Singh AK, Greaves MW, et al. Aquagenic pruritus associated with the idiopathic hypereosinophilic syndrome. *Br J Dermatol* 1990;122:103–106.

209. Van Den Hoogenband HM, Van Diggelen MW. PUVA therapy in the treatment of skin lesions of the hypereosinophilic syndrome. *Arch Dermatol* 1985;121:450.

210. Leckie M, ten Brinke A, Khan J, et al. Effects of an interleukin-5 blocking monoclonal antibody on eosinophils, airway hyper-responsiveness, and the late asthmatic response. *Lancet* 2000;356:2144–2148.

211. Gangur V, Oppenheim JJ. Are chemokines essential or secondary participants in allergic responses? *Ann Allergy Asthma Immunol* 2000;84:569–579.

212. Sabroe I, Peck MJ, Van Keulen BJ, et al. A small molecule antagonist of the chemokine receptors CCR1 and CCR3: potent inhibition of eosinophil function and CCR3-mediated HIV-1 entry. *J Biol Chem* 2000;275:25985–25992.

213. Ikemura T, Schwarze J, Makela M, et al. Type 4 phosphodiesterase inhibitors attenuate respiratory syncytial virus-induced airway hyper-responsiveness and lung eosinophilia. *J Pharmacol Exp Ther* 2000;294:701–706.

three six-carbon rings and a five-carbon ring (16). Hydrocortisone (cortisol) is the parent molecule from which other natural and synthetic GCs are derived. Essential features of the antiinflammatory GC consist of the following: (a) a two-carbon chain at the seventeenth position, (b) methyl groups at carbons 10 and 13, (c) a ketone oxygen at C3, (d) an unsaturated bond between C-4 and C-5, (e) a ketone oxygen at C-20, and (f) a hydroxyl group at C-11. Modifications of either the nucleus or the side chains produce different GC agents with varying antiinflammatory and mineralocorticoid activity as compared with cortisol. Further alterations at the C-17 and C-21 positions result in corticosteroids with high topical activity and minimal systemic adverse effects.

Cortisol secretion results from a cascade of stimulatory events in the hypothalamic-pituitary-adrenal (HPA) axis (17). The process begins in the hypothalamus with the secretion of corticotropin-releasing factor (CRF), which stimulates the release of adrenocorticotropic hormone (ACTH), a product of the basophil cells of the anterior pituitary gland. In turn, ACTH stimulates the production of GCs, which are primarily produced in the zona fasciculata of the adrenal cortex. Secretion of cortisol and ACTH normally reaches peak levels in the early morning and then declines throughout the day to a low point in the early to late evening (2). Daily secretion of cortisol is about 10 to 20 mg (28 to 55 μmol), but environmental stress or increased circulating levels of cytokines, such as interleukin-1 (IL-1), IL-2, IL-6, or tumor necrosis factor-α (TNF-α), can raise levels to as high as 400 to 500 mg (18).

At least 90% of circulating cortisol is protein bound, principally to cortisol-binding globulin or transcortin (16). The unbound fraction is biologically active and may bind to transcortin

(high affinity, low capacity) or to serum albumin (low affinity, high capacity). Transcortin has a binding capacity of only 0.7 μmol (250 μg) of cortisol per liter serum. Thus, at low concentrations, about 90% of cortisol is plasma protein bound, and at higher concentrations of cortisol, transcortin binding becomes saturated. Some synthetic GCs, such as dexamethasone, exhibit little or no binding to transcortin. Because pharmacologic actions, metabolism, and excretion of corticosteroids all relate to unbound steroid concentrations, the binding of circulating steroids to transcortin and albumin play important roles in modifying GC potency, half-life, and duration of effects (2).

The intrinsic pharmacokinetic properties of GCs are described by their volume of distribution, absorption, and clearance, which is dependent on metabolism, half-life, and excretion. For a specific corticosteroid, bioavailability is an important part of the equation (Tables 34.1 and 34.2).

Natural and synthetic steroids are lipophilic compounds readily absorbed after intravenous, oral, subcutaneous, or topical administration. However, lipophilicity varies among preparations. In general, the systemic availability of both oral and intravenous GC preparations is high and is limited by first-pass liver metabolism rather than by incomplete absorption. However, with inhaled GCs, the pharmokinetic profile and the method of delivery determine the extent and time of systemic absorption of a given GC. Unless rinsed out, a portion of a dose of ICS is swallowed and absorbed from the gastrointestinal (GI) tract. The rest reaches the lower airways and exerts the desired effect. The ratio of desirable to undesirable effects is dependent on three GC characteristics: the topical activity of drug in the

TABLE 34.1. *Pharmokinetic variables and equivalent doses of common oral glucocorticosteroids*

Oral glucocorticosteroids	Plasma half-life (hr)	Clearance (L/min)	Binding affinity	Volume of distribution (L/kg)	Systemic bioavailability (%)	Comparative dose (mg)
Cortisol	0.5	ND	0.04	1.4	40–70	20
Prednisone	1	0.2	1.6	2.5	25	5
Prednisolone	3.5	0.2	1.6	0.4–0.8	21	5
Methylprednisolone	3	0.4	4.2	0.8–1.1	39	4
Dexamethasone	3.5	0.4	1.0	0.7–1.4	20	0.75

TABLE 34.2. *Pharmokinetic variables of common inhaled and intranasal glucocorticosteroids*

Inhaled glucocorticosteroids	Plasma half-life (hr)	Clearance (L/min)	Binding affinity	Volume of distribution (L/kg)	Systemic bioavailability (%)	
					Inhaled	Oral
BDP	0.1–0.5	3.8	0.4	ND	20	<20
BUD	2.8	1.4	9.4	2.7–4.3	25	6–13
Flunisolide	1.6	1.0	1.8	1.8	39	21
FP	3.1–7.8	0.9–1.1	18.0	3.7–8.9	20	<1
MF						<1
TA	1.5	0.7–1.2	3.6	2.1	21	10–22

BDP, beclomethasone dipropionate; BUD, budesonide; FP, fluticasone propionate; MF, mometasone furoate; TA, triamcinolone acetonide.

airways (GC receptor–binding affinity); the ratio of oropharyngeal to lower airway deposition, and the systemic activity of drug after absorption by the GI tract or lungs and first-pass metabolism (19). Catabolism of corticosteroids primarily occurs in the liver, although other organs, such as the kidney, placenta, lung, muscle, and skin, may contribute to the metabolism of endogenous and synthetic GCs. Enzymatic coupling with a sulfate or glucuronic acid results in formation of water-soluble compounds, which facilitates renal excretion. There is minimal excretion through the biliary and fecal routes.

MOLECULAR AND ANTIINFLAMMATORY MECHANISMS OF GLUCOCORTICOID ACTION

Although synthetic corticosteroids have been in use for 50 years, the mechanisms by which GCs act in suppressing inflammation remain incompletely understood. Glucocorticoids exert their effects at the cellular level by binding to a single GC receptor in the cytoplasm of the target cell. The number of genes directly regulated by GC receptors in any given cell is unknown, but studies suggest that the number of steroid-responsive genes per cell ranges from 10 to 100 (20–22). The relative potency of GCs is dependent on plasma protein binding, intracellular receptor affinity, and intracellular proteins that inhibit steroid binding to the GC receptor. After activation, the GC receptor complex acts in a variety of ways. First, it acts directly, by inhibiting cytokine-induced production of proinflammatory proteins. It also acts indirectly, by upregulating or downregulating transcription factors to alter specific messenger ribonucleic acid (mRNA) production. This, in turn, results in increased production of antiinflammatory mediators and proteins and decreased production of proinflammatory mediators, including cytokines (23–25). It is also capable of repressing gene expression by inhibiting cytokine transcription factors, thus blocking their effects and decreasing the inflammatory response (26,27). This process could work both ways. Theoretically, high levels of transcription factors could suppress GC action by neutralizing receptors. This occurrence could be a potential mechanism of GC resistance (2).

These mechanisms are thought to be among the most important in explaining GC antiinflammatory action, but other factors come into play as well. GCs hinder the recruitment and activation of T lymphocytes, eosinophils, dendritic cells, macrophages, and other inflammatory cells. They also inhibit the survival of mast cells at the airway surface, although they do not prevent their activation (28). Airway epithelial cells are likely major targets for inhaled GCs because these cells release numerous inflammatory mediators.

GCs increase the synthesis of lipocortin-1, a protein that inhibits phospholipase A_2. This mechanism had been thought to inhibit the production of lipid mediators, such as prostaglandins, leukotrienes, and platelet-activating factor. However, recently published reports suggest that corticosteroids do not significantly reduce leukotriene production in patients treated with inhaled GCs (29–31).

CORTICOSTEROID THERAPY

Whatever the route of administration, a general rule of GC therapy has been that the lowest possible effective dose should be used for the shortest duration of time. Complications of GC therapy relate to the pharmacology of the agent, dose, dosing interval, and duration of use. Whenever possible, local administration—topical cutaneous or inhaled nasal or bronchial—is the preferred route to avoid or reduce systemic side effects. If possible, treatment should be with agents with little or no mineralocorticoid activity. Treatment of non–life-threatening disorders (e.g., atopic dermatitis) with long-term systemic GC therapy should be undertaken only after alternative and more conservative therapy has failed. Maximal doses of topical preparations should accompany prolonged courses of systemic GC therapy to permit rapid and safe reductions in the dose and use of the systemic preparations. Single-dose oral GCs should be given in the morning to minimize disruption of the HPA axis. One- to 2-week courses of moderate-dose daily systemic GC therapy for acute allergic disease exacerbations are usually safe and unlikely to lead to significant adverse effects. Alternate-day systemic GC therapy is best undertaken with oral agents with tissue half-lives in the 12- to 36-hour (intermediate) range, such as prednisone, prednisolone, and methylprednisone. Patients receiving GC therapy should undergo frequent reevaluation for the need for continued use of oral steroids. Children on continuous oral GC or high-dose ICS therapy should be regularly evaluated for growth. Adults should be monitored for osteopenia. Appropriate calcium and vitamin D intake should be encouraged.

Inhaled Corticosteroids and Asthma

As our knowledge of the mechanisms and inflammatory characteristics of asthma has grown, ICS therapy has become first-line treatment for chronic asthma, based on its ability to reduce symptoms, improve lung function, decrease bronchial hyperresponsiveness, reduce or eliminate the need for oral steroids, and improve quality of life. Numerous studies have documented the long-term efficacy of ICS therapy in reducing chronic inflammation in asthmatic airways in both adults and children with asthma of all severities (32–35).

Calpin and colleagues reviewed the literature and confirmed the beneficial effects of ICS on symptoms and peak expiratory flow (PEF) (36). In 24 studies that met review criteria, overall symptom scores were reduced by 50% with ICS; the as-needed use of β_2 agonists—an indirect marker of symptom severity—was reduced by 38%; and PEF increased by 38 L/min, or 11% of the predicted value. In addition to improvements in lung function, studies also suggest that low-dose ICS reduced the risk for death in asthma by 50% when patients use at least six canisters per year of ICS (37).

Recently, the trend has been toward earlier introduction and relatively high initial doses of ICS to gain maximum control quickly, after which the dose is reduced to the minimum needed to maintain control. This strategy is based in part on recent advances in our knowledge about the mechanisms of asthma. The classic definition of asthma included the term *reversible airway obstruction*, but there is a growing recognition that some patients with long-standing asthma may have some measure of irreversible airflow obstruction despite apparently appropriate treatment (38–44). Although the phenomenon is not completely understood, it is believed that structural changes, called *airway remodeling*, occur in conjunction with, or because of, chronic airway inflammation.

Although there is still much to be learned about airway remodeling, the current beliefs that irreversible damage can occur, even in patients with mild disease, and that permanent changes may be preventable have spurred the movement toward early introduction of ICS therapy in all patients with asthma. However, some authors suggest that it is still uncertain whether the costs and risks of continuous ICS therapy are justified in patients with only mild disease (11).

Inhaled Corticosteroid Preparations

Six ICS preparations are currently available for the treatment of asthma in the United States.

TABLE 34.3. *Comparison of drug deposition in lungs with metered-dose inhibitors (MDIs) and dry-powder inhalers (DPIs) (%)*

Drug	MDI (CFC)	MDI plus spacer[a] (CFC)	DPI[b]	HFA-MDI	Nebulizer
BDP	4–7.6	18.6	29.8	55–60	NA
BUD	15 (3–47)	14–36	32 (16–59)	NA	10–20
Flunisolide	32	NA	NA	44	NA
FP	26	NA	15	13–18	NA
MF	NA	NA	NA	NA	NA
TA	NA	12–22	NA	NA	NA

[a]BDP used a volumatic spacer; BUD used a Nebuhaler spacer; TA used a built-in spacer.
[b]BDP used Clickhaler; BUD used Turbuhaler; FP used Diskus.
CFC, chlorofluorocarbon; HFA, hydrofluoroalkane; BDP, beclomethasone dipropionate; BUD, budesonide; FP, fluticasone propionate; MF, mometasone furoate; TA, triamcinolone acetonide

They are beclomethasone dipropionate (BDP), flunisolide, fluticasone propionate (FP), triamcinolone acetonide (TA), budesonide (BUD), and mometasone furoate (MF). Pharmacokinetic variables are summarized in Table 34.2. Studies show differences in potencies and levels of adverse systemic effects, but these need to be interpreted with caution because adverse effects can be measured in several ways, and the results of different measurements do not always correspond. Comparisons are further complicated by a choice of inhaler delivery systems for one or more of the drugs (Table 34.3). The characteristics of the delivery device may greatly change the risk-to-benefit ratio of the ICS (45) (Table 34.4).

The ratio of doses producing undesirable effects to doses producing desirable effects (therapeutic index) is the most relevant measurement for comparing various inhaled steroids or a single drug in different formulations. Desirable topical effects depend on potency, the amount of drug delivered to the lungs, and probably also the local pharmacokinetics in target tissues and cells. Undesirable systemic effects derive from mineralocorticoid activity, rate of clearance from the body, and the bioavailability of the steroid after lung or gastrointestinal absorption and first-pass metabolism of the swallowed fraction of the dose (45).

Most newer ICS products have low oral bioavailability (Table 34.2), but BUD and FP have a lower oral bioavailability than BDP because of their extensive hepatic first-pass metabolism; therefore, BUD and FP appear to have fewer systemic effects than BDP at equivalent antiasthma doses. The relative antiinflammatory potency of the ICS, from most potent to least potent, can be summarized as follows: FP = mometasone > BUD = BDP > TA = flunisolide.

MF is the newest ICS. Its antiinflammatory properties are equivalent to those of FP, and it has a quick onset of action. Studies have shown that MF has the greatest binding affinity for glucocorticoid receptor (GR), followed by FP, BUD, and TA (46). Along with FP, MF appears to have substantially higher topical potency and lipid solubility but lower systemic bioavailability than do older compounds. Emerging data suggest that MF and FP may have potentially fewer systemic effects, particularly in children (47).

TABLE 34.4. *Comparison factors for risk/benefit ratios of glucocorticoids and delivery systems[a]*

Pharmacokinetics	Pharmacodynamics	Delivery device characteristics
Receptor affinity	Dose-response characteristics	Output
Plasma half-life	Duration of action	Particle-size distribution
Volume of distribution		Efficiency of lung delivery
Plasma clearance		Ease of use
Rate of first-pass metabolism		

[a]Cost could also be relevant.

Delivery Devices

There are a number of factors to consider when choosing an ICS and a delivery device (Tables 34.3 and 34.4). Devices that are easier to use lead to better compliance, as does less frequent dosing. There are three basic delivery systems for ICS therapy: the metered-dose inhaler (MDI), which is the most common, the dry-powder inhaler (DPI), and the nebulizer, which is used for infants and young children. Some devices have multidose capabilities (48). MDIs may be breath activated or pressurized, either using chlorofluorocarbon (CFC), which is being phased out, or hydrofluoroalkane (HFA) as the propellant. The HFA propellant has been shown to be more efficient in delivering the drug to the small airways (49). A spacer should be used with CFC- or HFA-propelled MDIs to reduce oropharyngeal deposition.

The dose of drug delivered to the lungs differs between MDIs and DPIs and among devices delivering different ICS preparations (Table 34.3), so these differences have to be considered when choosing a device. Nebulizers deliver relatively low doses of drug to the lungs. Although few controlled nebulizer studies exist for the age groups requiring nebulized treatment, recent reports indicate that only about 10% and 20% of the administered dose of BUD reaches the lungs of infants and young children, respectively (50).

Dose-Response Considerations

Although studies consistently demonstrate a clinical benefit of inhaled steroids, the dose-response curve for this benefit is apparently relatively flat in large population studies; in individual patients, the dose-response curve may be linear. In measurements of improved lung function, there seem to be few differences among doses, and most of the benefit appears to be obtained at the lowest doses used (34). In contrast, there is a much steeper dose-response curve relative to systemic effects. From this, we might infer that the slight improvement in lung function with higher doses would not be justified in light of a disproportionately greater increase in the risk for adverse side effects. However, measurements of

other parameters, such as reduction in bronchial hyperresponsiveness, prevention of asthma exacerbations and hospitalizations, and bronchial protection during exercise, do show greater improvement with higher doses (28). For example, Pauwels and colleagues found that inhaled BUD, 800 μg daily, had a significantly higher preventive effect on the occurrence of mild and severe asthma exacerbations than 200 μg daily (51).

It may be that pulmonary function tests have a relatively low sensitivity in the assessment of the effects of ICS (28). This possibility has implications for the interpretation of clinical comparisons among various inhaled steroids or inhalers, as does the degree of severity of the patient's asthma. Patients with very mild asthma have relatively minimal airflow obstruction and little room for improvement, so that low doses potentially provide maximal improvement. Patients with unstable or more severe asthma have significantly greater airflow obstruction and therefore may show a greater response to increasing doses.

Clinical Use of Inhaled Corticosteroid Therapy

Inhaled corticosteroid therapy is recommended as first-line treatment for all patients with persistent symptoms. The clinician should begin ICS in any patient who requires a β_2 agonist inhaler more than twice a week or uses more than two β_2-agonist canisters per year. The current approach is to start with a dose of ICS corresponding to the asthma severity classification based on the NAEPP 2 report (15) (Table 34.5 shows comparative doses for adults and children). Once control is achieved, the dose should be stepped down to the lowest possible dose necessary for optimal control, which is defined as best or normal lung function and only occasional need for a β_2-agonist inhaler. An MDI with a large-volume spacer or mouth rinsing after use of a DPI helps to reduce the risk of local and systemic effects. Twice-daily dosing is standard for older preparations, but in unstable asthma, four-times-daily dosing achieves better control (52), and once-daily dosing does not reduce efficacy

TABLE 34.5. *Comparative ICS dosages for adults (> 12 yr) and children*

Drug (μg per puff)	Low dose (μg)	Medium dose (μg)	High dose (μg)
Beclomethasone MDI 42, 84	Adults 168–504	Adults 504–840	Adults >840
	Children 84–336	Children 336–672	Children >672
Budesonide DPI 200	Adults 200–600	Adults 600–1,000	Adults >1,000
	Children 100–400	Children 400–800	Children >800
Respules 0.25 mg, 0.5 mg (1–8 yr)	0.5 mg	1.0 mg	>1.0 mg
Flunisolide MDI 250	Adults 500–1,000	Adults 1,000–2,000	Adults >2,000
	Children 500–750	Children 750–1,500	Children >1,500
Triamcinolone 100	Adults 400–1,000	Adults 1,000–2,000	Adults >2,000
	Children 400–600	Children 600–1,200	Children >1,200
Fluticasone MDI 44, 110, 220	Adults 88–264	Adults 264–660	Adults >660
DPI 50, 100, 250	Children 88–176	Children 176–440	Children >440
DPI 100, 200, 500/salmeterol			

MDI, metered-dose inhaler; DPI, dry-powder inhaler

for doses of 400 μg or less (53). The newer ICS preparations—FP and MF—may be given as once-daily doses.

Systemic Glucocorticoid Therapy and Acute Severe Asthma

In asthma, systemic GC therapy should be reserved for patients with acute, severe disease who do not respond to conservative treatment. Systemic GC use reduces hospitalization and prevents relapses, especially in patients at high risk for fatal asthma (54). Administration can be by oral, intravenous, or intramuscular routes. Commonly used intravenously administered GC preparations include hydrocortisone, methylprednisolone, and dexamethasone. There are no data to suggest that one compound is more efficacious than another in comparable doses (54), but there are differences in side effects and costs. Thus, methylprednisolone, because of its greater antiinflammatory potency, lower mineralocortoicoid activity, and lower price by comparison with hydrocortisone, may be the drug of choice for intravenous therapy (54).

For acutely ill asthmatic adults, 10 to 15 mg/kg per 24 hours intravenously of hydrocortisone (or its equivalent) is generally appropriate. This would equate to a comparable dose of 600 to 900 mg of hydrocortisone (4 to 6 mg/kg in children), 150 to 225 mg of prednisone (1 to 1.5 mg/kg in children), or 120 to 180 mg of methylprednisolone (1 mg/kg in children) per day for an average adult asthmatic patient. For

maximum therapeutic benefit, treatment should be maintained for 36 to 48 hours depending on the clinical response. Dosing intervals depend on the clinical condition of the acutely ill asthmatic patient. However, intervals may begin every 4 to 6 hours. When signs and symptoms improve, doses can be tapered to twice daily, then to a single morning daily dose. Patients who require intravenous GC can be switched to oral GC once stable. The total duration of intravenous therapy is dependent on both subjective and objective improvement in respiratory status and responsiveness to adrenergic bronchodilator therapy (54).

Oral GCs in moderately high doses may be required in severe chronic asthma or in acute exacerbations. In most hospitalized patients without risk for impending ventilatory failure, oral prednisone, prednisolone, or methylprednisolone are as effective as intravenous treatments (17). Prednisone, 40 to 60 mg/day (1 to 2 mg/kg/day in children), or methylprednisolone, 7.5 to 60 mg/day (0.25 to 2.0 mg/kg/day in children), may be given in single or divided doses. In patients with mild asthma, which is typically well controlled, an asthma exacerbation may require a 3- to 10-day course of oral GCs (55). Patients who need to continue oral GC treatment for longer periods should convert to alternate-day administration to reduce the risk for side effects. The clinician should attempt to reduce the dose by 5 to 10 mg every 2 weeks until the lowest clinically effective dose is reached. The goal is to discontinue systemic GC therapy if possible.

Intranasal Glucocorticoids and Allergic Rhinitis

Intranasal GCs are used widely for the treatment of both perennial and seasonal allergic rhinitis. In addition, intranasal GCs are used in the treatment of vasomotor rhinitis, nasal polyposis, rhinitis medicamentosa, and recurrent serous otitis media secondary to allergen-induced eustachian tube dysfunction. Pharmacologically, it would appear that newer compounds have substantially higher lipophilicity and topical potencies and lower systemic bioavailability than compounds developed earlier. In clinical use, however, all available intranasal GCs appear to be similarly efficacious in controlling symptoms (Table 34.2).

Intranasal corticosteroids have been reported to reduce nasal congestion, itching, sneezing, and rhinorrhea (56–60). The onset of action varies among the different preparations (61). However, the newer intranasal GCs, such as BUD, FP, and MF, appear to have a relatively rapid onset of action, within 12 hours (62–64). Ciclesonide is new GC that appears to have a rapid onset and effectively reduces symptoms without producing local or systemic side effects (65). Although TA and BDP appear to have some clinical activity within several hours, the maximal effects may not be evident for 3 to 7 days. Studies suggest that patients treated prophylactically before the allergy season have a significantly higher proportion of symptom-free days, and they experience reduced symptoms compared with placebo-treated groups.

Local adverse effects on the nasal mucosa include epistaxis, which occurs in up to 5% to 8% of patients and is usually self-limiting. Atrophy or thinning of the nasal tissue had been a concern with long-term use; however, with newer preparations (BUD, FP, MF), long-term use does not cause atrophy of the nasal mucosa or epithelial cell metaplasia. The greater safety margin of the newer intranasal GCs may make them preferable to older preparations, especially for use in children. The potential for systemic absorption and HPA axis suppression is critical in children because systemically absorbed GCS may interrupt or retard growth.

In two studies at the same institution, one study reported significantly slower growth rates after one year in children treated with intranasal BDP versus placebo, beginning as early as 1 month after treatment began (66), whereas the other reported no difference in placebo and treatment growth rates when children were treated with intranasal MF (67).

Corticosteroids for Other Allergic Diseases

Nasal Polyposis

Topical GCs are an accepted medical adjunct to surgery in patients who have nasal polyposis. Randomized trials have demonstrated the efficacy of topical corticosteroids, such as BDP nasal spray (68) and FP nasal drops (69,70), in ameliorating rhinitis symptoms and reducing polyp size. Flunisolide and BUD have also been shown to delay the recurrence of polyps after surgery (71). In mild cases, topical GCS can be used alone as long-term therapy. In more severe disease, they can be combined with systemic GCs, surgery, or both when necessary. A short (3-day) course of oral GC therapy in some patients with severe nasal polyposis may be necessary before topical nasal treatments can become effective.

Atopic Dermatitis

The use of high-potency topical GCS has led to improved treatment for dermatologic conditions with an inflammatory etiology, such as atopic dermatitis. Clobetasol propionate has proved safe and effective for limited-course treatment of inflammatory and pruritic symptoms of moderate-to-severe corticosteroid-responsive dermatoses (72), and the new compound, MF, appears to have even greater efficacy (73). The MF cream may also be used intermittently as a maintenance treatment to prevent recurrences of eczema (74).

In severe cases of atopic dermatitis, oral steroids may be used sparingly (75,76). Prednisone or prednisolone are recommended. Allergic contact dermatitis that fails to respond to topical treatment may improve with once-daily, then alternate-day oral prednisone at doses of 30 to 60 mg for 1 to 2 weeks.

Ocular Allergy

Nonsteroidal antiinflammatory agents, antihistamines, and mast cell stabilizers are the typical treatments for mild to moderate allergic conjunctivitis, but in severe cases, topical corticosteroids, preferably those with reduced side effects, may be necessary. Loteprednol etabonate (LE) has been reported to be effective for treating ocular allergy and inflammation (77). LE eye drops are available as either 0.5% or 0.2% suspensions, but several randomized trials confirm that the lower dose is effective in reducing redness and itching without causing significant changes in intraocular pressure (77–79), even with long-term use (80).

Treatments for vernal keratoconjunctivitis, a severe but transient form of ocular allergy, include fluorometholone 0.1%, nedocromil 2%, and sodium cromoglycate 2%. Atopic keratoconjunctivitis generally requires ocular corticosteroids. Ocular corticosteroids should be managed by an ophthalmologist experienced in their use. Because it potentiates the tendency for paclitaxel (Taxol) to induce full-thickness skin necrosis, fluorometholone should not be used in patients receiving treatment with paclitaxel (81).

Idiopathic Anaphylaxis

Idiopathic anaphylaxis in both adults and children has been successfully treated with systemic prednisone, hydroxyzine, and albuterol to control symptoms and induce remission (82). It should be noted, however, that systemic administration of steroids, notably methylprednisolone, can very rarely induce anaphylaxis (83).

Adverse Effects of Glucocorticoid Therapy

Potentially, there are many adverse effects associated with GC therapy (Table 34.6), particularly with oral and intravenous routes of administration (2,17,55,84). Patients on chronic steroid therapy should be monitored. Depending on signs and symptoms tests might include those for suppression of the HPA axis, cataracts, hyperglycemia, hypertension, and osteoporosis. Complications attributable to steroid use are directly

TABLE 34.6. *Potential adverse effects of glucocorticoids*

Hypertension
Osteoporosis; fractures
Diabetes
Peptic ulcer diseases
Immunosuppression
Glaucoma
Weight gain
Behavioral symptoms
Cataracts
Growth retardation
Pancreatitis
Hypoadrenalism
Avascular necrosis
Muscle wasting
Fluid retention
Cushing syndrome
Myopathy
Hypokalemia
Recurrent infections
Hypoglycemia
Nodular panniculitis
Poor wound healing
Hypothalamic-pituitary-adrenal axis suppression

related to dose, dosing schedule, route of administration, and duration of therapy (85–88).

Steroid-induced osteoporosis has been treated with alendronate, an antiresorptive agent (89), and ideally it is important to limit systemic steroid use as much as possible. Generally, short bursts of high-dose oral or intravenously administered GCs are not harmful, but risks for fracture or bone loss after numerous short bursts have been reported to be similar to risks with daily or alternate-day long-term steroid use (90). The risk for bone loss increases with concomitant use of some medications, notably excessive thyroid replacement treatment.

Treatment with GCs may cause HPA axis suppression by reducing ACTH production, which in turn results in decreased serum cortisol output by the adrenal gland. Prolonged therapy with systemic GC may result in adrenal gland atrophy. The degree of HPA suppression is dependent on the dose, duration, frequency, time of day, and route of administration of GC. Patients who develop acute adrenal insufficiency can present with dehydration, shock, electrolyte abnormalities, severe abdominal pain, and lethargy. This is a medical emergency that requires prompt diagnosis and rapid treatment with intravenous hydrocortisone (2 mg/kg followed by 1.5 mg/kg every 6 hours until the patient becomes stabilized and can tolerate oral therapy). All adrenally suppressed individuals should receive hydrocortisone at the time of any surgical procedure or at times of acute stress. Complete recovery from adrenal suppression can take as long as 12 months after cessation of long-term GC therapy for most patients.

The effect of ICS on linear growth in children is controversial. A review conducted by the Expert Panel Report 2 found that most studies did not demonstrate an effect on growth, but others did find growth delay (15). According to some reports, even moderate doses of ICS can slow childhood growth (91). In an analysis by Agertoft, long-term growth studies showed suppressive effects with 400 μg/day BUD, but there was no evidence to support any significant effects on final adult height (88). Recent studies with FP at doses below 200 μg/day did not significantly alter growth rates and velocity in children aged 4 to 11 years followed for 12 months. Similarly, a study of 5- to 12-year-old children treated with BUD (200 μg twice daily), who were followed for 4 to 6 years, found only a small, transient reduction in growth velocity (92). Because asthma itself appears to delay growth in some children (93,94), this issue remains controversial. Until it is clarified, physicians should be cautious, use step-down therapy when possible, and closely monitor children's growth rates.

The principal local adverse effects of ICS therapy include oral candidiasis, dysphonia, throat irritation, and cough. Oral candidiasis is directly related to dose frequency, and both it and hoarseness appear to be dose dependent. These problems are not sufficient reasons to discontinue ICS treatment. A spacer may alleviate both oral candidiasis and hoarseness, and the former responds to oral antifungal preparations, such as nystatin. Gargling and mouth rinsing after inhalation can reduce future occurrences. An alternative steroid could alleviate hoarseness, but simply resting the voice may help.

Steroid-resistant, Steroid-dependent Asthma

Most patients with asthma respond well to GC therapy, but a few are either steroid resistant or steroid-dependent; that is, they respond only to continuous high doses of oral GC. Inability to respond to the therapeutic effects of GC therapy is likely to arise from the same mechanisms in both populations (95).

Corticosteroid-resistant asthma is defined as failure to improve forced expiratory volume in 1 second (FEV_1) or PEF by more than 15% after treatment with oral prednisolone, 30 to 40 mg daily for 2 weeks. True GC-resistant asthmatic patients are rare (96). Much more commonly, patients require large oral or inhaled doses to control their asthma. A poor response to GC therapy could be related to noncompliance or abnormal metabolism or to defects in cellular or molecular action. Recent reports suggest that patients who are insensitive to GC therapy may have diminished GR ligand or DNA-binding affinity. Abnormal GR binding may be due to cytokine-driven alternative splicing of the GR pre-mRNA to a novel isoform called GR-β, which does not bind GC but antagonizes the transactivating activity of the typical GR (97). There is also evidence for excessive expression of the transcription factor AP-1. Further studies may reveal more about the mechanisms involved in steroid resistance or dependence. It is unknown whether there is any downregulation of GR in the airways with treatment with topical GC (98).

It is important to determine that the patient has asthma and not another disease, such as chronic obstructive pulmonary disease, or vocal cord dysfunction to avoid overtreatment with oral GCS. The clinician should also investigate the possibility of instigating factors, such as allergens at home, school, or work, other medications, or psychological problems that could increase the severity of asthma and its resistance to treatment.

Some alternative treatments are so-called corticosteroid-sparing drugs because they reduce GC requirements. These include methotrexate, oral gold, and cyclosporine. Methotrexate, an antimetabolite, has been extensively studied (99–103). Methotrexate has both immunosuppressive and antiinflammatory mechanisms, but there is little evidence of immunosuppressive effects at low doses, and its benefit for asthma has not been confirmed. Oral gold also has a history of use for steroid-resistant or steroid-dependent asthma but can cause proteinuria and a skin rash.

Cyclosporine has been less well studied (95). These treatments all have adverse effects that can cause problems of their own, so they have been recommended for treatment in asthma patients only when there is no alternative.

REFERENCES

1. Addison T. *On the constitutional and local effects of disease of the suprarenal capsules.* London: Samuel Higley, 1855.
2. Schleimer RP, Busse WW, O'Byrne PM. *Inhaled glucocorticoids in asthma, mechanisms and clinical actions.* New York: Marcel Dekker, 1997.
3. Hench PS, Kendall EC, Slocumb CH, et al. The effect of a hormone of the adrenal cortex (17-hydroxy-11-dehydrocortiscosterone; compound E) and of pituitary adrenocorticotropic hormone on rheumatoid arthritis. *Proc Staff Meet Mayo Clin* 1949;24:181.
4. Hench PS, Kendall EC, Slocumb CH, et al. Effects of cortisone acetate and pituitary ACTH on rheumatoid arthritis, rheumatic fever and certain other conditions. *Arch Intern Med* 1950;85:545.
5. Khoo BP, Leow YH, Ng SK, et al. Corticosteroid contact hypersensitivity screening in Singapore. *Am J Contact Dermatitis* 1998;9(2):87–91.
6. Gaddie J, Reid IW, Skinner C, et al. Aerosol beclomethasone dipropionate: a dose response study in chronic bronchial asthma. *Lancet* 1973;2:280–281.
7. Davies G, Thomas P, Broder I, et al. Steroid-dependent asthma treated with inhaled beclomethasone dipropionate: a long-term study. *Ann Intern Med* 1977;86:549–553.
8. Johnson CE. Aerosol corticosteroids for the treatment of asthma. *Drug Intell Clin Pharmacol* 1987;21(10):784–790.
9. Djukanovic R, Roche WR, Wilson JW, et al. State of the art: mucosal inflammation in asthma. *Am Rev Respir Dis* 1990;142:434–437.
10. Laitinen LA, Heino M, Laitinen A, et al. Damage of the airway epithelium and bronchial reactivity in patients with asthma. *Am Rev Respir Dis* 1985;131:599–606.
11. Boushey HA. Effects of inhaled corticosteroids on the consequences of asthma. *J Allergy Clin Immunol* 1998;102:S5–S16.
12. Kraan J, Koeter GH, van der Mark TW, et al. Changes in bronchial hyperreactivity induced by 4 weeks of treatment with antiasthmatic drugs in patients with allergic asthma: a comparison between budesonide and terbutaline. *J Allergy Clin Immunol* 1985;76:628–636.
13. Kerrebijn KF, van Essen-Zandvliet EEM, Neijens HJ. Effect of long-term treatment with inhaled corticosteroids and beta-agonists on the bronchial responsiveness in children with asthma. *J Allergy Clin Immunol* 1987;79:653–659.
14. National Asthma Education Program Expert Panel. *Guidelines for the diagnosis and management of asthma.* National Asthma Education Program/Expert Panel Report. NIH Publication No. 91-3042. Bethesda, MD: NIH/National Heart, Lung, and Blood Institute, 1991
15. National Asthma Education and Prevention Program. *Expert Panel Report 2: guidelines for the diagnosis and management of asthma.* NIH Publication No. 97-4051. Bethesda, MD: NIH/National Heart, Lung, and Blood Institute, April 1997.
16. Orth DN, Kovacs WJ, DeBold CR. The adrenal cortex. In: Wilson JD, Forster DW, eds. *Williams textbook of endocrinology.* 8th ed. Philadelphia: WB Saunders, 1991:489–619.
17. Jackson RV, Bowman RV. Corticosteroids. *Med J Aust* 1995;162:663–665.
18. Esteban NV, Laughlin T, Yergey AI, et al. Daily cortisol production rate in man determined by stable isotope dilution/mass spectrometry. *J Clin Endocrinol Metab*, 1991;72:39–45.
19. Pedersen S, O'Byrne P. A comparison of the efficacy and safety of inhaled corticosteroids in asthma. *Allergy* 1997;52[Suppl 39]:1–34.
20. Briehl MM, Flomerfelt FA, Wu XP, et al. Transcriptional analyses of steroid-regulated gene networks. *Mol Endocrinol* 1990;4:287–294.
21. Baughman G, Harrington MT, Campbell NF, et al. Genes newly identified as regulated by glucocorticoids in murine thymocytes. *Mol Endocrinol* 1991;5:637–644.
22. Owens GP, Hahn WE, Cohen JJ, et al. Identification of mRNAs associated with programmed cell death in immature thymocytes. *Mol Cell Biol* 1991;11:4177–4188.
23. Barnes PJ. Mechanisms of action of glucocorticods in asthma. *Am J Respir Crit Care Med* 1996;154[Suppl]:S21–S27.
24. Barnes PJ, Adcock I. Anti-inflammatory actions of steroids: molecular mechanisms. *Trends Pharmacol Sci* 1993;14:436–441.
25. Guyre PM, Girard MT, Morganelli PM, et al. Glucocorticoid effects on the production and action of immune cytokines. *J Steroid Biochem* 1988;30:89–93.
26. Scheinman RI, Cogswell PC, Lofquist AK, et al. Role of transcriptional activation of I kappa B alpha in mediation of immunosuppression by glucocorticoids. *Science* 1995;270:283–286.
27. Auphan N, DiDonato JA, Rosette C, et al. Immunosuppression by glucocorticoids: inhibition of NF-kappa B activity through induction of I kappa B synthesis. *Science* 1995;270:286–290.
28. Barnes PJ. Efficacy of inhaled corticosteroids in asthma. *J Allergy Clin Immunol* 1998;102:531–538.
29. Bisgaard H. Role of leukotrienes in asthma pathophysiology. *Pediatr Pulmonol* 2000;30(2):166–176.
30. Bosse M, Audette M, Laflamme G, et al. Eosinophil activation status and corticosteroid responsiveness in severe asthma. *Int Arch Allergy Immunol* 2000;122(3):200–208.
31. Kraft M. Corticosteroiids and leukotrienes: chronobiology and chronotherapy. *Chronobiol Int* 1999;16(5):683–693.
32. Barnes PJ. Inhaled glucorticoids for asthma. *N Engl J Med* 1995;332:868–875.
33. Kamada AK, Szefler SJ, Martin RJ, et al. Issues in the use of inhaled steroids. *Am J Respir Crit Care Med* 1996;153:1739–1748.
34. Barnes PJ, Pedersen S, Busse WW. Efficacy and safety of inhaled corticosteroids: an update. *Am J Respir Crit Care Med* 1998;157:S1–S53.
35. Pedersen W, Hjuler I, Bisgaard H. Nasal inhalation of budesonide from a spacer in children with perennial rhinitis and asthma. *Allergy* 1998;53(4):383–387.

36. Calpin C, Macarthur C, Stephens D, et al. Effectiveness of prophylactic inhaled steroids in childhood asthma: a systematic review of the literature. *J Allergy Clin Immunol* 1997;100:452–457.

37. Suissa S, Ernst P, Benayoun S, et al. Low-dose inhaled corticosteroids and the prevention of death from asthma. *N Engl J Med* 2000;343(5):332–336.

38. Sears MR. Consequences of long-term inflammation: the natural history of asthma. *Clin Chest Med* 2000; 21(2):315–329.

39. Djukanovic R. Asthma: a disease of inflammation and repair. *J Allergy Clin Immunol* 2000;105(2 Pt. 2):S522–S526.

40. Vignola AM, Chanez P, Bonsignore G, et al. Structural consequences of airway inflammation in asthma. *J Allergy Clin Immunol* 2000;105(2 Pt. 2):S514–S517.

41. Fahy JV, Corry DB, Boushey HA. Airway inflammation and remodeling in asthma. *Curr Opin Pulmon Med* 2000;6(1):15–20.

42. Fish JE, Peters SP. Airway remodeling and persistent airway obstruction in asthma. *J Allergy Clin Immunol* 1999;104(3 Pt. 1):509–516.

43. Homer RJ, Elias JA. Consequences of long-term inflammation: airway remodeling. *Clin Chest Med* 2000;21(2):331–343.

44. Carter PM, Heinly TL, Yates SW, et al. Asthma: the irreversible airways disease. *J Investig Allergol Clin Immunol* 1997;7(6):566–571.

45. O'Byrne PM, Pedersen S. Measuring efficacy and safety of different inhaled corticosteroid preparations. *J Allergy Clin Immunol* 1998;102:879–886.

46. Lumry WR. A review of the preclinical and clinical data of newer intranasal steroids used in the treatment of allergic rhinitis. *J Allergy Clin Immunol* 1999;104 (4 Pt. 1):S150–S158.

47. Corren J. Intranasal corticosteroids for allergic rhinitis: how do different agents compare? *J Allergy Clin Immunol* 1999;104(4 Pt. 1):S144–S149.

48. Ariyananda PL, Agnew JE, Clark SW. Aerosol delivery systems for bronchial asthma. *Postgrad Med J* 1996;72:151–156.

49. Tashkin DP. *Impact of emergency therapies on small airway inflammation in asthma.* Program and abstracts of the 1999 Annual Meeting of the American College of Allergy, Asthma, and Immunology, November 12–17, 1999, Chicago. Symposium: The use of inhaled corticosteroids in asthma: improving treatment goals for the millennium.

50. Lodrup Carlsen KC, Nikander K, Carlsen K-H. How much budesonide reaches infants and toddlers? *Arch Dis Child* 1992;67:1077–1079.

51. Pauwels RA, Lofdahl C-G, Postma DS, et al. Effect of inhaled formoterol and budesonide on exacerbations of asthma. *N Engl J Med* 1997;337:1412–1418.

52. Malo J, Cartier A, Merland N, et al. Four-times-a-day dosing frequency is better than twice-a-day regimen in subjects requiring a high-dose inhaled steroid, budesonide, to control moderate to severe asthma. *Am Rev Respir Dis* 1989;140:624–628.

53. Jones AH, Langdon CG, Lee PS, et al. Pulmicort Turbohaler once daily as initial prophylactic therapy for asthma. *Respir Med* 1994;88:293–299.

54. McFadden ER. Dosages of corticosteroids in asthma. *Am Rev Respir Dis* 1993;147:1306–1310.

55. Greenberger PA. Corticosteroids in asthma: rationale, use, and problems. *Chest* 1992;101[Suppl. 6]:418S–421S.

56. Gawchik SM, Lim J. Comparison of intranasal triamcinolone acetonide with oral loratadine in the treatment of seasonal ragweed-induced allergic rhinitis. *Am J Managed Care* 1997;3(7):1052–1058.

57. Condemi J, Schulz R, Lim J. Triamcinolone acetonide aqueous nasal spray versus loratadine in seasonal allergic rhinitis. *Ann Allergy Asthma Immunol* 2000;84(5):533–538.

58. Gehanno P, Desfougeres JL. Fluticasone propionate aqueous nasal spray compare with oral loratadine in patients with seasonal allergic rhinitis. *Allergy* 1997;52(4):445–450.

59. Adamopoulos G, Manolopoulos L, Giotakis I. A comparison of the efficacy and patient acceptability of budesonide and beclomethasone dipropionate aqueous nasals sprays in patients with perennial rhinitis. *Clin Otolaryngol* 1995;20(4):340–344.

60. Creticos P, Fireman P, Settipane G, et al. Intranasal budesonide aqueous pump spray (Rhinocort Aqua) for the treatment of seasonal allergic rhinitis. *Allergy Asthma Proc* 1998;19(5):285–294.

61. Day J, Carillo T. Comparison of the efficacy of budesonide and fluticasone propionate aqueous nasal spray for once daily treatment of perennial allergic rhinitis. *J Allergy Clin Immunol* 1998;102(6 Pt. 1):902–908.

62. Jen A, Baroody F, de Tineo M, et al. As-needed use of fluticasone propionate nasal spray reduces symptoms of seasonal allergic rhinitis. *J Allergy Clin Immunol* 2000;105(4):732–738.

63. Bronsky EA, Aaronson DW, Berkowitz RB, et al. Dose ranging study of mometasone furoate (Nasonex) in seasonal allergic rhinitis. *Ann Allergy Asthma Immunol* 1997;79(1):51–56.

64. Davies RJ, Nelson HS. Once-daily mometasone furoate nasal spray: efficacy and safety of a new intranasal glucocorticoid for allergic rhinitis. *Clin Ther* 1997;19(1):27–38.

65. Schmidt BM, Timmer W, Georgens AC, et al. The new topical steroid ciclesonide is effective in the treatment of allergic rhinitis. *J Clin Pharmacol* 1999;39(10):1062–1069.

66. Skoner DP, Rachelefsky GS, Meltzer EO, et al. Detection of growth suppression in children during treatment with intranasal beclomethasone dipropionate. *Pediatrics* 2000;105(2):E23.

67. Schenkel EJ, Skoner DP, Bronsky EA, et al. Absence of growth retardation in children with perennial allergic rhinitis after one year of treatment with mometasone furoate aqueous nasal spray. *Pediatrics* 2000;105(2):E22.

68. Irifune M, Ogino S, Harada T, et al. Topical treatment of nasal polyps with beclomethasone dipropionate powder preparation. *Auris Nasus Larynx* 1999;26(1):49–55.

69. Holmstrom M. Clinical performance of fluticasone propionate nasal drops. *Allergy* 1999;54[Suppl. 53]:21–25.

70. Pentilla M, Poulsen P, Hollingworth K, et al. Dose-related efficacy and tolerability of fluticasone propionate nasal drops 400 microg once daily and twice daily in the treatment of bilateral nasal polyposis: a placebo-controlled randomized study in adult patients. *Clin Exp Allergy* 2000;30(1):94–102.

71. Mygind N. Advances in the medical treatment of nasal polyps. *Allergy* 1999;54[Suppl 53]:12–16.

72. Gordon ML. The role of clobetasol propionate emollient 0.05% in the treatment of patients with dry, scaly, corticosteroid-responsive dermatoses. *Clin Ther* 1998;20(1):26–39.

73. Prakash A, Benfield P. Topical mometasone: a review of its pharmacological properties and therapeutic use in the treatment of dermatological disorders. *Drugs* 1998;55(1):145–163.

74. Veien NK, Olholm Larsen P, Thestrup-Pedersen K, et al. Long-term intermittent treatment of chronic hand eczema with mometasone furoate. *Br J Dermatol* 1999;140(5):882–886.

75. Walker C, Craig TJ. Atopic dermatitis: a clinical review for the primary care physician. *J Am Osteopath Assoc* 1999;99[Suppl. 3]:S5–S10.

76. Correale CE, Walker C, Murphy L, et al. Atopic dermatitis: a review of diagnosis and treatment. *Am Fam Physician* 1999;60(4):1191–1198, 1209–1210.

77. Abelson M, Howes J, George M. The conjunctival provocation test model of ocular allergy: utility for assessment of an ocular corticosteroid, loteprednol etabonate. *J Occup Pharmacol Ther* 1998;14(6):533–542.

78. Dell SJ, Lowry GM, Northcutt JA, et al. A randomized, double-masked, placebo-controlled parallel study of 0.2% loteprednol etabonate in patients with seasonal allergic conjunctivitis. *J Allergy Clin Immunol* 1998;102(2):251–255.

79. Shulman DG, Lothringer LL, Rubin JM, et al. A randomized, double-masked, placebo-controlled parallel study of loteprednol etabonate 0.2% in patients with seasonal allergic conjunctivitis. *Ophthalmology* 1999;106(2):362–369.

80. Novack GD, Howes J, Crockett RS, et al. Changes in intraocular pressure during long-term use of loteprednol etabonate. *J Glaucoma* 1998;7(4):266–269.

81. Aboolian A, Tornambe R, Ricci M. Skin necrosis in the presence of paclitaxel and fluorometholone. *Support Care Cancer* 1999;7(3):158–159.

82. Ditto AM, Krasnick J, Greenberger PA, et al. Pediatric idiopathic anaphylaxis: experience with 22 patients. *J Allergy Clin Immunol* 1997;100(3):320–326.

83. Schonwald S. Methylprednisolone anaphylaxis. *Am J Emerg Med* 1999;17(6):583–585.

84. Kelly HW, Murphy SM. Corticosteroids for acute, severe asthma. *Ann Pharmacother* 1991;25:72–79.

85. Barnes PJ, Pedersen S. Efficacy and safety of inhaled steroids in asthma. *Am Rev Respir Dis* 1993;148:S1–S26.

86. Kamada AK, Szefler SJ. The safety of inhaled corticosteroid therapy in children. *Curr Opin Pediatr* 1997;9:585–589.

87. Storms WW. Risk-benefit assessment of fluticasone propionate in the treatment of asthma and allergic rhinitis. *J Asthma* 1998;35(4):313–336.

88. Agertoft L, Pedersen S. Effect of long term treatment with inhaled budesonide on adult height in children with asthma. *N Engl J Med* 2000;343(15):1064–1069.

89. Saag KG, Emkey R, Schnitzer TJ, et al. Alendronate for the prevention and treatment of glucocorticoid-induced osteoporosis. *N Engl J Med* 1998;339:292–299.

90. Adinoff AD, Hollister JR. Steroid induced fractures and bone loss in patients with asthma. *N Engl J Med* 1983;309:265–268.

91. Allen DB. Influence of inhaled corticosteroids on growth: a pediatric endocrinologist's perspective. *Acta Paediatr* 1998;87(2):123–129.

92. The Childhood Asthma Management Program Research Group. Long-term effects of budesonide or nedocromil in children with asthma. *N Engl J Med* 2000;343(15):1054–1063.

93. Kamada AK, Szefler SJ. Glucocorticoids and growth in asthmatic children. *Pediatr Allergy Immunol* 1995;6:145–154.

94. Wolthers OD. Long-, intermediate-, and short-term growth studies in asthmatic children treated with inhaled glucocorticosteroids. *Eur Respir J* 1996;9:821–827.

95. Cypcar D, Busse W. Steroid-resistant asthma. *J Allergy Clin Immunol* 1993;92:362–372.

96. Barnes PJ, Greening AP, Crompton GK. Glucocorticoid resistance in asthma. *Am J Respir Crit Care Med* 1995;152:S125–S142.

97. Leung DY, Szefler SJ. New insights into steroid resistant asthma. *Pediatr Allergy Immunol* 1998;9(1):3–12.

98. Demoly P, Chung KF. Pharmacology of corticosteroids. *Respir Med* 1998;92:385–394.

99. Mullarkey MF, Webb DR, Pardee NE. Methotrexate in the treatment of steroid-dependent asthma. *Ann Allergy* 1986;56:347–350.

100. Mullarkey MF, Blumenstein BA, Andrade WP, et al. Methotrexate in the treatment of corticosteroid-dependent asthma. *N Engl J Med* 1988;318:603–607.

101. Mullarkey MF, Lammert JK, Blumenstein BA. Long-term methotrexate treatment in corticosteroid-dependent asthma. *Ann Intern Med* 1990;112:577–581.

102. Shiner RJ, Nunn AJ, Fan Chung K, et al. Randomized, double-blind, placebo-controlled trial of methotrexate in steroid-dependent asthma. *Lancet* 1990;336:137–140.

103. Dyer PD, Vaughan TR, Weber RW. Methotrexate in the treatment of steroid-dependent asthma. *J Allergy Clin Immunol* 1991;88:208–212.

35

β Agonists

Jacqueline A. Pongracic

Department of Pediatrics and Medicine, Northwestern University Medical School,
Department of Allergy, Children's Memorial Hospital, Chicago, Illinois

Since bronchoconstriction has long been regarded to be a hallmark of asthma, bronchodilation has become an important component of asthma therapy. Among the various agents available for this purpose, β-adrenergic agonists have played a prominent role. Rapid-acting β agonists have been used for many years. The availability of long-acting preparations has changed the way β agonists may be used. In addition, the newest agent in the β agonist family, an enantiomer, has provided additional options in asthma management.

HISTORICAL PERSPECTIVES

Although sympathomimetic agents have been used for asthma as far back as 3000 BC, it was only 60 years ago that the first β-adrenergic agonist, isoproterenol, appeared on the scene (1). As a potent, nonselective β agonist, isoproterenol was associated with many side effects. These toxicity issues led to the development of the β_2-selective agonist, albuterol, more than 30 years ago. Since then, a variety of other β_2-selective agonists have been developed as well. Pirbuterol, terbutaline, and fenoterol are short, rapidly acting agents. Fenoterol is potent, but less β_2 selective than the others, and it is not available in the United States. Salmeterol and formoterol are agonists with a significantly longer duration of action. In response to continued concerns about side effects, further examination and refinements

in these molecules have led to the production of an enantiomeric form of albuterol, called *levalbuterol*.

MECHANISM OF ACTION AND PHARMACOLOGY

β-Adrenergic agonists exert their effects through interactions with membrane-bound receptors. β-Adrenergic receptors are members of a superfamily of transmembrane G-protein–coupled receptors, which operate through signal transduction (2,3). An agonist drug, such as albuterol, binds to the extracellular domain of the receptor and induces a conformational change so that the intracellular regions of the receptor may bind to a G protein. As a result, adenylyl cyclase is activated and causes an increase in cyclic adenosine monophosphate (cAMP). cAMP acts as a second messenger by activating protein kinase A, which causes phosphorylation with resultant cellular effects, such as muscle relaxation. Three types of β-adrenergic receptors have been characterized: β_1, β_2, and β_3. β_1 Receptors predominate in the heart, whereas β_3 receptors are found in adipose tissue. β_2 Receptors are ubiquitous; in the lung, these receptors reside in smooth muscle, submucosal glands, epithelium, and alveoli as well as in smooth muscle and endothelium of the pulmonary arterial system. β_2 Receptors are also found on a variety of inflammatory cells, including mast cells, macrophages, neutrophils, eosinophils, and lymphocytes (3). It is interesting to note that these cells are commonly associated with asthma.

Review of the development of β-adrenergic agents clarifies the functional differences among these medications. The early β agonists were initially modeled after adrenaline and noradrenaline. Structural modifications of these catecholamines were noted to impart functional changes in these compounds. For example, substitutions in the hydroxyl groups on the benzene ring reduce inactivation by the gastrointestinal enzyme catechol *O*-methyltransferase, as is the case for metaproterenol and fenoterol. These specific alterations increase duration of action and allow for oral administration. Modifications of the side-chain increase β_2-receptor selectivity, reduce inactivation by monoamine oxidase, and extend duration of action, as is seen for albuterol, terbutaline, pirbuterol, and procaterol. Salmeterol and formoterol have much larger lipophilic side chains that account for their long-lasting β_2-selective effects. Despite their structural and functional similarities, salmeterol and formoterol have different mechanisms of action at the cellular level. Salmeterol binds to an exosite through its long side chain. This, in conjunction with ongoing stimulation of the receptor by the head of the molecule, accounts for its prolonged duration of action (4). In contrast, formoterol penetrates the plasma membrane and gradually leaches out (5).

RAPID-ACTING β AGONISTS

These agents have a quick onset of action, with bronchodilation occurring within minutes of administration. Commonly prescribed in the United States, albuterol begins to induce bronchodilation within 5 minutes of inhalation. Its pharmacologic effects peak after 60 to 90 minutes and last 4 to 6 hours. This class of agents acts primarily by relaxing smooth airway muscle (6). Because β_2 receptors are also found on a variety of inflammatory cells, investigators have postulated that β_2 agonists may also possess antiinflammatory effects. Albuterol inhibits histamine release from activated mast cells *in vitro* (7). Inhibitory effects have also been demonstrated on vascular leakage (8), eosinophils (9–12), lymphocytes (13–15), and neutrophils (16,17). *In vivo* studies of albuterol have failed to uphold an antiinflammatory effect and, in fact, show a potentiated late-phase response, elevation in sputum eosinophils, and increased number of activated eosinophils in bronchial biopsy specimens (18,19).

LONG-ACTING β AGONISTS

Salmeterol and formoterol are in clinical use, although formoterol is not available in the United States. Both drugs provide bronchodilation for 12 hours, much longer than that seen with rapid-acting agents (20,21). Interestingly, they differ in time to onset of action. Salmeterol effects are seen in 10 to 20 minutes, whereas formoterol actions begin in as little as 1 to 3 minutes (21,22). In addition to their bronchodilatory properties, salmeterol and formoterol have bronchoprotective effects. This has been shown for bronchoprovocation with methacholine (23–25), histamine (26), exercise (27), hyperventilation (28,29), sulfur dioxide (30), and distilled water (31).

Salmeterol and formoterol also inhibit allergen-induced early- and late-phase airway responses and accompanying bronchial hyperresponsiveness (32–34). This has led to speculation about potential antiinflammatory effects by long-acting β agonists. Salmeterol inhibits antigen-induced mediator release from human lung mast cell preparations (35) and thromboxane B_2 synthesis from human alveolar macrophages (36). Salmeterol and formoterol also inhibit neutrophil leukotriene B4 production (37). Several *in vivo* studies of salmeterol in humans have documented no antiinflammatory effect as measured by bronchoalveolar lavage (38,39), bronchial biopsy (40), sputum or circulating eosinophils or eosinophilic cationic protein (ECP) (41–43), or urinary leukotriene E4 excretion (44), despite improvements in peak expiratory flow rates and decreased need for rescue therapy. Other studies have documented reductions in sputum eosinophils (45), ECP in bronchoalveolar lavage (46), serum ECP (47), and airway mucosal mast cells and eosinophils (48). In a 12-week study, salmeterol, combined with inhaled corticosteroids, led to a reduction in eosinophils in the lamina propria (49). Most evidence suggests that despite their antiinflammatory effects *in vitro*, long-acting beta agonists do not exhibit significant antiinflammatory effects *in vivo*. It is important to note that these agents do not appear to enhance airway inflammation.

ENANTIOMERS

Until recently, all β_2 agonists in clinical use were racemic mixtures of two mirror-image enantiomers, called R and S, in equal parts. (R)-isomers appear to induce bronchodilator responses, whereas (S)-isomers do not (50). Studies performed in humans have demonstrated that regular use of racemic albuterol is associated with increases in airway responsiveness to allergen (18,51). Since then, evidence points to the stereoselectivity of β_2-adrenergic–mediated bronchodilation and in the development of airway hyperresponsiveness. *In vitro*, (R)-albuterol induces bronchodilation in isolated human trachea (52), whereas (S)-albuterol augments contractile responses to histamine and leukotriene C4 in bronchial tissue (53). In isolated smooth muscle cells, (S)-albuterol has been shown to increase calcium influx (54,55). (S)-albuterol has much less affinity for β_2 receptors than does (R)-albuterol (56). (S)-albuterol appears to have proinflammatory effects as well, with evidence of eosinophil activation demonstrated through elevations in superoxide and eosinophil peroxidase (57,58).

In vivo, the differences between (R)-albuterol and (S)-albuterol continue to exist. (S)-albuterol is metabolized 10 times more slowly than (R)-albuterol (59–61) and is detectable in the blood stream for up to 24 hours after administration of racemic albuterol (60). In 1999, a preservative-free formulation of (R)-albuterol, called levalbuterol, became commercially available for nebulized administration. Clinical studies have evaluated the safety and efficacy of levalbuterol in adults and children. A multicenter randomized study in 362 teenagers and adults with moderate to severe asthma reported that 0.63 mg of levalbuterol was as effective as

2.5 mg of racemic albuterol over 4 weeks of administration (62). Because of the flat dose-response curve, this study failed to show a significant difference with regard to efficacy between levalbuterol and racemic albuterol. In this study, levalbuterol use was associated with dose-dependent side effects similar to those seen for racemic albuterol. In a smaller study of levalbuterol and racemic albuterol in children, lower doses of levalbuterol were as effective as 2.5 mg of racemic albuterol, and all treatments were equally well tolerated in terms of side effects (63). Other studies have addressed whether levalbuterol has a bronchoprotective effect. Using methacholine challenge, a small randomized, double-blind, placebo-controlled study showed a small, sustained bronchoprotective effect for levalbuterol as compared with (S)-albuterol and racemic albuterol (64). A small increase in airway hyperresponsiveness was seen for (S)-albuterol. Other investigations have not confirmed this finding (65,66), yet regular treatment with (R)-albuterol and racemic albuterol results in partial loss of bronchoprotection after methacholine challenge (66).

CLINICAL USE OF β AGONISTS IN ASTHMA

Current national guidelines promote the regular daily use of antiinflammatory, or "controller," agents for persistent asthma (67,68). Despite the use of controller therapy, some individuals may develop breakthrough symptoms or acute exacerbations of their disease. Rapid-acting β agonists are recommended for the relief of mild or severe symptoms. β_2 Agonists are preferred over other bronchodilators, such as methylxanthines and anticholinergic agents, because β agonists exhibit faster onset of action without significant adverse effects when used appropriately. These guidelines also suggest that the frequency with which β agonists are needed for symptom relief serves as a useful marker of asthma control and of the need for adjusting antiinflammatory therapy.

Rapid-acting β agonists may also be used to confirm the diagnosis of asthma by establishing whether reversible bronchospasm exists (67).

These agents are also effective therapy for the prevention of symptoms, such as exercise-induced bronchospasm, when used 5 to 15 minutes before exercise (69–71). Given their short duration of action, rapid-acting agents are not well suited for the prevention of nocturnal symptoms.

The regular daily use of these agents is generally not recommended, but this has been a source of controversy for many years. Although some reports maintain that routine use of β_2 agonists is safe and effective (72), other studies have reported detrimental effects. Several studies have demonstrated a reduction in FEV_1 after regular β_2-agonist use (73–77). Increases in bronchial reactivity have also been noted (73–81). Although some prospective studies of regular inhaled β-agonist use failed to demonstrate deterioration in asthma (82–85), other studies have shown deleterious effects in as little as 3 weeks (86). Because there has been no evidence that regular use of rapid-acting β agonists improves long-term asthma control, their regular use is not advised. Consensus panel reports clearly state that antiinflammatory treatment should be considered when β agonists are needed on a frequent, regular basis (67,68,71).

The situation appears to be quite different for the long-acting class of agents. In light of their slower onset of action, long-acting β agonists are not recommended for relief of acute symptoms (87). These agents block exercise-induced bronchoconstriction (88,89) as well as cold air–induced responses (90) for up to 12 hours. Given their onset of action, they should be administered 30 to 60 minutes before exercise (91). This class is also better suited for control of nocturnal asthma (87,91). Despite the ability to prevent such symptoms, long-acting β agonists should be used as adjunctive therapy to inhaled corticosteroids and should not be used as monotherapy (67,87,91). In fact, several studies have demonstrated that the combined use of inhaled corticosteroids with salmeterol or formoterol is associated with improvements in pulmonary function and symptom control (92–98). Moreover, these results are superior to those seen after increasing the dose of inhaled corticosteroids. Although all groups improved, a similar study in children failed to demonstrate an additional benefit for salmeterol after 1 year of treatment (99). Based on the benefits demonstrated in these studies, long-acting β agonists should be used in conjunction with inhaled corticosteroids for the management of asthma that is inadequately controlled (100).

Levalbuterol has been approved for use by nebulization in patients aged 12 years or older for treatment of asthma. It may be administered every 6 to 8 hours, but, similar to the other rapid-acting agents, levalbuterol should not be used for maintenance therapy. Levalbuterol may be a suitable alternative for patients who experience unacceptable side effects from racemic β agonists, but further studies are needed to clarify the position of levalbuterol in the management of asthma.

ADVERSE EFFECTS

A variety of side effects have been described with the use of β agonists. It is important to note that most of the adverse effects associated with β agonists are reduced when these drugs are administered through inhalation. Tolerance to systemic (nonbronchodilator) effects occurs as well (101,102). Given the widespread distribution of β_2 receptors, many organ systems may be affected. The most common complaint is tremor, which is due to stimulation of β_2 receptors in skeletal muscle (103). Restlessness is also commonly reported (104). Often associated with oral or intravenous administration, tachycardia and palpitations are much less frequent when usual doses are administered through inhalation. Mediated by β vascular relaxation in skeletal muscle, cardiac stimulation occurs as a result of decreased peripheral resistance with resultant sympathetic output. It is also important to note that prolongation of QTc may lead to arrhythmias or myocardial ischemia in susceptible patients. Isoproterenol use is associated with alterations in coronary blood flow that may lead to subendocardial ischemia (105). Transient decreases in PaO_2 may occur when vascular dilation and increased cardiac output enhance perfusion to underventilated areas of lung (106). Abdominal complaints are sometimes seen in children receiving aggressive therapy for management of severe, acute asthma. Metabolic effects include hyperglycemia (due to glycogenolysis) and reductions in serum potassium and magnesium. Intracellular potassium shifts occur as a result of direct stimulation of the Na^+-K^+ pump. Magnesium also moves in this fashion, but increased urinary excretion further contributes to the reduction in this cation.

Paradoxical bronchospasm may occur after the use of β agonists. A review noted that despite the low frequency with which this occurs, these reactions may be quite severe, even life-threatening (107). This report found that warmth, flushing, pruritus, nasal obstruction, and laryngeal wheeze frequently accompanied acute bronchospasm. It has been suggested that a lack of efficacy to β agonists may also be attributed to this phenomenon. Paradoxical bronchospasm was associated with use of new metered-dose inhalers (MDIs) and bottles of nebulized solutions. Propellants have been implicated because they account for 58% to 99% of the composition of MDIs (107). For nebulized solutions, other possible factors have been suggested, such as acidity, osmolality, and preservatives, specifically benzalkonium chloride, ethylenediamine tetraacetic acid, and sulfites (108). Contamination of nebulized solutions, particularly from multidose bottles may also contribute to this problem. Finally, recent investigations suggest that the detrimental effects of (S)-albuterol may account for paradoxical bronchospasm (109).

Short-term loss of effectiveness, or tachyphylaxis, occurs for β agonists as it commonly does with agonist–cell surface receptor interactions. This occurs in response to continuous or frequent, repetitive use. Whether clinically relevant tachyphylaxis to bronchodilatory effect exists remains controversial (1). Tolerance has also been demonstrated in some, but not all, studies of long-term, inhaled β agonist use (110–114). Tolerance occurs after as little as 3 weeks of repeated use and appears to affect the duration rather than peak response (110–113).

β AGONISTS AND ASTHMA MORTALITY

Two major epidemics within the past 40 years prompted international concern and investigation into the relationships between β agonists and asthma deaths. As a result, the safety of β agonists has been hotly debated. The first epidemic occurred in the 1960s, when a 2- to 10-fold increase in asthma mortality rates were noted in six countries, including the United Kingdom and Norway (115). Initial evaluation did not find the rise to be related to changes in diagnosis, disease classification, or death certificate information (116). Because MDI β-agonist preparations had been introduced in the early 1960s, investigators pursued the possibility of a new treatment effect. A high-dose isoproterenol forte preparation was in use in the affected countries at the time (115), and the epidemics occurred only in those countries. Case series analysis revealed that many of those who died of asthma used excessive amounts of this high-dose product (117). Despite what had been learned, another epidemic occurred in New Zealand 10 years later (118). Epidemiologic studies found that the risk for asthma death was increased in those patients who had been treated with the potent but less $β_2$-selective agent fenoterol (119–121). Subsequent studies have attempted to address whether this is a specific effect of fenoterol or a class effect of rapid-acting β agonists. The Saskatchewan studies suggest a general class effect (122,123), although their methods have been contested (124–126). Other studies have demonstrated increased risk for death in asthmatic children receiving fenoterol (127).

A few studies have tried to assess similar risks for long-acting β agonists. The Serevent National Surveillance Project enrolled more than 25,000 adults but had insufficient power to establish relative risk because of the low number of deaths from asthma (128). Another large-scale study, which tracked prescription events, lacked a control group, and no causal association could be established between salmeterol and asthma death (129). A much smaller, case-control study of salmeterol and near-fatal asthma suggested that salmeterol confers no increased risk (130). More studies are clearly needed to clarify whether a relationship truly exists.

SUMMARY

β-Agonists have a pivotal role in asthma management. Refinements in their chemical structure have led to improvements in efficacy, safety, and tolerance. Rapid-acting agents are indicated for the treatment of mild, intermittent asthma and for initial management of acute asthma symptoms in patients with persistent asthma. Regular use of rapid-acting β agonists is not recommended. This class is also effective for the prevention of exercise-induced bronchospasm. Long-acting β agonists have a delayed, but prolonged, onset of action. Consequently, these agents are best used for prevention of symptoms. Long-acting β agonists should not be used as monotherapy for asthma, and current guidelines emphasize their position as adjunctive therapy in combination with inhaled corticosteroids. Levalbuterol, the enantiomer of racemic albuterol, may offer some benefit, but additional studies are needed to confirm and establish its position in the pharmacologic management of asthma.

REFERENCES

1. Pearce N, Hensley MJ. Epidemiologic studies of beta agonists and asthma deaths. *Epidemiol Rev* 1998; 20(2):173–186.
2. Liggett SB. Molecular and genetic basis of β_2-adrenergic receptor function. *J Allergy Clin Immunol* 1999;103:S42–S46.
3. Barnes PJ. Beta-adrenergic receptors and their regulation. *Am J Respir Crit Care Med* 1995;152:838–860.
4. Green SA, Spasoff AP, Colemen RA, et al. Sustained activation of a G protein-coupled receptor via 'anchored' agonist binding: molecular localization of the salmeterol exosite in the beta-2-adrenergic receptor. *J Biol Chem* 1996;271:24029–24035.
5. Anderson GP. Formoterol: pharmacology, molecular basis of agonism, and mechanism of long duration of a highly potent and selective beta2-adrenoceptor agonist bronchodilator. *Life Sci* 1993;52:2145–2160.
6. Barnes PJ. Neural control of human airways in health and disease. *Am Rev Respir Dis* 1986;134:1289–1314.
7. Church MK, Hiroi J. Inhibition of IgE-dependent histamine release from human dispersed lung mast cells by antiallergic drugs and salbutamol. *Br J Pharmacol* 1987;90:421–429.
8. Svensson C, Greiff L, Andersson M, et al. Antiallergic actions of high topical doses of terbutaline in human nasal airways. *Allergy* 1995;50:884–890.
9. Yukawa T, Ukena D, Chanez P et al. Beta-adrenergic receptors on eosinophils: binding and functional studies. *Am Rev Respir Dis* 1990;141:1446–1452.
10. Rabe KF, Giembycz MA, Dent G, et al. β2-Adrenoceptor agonists and respiratory burst activity in guinea pig and human eosinophils. *Fundam Clin Pharmacol* 1991;5:A402.
11. Munoz NM, Vita AF, Neely SP, et al. Beta adrenergic modulation of formyl-methionone-leucine-phenylalanine stimulate secretion of eosinophil peroxidase and leukotriene C4. *J Pharmacol Exp Ther* 1994;268:1339–1343.
12. Hadjokas NE, Crowley JJ, Bayer CR, et al. Beta-adrenergic regulation of the eosinophil respiratory burst as detected by lucigenin-dependent luminescence. *J Allergy Clin Immunol* 1995;95:735–741.
13. Didier M, Aussel C, Ferrua B, et al. Regulation of interleukin 2 synthesis by cAMP in human T cells. *J Immunol* 1987;139:1179–1184.
14. Feldman RD. β-Adrenergic receptor-mediated suppression of interleukin-2 receptors in human lymphocytes. *J Immunol* 1987;139:3355–3359.
15. Borger P, Hoekstra Y, Esselink MT, et al. Beta-adrenoceptor-mediated inhibition of IFN-gamma, IL-3, and GM-CSF mRNA accumulation in activated human T lymphocytes is solely mediated by the β_2-adrenoceptor subtype. *Am J Respir Cell Mol Biol* 1998;19: 400–407.
16. Busse WW, Sosman JM. Isoproterenol inhibition of isolated neutrophil function. *J Allergy Clin Immunol* 1984;73:404–410.
17. Bloemen PG, van den Tweel MC, Henricks PA, et al. Increased cAMP levels in stimulated neutrophils inhibit their adhesion to human bronchial epithelial cells. *Am J Physiol* 1997;272:L580–587.
18. Gauvreau GM, Jordana M, Watson RM, et al. Effect of regular inhaled albuterol on allergen-induced late responses and sputum eosinophils in asthmatic subjects. *Am J Respir Crit Care Med* 1997;156:1738–1745.
19. Manolitsas DN, Wang J, Devalia JL, et al. Regular albuterol, nedocromil sodium, and bronchial inflammation in asthma. *Am J Respir Crit Care Med* 1995;151:1925–1930.
20. Wallin A, Sandström R, Rosenhall L et al. Time course and duration of bronchodilatation with formoteral dry powder in patients with stable asthma. *Thorax* 1993;48:611–614.
21. Palmqvist M, Persson G, Lazer L, et al. Inhaled dry-powder formoterol and salmeterol in asthmatic patients: onset of action, duration of effect and potency. *Eur Respir J* 1997;10:2484–2489.
22. Van Noord JA, Smeets JJ, Raaijmakers JA, et al. Salmeterol versus formoterol in patients with moderately severe asthma: onset and duration of action. *Eur Respir J* 1996;9:1684–1688.
23. Ramsdale EH, Otis J, Kline PA, et al. Prolonged protection against methacholine-induced bronchoconstriction by the inhaled β_2-agonist formoterol. *Am Rev Respir Dis* 1991;143:998–1001.
24. Derom EY, Pauwels RA, Van Der Straeten MEF. The effect of inhaled salmeterol on methacholine responsiveness in subjects with asthma up to 12 hours. *J Allergy Clin Immunol* 1992;89:811–815.
25. Verberne AAPH, Hop WCJ, Bos AB, et al. Effect of a single dose of inhaled salmeterol on baseline airway caliber and methacholine-induced airway obstruction in asthmatic children. *J Allergy Clin Immunol* 1993;91:127–134.
26. Gongora HC, Wisniewski AFZ, Tattersfield AE. A single-dose comparison of inhaled albuterol and two formulations of salmeterol on airway reactivity in asthmatic subjects. *Am Rev Respir Dis* 1991;144:626–629.
27. Newnham DM, Ingram CG, Earnshaw J, et al. Salmeterol provides prolonged protection against exercise-induced bronchoconstriction in a majority of subjects with mild, stable asthma. *Respir Med* 1993;87: 439–444.

28. Malo J-L, Cartier A, Trudeau C, et al. Formoterol, a new inhaled $β_2$-adrenergic agonist, has a longer blocking effect than albuterol on hyperventilation-induced bronchoconstriction. *Am Rev Respir Dis* 1990;142:1147–1152.

29. Nowak D, Jorres R, Rabe KF, et al. Salmeterol protects against hyperventilation-induced bronchoconstriction over 12 hours. *Eur J Clin Pharmacol* 1992;43:591–595.

30. Gong H, Linn WS, Shamoo DA, et al. Effect of inhaled salmeterol on sulfur dioxide induced bronchoconstriction in asthmatic subjects. *Chest* 1996;110:1229–1235.

31. Bootsma GP, Dekhuijzen PNR, Festen J, et al. Sustained protection against distilled water provocation by a single dose of salmeterol in patients with asthma. *Eur Respir J* 1997;10:2230–2236.

32. Twentyman OP, Finnerty JP, Harris A, et al. Protection against allergen-induced asthma by salmeterol. *Lancet* 1990;336:1338–1342.

33. Pedersen B, Dahl R, Larsen BB, et al. The effect of salmeterol on the early and late phase reaction to bronchial allergen and postchallenge variation in bronchial reactivity, blood eosinophils, serum eosinophil cationic protein and serum eosinophil protein X. *Allergy* 1993;48:377–382.

34. Palmqvist M, Balder B, Lowhagen O, et al. Late asthmatic reaction decreased after pretreatment with salbutamol and formoterol, a new long-acting $β_2$-agonist. *J Allergy Clin Immunol* 1992;89:844–849.

35. Butchers PR, Vardey CJ, Johnson M. Salmeterol: a potent and long-acting inhibitor of inflammatory mediator release from human lung. *Br J Pharmacol* 1991;104:672–676.

36. Baker AJ, Palmer J, Johnson M, et al. Inhibitory actions of salmeterol on human airway macrophages and blood monocytes. *Eur J Pharmacol* 1994;264:301–306.

37. Johnson M. The pharmacology of salmeterol. *Lung* (Suppl.) 1990;168:115–119.

38. Gardiner PV, Ward C, Booth H, et al. Effect of eight weeks treatment with salmeterol on bronchoalveolar lavage inflammatory indices in asthmatics. *Am J Respir Crit Care Med* 1994;150:1006–1011.

39. Kraft M, Wenzel SE, Bettinger CM, et al. The effect of salmeterol on nocturnal symptoms, airway function, and inflammation in asthma. *Chest* 1997;111:1249–1254.

40. Roberts JA, Bradding P, Britten KM, et al. The long-acting $β_2$-agonist salmeterol xinafoate: effects on airway inflammation in asthma. *Eur Respir J* 1999;14:275–282.

41. Weersink EJM, Aalbers R, Koeter GH, et al. Partial inhibition of the early and late asthmatic response by a single dose of salmeterol. *Am J Respir Crit Care Med* 1994;150:1261–1267.

42. Pizzichini MMM, Kidney JC, Wong BJO, et al. Effect of salmeterol compared with beclomethasone on allergen-induced asthmatic and inflammatory responses. *Eur Respir J* 1996;9:449–455.

43. Turner MO, Johnston PR, Pizzichini E, et al. Antiinflammatory effects of salmeterol compared with beclomethasone in eosinophilic mild exacerbations of asthma: a randomized, placebo controlled trial. *Can Respir J* 1998;5(4):261–268.

44. Taylor IK, O'Shaughnessy KM, Choudry NB, et al. A comparative study in atopic subjects with asthma of the effects of salmeterol and salbutamol on allergen-

induced bronchoconstriction, increase in airway reactivity, and increase in urinary leukotriene E_4 excretion. *J Allergy Clin Immunol* 1992;89:575–583.

45. Dente FL, Bancalari L, Baaci E, et al. Effect of a single dose of salmeterol on the increase in airway eosinophils induced by allergen challenge in asthmatic subjects. *Thorax* 1999;54:622–624.

46. Dahl R, Pederson B. The influence of inhaled salmeterol on bronchial inflammation: a bronchoalveolar lavage study in patients with bronchial asthma. *Eur Respir Rev* 1991;1:277–285.

47. DiLorenzo G, Morici G, Norrito F, et al. Comparison of the effects of salmeterol and salbutamol on clinical activity and eosinophil cationic protein serum levels during the pollen season in atopic asthmatics. *Clin Exp Allergy* 1995;25:951–956.

48. Wallin A, Sandström T, Söderber M, et al. The effects of regular inhaled formoterol, budesonide, and placebo on mucosal inflammation and clinical indices in mild asthma. *Am J Respir Crit Care Med* 1998;158:79–86.

49. Li X, Ward C, Thien F, et al. An antiinflammatory effect of salmeterol, a long-acting $β_2$ agonist, assessed in airway biopsies and bronchoalveolar lavage in asthma. *Am J Respir Crit Care Med* 1999;160:1493–1499.

50. Hartley D, Middlemiss D. Absolute configuration of the optical isomers of salbutamol. *J Med Chem* 1971;14:895–899.

51. Cockroft DW, McParland CP, Britto SA, et al. Regular inhaled salbutaol and airway responsiveness to allergen. *Lancet* 1993;342:833–838.

52. Prior C, Leonard MB, McCullough JR. Effects of enantiomers of beta 2-agonists on Ach release and smooth muscle contraction in the trachea. *Am J Physiol* 1998;274:L32–38.

53. Templeton AGB, Chapman ID, Chilverws E, et al. Effect of (S)-albuterol on isolated human bronchus. *Pulm Pharmacol* 1998;11:1–6.

54. Yamaguchi H, McCullough J. S-albuterol exacerbates calcium responses to carbachol in airway smooth muscle cells. *Clin Rev Allergy Immunol* 1996;14:47–55.

55. Mitra S, Ugur M, Ugur O, et al. (S)-albuterol increases intracellular free calcium by muscarinic receptor activation and a phospholipase C-dependent mechanism in airway smooth muscle. *Mol Pharmacol* 1998;53:347–354.

56. Penn RB, Frielle T, McCullough JR, et al. Comparison of R-, S-, and RS-albuterol interaction with human beta 1- and beta 2-adrenergic receptors. *Clin Rev Allergy Immunol* 1996;14:37–45.

57. Volcheck GW, Gleich GJ, Kita H. Pro- and antiinflammatory effects of beta adrenergic agonists on eosinophil response to IL-5. *J Allergy Clin Immunol* 1998;101:S35.

58. Leff AR, Herrnreiter A, Naclerio RM, et al. Effect of enantiomeric forms of albuterol on stimulated secretion of granular protein from human eosinophils. *Pulm Pharmacol Ther* 1997;10:97–104.

59. Walle T, Eaton Ea, Walle UK, et al. Stereoselective metabolism of RS-albuterol in humans. *Clin Rev Allergy Immunol* 1996;14:101–113.

60. Gumbhir-Shah K, Kellerman D, DeGraw S, et al. Pharmacokinetics and pharmacodynamics of cumulative single doses of inhaled salbutamol enantiomers in asthmatic subjects. *Pulm Pharmacol Ther* 1999(12):353–362.

61. Koch P, McCullough JR, DeGraw SS, et al. Pharmacokinetics and safety of (R)-, (S)-, and (RS)-albuterol following nebulization in healthy volunteers. *Am J Respir Crit Care Med* 1997;155:A279.

62. Nelson HS, Bensch G, Pleskow WW, et al. Improved bronchodilation with levalbuterol compared with racemic albuterol in patients with asthma. *J Allergy Clin Immunol* 1998;102:943–952.

63. Gawchik SM, Saccar CL, Noonan M, et al. The safety and efficacy of nebulized levalbuterol compared with racemic albuterol and placebo in the treatment of asthma in pediatric patients. *J Allergy Clin Immunol* 1999;103:615–621.

64. Perrin-Fayolle M, Blum PS, Morley J, et al. Differential responses of asthmatic airways to enantiomers of albuterol. *Clin Rev Allergy Immunol* 1996;14:139–147.

65. Cockroft DW, Swystun VA. Effect of single doses of S-albuterol, R-albuterol, racemic albuterol, and placebo on the airway response to methacholine. *Thorax* 1997;52:845–848.

66. Cockroft DW, Davis BE, Swystun VA, et al. Tolerance to the bronchoprotective effect of β_2-agonists: comparison of the enantiomer of albuterol with racemic albuterol and placebo. *J Allergy Clin Immunol* 1999;103:1049–1053.

67. National Institutes of Health, National Heart, Lung and Blood Institute. *Expert Panel Report 2: guidelines for the diagnosis and management of asthma.* NIH Publication No. 97-4051, 1997.

68. American Academy of Allergy, Asthma and Immunology. *Pediatric asthma: promoting best guidelines.* 1999.

69. Anderson S, Seale JP, Ferais L, et al. An evaluation of pharmacotherapy for exercise induced asthma. *J Allergy Clin Immunol* 1979;64:612–624.

70. Godfrey S, Konig P. Inhibition of exercise-induced asthma by different pharmacological pathways. *Thorax* 1976;31:137–143.

71. National Institutes of Health, National Heart, Lung and Blood Institute. *Global initiative for asthma: global strategy for asthma management and prevention, NHLBI/WHO workshop report.* NIH Publication No. 95-3659, 1995.

72. Wanner A. Is the routine use of inhaled β-adrenergic agonists appropriate in asthma treatment? Yes. *Am J Respir Crit Care Med* 1995;151:597–599.

73. Vathenen AS, Knox AJ, Higgens JR, et al. Rebound increases in bronchial responsiveness after treatment with inhaled terbutaline. *Lancet* 1988;1(8585):554–558.

74. Sears MR, Taylor CG, Print DC, et al. Regular inhaled beta-agonist treatment in bronchial asthma. *Lancet* 1990;336:1391–1396.

75. Taylor DR, Sears MR, Herbison GP, et al. Regular inhaled beta agonists in asthma: effects on exacerbations and lung function. *Thorax* 1993;48:134–138.

76. Van Schayck CP, Dompeling E, van Herwaarden CLA, et al. Bronchodilator treatment in moderate asthma or chronic bronchitis: continuous or on demand? A randomised controlled study. *Br Med J* 1991;303:1426–1431.

77. Harvey JE, Tattersfield AE. Airway response to salbutamol: effect of regular salbutamol inhalation in normal, atopic and asthmatic subjects. *Thorax* 1982;37:280–287.

78. Wahedna I, Wong CS, Wisniewski AF, et al. Asthma control during and after cessation of regular

79. Van Schayck CP, Graafsma SJ, Visch MB, et al. Increased bronchial responsiveness after inhaling salbutamol during 1 year is not caused by subsensitization to salbutamol. *J Allergy Clin Immunol* 1990;86:793–800.

80. Kerrebijn KF, von Essen-Zandvliet EEM, Neijens JJ. Effect of long-term treatment with inhaled corticosteroids and beta agonists on the bronchial responsiveness in children with asthma. *J Allergy Clin Immunol* 1987;79:653–659.

81. Kraan JG, Koeter GH, Van der Mark TW, et al. Changes in bronchial hyperreactivity induced by 4 weeks of treatment with antiasthmatic drugs in patients with allergic asthma: a comparison between budesonide and terbutaline. *J Allergy Clin Immunol* 1985;76: 628–636.

82. Drazen JM, Israel E, Boushey HA, et al. Comparison of regularly scheduled with as-needed use of albuterol in mild asthma. *N Engl J Med* 1996;335:841–847.

83. Vandewalker ML, Kray KT, Weber RW, et al. Addition of terbutaline to optimal theophylline therapy: double blind crossover study in asthmatic patients. *Chest* 1986;90:198–203.

84. Pearlman DS, Chervinsky P, LaForce C, et al. A comparison of salmeterol with albuterol in the treatment of mild-to-moderate asthma. *N Engl J Med* 1992;327:1420–1425.

85. D'Alonzo GE, Nathan RA, Henochowicz S, et al. Salmeterol xinafoate as maintenance therapy compared with albuterol in patients with asthma. *JAMA* 1994;271:1412–1416.

86. Wahedna I, Wong CS, Wisniewski FZ, et al. Asthma control during and after cessation of regular beta$_2$-agonist treatment. *Am Rev Respir Dis* 1993;148:707–712.

87. Nelson HS. B-adrenergic bronchodilators. *N Engl J Med* 1995;333(8):499–506.

88. Kemp JP, Dockhorn RJ, Busse WW, et al. Prolonged effect of inhaled salmeterol against exercise-induced bronchospasm. *Am J Respir Crit Care Med* 1994;150:1612–1615.

89. Boner AL, Spezia E, Piovesan P, et al. Inhaled formoterol in the prevention of exercise-induced bronchoconstriction in asthmatic children. *Am J Respir Crit Care Med* 1994;149:935–939.

90. Nowak D, Jorres R, Rabe KF, et al. Salmeterol protects against hyperventilation-induced bronchoconstriction over 12 hours. *Eur J Clin Pharmacol* 1992;43:591–595.

91. Busse WW. Long- and short-acting β_2-adrenergic agonists effects on airway function in patients with asthma. *Arch Intern Med* 1996;156:1514–1520.

92. Greening AP, Ind PW, Northfield M, et al. Added salmeterol versus higher-dose corticosteroid in asthma patients with symptoms on existing inhaled corticosteroid. *Lancet* 1994;344:219–224.

93. Woolcock A, Lundback B, Ringdal N, et al. Comparison of addition of salmeterol to inhaled steroids with doubling the dose of inhaled steroids. *Am J Respir Crit Care Med* 1996;153:1481–1488.

94. Wilding P, Clark M, Coon JT, et al. Effect of long term treatment with salmeterol on asthma control: a double blind, randomised crossover study. *Br Med J* 1997;314:1441–1446.

95. Russell G, Williams DAJ, Weller P, et al. Salmeterol

xinafoate in children on high dose inhaled steroids. *Ann Allergy Asthma Immunol* 1995;75:423.

96. Pauwels RA, Lofdahl CG, Postma DS, et al. Effect of inhaled formoterol and budesonide on exacerbations of asthma. *N Engl J Med* 1997;337:1405–1411.

97. Condemi JJ, Goldstein S, Kalberg C, et al. The addition of salmeterol to fluticasone propionate versus increasing the dose of fluticasone propionate in patients with persistent asthma. *Ann Allergy Asthma Immunol* 1999;82:383–389.

98. Pearlman DS, Stricker W, Weinstein S, et al. Inhaled salmeterol and fluticasone: a study comparing monotherapy and combination therapy in asthma. *Ann Allergy Asthma Immunol* 1999;82:257–265.

99. Verberne AAPH, Frost C, Duiverman EJ, et al. Addition of salmeterol versus doubling the dose of beclomethasone in children with asthma. *Am J Respir Crit Care Med* 1998;158:213–219.

100. Jenkins CR. Long-acting β_2-agonists: the new symptom controllers for asthma. *Med J Aust* 1999;171:255–258.

101. Maconochie JG, Minton NA, Chilton JE, et al. Does tachyphylaxis occur to the non-pulmonary effects of salmeterol? *Br J Clin Pharmacol* 1994;37:199–204.

102. Newnham DM, Grove A, McDevitt DG, et al. Subsensitivity of bronchodilator and systemic β_2-adrenoceptor responses after regular twice daily treatment with eformoterol dry powder in asthmatic patients. *Thorax* 1995;50:497–504.

103. Bengtsson B. Plasma concentration and side-effects of terbutaline. *Eur J Respir Dis* (Suppl.) 1984;134:231–235.

104. White MV, Sander N. Asthma from the perspective of the patient. *J Allergy Clin Immunol* 1999;103:S47–52.

105. Winsor T, Mills B, Winbury MM, et al. Intramyocardial diversion of coronary blood flow: effects of isoproterenol-induced subendocardial ischaemia. *Microvasc Res* 1975;9:261–278.

106. Wagner PD, Dantzker DR, Iacovoni VE, et al. Ventilation-perfusion inequality in asymptomatic asthma. *Am Rev Respir Dis* 1978;118:511–524.

107. Nicklas RA. Paradoxical bronchospasm associated with the use of inhaled beta agonists. *J Allergy Clin Immunol* 1990;85:959–964.

108. Asmus MJ, Sherman J, Hendeles L. Bronchoconstrictor additives in bronchodilator solutions. *J Allergy Clin Immunol* 1999;104:S53–60.

109. Handley D. The asthma-like pharmacology and toxicology of (S)-isomers of β-agonists. *J Allergy Clin Immunol* 1999;104:S69–76.

110. Newnham DM, McDevitt DG, Lipworth BJ. Bronchodilator subsensitivity after chronic dosing with formoterol in patients with asthma. *Am J Med* 1984;97:29–37.

111. Weber RW, Smith JA, Nelson HS. Aerosolized terbutaline in asthmatics: development of subsensitivity wit long-term administration. *J Allergy Clin Immunol* 1982;70:417–422.

112. Repsher LH, Anderson JA, Bush RU, et al. Assessment of tachyphylaxis following prolonged therapy of asthma with inhaled albuterol aerosol. *Chest* 1984;85:34–38.

113. Georgopoulos D, Wong D, Anthonisen NR. Tolerance to β_2-agonists in patients with chronic obstructive pulmonary disease. *Chest* 1990;97:280–284.

114. Holgate ST, Baldwin CJ, Tattersfield AE. β-Adrenergic agonists resistance in normal human airways. *Lancet* 1977;2:375–377.

115. Stolley PD. Why the United States was spared an epidemic of deaths due to asthma. *Am Rev Respir Dis* 1972;105:883–890.

116. Speizer FE, Doll R, Heaf P. Observations on recent increases in mortality from asthma. *Br Med J* 1968;1:3359.

117. Fraser PM, Speizer FE, Waters DM, et al. The circumstances preceding death from asthma in young people in 1968 to 1969. *Br J Dis Chest* 1971;65:71–84.

118. Jackson RT, Beaglehole R, Rea HH, et al. Mortality from asthma: a new epidemic in New Zealand. *Br Med J* 1982;285:771–774.

119. Crane J, Pearch N, Flatt A, et al. Prescribed fenoterol and death from asthma in New Zealand, 1981–83: case-control study. *Lancet* 1989;1:917–922.

120. Pearce N, Grainger J, Atkinson M, et al. Case-control study of prescribed fenoterol and death from asthma in New Zealand, 1977–1981. *Thorax* 1990;45:170–175.

121. Grainger J, Woodman K, Pearch N, et al. Prescribed fenoterol and death from asthma in New Zealand, 1981–1987: a further case-control study. *Thorax* 1991;46:105–111.

122. Spitzer WD, Suissa S, Ernst P, et al. The use of beta agonists and the risk of death and near death from asthma. *N Engl J Med* 1992;326:501–506.

123. Suissa S, Ernst P, Boivin JF, et al. A cohort analysis of excess mortality in asthma and the use of inhaled β-agonists. *Am J Respir Crit Care Med* 1994;149:604–610.

124. Beasley R, Pearce N, Crane J, et al. B-agonists: what is the evidence that their use increases the risk of asthma morbidity and mortality? *J Allergy Clin Immunol* 1999;103:S18–30.

125. Pearce N, Hensley MJ. Epidemiologic studies of beta agonists and asthma deaths. *Epidemiol Rev* 1998;20:173–186.

126. Barrett TE, Strom BL. Inhaled beta-adrenergic receptor agonists in asthma: more harm than good? *Am J Respir Crit Care Med* 1995;151:574–577.

127. Matsui T. Asthma deaths and B2-agonists. In: Shimomiya K, ed. *Current advances in paediatric allergy and clinical epidemiology: selected proceedings from the 32nd Annual Meeting of the Japanese Society of Paediatric Allergy and Clinical Immunology.* Tokyo: Churchill Livingstone, 1996:161–164.

128. Castle W, Fuller R, Hall J, et al. Serevent nationwide surveillance study: comparison of salmeterol with salbutamol in asthmatic patients who require regular bronchodilator treatment. *Br Med J* 1993;306:1034–1037.

129. Mann RD, Kubota K, Pearch G, et al. Salmeterol: a study by prescription event monitoring in a UK cohort of 15,407 patients. *J Clin Epidemiol* 1996;49:247–250.

130. Williams C, Crossland L, Finnerty J, et al. Case-control study of salmeterol and near-fatal attacks of asthma. *Thorax* 1998;53:7–13.

36

Other Antiallergic Drugs: Cromolyn, Nedocromil, Antileukotrienes, Anticholinergics, and Theophylline

Carol A. Wiggins

*Department of Allergy and Immunology, Emory University School of Medicine
and Piedmont Hospital, Atlanta, Georgia*

CROMOLYN AND NEDOCROMIL

Cromolyn and nedocromil are chemically dissimilar drugs with similar pharmacologic and therapeutic properties. These drugs, collectively referred to as cromones, are nonsteroidal antiinflammatory medications with no significant adverse effects. Roger Altounyan and colleagues developed the cromones as synthetic analogues of the herbal remedy khellin. The remarkable safety of these drugs makes them appealing as first-line therapy for mild asthma. Although often classified as mast cell stabilizing drugs, the cromones possess a number of antiinflammatory properties.

Pharmacology

Cromolyn and nedocromil have low oral bioavailability, and all of their pharmacologic effects in asthma result from topical deposition in the lung. Cromolyn has a very short plasma half-life of 11 to 20 minutes (1). Nedocromil has a longer plasma half-life of 1.5 to 2 hours (2). There are no significant drug interactions with the cromones (1,2). Neither drug relieves bronchospasm; both must be used preventively, as maintenance medications or prior to exercise or allergen exposure.

Mechanism of Action

Recent studies have reported that the cromones block chloride transport channels in airway epithelial cells, neurons, and mucosal mast cells (3–6). Mast cell degranulation is dependent on calcium channel activation that is blocked by cromolyn and nedocromil. The chloride transport channels, which are blocked by the cromones, may provide the negative membrane potential necessary to maintain calcium influx and the sustained intracellular calcium elevation necessary for mast cell degranulation, and may allow for changes in cell tonicity and volume. The ability of the cromones to block chloride transport also may be the underlying mechanism for their other antiinflammatory effects (7,8).

The cromones have been reported to inhibit release of histamine, prostaglandin D_2, and tumor necrosis factor-α from human mast cells (8–11). The cromones inhibit antigen- and anti–immunoglobulin E (IgE)-induced mast cell degranulation as well as mediator release triggered by calcium ionophore, phospholipase A, substance P, and compound 48/80 (1,8). Cromolyn inhibits mast cell degranulation in some tissue types better than others. Mediator release from human mast cells obtained from bronchoalveolar lavage is inhibited by much lower concentrations of cromolyn than is required to inhibit release from mast cells from human lung fragments. Cromolyn and nedocromil also have been reported to inhibit mediator release from human peritoneal mast cells but not from skin mast cells (8).

The cromones suppress eosinophil chemotaxis and decrease eosinophil survival (12–16). Cromolyn and nedocromil have been reported to inhibit neutrophil activation and migration (13–16). The cromones also inhibit expression of adhesion molecules (16–20). Recent studies have demonstrated that cromolyn and nedocromil inhibit antigen-induced production of interleukin-5 (IL-5) from mast cells (12) and mononuclear cells from sensitized asthmatics (20), and inhibit granulocyte-macrophage colony-stimulating factor secretion (15). The cromones have been shown to antagonize the effects of the inflammatory neuropeptides substance P, bradykinin, and neurokinin A (21–26). Cromolyn and nedocromil also have been reported to inhibit IgE synthesis (27,28).

Challenge Studies

Inhalation challenge studies have determined that the cromones inhibit both the early and late asthmatic reactions when administered prior to allergen challenge (29–31). Nedocromil also inhibits the late phase of inflammation when administered after the onset of the early phase reaction (32). Cromolyn and nedocromil also inhibit bronchial hyperresponsiveness to other stimuli, including fog, exercise, cold air, and sulfur dioxide (33–36). The cromones do not inhibit bronchospasm induced by histamine or methacholine in the acute setting (37–41), but may inhibit bronchial hyperresponsiveness to methacholine after several weeks of therapy (41).

Efficacy

Cromolyn and nedocromil are useful controller medications for children and adults with mild asthma. Both drugs have been reported to improve clinical outcomes and lung function when started early in the course of the disease (42). They are effective in both nonallergic and allergic asthma. Although at least one study suggested that nedocromil is superior to cromolyn

(43), most studies have reported no significant difference in efficacy (44–47). However, nedocromil may be effective when used on a twice a day schedule; this would tend to improve patient compliance compared with cromolyn, which must be used four times daily for optimal benefit (48).

The cromones are less efficacious than inhaled corticosteroids in the treatment of asthma (49–52). Some studies have suggested that the cromones have modest corticosteroid-sparing properties (53–55); others have failed to demonstrate significant steroid-sparing effects (56,57). Studies have demonstrated that cromolyn and nedocromil are similar in efficacy to theophylline, with far fewer side effects (58–61). Cromolyn is less effective than inhaled β agonists for prevention of exercise-induced asthma (62).

There is a common perception that nedocromil may be particularly useful when cough is a major asthma symptom, presumably by virtue of inhibitory effects on neuropeptides. However, cromolyn also inhibits the effects of inflammatory neuropeptides. Inhaled corticosteroids are effective in reducing asthmatic cough, and there is no evidence that nedocromil is superior to inhaled corticosteroids in suppressing cough as an asthma symptom. The cromones may be helpful in reducing the cough associated with angiotensin-converting enzyme inhibitors when there is not an alternative to this class of drugs (63).

Safety and Drug Interactions

Cromolyn and nedocromil have no known drug interactions, toxicity, or clinically significant adverse effects. Cough or paradoxic bronchospasm may occur with inhalers. Some patients experience a bad taste with nedocromil. Both are pregnancy category B and generally recognized as safe for use in pregnancy. Cromolyn is the preferred first step therapy for mild persistent asthma in pregnancy according to recent national guidelines (64).

Dosing and Preparations

Cromolyn is available as a metered-dose inhaler that delivers 1 mg per actuation, and in 20-mg ampoules for nebulization. The recommended dose of cromolyn is two inhalations, or one ampoule every 4 hours, or 10 to 60 minutes prior to exercise or allergen exposure.

Cromolyn is also available as a nasal spray for treatment of allergic rhinitis. It is less effective than topical nasal steroids and must be used four to six times daily for optimal benefit. Cromolyn and nedocromil are available as ophthalmic preparations for treatment of allergic and vernal conjunctivitis. Cromolyn is also available as a capsule to be taken orally for systemic mastocytosis and eosinophilic gastroenteritis.

Nedocromil is available as a metered-dose inhaler that delivers 2 mg during actuation. The recommended dose for asthma or cough for children 6 years of age and older and adults is two inhalations up to 4 times daily.

Nedocromil is available for treatment of allergic conjunctivitis in a 2% solution.

ANTILEUKOTRIENES

When the leukotrienes were identified as important mediators of asthma, investigators began searching for compounds that would specifically inhibit the inflammatory activity of the leukotrienes. Three antileukotriene drugs are available in the United States: zileuton, zafirlukast, and montelukast.

Leukotriene Formation and Biologic Activity of the Leukotrienes

The leukotrienes are formed from arachidonic acid. The initial steps in this process are catalyzed by an enzyme complex containing 5-lipoxygenase (5-LO). Separate pathways lead to production of leukotriene B_4 (LTB_4) or the cysteinyl leukotrienes: leukotriene C_4 (LTC_4), leukotriene D_4 (LTD_4), and leukotriene E_4 (LTE_4) (65).

The cysteinyl leukotrienes have a common receptor that is distinct from the LTB_4 receptor. The cysteinyl leukotrienes are potent mediators of bronchoconstriction, airway responsiveness, microvascular permeability, and mucus secretion. LTB_4 is a well-recognized chemoattractant for neutrophils in the lung (66).

The leukotrienes appear to be important mediators of aspirin-sensitive asthma. Aspirin-sensitive asthmatics have increased baseline levels of leukotrienes compared with non–aspirin-sensitive asthmatics, and develop markedly enhanced levels of leukotrienes in their lungs, nasal secretions, and urine following aspirin challenge (67–70).

Mechanism of Action

The first antileukotriene to be approved was the 5-LO inhibitor zileuton. Zileuton directly inhibits the catalytic activity of 5-LO and inhibits production of LTB_4 as well as the cysteinyl leukotrienes. Zafirlukast and montelukast are competitive antagonists of the cysteinyl leukotriene receptor and therefore inhibit the activity of LTC_4, LTD_4, and LTE_4 (66).

The antileukotrienes have been reported to inhibit influx of eosinophils into the airways and to reduce blood eosinophil levels (71–75). In one study, zafirlukast also inhibited lymphocyte and basophil influx into bronchoalveolar lavage fluid following allergen challenge (76). Montelukast and zafirlukast have demonstrated bronchodilator activity (77–79).

Challenge Studies

Montelukast and zafirlukast inhibit both the early- and late-phase responses to allergen challenge (80,81). Zileuton does not significantly inhibit the airway response to allergen (82). The antileukotrienes have demonstrated protective effects against exercise-induced bronchoconstriction (83–86). Zafirlukast has been reported to inhibit sulfur dioxide–induced bronchospasm (87). Zafirlukast and zileuton inhibit bronchoconstriction by cold, dry air (88,89). Zileuton and montelukast have been reported to inhibit aspirin-induced bronchospasm in aspirin-sensitive asthma (90,91).

Efficacy for Asthma

Numerous studies have demonstrated that the antileukotrienes are well tolerated and superior to placebo in the treatment of mild to moderate bronchial asthma (92–100). A few studies have compared the antileukotrienes with other drugs. In one study comparing beclomethasone dipropionate to montelukast, beclomethasone dipropionate resulted in greater improvement in symptom control, number and duration of asthma exacerbations, and peak expiratory flow rates, although montelukast had a faster onset of action (101). In another study comparing low-dose fluticasone (88 μg twice daily) with zafirlukast, fluticasone was superior to zafirlukast in improving morning and evening peak flow rates, number of symptom-free days, use of β agonists, and forced expiratory volume in 1 second (FEV_1) (102).

Antileukotrienes may result in improved asthma control as additional therapy in patients not adequately controlled by inhaled corticosteroids. In one study, adding zafirlukast was as effective as doubling the dose of inhaled beclomethasone dipropionate in patients not adequately controlled with low doses (400 μg/day or less) of the inhaled corticosteroid (103). Another study reported that the addition of montelukast was superior to placebo in patients not adequately controlled by low-dose beclomethasone dipropionate (104).

There is some evidence that antileukotrienes may have steroid-sparing effects. In patients receiving moderate to high doses of inhaled corticosteroids, the addition of montelukast allowed a reduction of the inhaled corticosteroid by a mean value of 47% (105). The addition of pranlukast, a cysteinyl leukotriene antagonist available in Japan, allowed patients previously requiring high doses of beclomethasone dipropionate (1,500 μg/day or more) to halve their dose of beclomethasone dipropionate (106).

Zileuton and theophylline are comparable in efficacy and tolerability (107). Several studies have compared the antileukotrienes with salmeterol. The addition of salmeterol resulted in greater improvement in asthma control than did the addition of zafirlukast in patients with persistent asthma, most of whom were receiving inhaled corticosteroids (108). Two studies comparing montelukast with salmeterol found that montelukast provided superior protection from exercise-induced asthma when used as maintenance asthma therapy (109,110). One study compared zafirlukast with cromolyn; the two drugs were equally effective (111).

Safety and Drug Interactions

The antileukotrienes are generally safe and well tolerated. Zileuton can cause liver toxicity, and significant elevations of hepatic transaminases occurred in 4.6% of patients in long-term surveillance studies. Patients receiving zileuton should have serum alanine transaminase measured monthly for the first three months, quarterly for the next year, and at the discretion of the prescribing physician thereafter. The majority of transaminase elevations occur within the first 2 months of therapy (112). Zafirlukast and montelukast do not appear to cause hepatotoxicity at recommended doses.

There have been several reports of Churg-Strauss syndrome and eosinophilic pneumonia developing after initiation of therapy with cysteinyl leukotriene receptor antagonists. All of the patients reported were adults with severe asthma, and most had previously received systemic corticosteroids (113–115). The likely explanation for these occurrences is that vasculitis or eosinophilia was present but not recognized, and in many cases suppressed by systemic corticosteroids, prior to the initiation of antileukotriene therapy (115,116).

Zileuton and zafirlukast may prolong the prothrombin time in patients receiving warfarin (117,118). Zileuton may double serum theophylline levels and theophylline dosages should be reduced and serum levels monitored in patients taking both drugs (119). Montelukast has not demonstrated any clinically significant drug interactions.

Zileuton is a category C drug in pregnancy. Zafirlukast and montelukast are category B drugs in pregnancy; however, current guidelines recommend the use of medications with which there has been more experience in pregnancy (120).

Dosage and Preparations

Zileuton is available in 600-mg tablets that are taken four times daily. Zafirlukast is available in 20-mg tablets to be taken twice a day. Both are approved for ages 12 and above. Montelukast is available in 4- and 5-mg chewable tablets (for ages 2–6 and 6–15, respectively), and 10-mg tablets for ages 15 and older. Montelukast is administered once a day in the evening.

ANTICHOLINERGICS

The naturally occurring anticholinergics, most notably atropine, have been used for centuries to treat asthma and a variety of other medical conditions. The toxicity of these drugs has long been recognized, and is reflected in the common name *Atropa belladonna*, "deadly nightshade," the plant from which atropine is derived. Scopolamine, another naturally occurring anticholinergic, is now used primarily in the treatment of motion sickness. Ipratropium bromide, a synthetic congener of atropine, is the only anticholinergic now in common use for asthma and chronic obstructive pulmonary disease.

Cholinergic Mechanisms in Asthma

The autonomic innervation of the airways is supplied by branches of the vagus nerve, which are found primarily in large and medium-sized airways. The postganglionic terminals of the vagal fibers supply smooth muscles of the airways and vasculature. Release of acetylcholine from the parasympathetic postganglionic fibers, acting on muscarinic receptors, results in smooth muscle contraction and release of secretions from submucosal glands (121). The activity of the cholinergic fibers results in a constant, low level of tonic activity of the airways (122). A variety of stimuli, including irritants, exercise, cold dry air, histamine, and allergens can trigger irritant receptors of vagal afferent nerves, resulting in almost immediate reflex bronchoconstriction and mucus hypersecretion (123).

Mechanism of Action of Anticholinergics

The anticholinergic agents compete with acetylcholine at muscarinic receptors. There are three known subtypes of muscarinic receptors in the lung. M1 and M3 receptors promote bronchoconstriction and mucus secretion, whereas M2 receptors promote bronchodilatation (123). All of the currently available anticholinergics nonselectively inhibit all muscarinic receptor subtypes (124). The blockade of M2 receptors may potentiate bronchoconstriction, which antagonizes the bronchodilatory effect of M1 and M3 receptor blockade (125,126). This has led to a search for selective drugs that do not antagonize the bronchodilatory effects of M2 receptors, but none is currently available. Because muscarinic receptors are found primarily in the central airways, anticholinergic bronchodilatation occurs mostly in the larger airways (127,128).

The anticholinergics provide virtually complete protection against bronchoconstriction induced by cholinergic agonists such as methacholine (126,127). Anticholinergics provide varied or partial protection against bronchoconstriction induced by inflammatory mediators, including histamine, irritants, exercise, or allergens (128,129).

Pharmacology

Atropine is well absorbed from mucosal surfaces and reaches peak serum levels within an hour. The bronchodilatory effects last for 3 to 4 hours. Atropine relaxes smooth muscle in the airways, gastrointestinal tract, iris, and peripheral vasculature. It inhibits relaxation of the urinary sphincter. It causes bradycardia at low doses and tachycardia at high doses. It reduces salivary secretions and mucociliary clearance in the airways. Atropine crosses the blood–brain barrier and can cause central nervous system side effects. Scopolamine has similar pharmacologic properties, but is even more likely to cause central nervous system side effects at low doses (130).

Ipratropium bromide is a quaternary ammonium congener of atropine. The quaternary ammonium structure allows for poor absorption across respiratory and other mucous membranes (131). This results in a lack of significant anticholinergic side effects and allows ipratropium to remain in the airways longer than atropine. Ipratropium does not cross the blood–brain barrier or inhibit mucociliary clearance (131,132). Bronchodilatation induced by ipratropium bromide lasts 5 to 6 hours (126).

Efficacy

Anticholinergics are less effective bronchodilators than β-adrenergic agonists. Ipratropium bromide has a much slower onset of action than albuterol. Peak bronchodilatation occurs 30 to 90 minutes after inhalation of ipratropium, compared with 5 to 15 minutes after inhalation of albuterol (133). Ipratropium bromide has a longer duration of action than albuterol. Some patients may respond better to ipratropium than to albuterol, but there are no reliable predictors for which patients respond well to ipratropium (134,135). Anticholinergic agents are superior to β-adrenergic agonists in preventing bronchospasm induced by β blockers or psychogenic bronchospasm (135–138). Ipratropium bromide appears to improve outcomes when added to albuterol in emergency treatment of acute exacerbations of asthma, but the additional effect is not always large (139).

Ipratropium bromide nasal spray relieves rhinorrhea associated with allergic (140) or nonallergic rhinitis (141) and viral upper respiratory infections (142).

Safety and Drug Interactions

Atropine may cause significant side effects, even at therapeutic doses. Warmth and flushing of the skin, impairment of mucociliary clearance, gastroesophageal reflux, and urinary retention are common. Central nervous system effects ranging from irritability to hallucinations and coma may occur. Tahyarrhythmias may occur at low doses, and atrioventricular dissociation may occur at high doses. Atropine may trigger angle-closure glaucoma (130). Because of the frequency of side effects, potential for severe toxicity, and availability of drugs with superior safety and efficacy, there is no role for atropine in the management of asthma; it is mainly used to treat symptomatic bradycardia and reverse organophosphate poisoning.

Ipratropium bromide has no severe adverse effects or drug interactions and is very well tolerated. Rare cases of acute angle-closure glaucoma and blurred vision and dilatation of the pupil have occurred with nebulized ipratropium, presumably due to direct contact with the eye (143–145).

Dry mouth is a common side effect, and some patients complain of a bad taste or worsening bronchospasm with ipratropium (126). Ipratroprium is a category B drug in pregnancy.

Preparations and Dosing

Ipratropium bromide is available in a metered-dose inhaler, alone or in combination with albuterol, and is administered as two inhalations four times a day. Each actuation delivers 18 μg of ipratropium bromide. It is also available in unit dose vials for use in nebulizers as a 0.02% solution. Ipratropium bromide is available in a nasal spray, 0.03% for rhinitis and 0.06% for upper respiratory infections. The recommended dose is two sprays in each nostril two to three times a day.

Atropine and scopolamine in low doses are incorporated in combination tablets with antihistamines and decongestants to treat rhinitis symptoms.

THEOPHYLLINE

Theophylline was one of the first drugs to be used as maintenance therapy for asthma. However, the emphasis on treatment of inflammation in asthma, as well as the introduction of newer drugs with similar or superior efficacy and improved safety and tolerability, has led to decreased use of theophylline.

Pharmacology

Theophylline is a member of the methylxanthine family of drugs, which includes the naturally occurring alkaloid compounds caffeine and theobromine. The solubility of the methylxanthines is low unless they form salts or complexes with other compounds such as ethylenediamine (as in aminophylline). Theophylline is rapidly absorbed after oral, rectal, or parenteral administration, and maximum serum levels occur 2 hours after ingestion on an empty stomach. Most theophylline preparations in current use are sustained release and administered once or twice a day. Food generally slows the rate but not the amount of absorption (146).

The elimination rate of theophylline varies widely in individuals, depending on age, genetic, and environmental factors, as well as underlying diseases. Serum levels of theophylline are altered by many other medications. High-protein, low-carbohydrate diets and diets high in charcoal-grilled foods, as well as smoking tobacco and marijuana, may increase theophylline clearance and therefore decrease serum levels. Pregnancy, fever, older age, liver disease, congestive heart failure, and chronic obstructive pulmonary disease with chronic hypoxemia may increase serum theophylline levels (147,148).

Mechanism of Action

Theophylline inhibits cyclic adenosine monophosphate (cAMP)-specific phosphodiesterases at high concentrations, but its bronchodilation may result from being an antagonist for adenosine receptors (151). The clinical effects of theophylline are primarily relaxation of smooth muscle in pulmonary arteries and airways (150), increased respiratory drive during hypoxia (157), and decreased fatigue of diaphragmatic muscles (152). Theophylline also increases mucociliary clearance and decreases microvascular leakage of plasma into airways (153).

In recent years, modest antiinflammatory effects of theophylline have been reported. Theophylline inhibits eosinophil infiltration into the airways of asthmatics (154,155). Withdrawal of theophylline in patients treated with both theophylline and inhaled corticosteroids has been reported to result in increased numbers of total and activated eosinophils in the airways (156). Theophylline inhibits influx of CD8$^+$ T cells and leads to decreased IL-4 expression in asthmatic airways (157,158).

Challenge Studies

In several studies it is reported that theophylline inhibits bronchial hyperresponsiveness to methacholine (159–161). In other studies, theophylline inhibits the early-phase but not the late phase response to inhaled allergen (162–164).

Efficacy

Studies have demonstrated that theophylline is similar in efficacy but less well tolerated than cromolyn (165,166). A recent comparison study with the leukotriene antagonist zileuton found that it was as effective as theophylline and had fewer unpleasant side effects (167). Theophylline is more effective as maintenance therapy than long-acting oral albuterol or inhaled albuterol four times daily (168,169).

Inhaled beclomethasone dipropionate and inhaled fluticasone have superior efficacy to theophylline for moderate to severe bronchial asthma, and the inhaled corticosteroids have fewer adverse effects (170,171). The addition of theophylline to low-dose budesonide was as effective as doubling the dose of budesonide in one study of moderate asthma (172). Low-dose budesonide was superior to theophylline in the treatment of nocturnal asthma, and adding theophylline to budesonide provided no additional benefit (173). Theophylline is often used as prophylaxis for nocturnal asthma symptoms. However, salmeterol has similar efficacy and fewer side effects (174–177). In most comparison studies, more patients withdrew from theophylline treatment groups because of inability to tolerate the drug.

In the past, intravenous theophylline has been considered to be a standard therapy for status asthmaticus. However, recent studies in adults and children have reported that theophylline offers little additional benefit to corticosteroids and beta$_2$ agonists in hospitalized asthmatics (178–180).

Safety and Drug Interactions

Theophylline is a drug with a narrow therapeutic index. Serum levels should be monitored and maintained between 10 and 15 μg/mL. Many common drugs can double or triple serum theophylline levels. Severe and fatal toxicity may occur when serum levels exceed 25 μg/mL. In a 10-year prospective study of theophylline overdoses referred to the Massachusetts Poison Control Center, there were 356 cases in which the theophylline level was greater than 30 μg/mL. Seventy-four patients had arrhythmias, and 29 had seizures. Fifteen subjects died (181). Other toxic effects of theophylline include hypokalemia, hyperglycemia, encephalopathy, hyperthermia, and hypotension (182).

In addition to potentially life-threatening side effects, theophylline has unpleasant side effects that patients may find intolerable. Side effects such as headache, irritability, nausea, and insomnia may occur even when serum levels are within the therapeutic range.

Drugs that significantly elevate theophylline levels include clarithromycin, erythromycin, most of the quinolone antibiotics, cimetidine, disulfiram, estrogen, fluvoxamine, interferon-α, mexiletine, pentoxiphylline, propafenone, propranolol, tacrine, ticlopidine, thiabendazole, verapamil, and zileuton. Theophylline may decrease the effects of adenosine, diazepam, flurazepam, lithium, and pancuronium. Carbamazapine, phenobarbital, phenytoin, rifampin, and sulfinpyrazone may decrease theophylline levels (149). Theophylline is a category B drug in pregnancy.

Preparations and Dosing

Theophylline is usually prescribed in long-acting tablets or capsules, which come in a number of different dosages, to be administered once or twice a day. It is also available as uncoated tablets, encapsulated sprinkles, in suspension, and as a rectal suppository.

The dosage of theophylline is based on body weight. For children older than 6 months and adults, the starting dose should be 10 mg/kg up to a maximum initial dose of 300 mg/day. The dosage may be increased every 3 days, if tolerated, up to 16 mg/kg with a maximum dose of 600 mg/day. A serum level should be measured after at least 3 days at the maximum dose. The peak serum level occurs 8 to 13 hours after the sustained-release preparations and should be 10 to 15 μg/mL. Dosage requirements generally maintain stable, but concomitant medications and acute or chronic illness may alter serum levels (149).

REFERENCES

1. Murphy S, Kelly HW. Cromolyn sodium: a review of mechanisms and clinical use in asthma. *Drug Intel Clin Pharm* 1987;2(Part 1):22–35.
2. Parish RC, Miller L. Nedocromil sodium. *Ann Pharmacol* 1993;27:599–606.
3. Heinke S, Szucs G, Norris A, et al. Inhibition of volume-activated chloride currents in endothelial cells by cromones. *Br J Pharmacol* 1995;115:1393–1398.
4. Janssen LJ, Wattie J, Betti PA. Effects of cromolyn and nedocromil on ion currents in canine tracheal smooth muscle. *Eur Respir J* 1998;12:50–56.
5. Alton EW, Norris AA. Chloride transport and the actions of nedocromil sodium and cromolyn sodium in asthma. *J Allergy Clin Immunol* 1996;98(Part 2; suppl):102–105; discussion 105–106.
6. Alton EW, Kingsleigh-Smith DJ, Munkonge FM, et al. Asthma prophylaxis agents alter the function of an airway epithelial chloride channel. *Am J Respir Cell Mol Biol* 1996;14:380–387.
7. Norris AA, Alton EW. Chloride transport and the action of sodium cromoglycate and nedocromil sodium in asthma. *Clin Exp Allergy* 1996;26:250–253.
8. Okayama Y, Benyon RC, Rees PH, et al. Inhibition profiles of sodium cromoglycate and nedocromil sodium on mediator release from mast cells of human skin, lung, tonsil, adenoid and intestine. *Clin Exp Allergy* 1992;22:401–409.
9. Bissonette EY, Enisco JA, Befus AD. Inhibition of tumor necrosis factor release from mast cells by the anti-inflammatory drugs sodium cromoglycate and nedocromil sodium. *Clin Exp Immunol* 1995;102:78–84.
10. Flint KC, Leung KBP, Pearce FL. Human mast cells recovered by bronchoalveolar lavage: their morphology, histamine release and the effects of sodium cromoglycate. *Clin Sci* 1985;68:427–432.
11. Church MK, Young KO. The characteristics of inhibition of histamine release from human lung fragments by sodium cromoglycate, salbutamol, and chlorpromazine. *Br J Pharmacol* 1983;78:671–679.
12. Warringa RA, Mengelers HJ, Maikoe T, et al. Inhibition of cytokine-primed eosinophil chemotaxis by nedocromil sodium. *J Allergy Clin Immunol* 1993;9:802–809.
13. Manolitsas ND, Wang J, Devalia JL, et al. Regular albuterol, nedocromil sodium, and bronchial inflammation in asthma. *Am J Respir Crit Care Med* 1995;151:1925–1930.
14. Bruijnzeel PL, Waringa RA, Kok PT, et al. Effects of nedocromil sodium on in vitro induced migration, activation and mediator release from human granulocytes. *J Allergy Clin Immunol* 1993;92(Part 2):159–164.
15. Roca-Ferrer J, Mullol J, Lopez E, et al. Effect of topical anti-inflammatory drugs on epithelial cell-induced eosinophil survival and GM-CSF secretion. *Eur Respir J* 1997;10:1489–1495.
16. Hoshino M, Nakamura Y. The effect of inhaled sodium cromoglycate on cellular infiltration into the bronchial mucosal and the expression of adhesion molecules in asthmatics. *Eur Respir J* 1997;10:858–65.
17. Klein LM, Lavaker RM, Matis WL, et al. Degranulation of human mast cells induces an endothelial antigen central to leukocyte adhesion. *Proc Natl Acad Sci USA* 1989;86:8972–8976.
18. Sacco O, Lantero S, Scarso L, et al. Modulation of HLA-DR antigen and ICAM-1 molecule expression on airway epithelial cells by sodium nedocromil. *Gen Pharmacol* 1998;31:545–552.
19. Jahnova E, Horvathova M, Gazdik F: Expression of adhesion molecules and effects of disodium cromoglycate treatment in asthmatics. *Physiol Res* 1998;47:439–443.

20. Matsuse H, Shimoda T, Matsuo N, Obase Y, et al. Sodium cromoglycate inhibits antigen-induced cytokine production by peripheral blood mononuclear cells from atopic asthmatics in vitro. *Ann Allergy Asthma Immunol* 1999;83(Part 1):522–525.

21. Louis RE, Radermeker MF. Substance P–induced histamine release from human basophils, skin, and lung fragments: effect of nedocromil sodium and theophylline. *Int Arch Allergy Appl Immunol* 1990 92:329–333.

22. Heiman AS, Newton L. Effect of hydrocortisone and disodium cromoglycate on mast cell-mediator release induced by substance P. *Pharmacology* 1995;50:218–228.

23. Yamawaki I, Tomaoki J, Takeda Y, et al. Inhaled cromoglycate reduces airway neurogenic inflammation via tachykinin antagonism. *Res Commun Mol Pathol Pharmacol* 1997;98:265–272.

24. Dixon CM, Barnes PJ. Bradykinin-induced bronchoconstriction: inhibition by nedocromil sodium and sodium cromoglycate. *Br J Pharmacol* 1989;27:831–836.

25. Barnes PJ. Effect of nedocromil sodium on airway sensory nerves. *J Allergy Clin Immunol* 1993;92(Part 2):182–186.

26. Crimi N, Palermo F, Oliveri R, et al. Protection of nedocromil sodium on bronchoconstriction induced by inhaled neurokinin A (NKA) in asthmatic patients. *Clin Exp Allergy* 1992;22:75–81.

27. Loh RK, Jabara HH, Geha RS. Disodium cromoglycate inhibits $S_\mu \to S_\epsilon$ deletion and switch recombination and IgE synthesis in human B cells. *J Exp Med* 1994;180:663–671.

28. Loh RK, Jabara HH, Geha RS. Mechanisms of Inhibition of IgE synthesis by nedocromil sodium: nedocromil sodium inhibits deletional switch recombination in human B cells. *J Allergy Clin Immunol* 1996;97:1141–1150.

29. Pelikan Z, Pelikan-Filipek M, Schoemaker MC, et al. Effects of disodium cromoglycate and beclomethasone dipropionate on the asthmatic response to allergen challenge I. Immediate response (IAR). *Ann Allergy* 1988;60:211–6.

30. Pelikan Z, Pelikan-Filipek M, Remijer L. Effects of disodium cromoglycate and beclomethasone dipropionate on the late asthmatic response to allergen challenge II. Late allergic response (LAR). *Ann Allergy* 1988;60:217–225.

31. Calhoun WJ, Jarjour NN, Gleich GJ, et al. Effect of nedocromil sodium pretreatment on the immediate and late responses of the airway to segmental antigen challenge. *J Allergy Clin Immunol* 1996;98(Part 2; suppl):46–50.

32. Pelikan Z, Knotternerus I. Inhibition of the late asthmatic response by nedocromil sodium administered more than two hours after allergen challenge. *J Allergy Clin Immunol* 1993;92(Part 1):19–28.

33. del Bufalo C, Fasano L, Patalano F, et al. Inhibition of fog-induced bronchoconstriction by nedocromil sodium and sodium cromoglycate in intrinsic asthma: a double-blind, placebo controlled study. *Respiration* 1989;55:181–5.

34. Davies SE. Effect of sodium cromoglycate on exercise-induced asthma. *BMJ* 1968;3;593–599.

35. Breslin FJ, McFadden ER, Ingram RH. The effects of cromolyn sodium on the airway response to hyperpnea and cold air in asthma. *Am Rev Respir Dis* 1980;122: 11–16.

36. Ryo UY, Kang B, Townley RG. Cromolyn therapy in patients with bronchial asthma. Effect on inhalation challenge with allergen, histamine, and methacholine. *JAMA* 1976;236;927–931.

37. Patel KR. Sodium cromoglycate in histamine and methacholine reactivity in asthma. *Clin Allergy* 1984;14;143–145.

38. Griffin MP, Macdonald N, McFadden ER. Short- and long-term effect of cromolyn sodium on the airway of asthmatics. *J Allergy Clin Immunol* 1983;71:331–338.

39. Crimi E, Brusasco V, Brancatisano M, et al. Effect of nedocromil sodium on adenosine- and methacholine-induced bronchospasm in asthma. *Clin Allergy* 1987;17:135–141.

40. Bel EH, Timmers MC, Hermans J, et al. The long-term effects of nedocromil sodium and beclomethasone dipropionate on bronchial hyperresponsiveness to methacholine in nonatopic asthmatic subjects. *Am Rev Respir Dis* 1990;141:21–28.

41. Orefice U, Struzzo P, Dorigo R, et al. Long term treatment with sodium cromoglycate, nedocromil sodium and beclomethasone dipropionate reduces bronchial hyperresponsiveness in asthmatic subjects. *Respiration* 1992;59:97–101.

42. Konig P. The effects of cromolyn sodium and nedocromil sodium in early asthma prevention. *J Allergy Clin Immunol* 2000;105(Part 2):575–581.

43. Lal S, Dorow PD, Venho KK, et al. Nedocromil sodium is more effective than cromolyn sodium for the treatment of chronic reversible obstructive airway disease. *Chest* 1993;104:438–447.

44. Boldy DA, Ayers JG. Nedocromil sodium and sodium cromoglycate in patients aged over 50 years with asthma. *Respir Med* 1993;87:517–523.

45. Schwartz HJ, Blumenthal M, Brady R, et al. A comparative study of nedocromil sodium and placebo. How does cromolyn sodium compare as an active control treatment? *Chest* 1996;109:945–952.

46. Konig P, Hordvik NL, Kreutz C. The preventive effect and duration of action of nedocromil sodium and cromolyn sodium on exercise-induced asthma (EIA) in adults. *J Allergy Clin Immunol* 1987;79:64–68.

47. De Benedictis FM, Tuteri G, Pazelli P, et al. Cromolyn versus nedocromil: duration of action in exercise-induced asthma in children. *J Allergy Clin Immunol* 1995;96:510–514.

48. Creticos P, Burk J, Smith L, et al. The use of twice daily nedocromil sodium in the treatment of asthma. *J Allergy Clin Immunol* 1995;95:829–836.

49. Svendsen UG, Frolund L, Madsen F, et al. A comparison of the effects of sodium cromoglycate and beclomethasone dipropionate on pulmonary function and bronchial hyperreactivity in subjects with asthma. *J Allergy Clin Immunol* 1987;80:68–74.

50. Svendsen UG, Frolund L, Madsen F, et al. A comparison of the effects of nedocromil sodium and beclomethasone dipropionate on pulmonary function, symptoms and bronchial responsiveness in patients with asthma. *J Allergy Clin Immunol* 1989;84:224–231.

51. Peden DB, Bergen WE, Noonan MJ, et al. Inhaled fluticasone proprionate delivered by means of two different multidose powder inhalers is effective and safe in a large

pediatric population with persistent asthma. *J Allergy Clin Immunol* 1998;102:32–38.

52. Jarvis B, Faulds D. Inhaled fluticasone proprionate: a review of its therapeutic efficacy at dosages < or = 500 microg/day in adults and adolescents with mild to moderate asthma. *Drugs* 1999;57:769–803.

53. Boulet LP, Cartier A, Cockcroft DW, et al. Tolerance to reduction of oral steroid dosage in severely asthmatic patients receiving nedocromil sodium. *Respir Med* 1990;84:317–323.

54. Wong CS, Cooper S, Britton JR, et al. Steroid sparing effect of nedocromil sodium in asthmatic patients on high doses of inhaled steroids. *Clin Exp Allergy* 1993;23:370–376.

55. O'Hickey SP, Rees PJ. High-dose nedocromil sodium as an addition to inhaled corticosteroids in the treatment of asthma. *Respir Med* 1994;88:499–502.

56. Bone R, Kubik MM, Keany NP, et al. Nedocromil sodium in adults with asthma dependent on inhaled corticosteroids: a double blind, placebo controlled study. *Thorax* 1989;44:654–659.

57. Goldin JG, Bateman E. Does nedocromil sodium have a steroid sparing effect in adult asthmatic patients requiring maintenance oral corticosteroids? *Thorax* 1988;43:982–986.

58. Furakawa CT, Shapiro GG, Bierman CW, et al. A double-blind study comparing the effectiveness of cromolyn sodium and sustained release theophylline in childhood asthma. *Pediatrics* 1984;74:453–459.

59. Callaghan B, Teo NC, Clancy L. Effects of the addition of nedocromil sodium to maintenance bronchodilator therapy in the management of chronic asthma. *Chest* 1992;101:787–792.

60. Crimi E, Orefice U, De Beneditto F, et al. Nedocromil sodium versus theophylline in the treatment of reversible obstructive airway disease. *Ann Allergy Asthma Immunol* 1995;74:501–508.

61. Hendeles L, Harman E, Huang D, et al. Theophylline attenuation of airway response to allergen: comparison with cromolyn metered-dose inhaler. *J Allergy Clin Immunol* 1995;95:505–514.

62. Rohr AS, Siegel SC, Katz RM, et al. A comparison of inhaled albuterol and cromolyn in the prophylaxis of exercise-induced bronchospasm. *Ann Allergy* 1987;59:107–109.

63. Hargreaves MR, Benson MK. Inhaled cromoglycate in angiotensin-converting enzyme inhibitor cough. *Lancet* 1995;345:13–16.

64. National Asthma Education Program Expert Panel Report 2. Guidelines for the diagnosis and management of asthma. NHLBI, NIH Publication No. 97-4051, April 1997.

65. Samuelsson B, Dahlen SE, Lindgren JA, et al. Leukotrienes and lipoxins: structures, biosynthesis, and biological effects. *Science* 1987;237:1171–1176.

66. Holgate ST, Bradding P, Sampson AP. Leukotriene antagonists and synthesis inhibitors: new direction in asthma therapy. *J Allergy Clin Immunol* 1996;98:1–13.

67. Christie PE, Tagari P, Fordhutchinson AW, et al. Urinary leukotriene-E4 concentrations in aspirin-sensitive asthmatic subjects. *Am Rev Respir Dis* 1991;143 (Part 1):1025–1029.

68. Israel E, Fischer AR, Rosenberg MA, et al. The pivotal role of 5-lipoxygenase products in the reaction of aspirin-sensitive asthmatics to aspirin. *Am Rev Respir Dis* 1993;148(Part 1):1447–1451.

69. Cowburn AS, Sladek K, Soja J, et al. Overexpression of leukotriene C4 synthetase in bronchial biopsies from patients with aspirin-intolerant asthma. *J Clin Invest* 1998;101:834–846.

70. Ferreri NR, Howland WC, Stevenson DD, et al. Release of leukotrienes, prostaglandins, and histamine into nasal secretions of aspirin-sensitive asthmatics during reactions to aspirin. *Am Rev Respir Dis* 1988;137:847–854.

71. Wenzel SE, Trudeau JB, Kaminsky DA, et al. Effect of 5-lipoxygenase inhibition on bronchoconstriction and airway inflammation in nocturnal asthma. *Am J Respir Crit Care Med* 1995;152:879–905.

72. Kane GC, Pollice M, Kim CJ, et al. A controlled trial of the effect of the 5-lipoxygenase inhibitor zileuton on lung inflammation produced by segmental antigen challenge in human beings. *J Allergy Clin Immunol* 1996;97:646–654.

73. Munoz NM, Douglas I, Mayer D, et al. Eosinophil chemotaxis inhibited by 5-lipoxygenase blockade and leukotriene antagonism. *Am J Respir Crit Care Med* 1997;155:1398–1403.

74. Pizzichini E, Leff JA, Reiss TF, et al. Montelukast reduces airway eosinophilic inflammation in asthma. *Eur Respir J* 1999;14:12–18.

75. Volvovitz B, Tabachnik E, Nussinovitch M, et al. Montelukast, a leukotriene receptor antagonist, reduces the concentration of leukotrienes in the respiratory tract of children with persistent asthma. *J Allergy Clin Immunol* 1999;104:1162–1167.

76. Calhoun WJ, Lavins BJ, Minkwitz et al. Effect of zafirlukast (Accolate) on cellular mediators of inflammation: bronchoalveolar lavage fluid findings after segmental antigen challenge. *Am Rev Respir Crit Care Med* 1998;157(Part 1):1381–1389.

77. Taylor IK, O'Shaunessey KM, Fuller RW, et al. Effect of cysteinyl- leukotriene receptor antagonist ICI 204.219 on allergen-induced bronchoconstriction and airway hyperreactivity in atopic subjects. *Lancet* 1991;337:690–694.

78. Gaddy JN, Margoskee DJ, Bush RK, et al. Bronchodilation with a potent and selective leukotriene D4 (LTD4) receptor antagonist (MK-571) in patients with asthma. *Am Rev Respir Dis* 1992;146:358–363.

79. Reiss TF, Sorkness CA, Stricker W, et al. Effects of montelukast (MK-0476); a potent cysteinyl leukotriene receptor antagonist, on bronchodilation in asthmatic subjects treated with and without corticosteroids. *Thorax* 1997;52:45–48.

80. Findlay SR, Barden JM, Easley CB, et al. Effect of the oral leukotriene antagonist ICI 204.219 on antigen-induced bronchoconstriction in subjects with asthma. *J Allergy Clin Immunol* 1992;89:1040–1045.

81. Diamant Z, Grootendorst DC, Veselic-Charvat M, et al. The effect of montelukast (MK-0476), a cysteinyl leukotriene receptor antagonist, on allergen-induced airway responses and sputum cell counts in asthma. *Clin Exp Allergy* 1999;2:42–51.

82. Hui KP, Taylor GW, Rubin P. Effect of a 5-lipoxygenase inhibitor on leukotriene generation and airway responses after allergen challenge in asthmatic patients. *Thorax* 1991;46:184–189.

83. Manning PJ, Watson RM, Margolskee DJ, et al. Inhibition of exercise-induced bronchoconstriction by MK-571, a potent leukotriene D4 receptor antagonist. *N Engl J Med* 1990;323:1736–1739.

84. Finnerty JP, Wood-Baker R, Thompson H, et al. Role of leukotrienes in exercise-induced asthma. Inhibitory effect of ICI 204.219, a potent leukotriene D_4 receptor antagonist. *Am Rev Respir Dis* 1992;145(Part 1):746–749.

85. Reiss TF, Hill JB, Harman E, et al. Increased urinary excretion of LTE_4 after exercise and attenuation of exercise-induced bronchospasm by montelukast, a cysteinyl leukotriene receptor antagonist. *Thorax* 1997;52:1030–1035.

86. Meltzer SS, Hasday JD, Cohn J, et al. Inhibition of exercise-induced bronchospasm by zileuton: a 5-lipoxygenase inhibitor. *Am J Respir Crit Care Med* 1996;153:931–935.

87. Lazarus SC, Wong HH, Watts MJ, et al. The leukotriene receptor antagonist zafirlukast inhibits sulfur dioxide–induced bronchoconstriction in patients with asthma. *Am J Respir Crit Care Med* 1997;156:1725–1730.

88. Richter K, Jorres RA, Magnussen H. Efficacy and duration of the antileukotriene zafirlukast on cold air-induced bronchoconstriction. *Eur Respir J* 2000;15:693–699.

89. Israel E, Demarkarian R, Rosenberg M, et al. The effects of a 5-lipoxygenase inhibitor on asthma induced by cold, dry air. *N Engl J Med* 1990;323:1140–1144.

90. Israel E, Fischer AR, Rosenberg MA, et al. The pivotal role of 5-lipoxygenase products in the reaction of aspirin-sensitive asthmatics to aspirin. *Am Rev Respir Dis* 1993;148(Part 1):1447–1451.

91. Dahlen B, Kumlin M, Margolskee DJ, et al. The leukotriene-receptor antagonist MK-0679 blocks airway obstruction induced by inhaled lysine-aspirin in aspirin-sensitive asthmatics. *Eur Respir J* 1993;6:1018–1026.

92. Leff JA, Busse WW, Pearlman D, et al. Montelukast, a leukotriene-receptor antagonist, for the treatment of mild asthma and exercise-induced bronchoconstriction. *N Eng J Med* 1998;339:147–152.

93. Israel E, Cohn J, Dube L, et al. Effect of treatment with zileuton, a 5-lipoxygenase inhibitor, in patients with chronic asthma. A randomized controlled trial. Zileuton Clinical Trial Group. *JAMA* 1996;275:931–936.

94. Liu MC, Dube LM, Lancaster J. Acute and chronic effects of a 5-lipoxygenase inhibitor in asthma: a 6-month randomized multicenter trial. Zileuton Study Group. *J Allergy Clin Immunol* 1996;98(Part 1):859–871.

95. Nathan RA, Bernstein JA, Bonuccelli, et al. Zafirlukast improves asthma and quality of life in patients with moderate reversible airflow obstruction. *J Allergy Clin Immunol* 1998;102(Part 1):935–942.

96. Kemp JP, Minkwitz MC, Bonuccelli CM, et al. Therapeutic effect of zafirlukast as monotherapy in steroid-naïve patients with severe persistent asthma. *Chest* 1999;115:336–342.

97. Grossman J, Smith LJ, Wilson AM, et al. Long-term safety and efficacy of zafirlukast in the treatment of asthma: interim results of an open-label trial. *Ann Allergy Immunol* 1999;82:361–369.

98. Altman LC, Munk Z, Seltzer J, et al. A placebo-controlled, dose-ranging study of montelukast, a cysteinyl leukotriene-receptor antagonist. Montelukast Asthma Study Group. *J Allergy Clin Immunol* 1998;102:50–56.

99. Reiss TF, Chervinsky P, Dockhorn RJ, et al. Montelukast, a once-daily leukotriene antagonist, in the treatment of chronic asthma: a multicenter, randomized, double-blind trial. Montelukast Clinical Research Study Group. *Arch Intern Med* 1998;158:1213–1220.

100. Knorr B, Maltz J, Bernstein JA, et al. Montelukast for chronic asthma in 6- to 14-year old children: a randomized, double-blind trial. Pediatric Montelukast Study Group. *JAMA* 1998;279:1181–1186.

101. Malmstrom K, Rodriguez-Gomez G, Guerra J, et al. Oral montelukast, inhaled beclomethasone, and placebo for chronic asthma. A randomized, controlled trial. Montelukast/Beclomethasone Study Group. *Ann Intern Med* 1999;130:487–495.

102. Bleeker ER, Welch MJ, Weinstein SF, et al. Low-dose inhaled fluticasone proprionate versus oral zafirlukast in the treatment of persistent asthma. *J Allergy Clin Immunol* 2000;105(Part 1):1123–1129.

103. Nayak AS, Anderson PJ, Charous BL, et al. Addition of zafirlukast compared with a doubled dosage of inhaled corticosteroids in asthmatic patients with symptoms on inhaled corticosteroids [Abstract]. *Eur Respir J* 1998;12(Suppl 28):361.

104. Laviolette M, Malmstrom K, Lu S, et al. Montelukast added to inhaled beclomethasone in treatment of asthma. Montelukast/Beclomethasone Additivity Group. *Am J Respir Crit Care Med* 1999;160:1862–1868.

105. Lofdahl CG, Reiss TF, Leff JA, et al. Randomised, placebo controlled trial of effect of a leukotriene receptor antagonist, montelukast, on tapering inhaled corticosteroids in asthmatic patients. *BMJ* 1999;319:87–90.

106. Tamaoki J, Kondo M, Sakai N, et al. Leukotriene antagonist prevents exacerbation of asthma during reduction of high-dose inhaled corticosteroid. The Tokyo Joshi-Idai Asthma Research Group. *Am J Respir Crit Care Med* 1997;155:1235–1240.

107. Schwartz HJ, Petty T, Dube LM, et al. A randomized controlled trial comparing zileuton with theophylline in moderate asthma. *Arch Intern Med* 1998;158:141–148.

108. Busse W, Nelson H, Wolfe J, et al. Comparison of inhaled salmeterol and oral zafirlukast in patients with asthma. *J Allergy Clin Immunol* 1999;103:1075–1080.

109. Villaran C, O'Neill SJ, Helbling A, et al. Montelukast versus salmeterol in patients with asthma and exercise-induced bronchoconstriction. Montelukast/Salmeterol Study Group. *J Allergy Clin Immunol* 1999;104(Part 1):547–553.

110. Edelman JM, Turpin JA, Bronsky EA, et al. Oral montelukast compared with inhaled salmeterol to prevent exercise-induced bronchoconstriction. A randomized, double-blind trial. Exercise Study Group. *Ann Intern Med* 2000;132:97–104.

111. Nathan RA, Minkwitz MC, Bonuccelli CM. Two first-line therapies in the treatment of mild asthma: use of peak flow variability as a predictor of effectiveness. *Ann Allergy Asthma Immunol* 1999;82:497–503.

112. Zyflo Filmtab (zileuton tablets). In: *Physicians' desk reference,* 53rd ed. Montvale, NJ: Medical Economics Co., 1999:481–483.

113. Wechsler ME, Garpestad E, Flier SR, et al. Pulmonary infiltrates, eosinophilia, and cardiomyopathy following corticosteroid withdrawal in patients with asthma receiving zafirlukast. *JAMA* 1998;279:455–457.

114. Franco J, Artes MJ. Pulmonary eosinophilia associated with montelukast. *Thorax* 1999;54:558–560.

115. Wechsler ME, Finn D, Gunwardena D, et al. Churg-Strauss syndrome in patients receiving montelukast as treatment for asthma. *Chest* 2000;117:708–713.

116. Wechsler ME, Pauwels R, Drazen JM. *Drug Saf* 1999;21:241–251.

117. Awni WM, Hussein Z, Granneman GR, et al. Pharmacodynamic and stereoselective pharmacokinetic interactions between zileuton and warfarin in humans, *Clin Pharmacokinet* 1995;29(suppl 2):67–76.

118. Adkins JC, Brogden RN. Zafirlukast. A review of its pharmacology and therapeutic potential in the management of asthma. *Drugs* 1998;55:121–144.

119. Granneman GR, Braeckman RA, Locke CS, et al. Effect of zileuton on theophylline kinetics. *Clin Pharmacokinet* 1995;29(suppl 2):77–83.

120. American College of Obstetrics and Gynecology and American College of Allergy Asthma Immunology. The use of newer allergy and asthma medications during pregnancy. *Ann Asthma Allergy Immunol* 2000;84:476–480.

121. Barnes PJ. Neural control of human airways in health and disease. *Am Rev Respir Dis* 1986;134:1289–1314.

122. Ingram RH, Wellman JJ, McFadden ER, et al. Relative contributions of large and small airways to flow limitation in normal subjects before and after atropine and isoproterenol. *J Clin Invest* 1977;59:696–703.

123. Barnes PJ. Cholinergic control of airway smooth muscle. *Am Rev Respir Dis* 1987;136(Part 2):542–545.

124. Fryer AD, el-Fakahany EE. Identification of three muscarinic receptor subtypes in rat lung using binding studies with selective antagonists. *Life Sci* 1990;47:611–618.

125. Fryer AD, Maclagan J. Ipratropium bromide potentiates bronchoconstriction induced by vagal nerve stimulation in the guinea pig. *Eur J Pharmacol* 1987;139:187–191.

126. Gross NJ. Ipratropium bromide. *N Engl J Med* 1988;319:486–494.

127. Hensley MJ, O'Cain CF, McFadden ER, et al. Distribution of bronchodilatation in normal subjects: beta agonist versus atropine. *J Appl Physiol* 1978;45:778–782.

128. Morris HG. Review of ipratropium bromide in induced bronchospasm in patients with asthma. *Am J Med* 1986;81:36–44.

129. deVries K. The protective effect of Sch 1000 MDI on bronchoconstriction induced by serotonin, histamine, acetylcholine and propranolol [Abstract]. *Postgrad Med J* 1975;51(Suppl 77):106.

130. Brown JH, Taylor P. Muscarinic receptor agonists and antagonists. In: Hardman JG, Gilman AG, Limbird LE, eds. *Goodman and Gilman's the pharmacological basis of therapeutics,* 9th ed. New York: McGraw Hill, 1996:144–160.

131. Ali-Melkkila T, Kanto J, Iisalo E. Pharmacokinetics and related pharmacodynamics of anticholinergic drugs. *Acta Anaesthesiol Scand* 1993;37:633–642.

132. Wanner A. Effect of ipratropium bromide on mucociliary clearance. *Am J Med* 1986;81:23–27.

133. Ruffin RE, Fitzgerald JD, Rebuck AS. A comparison of the bronchodilator activity of Sch 1000 and salbutamol. *J Allergy Clin Immunol* 1977;59:136–141.

134. Burge PS, Harries MG, I'Anson E. Comparison of atropine with ipratropium bromide in patients with reversible airways obstruction unresponsive to salbutamol. *Br J Dis Chest* 1980;74:259–262.

135. Brown IG, Chan CS, Kelley CA, et al. Assessment of the clinical usefulness of nebulized ipratropium bromide in patients with chronic airflow limitation. *Thorax* 1984;39:272–276.

136. Ind PW, Dixon CMS, Fuller RW, et al. Anticholinergic blockade of beta-blocker induced bronchoconstriction. *Am Rev Respir Dis* 1989;139:1390–1394.

137. McFadden ER, Luparello T, Lyons HA, et al. The mechanism of action of suggestion in the induction of acute asthma attacks. *J Psychosom Med* 1969;31:134–143.

138. Neild JE, Cameron IR. Bronchoconstriction in response to suggestion: its prevention by an anticholinergic agent. *BJM* 1985;290:674.

139. Stoodley RG, Aaron SD, Dales RE. The role of ipratropium bromide in the emergency management of acute asthma exacerbation: a metaanalysis of randomized clinical trials. *Ann Emerg Med* 1999;34:8–18.

140. Kaiser HB, Findlay SR, Georgitis JW, et al. Long-term treatment of perennial allergic rhinitis with ipratropium bromide nasal spray 0.06%. *J Allergy Clin Immunol* 1995;95(Part 2):1128–1132.

141. Georgitis JW, Banov C, Boggs PB, et al. Ipratropium bromide nasal spray in non-allergic rhinitis: efficacy, nasal cytological response and patient evaluation on quality of life. *Clin Exp Allergy* 1994;24:1049–1055.

142. Hayden FG, Diamond L, Wood PB, et al. Effectiveness and safety of intranasal ipratropium bromide in common colds. *Ann Intern Med* 1996;125:89–97.

143. Hall SK. Acute angle-closure glaucoma as a complication of combined beta- agonist and ipratropium bromide therapy in the emergency department. *Ann Emerg Med* 1994;23:884–887.

144. Kizer KM, Bess DT, Bedford NK. Blurred vision from ipratropium bromide inhalation. *Am J Health Syst Pharm* 1999;56:941.

145. Cabana MD, Johnson H, Lee CK, et al. Transient anisocoria secondary to nebulized ipratropium bromide. *Clin Pediatr* 1998;31:445–447.

146. Serafin WE. Drugs used in the treatment of asthma: methylxanthines. In: Hardman JG, Gilman AG, Limbird LE, eds. *Goodman and Gilman's the pharmacological basis of therapeutics,* 9th ed. New York: McGraw Hill, 1996: 659–682.

147. Jusko WJ, Gardner MJ, Mangione A, et al. Factors affecting theophylline clearances: age, tobacco, marijuana, cirrhosis, congestive heart failure, obesity, oral contraceptives, benzodiazapines, and ethanol. *J Pharm Sci* 1979;68:1358–1366.

148. Jenne JW. Effect of disease states on theophylline elimination. *J Allergy Clin Immunol* 1986;78(Part 2):727–735.

149. Weinberger M, Hendeles L. Theophylline in asthma. *N Engl J Med* 1996;334:1380–1388.

150. Rabe KF, Magnussen H, Dent G. Theophylline and selective PDE inhibitors as bronchodilators and smooth muscle relaxants. *Eur Respir J* 1995;8:637–642.

151. Easton PA, Anthionisen NR. Ventilatory response to sustained hypoxia after pretreatment with aminophylline. *J Appl Physiol* 1988;64:1445–1450.

152. Murciano D, Aubier M, Lecocguic Y, et al. Effects of theophylline on diaphragmatic strength and fatigue in patients with chronic obstructive pulmonary disease. *N Engl J Med* 1984;311:349–353.

153. Cotromanes E, Gerrity TR, Garrard CS, et al. Aerosol penetration and mucociliary transport in the healthy human lung: effect of low serum theophylline levels. *Chest* 1985;88:194–200.

154. Aizawa H, Iwanaga T, Inoue H, et al. Once-daily theophylline reduces serum eosinophil levels in induced

sputum of asthmatics. *Int Arch Allergy Immunol* 2000;121:123–128.

155. Horiguchi T, Tachikawa S, Kasahara J, et al. Suppression of airway inflammation by theophylline in adult bronchial asthma. *Respiration* 1999;66:124–127.

156. Minoguchi K, Kohno Y, Oda N, et al. Effect of theophylline withdrawal on airway inflammation in asthma. *Clin Exp Allergy* 1998;28(suppl 3):57–63.

157. Finnerty JP, Lee C, Wilson S, et al. Effects of theophylline on inflammatory cells and cytokines in asthmatic subjects: a placebo-controlled parallel group study. *Eur Respir J* 1996;9:1672–1677.

158. Dujanovic R, Finnerty JP, Lee C, et al. The effects of theophylline on mucosal inflammation in asthmatic airways: biopsy results. *Eur Respir J* 1995;8:831–833.

159. McWilliams BC, Menendes R, Kelley HW, et al. Effects of theophylline on inhaled methacholine and histamine in asthmatic children. *Am Rev Respir Dis* 1984;130:193–197.

160. Magnussen H, Reuss G, Jorres R. Theophylline has a dose-related effect on the airway response to inhaled methacholine in asthmatics. *Am Rev Respir Dis* 1987;136:1163–1167.

161. Koeter GH, Kraan J, Boorsma M, et al. Effect of theophylline and enprophylline on bronchial hyperresponsiveness. *Thorax* 1989;44:1022–1026.

162. Cockcroft DW, Murdock KY, Gore BP, et al. Theophylline does not inhibit allergen-induced increase in airway responsiveness to methacholine. *J Allergy Clin Immunol* 1989;83:913–920.

163. Hendeles L, Harman E, Huang D, et al. Theophylline attenuation of airway responses to allergen: comparison with cromolyn metered-dose inhaler. *J Allergy Clin Immunol* 1995;95:505–514.

164. Kraft M, Pak J, Martin RJ. Theophylline's effect on neutrophil function and the late asthmatic response. *J Allergy Clin Immunol* 1996;98:251–257.

165. Hambleton G, Weinberger M, Ginchansky E, et al. Comparison of cromoglycate and theophylline in controlling symptoms of chronic asthma. *Lancet* 1977;1:381–385.

166. Furakawa CT, Shapiro GG, Bierman CW. A double-blind study comparing the effectiveness of cromolyn sodium and sustained-release theophylline in childhood asthma. *Pediatrics* 1984;74:453–459.

167. Schwartz HJ, Petty T, Dube LM, et al. A randomized controlled trial comparing zileuton with theophylline in moderate asthma. *Arch Intern Med* 1998;158:141–148.

168. Pierson WE, Laforce CF, Bell TD, et al. Long-term, double-blind comparison of controlled-release albuterol versus theophylline in adolescents and adults with asthma. *J Allergy Clin Immunol* 1990;85:618–626.

169. Rivington RN, Boulet LP, Cote J. Efficacy of uniphyl,

salbutamol, and their combination in asthmatic patients on high-dose inhaled steroids. *Am J Respir Crit Care Med* 1995;151(Part 1):325–332.

170. Reed CE, Offord KP, Nelson HS, et al. Aerosol beclomethasone dipropionate spray compared with theophylline as primary treatment for chronic mild-to-moderate asthma. The American Academy of Allergy, Asthma and Immunology Beclomethasone-Theophylline Study Group. *J Allergy Clin Immunol* 1998; 101(Part 1):14–23.

171. Gallant SP, Lawrence M, Meltzer EO, et al. Fluticasone proprionate compared with theophylline for mild-to-moderate asthma. *Ann Allergy Asthma Immunol* 1996;77:112–118.

172. Evans DJ, Taylor DA, Zetterson O, et al. A comparison of low-dose inhaled budesonide plus theophylline and high-dose budesonide for moderate asthma. *N Engl J Med* 1997;337:1412–1418.

173. Youngchaiyud P, Permpikul C, Suthamsmai T, et al. A double-blind comparison of inhaled budesonide, long-acting theophylline, and their combination in treatment of nocturnal asthma. *Allergy* 1995;50:28–33.

174. Fjellbirkeland L, Gulsvik A, Palmer JB. The efficacy and tolerability of inhaled salmeterol and individually dose-titrated, sustained-release theophylline in patients with reversible airways disease. *Respir Med* 1994;88:599–607.

175. Pollard SJ, Spector SL, Yancey SW, et al. Salmeterol versus theophylline in the treatment of asthma. *Ann Allergy Clin Immunol* 1997;78:457–464.

176. Selby C, Engleman HM, Fitzpatrick MF, et al. Inhaled salmeterol or oral theophylline in nocturnal asthma? *Am J Respir Crit Care Med* 1997;155:104–108.

177. Davies B, Brooks G, Devoy M. The efficacy and safety of salmeterol compared to theophylline: meta-analysis of nine controlled studies. *Respir Med* 1998;92:256–263.

178. Self TH, Abou-Shala N, Burns R, et al. Inhaled albuterol and oral prednisone therapy in hospitalized asthmatics. Does aminophylline add any benefit? *Chest* 1990;98:1317–1321.

179. Carter E, Cruz M, Chesrown S, et al. Efficacy of intravenously administered theophylline in children hospitalized with severe asthma. *J Pediatr* 1993;122:470–476.

180. Murphy DG, McDermott MF, Rydman RJ, et al. Aminophylline in the treatment of acute asthma when β_2-adrenergics and steroids are provided. *Arch Intern Med* 1993;153:1784–1788.

181. Shannon M. Life-threatening events after theophylline overdose: a 10-year prospective analysis. *Arch Intern Med* 1999;159:989–994.

182. Sessler CN. Theophylline toxicity: clinical features of 116 consecutive cases. *Am J Med* 1990;88:567–576.

37

Delivery Devices for Inhaled Medications

Theodore M. Lee

Peachtree Allergy and Asthma Clinic, P.C., and Emory University School of Medicine, Atlanta, Georgia

INTRODUCTION

History of Inhalation Therapy

Inhalation therapy for bronchial disorders has been used since ancient times, initially in the form of cigarettes containing stramonium, a botanically derived antimuscarinic agent. The stramonium cigarette was smoked as a treatment for acute asthma (1,2). In the early part of the 20th century, hand-held glass atomizers driven by rubber bulbs were used to aerosolize bronchodilator medications such as epinephrine (3). Nebulizers incorporating an internal baffle to remove excessively large particles were introduced in the 1930s; subsequently, a continuous air supply was obtained by attaching pumps to the nebulizer. A few years later, a smaller, easier to use nebulizer apparatus were marketed (4). Pressurized metered-dose inhalers (MDIs) containing isoproterenol or epinephrine in an inert propellant were introduced in the 1950s (5). The first dry powder inhaler (DPI) was launched in the 1970s as the delivery device for cromolyn sodium.

Inhalation devices in use today include conventional pressurized MDIs, used with or without holding chambers, breath-actuated MDIs, nebulizers, and a variety of DPIs.

Particle Size

A synopsis of the significance of particle size in inhalation therapy is a necessary preface to a clinically oriented discussion of aerosol devices. The desirable size for pharmaceutical aerosols is 2 to 5 μm. Particles larger than 5 μm penetrate into the bronchi poorly, but are potentially systemically absorbed if swallowed. Particles under 2 μm are not deposited into the airways and are either exhaled or are deposited in alveoli (6,7) (Table 37.1) with minimal if any clinical benefit in the usual applications, but with occurrence of systemic absorption. The term *fine particle mass* is used for the percentage of the emitted dose that is in the respirable range, less than or equal to 5 μm (8). With most devices used for aerosol therapy, fine particle mass typically ranges from 10% to 25%. Deposition into peripheral airways relative to central airways is maximal at 2 to 3 μm (9).

METERED-DOSE INHALERS

Propellants

Until recently, the propellants used in all pressurized MDIs have been chlorofluorocarbons known as Freon compounds. A mixture of several structurally similar compounds is used to obtain desired aerosol characteristics. Freon compounds are nonflammable and are unreactive under usual circumstances, characteristics favorable for their use as aerosol propellants and in their major historical application, refrigerator technology. However, it has become apparent that Freon compounds have serious negative effects on the environment. After release into the atmosphere, they rise to the stratosphere where they are eventually decomposed by ultraviolet solar radiation (10).

TABLE 37.1. *Deposition of aerosols*

Particle diameter (μm)	Percentage deposition			
	Oropharynx	Tracheobronchial	Alveolar	Exhaled
1	0	0	16	84
2	0	2	40	58
3	5	7	50	38
4	20	12	42	26
5	37	16	30	17
6	52	21	17	10
7	56	25	11	8
8	60	28	5	7

Adapted from references 6, 7, and 92; with permission.

As a result of the decomposition, chlorine radicals are released that react with and deplete stratospheric ozone (11). An intact stratospheric ozone layer shields the earth's surface from ultraviolet radiation. Increased penetration of ultraviolet radiation occurring as a consequence of ozone depletion has several harmful effects, which include increased incidence of skin cancers and cataracts (12). For these reasons an international protocol for reduction in production of Freon compounds was signed in Montreal in 1987 (13); this was later expanded into an agreement for total elimination of Freon compounds. These events have stimulated interest in alternatives, including non–chlorofluoro-hydrocarbon propellants, and in DPIs, which do not use propellants.

Chlorine-free aerosol hydrofluoroalkane (HFA) propellants known as HFA-134a (GR 106642X) and HFA-227 (14,15) have been developed to avoid environmental issues. These propellants generally appear to be safe and effective alternatives (16,17), although they are not necessarily absolutely interchangeable with chlorofluorocarbon (CFC) propellants. For example, beclomethasone dipropionate is in solution in HFA propellants, whereas CFC formulations are suspensions (18). Beclomethasone dipropionate is at least twice as potent when administered in conjunction with HFA propellants, compared with the CFC formulation, and the aerosol properties are much more favorable for pulmonary deposition (19).

Although HFA substances do not contribute to stratospheric ozone depletion, they are not totally environmentally benign. HFAs are greenhouse gases that can trap heat in the atmosphere, contributing to global warming. However, HFA used in MDIs accounts for only a tiny fraction of total emission of greenhouse gases (20).

Aside from environmental concerns, paradoxical bronchospasm, a rare occurrence, has been attributed to Freon compounds (21–23), although other propellant excipients also may be implicated.

Another infrequently encountered issue associated with propellant excipients in MDIs concerns major elevation of breath ethanol measurements shortly after use of those MDIs that contain ethanol as a dispersing agent. This problem may be avoided by introducing a 10-minute interval between the use of an MDI and breath alcohol testing (24).

Technique of Use of Metered-Dose Inhalers

Figure 37.1 shows a schematic diagram of the operation of an MDI. Prior to actuation, the propellant-drug formulation for the subsequent single dose is contained within the small metering chamber inside the MDI cannister. During actuation, the metering chamber briefly communicates with the atmosphere but is sealed off from the remainder of the formulation within the cannister; at this time, the dose within the metering chamber exits the inhaler through the valve stem. Immediately after the dose is released, however, the valve blocks the connection of the metering chamber to the atmosphere but permits the chamber to communicate with the interior of the cannister, allowing refilling of the metering chamber.

In most cases the active drug is not soluble in the propellant; therefore, micronized drug

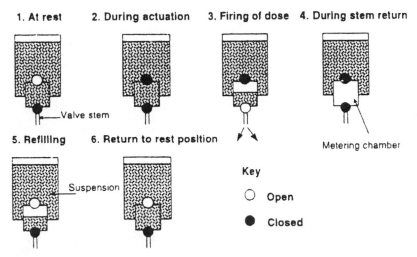

FIG. 37.1. The operation of a propellant metered-dose inhaler valve. (Adapted from Purewal TS. Formulation of metered dose inhalers. In: Purewal TS, Grant DJW, eds. *Metered dose inhaler technology.* Buffalo Grove, IL: Interpharm, 1998:9–68; with permission.)

particles within the cannister are in suspension rather than in solution. Shaking the canister prior to each actuation is essential to ensure that drug particles that may have "creamed" to the upper surface of the propellant or settled out toward the bottom of the device are resuspended (25). If the inhaler is not shaken prior to each actuation, the aliquot of propellant that enters the metering chamber from the canister may not be a homogenous suspension and therefore may not contain the expected amount of suspended drug. Inattention to shaking a budesonide MDI prior to actuation has been documented to result in a significant reduction in drug delivery to the airways (26).

The likelihood that the drug-propellant suspension drawn into the metering chamber will remain homogenous decreases if the pause between shaking and actuation is too long. MDIs are tested to ensure that their suspension is sufficiently stable so that small variations in the pause interval will not produce a major impact on drug delivery. Because the surfactants used to stabilize suspensions in CFC-containing MDIs are not compatible with HFA propellants, ensuring suspension stability has been a significant challenge in the development of non-CFC MDIs (25).

Several other details are important for proper use of an MDI. The canister must be held still and in the vertical position until the valve has completely returned to its rest position. If shaking is started while the valve is still compressed, or if the canister is tilted to the side while the metering chamber is refilling, some or all of the chamber may be filled with propellant vapor rather than with drug-containing suspension. The likelihood of such problems increases toward the end of the canister life, when the volume of suspension remaining in the canister is low (27).

When a period of time elapses between actuations of an MDI, the suspension that entered the metering chamber at the time of the last actuation may lose homogeneity, with some drug sticking to the walls of the metering chamber. Shaking usually will not be adequate to resuspend drug partitioned within the chamber. When this occurs, the amount of drug delivered with the next actuation will be reduced (27,28). This problem, termed *loss of prime*, has been documented to be a significant issue with generic albuterol inhalers using CFC propellants. The patient can compensate for this phenomenon by discarding the first two puffs prior to each therapeutic use of the MDI, a procedure termed *priming* the inhaler (29). Loss of prime appears to be a less significant issue with the newer HFA inhalers as a result of systematic improvements in device design implemented to ensure dose consistency (30).

Breath holding increases drug deposition in the airways by providing more time for the particles to settle onto the airways. Greater bronchodilatation is found with a 10-second pause compared with a 4-second pause, but a 20-second period of breath holding appears to produce no further benefit (31).

When an MDI is used without a holding chamber, the issue of whether the lips should be closed around the inhaler mouthpiece or instead held several centimeters from the open mouth (32,33) is open to debate. Comparisons between the two techniques have not shown consistent superiority of either technique over the other (31,34,35).

Another issue relevant to optimal inhaler technique regards the lung volume at which inhalation begins. Although it has been proposed that inhalation from functional residual capacity yields improved results as compared with inhalation from residual volume (36), the difference is probably minor (37).

Limitations of Metered-Dose Inhalers as a Delivery System for Inhaled Medications

Many studies have documented the prevalence of errors in patients' use of MDIs (38–54). These are summarized in Table 37.2 (38–50). Moreover, health-care professionals often are not familiar

TABLE 37.2. *Errors in patient use of metered-dose inhalers*

	% of Patients
Common errors	
Coordination of actuation	27
Breath-hold too short	26
Excessively rapid inspiratory flow rate	19
Improper shaking	13
Less common errors	
Inspiratory halt	6
Initiating the inhalation at total lung capacity	4
Nasal inhalation	2
Multiple actuations but one inhalation	3
Unusual errors (each less than 1% of patients)	
Exhale during activation	
Wrong end of inhaler in mouth	
Wrong position	
Failure to remove cap	

Data were compiled from 13 published studies involving 1,926 patients.
Adapted from references 38–50; with permission.

with the appropriate use of the devices (51). Despite training, around 15% of individuals are not able to use inhalers properly without assistive devices (40,43). Of patients with initially inadequate technique who master proper technique with training, around 50% subsequently again develop significant deficiencies in technique over time (43,52). When patients who are initially competent with MDI use are examined at follow-up, as many as 20% demonstrate incorrect usage at a later date (52). In addition to the suboptimal response to treatment with inhaled medications resulting from incorrect inhaler technique, there is significant direct economic cost as a result of wasted aerosol medication (54).

Holding Chambers: Adjuncts to Metered-Dose Inhalers

Holding chambers (also frequently referred to as spacers) are inhalation aids designed to overcome coordination difficulties and enhance aerosol deposition in the lower airways. There are three categories of holding chambers: (a) tubes without valves, (b) tubes or reservoirs incorporating one-way flap valves near the mouthpiece (with either mask or mouthpiece attached to the device), and (c) collapsible bags (55–57). Figure 37.2 illustrates a variety of holding chambers available in the United States.

The valved devices are particularly advantageous for use in young children who might otherwise exhale into the device, causing dissipation of the medication that had been delivered into the holding chamber from an MDI (58,59). For those patients, typically infants and children under 3 years of age who are not able to seal their lips around the mouthpiece of the holding chamber, valved holding chambers fitted with face masks designed to produce a tight seal over the patient's mouth and nose are available (60).

When an MDI and holding chamber are used, slow inspiratory flow rates have been documented to result in improved efficacy of inhaled medications, probably as a result of reduced impact in the oral cavity, pharynx, and large central airways, with greater homogeneity of lung deposition (31,61). Laube et al., using radiolabeled cromolyn sodium, found that a mean of 11.8% of

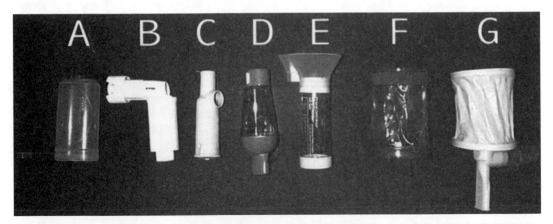

FIG. 37.2. Various holding chambers. **A:** Tube holding chamber (Ellipse, Allen & Hanburys Division of Glaxo Wellcome). **B:** Tube holding chamber integrated with metered-dose inhaler actuator (Azmacort, Aventis Pharmaceuticals). **C:** Valved holding chamber with mouthpiece (Optihaler, HealthScan Products). **D:** Valved holding chamber with mouthpiece (Easivent, DEY). **E:** Valved holding chamber with mask (Aerochamber with Mask, Monoghan Medical Corp.). **F:** Large-volume collapsible bag holding chamber (E-Z Spacer WE Pharmaceuticals). **G:** Large-volume collapsible bag holding chamber with inspiratory flow auditory monitor (InspirEaze, Key Pharmaceuticals).

radiolabeled aerosol was deposited into the lungs with slow inspiration using a large-volume holding chamber, as compared with a mean of 8.6% with faster inspiration (61). Some holding chamber devices incorporate a whistle to alert patients when inspiratory flow is excessive; the patient is instructed to inhale slowly so that the whistle does not emit any sound (56).

Clinicians differ in their preferences regarding whether or not holding chambers are routinely prescribed with MDIs for all patients. When moderate or high dosages of inhaled corticosteroids are administered via MDI, it is usual practice to routinely administer these via a holding chamber. As a result of reduced oropharyngeal-laryngeal deposition, local adverse effects of candidiasis and hoarseness are minimized (62). With those inhaled corticosteroids that have higher oral bioavailability (e.g., beclomethasone dipropionate as contrasted with fluticasone), the use of the spacer reduces potential systemic effects as well, because reduction in swallowed (and subsequently systemically available) medication results from a decrease in oral deposition (63). The decrease in systemic bioactivity because of reduced oral deposition exceeds the increase in systemic bioactivity resulting from increased pulmonary deposition as a consequence of use

of the spacer. The net effect of the spacer in this situation is reduced systemic bioactivity. However, when inhaled steroids with minimal oral bioavailability (e.g., fluticasone) are used with a large-volume spacer, the net effect of the spacer may instead result in increased systemic bioactivity, because there is little further decrease in gastrointestinal absorption as a result of the spacer, but increased pulmonary deposition of the inhaled steroid preparation with subsequent increased absorption (64). It should be noted that much of the clinical trial data evaluating the effects of many inhaled corticosteroids at specific dosages have been generated without the use of holding chambers. The conclusions obtained from of these studies with regard to efficacy and systemic effects of a particular inhaled steroid MDI preparation at a specific dosage used without a holding chamber cannot necessarily be generalized to administration of the same preparation through a holding chamber.

Whether bronchodilator MDIs should always be administered in conjunction with a holding chamber is open to debate. Clearly, use of a holding chamber with medication delivered via MDI is absolutely necessary in young children (65) and during acute bronchospastic episodes (66). In adults and older children who have excellent inhaler technique and coordination of actuation of the MDI with inhalation, data have indicated that in maintenance therapy the holding chamber provides only minimal additional clinical benefit compared with use of the MDI alone (41,67). However, use of these devices does result in additional bronchodilatation or bronchoprotection in those patients whose inhaler technique is suboptimal. These data suggest that use of holding chambers is not always essential with the routine use of MDI bronchodilator medications. When routine use of a holding chamber is not prescribed, however, it is critical to assess and unequivocally confirm that a patient's inhalation technique and coordination are excellent at each clinic visit and to provide the patient with a holding chamber for use during acute episodes of airflow reduction. To diminish uncertainties of drug delivery, many clinicians do advise the routine use of holding chambers with MDIs.

Drug particles may become charged when they are emitted by an MDI. Static electricity accumulates on plastic holding chambers, which may attract and bind the drug particles on the holding chamber's surface, thus reducing the delivered dose. Metal devices or those with an antistatic lining may reduce this effect (68). Washing the holding chamber before use is a simple way to minimize any charge present on the device (69,70); the charge may subsequently reaccumulate, however.

Patients must be instructed to actuate each individual puff of the MDI into the holding chamber and inhale it separately from subsequent puffs. Inhalation of each puff should immediately follow actuation. Errors in this technique may have significant clinical ramifications. In one study it was demonstrated that a single puff of beclomethasone dipropionate correctly actuated into a large-volume holding chamber and inhaled immediately will deliver a similar dose to the patient as five puffs actuated repetitively into the same chamber followed by inhalation (71). A delay of 20 seconds between actuation of an MDI and inhalation may reduce the available fine particle mass by 80% (72).

The use of valved holding chambers with mask to deliver medications to infants and toddlers via tidal breathing differs considerably from the considerations that apply to the usual administration to older children and adults. Based on radionuclide studies conducted by Tal et al., in this situation only around 2% of the dose placed into the holding chamber is deposited into the patient's lungs, a roughly 10-fold reduction from what is typically observed in older patients. However, if the patient is crying during the administration of the aerosol, lung deposition of less than 0.35% was observed. Ideally inhalation should be administered when the patient is calm or asleep. The mask should remain sealed over the patient's face for 20 to 30 seconds of tidal breathing after actuation of the MDI. Tal et al. (using a plastic spacer without special precautions to reduce electrostatic charge) found longer periods of time to be useless because the aerosol adhered to the spacer after 30 seconds. Because of the expected 10-fold reduction in pulmonary deposition, the full adult dose of aerosol medication, typically at least two puffs, is administered (73). It may be appropriate to start with several puffs, a dose larger than would be typically used in older children and adults, then to reduce the dose once it is clear that the treatment is effective (74).

Despite the widespread popularity of the small-volume jet nebulizer in the treatment of acute asthma in children and adults, in the clinic and emergency department as well as at home, nearly all published data addressing this issue indicate the equivalence of MDI delivered with the holding chamber. In some studies, the use of an MDI with a valved holding chamber has been demonstrated to produce a more rapid onset of effect and a lesser degree of systemic adrenergic adverse effects (75–77). The use of an MDI with a holding chamber is also cost effective as compared with nebulizer therapy in both acute and maintenance therapy (75), and a larger variety of medications are available in MDI than in nebulizer solutions. However, in acute bronchospasm with respiratory distress and hypoxemia, when concomitant emergent administration of high concentrations of ambient oxygen and bronchodilators is necessary, use of a nebulizer driven by oxygen may be advantageous. Some infants and small children (and their parents) dislike and do not tolerate the facial pressure and tight seal necessary with the holding chamber–mask devices. Use of nebulized delivery of medications is preferable in these instances.

Breath-Actuated Metered-Dose Inhalers

The breath-actuated inhaler is an alternative to holding chambers, and was developed to improve coordination of actuation of the MDI with inhalation. Prior to actuation, the patient moves a lever on the device upward, which compresses a spring within the device. A conventional MDI is contained within the device and is triggered by the spring when the patient inhales through the mouthpiece at an inspiratory flow rate exceeding 22 to 36 L/min (78). Although the device is of little additional benefit to patients with good inhaler coordination, its use in those with poor coordination increased the deposition of radiolabeled aerosol into the lungs from a mean of 7.2% with a conventional MDI to a mean of 20.8% with the breath-actuated inhaler; there was a corresponding dramatic improvement in change in forced expiratory volume in 1 second (FEV_1) after inhaler use as compared with that measured after conventional MDI in these patients (79).

The dependence on inspiratory flow has been a theoretical drawback of the breath-actuated inhaler. At least one case has been documented in which a patient experiencing acute severe airway obstruction was not able to generate sufficient inspiratory flow to activate the device with subsequent respiratory arrest (80), indicating that in rare instances this problem is of serious clinical significance. In the United States in the year 2000, the β agonist pirbuterol is the only medication available in a breath-actuated inhaler.

DRY POWDER INHALERS

The primary clinical advantage of DPIs as compared with MDIs is that DPIs are inherently breath actuated; thus, with DPIs, in contrast to MDIs, it is not necessary for the patient to master simultaneous coordination of inhalation with actuation of the device. Thus, administration is simplified without the need for inspiratory flow sensors or the additional bulk and complexity of holding chambers. Overall pulmonary deposition is similar to that of an MDI with spacer; fine particle mass is around 20% with the available DPIs at the usual inspiratory flow rates (81,82). Another positive feature of some DPIs is the incorporation of a counter in the device, with

discrete-dose DPIs the counter will show an exact count of the number of doses remaining in the device. Because the DPIs do not use propellants, environmental problems and other issues relating to potential problems with propellant excipients are avoided. The primary disadvantage of currently available DPIs is their dependency on patient effort and inspiratory flow to provide delivery of medication.

Commonly used multiple-use DPIs include the Turbuhaler, a reservoir device in which each dose is loaded for inhalation from a reservoir in the device (Fig. 37.3), and the Diskus, in which each of multiple discrete doses is contained within the device within a separate packet (Fig. 37.4). The

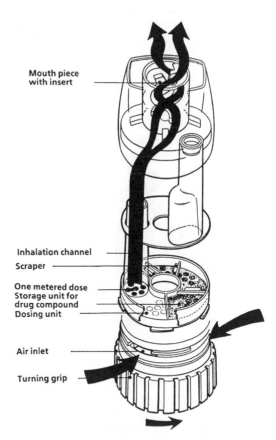

Mouth piece with insert

Inhalation channel
Scraper
One metered dose
Storage unit for drug compound
Dosing unit
Air inlet
Turning grip

FIG. 37.3. Turbuhaler is a cylindrical, multidose dry powder inhaler device. The dosing is achieved by twisting the turning grip back and forth followed by deep inhalation. It contains 200 metered doses and is equipped with a dosage window. (From Vaswani SK, Creticos PS. Metered dose inhaler: past, present, and future. *Ann Allergy Asthma Immunol* 1998;80:11–21; with permission.)

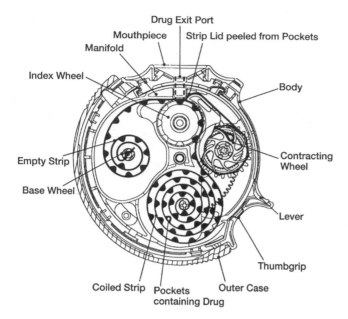

FIG. 37.4. Diskus is a disk-shaped, pocket-size, multidose dry powder inhaler device. During inhalation, air is drawn through the device delivering the dose via the mouthpiece. It contains 60 metered doses and has a built-in dosage counter. (From Vaswani SK, Creticos PS. Metered dose inhaler: past, present, and future. *Ann Allergy Asthma Immunol* 1998;80:11–21; with permission.)

Rotahaler is an older DPI that requires each dose to be loaded separately into the inhaler prior to administration. The Spinhaler, the first DPI marketed in the early 1970s as a delivery device for cromolyn sodium, is no longer available. The Diskhaler contains a small number of discrete doses; it has not achieved wide acceptance as a delivery system for asthma medications.

Inspiratory Flow Dependency of Dry Powder Inhaler Devices

The currently available DPIs require an inspiratory flow rate of at least 60 L/min for optimal dispersion of the powdered medication into respirable particles (82); below 30 L/min, the fine particle output may be reduced by as much as 50% (83). Because of this inspiratory flow dependency of the proper functioning of the DPI devices, there may be uncertainty regarding adequacy of drug delivery during asthma exacerbations, when flow rates are diminished. However, in one series of adult patients hospitalized with asthma exacerbation, 98% could generate an adequate inspiratory flow (84). In another adult study, treatment of acute asthma with albuterol delivered by DPI was as effective as treatment using a nebulizer or MDI with holding chamber (85).

A related issue pertains to whether flow rates generated by the inspiratory efforts of small children can effectively and reliably actuate these devices. In one study, only 40% of preschool children with acute wheezing could generate an inspiratory flow rate exceeding 28 L/min, although around 75% could exceed this inspiratory flow rate during periods of stable asthma (86). These considerations suggest caution in using available DPIs in preschool children, especially for rapid-onset bronchodilators such as albuterol. In another study, 80% of 6-year-old children could use a Turbuhaler effectively (87). In some instances, the flow-volume loop generated by a computerized spirometer may be useful in the clinic to ascertain whether or not a child's inspiratory flow rate, measured during a period of clinical stability, is sufficient for effective maintenance use of DPIs (74).

The deposition site of aerosol generated by DPIs is more central than with MDI or nebulizer administration. The clinical significance of this is uncertain; in one study comparing the effects of different delivery systems for albuterol, bronchodilation correlated more closely with total lung deposition than with peripheral distribution within the lung (88).

An investigational battery-powered, breath-actuated DPI is of interest because it is not dependent on inspiratory flow for adequate dispersion (89–91).

Future Directions in Dry Powder Inhaler Therapy

At this writing, the variety of medications available in multiple-use DPI devices in the United States is limited. Although somewhat more medications are available in single-use formulations, the additional complexity of these devices and the additional time involved in their use makes them generally less attractive for most patients than alternatives. The popularity of DPIs as the preferred device for administration of asthma medications to older children and adults is likely to significantly increase as pharmaceutical manufacturers provide more drugs in multiple-use DPI devices.

NEBULIZERS

A device that simply sprays gas through a liquid resulting in aerosolization is termed an atomizer. In contrast, nebulizers are more complex devices, which, by the incorporation of baffles, selectively remove particles that are too large to enter the lower airways. Most nebulizers used in aerosol drug therapy are jet nebulizers driven by air compressors. In the jet nebulizer, the compressed air moves through a narrow hole known as a Venturi. Negative pressure pulls liquid up to the Venturi by the Bernoulli effect; at the Venturi, the liquid is subsequently atomized. Many of the droplets initially atomized are much larger than the 5 mm maximum necessary for them to enter the smaller lower airways. These large particles impact on the nebulizer's baffles or the internal wall of the nebulizer and return to the reservoir for renebulization. Details of the baffle design have a major effect on the sizes of the particles produced. Ultrasonic nebulizers use a rapidly vibrating piezoelectric crystal to generate aerosol. Vibrations from the crystal are transmitted to the surface of the liquid in the nebulizer, where standing waves are formed. Droplets released from the crests of these waves produce the aerosol. The ultrasonic nebulizers are quieter and usually smaller than jet nebulizers but have the drawback

of not nebulizing drug suspensions efficiently (92).

Many clinicians are surprised to learn that most of the drug placed into a nebulizer chamber never reaches the lungs. Around 50% to 70% of the dose never leaves the nebulizer. Of the approximately 30% to 50% that is emitted, some particles are too large to enter the lungs, and some are so small that they are not deposited into the airways but are exhaled. With many nebulizer designs, much of the nebulized medication is released during expiration and is therefore dispersed into the room air. Typically, only 7% to 25% of medication placed into the nebulizer is delivered to the patient's airway (92,93).

For drugs that are relatively inexpensive and have a high therapeutic index such as bronchodilators, it is simple and effective to compensate for these issues by placing a large dose of medication into the nebulizer, provided that the dosage delivered to the patient is within the flat range of the dose-response curve, the precision and efficiency of delivery may not be a critical issue. However, these factors may become meaningful when medications that are expensive and have a greater potential for significant dose-dependent adverse effects, such as corticosteroids, are used. Such issues have served as an impetus for modifications in nebulizer design.

The traditional nebulizer design provides continuous flow of gas from the compressor into the nebulizer; the rate of aerosol outflow from the nebulizer is equal to the inflow rate from the compressor and does not change with the phases of respiration (Fig. 37.5). Modifications to the conventional design include the open vent design, the dosimetric design with a manually operated valve to interrupt gas flow into the nebulizer during expiration, combinations of the open vent and dosimetric features, and the more recent breath-assisted open vent nebulizers designed to combine the advantages of the open vent design with the convenience of continuous operation and the efficiency of intermittent nebulization excluding the expiratory phase (92).

Open vent nebulizers provide a vent from the open atmosphere into the nebulizer. Negative pressure generated as compressed air expands at the Venturi and draws air in through the

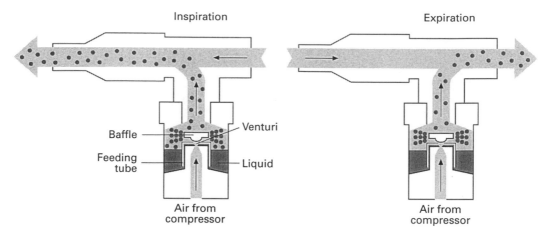

FIG. 37.5. Conventional nebulizer design. Air from the compressor passes through a small hole (Venturi). Rapid expansion of air causes a negative pressure, which sucks fluid up the feeding tube system, where it is atomized. Larger particles impact on baffles and the walls of the chamber and are returned for renebulization. Small aerosol particles are released continuously from the nebulizer chamber. On expiration, the nebulizer continues to generate aerosol, which is wasted. [From O'Callaghan C, Barry PW. The science of nebulized drug delivery. *Thorax* 1997;52(suppl 2):31–44; with permission.]

open vent, resulting in more airflow through the chamber than provided by the compressor; therefore more aerosol is generated in a given period of time. This nebulizer design has been combined with a manual interrupter that the patient operates to allow aerosol generation only during inspiration. For a given medication dose placed into the nebulizer, the use of the manual interrupter results in greater delivery to the airways but with prolongation of the nebulization time (92).

With the breath-assisted open vent nebulizers, the vent is designed to be open only during inspiration, enhancing aerosol generation only during the inspiratory phase. Aerosol generation continues as a result of the continuous gas flow from the compressor during expiration, but is not enhanced by the vent, which is closed during expiration (Fig. 37.6). The primary advantages of this design include significantly improved delivery of drug placed into the nebulizer into the airway and the convenience of continuous operation without the need for patient coordination of actuation of a manual interrupter. Other benefits include the generation of a greater fraction of smaller particles due to increased evaporation from droplets due to the additional airflow, and the need for less powerful compressors with this category of nebulizer (92).

For a single drug preparation, various nebulizers may give widely differing drug delivery that further varies depending on the patient's tidal volume during nebulization. In one study using nebulized budesonide, four different nebulizer devices, and tidal volumes ranging from 75 to 600 mL, the estimated percentage of the dosage placed into the nebulizer to be inhaled by the patient varied over a fourfold range depending on these factors (94).

A common error in the use of nebulized medications in young children is to wave the face mask in front of the child's face instead of keeping it in direct contact with the face. Although the child's acceptance of the treatment may be improved, drug delivery to the airways is almost negligible with such an improper technique. With proper use, the mask (or mouthpiece) with its attached tubing provides a critical function as a reservoir containing aerosol-laden air from the nebulizer. During each tidal inhalation, much of the air that the patient inspires comes from this reservoir. The reservoir is continuously refilled by the flow of aerosol-laden air entering it at a flow rate much less than the patient's inspiratory flow rate. Without the reservoir, nearly all of the air that the patient inhales is unmedicated room air; nearly all of the aerosol simply escapes into

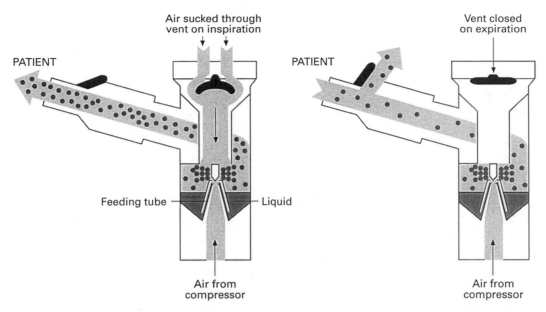

FIG. 37.6. An example of a breath-assisted, open vent nebulizer, the Pari LC Jet Plus. On inspiration the valve located at the top of the chamber opens, allowing extra air to be sucked through the vent on inspiration. The main effect of this is to pull more aerosol from the nebulizer on inspiration, increasing the dose to the patient. On expiration the vent closes and aerosol exits via a one-way valve near the mouthpiece. Aerosol lost from the nebulizer on expiration is thus proportionally less than that from a conventional nebulizer. Nebulization times will be faster and the drug dose received by the patient will be significantly greater than with conventional nebulizers but not as fast as with the open vent nebulizer. [From O'Callaghan C, Barry PW. The science of nebulized drug delivery. *Thorax* 1997;52(suppl 2):31–44; with permission.]

the atmosphere. One study demonstrated that the dose of inspired drug when the mask is moved 1 cm from the child's face is only 50% of that when the mask is in contact with the face, and a distance of 2 cm resulted in an 80% reduction (94). Even with proper use of a mask or mouthpiece, significant entrainment of room air occurs (95).

When nebulizers are used in older children and adults, the use of a mouthpiece in preference to face mask may reduce unwanted systemic effects (96).

Most drugs used for nebulization are now supplied in single-use ampoules, largely eliminating the need for preservative additives, some of which have been documented to have significant bronchoconstrictor effects. When multiple use vials are used, the clinician should be aware of the additives present and any bronchoconstrictor potential that they may have with repetitive dosing (97).

SUMMARY

Device Recommendations in Specific Clinical Settings

In adults and older children with long-established asthma who consistently demonstrate excellent technique with MDIs used either with or without holding chambers, there is in general nothing to be gained by a universal recommendation for a change in their delivery system. As CFC-containing devices are phased out, the HFA-containing devices for delivery of similar medications can be easily substituted. Some patients who use holding chambers with MDIs may desire to change to DPIs because of the more compact nature of the DPI devices.

In infants and toddlers the choice for aerosol therapy is between nebulizer versus MDI used in conjunction with valved holding chamber and mask. This selection of device often depends on the preference of the patient's caregiver.

Although MDIs used with valved holding chambers are faster, use less costly medication, and are clearly at least as effective as nebulized delivery when properly administered, there is a risk that the medication will not be adequately delivered if the patient is crying during the procedure. Therefore, under typical circumstances of home administration to infants and toddlers, nebulized delivery may be more reliable and in certain situations may be preferable to MDI with valved holding chamber. Choice of nebulizer is important when corticosteroid suspensions are administered, but is less critical with other medications used in the treatment of asthma.

Preschool children generally should be treated with MDIs and holding chamber with mouthpiece. Age 3 to 4 is usually the appropriate time to "wean" children who first developed asthma at a younger age from nebulized therapy. DPIs may be considered for maintenance therapy in this age group in specific cases.

In acute severe airflow obstruction, MDI alone (even in subjects with excellent inhaler technique) is often unsatisfactory. Although nebulizer therapy has traditionally been used in this situation, it has been clearly demonstrated that MDI with holding chamber (a valved chamber should be used with small children) is faster and at least equally efficacious. For clinic and emergency room use in this situation, the choice between the two modalities depends on the preferences of the staff and the equipment available.

For adults and older children with newly diagnosed asthma or other bronchial disorders, a case can be made for the routine institution of therapy with inhaled medications using multiple-use DPI formulations. The technique is easier to learn than with an MDI, a dose indicator is present, and the additional bulk and complexity of a spacer device is eliminated. At this writing, however, no multiple-use, rapid-acting bronchodilator is commercially available in the United States in DPI form. Consequently, at this time the DPIs can be effectively used only for administration of maintenance "controller" medications—inhaled steroids and the long-acting bronchodilator salmeterol. However, all patients for whom inhaled controller medications are prescribed also require a rescue bronchodilator (98). Thus, the patient must be instructed in two inhaler techniques: a rapid inspiratory effort with the DPIs and the slow inspiratory effort most efficacious for delivery of aerosol medication from the MDI used to administer the rapid-acting rescue bronchodilator, with or without a holding chamber. The advent of rapid-acting bronchodilator DPIs in the United States, expected within the next few years, will be a welcome solution to this dilemma. Comments similar to these regarding DPIs are also applicable to the breath-actuated inhaler, which, although compact and simple to use, currently is available for use with only one medication in the United States. Whether or not the potential benefit of the currently investigational battery-driven breath-actuated DPI devices (which possibly are more reliable than both conventional DPIs and breath-actuated MDIs for delivery of rapid-acting bronchodilators during sudden episodes of life-threatening airway obstruction with severely reduced inspiratory flow rates) will outweigh their inherent additional complexity remains to be seen.

Priorities for Inhaled Drug Delivery in Clinical Practice

For the busy clinician barraged by competing claims from marketers of various modalities of delivery of inhaled medication, the practical issue to be addressed is summarized by the following question: "is there a delivery system that is clearly clinically superior to the others?" This straightforward query cannot be answered simply. As the preceding discussion and references indicate, there are well-documented differences in the characteristics of various devices in terms of delivery of drug to the airways, but consistent clinically relevant ramifications of these differences are more difficult to establish. A delivery system that is clinically highly efficacious for delivery of one drug formulation may show inferior performance with a different drug or formulation. Data comparing clinical effects of specific drug formulations administered via specific delivery devices in side-by-side trials must be evaluated to conclusively prove the relative merits of one drug–device combination over another. Preferences of individual patients, as well as economic considerations, must be taken into account; in many situations such issues may supersede recommendations based on purely scientific considerations. Many patients adhere poorly to complicated treatment programs involving multiple inhaled medications, each administered with a different type of device on a different schedule. Attention directed to minimizing the number of daily doses administered and the number of different categories of devices used for such patients is often dramatically effective in restoring adherence with resultant attainment of satisfactory asthma control.

REFERENCES

1. Cooper S. A dissertation on the properties and effects of the *Datura stramonium*, or common thornapple [Dissertation]. Philadelphia: Smith, 1797:39.
2. Gandevia B. Historical review of the use of parasympatholytic agents in the treatment of respiratory disorders. *Postgrad Med J* 1975;51(suppl 7):13 20.
3. Graeser JB, Rowe AH. Inhalation of epinephrine for relief of asthmatic symptoms. *J Allergy Clin Immunol* 1935;6:415.
4. Wright BM. A new nebuliser. *Lancet* 1958;2:24–25.
5. Freedman T. Medihaler therapy for bronchial asthma: a new type of aerosol therapy. *Postgrad Med* 1956; 20:667–673.
6. Stalhofen W, Gebbert J, Heyder J. Experimental determination of the regional deposition of aerosol particles in the human respiratory tract. *Am Ind Hyg Assoc J* 1980;41:385–399.
7. Task Group on Lung Dynamics. Deposition and retention models for internal dosimetry of the human respiratory tract. *Health Physics* 1966;12:173–208.
8. Sheth KA, Kelly HW, Mitchell BH. *Innovations in dry powder inhalers.* Meniscus Ltd., 2000.
9. Rudolph G, Kobrich R, Stalhofen W. Modeling and algebraic formulation of regional aerosol deposition in man. *J Aerosol Sci* 1990;21(suppl 1):306–406.
10. Newman SP. Metered dose pressurized aerosols and the ozone layer. *Eur Respir J* 1990;3:495–497.
11. Molina MJ, Rowland FS. Stratospheric risk for chlorofluoromethanes: chlorine atom-catalyzed destruction of ozone. *Nature* 1974;249:810–812.
12. Jones RR. Ozone depletion and cancer risk. *Lancet* 1987;2;443–445.
13. Technology Review Panel/Technical Options Committee on Aerosols, Sterillants and Miscellaneous Uses (pursuant to the Montreal Protocol). Nairobi, Kenya, United Nations Environment Programme, 1989.
14. Leach CL. Preclinical safety of propellant HFA-134a and Airomir. *Br J Clin Pract* 1995;79(suppl);10–12.
15. Taggart SCO, Custovic A, Richards DH, et al. GR106642X: a new non- ozone depleting propellant for inhalers. *BMJ* 1995;310:1639–1640.
16. Dockhorn R, Vanden Burgt J, Ekholm B, et al. Clinical equivalence of a novel non–chlorofluorocarbon-containing salbutamol sulfate metered-dose inhaler and a conventional chlorofluorocarbon inhaler in patients with asthma. *J Allergy Clin Immunol* 1995; 96:50–56.
17. Parameswaran K. Concepts of establishing clinical bioequivalence of chlorofluorocarbon and hydrofluoroalkane B-agonists. *J Allergy Clin Immunol* 1999; 104(suppl):243–245.
18. Borgstrom L. The pharmacokinetics of inhaled hydrofluoroalkane formulations. *J Allergy Clin Immunol* 1999;104(suppl):246–249.
19. Leach CL. Effect of formulation parameters on hydrofluoroalkane-beclomethasone dipropionate drug deposition in humans. *J Allergy Clin Immunol* 1999;104(suppl):250–252.
20. Forte R, Dibble JD. The role of international environmental agreements in metered dose inhaler technology changes. *J Allergy Clin Immunol* 1999;104(suppl):217–220.
21. Yarbrough J, Mansfield LE, Ting S. Metered dose inhaler induced bronchospasm in asthmatic patients. *Ann Allergy* 1985;55:25–27.
22. Wilkinson JRW, Roberts JA, Bradding P, et al. Paradoxical bronchoconstriction in asthmatic patients after salmeterol by metered dose inhaler. *BMJ* 1992;305:931–932.
23. Vaswani SK, Creticos P. Metered dose inhaler: past, present, and future. *Ann Allergy Asthma Immunol* 1998; 80:11–21.
24. Gomez HF, Moore L, McKinney P, et al. Elevation of breath ethanol measurements by metered-dose inhalers. *Ann Emerg Med* 1995;25:608–611.
25. Brindley A. The chlorofluorocarbon to hydrofluoroalkane transition: the effect on pressurized metered dose inhaler suspension stability. *J Allergy Clin Immunol* 1999;104(suppl):221–226.
26. Thorsson L, Edsbacker S. Lung deposition of budesonide from a pressurized metered dose inhaler attached to a spacer. *Eur Respir J* 1998;12:1340–1345.
27. Cummings RH. Pressurized metered dose inhalers; chlorofluorocarbon to hydrofluoroalkane transition-valve performance. *J Allergy Clin Immunol* 1999;104 (suppl):230–235.
28. Cyr TD, Graham SJ, Li R, Lovering HG. Low first-spray drug content in albuterol metered-dose inhalers. *Pharmacol Rev* 1991;8:658–560.
29. Blake KV, Harman E, Hendeles L. Evaluation of a generic albuterol metered-dose inhaler: importance of priming the MDI. *Ann Allergy* 1992;68:169–174.
30. Ross DL, Gabrio BJ. Advances in metered-dose inhaler technology with the development of a chlorofluorocarbon-free drug delivery system. *J Aerosol Med* 1999;12:151–160.
31. Newman SP, Pavia D, Clarke SW. How should a pressurized beta-adrenergic bronchodilator be inhaled? *Eur J Respir Dis* 1981;62:3–21.
32. Connolly CK. Methods of using pressurized aerosols. *BMJ* 1975;2:21.
33. Dolovich M, Ruffin RE, Roberts RE, et al. Optimal delivery of aerosols from metered dose inhalers. *Chest* 1981;80(suppl):911–915.
34. Lawford P, McKenzie D. Pressurized bronchodilator aerosol technique: influence of breath holding time and relationship of inhaler to mouth. *Br J Dis Chest* 1982;76:229–233.

35. Thompson A, Traver GA. Comparison of three methods of administering a self- propelled bronchodilator [Abstract]. *Am Rev Respir Dis* 1982;125(suppl 4):140.

36. Riley DJ, Liu RT, Edelman NH. Enhanced responses to aerosolized bronchodilator therapy in asthma using respiratory maneuvers. *Chest* 1979;76:501–507.

37. Newman SP, Clarke SW. The proper use of metered dose inhalers. *Chest* 1984;86:342–344.

38. McFadden ER. Improper patient techniques with metered dose inhalers: clinical consequences and solutions to misuse. *J Allergy Clin Immunol* 1995;96:278–283.

39. Lindgren S, Bake B, Larsson S. Clinical consequences of inadequate inhalation technique in asthma therapy. *Eur J Respir Dis* 1987;70:93–98.

40. Coady TJ, Stewart CJ, Davies HJ. Synchronization of bronchodilator release. *Practitioner* 1976;217:273–275.

41. Epstein SW, Manning CPR, Ashley MJ, et al. Survey of the clinical use of pressurized aerosol inhalers. *CMAJ* 1979;120:813–816.

42. Shim C, Williams MH. The adequacy of inhalation of aerosol from canister nebulizers. *Am J Med* 1980;69:891–894.

43. Crompton GK. Problems patients have using pressurized aerosol inhalers. *Eur J Respir Dis* 1982; 63:101–104.

44. Lee HS. Proper aerosol inhalation technique for delivery of asthma medications. *Clin Pediatr* 1983; 22:440–443.

45. Agusti AGN, Ussetti P, Roca, et al. Letter. *Chest* 1985;88:159–160.

46. Pedersen S, Frost L, Arnfred T. Errors in inhalation technique and efficiency in inhaler use in asthmatic children. *Allergy* 1986;41:118–124.

47. Allen SC, Prior A. What determines whether an elderly patient can use a metered dose inhaler correctly? *Br J Dis Chest* 1986;80:45–49.

48. Armitage JM, Williams SJ. Inhaler technique in the elderly. *Age Aging* 1988;17:275–278.

49. Manzella BA, Brooks CM, Richards JM, et al. Assessing the use of metered dose inhalers by adults with asthma. *J Asthma* 1989;26:223–230.

50. Diggory P, Bailey R, Vallon A. Effectiveness of inhaled bronchodilator delivery systems for elderly pa;tients. *Age Aging* 1991;20:379–382.

51. Hanania NA, Wittman R, Kesten S, et al. Medical personnel's knowledge of and ability to use inhaling devices: metered-dose inhalers, spacing chambers, and breath actuated dry powder inhalers. *Chest* 1994;105:111–116.

52. De Blaquiere P, Christensen DB, Carter WB, et al. Use and abuse of metered dose inhalers by patients with chronic lung disease. *Am Rev Respir Dis* 1989;140:910–916.

53. Orehek J, Gayard P, Grimaud CH, et al. Patient error in use of bronchodilator metered aerosols. *BMJ* 1976;1;76.

54. King D, Earnshaw, Delaney JC. Pressurized aerosol inhalers: the cost of misuse. *Br J Clin Pract* 1991;45:10–11.

55. Tobin MJ. Use of bronchodilator aerosols. *Arch Intern Med* 1985;145;1659–1663.

56. Tobin MJ, Jenouri G, Danta I, et al. Response to bronchodilator drug administration by a new reservoir aerosol delivery system and a review of other auxiliary

delivery systems. *Am Rev Respir Dis* 1982;126:670–675.

57. Dalby RN, Somaraju S, Chavan VS, et al. Evaluation of aerosol drug output from the Optichamber and Aerochamber spacers in a model system. *J Asthma* 1998;35:173–177.

58. Dolovich M, Ruffin R, Corr D, et al. Clinical evaluation of a simple demand inhalation MDI aerosol delivery device. *Chest* 1983;84:36–41.

59. Hodges IGC, Milner AD, Stokes GM. Assessment of a new device for delivering aerosol drugs to asthmatic children. *Arch Dis Child* 1981;56:787–800.

60. Conner WT, Dolovich MB, Frame RA, et al. Reliable salbutamol administration in 6 to 36-month-old children by means of a metered dose inhaler and Aerochamber with mask. *Pediatr Pulmonol* 1989;6;263–267.

61. Laube BL, Edwards AM, Dalby RD, et al. The efficacy of slow versus faster inhalation of cromolyn sodium in protecting against allergen challenge in patients with asthma. *J Allergy Clin Immunol* 1998;101;475–483.

62. Toogood JH, Baskerville J, Jenning B, et al. Use of spacers to facilitate inhaled corticosteroid treatment of asthma. *Am Rev Respir Dis* 1984;129:723–729.

63. Brown PH, Blundell G, Greening AP, et al. Do large volume spacer devices reduce the systemic effects of high dose inhaled corticosteroids? *Thorax* 1990;45:736–739.

64. Dempsey OJ, Wilson AM, Coutie WJ, et al. Evaluation of the effect of a large volume spacer on the systemic bioactivity of fluticasone propionate metered-dose inhaler. *Chest* 1999;116:935–940.

65. Pedersen S. Aerosol treatment of bronchoconstriction in children with or without a tube spacer. *N Engl J Med* 1983;803:1328–1330.

66. McFadden ER. Therapy of acute asthma. *J Allergy Clin Immunol* 1989;84:151–158.

67. Giannini D, DiFranco A, Bacci E, et al. The protective effect of salbutamol inhaled using different devices on methacholine bronchoconstriction. *Chest* 2000;117:1319–1323.

68. Bisgaard H, Anhoi J , Klug B, et al. A non-electrostatic spacer for aerosol delivery. *Arch Dis Child* 1995;73:226–230.

69. Barry PW, O'Callaghan C. The level of static charge on spacer devices used with inhalational drugs. *Pediatr Rev* 1995;8:210.

70. Wildhaber JH, Devadason SG, Eber E, et al. Effect of electrostatic charge, flow decay and multiple actuations in the in vitro delivery of salbutamol from different small volume spacers for infants. *Thorax* 1996;51:985–988.

71. O'Callaghan C, Cant M, Robertson C. Delivery of beclomethasone dipropionate from a spacer device: what dose is available for inhalation? *Thorax* 1994;49:961–964.

72. Barry PW, Robertson CF, O'Callaghan C. Optimum use of a spacer device. *Arch Dis Child* 1993;69:693–694.

73. Tal A, Golan H, Grauer N, et al. Deposition pattern of radiolabeled salbutamol inhaled from a metered-dose inhaler by means of a spacer with mask in young children with airway obstruction. *J Pediatr*;128:479–484.

74. Gillies J. Overview of delivery system issues in pediatric asthma. *Pediatr Pulmonol* 1997;(suppl 15):55–58.

75. Leversha AM, Campanella SG, Aickin RP, et al. Costs and effectiveness of spacer versus nebulizer in

young children with moderate and severe acute asthma. *J Pediatr* 2000;136:497–502.

76. Idris AH, McDermott MF, Raucci JC, et al. Emergency department treatment of severe asthma. Metered-dose inhaler plus holding chamber is equivalent in effectiveness to nebulizer. *Chest* 1993;103:665–672.

77. Newhouse MT. Asthma therapy with aerosols: Are nebulizers obsolete? A continuing controversy. *J Pediatr* 1999;135:5–8.

78. Baum EA, Bryant AM. The development and laboratory testing of a novel breath-actuated pressurized inhaler. *J Aerosol Med* 1988;1:219–220.

79. Newman SP, Weisz AWB, Talace N, et al. Improvement of drug delivery with a breath actuated pressurised aerosol for patients with poor inhaler technique. *Thorax* 1991;46:712–716.

80. Hannaway PJ. Failure of a breath-actuated bronchodilator inhaler to deliver aerosol during a bout of near fatal asthma [Letter]. *J Allergy Clin Immunol* 1996;98: 853.

81. Bisgaard H. Drug delivery from inhaler devices. *BMJ* 1996;313:895–896.

82. Ollson B. Aerosol particle generation from dry powder inhalers: can they equal pressurized metered dose inhalers? *J Aerosol Med* 1995;8(suppl 3):13–18.

83. Prime D, Grant AC, Slater AL, et al. A critical comparison of the dose delivery characteristics of four alternative inhalation devices delivering salbutamol: pressurized metered dose inhaler, Diskus inhaler, Diskhaler inhaler, and Turbuhaler inhaler. *Aerosol Med* 1999;12: 75–84.

84. Brown PH, Ning AC, Greening AP, et al. Peak inspiratory flow through a Turbuhaler in acute asthma. *Eur Respir J* 1995;8:1940–1941.

85. Raimondi AC, Schottlender J, Lombardi D, et al. Treatment of acute severe asthma with inhaled albuterol delivered via jet nebulizer, metered dose inhaler with spacer, or dry powder. *Chest* 1997;112:24–28.

86. Pedersen S, Hansen OR, Fuglsang G. Influence of inspiratory flow rate upon the effect of a Turbuhaler. *Arch Dis Child* 1990;65:308–310.

87. Goren A, Noviski N, Avital A, et al. Assessment of the ability of young children to use a powder inhaler device (Turbuhaler). *Pedatr Pulmonol* 1994;18:77–80.

88. Zainudin BMZ, Biddiscombe M, Tolfree SEJ, et al. Comparison of bronchodilator responses and deposition patterns of salbutamol inhaled from a pressurized metered dose inhaler, as a dry powder, and as a nebulised solution. *Thorax* 1990;45:469–473.

89. Spiros inhaler and albuterol metered-dose inhaler in asthma. *Chest* 1999;115:329–335.

90. Geoffroy P, Lalonde RL, Ahrens R, et al. Clinical comparability of albuterol delivered by the breath actuated inhaler (Spiros) and albuterol by MDI in patients with asthma. *Ann Allergy Asthma Immunol* 1999;82:377–382.

91. Ahrens RC, Hendeles L, Clarke W, et al. Therapeutic equivalence of Spiros dry powder inhaler and Ventolin metered dose inhaler. *Am J Respir Crit Care Med* 1999;160:1238–1243.

92. O'Callaghan C, Barry W. The science of nebulised drug delivery. *Thorax* 1997;52(suppl 2):31–44.

93. Szefler S. Pharmacodynamics and pharmacokinetics of budesonide: a new nebulized corticosteroid. *J Allergy Clin Immunol* 1999;104(suppl);175–183.

94. O'Callaghan C. Delivery systems: the science. *Pediatr Pulmonol* 1997;(suppl) 15:51–54.

95. Collis GG, Cole CH, Le Souef PN. Dilution of nebulized aerosols by air entrainment in children. *Lancet* 1990;336:341–343.

96. Lowenthal D, Kattan M. Facemasks versus mouthpieces for aerosol treatment of asthmatic children. *Pediatr Pulmonol* 1992;14:192–196.

97. Asmus MJ, Sherman J, Hendeles L. Bronchoconstrictor additives in bronchodilator solutions. *J Allergy Clin Immunol* 1999;104(suppl):53–60.

98. National Asthma Education and Prevention Program. *Expert Panel Report 2: Guidelines for the Diagnosis and Management of Asthma.* Publication 97-4051. Bethesda, MD: National Heart, Lung, and Blood Institute, U.S. Department of Health and Human Services, 1997.

38

Novel Immunologic Therapies

Leslie C. Grammer

*Division of Allergy-Immunology, Department of Medicine, Northwestern University
Medical School, Chicago, Illinois*

There are a variety of novel immunologic approaches to the therapy of allergic diseases that afflict up to 20% of the American population. These approaches generally can be divided into three categories. One such approach is to administer monoclonal antibodies against proteins that have been reported to be key in mediating allergic inflammation. Another is to administer other monoclonal proteins that will interfere with the allergic inflammatory process. A final approach is modifying allergen immunotherapy using innovative approaches to reduce allergenicity while maintaining immunogenicity.

MONOCLONAL ANTIBODIES

Monoclonal Anti–Immunoglobulin E

The elimination of immunoglobulin E (IgE) to provide a definitive therapy for allergic diseases is based on the importance of IgE in allergic disease, both in early- and late-phase reactions (1,2). Various strategies have been used to interfere with the binding of IgE to its receptor, thus abrogating allergic disease. Examples include inhibiting IgE production, use of IgE fragments to occupy the receptor, administration of soluble receptors to bind free IgE, and neutralizing antibodies against IgE. Polyclonal and monoclonal anti-IgE antibodies have been produced to study mechanisms of allergic disease (3).

Anti-IgE recombinant humanized monoclonal antibody rhuMAb-E25 is being studied in phase III clinical trials for treatment of allergic asthma and allergic rhinitis. Several studies have reported information on the safety and efficacy of this approach (4–7). In one parallel group randomized placebo controlled trial in humans with mild asthma, both early and late responses were attenuated in some individuals (4). Skin test responses were unaffected. In a similar study, there was a statistically significant, clinically modest reduction in airway responsiveness to methacholine (5). The cutaneous response was not affected. Similarly, in a multicenter trial of more severe asthma, a modest improvement in asthma symptoms was observed (6). In a ragweed rhinitis trial, some symptomatic improvement was described in patients who had markedly reduced free IgE levels and markedly increased bound IgE levels (7).

Thus far, rhuMAb-E25 has not induced an antibody response in humans. The most common side effect has been the development of urticarial eruptions. All occurred after initial administration and were easily controlled (8).

Anti–Interleukin-5

Interleukin-5 (IL-5) is a helper T cell type 2 (T_H2) cytokine that is reported to be essential for the recruitment of eosinophils in the allergic inflammatory response (9). In animal models, an anti–IL-5 blocking antibody has been reported to inhibit eosinophil recruitment from the bone marrow into tissue. This effectively ablates any late-phase response in these animal models. A humanized anti–IL-5 blocking antibody

(SB-240563) has been studied (10). When administered intravenously to allergic subjects, it reduced both blood and sputum eosinophilia, but was not as successful at reducing airway hyperresponsiveness or allergen-induced late-phase response (11). These results question the association between IL-5 and allergic disease, but do not preclude its importance in disorders that are known to be eosinophil mediated (12).

Anti–CCR-3

Another important target for intervening in allergic disease emerged with the discovery that a cluster of cytokines belonging to the CC chemokine family (which includes RANTES and MCP-1, -3, and -4) are potent eosinophil chemoattractants that use a common receptor, CCR-3 (12).

A monoclonal antibody to CCR-3 has been reported to cause inhibition of eosinophil migration (13). Using bacteriophage expression libraries and combinatorial chemistry, highly selective CCR-3 antagonists are being discovered. There are reports that CCR-3 works synergistically with IL-5 to recruit eosinophils to allergic inflammation in target tissues (12).

OTHER MONOCLONAL PROTEINS

Soluble Interleukin-4 Receptor

Interleukin-4 plays an important proinflammatory role in asthma through several mechanisms, including stimulation of T_H2 lymphocytes, which results in production of IL-5, IL-13, and more IL-4. When IL-4 is absent, T_H2 lymphocyte differentiation is inhibited. Several studies have reported the results of using soluble IL-4 receptor (sIL-4R) as a treatment for allergic disease.

In one such randomized, placebo-controlled trial of 25 moderate asthmatics, all requiring inhaled corticosteroids, there was improvement in forced expiratory volume in 1 second (FEV_1) on the fourth day of aerosolized sIL-4R treatment in the high-dose group (14). There were no serious side effects of sIL-4R. Possible immune effects of long-term IL-4 blockade remain potential concerns.

Engineered Recombinant Allergenic Proteins

The major advantage of recombinant DNA technology is the ability to produce single allergens of identical structure. The use of single allergens, instead of the currently available allergenic vaccines, would allow a potentially more precise diagnosis and patients could receive immunotherapy only with the proteins to which they are allergic. On the other hand, one advantage of natural vaccines is in their antigenic completeness. Isoforms are proteins with similar amino acid sequences that have very different allergenicity. Overcoming the problems of isoform variability will present difficulties using recombinant technology (15,16).

The real innovation that would be possible with recombinant technology is to use it to develop new forms of treatment. Recombinant allergens can be engineered by site-directed mutagenesis to produce "hypoallergens" that no longer bind IgE but do retain T-cell epitopes (17). Among the hypoallergens that have been reported are a grass allergen (Ph1 p 5), group 2 mite allergens, and a peanut allergen (Ara h 2) (18–20).

Interferons

Recombinant interferon-γ (IFN-γ) is available as a therapy approved by the U.S. Food and Drug Administration for chronic granulomatous disease. This cytokine is known to suppress IgE production (21) and to downregulate the function and proliferation of $CD4^+$ T_H2 cells (22). The role of interferons in IgE-mediated diseases probably will be restricted to very severely affected patients because the risk for side effects, including fever, chills, headache, and rash, generally outweigh any possible benefit (23,24).

Novel Modified Allergen Immunotherapy

Allergen–Antibody Complexes

A novel approach to specific allergen desensitization—administering allergen–antibody complexes—has been proposed by SaintRemy and colleagues (25). The scientific rationale for this approach is that, under certain conditions, immune complexes can suppress the immunologic response to the antigen they contain (26). In several studies, efficacy and safety have been reported (27). These impressive results have only been reported by one center, and thus require confirmation by other investigative groups.

T Cell Peptides

T cells and B cells recognize different epitopes on the same protein. Whereas B cells recognize conformational epitopes via their immunoglobulin receptors, T cells recognize linear epitopes 8 to 22 amino acids in length via their T-cell receptors. These peptide fragments are associated with products of the major histocompatibility complex (MHC) expressed on the surface of antigen-presenting cells. CD4+ T cells regulating IgE response by B cells are MHC class II restricted. At least 100 allergens have been sequenced, and identification of T-cell epitopes is a rapidly progressing endeavor (28).

The tolerizing property of T-cell peptides was tested in a murine model using *Fel d I*. In animals with a preexisting immune response to *Fel d I*, subcutaneous injections of T-cell epitopes resulted in tolerance as measured by decreased IL-2 production when spleen cells were cultured with antigen (29).

Several clinical trials have been initiated. In a 10-center trial of mixed cat peptides in 270 patients, patients were randomized to placebo or one of several doses. There was a dose response. Scores were significantly decreased in the high-dose group compared with placebo. No serious side effects were reported (30). In a trial of T-cell epitopes of bee venom phospholipase A2, induction of anergy was reported in bee sting–allergic patients (31). Unfortunately some of the 16 or 17 amino acid peptide vaccines cause delayed bronchoconstriction without evidence of enhanced inflammation (32,33). These reactions are IgE independent and MHC restricted. This potential side effect may be obviated if longer peptides of 25 or 26 amino acids are used for therapy (34,35).

Immunotherapy Affecting Dendritic Cells

Immunotherapy could be aimed at inducing a T_H1 response to allergens using dendritic cells. The ideal dendritic cell would be one that is producing high levels of IL-12 (36). There are various ways that IL-12 production by dendritic cells can be increased. One *in situ* possibility is to add a recall antigen, such as tetanus toxoid, to the allergen of interest. The presentation of recall antigen by dendritic cells results in stimulation of specific CD4+ memory cells that rapidly upregulate CD40L, effectively conditioning the dendritic cell to increase its IL-12 production *in vivo* (37). T-cell activity after dendritic cell vaccination is dependent on the type of antigen and mode of delivery (38).

Immunostimulatory DNA Sequence Oligodeoxynucleotides

Another method of triggering maturation of dendritic cells and upregulation of their production of IL-12 is to administer CpG immunostimulatory DNA sequence oligodeoxynucleotides (ISS-ODNs) (39). Bacterial DNA contains a relatively high frequency of unmethylated CpG dinucleotides that exist at a much lower frequency and are methylated in the DNA of vertebrates (40). It appears that the innate human immunologic system has evolved pattern recognition receptors that distinguish procaryotic DNA from vertebrate DNA by detecting these unmethylated CpG dinuleotides, also called CpG motifs. CpG DNA activates not only dendritic cells but macrophages to increase expression of costimulatory molecules and to produce a variety of chemokines and cytokines, including IL-12, IL-18, and IFN-α. When natural killer cells are activated by CpG motifs, they produce IFN-γ, further intensifying the T_H1 response (41).

The effect of administering ISS-ODNs with cedar pollen allergens has been studied in mice with established sensitization. In this animal model, there was a clear shift from a T_H2 to a T_H1 immunologic response (42). Of interest is that in studies of mice genetically deficient in IFN-γ or IL-12, neither cytokine is required for the immunotherapeutic activity of CpG. This is a surprising finding which suggests that additional or redundant mechanisms must be operative (43). *In vitro* studies of human immune cell responses to CpG DNA show results comparable with murine studies (44–46). However, the optimal flanking bases around the CpG nucleotide and the number and arrangement of CpG dinucleotides are somewhat different for activating murine cells as compared with activating human cells.

In studies of subhuman primates, including apes, there have been several reports that CpG motifs are potent adjuvants (47–49). Human trials using CpG as a vaccine adjuvant began in Canada in 1999. Clinical trials using CpG DNA for cancer immunotherapy started in the United States in 2000. Clinical trials are expected to start soon for the treatment of human allergic disease in Germany. In the next few years, the potential role of CpG DNA in the immunotherapy of allergic disease should become much clearer.

DNA Vaccines

There are many viral diseases for which efficient vaccines are not available. Using DNA that encodes for viral proteins results in a robust response in many situations. Swine immunized with naked DNA vaccines for the highly virulent foot-and-mouth disease were protected on subsequent exposure (50). In a phase I study of vaccination with a plasmid containing DNA encoding for hepatitis D surface antigen, a booster response but not a primary response was reported (51). A DNA vaccine for hepatitis E virus has been reported to be effective in mice (52). Finally, an important disease in cultured rainbow trout is viral hemorrhagic septicemia (VHS). In a dose ranging study, even the smallest dose of plasmid containing VHS DNA resulted in protection from an immersion challenge with the virus (53). Although these results are encouraging, the possibility of the DNA being incorporated into the genome at an inopportune position that might activate a promoter or oncogene is of concern.

CONCLUSION

Novel immunologic therapies offer the hope of true revolutions in treatment of asthma and allergic-immunologic disorders. Knowledge gained from basic research has led to potential therapies, but the clinical effectiveness remains to be established. When an antagonist or biologic modifier becomes available, its administration helps to reinforce or minimize the contribution of the agonist or biologic reactant to disease processes. For example, platelet-activating factor (PAF) is known to be a bronchoconstrictor agent and is a potent chemotactic factor for eosinophils. To date, PAF antagonists have had modest effects on inhibiting allergen-induced as opposed to PAF-induced bronchial responses. Thus, the contribution of PAF to allergen-induced bronchial responses seems less than initially anticipated based on the potency of PAF as a bronchoconstrictor agonist.

Novel therapies need to be safe if widespread use is planned. Physicians will need to be aware of possible unexpected positive or negative effects when new therapies are used. For example, administration of novel immunologic therapy for patients with asthma and allergic rhinitis might concurrently exacerbate the patient's rheumatoid arthritis or vice versa. There will be opportunities to revolutionize therapy, and learning how best to use the novel agents will involve pharmacologic studies, clinical trials, effectiveness studies, and postlicensing surveillance.

REFERENCES

1. Ishizaka K, Ishizaka T. Identification of gamma-E antibodies as a carrier of reaginic activity. *J Immunol* 1967;99:1187–1198.
2. Solley GO, Gleich GJ, Jordan RE, et al. The late phase of the immediate wheal and flare skin reaction. Its dependence upon IgE antibodies. *J Clin Invest* 1976;58:408–420.
3. Lichtenstein LM, Levy DA, Ishizaka K. In vitro reverse anaphylaxis. *Immunology* 1970;19:831–842.
4. Fahy J, Fleming H, Wong H, et al. The effect of an anti-IgE monoclonal antibody on the early-and late-phase responses to allergen inhalation in asthmatic subjects. *Am J Respir Crit Care Med* 1997;155:1828–1834.
5. Boulet L, Chapman K, Cote J, et al. Inhibitory effects of an anti-IgE antibody E25 on allergen-induced early asthmatic responses. *Am J Respir Crit Care Med* 1997;155:1835–1840.
6. Jardieu PM, Fick RB Jr. IgE inhibition as a therapy for allergic disease. *Int Arch Allergy Immunol* 1999;118:112–115.
7. Casale TB, Bernstein IL, Busse W, et al. Use of anti-IgE humanized monoclonal antibody in ragweed-induced

allergic rhinitis. *J Allergy Clin Immunol* 1997;100:100–110.

8. Togias A, Corren J, Shapiro G, et al. Anti-IgE treatment reduces skin test (ST) reactivity. *J Allergy Clin Immunol* 1998;101(suppl):171.

9. Jagels MA, Daffern PJ, Zuraw BL, et al. Mechanisms and regulation of polymorphonuclear leukocyte and eosinophil adherence to human airway epithelial cells. *Am J Respir Cell Mol Biol* 1999;21:418–427.

10. Danzig M, Cuss F. Inhibition of interleukin-5 with a monoclonal antibody attenuates allergic inflammation. *Allergy* 1997;52:787–794.

11. Leckie MJ, ten Brinke A, Khan J, et al. Effects of an interleukin-5 blocking monoclonal antibody on eosinophils, airway hyper-responsiveness, and the late asthmatic response. *Lancet* 2000;356:2144–2148.

12. Teran C. Chemokines and IL-5: major players of eosinophil recruitment in asthma. *Clin Exp Allergy* 1999;29:287–290.

13. Heath H, Zin S, Rao P, et al. The importance of CCR-3 demonstrated using an antagonistic monoclonal antibody. *J Clin Invest* 1997;99:178–184.

14. Borish LC, Nelson HS, Lanz MF, et al. Interleukin-4 receptor in moderate atopic asthma: a phase I/II randomized, placebo-controlled trial. *Am J Respir Crit Care Med* 1999;160:1816–1823.

15. Breiteneder H, Ferreira F, Hoffmann-Sommergruber K, et al. Four recombinant isoforms of Cor a 1, the major allergen of hazel pollen, show different IgE-binding properties. *Eur J Biochem* 1993;212:355–362.

16. Schenk S, Hoffmann-Sommergruber K, Breiteneder H, et al. Four recombinant isoforms of Cor A 1, the major allergen of hazel pollen, show different reactivity with allergen- specific T-lymphocyte clones. *Eur J Biochem* 1994;224:717–722.

17. Ferreira F, Ebner C, Kramer B, et al. Modulation of IgE reactivity of allergens by site- directed mutagenesis: potential use of hypoallergenic variants for immunotherapy. *Fed Am Soc Exp Biol* 1998;12:231–242.

18. Schramm G, Kahlert H, Suck R, et al. "Allergen engineering": variants of the timothy grass pollen allergen Phl p 5b with reduced IgE-binding capacity buy conserved T cell reactivity. *J Immunol* 1999;162:2406–2414.

19. Smith AM, Chapman MD. Reduction in IgE binding to allergen variants generated by site-directed mutagenesis: contribution of disulfide bonds to the antigenic structure of the major house dust mite allergen, Der p2. *Mol Immunol* 1996;33:399–405.

20. Burks W, Bannon BA, Sicherer S, Sampson HA. Peanut-induced anaphylactic reactions. *Int Arch Allergy Immunol* 1999;119:165–172.

21. Péne J, Rousset F, Briére F, et al. IgE production by normal human lymphocytes is induced by interleukin 4 and suppressed by interferons gamma and alpha and prostaglandin E2. *Proc Natl Acad Sci USA* 1988;85:6880–6884.

22. Gajewski TF, Fitch FW. Anti-proliferative effect of IFN-gamma in immune regulation. I. IFN-gamma inhibits the proliferation of Th2 but not Th1 murine helper T lymphocyte clones. *J Immunol* 1988;140:4245–4252.

23. Pung YH, Vetro SW, Bellanti JA. Use of interferons in atopic (IgE-mediated) diseases. *Ann Allergy* 1993;71:234–238.

24. *Physicians desk reference,* 54th ed. Montvale NJ: Medical Economics Co., 2000:1441–1443.

25. Leroy BP, Lachapelle JM, Jacquemin M, et al. Treatment of atopic dermatitis by allergen-antibody complexes: long-term clinical results and evolution of IgE antibodies. *Dermatology* 1992;184:271–274.

26. Taylor RB, Tite JP, Manzo C. Immunoregulatory effects of a covalent antigen-antibody complexes. *Nature* 1979;281:488–490.

27. Leroy BP, Boden G, Lachapelle JM, et al. A novel therapy for atopic dermatitis with allergen-antibody complexes: a double-blind, placebo controlled study. *J Am Acad Dermatol* 1993;28:232–239.

28. de Weck AL. Allergen standardization at a crossroads. *Allergy Clin Immunol Int* 1997;9:25–30.

29. Briner TJ, Kuo M-C, Keating KM, Rogers BL. Peripheral T-cell tolerance induced in naive and primed mice by subcutaneous injection of peptides from the major cat allergen Fel d I. *Proc Natl Acad Sci U S A* 1993;90:7608–7612.

30. Norman PS, Nicodemus CF, ALLERVAX Cat Study Group. Multicenter study of several doses of ALLERVAX Cat peptides in the treatment of cat allergy. *J Allergy Clin Immunol* 1997;99(suppl):127.

31. Müller UR, Akdis AC, Fricker M, et al. Successful immunotherapy with T cell epitope peptides of bee venom phospholipase A2 induces specific T cell anergy in bee sting allergic patients. *J Allergy Clin Immunol* 1998;101:747–754.

32. Haselden BM, Kay AB, Larché M. Immunoglobulin E—dependent major histocompatibility complex–restricted T cell peptide epitope-induced late asthmatic reactions. *J Exp Med* 1999;189:1885–1894.

33. Larche M, Haselden BM, Oldfield WL, et al. Mechanisms of T cell peptide epitope-dependent late asthmatic reactions. *Int Arch Allergy Immunol* 2001;124:272–275.

34. Oldfield WLG, Shirley KE, Larché M, et al. A double-blind, placebo-controlled study of short peptides derived from Fel D 1 in cat-allergic subjects [Abstract]. *J Allergy Clin Immunol* 2001;107(suppl):216.

35. Alexander C, Oldfield WLG, Shirley KE, et al. A dosing protocol of allergen-derived T-cell peptide epitopes for the treatment of allergic disease [Abstract]. *J Allergy Clin Immunol* 2001;107(suppl):217.

36. Macatonia SE, Hosken NA, Litton M, et al. Dendritic cells produce IL-12 and direct the development of Th 1 cells from naive CD4(+) T cells. *J Immunol* 1995;154:5071–5079.

37. Cella M, Scheidegger D, Palmer-Lehmann K, et al. Ligation of CD40 on dendritic cells triggers production of high levels of interleukin-12 and enhances T cell stimulatory capacity: T-T help via APC activation. *J Exp Med* 1996;184:747–752.

38. Serody JS, Collins EJ, Tisch RM, et al. T cell activity after dendritic cell vaccination is dependent on both the type of antigen and the mode of delivery. *J Immunol* 2000;164:4961–4967.

39. Sparwasser T, Koch ES, Vabulas RM, et al. Bacterial DNA and immunostimulatory CpG oligonucleotides trigger maturation and activation of murine dendritic cells. *Eur J Immunol* 1998;28:2045–2054.

40. Krieg AK, Yi AK, Matson S, et al. CpG motifs in bacterial DNA trigger direct B-cell activation. *Nature* 1995;374:546–549.

41. Krieg AM, Hartmann G, Yi A-K. Mechanisms of action of CpG DNA. In: Wagner H, ed. *Current topics in microbiology and immunology* (in press).

42. Kohama Y, Akizuki O, Hagihara K, et al. Immunostimulatory oligodeoxynucleotide induces T_{H1} immune response and inhibition of IgE antibody production to cedar pollen allergens in mice. *J Allergy Clin Immunol* 1999:104:1231–1238.

43. Kline JN, Krieg AM, Waldschmidt TJ, et al. CpG oligodeoxynucleotides do not require Th1 cytokines to prevent eosinophilic airway inflammation in a murine model of asthma. *J Allergy Clin Immunol* 1999;104:1258–1264.

44. Hartmann G, Krieg AM. CpG DNA and LPS induce distinct patterns of activation in human monocytes. *Gene Ther* 1999;6:893–903.

45. Hartmann G, Krieg AM. Mechanism and function of a newly identified CpG DNA motif in human primary B-cells. *J Immunol* 2000;164:944–953.

46. Hartmann G, Weiner G, Krieg AM. CpG DNA as a signal for growth, activation and maturation of human dendritic cells. *Proc Natl Acad Sci U S A* 1999;96:9305–9310.

47. Jones TR, Obalidia N III, Gramzinski RA, et al. Synthetic oligodeoxynucleotides containing CpG motifs enhance immunogenicity of a peptide malaria vaccine in Aotus monkeys. *Vaccine* 1999;17:3065–3071.

48. Davis HL, Suparto I, Weeratna R, et al. Vaccination of orangutans at risk for hepatitis B infection: hyporesponsiveness to hepatitis B surface antigen overcome by CpG DNA. *Vaccine* (in press).

49. Hartmann G, Weeratna RD, Ballas ZK, et al. Delineation of a CpG phosphorothioate oligodeoxynucleotide for activation primate immune responses *in vitro* and *in vivo*. *J Immunol* (in press).

50. Beard C, Ward G, Reider E, et al. Development of DNA vaccines for foot-and-mouth disease, evaluation of vaccines encoding replication and non-replication nucleic acids in swine. *J Biotechnol* 1999;73:243–249.

51. Tacket CO, Roy MJ, Widera G, et al. Phase I safety and immune response studies of a DNA vaccine encoding hepatitis B surface antigen delivered by a gene delivery device. *Vaccine* 1999;17:2826–2869.

52. He J, Binn LN, Caudill JD, et al. Antiserum generated by DNA vaccine binds to hepatitis E virus (HEV) as determined by PCR and immune electron microscopy (IEM): application for HEV detection by affinity-capture RT-PCR. *Virus Res* 1999;62:59–65.

53. Lorenzen N, Lorenzen E, Einer-Jensen K, et al. Genetic vaccination of rainbow trout against viral hemorrhagic septicaemia virus: small amounts of plasmic DNA protect against a heterologous serotype. *Virus Res* 1999;63:19–25.

39

Management of the "Difficult" Patient

Howard L. Alt

Department of Psychiatry, Northwestern University Medical School, Chicago, Illinois

There are models of understanding, as well as strategies of management, of the "difficult" patient treated for allergic diseases such as asthma. What is the so-called difficult patient? There are several characteristics that define these patients. First, they consume more of the physician's time than other patients. They are the ones physicians do not want to see when scheduled and are happy when they cancel. They tend to upset physicians, make them feel angry, frustrated, helpless, guilty, and at a loss for how to apply treatment. These patients have difficulties complying with the treatment plan; as examples, they do not take their prescribed medications, they do not follow recommendations that would help the course of their disease, and they make frequent demands for changes in the treatment plan.

It is useful for physicians to have a framework for understanding the various psychiatric disorders, including depression, anxiety, bipolar disorder, personality disorders, obsessive-compulsive states, and psychotic illnesses (1). A detailed discussion of these diagnoses is beyond the scope of this text. Table 39.1 lists cardinal features of each of the above mental disorders. Causation of many of these diagnoses is not totally clear; however, alterations in neurotransmitters and genetic factors are implicated. Environmental factors may play a contributory role.

Having a knowledge of the diagnoses in Table 39.1 should help in differentiating difficult patient issues from situations in which psychiatric or psychopharmacological treatment is necessary. When psychiatric referral or consultation is required, it is important to understand how this can best be accomplished in a way that maintains the treatment alliance with the patient and does not lead to feelings of abandonment.

The majority of so-called difficult patients are understood better by considering their personality styles. Issues of anger, dependency, control, idealization/depreciation, denial, self-esteem, fear, effects of life losses, mourning, and narcissism are common. When structured around a personality disorder, they become more problematic. There are a variety of ways of understanding these styles and strategies of working with them. With the available time in the medical setting limited, physicians need to know how to best respond to these patients, build an effective treatment alliance, and use the power of the patient's attachment to the treating physician.

IMPORTANCE OF THE CHILD–CAREGIVER RELATIONSHIP

A concept that is important for the physician and other health-care providers is the developmental unfolding of the relationship of mutuality that should form between the child and the caregiver (2,3). Unfortunately, this does not always happen; there are healthy and unhealthy modes of caregivers relating to children. Whether in relationships with parents, siblings, teachers, friends, lovers, or spouses, we see the critical importance of this early connection throughout life. This early child–caregiver relationship is also what leads to the ability to form a good treatment alliance with a physician. If this developmental process is unhealthy, it often results in unhealthy

TABLE 39.1. *Characteristics of mental disorders*

Psychosis: severe symptoms of delusions, hallucinations, disorganization of thought, emotion, and behavior
Neurosis: presence of strong negative feelings such as anxiety or depression; personality intact; can recognize and objectively evaluate reality
Schizophrenia: principal clinical symptoms are delusions, hallucinations, withdrawal from reality; inability to feel normal emotions; flat affect
Affective disorders: these affect two abnormalities of mood—depression and elation (mania)
　Major affective disorders
　　Major depression: hopeless mood, pessimistic thinking, loss of enjoyment, reduced energy, slowness of thought
　　Manic depressive psychosis: discrete episodes of depression (as described in major depression) and then of mania characterized by euphoria, loud speech, quickened thought, excitement, and reduced need for sleep
　Minor affective disorders
　　Melancholia: a depressive syndrome characterized by early morning awakening, depression most severe in the morning, loss of appetite and libido
　　Cyclothymia: less severe illness than manic depressive psychosis; personality disorder of the affective type characterized by extreme mood swings
　　Depressive neurosis: also called dysthymic disorder; usually a situational depression but the mood change is disproportionately severe or prolonged for the loss; often occurs with other symptoms such a phobia or anxiety
Anxiety disorders: feeling of fear, dread, or apprehension without an appropriate justification
　Phobia: inappropriate fear of certain objects or situations
　Panic attacks: symptoms arise from overactivity of the sympathetic nervous system—palpitations, dry mouth, sweating, dyspnea, dilated pupils, trembling
Obsessive–compulsive disorder: obsessions are recurring thoughts, words, or ideas that an individual cannot voluntarily suppress; compulsions are impulses to perform repetitive acts that are apparently unnecessary and stereotypical, such as checking multiple times to see if the door is locked
Posttraumatic stress disorder: an individual reexperiences a terrifying event (rape, torture) as nightmares and even as daydreams
Somatiform disorder: multiple physical complaints such as dizziness, indigestion, back pain, with no organic cause
Dissociative disorder: some mental processes are split off from the rest of the psyche; the patient experiences sudden, temporary alterations in consciousness, memory, and motor behavior
Personality disorders: maladaptive, inflexible pattern of thinking, feeling, and behaving that impairs social functioning
　Paranoid: pervasive unjustified suspiciousness and mistrust of others
　Affective: mood disturbances, including anxiety, depression, and elation
　Schizoid: likes to be alone; prefers interacting with things, rather than with people
　Schizotypical: eccentricities of thought, speech or behavior, but not severe enough to be labeled schizophrenic
　Explosive: emotional rage and tantrums precipitated by minor frustration
　Compulsive: overscrupulous, perfectionistic, preoccupied with rules; unable to express loving emotions
　Histrionic: overly dramatic behavior, enjoys being the center of attention, highly reactive and excitable
　Dependent: lacks mental energy; allows others to control their life
　Antisocial: violate other people's rights; have no sense of remorse or guilt; never learn from past mistakes
　Passive–aggressive: responds negatively to demands placed on them by using passive means such as dawdling or intentional forgetfulness
　Narcissistic: grandiose sense of self-importance; can't withstand any criticism
　Borderline: angry outbursts; unstable intense relationships; frantic efforts to avoid abandonment

configurations a patient can set up with the physician, which could be called the difficult patient syndrome.

HEALTHY CHILD–CAREGIVER RELATIONSHIPS

In the optimal unfolding of the child's needs, both physical and psychological, there is a sense of well-being both in the child and the caregiver. In a healthy relationship between a child and his or her caregiver, there is communicative matching (4), the mutual attunement of the caregiver and child, the emotional sense of understanding the other. Jessica Benjamin (5) has written about the mutuality of relating that occurs wherein both caregiver and child feel known and responded to. The child may feel hungry, need to be changed, or have some other sense of discomfort or bodily pain. When the caregiver is able to understand the need and be responsive, the child begins to develop a sense of trust, well-being, and security toward him or her. The caregiver can sense what the child needs, respond to that need, and effect a transaction in which the child is soothed and comforted. As the child grows up, this dance of attunement grows more complex. The mother and father both play roles in eventually allowing the child to grow, individuate, and attain relative independence as they offer experiences of security, connection, and an adventuresome introduction to the world. From this accurate understanding and effective responsiveness, a capacity for love develops that is the base of the child's connection to others throughout life (6).

A healthy relationship between child and caregiver is vitally important for the future relationship between patient and physician. The trust and ability to let another be helpful is central to this relationship. When there is a failure in these early experiences, the sense of trust, alliance, and connection with the physician becomes impaired.

UNHEALTHY RELATIONSHIPS

A number of unhealthy child–caregiver relationships can result in future relationship problems. One example is a relationship in which the child's needs are not met (7). These needs include touching and holding, affirmations, and having the child's love accepted by the caregiver. When these basic needs go unmet, they result in negative feelings such as shame. When these experiences occur too often, shame is internalized and made a permanent part of the child's self. That is, it no longer requires an external trigger to produce shame. The first response to shame is anger, which is then strategically handled in a variety of ways—attacking the other, contempt, striving for power, attacking the self—resulting in low self-esteem or striving for perfection. These unmet needs lead to a rupture of the interpersonal bridge between caregiver and child.

Heinz Kohl, the developer of a model of narcissism and disorders of the self, states that there is a basic need of the developing child for someone to admire and idealize (8). When these needs are met, the child's self becomes strong, cohesive, and able to withstand appropriate injuries that growing up in the world inevitably presents. Then a child can tolerate occasional disillusionment with the important others in the child's life. There may be some reaction of anger or hurt, but with quick recovery. However, when these needs have not been sufficiently addressed, the child is much more vulnerable to psychological insult and the need to idealize and then devalue the other. There may be rage attacks, meltdowns, depression, or withdrawal. This can even become an entrenched personality style. When these individuals are responded to in an empathic and understanding manner, they begin to perk up again and recover.

Aaron Beck, the founder of cognitive psychology, emphasizes that an individual's underlying views and assumptions of the world inform that person's emotional life (9). Differences in the quality of life can occur with an individual's success at being able to work with difficult emotional states of anger, depression, worry, and obsession. The ability to let go of anger and get on with other activities can make the difference between suffering through the whole day versus using the day in positive, satisfying ways. If the caregiver does not teach the child how to handle negative emotions, a child may not be able to recover from a disagreement with a playmate; these children are not able to let go of the anger and reinvest in new play. This may be true for worries and shame as well. When a child has been effectively soothed, loved, and redirected toward new activities, the child is better able to internalize these behaviors throughout life. The child has learned strategies for defusing, distracting, and reinvolving with less emotional upset. These are basic principles of cognitive therapy. They are also the basis for Buddhist psychology in which the skill of becoming less identified with difficult feelings is developed (10).

Anxiety can have a powerful influence on the quality and enjoyment of life. Dr. David Barrow has written extensively on the anxiety disorders (11). He uses the analogy of a spring that becomes more tightly wound as the level of anxiety increases. The higher this gets, the less it takes to develop into a full-blown anxiety attack. Some patients are hypervigilant to internal bodily cues. The patient is acutely focused on aspects of his or her physicality. This hypervigilance leads to a vicious cycle of more adrenaline being released, more anxiety, and more vigilance. In asthma, the hypervigilance could be focused on the nature and level of breathing or wheezing.

Each of these unhealthy relationships between caregiver and child can result in the so-called difficult patient. Considering these unhealthy early relationships, it is possible for physicians to postulate the causes of the difficulties and to experiment with strategies that may help the treatment alliance. In *The Body in Pain*, Elaine Scary writes "there have always been . . . physicians whose daily work was premised on both a deep affection for the human body and a profound respect for the human voice." She underscores the importance of deeply listening to the patient sitting across from us (12). Even though the physician does not have a great deal of time to spend with each patient, it is important to approach the patient with caring, respect, interest, and a curiosity both to the physical and psychological characteristics.

A deep interest in understanding is an essential aspect of treating and healing the patient. A failure in child–caregiver interactions in prior experiences is often what has gone wrong in the so-called difficult patient. By focusing on these issues of connection, the physician can begin to soften the patient's negativity as strategies are formulated to help the patient. Whether the issues pertain to shame, fear, depression, loss, low self-esteem, or narcissistic injury, this understanding approach to the patient is most useful.

ADJUSTMENT REACTIONS TO ILLNESS

There are significant effects of a chronic illness, such as asthma, on a developing child. How a caregiver responds to these effects can result in teaching the child healthy or unhealthy relationships. The illness presents discomfort and anxiety for the child. When the caregiver is able to respond effectively to the discomfort of a child, there is a foundation of security, trust, and well-being. The child feels better and develops a sense of the caregiver's competence in being able to respond. On the other hand, the caregiver may become frustrated or anxious about the illness and can overrespond or even withdraw. The caregiver may feel helpless, resulting in behaviors that are excessively lenient or excessively controlling.

In the adult, asthma may lead to psychological dynamics. The sense of control over one's life is affected because of the unpredictability of when an asthma exacerbation will occur. In some personality styles, the individual needs to maintain a great amount of control and can become very disturbed by lack of control. As in any chronic illness, depression, and loss of self-esteem also may occur in asthma.

In the situation in which there is curtailment of previous activities, the patient may experience feelings of loss, anger, and depression. What is most helpful is to further the dialogue about these situations. Talking to someone who is interested and will be empathic to these feelings helps the patient to feel less alone, to express anger and frustration, and, most important, to do the mourning work around the losses of physical integrity and functioning. Some of problems with the so-called difficult patient arise when this talking process is not encouraged.

CHARACTER PATTERNS OF DIFFICULT PATIENTS

To begin to lay a psychological and dynamic foundation for understanding these patients, it is essential to introduce the concept of character patterns, also called personality styles. They are characteristic ways that people think, feel, and behave as they grow up in dealing with the significant others around them, their internal feelings and thoughts, and their self-esteem and self-concept. These personality styles are primarily formed in the relationships that children have with their caregivers. These relationships are very intense; how children are responded to in daily activities defines how they feel about themselves, their self-esteem, their sense of being loved, and how they believe they should treat other people. When there are failures in these early interactions the character styles become character disorders. These personality disorders include dependent, passive-aggressive, explosive, histrionic, antisocial, schizoid, obsessive-compulsive, borderline, paranoid, and narcissistic states. These patients consume a lot of the treatment team's time and are often noncompliant. They present to the treatment team with anger, blaming, helplessness, failure to take responsibility, and denial. The physician does not look forward to appointments with the so-called difficult patient because the physician feels angry, helpless, and guilty. Physicians feel best when they are helping their patients. These patients make physicians feel defeated in that regard. Physicians often either withdraw from the patient emotionally or become angry. These patients are often discharged from the practice for noncompliance or referred out of the system. There appears to be a perverseness about their behavior. Physicians give their best efforts and attempt to help the difficult patient who is frustrating and defeating them. But just as the physician pulls away, the difficult patient may entreat the physician to help. Some difficult patients seem to become angry or withdrawn with no clear reason, in response to something we have said. By looking more closely at a psychodynamic understanding of the borderline personality disorder and the narcissistic personality disorder, we can better understand the mystery of these reactions.

The Borderline Personality Disorder

The Diagnostic and Statistical Manual for Mental Disorders (1) describes the following aspects of borderline personality disorder: intense angry outbursts, empty feelings, unstable self-image, emotional hyperreactivity, unstable and intense relationships, frantic efforts to avoid abandonment, issues around idealization and devaluation, impulsivity, and suicidal threats. There is debate around the etiology of this disorder. The various theories include genetic predisposition and childhood trauma and abuse, as well as a psychodynamic model based on early childhood relationships.

A model has been developed by Margaret Mahler, *The Psychological Birth of the Human Infant*, and by James Masterson (13) in *The Search for the Real Self: Unmasking the Personality Disorders of Our Time*. Mahler calls her model of development *separation/individuation*. She evaluated how children use their parents to

develop independence and relative separation. At first children are unaware of their vulnerability and the need for the parent. They play and explore the world with joy and lack of fear. Gradually, by 18 months, they begin to realize that they are vulnerable and need their parent. Finally, at about 36 months, they achieve, if all has gone well, a sense of independence and authentic individuation. They believe that they are individuals, both different and similar to their parents.

The crucial phase for the development of problems is around the vulnerable 18-month-old stage. Children need the mother to be sensitive to both the needs for dependence and independence. If both can be sensitively responded to, children can continue their quest for selfhood. However, parents may have their own needs that impinge on the child. For example, parents may need the child to depend and be attached to them and may be threatened by the push for emancipation. They may then punish efforts toward independence and reward dependent behaviors. Alice Miller (14), in *Prisoners of Childhood*, describes how the parents' use of the child for their own needs is destructive to the child. The child is vulnerable and influenced by this and does damage to his or her own development to keep the mother connected.

Alternatively, the mother may have conflicts around being needed. This may make her uncomfortable with the child's dependency, and she may reward only the independent side. Again the child feels abandoned because he or she still needs the mother. Masterson characterizes selectively rewarding and punishing these needs as leading to an "abandonment depression." The developmental need of the child is not met by either behavior of the parent. This can be described as the "need/fear dilemma." The child both needs and fears the connection with the parent. He or she may fear overinvolvement or intrusiveness, but also withdrawal and abandonment.

Whatever difficulties so-called difficult patients had in their child–caregiver relationships will likely also occur in the patient–physician relationship. There are powerful issues of connection, abandonment, idealization, and devaluation at play. Patients come to the physician with a readiness to admire, connect, and be helped. However, they then begin to fear the dependency

in the patient, we will just react to the behaviors. If we train ourselves to become mindful about our reactions, we can begin to develop strategies and a curiosity about the situation. This also helps to open up some perspective on how to help our patients.

Once physicians begin to step back and become curiously mindful about how they are feeling, they can begin to fit the patient's behaviors into the patterns discussed above. They can classify their patient as a dependent personality, a narcissistic personality, a borderline personality, or some other type of personality disorder.

It is important for the physician to treat the patient with respect, caring, and empathic listening. After the diagnosis and formulation of a treatment plan, the physician can explain the nature of the illness, what helps it and what does not, the course, and the treatment plan. It is helpful to write this out and keep a copy in the hands of both the patient and doctor. It is also useful to point out that treatment will take time to become optimally adjusted, effective, and may not completely eliminate the symptoms. The goal is to reach the maximum improvement possible.

The physician should expect that the "difficult" patient will be difficult. By approaching the patient's behavior with curiosity, detachment, and caring, the physician can set up the most constructive alignment with the patient to conduct the treatment. If the physician can avoid personalizing the patient's behavior, if he or she can maintain the caring connection with a useful distance, then the borderline patient's destructive behavior can be reduced.

The physician's first tendency is to withdraw from patients who are being very demanding. This only increases the anxiety and behavioral maneuvers. By being easily accessible and yet limiting the time, patients do not feel abandoned. Patients also are reassured by our response to the sense of crisis they carry with them. Physicians care, are appropriately available, encourage a vigorous relationship with reality around their illness, and set firm and understandable limits based on what's best for the patient, not out of anger or retaliation. They are reassured by the doctor remaining present in a caring manner.

One can direct statements back to patients about their illness and how they are taking care of themselves. For example, the physician might say, "If this recommendation would help you, why wouldn't you want to do it?" This shifts the role of the doctor to one of consultant rather than the all-powerful controller or the defeated helpless one. It removes the physician from the destructive interpersonal drama with these patients, and allows the physician to be an advisor.

The handling of a referral of a patient to a psychiatrist requires a high degree of sensitivity. Patients may feel that they are being told they are crazy or their problems are "all in their head." They also may feel that the primary doctor is trying to abandon them. From the physician's side, if the referral is in response to negative feelings evoked by the difficult patient, then it is often doomed. The patient feels the referral to a psychiatrist is an abandonment or punishment. Patients who have borderline or narcissistic disorders are especially prone to these reactions due to their issues around dependency, abandonment, and personal slights. For these reasons the best model is when the psychiatrist is an ongoing part of the treatment team. The doctor can say to the patient that the referral will help the doctor and patient to work even better as the allergic disease is treated. The doctor can make sure to set an appointment with the patient after his or her scheduled time to see the psychiatrist. The role of the psychiatrist to treat any underlying psychiatric disorders such as depression or anxiety can help the patient focus with the allergist on what needs to happen to help the allergic disease.

Differentiate the behaviors from the person. A person may present for treatment and have some obnoxious ways of relating. These are there for some function and not equivalent to the essential person inside that hurts, suffers, hates, loves, and wants to be loved. This is inherent in being a physician, where the challenge is to aid individuals with their problems. It is important to maintain a sense of respect and understanding for our patients. By training the ability to truly listen and understand what the patient is experiencing, the physician can wisely and firmly respond.

REFERENCES

1. American Psychiatric Association. *Diagnostic and statistical manual of mental disorders,* 4th ed. Washington, DC: American Psychiatric Association, 1994.
2. Winnicott DW. Hate in the Countertransference. *Int J Psychoanalysis* 1949;30:69–74.
3. Masterson JF. *The search for the real self: unmasking the personality disorders of our age.* New York: Free Press, 1988.
4. Masterson JF. *The narcissistic and borderline disorders: an integrated developmental approach.* New York: Brunner Mazel, 1981.
5. Benjamin J. *The bonds of love.* New York: Pantheon, 1988.
6. Mahler MS. *The psychological birth of the human infant: symbiosis and individuation.* London: Hutchinson, 1975.
7. Kaufman G. *Shame, the power of caring.* Rochester, NY: Shenkman Books, 1992.
8. Kohl H. *The analysis of the self. A systematic approach to the psychoanalytic treatment of narcissistic personality disorders.* New York: International University Press, 1971.
9. Beck AT, Emery G. *Anxiety disorders and phobias: a cognitive perspective.* New York: Basic Books, 1985.
10. Epstein M. *Thoughts without a thinker, psychotherapy from a Buddhist perspective.* New York: Basic Books, 1995.
11. Barrow DH. *Anxiety and its disorders: the nature and treatment of anxiety and panic.* New York: Guilford, 1988.
12. Scary E. *The body in pain.* New York: Oxford University Press, 1985.
13. Masterson J, Masterson JF. *The search for the real self: unmasking the personality disorders of our age.* New York: Free Press, 1988.
14. Miller A. *Prisoners of childhood.* New York: Basic Books, 1981.
15. Groves JE. Taking care of the hateful patient. *N Engl J Med* 1978;298:883–887.
16. Winnicott DW. Hate in the countertransference. *Int J Psychoanalysis* 1949;30:69–74.
17. Adler G. Helplessness in the helpers. *Br J Med Psychol* 1972;45:315–326.

40

Chronic Sinusitis: Role of Rhinoscopy and Surgery

Rakesh K. Chandra, David B. Conley, and Robert C. Kern

Department of Otolaryngology–Head and Neck Surgery, Northwestern University Medical School and Northwestern Memorial Hospital, Chicago, Illinois

INTRODUCTION AND HISTORICAL PERSPECTIVE

Chronic sinusitis affects an estimated 31 million people in the United States. Management of this disorder, which accounts for approximately 16 million patient visits per year, has changed dramatically in the past 50 years. This is due to new insights into the pathophysiology of sinusitis, advances in rhinoscopy (nasal endoscopy), improved radiographic imaging, and availability of antibiotics (1). Technical advances in endoscopic instrumentation have defined a new era in the office diagnosis and surgical management of sinusitis, permitting an unprecedented level of precision. Understanding the indications as well as the technical limitations of diagnostic and therapeutic rhinoscopy is now essential for practitioners who manage chronic sinusitis.

Hirschman performed the first fiberoptic nasal examination using a modified cystoscope (2). Refinements in instrumentation after World War II allowed the development of smaller scopes that provided better illumination. In the early 1950s, investigators at Johns Hopkins University designed a series of endoscopes with relatively small-diameter, wide-field, high-contrast optics, and adequately bright illumination. At this time W. Messerklinger of Graz began to use this technology for systematic nasal airway evaluation. He reported that primary inflammatory processes in the lateral nasal wall, particularly in the middle meatus, result in secondary disease in the maxillary and frontal sinuses (2). This region, which represents a common drainage site for the maxillary, frontal, and anterior ethmoid sinuses, is termed the osteomeatal complex. Messerklinger found that small anatomic variations or even minimal inflammatory activity in this area could result in significant disease of the adjacent sinuses as a result of impaired ventilation and drainage. With this observation, he used endoscopes to develop a surgical approach to relieve the obstruction in such a way that normal sinus physiology was preserved. Specifically, he demonstrated that even limited surgical procedures directed toward the osteomeatal complex and the anterior ethmoid air cells could relieve obstruction of drainage from the frontal and maxillary sinuses. This philosophy was markedly different from the ablative sinus procedures advocated in the past, such as Caldwell-Luc, in that cilia and sinus mucosal function were preserved. Hence these procedures were termed functional endoscopic sinus surgery (FESS); Stammberger and Kennedy further refined these techniques in the 1980s.

ANATOMY AND PHYSIOLOGY OF THE NOSE AND PARANASAL SINUSES

The frontal, maxillary, ethmoid, and sphenoid sinuses are formed early in development as

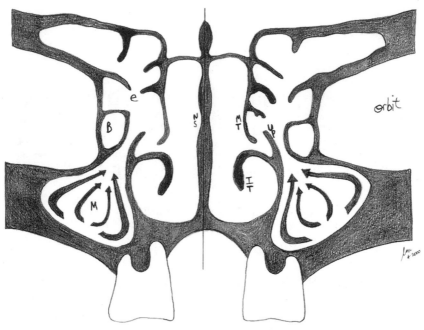

FIG. 40.1. A schematic view of sinonasal anatomy in the coronal plane. The maxillary sinus (*M*), ethmoid labyrinth (*e*) and bulla (*B*), uncinate process (*up*), nasal septum (*NS*), and middle (*MT*) and inferior (*IT*) turbinates are identified. The arrows demonstrate mucociliary clearance patterns in the maxillary sinuses. Cilia drive mucus toward the natural ostium.

evaginations of nasal respiratory mucosa into the facial bones. The ethmoid sinus develops into a labyrinth of 3 to 15 small air cells; however, the other sinuses exist as a single bony cavity on each side of the facial skeleton. The ethmoid and maxillary sinuses are present at birth and can be imaged in infancy. The frontal sinuses develop anatomically by 12 months and can be evaluated radiographically at 4 to 6 years. Sphenoid sinuses develop by the age of 3 but cannot be imaged until a child is 9 or 10 years of age. The point at which mucosal outpouching occurs persists as the sinus ostium, through which the sinus drains (3).

Diagnostic rhinoscopy offers a wealth of information regarding the distribution of inflammatory foci within the sinonasal labyrinth and the associated anatomic variations that may impair physiologic sinus drainage. It is usually performed in an office setting with the aid of topical decongestants and topical anesthesia. It is essentially an extension of the physical examination that helps confirm the diagnosis, gain insight into the pathophysiologic factors at work, and guide medical or surgical therapy. The princi-

ples of diagnostic and therapeutic rhinoscopy are based on a firm understanding of the anatomy and physiology of the nose and sinuses (Fig. 40.1). The lateral nasal walls are each flanked by three turbinate bones, designated the superior, middle, and inferior turbinates. The region under each turbinate is known respectively as the superior, middle, and inferior meatus. The anatomy of the lateral nasal wall is of key importance for the understanding of sinonasal physiology and the principles of FESS, because the ostium of each sinus drains into an anatomically specific location. The frontal, maxillary, and anterior ethmoid sinuses drain on the lateral nasal wall in a region within the middle meatus, known as the osteomeatal complex. This is an anatomically narrow space where even minimal mucosal disease can result in impairment of drainage from any of these sinuses. The posterior ethmoid sinuses drain into the superior meatus but are often aerated via the middle meatus during FESS. The sphenoid sinus drains into a region known as the sphenoethmoidal recess, which lies at the junction of the sphenoid and ethmoid bones in the posterior superior nasal cavity. The nasolacrimal duct courses anteriorly to the maxillary sinus ostium and drains into the inferior meatus.

The ethmoid bone is the most important component of the osteomeatal complex and lateral nasal wall. It is a T-shaped structure, of which the horizontal portion forms the cribriform plate of the skull base. The vertical part forms most of the lateral nasal wall and consists of the superior and middle turbinates, as well as the ethmoid sinus labyrinth. Within the middle meatus, a sickle-shaped projection of the ethmoid bone, known as the uncinate process, forms a recess, called the infundibulum, into which the maxillary sinus drains (4). A collection of anterior ethmoid air cells forms a bulla, which is suspended from the remainder of the ethmoid bone, and hangs just superiorly to the opening of the infundibulum into the meatus. The drainage duct for the frontal sinus courses inferiorly such that its ostium lies anterior and medial to the anteriormost ethmoid air cell. Therefore, the main components of the osteomeatal complex are the maxillary sinus ostium/infundibulum, the anterior ethmoid cells/bulla, and the frontal recess. The infundibulum and frontal recess exist as narrow clefts; thus, it is possible that minimal inflammation of the adjacent ethmoidal mucosa can result in secondary obstruction of the maxillary and frontal sinuses.

The paranasal sinuses are lined by pseudostratified-ciliated columnar epithelium, over which lays a thin blanket of mucus. The cilia beat in a predetermined direction such that the mucous layer is directed toward the natural ostium and into the appropriate meatus of the nasal airway. This is the process by which microbial organisms and debris are cleared from the sinuses (4). This principle of mucociliary flow is analogous to the "mucociliary elevator" described for the tracheobronchial tree. The maxillary ostium and infundibulum are located superior and medial to the sinus cavity itself. Therefore, mucociliary in the maxillary sinus must overcome the tendency for mucus to pool in dependent areas of the sinus. Successful FESS entails enhancement of drainage via the natural ostium. Antrostomies placed in dependent portions of the sinus are not effective because they interfere with normal sinus physiology.

Pathophysiology of Chronic Sinusitis

The American Academy of Otolaryngology–Head and Neck Surgery Task Force on Rhinosinusitis defines sinusitis as a condition "manifested by an inflammatory response involving the following: the mucous membranes (possibly including the neuroepithelium) of the nasal cavity and paranasal sinuses, fluids within these cavities, and/or underlying bone" (5). *Rhinosinusitis,* rather than *sinusitis,* is the more appropriate term, because sinus inflammation is often preceded by rhinitis and rarely occurs without coexisting rhinitis. Primary inflammation of the nasal membranes, specifically in the region of the osteomeatal complex, results in impaired sinus drainage and bacterial superinfection, resulting in further inflammation (Fig. 40.2). In most patients, a variety of host and environmental factors serve to precipitate initial inflammatory changes. Host factors include systemic processes such as allergic and immunologic conditions, various genetic disorders (e.g., immotile cilia syndrome and cystic fibrosis), and metabolic/endocrine disorders. Host variations in sinonasal anatomy also occur, predisposing some to ostial obstruction with even minimal degrees of mucosal inflammation. Neoplasms of the nose and maxilla and nasal polyps also may cause anatomic obstruction. Environmental factors play a vital role, including infectious agents, allergens, medications, trauma, and noxious fumes such as tobacco smoke (5). The pathophysiology of chronic sinusitis can be influenced by sinonasal anatomy, infection, and allergic/immunologic disorders. Rhinoscopy can provide significant insight into the relative importance of these elements in an individual patient. The infectious, allergic, and immunologic elements of chronic sinusitis are typically subjected to intense pharmacologic treatment. A failure of these therapies may indicate the need for surgery in the management of this problem.

Nasal and Sinus Anatomy

Anatomic variations can contribute to the pathophysiology of chronic sinusitis, including congenital, surgical, traumatic, or postinflammatory alterations in the normal structure. These include

Immune Deficiency

Immune deficiencies also play a role in sinusitis. Some individuals with recurrent acute or chronic sinusitis may have an immune deficiency. The most common is IgA deficiency, but IgG deficiency also may occur. Antibody defects predispose the patient to infection with encapsulated gram-positive and some gram-negative organisms. This is in contrast to T-cell deficiencies, which render the patient more susceptible to viral, fungal, and protozoal infections. Terminal complement component defects are associated with neisserial infections. Thus, the particular type of immune deficiency dictates the nature of the infectious organisms (9). These observations are particularly important in this era of widespread acquired immunodeficiency in which sinusitis can be more atypical than in the general population. Rhinoscopically directed cultures may be useful in the diagnosis and management of atypical infections.

Allergic Fungal Sinusitis

Allergic fungal sinusitis is a pathologic entity distinct from invasive fungal sinusitis. The latter is a fulminant infectious process with tissue invasion; chronicity is rare. In AFS, however, chronic hypersensitivity to dematiaceous fungi is associated with nasal polyposis, obstruction, and multiple sinus involvement. The immunologic processes at work in AFS may involve type I, type III, and type IVa_2 hypersensitivity, which are also observed in allergic bronchopulmonary aspergillosis (12). More recent studies, however, have suggested that the process in AFS is partially mediated by eosinophils (13).

The classic rhinoscopic finding in AFS is thick, tenacious "peanut butter"–like inspissated mucus within one or more paranasal sinuses. Histologic examination of this "allergic mucin" reveals embedded eosinophils, Charcot-Leydin crystals (eosinophil breakdown products), and extramucosal fungal hyphae. Although bone destruction and expansion may occur, the disease most often follows a slow, progressive course and thus represents a unique form of chronic sinusitis.

In fact, AFS may occur in up to 7% of patients with chronic sinusitis (14). The incidence of nasal polyposis in this disorder is high and, by some definitions, is required for diagnosis. Polyps, in combination with allergic mucin, often lead to secondary osteomeatal obstruction.

Any combination of the previously discussed inflammatory and anatomic factors can result in the histopathologic picture of chronic sinusitis, a proliferative process associated with fibrosis of the lamina propria and an inflammatory infiltrate of eosinophils, lymphocytes, and plasma cells. Chronic mucosal inflammation also may induce osteitic changes of the ethmoid bone (5). Although the precipitating and potentiating causes for chronic rhinosinusitis are multifactorial, the common outcome is a cycle by which ostial obstruction leads to stasis of secretions, microbial colonization, and further inflammatory changes and polyp formation in susceptible individuals.

THE DIAGNOSIS OF CHRONIC SINUSITIS

Classification

Working definitions for acute rhinosinusitis, subacute rhinosinusitis, chronic rhinosinusitis, recurrent acute rhinosinusitis, and acute exacerbation of chronic rhinosinusitis have been established by the Task Force on Rhinosinusitis sponsored by the American Academy of Otolaryngology–Head and Neck Surgery. This group also identified clinical factors that are associated with the diagnosis of sinusitis. These are grouped into two categories: major factors and minor factors (Table 40.1) (5). The presence of two or more major factors or one major and two minor factors is considered a "strong history for sinusitis." Nasal purulence alone is considered diagnostic of sinusitis, and rhinoscopic examination clearly can document this physical sign. A stream purulent of mucus may be apparent draining from beneath the middle turbinate. Endoscopically directed cultures of this drainage may be of particular value in guiding antibiotic therapy (5).

TABLE 40.1. *Major and minor factors in the diagnosis of sinusitis*

Major factors	Minor factors
Facial pain/pressure	Headache
Facial congestion/fullness	Fever (all nonacute forms of sinusitis)
Nasal obstruction/blockage	Halitosis
Nasal discharge/purulence	Fatigue
Discolored post nasal drip	Dental pain
Hyposmia/anosmia	Cough
Purulence in nasal cavity	Ear pain/pressure/ fullness
Fever (acute sinusitis only)	

Adapted from Lanza DC, Kennedy DW. Adult rhinosinusitis defined. *Otolaryngol Head Neck Surg* 1997;117 (suppl):1–7; with permission.

Classification of sinusitis as acute, subacute, recurrent acute, or chronic is dependent on temporal patterns. A diagnosis of chronic sinusitis requires that signs and symptoms consistent with a "strong history for sinusitis" persist for longer than 12 weeks. Patients also may have acute exacerbations of chronic sinusitis in which they experience worsening of the chronic baseline signs and symptoms or the development of new ones. These patients do not have complete resolution of symptoms between exacerbations, in contrast to those with recurrent acute sinusitis. Given the multifactorial nature of its etiology and the diversity of signs and symptoms, chronic sinusitis can be considered a syndrome. Generally, chronic sinusitis is the most common indication for FESS;

the goal of surgery is to remove symptomatic anatomic obstruction that has failed to respond to aggressive medical therapy. The resulting improvement in sinus ventilation and drainage often promotes relief of inflammation and resolution of symptoms.

Rhinoscopic Diagnosis

Nasal endoscopy is an extension of the physical examination that offers significant insight into the pathologic factors at work in chronic sinusitis. For centuries, the standard of diagnosis was visualization anteriorly using a nasal speculum and posteriorly using an angled mirror placed in the pharynx. Rhinoscopy using a rigid fiberoptic telescope, however, is considered more accurate and thorough, and can be performed at a reasonable cost (15). Several scopes are available to provide visualization with different angles of deflection (Fig. 40.5). The zero degree telescope, for example, gives a direct and magnified view of structures directly in front of the tip of the scope. In contrast, the 30 degree scope evaluates structures located at a 30 degree inclination from the long axis of the instrument in the direction of the bevel. Flexible endoscopy is preferable for patient comfort prior to the performance of endoscopy, the nose is often topically decongested and anesthetized with a combination of phenylephrine or oxymetazoline (for decongestion),

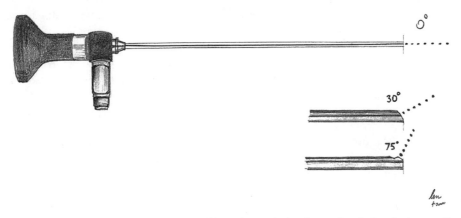

FIG. 40.5. Representative rhinoscopes. Note the variation in angle of view between the 0, 30, and 75 degree tips.

and lidocaine or pontocaine (for anesthesia). These are administered in aerosolized spray form. Decongestion temporarily shrinks the inflamed nasal mucosa, allowing the scope greater access to critical areas. The topical anesthesia improves patient comfort and compliance during the examination. Most endoscopists examine the key areas in a systematic sequence. Regardless of the order, attempts should be made to visualize the following: nasal septum, inferior turbinate and meatus, middle turbinate and meatus, superior meatus, sphenoethmoidal recess (15), and the presence of accessory ostia (Fig. 40.3).

In examining patients who have a history consistent with sinusitis, specific pathology that is not evident by a speculum examination may be detected by fiberoptic rhinoscopy. These include middle meatal polyps, pus, turbinate pathology, alterations in mucous viscosity, and synechiae (scar bands). In AFS, allergic mucin may be apparent in addition to polyps. Anatomic abnormalities of the septum, turbinates, or meatus are noted. These may contribute to the development of chronic sinusitis by causing ostial obstruction. In the absence of symptoms and mucosal inflammatory changes, findings such as a deviated septum or a concha bullosa are considered incidental. In each particular case, the surgeon must assess the degree of pathology and the contribution of anatomic abnormalities to that pathology. Those factors that appear to affect sinus drainage can then be addressed.

An additional role of diagnostic rhinoscopy is to rule out the presence of benign or malignant neoplasms of the nose and paranasal sinuses. These pathologies can cause anatomic obstruction of sinus drainage and thus produce symptoms of chronic sinusitis. Suspicious lesions observed rhinoscopically can be examined via biopsy with endoscopic guidance, often in the office setting. The differential diagnosis of sinonasal masses includes benign and malignant salivary gland tumors, inverting papilloma, and sinonasal carcinoma. These entities are relatively rare; their discussion is beyond the scope of this chapter. It is nonetheless important that to note that rhinoscopic examination may reveal pathology that may not be suspected on the initial history and physical examination in a patient with symptoms of chronic sinusitis.

Radiologic Diagnosis

Imaging has become a critical element in the diagnosis of sinusitis, the extent of inflammatory disease, and the evaluation of sinonasal anatomy. By the time FESS was introduced in the United States in 1984, computed tomography (CT) had become the modality of choice for diagnosis of sinusitis. Prior to this, imaging studies for sinusitis were conventional radiography and polytomography. CT has continued to be the gold standard, and its advantages continue to grow. At many institutions the cost of a screening coronal sinus CT scan limited sinus series is comparable with that of a plain film sinus series and provides far more clarity of bony detail. With improved technology, CT is being performed more quickly and with lower radiation doses. Therefore, CT stands as a cost-effective, efficient, safe, and informative modality. CT is also being used with ever-increasing frequency for image-guided surgery. In this practice, CT data are digitized into a computer system that allows the surgeon to correlate endoscopic anatomic points with those on the digitized CT scan (16).

Magnetic resonance imaging (MRI) has become more widespread, accessible, and affordable during recent years. Its utility in sinonasal imaging, however, is limited secondary to its inability to display fine bony detail. MRI, nonetheless, is useful in the detection of disease extension into adjacent compartments such as the brain and orbit. Compared with CT, MRI may better distinguish neoplastic from inflammatory processes and may more accurately distinguish fungal disease from other inflammatory conditions (16).

Computed tomography accurately demonstrates mucosal thickening within the sinus cavities and deep in the osteomeatal complex (16), the degree of bony thickening, and the presence of polyps, air-fluid levels, or sinus opacification (Fig. 40.4). The number and location of the involved sinuses also can be determined. In fact, several staging systems have been developed attempting to grade the severity of sinusitis based on these variables (17). The presence of bony anatomic variations that may contribute to the pathology of chronic sinusitis also can be detected. The CT scan should be viewed as an adjunct to rhinoscopy rather than a replacement for this procedure. Most importantly, the CT scan confirms and documents osteomeatal obstruction. A patient with sinusitis symptoms despite aggressive medical therapy who has sinus outflow obstruction on a CT scan is a typical candidate for FESS.

FUNCTIONAL ENDOSCOPIC SINUS SURGERY

Indications

Initial treatment for chronic sinusitis is medical. This may include any combination, depending on underlying causes, of topical steroid nasal sprays, oral steroids, antihistamines, decongestants, antibiotics, and nasal saline irrigations. Identification and avoidance of causative allergies is also indicated. Medical therapy should usually be the first-line treatment in uncomplicated cases, with an antibiotic course generally recommended for a minimum duration of 4 to 6 weeks. Surgical indications include chronic or recurrent acute pansinusitis, frank nasal polyposis, mucocele, pending orbital or cranial complications, mycotic infections, debilitating headache, and olfactory dysfunction (18,19). The most common clinical setting for FESS is persistent sinusitis symptoms despite an extended course of comprehensive medical therapy coupled with a CT scan demonstrating osteomeatal obstruction. There are some data to suggest that FESS can reduce significantly both the number of infections requiring antibiotics and the severity of facial pain or headache in patients with recurrent acute sinusitis who have normal CT scans; this subset of patients is thought to have reversible nasal mucosal disease (20). Although FESS may have a role in the management of carefully selected symptomatic patients with normal CT scans, the exact indications for surgery in this patient population are unclear.

Cystic fibrosis may be etiologic in children with nasal polyposis, and this scenario is a strong indication for FESS (21). In cases of extensive polyp disease, surgery is not curative but does improve symptoms. These patients often require revision surgery and are committed to long-term topical or oral steroid therapy. Thus, surgery is considered palliative in these cases because it cannot address the underlying pathophysiologic process (18). Uncomplicated pediatric chronic sinusitis that is refractory to medical management is only considered a relative indication for FESS. In these cases, adenoidectomy is first-line surgical therapy if the adenoid pad is enlarged (21).

Preoperative Imaging

The importance of preoperative CT scanning cannot be understated. This is crucial prior to the performance of FESS, not only for diagnostic purposes, but to demonstrate the relationships between the paranasal sinuses and critical surrounding structures such as the brain, orbit, and carotid artery. The ethmoid sinus system forms the skull base, and the frontal, maxillary, and ethmoid sinuses surround the orbit (Figs. 40.1 and 40.4). Anatomic details vary from patient to patient and must be correlated with endoscopic data for the safe performance of FESS (16). It is important to remember, however, that the CT scan represents only one point in time, and thus does not always predict the extent of inflammatory disease that will be encountered at surgery.

Unless orbital or intracranial complications are pending, it is preferable to avoid operating in the setting of acute symptom exacerbations in order to minimize the risks of perioperative bleeding and other complications. Also, the use of aspirin and other nonsteroidal antiinflammatory drugs is discouraged within 2 weeks of surgery. The usual preoperative studies, including laboratory studies, chest radiography, electrocardiography, and cardiac/pulmonary consultation, are obtained as indicated. Finally, the potential complications of FESS are discussed with the patient, and informed consent is obtained.

Intraoperative Procedure

After the administration of general anesthesia or sedation, topical anesthetics and vasoconstrictors are applied. Under endoscopic visualization, lidocaine with epinephrine is injected submucosally at key points. This provides vasoconstriction and obviates the need for deeper planes of systemic anesthesia.

When it is deemed that septal deviation contributes to ostial obstruction, a septoplasty (straightening of the septum) is performed. In some instances, septoplasty is necessary to allow surgical access (passage of the endoscope and forceps) to posterior areas in the nasal cavity. Also, the middle turbinate may be collapsed onto the lateral nasal wall and must be fractured medially, or even partially resected, for access to the osteomeatal complex. The same situation can exist if the turbinate is hypertrophic or pneumatized concha bullosa.

Any polyps are removed, and the uncinate process (Fig. 40.3) is resected to open the infundibulum. The goal of FESS is to resect the inflamed ethmoidal tissue (Fig. 40.6) and to reestablish ventilation in the diseased larger sinuses by enlargement of their natural ostia, thus breaking the cycle of inflammation described above. Bony and mucosal septations between ethmoid cells are removed to create an unobstructed cavity.

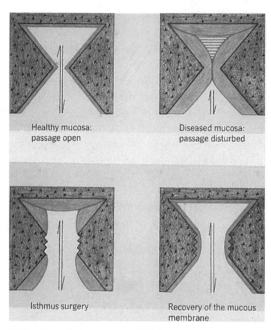

FIG. 40.7. Principle of FESS. After mucosal recovery, the result is a dilated natural ostium. (Reprinted from Wigand ME. *Endoscopic surgery of the paranasal sinuses and anterior skull base.* New York: Thieme, 1990; with permission.)

Subsequent mucous membrane recovery reestablishes mucociliary clearance via the newly enlarged physiologic ostia (Fig. 40.7) (22). Any purulent material encountered intraoperatively may be sent for culture to guide future antibiotic therapy, and resected tissue is sent to pathology for histologic evaluation.

The operation may be performed unilaterally or bilaterally, depending on the extent of disease. Each side takes 5 to 20 minutes in skilled hands (23). In children, the frontal and sphenoid sinuses are often underdeveloped; therefore, only limited anterior ethmoid and maxillary work is generally necessary. As a consequence of the smaller anatomy, pediatric FESS requires a more meticulous technique (21).

Postoperative Management

The patient may be discharged on the evening of surgery or observed overnight in the hospital. Antibiotic prophylaxis against toxic shock syndrome is necessary if nasal tampons are placed. Approximately 1 to 2 days after the

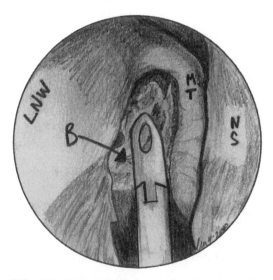

FIG. 40.6. Intraoperative view into the right middle meatus. The uncinate process has been removed, and the ethmoid bulla (*B*) is being resected with biting forceps. The middle turbinate (*MT*), nasal septum (*NS*), and lateral nasal wall (*LNW*) are identified.

operation, any tampons are removed and the postsurgical cavity is cleaned of crusted secretions and blood under endoscopic guidance in the office. The role for sinonasal endoscopy therefore extends into the postoperative period. This debridement is repeated two or three more times during the first postoperative weeks, at which time the ethmoid cavity begins to mucosalize. The larger sinuses may require up to 6 weeks to heal, particularly in the setting of nasal polyposis (19). During recovery, topical nasal steroid sprays and saline sprays are often recommended. Patients are told to refrain from exercise and heavy lifting for 1 to 2 weeks postoperatively. After the initial series of debridements, further office visits for diagnostic rhinoscopy are performed at 3-month intervals (18).

Complications

The incidence of major complications from FESS is 0% to 5%. These include cerebrospinal fluid (CSF) leak, nasolacrimal duct injury, hemorrhage requiring transfusion, blindness, and meningitis. Minor complications occur in 4% to 29% of cases and include synechiae, orbital entry, ecchymosis, orbital emphysema, and minor hemorrhage (24).

Synechiae are considered the most common complication overall and occur in up to 8% of patients. Of the affected patients, however, only 15% experience persisting symptoms as a result. These scar bands are usually found between the anterior portion of the middle turbinate and the lateral nasal wall, where they may cause functional stenosis of the middle meatus (19).

The incidence and severity of postoperative hemorrhage is reported to be increased in patients with acquired immunodeficiency syndrome and diffuse polyp disease, and in revision cases (19). Fortunately, intraoperative bleeding is usually controlled by local anesthetic or cautery and is seldom a problem. If bleeding impairs the surgeon's visualization, however, the procedure is terminated and the nose is packed. Generally the average blood loss is less than 30 mL (19).

Orbital penetration occurs in 2% to 4% of cases, and in up to one third of these cases there is also orbital emphysema. Blindness, fortunately, is rare, with an incidence as low as zero in several large series (18,19,24). CSF leakage may occur in up to 1.4% of cases (19), but in skilled hands the incidence is lower than 0.01% in large series (19,24).

Prognosis

Overall, FESS is considered successful in 80% to 90% of cases after at least 2 years of follow-up (18,19). However, FESS is only a palliative procedure in patients with diffuse polyp disease. One study reported that 55% of patients with preoperative nasal polyps had persistent disease at long-term follow-up, average 3 years and 5 months (18). Nonetheless, it is clear that surgery has a definite role in these patients because over half of the patients were asymptomatic or significantly improved and none were worse. As may be expected, however, results were better in those with a lesser degree of preoperative polyp disease (18).

Most experts believe there is a link between asthma and chronic sinusitis, although the details of this relationship are unclear. Recent studies have reported that chronic sinusitis patients with steroid-dependent asthma have dramatically reduced steroid requirements after FESS. The patients studied required an average of 1,300 mg less steroid and 21 fewer days of treatment in the year after FESS compared with the year before. Antibiotic use also was significantly reduced after FESS in these patients (25). Other trials have reported similar results. For example, in one study 40% of patients with asthma were able to discontinue steroids after intranasal polypectomy (26), and another group demonstrated that 90% of patients had improvement in asthma symptoms 6.5 years after FESS (27).

SUMMARY

Chronic sinusitis is a clinical syndrome associated with persistent, symptomatic inflammatory changes in the sinonasal mucosa. Rhinoscopy and sinus CT scans may demonstrate associated mucus outflow obstruction. The role of surgery is primarily reserved for the management of patients who fail medical therapy necessitating reversal of congenital and acquired sinus outflow obstruction and restoration of normal nasal physiology. Technologic advances in rhinoscopic instrumentation have improved the accuracy of the office diagnosis and the precision of the surgery. Prior to the advent of surgical telescopes, sinus procedures were destructive in nature, with permanent alteration of sinus physiology. The precision afforded by the current technology permits less invasive surgical intervention that restores normal function to obstructed sinus cavities.

REFERENCES

1. Kern RC, Conley DB. Management of sinusitis: current perspectives. *Allergy Proc* 1994;15:201–202.
2. Messerklinger W. Background and evolution of endoscopic sinus surgery. *Ear Nose Throat J* 1994;73:449–450.
3. Bolger WE, Kennedy DW. Changing concepts in chronic sinusitis. *Hosp Pract* 1992;27:20–22, 26–28.
4. McCaffrey TV. Functional endoscopic sinus surgery: an overview. *Mayo Clin Proc* 1993;68:571–577.
5. Lanza DC, Kennedy DW. Adult rhinosinusitis defined. *Otolaryngol Head Neck Surg* 1997;117(suppl):1–7.
6. Hamilos DL. *Chronic sinusitis.* St. Louis, MO: Division of Allergy Immunology, Washington University School of Medicine, 2000.
7. Fairbanks DNF, ed. *Antimicrobial therapy in otolaryngology-head and neck surgery,* 9th ed. Alexandria, VA: American Academy of Otolaryngology-Head and Neck Surgery Foundation, 1999.
8. Brook I, Thompson DH, Frazier EH. Microbiology and management of chronic maxillary sinusitis. *Arch Otolaryngol Head Neck Surg* 1994;120:1317–1320.
9. Ferguson BJ, Mabry RL. Laboratory diagnosis. *Otolaryngol Head Neck Surg* 1997;117(suppl):12–26.
10. Stammberger H. Surgical treatment of nasal polyps: past, present, and future. *Allergy* 1999;54(suppl 53):7–11.
11. Johnson JT, Kohut RI, Pillsbury HC, et al., eds. *Byron J. Bailey head and neck surgery-otolaryngology,* 1st ed. Philadelphia: JB Lippincott, 1993.
12. Osguthorpe JD, Derebery MJ, eds. Allergy management for the otolaryngologist. *Otolaryngol Clin North Am* 1998.
13. Ponikau JU, Sherris DA, Kern EB, et al. The diagnosis and incidence of allergic fungal sinusitis. *Mayo Clin Proc* 1999:74:877–884.
14. Ence BK, Gourley DS, Jorgensen NL, et al. Allergic fungal sinusitis. *Am J Rhinol* 1990;4:169–178.
15. Levine HL. The office diagnosis of nasal and sinus disorders using rigid nasal endoscopy. *Otolaryngol Head Neck Surg* 1990;102:370–373.
16. Zinreich SJ. Rhinosinusitis: radiologic diagnosis. *Otolaryngol Head Neck Surg* 1997;117(suppl):27–34.
17. Lund VJ, Kennedy DW. Staging for rhinosinusitis. *Otolaryngol Head Neck Surg* 1997;117(suppl):35–40.
18. Danielsen A, Olofsson J. Endoscopic endonasal surgery—a long-term follow-up study. *Acta Otolaryngol* 1996;116:611–619.
19. Stammberger H, Posawetz W. Functional endoscopic sinus surgery. Concept, indications, and results of the Messerklinger technique. *Eur Arch Otorhinolaryngol* 1990;247:63–76.
20. Cook PR, Nishioka GJ, Davis WE, et al. Functional endoscopic sinus surgery in patients with normal computed tomography scans. *Otolaryngol Head Neck Surg* 1994;110:505–509.
21. Lusk RP, Stankiewicz JA. Pediatric rhinosinusitis. *Otolaryngol Head Neck Surg* 1997;117(suppl):53–57.
22. Wigand ME. *Endoscopic surgery of the paranasal sinuses and anterior skull base,* 1st ed. New York: Thieme, 1990.
23. Stammberger H. *Endoscopic endonasal surgery—concepts in treatment of recurring rhinosinusitis.* Part II. Surgical technique. *Otol Head Neck Surg* 1986;94:147–156.
24. Ramadan HH, Allen GC. Complications of endoscopic sinus surgery in a residency training program. *Laryngoscope* 1995;105:376–379.
25. Palmer JN, Conley DB, Dong DG, et al. Efficacy of endoscopic sinus surgery in the management of patients with asthma and chronic sinusitis. *Am J Rhinol* 2001;15:49–53.
26. English G. Nasal polypectomy and sinus surgery in patients with asthma and aspirin idiosyncrasy. *Laryngoscope* 1986;96:374–380.
27. Senior BA, Kennedy DW, Tanabodee J, et al. Long-term impact of functional endoscopic sinus surgery on asthma. *Otol Head Neck Surg* 1999;121:66–68.

41

The Wheezing Infant

Mary Beth Hogan and Nevin W. Wilson

Section of Pediatric Allergy and Immunology, Department of Pediatrics, School of Medicine, West Virginia University, Morgantown, West Virginia

Recurrent wheezing is a common problem among infants and young children. The pathogenesis of recurrent wheezing, its relationship to the development of asthma, and ultimately its treatment options are poorly understood. The purpose of this chapter is to review the factors important in the development of infantile asthma. The current difficulties of evaluation and management of wheezing in very young children also are discussed. In this chapter, bronchiolitis is defined as a viral illness in infants and young children with their first or second episode of wheezing and cough. Infantile asthma refers to asthma in children under 3 years of age with three or more episodes of wheezing. These episodes improve with bronchodilators or antiinflammatory medications and may or may not be associated with viral infections.

EPIDEMIOLOGY

The prevalence rate for asthma in infants and young children is increasing, particularly in westernized countries (1). Atopy and possibly less frequent infectious events may be contributing factors (2). Hospital admission rates are climbing for infants with asthma (3). Asthmatic children under 24 months of age are four times more likely to be admitted to the hospital than teenagers with asthma (4). In Norway, 75% of all children hospitalized for asthma are under 4 years of age (5). Although the number of days in the hospital is declining in older children, hospital length of stay for infants is not changing

(6). In addition, infants are more likely to require emergency room assistance for asthma exacerbations (7). Ten percent of all childhood mortality from asthma occurs in children under 4 years of age (8). Overall, it appears that hospitalization rates may be improving for older children, but no real progress has been made in improving the quality of life of asthmatic infants.

TRIGGERS OF WHEEZING IN INFANTS

Gastroesophageal Reflux

Gastroesophageal reflux (GER) is a common cause of wheezing in infants under 1 year of age. Sheikh et al. (9) reported that 64.8% of infants with pH probe–diagnosed GER were able to discontinue asthma medications when GER was treated compared with an untreated placebo group. In another study, only 10% of the GER treatment group required pharmacologic intervention for wheezing, compared with 44% in the placebo group (10). Treatment of GER improves pulmonary function parameters in some wheezing infants (11). However, infants with GER and wheezing are less likely to respond to bronchodilator therapy (12).

Passive Smoke Inhalation

Parental smoking is a profound trigger for infantile asthma. Passive smoking increases airway responsiveness in normal 4 1/2-week-old infants (13). Maternal smoking during the first year of life is linked to exercise-induced bronchial responsiveness later in childhood (14). Overall as much as 13% of asthma in children under 4 years of age is estimated to be secondary to maternal smoking (15). In lower socioeconomic households, children of mothers who smoke 10 cigarettes or more per day are at increased risk of asthma (16). The likelihood of infantile asthma increases with increasing exposure to smoke by-products (17). Parents of asthmatics often underestimate how much smoke their children are actually exposed to when urinary nicotine metabolites are compared with parental history (18).

Fetal smoke exposure during pregnancy is linked to childhood asthma (19) and may play a larger role in the development of childhood asthma than postnatal exposure (20). Prenatal exposure to smoke is associated with decreased peak expiratory flow, mid-expiratory flow, and forced expiratory flow rates in school-aged children (21). In fact, this decrease in pulmonary function is noted shortly after birth in apparently normal infants. The most discouraging aspect to this public health problem is that maternal smoking during pregnancy is an entirely preventable cause of asthma.

Outdoor and Indoor Air Pollution

Outdoor air pollution exacerbates asthma. Increased emergency room visits, hospitalizations, and asthma severity among children with asthma are associated with elevated pollution levels (22). Infants with asthma also are affected by outdoor air pollution (23). Indoor air pollution is an additional important trigger for asthma in this age group. Frequent use of humidifiers is associated with increased wheezing. Damp housing increases the likelihood of a diagnosis of asthma in infants and increases the hospitalization rate (24). Wood burning stoves also are linked to increased respiratory symptoms in infants due to increased airborne particulate matter (25).

Allergy

Until recently, allergy was not considered a risk factor for the development of wheezing in infants

and very young children. Bernton and Brown (26) skin tested allergic children to cockroach allergen in 1967 and found no child under 4 years of age with a positive skin test. Other early studies also suggested that immunoglobulin E (IgE)-mediated allergy did not act as a trigger for infantile asthma (27). In more recent studies, allergy is commonly found in infants. Delacourt et al. (28) reported that 25% of infants with recurrent wheezing had positive skin test results to either dust mites or cat allergen. The prevalence rate for reactivity to one inhalant in a general population of 1-year-olds is 11%, and 30% by the age of 6 (29). Wilson et al. evaluated 196 children under 3 years of age with infantile asthma for allergy (30). Forty-five percent of the infants tested to indoor inhalant allergens had at least one positive skin test result. For the 49 children who were under 1 year of age, 28.5% were positive to cockroach and 10.2% were positive to dust mites.

Investigators are searching for factors that enhance the possibility of developing infantile atopy and asthma. Familial history of bronchial responsiveness and atopy appear to be independent risk factors for asthma severity among infants (31). Atopic dermatitis and food allergy are risk factors for later asthma (32). Urban children are at higher risk than rural children, and location of residence is of particular importance during the first 2 years of life (33). Allergic siblings are a strong predictor for the development of atopy (34).

Environmental factors affect the development of atopy in wheezing infants. Increased cockroach allergen in family rooms is associated with wheezing in the first year of life (35). A dose relationship exists between the amount of cat exposure and subsequent sensitization to cats in infancy (36). Children who are sensitized to cat or dust mite allergen by the age of 3 are exposed to significantly higher levels of these allergens than their nonatopic counterparts (37). High levels of allergen in the bedroom appear to be particularly important (38). Although lower levels of indoor allergens are associated with lower rates of sensitization, even very low levels are capable of causing allergy in infants with a family history of atopy (39).

Viral Infections

In infants, viral respiratory illnesses are a major trigger for asthma. A viral etiology for status asthmaticus is found in 86% of hospitalized infants (40). Respiratory syncytial virus (RSV) is the predominant viral organism causing wheezing in infants who present to an emergency department for care (41). Children in day care with a family history of atopy have a higher risk for developing respiratory illnesses than children without a family history of atopy (42).

Infants with RSV infection severe enough to result in hospitalization have a higher risk of atopy and asthma (43). Immunologic variation seems to account for the children who develop asthma after RSV infection. Children with RSV infection and elevated total serum IgE levels are at increased risk for persistent wheezing compared with RSV-infected children without elevated IgE levels (44). In addition, infants with RSV infection and eosinophilia were more likely to persistently wheeze afterward (45). In hospitalized infants, eosinophilia at the time of RSV infection is predictive of wheezing at the age of 7 (46). An RSV-specific IgE response after bronchiolitis also is associated with subsequent asthma (47). Evidence suggests that RSV is capable of inducing a helper T cell type 2 (T_H2) response from some children. Interferon-γ levels are almost absent in ventilated infants with RSV infection (48). Elevated interleukin-10 (IL-10) levels during the convalescent stage after RSV infection are associated with the development of asthma (49).

PREVENTION OF INFANTILE ASTHMA

Smoke avoidance is an obvious means to decreasing wheezing in infants and should be instituted for all exposed infants. Some investigators have noted that breast-feeding to 4 to 6 months of age is associated with decreased asthma in children (50). However, others have noted that breast-feeding is only protective against the development of severe asthma, but does not seem to affect the age at which asthma presents (51). Allergen avoidance seems to decrease atopy, but does not seem to affect the prevalence of childhood asthma (52). Prophylactic ketotifen may decrease the development of asthma in at-risk infants (53). To date, there is no clear recommendation for the prevention of asthma in at-risk children, other than there should be no pre- or postnatal smoke exposure.

EVALUATION OF THE PERSISTENTLY WHEEZING INFANT

Infants and small children with repeated episodes of wheezing require a complete history and physical examination. The frequency of hospitalizations and emergency room visits helps indicate the severity of the problem. Response to bronchodilators or steroids may provide clues supportive of a diagnosis of asthma. Coughing and wheezing associated with triggers other than viral infections suggest asthma. A history of wheezing with exposure to pets, foods, or indoor or outdoor allergens suggests the need for skin testing. Factors important in the history of the wheezing infant are listed in Table 41.1. In taking

TABLE 41.1. *Important factors in the history of the wheezing infant*

History	Potential etiology
Sudden onset	Foreign object
Intubation at birth	Subglottic stenosis, bronchopulmonary dysplasia
Maternal papillomatosis	Laryngeal papilloma
Forceps delivery	Vocal cord injury
Difficulty feeding	Congenital heart defect Neurogenic defect
Irritability, regurgitation, torticollis	Sandifer syndrome (gastroesophageal reflux)
Recurrent pneumonia	Aspiration Tracheoesophageal fistula Cystic fibrosis Ciliary dyskinesia Immunodeficiency Human immunodeficiency virus infection
Formula changes	Milk or soy allergy
Isolated episode	Tuberculosis Respiratory syncytial virus Adenovirus Histoplasmosis Parainfluenza virus
Eczema, urticaria	Atopic diseases associated with asthma
Severe or recurrent infections	Immunodeficiencies

an environmental history, one should remember that many infants spend significant amounts of time in more than one household.

The differential diagnosis of infantile wheezing may be complex (Table 41.2). Asthma in a child under 1 year of age is a diagnosis of exclusion because congenital defects are more prevalent in this age group. The height and weight should be compared with standard norms to determine the growth pattern. On auscultation, the presence of inspiratory wheezing may indicate extrathoracic obstruction. Wheezing due to asthma occurs throughout the entire expiratory phase. Specifically, expiratory stridor mimicking wheezing will not carry through to the end of expiration. Rales or rhonchi may indicate atelectasis or pneumonia.

TABLE 41.2. *Differential diagnosis of wheezing in infants*

Congenital disorders
Cystic fibrosis
Tracheoesophageal fistula
Primary ciliary dyskinesia
Immunodeficiency
Sickle cell disease (acute chest syndrome)
Diaphragmatic hernia
Bronchopulmonary dysplasia
α_1-antitrypsin deficiency
Pulmonary lymphangiectasia

Congenital heart disease
Aberrant left coronary artery
Chronic heart failure

Upper airway disorders
Foreign body
Laryngotracheomalacia
Vocal cord dysfunction/paralysis
Laryngeal web, papillomatosis, cleft
Subglottic or tracheal stenosis
Hemangioma

Lower airway disorders
Bronchial stenosis
Foreign object
Bronchial casts
Asthma
Bronchomalacia

Infectious/postinfectious
Epiglottitis
Croup
Tracheitis
Bronchiolitis
Diphtheria
Chlamydia
Pneumocytisis carnii
Histoplasmosis
Retropharyngeal abscess
Bronchiolitis obliterans

Compression syndromes
Tuberculosis
Lymphadenopathy
Vascular ring
Pulmonary sling
Mediastinal masses
Congenital goiter
Thyroglossal duct cyst
Teratoma
Aspiration syndromes
Neurogenic
Gastroesophageal reflux

Other
Munchausen syndrome by proxy
Neurofibroma

ALLERGY AND OTHER TESTS

Allergy appears to be a more common trigger in this population than previously appreciated. Skin testing using the prick-puncture technique to indoor allergens should be considered in infants and young children with asthma. Appropriate environmental control measures can then be instituted for those who are found to have evidence of atopy.

Infants under 1 year of age with persistent wheezing, and older children with a suggestive history, should be evaluated for GER, anatomic abnormalities, and feeding disorders. An upper gastrointestinal series performed after consultation with a radiologist will provide information about anatomic abnormalities (tracheoesophageal fistulas, vascular rings) and may provide evidence of GER if it occurs during the examination. Feeding disorders may be diagnosed with a modified barium swallow. The most helpful and accurate study for the evaluation of GER in infants and small children is a 24-hour esophageal pH monitoring. Bronchoscopy may be necessary if the presence of a foreign body or ciliary dyskinesia is suspected.

Standard pulmonary function testing such as spirometry or peak flow monitoring is not applicable to this population because they are not capable of performing the required maneuvers. Involuntary methods of assessing pulmonary function in small infants have been used for experimental purposes but are not generally available to clinicians. Methacholine provocation tests in very young children also have been studied experimentally but are not routinely performed.

A chest film should be performed the first time an infant has an acute episode of wheezing. Repeated radiographs for each subsequent episode of wheezing are not necessary. A sweat chloride test to exclude cystic fibrosis should be considered in any infant under 1 year of age with repeated episodes of wheezing or respiratory distress. Wheezing associated with increased numbers of severe or unusual infections should lead to evaluation for immune deficiency.

TREATMENT

The treatment of asthmatic infants is similar to that in older children and consists of avoiding identified triggers of wheezing, regular use of an antiinflammatory medication, and a bronchodilator for symptomatic relief. Treatment of this age group does pose certain challenges. Many medications and delivery systems for asthma have been inadequately tested in this population or there is conflicting data concerning their use. Monitoring the effectiveness of treatment in infants is more difficult without pulmonary function testing. Compliance with daily treatment is difficult due to the poor cooperation inherent in this age group as well as the reluctance of parents to have their children on medications when they are asymptomatic. Fortunately, the newer medications for asthma in infants promise better control of wheezing with improved safety and convenience. A summary of current asthma medications for infants is listed in Table 41.3.

β Agonists

The National Institutes of Health (NIH) National Asthma Education and Prevention Program Expert Panel Report (54) recommends the use of β agonists in infants and young children for acute wheezing. Side effects of these medications may include tremors, irritability, sleep disturbances, behavioral problems, and, at higher doses, tachycardias, agitation, hypokalemia, and hyperglycemia. Oral preparations are more likely to produce side effects than inhaled ones. Continuous nebulized albuterol has been successfully administered to infants with severe wheezing (55).

Debate continues as to how effective β agonists are for treating wheezing infants. Early

TABLE 41.3. *Medications for the treatment of infantile asthma*

Medication	Dosage
Prednisolone Prelone 15 mg/5 mL Pediapred 5 mg/5 mL, 15 mg/5 mL	1–2 mg/kg/day orally
Dexamethasone acetate	1.7 mg/kg i.m.
Cromolyn sodium	1 ampule t.i.d.–q.i.d. 2 puffs t.i.d.–q.i.d.
Nedocromil	2 puffs b.i.d.–q.i.d.
Montelukast	4 mg orally daily
Beclomethasone	Low dose: 84–336 μg/day Medium dose: 336–672 μg/day High dose: >672 μg/day
Budesonide	0.25 mg, 0.5 mg, 1 ampule daily
Fluticasone	Low dose: 88–175 μg/day Medium dose: 176–440 μg/day High dose: >440 μg/day
Albuterol	0.05 mg/kg every 4–6 h Minimum 1.25 mg, maximum 2.5 mg
Ipratropium	0.25 mg every 6 h

studies did not demonstrate clinical efficacy in infants under 18 months of age (56,57). However these studies used a mixed population of infants with asthma and bronchiolitis. Despite these studies, infants do have functioning β receptors (58), and recent studies in infants specifically diagnosed with asthma suggest that β agonists decrease wheezing as well as improve pulmonary functions. This improvement is noted both for nebulized medications and metered-dose inhalers (MDIs) with face mask spacer devices (59,60). It is prudent to administer a trial of inhaled β agonists to all wheezing infants regardless of the underlying etiology to determine whether there is any improvement. Infants with true asthma should be given inhaled β agonists as needed for wheezing during acute exacerbations of their disease.

Anticholinergics

Ipratropium bromide is a quaternary isopropyl derivative of atropine available as a nebulizer solution. In some infants with wheezing it has been found to improve pulmonary functions (61). In a double-blind crossover placebo-controlled trial, ipratropium was considered superior by parents (62). A pediatric asthma consensus group suggests that ipratropium may be useful as a second- or third-line medication in severe infantile asthma (63). A recent metaanalysis of clinical trials of ipratropium for wheezing in children under the age of 2 concluded that there is not enough evidence to support the uncritical use of anticholinergic therapy for wheezing infants (64).

Cromolyn Sodium

Cromolyn sodium (sodium cromoglycate) is an antiinflammatory medication that inhibits the degranulation of mast cells and inhibits early- and late-phase asthmatic reactions to allergen. It is not a bronchodilator but a prophylactic medication that must be used on a regular basis to have an effect. Its safety and lack of toxicity make it particularly attractive as a first-line therapy for the prevention of wheezing in this age group (65).

A study reported that cromolyn is no more effective than placebo in children under 1 year of age or in children 1 to 4 years of age using MDIs with a face mask spacer device (66). However, nebulized cromolyn in infants over 12 months of age is effective for treating asthma (67). Cromolyn is recommended by the NIH Expert Panel Report (54) as the first-line antiinflammatory medication for infants and small children with chronic asthma symptoms. Cromolyn is a medication that is not effective in all patients and optimally must be administered regularly three to four times per day (68). This daily treatment for any length of time in an uncooperative infant or toddler may become tedious for parents, adversely affecting compliance. Nevertheless, due to its high safety profile, cromolyn remains one of the most important prophylactic medications currently available for the prevention of wheezing in this age group.

Leukotriene Antagonists

Leukotrienes are chemical mediators that produce bronchospasm and eosinophilia, stimulate mucus secretion, and increase vascular permeability, all critical features of asthma. Leukotriene antagonists block these inflammatory effects. Montelukast is approved for children as young as age 2 by the U.S. Food and Drug Administration. So far, these medications appear to have a good safety profile and are well tolerated (69,70). Further studies in infants under 2 years of age are pending. Because it can be taken as a tablet once daily, the relative ease of administration of montelukast and its high safety profile makes it particularly attractive for this age group as a first-line controller medication for infantile asthma. However, until long-term exposure data are available, use as first-line controller medications will be limited.

Theophylline

Despite its long use and popularity in this age group, few data are available on theophylline effectiveness in infants. Studies comparing theophylline to sodium cromolyn in children under 5 years of age (71) have reported that cromolyn is superior to theophylline in controlling symptoms. However, theophylline is superior to ketotifen and placebo in controlling symptoms in this age group (72). Concern about theophylline side effects ranging from mild nausea, insomnia, and agitation to life-threatening cardiac arrhythmias and encephalopathic seizures have limited its use now that safer medications are available (73). Checking serum concentrations of theophylline is necessary to achieve maximal benefits without significant side effects, and minor symptoms are not predictive of elevated levels (74). Most serious side effects occur when the serum concentration of theophylline exceeds 20 mg/dL. Age, diet, fever, viral infections, and drug interactions may affect the metabolism of this medication. Drugs that increase serum theophylline concentrations include certain antibiotics such as ciprofloxacin, clarithromycin, and erythromycin, as well as cimetidine, verapamil, propranolol, and thiabendazole (75).

Corticosteroids

Corticosteroids are potent antiinflammatory medications that have profound effects on asthma. They decrease inflammatory mediators, reduce mucus production, decrease mucosal edema, and increase β-adrenergic responsiveness. Clinically, they improve lung function, reduce airway hyperreactivity, and modify the late-phase asthmatic response.

The use of oral or intravenous corticosteroids for acute exacerbations of wheezing in infants is controversial. Numerous studies clearly do not demonstrate an effect when these drugs are used for bronchiolitis (76,77), and some studies do not show an effect in a broad population of wheezing infants under 18 months of age (78). However, the efficacy of steroids in treating true infantile asthma is known. Asthmatic infants treated with steroids have a significantly reduced need for hospitalization (79) and markedly improved symptom scores when compared with placebo (80). As with all studies involving treatment of wheezing in this age group, the heterogeneity of the underlying cause of the acute wheezing is probably the reason for the wide discrepancy seen in results. It appears evident that the younger the infant, the less likely that steroids will have an effect, and that those with true bronchiolitis do not respond as well to steroid treatment. Despite these inconclusive data, infants with acute wheezing who have a history consistent with infantile asthma should be treated with systemic steroids. Intramuscular dexamethasone may be used in those infants who do not tolerate oral steroids (81).

Inhaled steroids provide many of the beneficial antiinflammatory properties of corticosteroids without numerous unwanted side effects. As infant-sized spacers with masks have become more available, attention has turned to the commercially available MDI steroids. Beclomethasone dipropionate MDI inconsistently demonstrates improvement when compared with placebo in asthmatic infants (82). However, newer inhaled steroids such as fluticasone (83) and budesonide are reported to be effective in this age group. Budesonide reduces wheezing, cough, dyspnea, acute exacerbations, use of β agonists, use of oral steroids, and hospital stays (84,85). It also increases pulmonary function results (86). Treatment of 1- to 3-year-old children with inhaled budesonide using a face mask spacer for 10 days at the first sign of a viral upper respiratory infection leads to a significant decrease in wheezing, cough, noisy breathing, and breathlessness (87).

Studies of short-term linear growth in children on inhaled steroids suggest some decrease in growth velocity. However, the long-term effects on adult height remain unknown because catchup growth may occur during puberty (88,89). There is no evidence of altered adrenal function due to inhaled steroids in infants or small children except in very low birth weight premature infants (90).

The use of inhaled steroids and the recent increased availability of nebulized inhaled steroids (such as with budesonide) offer a significant advance in the management of infantile asthma. However, the potential for growth effects and other problems due to systemic absorption in these considerably smaller patients could be increased. For these reasons, these medications should be reserved for those infants who have failed nonsteroidal antiinflammatory medications.

NATURAL HISTORY

Several studies have investigated whether pulmonary function tests obtained shortly after birth can predict which infants go on to wheeze later in life. Pulmonary function tests demonstrate that infants exposed to passive smoke *in utero* have decreased lung functions after birth (91). This may partially explain why these infants are at higher risk for wheezing during infancy. Infants with low compliance values were significantly more likely to go on to wheeze in the first 2 years of life compared with nonwheezing infants (92). Infants genetically predisposed to asthma or exposed to passive smoking have decreased compliance at 1 month of age. Increased pulmonary function measurements are noted in those infants who started wheezing in the first year of life and then improve compared with those who continue to wheeze (93). Availability of infant pulmonary function tests in the future may help diagnose asthma in infants and assist in therapeutic decision making.

Most studies have focused on determining clinical risk factors for persistent asthma in children. Maternal asthma and a history of atopic dermatitis or allergic rhinitis are associated with late onset or persistent wheezing (93). Persistent wheezing is associated with decreased lung functions and atopy (94). In fact, childhood bronchial reactivity and poorer lung functions are highly correlated with adult bronchial hyperreactivity and decreased lung functions (95). The loss of bronchial reactivity in childhood may be a key factor in "outgrowing asthma" (96). Early transiently wheezing children tend to have nonasthmatic mothers who smoke, were in day care, were not atopic, and had depressed eosinophil counts during viral respiratory illnesses (44,97). Overall, one third of asthmatic children present with symptoms prior to 18 months of age and one half of asthmatic children present prior to 3 years of age (98). Other investigators note a strong association with asthma in children who continue to wheeze or present with wheezing after 3 years of age (99).

REFERENCES

1. Beasley R, Crane J, Lai CKW, et al. Prevalence and etiology of asthma. *J Allergy Clin Immunol* 2000;105 (Part 2; suppl):466–472.
2. Shamssain MH, Shamsian N. Prevalence and severity of asthma, rhinitis, and atopic eczema: the north east study. *Arch Dis Child* 1999;81:313–317.
3. Lin S, Fitzgerald E, Hwang SA, et al. Asthma hospitalization rates and socioeconomic status in New York State (1987–1993). *J Asthma* 1999;36:239–251.
4. Goodman DC, Stukel TA, Chang CH. Trends in pediatric asthma hospitalization rates: regional and socioeconomic differences. *Pediatrics* 1998;101:208–213.
5. Jonasson G, Lodrup Carlsen KC, Leegaard J, et al. Trends in hospital admissions for childhood asthma in Oslo Norway, 1980–1995. *Allergy* 2000;55:232–239.
6. Wennergren G, Krisjansson S, Strannegard IL. Decrease in hospitalization for the treatment of asthma with increased use of anti-inflammatory treatment, despite an increase in prevalence of asthma. *J Allergy Clin Immunol* 1996;97:742–748.
7. Schaubel D, Johansen H, Mao Y, et al. Risk of preschool asthma: incidence, hospitalization, recurrence, and readmission probability. *J Asthma* 1996;33:97–103.
8. Weitzman JB, Kanarek NF, Smialek JE: Medical examiner asthma death autopsies: a distinct subgroup of asthma deaths with implications for public health preventive strategies. *Arch Pathol Lab Med* 1998;122:691–699.
9. Sheikh S, Stephen T, Howell L, et al. Gastroesophageal reflux in infants with wheezing. *Pediatr Pulmonol* 1999;28:181–186.
10. Ibero M, Ridao M, Artigas R, et al. Cisapride treatment changes the evolution of infant asthma with gastroesophageal reflux. *J Invest Allergol Clin Immunol* 1998;8:176–179.
11. Eid NS, Shepher RW, Thomson MA. Persistent wheezing and gastroesophageal reflux in infants. *Pediatr Pulmonol* 1994;18:39–44.
12. Sheikh S, Goldsmith LJ, Howell L, et al. Lung function in infants with wheezing and gastroesophageal reflux. *Pediatr Pulmonol* 1999:27:236–241.
13. Young S, Le Souef PN, Geelhoed GC, et al. The influence of a family history of and parental smoking on airway responsiveness in early infancy. *N Engl J Med* 1991;324:1168–1173.
14. Frischer T, Kuehr J, Meinert R, et al. Maternal smoking in early childhood: a risk factor for bronchial responsiveness to exercise in primary-school children. *J Pediatr* 1992;121:17–22.
15. Lister SM, Jorm LR. Parental smoking and respiratory illness in Australian children aged 0–4 years: ABS 1989–90 National Health Survey results. *Aust N Z J Public Health* 1998;22:781–786.
16. Martinez FD, Cline M, Burrows B. Increased incidence of asthma in children of smoking mothers. *Pediatrics* 1992;89:21–26.
17. Ehrlich RI, Du Toit D, Jordaan E, et al. Risk factors for childhood asthma and wheezing. Importance of maternal and household smoking. *Am J Respir Crit Care Med* 1996;154:681–688.
18. Kohler E, Sollich V, Schuster R, et al. Passive smoke exposure in infants and children with respiratory tract diseases. *Hum Exp Toxicol* 1999;18:212–217.
19. Hu FB, Persky V, Flay BR, et al. Prevalence of asthma and wheezing in public schoolchildren: association with maternal smoking during pregnancy. *Ann Allergy Asthma Immunol* 1997;79:80–84.
20. Stein RT, Holberg CJ, Sherrill D, et al. Influence of parental smoking on respiratory symptoms during the first decade of life: the Tucson Children's Respiratory Study. *Am J Epidemiol* 1999;149:1030–1037.
21. Gilliland FD, Berhane K, McConnell R, et al. Maternal smoking during pregnancy, environmental tobacco smoke exposure and childhood lung function. *Thorax* 2000;55:271–276.
22. Tseng RY, Li CK, Spinks JA. Particulate air pollution and hospitalization for asthma. *Ann Allergy* 1992;68:4225–4232.
23. Lindfors A, Wickman M, Hedlin G, et al. Indoor environmental risk factors in young asthmatics: a case-control study. *Arch Dis Child* 1995;73:408–412.
24. Wever-Hess J, Kowenberg JM, Duiverman EJ, et al. Risk factors for exacerbations and hospital admissions in asthma of early childhood. *Pediatr Pulmonol* 2000;29:250–256.
25. Honicky RE Osborn JS 3rd, Akpom CA. Symptoms of respiratory illness in young children and the use of wood-burning stoves for indoor heating. *Pediatrics* 1985;75:587–593.
26. Bernton HS, Brown H. Cockroach allergy: age of onset of skin reactivity. *Ann Allergy* 1970;28:420–422.
27. Rowntree S, Cogswell JJ, Platts-Mills TAE, et al. Development of IgE and IgG antibodies to food and inhalant

allergies in children at risk of allergic disease. *Arch Dis Child* 1985;75:633–637.

28. Delacourt C, Labbe D, Vassault A, et al. Sensitization to inhalant allergens in wheezing infants is predictive of the development of infantile asthma. *Allergy* 1994;49:843–847.

29. Kulig M, Bergmann R, Klettke U, et al. Natural course of sensitization to food and inhalant allergens during the first 6 years of life. *J Allergy Clin Immunol* 1999; 103:1173–1179.

30. Wilson NW, Robinson NP, Hogan MB. Cockroach and other inhalant allergies in infantile asthma. *Ann Allergy Asthma Immunol* 1999;83:27–30.

31. Wilson NM, Dore CJ, Silverman M. Factors relating to the severity of symptoms at 5 yrs in children with severe wheeze in the first 2 yrs of life. *Eur Respir J* 1997;10:346–353.

32. Kulig M, Bergmann R, Tacke U, et al. Long-lasting sensitization to food during the first two years precedes allergic airway disease. The MAS Study Group, Germany. *Pediatr Allergy Immunol* 1998;9:61–67.

33. Nilsson L, Castor O, Lofman O, et al. Allergic disease in teenagers in relation to urban or rural residence at various stages of childhood. *Allergy* 1999;54:716–721.

34. Tariq SM, Matthew SM, Hakim EZ, et al. The prevalence of and risk factors for atopy in early childhood: a whole population birth cohort study. *J Allergy Clin Immunol* 1998;101:587–593.

35. Gold DR, Burge HA, Carey V, et al. Predictors of repeated wheeze in the first year of life. The relative roles of cockroach, birth weight, acute lower respiratory illness, and maternal smoking. *Am J Respir Crit Care Med* 1999;160:227–236.

36. Lindfors A, van Hage-Hamsten M, Rietz H, et al. Influence of interaction of environmental risk factors and sensitization in young asthmatic children. *J Allergy Clin Immunol* 1999;104:755–762.

37. Wahn U, Lau S, Bergmann R, et al. Indoor allergen exposure is a risk factor for sensitization during the first three years of life. *J Allergy Clin Immunol* 1997;99: 763–769.

38. Eggleston PA, Rosenstreich D, Lynn H, et al. Relationship of indoor allergen exposure to skin test sensitivity in inner-city children with asthma. *J Allergy Clin Immunol* 1998;102:563–570.

39. Munir AKM, Kjellman N-IM, Bjorksten B. Exposure to indoor allergens in early infancy and sensitization. *J Allergy Clin Immunol* 1997;100:177–181.

40. Freymuth F, Vabret A, Brouard J, et al. Detection of viral, *Chlamydia pneumoniae* and *Mycoplasma pneumoniae* infections in exacerbations of asthma in children. *J Clin Virol* 1999;13:131–139.

41. Rakes GP, Arruda E, Ingram JM, et al. Rhinovirus and respiratory syncytial virus in wheezing children requiring emergency care. IgE and eosinophil analyses. *Am J Respir Crit Care Med* 1999;159:785–790.

42. Celedon JC, Litonjua AA, Weiss ST, et al. Day care attendance in the first year of life and illnesses of the upper and lower respiratory tract in children with a familial history of atopy. *Pediatrics* 1999;104:495–500.

43. Sigurs N, Bjarnason R, Sigurbergsson F, et al. Respiratory syncytial virus bronchiolitis in infancy is an important risk factor for asthma and allergy at age 7. *Am J Respir Crit Care Med* 2000;161:1501–1507.

44. Martinez FD, Stern DA, Wright Al, et al. Differential immune responses to acute lower respiratory illness in early life and subsequent development of persistent wheezing and asthma. *J Allergy Clin Immunol* 1998;102: 915–920.

45. Ehlenfield DR, Cameron K, Welliver RC. Eosinophilia at the time of respiratory syncytial virus bronchiolitis predicts childhood reactive airway disease. *Pediatrics* 2000;105:79–83.

46. Welliver RC, Duffy L. The relationship of RSV-specific immunoglobulin E antibody responses in infancy, recurrent wheezing, and pulmonary function at age 7–8 years. *Pediatr Pulmonol* 1993;15:19–27.

47. Bont L, Jeijnen CJ, Kavelaars A, et al. Peripheral blood cytokine responses and disease severity in respiratory syncytial virus bronchiolitis. *Eur Respir J* 1999;14:144–149.

48. Bont L, Jeijnen CJ, Davelaars A, et al. Monocyte IL-10 production during respiratory syncytial virus bronchiolitis is associated with recurrent wheezing in a one-year follow-up study. *Am J Respir Crit Care Med* 2000;161:1518–1523.

49. Noma T, Mori A, Yoshizawa I. Induction of allergen-specific IL-2 responsiveness of lymphocytes after respiratory syncytial virus infection and prediction of onset of recurrent wheezing and bronchial asthma. *J Allergy Clin Immunol* 1996;98:1–28.

50. Oddy WH, Holt PG, Sly PD, et al. Association between breast feeding and asthma in 6 year old children: findings of a prospective birth cohort study. *BMJ* 1999;319:815–819.

51. Wafula EM, Limbe MS, Onyango FE, et al. Effects of passive smoking and breastfeeding on childhood bronchial asthma. *East Afr Med J* 1999;76:606–609.

52. Hide DW, Matthew S, Matthews L, et al. Effect of allergen avoidance in infancy on allergic manifestations at age two years. *J Allergy Clin Immunol* 1994;93:842–846.

53. Bustos GJ, Bustos D, Bustos GJ, et al. Prevention of asthma with ketotifen in preasthmatic children: a three year follow-up study. *Clin Exp Allergy* 1995;25:568–573.

54. National Heart, Lung, and Blood Institute, National Asthma Education and Prevention Program Expert Panel Report. Guidelines for the diagnosis and management of asthma. NIH Publication No. 97-4051A. National Institutes of Health, 1997.

55. Katz RW, Kelly HW, Crowley MR, et al. Safety of continuous nebulized albuterol for bronchospasm in infants and children. *Pediatrics* 1993;92:666–669.

56. Prendiville A, Green S, Silverman M. Airway responsiveness in wheezy infants: evidence for functional beta adrenergic receptors. *Thorax* 1987;42:100–104.

57. Prendiville A, Green S, Silverman M. Paradoxical response to nebulized salbutamol in wheezy infants, assessed by partial expiratory flow-volume curves. *Thorax* 1987;42:86–91.

58. Lenney W, Milner AD. Alpha and beta adrenergic stimulants in bronchiolitis and wheezy bronchitis in children under 18 months of age. *Arch Dis Child* 1978;53:707–709.

59. Bentur L, Canny GJ, Shields MD, et al. Controlled trial of nebulized albuterol in children younger than 2 years of age with acute asthma. *Pediatrics* 1992;89:133–137.

60. Kraemer R, Frey U, Sommer CW, et al. Short-term effect of albuterol, delivered via a new auxiliary device, in wheezy infants. *Am Rev Respir Dis* 1991;144:347–351.

61. Hodges IGC, Groggins RC, Milner AD, et al. Bronchodilator effect of inhaled ipratropium bromide in wheezy toddlers. *Arch Dis Child* 1981;56:729–732.

62. Schuh S, Johnson D, Canny G, et al. Efficacy of adding nebulized ipratropium bromide to nebulized albuterol therapy in acute bronchiolitis. *Pediatrics* 1992;90:920–923.

63. Warner JO, Gotz M, Landau LI, et al. Management of asthma: a consensus statement. *Arch Dis Child* 1989;64:1065–1079.

64. Everard ML, Bara A, Kurian M. Anti-cholinergic drugs for wheeze in children under the age of two years. *Cochrane Database of Systematic Review* 2000:CD001279.

65. Brugman SM, Larson GL. Asthma in infants and small children. *Clin Chest Med* 1995;16:637–656.

66. Tasche MJ, van der Wouden JC, Uijen JH, et al. Randomised placebo-controlled trial of inhaled sodium cromoglycate in 1–4-year-old children with moderate asthma. *Lancet* 1997;350:1060–1064.

67. O'Callahan C, Milner AD, Swarbrick A. Nebulized sodium cromoglycate in infancy: airway protection after deterioration. *Arch Dis Child* 1990;65:404–406.

68. Zeiger RS. Special considerations in the approach to asthma in infancy and early childhood. *J Asthma* 1983;20:341–359.

69. Becker A. Leukotriene receptor antagonists: efficacy and safety in children with asthma. *Pediatr Pulmonol* 2000;30:183–186.

70. Grossman J, Smith LJ, Wilson AM, et al. Long-term safety and efficacy of zafirlukast in the treatment of asthma: interim results of an open-label extension trial. *Ann Allergy Asthma Immunol* 1999;82:361–369.

71. Glass J, Archer LN, Adams W, et al. Nebulized cromoglycate, theophylline, and placebo in preschool asthmatic children. *Arch Dis Child* 1981;56:648–651.

72. Carswell F, Stratton D, Hughes AO, et al. A controlled comparison of slow release theophylline, ketotifen, and placebo in the prophylaxis of asthma in young children. *Agents Actions Suppl* 1983;13:141–144.

73. Hendeles L, Weinberger M, Szefler S, et al. Safety and efficacy of theophylline in children with asthma. *J Pediatr* 1992;120:177–183.

74. Melamed J, Beaucher WN. Minor symptoms are not predictive of elevated theophylline levels in adults on chronic therapy. *Ann Allergy Asthma Immunol* 1995;75:516–520.

75. Weinberger M, Hendeles L. Theophylline in asthma. *N Engl J Med* 1996;334:1380–1388.

76. Dabbous JA, Tkachyk JS, Stamm SJ. A double blind study in the effects of corticosteroids in the treatment of bronchiolitis. *Pediatrics* 1966;37:477–484.

77. Berger I, Argaman Z, Schwartz SB, et al. Efficacy of corticosteroids in acute bronchiolitis: short-term and long-term follow-up. *Pediatr Pulmonol* 1998;26:162–166.

78. Webb MS, Henry RL, Milner AD. Oral corticosteroids for wheezing attacks under 18 months. *Arch Dis Child* 1986;61:15–19.

79. Fox GF, Marsh MJ, Milner AD. Treatment of recurrent acute wheezing episodes in infancy with oral salbutamol and prednisolone. *Eur J Pediatr* 1996;155:512–516.

80. Tal A, Levy N, Bearman JE. Methylprednisolone therapy for acute asthma in infants and toddlers: a controlled clinical trial. *Pediatrics* 1990;86:350–356.

81. Gries DM, Moffitt DR, Pulos E, et al. A single dose of intramuscularly administered dexamethasone acetate is as effective as oral prednisone to treat asthma exacerbations in young children. *J Pediatr* 2000;136:298–303.

82. Calpin C, Macarthur C, Stephens D, et al. Effectiveness of prophylactic inhaled steroids in childhood asthma: a systemic review of the literature. *J Allergy Clin Immunol* 1997;100:452–457.

83. Bisgaard H, Gillies J, Groenewald M, et al. The effect of inhaled fluticasone propionate in the treatment of young asthmatic children: a dose comparison study. *Am J Respir Crit Care Med* 1999;160:126–131.

84. Connett GJ, Warde C, Wooler E, et al. Use of budesonide in severe asthmatics aged 1-3 years. *Arch Dis Child* 1993;69:351–355.

85. Noble V, Ruggins NR, Everard ML, et al. Inhaled budesonide for chronic wheezing under 18 months of age. *Arch Dis Child* 1992;67:285–288.

86. Mellon M. Efficacy of budesonide inhalation suspension in infants and young children with persistent asthma. Budesonide Inhalation Suspension Study Group. *J Allergy Clin Immunol* 1999;104(Part 2):191–199.

87. Svedmyr J, Nyberg E, Thunqvist P, et al. Prophylactic intermittent treatment with inhaled corticosteroids of asthma exacerbations due to airway infections in toddlers. *Acta Paediatr* 1999;88:42–47.

88. Sharek PJ, Bergman DA. The effect of inhaled steroids on the linear growth of children with asthma: a meta-analysis. *Pediatrics* 2000;106:E8.

89. Price JF: Inhaled corticosteroids: clinical relevance of safety measures. *Pediatr Pulmonol Suppl* 1997;15:40–45.

90. Cole CH, Shah B, Abbasi S, et al. Adrenal function in premature infants during inhaled beclomethasone therapy. *J Pediatr* 1999;135:65–70.

91. Young S, Sherrill Dl, Arnott J, et al. Parental factors affecting respiratory function during the first year of life. *Pediatr Pulmonol* 2000;29:331–340.

92. Yau KI, Fang LJ, Shieh KH. Factors predisposing infants to lower respiratory infection with wheezing in the first two years of life. *Ann Allergy Asthma Immunol* 1999;82:165–170.

93. Rusconi F, Galassi C, Corbo GM, et al. Risk factors for early, persistent, and late-onset wheezing in young children. *Am J Respir Crit Care Med* 1999;160:1617–1622.

94. Brooke AM, Lambert PC, Burton PR, et al. The natural history of respiratory symptoms in preschool children. *Am J Respir Crit Care Med* 1995;152:1872–1878.

95. Jan Roorda R, Gerritsen J, Van Aalderen WMC, et al. Follow-up of asthma from childhood to adulthood: influence of potential childhood risk factors on the outcome of pulmonary function and bronchial responsiveness in adulthood. *J Allergy Clin Immunol* 1994;93:575–584.

96. Kondo S. Spontaneous improvement in bronchial responsiveness and its limit during preadolescence and early adolescence in children with controlled asthma. *Chest* 1993;104:1359–1363.

97. Martinez FD, Wright AL, Taussig LM, et al. Asthma and wheezing in the first six years of life. *N Engl J Med* 1995;332:133–138.

98. Croner S, Kjellman NI. Natural history of bronchial asthma in childhood. A prospective study from birth up to 12–14 years of age. *Allergy* 1992;47:150–157.

99. Dodge R, Martinez FD, Cline MG, et al. Early childhood respiratory symptoms and the subsequent diagnosis of asthma. *J Allergy Clin Immunol* 1996;98: 48–54.

42

Sleep Disorders in the Allergic Patient

Lisa F. Wolfe

*Division of Pulmonary and Critical Care Medicine and The Center for Sleep and Circadian Biology,
Northwestern University, Chicago, Illinois*

In the fourth century, biblical scholars believed that sleep was "the incomplete experience of death" (1). The modern understanding that sleep is an active, complex, and essential behavior did not begin until the use of electroencephalography (EEG), which highlighted differences between wake and sleep (2).

SLEEP ARCHITECTURE

Electroencephalography has been used to identify the hallmarks of sleep and categorize stages of sleep. For ease of communication, sleep is divided into either rapid eye movement (REM) or non-REM stages. Although the eye movements of REM sleep were first discovered in 1953 (3), it was not until 1957 that REM sleep was first described using EEG and the classic architecture of a full night's sleep was first reported (4). These papers noted that REM sleep was associated with dreaming, and heart rate variability, and the episodes recurred about three to four times per night. Ultimately, in 1968, a formal protocol was developed for scoring sleep stages combining EEG, electrooculography (EOG), and chin electromyography (EMG) (5).

Typical adult sleep architecture is demonstrated in Fig. 42.1. Sleep onset is associated with non-REM sleep. Non-REM sleep is composed of four stages. Stages 3 and 4 are referred to as slow wave sleep (SWS). During sleep onset, stage 1 sleep is seen with its characteristic slow rolling eye movements and easy arousability. Stage 2 sleep is seen soon after and is defined by a specific EEG pattern (referred to as K complexes and spindles), and it becomes more difficult to awaken the sleeper. Stage 2 sleep lasts for up to 25 minutes, followed by stages 3 and 4 sleep, with the hallmark EEG slow waves. SWS lasts from 20 to 40 minutes, and physiologic events include endocrine changes such as growth hormone release (6). SWS terminates with an arousal, and as sleep is reinitiated, early non-REM sleep becomes a bridge to initiate REM sleep. REM sleep is associated with reduced muscle tone and ventilatory variability (7), and episodes can last up to 1 hour.

A complete cycle of non-REM to REM sleep lasts approximately 90 minutes, and there are three to four cycles per night. Throughout the night the composition of the cycle changes. SWS predominates the beginning of the night and is virtually gone by the final cycle. REM sleep is minimal during the first cycle and concentrated in the early morning. Maturity also affects the architecture of sleep. Most prominent are the significant reductions in SWS and sleep continuity. SWS decreases from 24% to 30% of the sleep period to 16%, and wake after sleep onset (WASO) time increases from 2% to 4% of the sleep period to 17% (8). The percentage of REM sleep remains stable at about 20% of the total sleep time (TST).

DETERMINATES OF SLEEP REGULATION

There are two processes that regulate the occurrence of sleep and the architecture of sleep

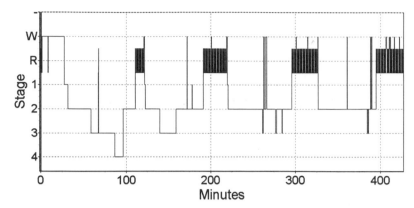

FIG. 42.1. A representative sample of sleep from a healthy young adult without sleep complaints. *W*, wake; *1*, stage 1 sleep; *2*, stage 2 sleep; *3*, stage 3 sleep; *4*, stage 4 sleep; *R*, REM sleep.

periods. The homeostatic drive quantifies the physiologic need to sleep, and the circadian pacemaker ensures proper timing of the sleep process. Additionally, the circadian pacemaker is influential in the architecture and in non-REM/REM distribution sleep stages throughout the night.

Circadian Rhythms

The word *circadian* is derived from Latin roots *circa* (about) and *diem* (a day). The term *circadian rhythm* refers to any behavior or physiologic process that is known to vary in a predictable pattern over a 24-hour period. This internal process is governed by a three-component mechanism. First, inputs such as light and activity help synchronize (entrain) to the environment. These inputs are called zeitgebers, which is German for "time giver." Next, information from zeitgebers is transferred to an internal clock, which acts as a pacemaker, setting the rate and timing of output pathways. Examples of these output pathways include lung function (9), sympathetic tone (10), and urine production (11), all of which vary over a 24-hour period so that optimum performance occurs during the daytime. Circadian rhythm regulation plays a role in controlling both the timing of sleep initiation as well as the character of sleep architecture, SWS predominating early in the night and REM sleep dominating the early morning.

Recent investigations have illuminated much about the site of the circadian pacemaker. It is a hypothalamic structure, the suprachiasmatic nucleus (SCN). In animal models, surgical lesions of the SCN halt circadian behavior such as drinking (12). The genes that create rhythms in the SCN have been identified. This apparatus is contained in all cells (13); however, the importance of these genes outside the SCN is of unknown significance. There are nine currently identified genes that participate in a feedback system to regulate circadian processes. The mammalian circadian genes period (*per 1, per 2,* and *per 3*), clock (*clock*), B-mal (*B-mal 1*), timeless (*tim*), casein kinase I epsilon (*CK1e*), and cryptochrome (*cry1* and *cry2*) have homologies and are highly conserved throughout many systems such as the mouse and fly (14). In animal models, significant modifications of these genes alter rhythms of sleep and activity (15), and there is a human disorder advanced sleep phase syndrome characterized by sleep which itself is normal but is temporally displaced (16).

Sleep as a Homeostatic Process

Homeostasis is the process by which the body maintains stability. Thirst, hunger, and temperature are all processes that are carefully regulated to ensure optimal function. Sleep can be thought of as kin to these processes, and investigations in sleep deprivation have been the main tool for understanding the body's drive/need to sleep. Initial studies revealed that sleep deprivation resulted in reduced daytime cognitive performance and shorter sleep latency, or time to falling asleep, as measured by EEG. These types of studies highlighted the use of a daytime multiple sleep latency test to quantitate sleepiness by measuring several times over the course of a day how quickly a subject could willingly fall asleep (17). Soon after, studies that used a spectral analysis of EEG performed after sleep deprivation found that slow wave activity was a significant hallmark of sleep debt, and as that debt was repaid by sleeping, slow wave activity was reduced (18). The goal of the sleep homeostatic process is not well defined or understood; however, current models hypothesize that maintenance and remodeling of synaptic connections may be involved (19).

Two-Process Model

The two-process model of sleep regulation has been used to explain the relationship between circadian rhythm regulation of sleep (process C) and the homeostatic drive to sleep (process S). Both processes S and C have an impact on sleep regulation, and to promote optimum sleep quality, maximum sleep debt should intersect with appropriate circadian time (20,21).

SLEEP AND THE PHYSIOLOGY OF THE IMMUNE SYSTEM

Both sleep homeostasis and circadian rhythms modulate the expression of immune molecules and cells. Cytokines such as interleukin-2 (IL-2), tumor necrosis factor α, and granulocyte-macrophage colony-stimulating factor cycle in a circadian manner, each with a unique pattern of expression (22). IL-6 on the other hand appears to be linked more to the sleep homeostatic process, and levels peak in relationship to the degree of sleep deprivation (23). Immune cells such as lymphocytes, monocytes, and natural killer cells all have a circadian rhythm of expression, but this rhythm is modified by the sleep process (24). The impact of sleep deprivation on human immune function has yet to be fully investigated,

but from animal studies it appears that sleep deprivation limits the ability of the immune system to function and respond to an influenza vaccine challenge (25).

SLEEP DEPRIVATION

Epidemiology

In 2001 the National Sleep Foundation survey of American sleep habits found that 63% of adults get 8 hours of sleep per night, and 40% have significant sleepiness at least a few days a month. Two thirds of those who are sleepy responded that they "just keep going" when sleepy. One great risk of sleepiness is the risk of car accidents, and 19% of adults admitted that they have fallen asleep at the wheel during the past year (26).

Health Impact

The health impacts of sleep deprivation are diverse. The National Highway Transportation Safety Administration estimates that every year in the United States, falling asleep while driving is responsible for at least 100,000 automobile crashes, 40,000 injuries, and 1,550 fatalities. Due to underreporting, these figures represent a conservative estimate, and the groups most likely to be affected are young people (16–25 years of age), shift workers, and those with sleep disorders (27). Endocrine function is affected by sleep deprivation, including impaired glucose tolerance and elevations in cortisol levels and sympathetic tone (28). Sleep deprivation also can contribute to cardiac disease and sleep apnea (29,30).

SLEEP DISORDERS IN THE ALLERGY PATIENT

Daytime sleepiness frequently can persist in the face of adequate sleep. The most common, but by no means only, cause of daytime sleepiness in the face of sufficient sleep is poor-quality nocturnal sleep. Polysomnography (PSG) is the tool by which nocturnal sleep quality is investigated. During an overnight study,

EEG, electrocardiography (EKG), chin EMG, leg EMG, EOG, respiratory effort, pulse oximetry, tracheal sound, and nasal and oral airflow are measured (31). Traditionally, PSG is performed in an attended fashion, in a formal sleep laboratory. However, unattended home sleep studies are now more common, and although reservations persist, these studies can be helpful if they are performed for diagnostic proposes by well-trained sleep professionals (32). Although PSG may be used to investigate many causes of poor-quality sleep, it is most frequently used in the diagnosis and treatment of sleep-disordered breathing.

Snoring

Until recently, it was commonly assumed that snoring was a benign annoyance, not associated with negative health outcomes. Recent data have proven this not to be true. In adults, snoring is associated with daytime sleepiness (33), pregnancy-induced hypertension, and intrauterine growth retardation (34). In children, it is associated with poor school performance (35), sleep problems such as parasomnias, and upper respiratory infections (36).

Sleep Apnea

Definition

Sleep apnea is a term that relates to a pause in respiration that can occur for many reasons. Central sleep apnea describes respiratory pauses that occur because of failure of the central nervous system to trigger a respiratory effort. Alternatively, when a respiratory effort has been triggered, but a partial or complete obstruction of the upper airway prevents ventilation, an obstructive event has occurred. These obstructive events vary. An obstructive apnea is an event during which no ventilation occurs. An obstructive hypopnea is an event during which ventilation is reduced. The exact definition of a hypopnea can vary from laboratory to laboratory, and this variation does significantly affect outcome (37). However, commonly a 50% reduction in flow must be seen in combination with either an arousal or de-

saturation. Sleep can be disturbed by respiratory events during which there is no reduction in flow but an elevation of resistance through the upper airway that impairs normal respiration, requiring an increase in respiratory effort and resultant arousal (38). These events are referred to as respiratory event-related arousals (RERA). The number of apneas plus hypopneas per hour is reported as the apnea hypopnea index, and current standards suggest that more than five events per hour is abnormal in an adult (American Sleep Disorders Association, Diagnostic Classification Steering Committee, 1990, 29) and consistent with the diagnosis of obstructive sleep apnea syndrome (OSAS) if reported in association with daytime sleepiness. Although not routinely measured or reported in most sleep laboratories, RERAs at a rate of 10 or more per hour are associated with daytime sleepiness and are known as the upper airway resistance syndrome (39).

How to Interpret a Sleep Study Report

Although there are no published algorithms for evaluation of a PSG report, the following outlines one approach:

1. TST: Unlike the total recording time, the TST is a marker of sample size, and less then 2 to 4 hours of recording time is not adequate for a diagnostic study (40).
2. Sleep stages: Failing to display REM sleep or SWS is not uncommon due to effects of medications or aging. Because sleep apnea may predominate or worsen in REM sleep, a study is not complete without it (41).
3. Body position: A complete study should include both supine and lateral sleeping positions. Supine sleep may worsen apnea (41), whereas isolated supine apnea may be treated with positional therapy alone.
4. Sleep-disturbed breathing: Changes in technology have improved measurements of airflow. Traditionally, thermistry has been used, but nasal pressure transduction has improved sensitivity, the impact of which is still being debated (42).
5. Periodic limb movements: Events that occur at a rate of greater than eight per

hour are significant (43) and require further investigation.

6. EEG: The EEG may have findings such as "alpha delta sleep" or "alpha intrusions." This rhythm is associated with nonrestorative sleep (44); however, no specific treatments are available.

7. Cardiac: Treatment of the underlying sleep-disturbed breathing is an important reason for treating apnea associated arrhythmias (45).

Epidemiology of Obstructive Sleep Apnea

The most commonly cited risk factors for the development of OSAS are male sex, increasing age, and obesity. In a large prospective study of an unselected population of working adults, OSAS was reported in 2% of women and 4% of men (46); however, it should be noted that in particular communities such as African Americans (47), Hispanics (48), and Asians (49), the rate may be higher.

Impact of Obstructive Sleep Apnea on Health Outcomes

Obstructive sleep apnea not only impairs quality of life (50), but reduces neurocognitive function (51) and increases the risk of being involved in motor vehicle accidents (52). OSA is an independent risk factor in the development of hypertension (53,54), and it has been associated with increased mortality from coronary artery disease (55). In addition, patients with heart failure benefit from the treatment of both central (56) and obstructive apneas (57).

Treatment

There are many effective treatments of OSA. Positional therapy consists of training the patient to sleep in a decubitus rather then supine position. Wedge pillows or balls, either in a backpack or tee shirt, have been used for this purpose, and in the setting of isolated supine apnea this therapy is sufficient treatment (58). Dental devices also have been used to treat both snoring and sleep apnea. These devices increase the size of the pharynx by either mandibular or tongue

advancement. The effectiveness of these devices is inversely correlated to the severity of disease, being quite effective in the treatment of snoring but ineffective in relieving severe apnea (59). For patients with mild to moderate OSA, anatomic measurements are not effective in predicting therapy success. However, when effective, patients prefer these appliances when compared with nasal continuous positive airway pressure (CPAP) therapy (60). Surgical therapies are also available to treat both snoring and OSA. Tracheostomy is most successful, because the collapsible portion of the airway is bypassed, but the associated medical complications and cosmetic effect reduce the usefulness of the procedure. Cardiac disease such as pulmonary hypertension remains an indication for tracheostomy (61). Pharyngeal, palatal, and maxillofacial surgeries in the treatment of OSA have had extensive review recently (62–64). These procedures can be performed in stages. The phase I pharyngeal and palatal procedures are tailored to the individual, and design is guided by fiberoptic and cephalometric examinations. Phase II procedures emphasize maxillofacial surgery (65), and this aggressive surgical approach can increase the success rate of surgery from 25% to 50% in phase I procedures alone (66), up to as high as 75% after phase II (67). The use of laser and radiofrequency ablation has expanded the repertoire of surgical options for both snoring and mild apnea (68–70). The experience with radiofrequency ablation is limited but is promising because it is associated with a reduction in postoperative pain (71). Lastly, there is concern because traditional uvulopalatopharyngoplasty may be associated with an increase in CPAP intolerance (72). One surgery that is frequently overlooked is gastric bypass surgery, because even moderate weight loss can reduce apnea (73,74).

Although first described in 1981 (75) nasal CPAP therapy for OSA was not widely available until the late 1980s. Once therapy was available, the striking improvements, especially in daytime sleepiness, led to an explosion in research, and many of the studies of OSA and the benefits of CPAP therapy did not have adequate control groups. There was a striking lack of appropriate placebo models with which to design

TABLE 42.1. *Types of home nocturnal positive airway pressure devices*

Type of device	Pressure delivery	Indication	Mechanism
Continuous pressure	Unchanged through the night	OSA	Prevents upper airway obstruction
Bilevel pressure	Separate inspiratory and expiratory pressure	OSA Ventilatory failure	In OSA may increase patient comfort and compliance
Auto pressure	Delivered pressure changes breath to breath	Estimating CPAP requirements in OSA Improving OSA patient comfort and compliance	Measurement of changes in flow are compensated for by increased pressure delivered on a breath-to-breath basis

OSA, obstructive sleep apnea; CPAP, continuous positive airway pressure.

blinded control studies. The efficacy of CPAP was not convincingly demonstrated, and in 1997 this issue was brought to light (76) and many health-care providers began to question the need for CPAP therapy. During the past few years the development of placebos including sham CPAP has allowed the collection of data revealing the true efficacy of nasal CPAP as therapy for OSA (77). At this time it is considered standard treatment for those with moderate or severe sleep apnea (78). CPAP is effective because the pressure delivered is capable of preventing collapse along the entire upper airway, assuring patency that prevents obstruction. Many devices are currently available for delivery of positive pressure to the airway (Table 42.1). These devices can be classified into three categories. Continuous pressure machines are the mainstays of therapy in the treatment of OSA. Bi-level pressure can be used for nocturnal noninvasive ventilation in the setting of chronic ventilatory compromise such as end-stage neuromuscular disease. In the setting of OSA, bi-level ventilation is an option in patients who fail continuous pressure therapy due to discomfort, but there is no benefit to using bi-level as the standard therapy in all patients (79). Autotitrating positive airway pressure devices provide breath-to-breath changes in the amount of CPAP delivered to the patient. Variations in airflow such as seen in hypopneas or UAR events, vibrations consistent with snoring, and apneas such as seen in obstructive or central (open airway) sleep apnea are components of differing software algorithms in these machines (80). These devices currently are used to both aid in initial CPAP titrations in sleep laboratories (81) and in homes to improve compliance in some patients who have failed to tolerate standard CPAP (82).

ALLERGY, ASTHMA, RHINITIS, AND SLEEP-DISORDERED BREATHING

Allergic conditions have an intricate relationship with OSA. Radioallergosorbent testing is positive in 40% of children who snore and in 57% of children with sleep apnea (83). Nasal inflammation as assessed by polymorphonuclear cells, bradykinin, and vasoactive intestinal peptide are increased in nasal samples of patients with OSA who do not have allergic rhinitis (84). Mechanical nasal obstruction itself can induce nocturnal apneic events in individuals without underlying OSA (85). Patients with allergic rhinitis are more likely than matched controls to have snoring, disturbed sleep, sleep apnea, and daytime sleepiness (86). Occupational allergy to guar gum has been reported to cause both rhinitis and OSA, which resolved after exposure ended (87). Lastly, CPAP itself is associated with the development of nasal congestion and rhinorrhea that can decrease compliance with treatment. Nasal resistance can be worsened by "mouth leak." This kind of mouth leak can be prevented by the use of a chinstrap, and heated humidity can help to further reduce nasal symptoms and improve CPAP compliance (88,89).

Obstructive sleep apnea can complicate the management of asthma. By self-report, in a large nonselected population, asthma is associated with a 2.5-fold increase in the prevalence of OSA, and patients with asthma and OSA may

TABLE 42.2. *Nonpharmacologic therapy for insomnia*

Sleep hygiene
  Eliminate caffeine, alcohol, tobacco
  Quiet, dark, comfortable bedroom
  Regular sleep and rise times
  Exercise several hours before bed
Somatic relaxation
  Progressive muscle relaxation
  Cognitive relaxation, positive imagery
Behavioral therapies
  Do not go to bed unless sleepy
  The bedroom should be used for sleep and sex only
  If laying in bed awake and unable
    to sleep after 20 minutes, get out of bed until
    sleepy
  Avoid napping

have more nocturnal hypoxemia then patients with OSA alone (90). Treatment of OSA can improve control of asthma symptoms (91) and reduce airway hyperreactivity as measured by methacholine responsiveness (92). One potential reason that OSA may worsen asthma is that OSA is associated with airway inflammation. Exhaled pentane and nitric oxide levels are increased after sleep in patients with moderate to severe OSA (93).

THE ALLERGY PATIENT AND INSOMNIA

Although sleep disturbance from asthma classically has been associated with daytime sleepiness, epidemiologic studies have found that insomnia may be more common. In one study of patients with active asthma, 52% reported insomnia, whereas only 22% reported daytime sleepiness. Even when symptom free, 28% of asthmatics report insomnia (94). Many factors such as medication side effects and psychological factors may contribute to the persistence of insomnia. Medications used to treat asthma patients such as theophylline, pseudoephedrine, and corticosteroids are associated with insomnia, and when combined the effect is magnified (95,96). Exploration of alternative medications or dosing regimens that avoid dosing late in the day should be first-line management. Psychophysiologic factors may perpetuate this insomnia. The hallmarks of psychophysiologic insomnia include chronic

insomnia lasting over a month, and although there may have been an initial trigger, the insomnia symptoms persist even though the inciting event has been resolved. These patients have anxiety about going to bed but are able to fall asleep at other locations and times. Improvements in sleep hygiene along with behavioral and relaxation therapy may be helpful (Table 42.2) (97). Short-term use of short-acting benzodiazepines can be a helpful adjunct but should be initiated with caution in the setting of theophylline, which increases their elimination (98).

SUMMARY

Sleep is a process that occurs as the result of the interaction between circadian rhythms and sleep homeostasis. An adequate amount of quality sleep is required for health and well-being. Complete care of the allergy patient requires attention to the commonly coexistent sleep disorders that impact the quality of life of both children and adults with asthma and rhinitis. Taking a routine sleep history that allows a patient to discuss issues of daytime sleepiness, snoring, apnea, or insomnia that will allow caregivers to coordinate care for these important issues.

REFERENCES

1. Baron JL. *A treasury of quotations.* New York: Crown, 1956.
2. Canton R. The electric currents of the brain. *BMJ* 1875;2:278.
3. Aserinsky E. Regularly occurring periods of eye motility, and concomitant phenomena, during sleep. *Science* 1953;118:273–274.
4. Dement W, Kleitman N. Cyclic variations in EEG during sleep and their relation to eye movements, body motility, and dreaming. *Electroencephalogr Clin Neurophysiol* 1957;9:673–690.
5. Rechtschaffen A, Kales A. *A manual of standardized terminology: techniques and scoring system for sleep stages of human subjects.* Los Angeles: UCLA Brain Research Information Service/ Brain Research Institute, 1968.
6. Holl RW, Hartman ML, Veldhuis JD, et al. Thirty-second sampling of plasma growth hormone in man: correlation with sleep stages. *J Clin Endocrinol Metab* 1991;72:854–861.
7. Orem J, Netick A, Dement WC. Breathing during sleep and wakefulness in the cat. *Respir Physiol* 1977;30:265–289.
8. Boselli M, Parrino L, Smerieri A, et al. Effect of age on EEG arousals in normal sleep. *Sleep* 1998;21:351–357.

9. Spengler CM, Shea SA. Endogenous circadian rhythm of pulmonary function in healthy humans. *Am J Respir Crit Care Med* 2000;162:1038–1046.

10. Burgess HJ, Trinder J, Kim Y, et al. Sleep and circadian influences on cardiac autonomic nervous system activity. *Am J Physiol* 1997;273:H1761–H1768.

11. Koopman MG, Koomen GC, Krediet RT, et al. Circadian rhythm of glomerular filtration rate in normal individuals. *Clin Sci (Colch)* 1989;77:105–111.

12. Stephan FK, Zucker I. Circadian rhythms in drinking behavior and locomotor activity of rats are eliminated by hypothalamic lesions. *Proc Natl Acad Sci U S A* 1972;69:1583–1586.

13. Balsalobre A, Damiola F, Schibler U. A serum shock induces circadian gene expression in mammalian tissue culture cells. *Cell* 1998;93:929–937.

14. Young MW. Circadian rhythms. Marking time for a kingdom. *Science* 2000;288:451–453.

15. Vitaterna MH, King DP, Chang AM, et al. Mutagenesis and mapping of a mouse gene, Clock, essential for circadian behavior. *Science* 1994;264:719–725.

16. Toh KL, Jones CR, He Y, et al. An hPer2 phosphorylation site mutation in familial advanced sleep phase syndrome. *Science* 2001;291:1040–1043.

17. Carskadon MA, Dement WC. Effects of total sleep loss on sleep tendency. *Percept Mot Skills* 1979;48:495–506.

18. Borbely AA, Baumann F, Brandeis D, et al. Sleep deprivation: effect on sleep stages and EEG power density in man. *Electroencephalogr Clin Neurophysiol* 1981;51:483–495.

19. Benington JH. Sleep homeostasis and the function of sleep. *Sleep* 2000;23:959–966.

20. Daan S, Beersma DG, Borbely AA. Timing of human sleep: recovery process gated by a circadian pacemaker. *Am J Physiol* 1984;246:R161–R183.

21. Borbely AA. A two process model of sleep regulation. *Hum Neurobiol* 1982;1:195–204.

22. Young MR, Matthews JP, Kanabrocki EL, et al. Circadian rhythmometry of serum interleukin-2, interleukin-10, tumor necrosis factor-alpha, and granulocyte-macrophage colony-stimulating factor in men. *Chronobiol Int* 1995;12:19–27.

23. Vgontzas AN, Papanicolaou DA, Bixler EO, et al. Circadian interleukin-6 secretion and quantity and depth of sleep. *J Clin Endocrinol Metab* 1999;84:2603–2607.

24. Born J, Lange T, Hansen K, et al. Effects of sleep and circadian rhythm on human circulating immune cells. *J Immunol* 1997;158:4454–4464.

25. Renegar KB, Floyd R, Krueger JM. Effect of sleep deprivation on serum influenza-specific IgG. *Sleep* 1998;21:19–24.

26. National Sleep Foundation. *2001 Sleep in America Poll.* Washington, DC: National Sleep Foundation, 2001.

27. NCSDR/National Highway Transportation Administration Expert Panel on Driver Fatigue and Sleepiness. *Drowsy driving and automobile crashes.* Washington, DC: National Highway Transportation Administration, 2000.

28. Spiegel K, Leproult R, Van Cauter E. Impact of sleep debt on metabolic and endocrine function. *Lancet* 1999;354:1435–1439.

29. Boggild H, Burr H, Tuchsen F, et al. Work environment of Danish shift and day workers. *Scand J Work Environ Health* 2001;27:97–105.

30. Persson HE, Svanborg E. Sleep deprivation worsens obstructive sleep apnea. Comparison between diurnal and nocturnal polysomnography. *Chest* 1996;109:645–650.

31. Polysomnography Task Force, American Sleep Disorders Association Standards of Practice Committee. Practice parameters for the indications for polysomnography and related procedures. *Sleep* 1997;20:406–422.

32. Committee CPR. Indications for the clinical use of unattended portable recording for the diagnosis of sleep-related breathing disorders. *Am Sleep Disord Assoc News* 1999:19–20,22.

33. Gottlieb DJ, Yao Q, Redline S, et al. Does snoring predict sleepiness independently of apnea and hypopnea frequency? *Am J Respir Crit Care Med* 2000;162:1512–1517.

34. Franklin KA, Holmgren PA, Jonsson F, et al. Snoring, pregnancy-induced hypertension, and growth retardation of the fetus. *Chest* 2000;117:137–141.

35. Gozal D, Pope DW Jr. Snoring during early childhood and academic performance at ages thirteen to fourteen years. *Pediatrics* 2001;107:1394–1399.

36. Ferreira AM, Clemente V, Gozal D, et al. Snoring in Portuguese primary school children. *Pediatrics* 2000;106:E64.

37. Tsai WH, Flemons WW, Whitelaw WA, et al. A comparison of apnea-hypopnea indices derived from different definitions of hypopnea. *Am J Respir Crit Care Med* 1999;159:43–48.

38. Guilleminault C, Stoohs R, Clerk A, et al. A cause of excessive daytime sleepiness. The upper airway resistance syndrome. *Chest* 1993;104:781–787.

39. Rees K, Kingshott RN, Wraith PK, et al. Frequency and significance of increased upper airway resistance during sleep. *Am J Respir Crit Care Med* 2000;162:1210–1214.

40. American Thoracic Society. Medical Section of the American Lung Association. Indications and standards for cardiopulmonary sleep studies. *Am Rev Respir Dis* 1989;139:559–568.

41. Oksenberg A, Silverberg DS, Arons E, et al. The sleep supine position has a major effect on optimal nasal continuous positive airway pressure: relationship with rapid eye movements and non-rapid eye movements sleep, body mass index, respiratory disturbance index, and age. *Chest* 1999;116:1000–1006.

42. Norman RG, Ahmed MM, Walsleben JA, et al. Detection of respiratory events during NPSG: nasal cannula/pressure sensor versus thermistor. *Sleep* 1997;20:1175–1184.

43. Montplaisir J, Boucher S, Nicolas A, et al. Immobilization tests and periodic leg movements in sleep for the diagnosis of restless leg syndrome. *Mov Disord* 1998;13:324–329.

44. Moldofsky H, Scarisbrick P, England R, et al. Musculoskeletal symptoms and non-REM sleep disturbance in patients with "fibrositis syndrome" and healthy subjects. *Psychosom Med* 1975;37:341–351.

45. Harbison J, O'Reilly P, McNicholas WT. Cardiac rhythm disturbances in the obstructive sleep apnea syndrome: effects of nasal continuous positive airway pressure therapy. *Chest* 2000;118:591–595.

46. Young T, Palta M, Dempsey J, et al. The occurrence of sleep-disordered breathing among middle-aged adults. *N Engl J Med* 1993;328:1230–1235.

47. Redline S, Tishler PV, Hans MG, et al. Racial differences in sleep-disordered breathing in African-Americans and

Caucasians. *Am J Respir Crit Care Med* 1997;155:186–192.

48. Schmidt-Nowara WW, Coultas DB, Wiggins C, et al. Snoring in a Hispanic-American population. Risk factors and association with hypertension and other morbidity. *Arch Intern Med* 1990;150:597–601.

49. Ip MS, Lam B, Lauder IJ, et al. A community study of sleep-disordered breathing in middle-aged Chinese men in Hong Kong. *Chest* 2001;119:62–69.

50. Yang EH, Hla KM, McHorney CA, et al. Sleep apnea and quality of life. *Sleep* 2000;23:535–541.

51. Findley LJ, Barth JT, Powers DC, et al. Cognitive impairment in patients with obstructive sleep apnea and associated hypoxemia. *Chest* 1986;90:686–690.

52. Teran-Santos J, Jimenez-Gomez A, Cordero-Guevara J. The association between sleep apnea and the risk of traffic accidents. Cooperative Group Burgos-Santander. *N Engl J Med* 1999;340:847–851.

53. Nieto FJ, Young TB, Lind BK, et al. Association of sleep-disordered breathing, sleep apnea, and hypertension in a large community-based study. Sleep Heart Health Study. *JAMA* 2000;283:1829–1836.

54. Peppard PE, Young T, Palta M, et al. Prospective study of the association between sleep-disordered breathing and hypertension. *N Engl J Med* 2000;342:1378–1384.

55. Peker Y, Hedner J, Kraiczi H, et al. Respiratory disturbance index: an independent predictor of mortality in coronary artery disease. *Am J Respir Crit Care Med* 2000;162:81–86.

56. Sin DD, Logan AG, Fitzgerald FS, et al. Effects of continuous positive airway pressure on cardiovascular outcomes in heart failure patients with and without Cheyne-Stokes respiration. *Circulation* 2000;102:61–66.

57. Javaheri S, Parker TJ, Liming JD, et al. Sleep apnea in 81 ambulatory male patients with stable heart failure. Types and their prevalences, consequences, and presentations. *Circulation* 1998;97:2154–2159.

58. Jokic R, Klimaszewski A, Crossley M, et al. Positional treatment vs continuous positive airway pressure in patients with positional obstructive sleep apnea syndrome. *Chest* 1999;115:771–781.

59. Schmidt-Nowara W, Lowe A, Wiegand L, et al. Oral appliances for the treatment of snoring and obstructive sleep apnea: a review. *Sleep* 1995;18:501–510.

60. Ferguson KA, Ono T, Lowe AA, et al. A randomized crossover study of an oral appliance vs nasal-continuous positive airway pressure in the treatment of mild- moderate obstructive sleep apnea. *Chest* 1996;109:1269–1275.

61. Guilleminault C, Simmons FB, Motta J, et al. Obstructive sleep apnea syndrome and tracheostomy. Long-term follow-up experience. *Arch Intern Med* 1981;141:985–988.

62. Coleman J, Bick PA. Suspension sutures for the treatment of obstructive sleep apnea and snoring. *Otolaryngol Clin North Am* 1999;32:277–285.

63. Coleman J, Rathfoot C. Oropharyngeal surgery in the management of upper airway obstruction during sleep. *Otolaryngol Clin North Am* 1999;32:263–276.

64. Coleman J. Oral and maxillofacial surgery for the management of obstructive sleep apnea syndrome. *Otolaryngol Clin North Am* 1999;32:235–241.

65. Riley RW, Powell NB, Guilleminault C. Obstructive sleep apnea syndrome: a review of 306 consecutively treated surgical patients. *Otolaryngol Head Neck Surg* 1993;108:117–125.

66. Conway W, Fujita S, Zorick F, et al. Uvulopalatopharyngoplasty. One-year followup. *Chest* 1985;88:385–387.

67. Bettega G, Pepin JL, Veale D, et al. Obstructive sleep apnea syndrome. fifty-one consecutive patients treated by maxillofacial surgery. *Am J Respir Crit Care Med* 2000;162:641–649.

68. Boudewyns A, Van De Heyning P. Temperature-controlled radiofrequency tissue volume reduction of the soft palate (somnoplasty) in the treatment of habitual snoring: results of a European multicenter trial. *Acta Otolaryngol* 2000;120:981–985.

69. Powell NB, Riley RW, Troell RJ, et al. Radiofrequency volumetric tissue reduction of the palate in subjects with sleep-disordered breathing. *Chest* 1998;113:1163–1174.

70. Walker RP, Grigg-Damberger MM, Gopalsami C, et al. Laser-assisted uvulopalatoplasty for snoring and obstructive sleep apnea: results in 170 patients. *Laryngoscope* 1995;105:938–943.

71. Troell RJ, Powell NB, Riley RW, et al. Comparison of postoperative pain between laser-assisted uvulopalatoplasty, uvulopalatopharyngoplasty, and radiofrequency volumetric tissue reduction of the palate. *Otolaryngol Head Neck Surg* 2000;122:402–409.

72. Mortimore IL, Bradley PA, Murray JA, et al. Uvulopalatopharyngoplasty may compromise nasal CPAP therapy in sleep apnea syndrome. *Am J Respir Crit Care Med* 1996;154:1759–1762.

73. Smith PL, Gold AR, Meyers DA, et al. Weight loss in mildly to moderately obese patients with obstructive sleep apnea. *Ann Intern Med* 1985;103:850–855.

74. Peiser J, Lavie P, Ovnat A, et al. Sleep apnea syndrome in the morbidly obese as an indication for weight reduction surgery. *Ann Surg* 1984;199:112–115.

75. Sullivan CE, Issa FG, Berthon-Jones M, et al. Reversal of obstructive sleep apnoea by continuous positive airway pressure applied through the nares. *Lancet* 1981;1:862–865.

76. Wright J, Johns R, Watt I, et al. Health effects of obstructive sleep apnoea and the effectiveness of continuous positive airways pressure: a systematic review of the research evidence. *BMJ* 1997;314:851–860.

77. Davies RJ, Stradling JR. The efficacy of nasal continuous positive airway pressure in the treatment of obstructive sleep apnea syndrome is proven. *Am J Respir Crit Care Med* 2000;161:1775–1776.

78. Loube DI, Gay PC, Strohl KP, et al. Indications for positive airway pressure treatment of adult obstructive sleep apnea patients: a consensus statement. *Chest* 1999;115:863–866.

79. Reeves-Hoche MK, Hudgel DW, Meck R, et al. Continuous versus bi-level positive airway pressure for obstructive sleep apnea. *Am J Respir Crit Care Med* 1995;151:443–449.

80. Gugger M, Mathis J, Bassetti C. Accuracy of an intelligent CPAP machine with in-built diagnostic abilities in detecting apnoeas: a comparison with polysomnography. *Thorax* 1995;50:1199–1201.

81. Lloberes P, Ballester E, Montserrat JM, et al. Comparison of manual and automatic CPAP titration in patients with sleep apnea/hypopnea syndrome. *Am J Respir Crit Care Med* 1996;154:1755–1758.

82. Hudgel DW, Fung C. A long-term randomized, cross-over comparison of auto-titrating and standard nasal continuous airway pressure. *Sleep* 2000;23:645–648.

83. McColley SA, Carroll JL, Curtis S, et al. High prevalence

of allergic sensitization in children with habitual snoring and obstructive sleep apnea. *Chest* 1997;111:170–173.

84. Rubinstein I. Nasal inflammation in patients with obstructive sleep apnea. *Laryngoscope* 1995;105:175–177.

85. Zwillich CW, Pickett C, Hanson FN, et al. Disturbed sleep and prolonged apnea during nasal obstruction in normal men. *Am Rev Respir Dis* 1981;124:158–160.

86. Young T, Finn L, Kim H. Nasal obstruction as a risk factor for sleep-disordered breathing. The University of Wisconsin Sleep and Respiratory Research Group. *J Allergy Clin Immunol* 1997;99(suppl):757–762.

87. Leznoff A, Haight JS, Hoffstein V. Reversible obstructive sleep apnea caused by occupational exposure to guar gum dust. *Am Rev Respir Dis* 1986;133:935–936.

88. Richards GN, Cistulli PA, Ungar RG, et al. Mouth leak with nasal continuous positive airway pressure increases nasal airway resistance. *Am J Respir Crit Care Med* 1996;154:182–186.

89. Massie CA, Hart RW, Peralez K, et al. Effects of humidification on nasal symptoms and compliance in sleep apnea patients using continuous positive airway pressure. *Chest* 1999;116:403–408.

90. Hudgel DW, Shucard DW. Coexistence of sleep apnea and asthma resulting in severe sleep hypoxemia. *JAMA* 1979;242:2789–2790.

91. Chan CS, Woolcock AJ, Sullivan CE. Nocturnal asthma: role of snoring and obstructive sleep apnea. *Am Rev Respir Dis* 1988;137:1502–1504.

92. Lin CC, Lin CY. Obstructive sleep apnea syndrome and bronchial hyperreactivity. *Lung* 1995;173:117–126.

93. Olopade CO, Christon JA, Zakkar M, et al. Exhaled pentane and nitric oxide levels in patients with obstructive sleep apnea. *Chest* 1997;111:1500–1504.

94. Klink ME, Dodge R, Quan SF. The relation of sleep complaints to respiratory symptoms in a general population. *Chest* 1994;105:151–154.

95. Bailey WC, Richards JM Jr, Manzella BA, et al. Characteristics and correlates of asthma in a university clinic population. *Chest* 1990;98:821–828.

96. Weinberger M, Bronsky E, Bensch GW, et al. Interaction of ephedrine and theophylline. *Clin Pharmacol Ther* 1975;17:585–592.

97. Rakel ER, McCall WV. *A practical guide to insomnia.* Minneapolis: McGraw-Hill Healthcare Information, 1999.

98. Henauer SA, Hollister LE, Gillespie HK, et al. Theophylline antagonizes diazepam-induced psychomotor impairment. *Eur J Clin Pharmacol* 1983;25:743–747.

Subject Index

Page numbers followed by f indicate figure; page numbers followed by t indicate tables